The Urinary Sphincter

The Urinary Sphincter

edited by
Jacques Corcos
*McGill University and
Jewish General Hospital
Montreal, Quebec, Canada*

Erik Schick
*University of Montreal and
Maisonneuve–Rosemont Hospital
Montreal, Quebec, Canada*

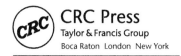
CRC Press
Taylor & Francis Group
Boca Raton London New York

CRC Press is an imprint of the
Taylor & Francis Group, an **informa** business

CRC Press
Taylor & Francis Group
6000 Broken Sound Parkway NW, Suite 300
Boca Raton, FL 33487-2742

First issued in paperback 2019

© 2001 by Taylor & Francis Group, LLC
CRC Press is an imprint of Taylor & Francis Group, an Informa business

No claim to original U.S. Government works

ISBN-13: 978-0-8247-0477-3 (hbk)
ISBN-13: 978-0-367-39700-5 (pbk)

Visit the Taylor & Francis Web site at
http://www.taylorandfrancis.com

and the CRC Press Web site at
http://www.crcpress.com

Foreword

The urinary sphincter is the key to understanding both normal and abnormal function of the lower urinary tract. Its relationships with the bladder, the pelvic floor, and the bony structures of the pelvis are complex and incompletely understood. This textbook, edited by Jacques Corcos and Erik Schick, presents a detailed and systematic account of our current knowledge on the anatomy, physiology, functional relationships and range of dysfunctions that affect the urinary sphincter. This methodical approach is continued in the chapters on the evaluation of sphincter function and the range of treatments available for the principal types of sphincter dysfunction.

This volume builds on the pioneering work of individuals such as Gosling and De Groat, who have taught us so much about the anatomy and physiology of the lower urinary tract in general, and the urinary sphincter in particular. It is important in any area of medicine, from time to time, to set down our current state of knowledge and ignorance, and the editors have assembled a highly expert group of basic scientists and clinicians who have done just that. When a monograph records knowledge systematically, the gaps in our understanding become clearly defined and enable us to construct research applications and projects capable of closing the gaps.

The advances in our knowledge of the basic science aspects always fuel the thinking of clinicians anxious to solve clinical conundrums such as: "What is the urinary sphincter's role in flooding incontinence?" or "Is giggle incontinence a sphincter problem rather than a bladder problem?" By juxtaposing the latest thinking on basic science with that in clinical research, new practical and effective solutions to difficult and unsatisfactorily managed patient problems are developed.

Paul Abrams, M.D., F.R.C.S.
Professor of Urology
Bristol Urological Institute
     and Southmead Hospital
Bristol, England

Preface

Imagination is more important than science.
Albert Einstein

A number of books on urinary incontinence have been published in the last 10 to 15 years. It would have been easier for us to write just another volume dealing with incontinence. It was not to be provocative or to make our work harder that we chose this apparently very limited topic: the urinary sphincter.

Since we deal with bladder dysfunction, incontinence, dyssynergia, retention, and the entire spectrum of lower urinary tract symptoms, we have learned the key position the urinary sphincter occupies in lower urinary tract function. It is becoming increasingly evident that normal and abnormal functioning of the urethra may have a tremendous impact on the functioning of the lower urinary tract and, by extension via the bladder, ultimately on the upper urinary tract as well. It appears that dysfunction of the urethral sphincteric mechanism will often influence bladder function, but the inverse is not inevitably the case. In other words, the urethral sphincter seems to have the predominant role in urethrovesical function.

Probably for didactic reasons, we are used to dividing the urethral sphincter into internal and external, proximal and distal, lisso-sphincter and rhabdosphincter, and so on. As we now know, there is no urinary sphincter, as such, in the sense of an anatomical structure made up of circular muscle fibers. Evidently, it would be much better to design the urethra as a unique *sphincteric mechanism* built with different muscular, nervous, vascular, connective, and epithelial structures that act together as a single functional unit. Its unique physiological role is to close the bladder outlet during the filling phase, ensuring continence, and to open up during voiding, allowing bladder emptying. This apparently simple anatomical structure, however, represents a highly sophisticated and complex functional unit. It is in structural continuity with the bladder and functionally integrated within the pelvic floor.

The book is divided into six parts. The first describes the anatomy and function of the male and female sphincteric mechanism as well as its interconnections with the pelvic floor. References to embryology and observations in infancy contribute to a better understanding of different pathological phenomena in adults and elderly subjects.

The second part, after a review of the epidemiology of the dysfunctional sphincter, analyzes in detail the pathophysiology of three possible functional abnormalities of the urinary sphincter—incompetency, hypertony, and dyssynergia—as well as the behavior of the sphincter when associated with genital prolapse in females.

Evaluation of sphincter competency is not an easy task. Clinical, urodynamic, electrophysiological, and imaging techniques are developed extensively in the third part of the book. Most of these tools explore the very close dynamics existing between the bladder and the urethra. The multiplicity of exploratory techniques reflects the difficulty we have in assessing sphincter function. Diagnosis of bladder-striated sphincter dyssynergia is not very difficult most of the time. Demonstrating sphincter incompetence is often challenging when, for example, decreased bladder compliance is one of the factors responsible for incontinence.

Treatment options are fully described in the fourth part of the book. A great deal of information is provided on lifestyle interventions, physiotherapy, disposable devices, pharmacological therapy, and the technique that "changed the face of the urological world," intermittent catheterization. It is important to be familiar with these techniques, their indications, and the results to expect from each, because most of the time they will be the first line of treatment. The surgical approach constitutes a large part of this section, including recent techniques, such as injectables, and different sling procedures that have now been widely adopted by the scientific community. The issue of autologous versus cadaveric or artificial slings is not yet settled. Injectables probably represent the greatest progress made in the last two decades in the treatment of sphincteric incompetence, even if we do not fully understand their mechanism of action. At present, the artificial sphincter seems to be the gold standard for the treatment of male intrinsic sphincter deficiency. All stents, sphincters, slings, and similar devices are the result of well-thought-out engineering work and bring viable solutions to otherwise hopeless patients, substantially improving their quality of life.

Finally, neurostimulators and neuromodulators have been developed as a result of extensive and remarkable animal work, in conjunction with the high-tech industry. They represent a major step forward in controlling sphincteric dysfunction. We are now able to modulate sphincteric activity to make it more efficient and better coordinated with bladder function. Progress in the neurocontrol of urethrovesical function will probably represent a major urological revolution in the twenty-first century. The control units of these neuromodulators will become as popular and widely used in the next 20 years as are cardiac pacemakers today.

The fifth part of the book is a synthesis of the treatment of three possible sphincteric dysfunctions: the incompetent, the dyssynergic, and the overactive sphincter. The reader will find a practical clinical approach to these problems with some algorithms that may be useful for students, teachers, and practicing physicians.

Finally, the sixth part of the book is a compilation of reports published so far on the standardization of terminology, methodology, and outcome measures elaborated by the International Continence Society. These reports are invaluable aids for those who are interested and actively involved in the study of urethrovesical function and dysfunction. They are the result of years of work and consultation and reflect the thoughts of two generations of highly specialized physicians.

We would like to thank each and every contributor who agreed to participate with us in this venture. They did some truly remarkable work and are principally responsible for the high quality of the book.

We also want to thank Carol Goldberg, who was responsible for the difficult secretarial support required in such an enterprise; Micheline Risler and Catherine Schick, who reviewed and corrected all references to adapt them to our standards; Raymond Bourdeau, who drew and modified the illustrations to provide uniformity throughout the book; and Ovid Da Sylva and his team, who corrected our numerous grammatical and vocabulary mistakes.

Finally, our warmest gratitude goes to our wives, Sylvie and Micheline, who sacrificed part of their family life during the long preparation of this book. Their constant encouragement allowed us to say "mission accomplished!"

Jacques Corcos
Erik Schick

Contents

Foreword   Paul Abrams   *iii*

Preface   *v*

Part 1   ANATOMY AND PHYSIOLOGY

A. The Urinary Sphincter as Part of an Anatomical Entity

1. Embryogenesis of the Sphincter   1
    Barry A. Kogan and Penelope A. Longhurst

2. Functional Anatomy of the Bladder and Urethra in Females   15
    François Haab, Philippe Sebe, Fabrice Mondet, and Calin Ciofu

3. The Male Striated Urethral Sphincter   25
    Robert P. Myers

B. The Urinary Sphincter as Part of a Functional Entity

4. Physiology of the Smooth Muscles of the Bladder and Urethra   43
    William H. Turner

5. Physiology of the Striated Muscles of the Pelvic Floor   71
    John F. B. Morrison

6. The Neural Control of Micturition and Urinary Continence   89
    Bertil F. M. Blok and Gert Holstege

C.   The Urinary Sphincter as Part of the Pelvic Floor

7.   The Pelvic Floor: Lessons from Our Past   101
     Richard A. Schmidt

8.   The Role of Connective Tissue at the Level of the Pelvic Floor   111
     Atsuo Kondo and Momokazu Gotoh

9.   The Pelvic Floor in Infancy and Childhood   133
     Patrick H. McKenna and C. D. Anthony Herndon

10. The Aging Pelvic Floor   175
     Cara Tannenbaum, Louise Perrin, and George A. Kuchel

Part 2   DYSFUNCTIONAL URINARY SPHINCTER

11. Epidemiology of the Dysfunctional Urinary Sphincter   183
     Andrew K. Chung, Kenneth M. Peters, and Ananias C. Diokno

12. Pathophysiology of the Incompetent Urinary Sphincter   193
     Firouz Daneshgari and Philippe E. Zimmern

13. Pathophysiology of the Hypertonic Sphincter or Hyperpathic Urethra   201
     Dirk-Henrik Zermann, Manabu Ishigooka, and Richard A. Schmidt

14. The Dyssynergic Sphincter   223
     Gérard Amarenco, Samer Sheikh Ismael, and Jean Marc Soler

15. Prolapse and Urethral Sphincteric Dysfunction   231
     Serge Peter Marinkovic, Kaven Baessler, and Stuart L. Stanton

Part 3   EVALUATION OF THE URINARY SPHINCTER

A.   Clinical Evaluation

16. Clinical History   241
     Line Leboeuf and Erik Schick

17. Physical Examination   251
     Erik Schick

18. The Voiding Diary   261
     Martine Jolivet-Tremblay and Erik Schick

19. Detection and Quantification of Urine Loss: The Pad-Weighing Test   275
     Erik Schick and Martine Jolivet-Tremblay

B.   Urodynamic Evaluation

20. Uroflowmetry and Postvoid Residual   285
     Jerzy B. Gajewski and Mostafa E. Abdelmagid

21. Urethral Pressure Profile   295
     Jerzy B. Gajewski

Contents   xi

22. Leak Point Pressure   303
    Jerzy B. Gajewski

23. Multichannel Urodynamic and Videourodynamic Testing   311
    Victor W. Nitti and Young H. Kim

24. Ambulatory Urodynamic Monitoring   335
    Stephen C. Radley, Derek J. Rosario, and Christopher R. Chapple

 C. Imaging and Electrophysiological Evaluation

25. Ultrasound Imaging of the Female Urinary Sphincter   357
    Bernard Jacquetin

26. Voiding Cystourethrography and Magnetic Resonance Imaging of
    the Lower Urinary Tract   407
    Gary E. Lemack and Philippe E. Zimmern

27. Electrophysiological Evaluation of Genitourinary Nervous Pathways   423
    Reinier-Jacques Opsomer

Part 4   TREATMENTS

 A. Nonsurgical Treatments

28. Lifestyle Interventions in the Treatment of Urinary Incontinence   437
    Ingrid Nygaard

29. Pelvic Floor Muscle Exercises   443
    Kari Bø

30. Pelvic Floor Reeducation: A Practical Approach   459
    Claudia Brown

31. Intermittent Catheterization   475
    Ananias C. Diokno and Bruce E. Lundak

32. Treatment of the Sphincter: Medical Therapy   483
    Scott E. Litwiller

33. Urethral Injection Treatment for Stress Urinary Incontinence   497
    Elmer B. Pineda, Jr., and H. Roger Hadley

34. The Artificial Urinary Sphincter   517
    Steven E. Mutchnik and Timothy B. Boone

35. Intravaginal and Intraurethral Devices for Stress Incontinence   535
    David R. Staskin, Roxane Gardner, and Matthew L. Lemer

36. Sacral Nerve Neuromodulation and Its Effects on
    Urinary Sphincter Function   541
    J. L. H. Ruud Bosch

37. Neurostimulation   553
    Philip E. V. Van Kerrebroeck

B.   Surgical Treatments

38. Sphincterotomy and Sphincter Stent Prosthesis Placement   565
     David A. Rivas and Michael Chancellor

39. Surgery for the Incompetent Urethral Sphincter: Bladder Neck
     Suspension Procedures   583
     Daniel S. Blander and Philippe E. Zimmern

40. Surgical Reconstruction of the Bladder Neck   605
     Marc Cendron

41. The Use of Artificial Material in Sling Surgery   615
     Matthew L. Lerner, Jong Myun Choe, and David R. Staskin

42. Fascial Slings   635
     Kathleen C. Kobashi and Gary E. Leach

Part 5   SYNTHESIS

43. Management of the Incompetent Sphincter: A Synthesis   651
     Jacques Corcos and Erik Schick

44. Management of the Dyssynergic Sphincter: A Synthesis   661
     Erik Schick and Jacques Corcos

45. Management of the Hypertonic Sphincter or Hyperpathic Urethra   679
     Dirk-Henrik Zermann, Manabu Ishigooka, and Richard A. Schmidt

Part 6   ICS REPORTS ON STANDARDIZATION

46. Overview of the ICS Standardization Reports   687
     Erik Schick

47. List of the Reports of the ICS Committee on Standardization of
     Terminology of Lower Urinary Tract Function   691

     Appendix: Reports of the ICS Committee

     Standardization of Terminology of Lower Urinary Tract Function:
        Synthesis of First Six Reports   *695*

     Seventh Report: Lower Urinary Tract Rehabilitation Techniques   *718*

     Standardization of Terminology of Female Pelvic Organ Prolapse
        and Pelvic Floor Dysfunction   *729*

     Intestinal Reservoirs   *742*

     Standardization of Terminology of Lower Urinary Tract Function:
     New Report on Evaluation of Micturition   *754*

Neurogenic Bladder Dysfunction 763

Report on Ambulatory Urodynamic Monitoring 782

Outcome Studies: General Principles 795

Outcome Studies: Adult Female 800

Outcome Studies: Adult Male 808

Outcome Studies: Frail Older People 817

Technical Report: Urodynamic Equipment 826

Technical Report: Digital Exchange of Pressure–Flow Study Data 839

Index 849

Contributors

Mostafa E. Abdelmagid, M.Sc., M.D., M.Sc., M.B., B.Ch.   Associate Professor, Department of Urology, Faculty of Medicine, Al-Azhar University, Cairo, Egypt

Gérard Amarenco, M.D.   Chief, Neurological Rehabilitation, Rothschild Hospital, Paris, France

Kaven Baessler, M.D.   Clinical Research Fellow, Urogynecology Unit, St. George's Hospital Medical School, London, England

Daniel S. Blander, M.D.   Southern California Permanente Medical Group, Irvine, California

Bertil F. M. Blok, M.D., Ph.D.   Department of Urology, Academic Medical Center, University of Amsterdam, Amsterdam, The Netherlands

Kari Bø, Ph.D., P.T.   Professor and Exercise Scientist, Institute for Sports and Biological Science, Norwegian University of Sports and Physical Education, Oslo, Norway

Timothy B. Boone, M.D., Ph.D.   Russell and Mary Hugh Scott Professor and Chairman, Scott Department of Urology, Baylor College of Medicine, Houston, Texas

J. L. H. Ruud Bosch, M.D., Ph.D.   Professor, Faculty of Medicine, Erasmus University Rotterdam, and Department of Urology, Academic Hospital Rotterdam, Rotterdam, The Netherlands

Claudia Brown, B.Sc., P.T.   Physiotherapist, Physiothérapie Polyclinique Cabrini, Montreal, Quebec, Canada

Marc Cendron, M.D.   Associate Professor of Surgery and Pediatrics, Division of Urology, Dartmouth–Hitchcock Medical Center, Lebanon, New Hampshire

Michael B. Chancellor, M.D.   Associate Professor, Department of Urology, University of Pittsburgh, Pittsburgh, Pennsylvania

Christopher R. Chapple, B.Sc., M.D., F.R.C.S.(Urol)   Consultant Urological Surgeon, Department of Urology, Central Sheffield University Hospitals, Sheffield, England

Jong Myun Choe, M.D.   Assistant Professor and Director of Continence Program and Urodynamics, Department of Urology, University of Cincinnati College of Medicine, Cincinnati, Ohio

Andrew K. Chung, M.D.   Department of Urology, William Beaumont Hospital, Royal Oak, Michigan

Calin Ciofu, M.D.   Department of Urology, Saint Antoine University, and Tenon Hospital, Paris, France

Jacques Corcos, M.D.   Associate Professor, Department of Urology, McGill University, and Chief, Department of Urology, Jewish General Hospital, Montreal, Quebec, Canada

Firouz Daneshgari, M.D., F.A.C.S.   Assistant Professor and Director of Female Urology, Department of Urology, University of Colorado Health Sciences Center, Denver, Colorado

Ananias C. Diokno, M.D.   Chief, Department of Urology, William Beaumont Hospital, Royal Oak, Michigan

Jerzy B. Gajewski, M.D., F.R.C.S.(C)   Professor, Department of Urology, Dalhousie University, Halifax, Nova Scotia, Canada

Roxane Gardner, M.D., M.P.H.   Department of Obstetrics and Gynecology, Brigham and Women's Hospital, Boston, Massachusetts

Momokazu Gotoh, M.D., Ph.D.   Assistant Professor, Department of Urology, Nagoya University School of Medicine, Nagoya City, Japan

François Haab, M.D.   Assistant Professor, Department of Urology, Saint Antoine University, and Tenon Hospital, Paris, France

H. Roger Hadley, M.D.   Professor and Chief, Division of Urology, Department of Surgery, Loma Linda University Medical Center, Loma Linda, California

C. D. Anthony Herndon, M.D.   Department of Urology, University of Connecticut, Farmington, Connecticut

Gert Holstege, M.D., Ph.D.   Professor, Department of Anatomy, Groningen University Medical School, Groningen, The Netherlands

Manabu Ishigooka, M.D.   Department of Urology, Yamagata University School of Medicine, Yamagata, Japan

Samer Sheikh Ismael, M.D.   Consultant, Neurological Rehabilitation, Rothschild Hospital, Paris, France

Bernard Jacquetin, M.D.   Professor, Auvergne University, Clermont I, and Head, Department of Urogynecology, Hotel-Dieu Maternity, Auvergne University Hospital, Clermont-Ferrand, France

Martine Jolivet-Tremblay, M.D., F.R.C.S.C.   Department of Urology, University of Montreal, and Maisonneuve–Rosemont Hospital, Montreal, Quebec, Canada

Young H. Kim, M.D.   Assistant Professor, Division of Urology, Department of Surgery, Brown University School of Medicine, Providence, Rhode Island

Kathleen C. Kobashi, M.D.   Department of Urology, Virginia Mason Medical Center, Seattle, Washington

Barry A. Kogan, M.D., F.A.A.P., F.A.C.S. Professor, Department of Urology and Pediatrics, and Chief, Division of Urology, Department of Surgery, Albany Medical College, Albany, New York

Atsuo Kondo, M.D., Ph.D. Vice President, Department of Urology, Komaki Shimin Hospital, Komaki, Japan

George A. Kuchel, M.D., F.R.C.P.(C) Travelers Chair in Geriatrics and Gerontology, Director, University of Connecticut Center on Aging, and Director, Division of Geriatric Medicine, University of Connecticut Health Center, Farmington, Connecticut

Gary E. Leach, M.D. Clinical Professor of Urology, University of Southern California Medical School, and Director, Tower Urology Institute for Continence, Cedars-Sinai Medical Center, Los Angeles, California

Line Leboeuf, M.D. Resident, Department of Urology, University of Montreal, and Maisonneuve–Rosemont Hospital, Montreal, Quebec, Canada

Gary E. Lemack, M.D. Assistant Professor, Department of Urology, The University of Texas Southwestern Medical Center at Dallas, Dallas, Texas

Matthew L. Lemer, M.D. Assistant Professor, Department of Urology, College of Physicians and Surgeons of Columbia University, New York, New York

Scott E. Litwiller, M.D., F.A.C.S. Clinical Professor, Department of Urology, Oklahoma University, and Director, Oklahoma Continence Center, St. Francis Memorial Hospital, Tulsa, Oklahoma

Penelope A. Longhurst, Ph.D. Research Associate Professor, Department of Basic and Pharmaceutical Sciences, Albany College of Pharmacy, Albany, New York

Bruce E. Lundak, M.D. Department of Urology, Bergen Mercy Hospital, Omaha, Nebraska

Serge Peter Marinkovic, M.D. Fellow, Urogynecology and Pelvic Reconstructive Surgery, St. George's Hospital Medical School, London, England

Patrick H. McKenna, M.D., F.A.C.S., F.A.A.P. Professor and Chief, Division of Urology, Department of Surgery, Southern Illinois University School of Medicine, Springfield, Illinois

Fabrice Mondet, M.D. Department of Urology, Saint Antoine University, and Tenon Hospital, Paris, France

John F. B. Morrison, M.B.Ch.B., B.Sc., Ph.D., F.R.C.S.Ed., F.I.Biol. Professor, Department of Physiology, Faculty of Medicine and Health Sciences, United Arab Emirates University, Al Ain, United Arab Emirates

Steven E. Mutchnik, M.D. Fellow, Neurourology and Urodynamics, Department of Urology, Baylor College of Medicine, Houston, Texas

Robert P. Myers, M.D., M.S. Professor of Urology, Mayo Graduate School of Medicine, and Consultant, Department of Urology, Mayo Clinic, Rochester, Minnesota

Victor W. Nitti, M.D., F.A.C.S. Associate Professor and Vice-Chairman, Department of Urology, New York University School of Medicine, New York, New York

Ingrid Nygaard, M.D. Associate Professor, Department of Obstetrics and Gynecology, University of Iowa College of Medicine, Iowa City, Iowa

Reinier-Jacques Opsomer, M.D. Professor, Department of Urology, Cliniques Saint-Luc, University of Louvain, Brussels, Belgium

Louise Perrin, B.Sc., P.T.   Division of Geriatric Medicine, School of Physiotherapy and Occupational Therapy, McGill University, Montreal, Quebec, Canada

Kenneth M. Peters, M.D.   Director of Research, Department of Urology, William Beaumont Hospital, Royal Oak, Michigan

Elmer B. Pineda, M.D.   Division of Urology, Department of Surgery, Loma Linda University Medical Center, Loma Linda, California

Stephen C. Radley, F.R.C.S.(Gyn), M.R.C.O.G.   Consultant, Department of Gynecology and Urology, Central Sheffield University Hospitals, Sheffield, England

David A. Rivas, M.D.   Associate Professor, Department of Urology, Jefferson Medical College, Thomas Jefferson University, Philadelphia, Pennsylvania

Derek J. Rosario, M.B.Ch.B., F.R.C.S.(Urol)   Department of Urology, Central Sheffield University Hospitals, Sheffield, England

Erik Schick, M.D.(Louvain), L.M.C.C., F.R.C.S.C.   Clinical Professor of Urology, Department of Surgery, University of Montreal, and Chief, Department of Urology, Maisonneuve–Rosemont Hospital, Montreal, Quebec, Canada

Richard A. Schmidt, M.D.   Professor of Neurourology, Department of Urology, University of Colorado Medical School, and Rose Hospital, Denver, Colorado

Philippe Sebe, M.D.   Department of Urology, Saint Antoine University, and Tenon Hospital, Paris, France

Jean Marc Soler, M.D.   Consultant, Urodynamics Laboratory, Bouffard-Vercelli Medical Center, Cerbere, France

Stuart L. Stanton, F.R.C.S., F.R.C.O.G.   Professor, Department of Pelvic Reconstruction and Urogynecology, St. George's Hospital Medical School, London, England

David R. Staskin, M.D.   Assistant Professor of Surgery, Department of Urology, Harvard Medical School, and Director, Beth Israel Deaconess Medical Center Continence Center, Boston, Massachusetts

Cara Tannenbaum, M.D., F.R.C.P.   Assistant Professor of Medicine, Division of Geriatric Medicine, McGill University Health Centre, Montreal, Quebec, Canada

William H. Turner, M.D., F.R.C.S.(Urol)   Consultant Urologist, Department of Urology, Addenbrooke's Hospital, Cambridge, England

Philip E. V. Van Kerrebroeck, M.D., Ph.D., Fellow E.B.U.   Professor and Chairman, Department of Urology, University Hospital Maastricht, Maastricht, The Netherlands

Dirk-Henrik Zermann, Priv.-Doz. Dr. med. habil.   Department of Urology, University Hospital, Friedrich-Schiller-University, Jena, Germany

Philippe E. Zimmern, M.D., F.A.C.S.   Professor, Department of Urology, The University of Texas Southwestern Medical Center at Dallas, Dallas, Texas

1

Embryogenesis of the Sphincter

BARRY A. KOGAN

Albany Medical College, Albany, New York

PENELOPE A. LONGHURST

Albany College of Pharmacy and Albany Medical College, Albany, New York

I. INTRODUCTION

The structure and function of an organ can be understood best in the context of its embryogenesis. Hence, it is surprising that relatively little is known about the development of the urinary sphincter. In reviewing numerous embryology texts, there are extensive discussions of renal, ureteral, bladder, and even prostatic development, but virtually nothing is written about the urinary sphincter. Furthermore, the limited published literature includes both animal and human studies, with this distinction being important because of the variations in voiding purposes and patterns in differing species. In addition, few of the studies beyond simple histology are gender-specific and the recent recognition of high-pressure voiding in human male neonates suggests that there may be gender-specific development of the sphincter.

The sphincter can be broken down anatomically into the striated (external) sphincter, smooth (internal) sphincter, and the pelvic floor. In this discussion, we will concentrate on the external and internal sphincters.

II. HISTOLOGY OF THE EMBRYONIC EXTERNAL SPHINCTER BEFORE SEXUAL DIFFERENTIATION (INDIFFERENT STAGE)

Several authors have studied the histology of the cloaca and lower urinary tract during embryonic development. Bourdelat et al. noted undifferentiated mesenchyme anterior to the urethra at a crown–rump length (CRL) of 12–15 mm (5th week) (1). Tichy noted similar findings at the 18 mm-stage (2). Interestingly, as late as the 24-mm stage (6th week), Mat-

1

suno found striated muscle in the abdominal wall, smooth muscle in the intestinal tract, but no differentiated muscle in the urinary tract (3); however by the 31- (1) and 45-mm stage (2), this condensation ventral to the urethra appears to be intimately related to the puborectalis muscle near the bladder neck (Fig. 1) (1) and extends as a loop distally, demonstrated as paired condensations of undifferentiated mesenchymal cells laterally on either side of the urethra on more distal sections (Fig. 2) (2). It is important to note that at this stage, although the periurethral musculature remains undifferentiated, the puborectalis, levator ani, and bulbocavernosus muscles have differentiated striated muscle cells. One explanation for this lack of muscular differentiation in the embryonic urinary sphincter is that at this early stage urine production is minimal; hence, there is no need for a striated external sphincter.

A. Histology of the Fetal Female External Sphincter

By the 60-mm stage, the thickening mesenchyme extends, caudal to the mullerian tubercle, to surround the urethra completely (Fig. 3) (4,5). By the 65-mm stage (12th week) clear striations are seen in muscle cells that extend from the anterior abdominal wall obliquely with a U-shaped configuration in a caudal direction around the urethra, clearly separate from the pelvic floor muscles (3). Smooth-muscle primordia are seen between the urethra and this developing striated sphincter (Fig. 4) (1). Although Kokoua and co-workers report that no distinguishable sphincteric structures can be detected at 14 weeks of gestation (6), by the 115-mm (16th-week) stage, the thickened striated muscle completely encloses the urethra at the level of the urogenital diaphragm (3). Interestingly, this circular configuration is prevented by the vagina caudally and the fibers seem to merge with the lateral wall of the vagina (2). Even at this stage it is clear that these striated muscle cells are distinctly smaller than their counterparts in the pelvic floor (Fig. 5; see color insert) (7). The distinct phenotype of these muscles that distinguishes them from smooth muscle and other nearby striated muscle cells, suggests a specialized purpose for this developing urinary sphincter, and may be related to differences between fast-twitch and slow-twitch muscle types. de Leval

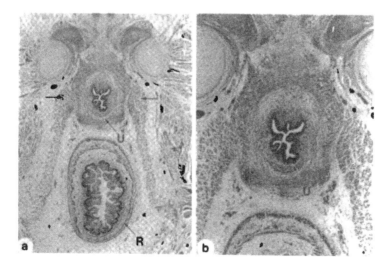

Figure 1   Transverse section of a 31-mm human embryo at (a) low and (b) high magnification: The anterior parts of the m. pubo-rectalis (arrows) are very closely related to the urethra (U). (From Ref. 1.)

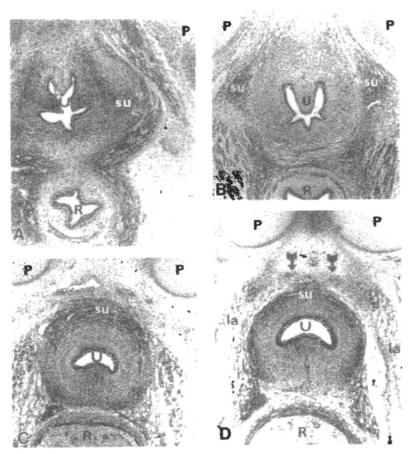

Figure 2 Transverse sections of the pelvis of a fetus (45-mm CRL) made in different levels of m. sphincter urethrae primordium demonstrate its shape and relation to the neighboring structures: (A) a section at urogenital diaphragm level exhibiting a typical stellate shape of the urethra (U). The most distal margin of the m. sphincter urethrae primordium (su), represented at this level by paired condensations of cells, is situated lateral to the urethra (U) and proximal to the upper margin of the bulbocavernosus muscle primordium (bc), dorsally joining the rudiments of the m. sphincter ani externus (sae): R, rectum; P, pubic bone; (B) more proximally, the primordium of the m. sphincter urethrae (su) is made up of clusters of cells situated lateral to the urethra (U) and projecting ventrally: R, rectum; P, pubic bone; la, levator ani; (C) still more proximally, the m. sphincter urethrae primordium (su) forms an arch on the anterior wall of the urethra (U) integrated in its wall. The ventral margin of the puborectal part of m. levator ani (la) primordium is on either side of the urethra: R, rectum; P, pubic bone; (D) The primordium of the m. sphincter urethrae (su) is discernibly thinner at the vesicourethral junction level. The primordium of the sphincter lies between the arms of the primordium of the puborectal portion of the m. levator ani (la). Part of the levator fibers projects from the condensation of the connective tissue plate (arrows) outside the urethra (U): R, rectum; P, pubic bone. (hematoxylin and eosin [H&E], × 80). (From Ref. 2.)

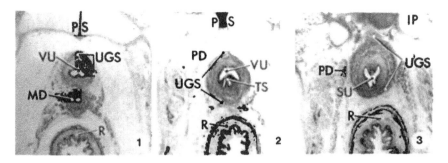

Figure 3 Cross section of a female urethra in a 60-mm–CRL fetus: (left panel) just caudal to the bladder; (center panel) at the level of the tuberculum sinuale; (right panel) through the urogenital sinus. Note the position of the pelvic diaphragm. IP, ischiopubic ramus; MD, fused paramesonephric ducts; PD, pelvic diaphragm; PS, pubic symphysis; R, rectum; SU, urogenital sinus; TS, tuberculum sinuale (müllerian tubercle); UGS, urogenital sphincter primordium; VU, vesicourethral canal (trichrome × 17). (From Ref. 4.)

has suggested that the narrow caliber muscles in this portion of the sphincter are exclusively slow-twitch (8).

By 40 weeks of gestation the striated sphincter is obvious as a ring-shaped muscle at the level of the membranous urethra (6). The shape and configuration in these muscles remains as described until well after birth (Fig. 6) (2). Kokoua and co-workers have reported that the striated muscle is no longer seen posteriorly; hence, this external sphincter assumes a horseshoe or omega conformation sometime during the first year of life (6). However, other investigators did not find this alteration in configuration, which may be explained by the fact that sections taken in only a transverse plane might fail to identify muscle fibers that are oriented obliquely from the bladder neck down along the urethra to the membranous urethra.

B. Histology of the Fetal Male External Sphincter

At the 60-mm stage, the undifferentiated mesenchyme of the striated sphincter is clearly visible above the bulbospongiosus muscle (9). It is circular, but particularly thick anteriorly. On the dorsal side it is thinner, especially toward the bladder base, leading to a "signet-ring" type configuration (Fig. 7). In the 94-mm fetus, the prostatic buds are identified, growing within the undifferentiated mesenchyme, further thinning the mesenchyme dorsally (9). In the 115-mm male fetus, striations are seen in the mesenchyme, which now extends to contact the smooth muscle of the rectum (9). Although the ventral aspect of this developing external sphincter extends from the bladder base down to the corpus spongiosum, the dorsal side is limited to that portion distal to the developing prostate (9). Kokoua and co-workers could find no identifiable striated sphincter in a 19-week male fetus, but report that striated fibers were visible around the urethra by 20 to 21 weeks (6). By the 245-mm stage, the smooth and striated muscles are fully differentiated, as are the fascial planes of the pelvis (9). Interestingly, the striated sphincter intermingles with the smooth muscle of the urethra where they contact, with no fascia separating the two. This basic arrangement of anterior sphincteric fibers that extend along the entire prepenile urethra, but continue posterolaterally around the prostate only below it, results in a horseshoe configuration above and a circular configuration below the prostate (see Fig. 7). Most investigators have observed this

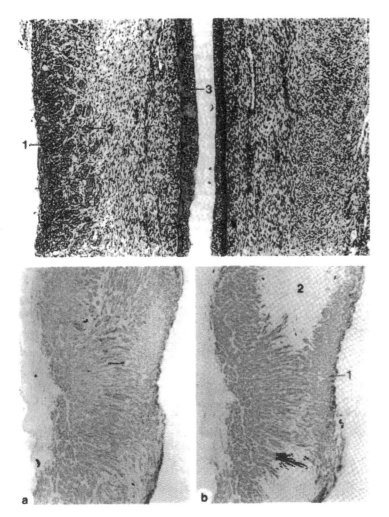

Figure 4 Sagittal section of the urethra in a $16\frac{1}{2}$-week-old female fetus (top panels): 1, striated muscle layer; 2, smooth muscle layer; 3, epithelium; parasagittal sections of the urethra in a 28-week-old fetus (lower panels), incubated with antibodies against (a) desmin and (b) titin. The external striated muscle fibers (1) express both desmin and titin, whereas the internal smooth muscle fibers (2) express only desmin. (From Ref. 1.)

configuration throughout life. As the prostate and bladder neck will continue to provide continence at most times, one might hypothesize that this horseshoe-type configuration maintains the pelvic anatomy by fixing the striated external sphincter in position relative to the pubic symphysis.

Kokoua et al. describe a tail-like structure extending from the dorsal aspect of the striated sphincter in the male down toward the perineal body (6). They hypothesize that this tail, which later disappears, may be a precursor of the rectourethralis. They describe that the disappearance of the tail during development coincides with splitting of the dorsal sphincter. However, others have not found this splitting; this, again, may relate to the technique of sectioning.

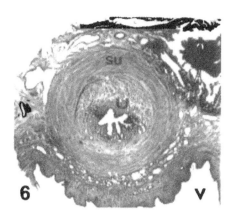

Figure 6   Transverse section of the upper portion of m. sphincter urethrae (su) in a 10-year-old girl: The sphincter forms a concentric circle around urethra (U); V, vagina (H & E stain). (From Ref. 2.)

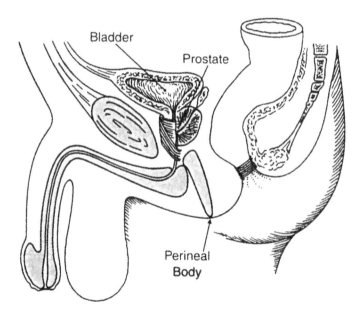

Figure 7   Diagrammatic representation of "signet-ring" configuration of striated sphincter in a male fetus.

C.   Differentiation of the Striated Muscle Cells of the Sphincter

The striated external sphincter develops from undifferentiated mesenchyme. A study by Borirakchanyavat et al. using male and female Fisher 344 rats demonstrated a surprising pattern of differentiation of these muscle cells (10). The first marker noted in this undifferentiated mesenchyme (at day 14 of 21 days gestation) was α-smooth muscle actin. Surprisingly, from days 14–18 of gestation, no striated muscle markers were noted, although the muscle was located in the typical anatomical location for the external striated sphincter, and continued to stain for α-smooth-muscle actin. It was not until postnatal day 1 that striations were visualized and staining for α-sarcomeric actin, a striated muscle marker, was present, in addition to continued staining for α-smooth muscle actin. This is in contrast to the levator ani muscle in which a striated phenotype is present by day 16 of gestation (similar to the afore described finding in humans) (3). By maturity, the striated phenotype is clear, and there is no staining for α-smooth-muscle actin in the external sphincter (10). Similar findings have been seen in the esophageal sphincter (11) and in cardiac muscle (12). The most intriguing hypothesis to explain these findings is that there is transdifferentiation of a smooth muscle-like mesenchyme to a striated phenotype. This highlights the multipotential nature of developing mesenchymal cells.

III. HISTOLOGY OF THE INTERNAL SPHINCTER

Histological studies in the human fetus allow clear differentiation of the smooth-muscle fibers in the bladder starting at 27-mm–CRL (7th week of gestation) (3). This early fine muscular development progresses and extends around the bladder, and by the 65-mm–CRL stage (12 weeks) seems to form a more mature meshwork of bundles that stain positively for cholinesterases (13). In contrast, the smooth-muscle primordium of the urethra is relatively undifferentiated and fails to stain for cholinesterases (Fig. 8) (13). Finally, in the 112-mm–CRL stage, histologically distinct smooth-muscle cells are identifiable (13). The trigone develops during this stage as well, and an inner longitudinal layer and a second circular layer are clearly seen (5). These layers are contiguous with the urethral smooth muscle. This is especially true of the longitudinal component. The circular layer develops into the bladder neck in the male and, in the female, extends well down the urethra, although it is much less prominent (13). In the male the circular layer is seen primarily ventrally over the prostate, but a horseshoe-like configuration is observed by following these fibers to the region of the membranous urethra, inside the similarly developing striated muscles (5). Although these smooth-muscle cells appear identical with bladder smooth-muscle cells, Gilpin and Gosling have shown that even at this stage of fetal development, both the trigonal and urethral smooth-muscle cells form smaller muscle bundles with a more extensive extracellular matrix than seen in the bladder (13). Furthermore, they are functionally distinct, as they have very limited cholinesterase staining, in contrast to bladder smooth-muscle cells (see Fig. 8). Obviously, this emphasizes the different role these muscles play functionally. In addition, the gender differences in the circular smooth-muscle development may be accounted for by the necessity of bladder neck closure during ejaculation. Failure of this muscle to achieve full functionality may account for the gender differences noted in neonatal voiding, with males having higher voiding pressures and more of an obstructed picture.

IV. INNERVATION

Information on the innervation of the developing urethral sphincter is sparse, and generally neither gender-specific nor correlated with duration of gestation. Frequently, the sphincter is not specifically identified, and the area described broadly covers the bladder base or neck region, or urethra, or both. In a study of gross anatomical dissections of male and female human fetuses of 110 to 290-mm CRL, the external sphincter was reported to be innervated (anatomically, as this study did not assess function) by the perineal nerve and probably also pelvic splanchnic nerves arising from ventral branches of S2–S4 spinal nerves (14). More

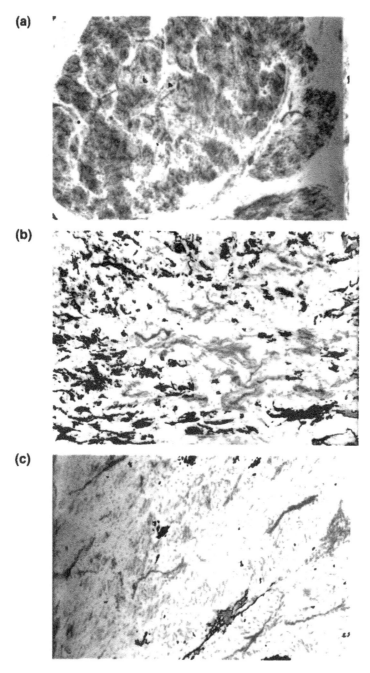

Figure 8 (a) Posterior wall of bladder from an 18-day-old postnatal male: Acetylcholin-esterase activity is evident in both the smooth-muscle cells and the interfascicular nerves (arrows); middle portion of the urethra from a 33-cm–CRL female. (b) Numerous acetyl-cholinesterase-positive nerves accompany the smooth-muscle bundles; (c) the smooth muscle of the proximal (preprostatic) urethra from a 20.6-cm–CRL male has relatively fewer acetylcholinesterase-containing nerves compared with the female specimen in (b) (× 175). (From Ref. 13.)

recently, Shafik and Doss described the gross anatomy of pudendal nerve branches in the bladder neck and proximal urethra from six fully mature neonates (15). Within the pudendal canal the pudendal nerve gave rise to the inferior rectal nerve and divided into two terminal branches: the perineal and dorsal nerves. When the perineal nerve exits the canal it divides into terminal scrotal lateral and striated urethral sphincter medial (muscular) branches (Fig. 9) (15). The upper muscular branch innervates the bulbocavernosus muscle and the lower branch the urethral sphincter. The bulbocavernosus branch courses medial and downward medial to the sphincter branch and terminates in the bulbocavernosus muscle. The nerve to the striated external sphincter enters the deep perineal pouch near the penile bulb and divides into multiple branches that penetrate the striated sphincter laterally at the 3- and 9-o'clock positions (15). These investigations demonstrate that the neural connections are grossly present, but do not confirm that neural control is present or mature.

Immunohistochemistry has been used to identify transmitters and investigate colocalization of neuropeptides and enzymes responsible for synthesis of neurotransmitter substances in nerves and ganglia of human bladder and bladder neck. In male infants, Dixon and co-workers found that 60% of the intramural neurons in the bladder neck were nonimmunoreactive to the enzyme tyrosine hydroxylase, a marker for catecholaminergic neurons (16). This population of neurons contains calcitonin gene-related peptide, neuropeptide Y,

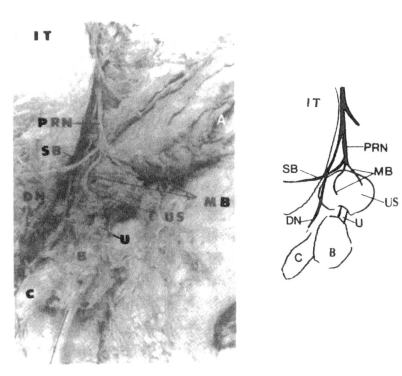

Figure 9   Dissected cadaveric specimen and schema of perineal nerve after removal of perineal membrane showing striated sphincter and part of membranous urethra, which demonstrates muscular branch penetrating sphincter: IT, ischeal tuberosity; PRN, perineal nerve; SB, scrotal branch; MB, muscular branches of upper to bulbocavernosus muscle and lower to urethral sphincter; US, striated urethral sphincter; U, urethra; DN, dorsal nerve of penis; B, bulbocavernosus muscle; C, crus penis; A, anus. (From Ref. 15.)

nitric oxide synthase, somatostatin, and vasoactive intestinal polypeptide. The remaining 40% of neurons were tyrosine hydroxylase- and dopamine β-hydroxylase–immunoreactive and, therefore, adrenergic. The tyrosine hydroxylase-immunoreactive nerves also contained calcitonin gene-related peptide, neuropeptide Y, nitric oxide synthase, somatostatin, vasoactive intestinal polypeptide, and bombesin. Only a few nerves were immunoreactive for substance P and *met*-enkephalin. In a further study using younger, 13- to 20-week-old male fetuses, Dixon found large clusters of paraganglion cells that were dopamine β-hydroxylase–immunoreactive, but lacked tyrosine hydroxylase, nitric oxide synthase, and the other neuropeptides (Fig. 10) (17). These cells were lateral to the urinary bladder and prostate, in close proximity to autonomic ganglia or thick bundles of nerve fibers. Paraganglia were confined to the adventitial connective tissue of the bladder neck in 13- and 16-week specimens, but at 17 weeks and in all older fetuses, clusters of paraganglion cells were also found in the bladder wall. von Heyden and co-workers identified norepinephrine in both smooth and striated urethral sphincter muscle from a 31-week-gestation male fetus and a 41-week-gestation female fetus. The relative amounts of norepinephrine were graded as numerous in the smooth sphincter from the male fetus and rare in the smooth sphincter from the female fetus and striated sphincter of both male and female (18). Numerous neuropeptide Y-positive nerves were identified in the smooth sphincter and rare neuropeptide Y-positive nerves identified in the striated sphincter in both the male and female fetus, and galanin staining was numerous in the smooth sphincter and negative in the striated sphincter of the female fetus, and rare in preparations from the male fetus. These characteristics did not appear to be much different from what was reported in tissues from adult cadavers (18). The presence or distribution of acetylcholine-containing cholinergic nerves was not examined in the fetal specimens, but acetylcholine staining was abundant in striated sphincter from male and female adults. These findings emphasize the wide variety and complexity of the neural connections in this region, even in the fetus. Much additional work is needed to sort out the functional consequences of this complex system.

V.   IN VITRO PHARMACOLOGY

Andersson and co-workers carried out in vitro studies examining the responsiveness of urethral tissue from human fetuses (gestational age 16–22 weeks) to acetylcholine, norepinephrine, and prostaglandins (19). Although both male and female fetuses were used, no gender-specific observations were made. Approximately 10 mm of the urethra attached to the bladder base was used. A small portion of the bladder was tied over a PE 190 catheter, such that the catheter could be used for perfusion through the urethral lumen. The preparation was mounted in an organ bath and the distal end of the urethra was attached to a force displacement transducer for recording of longitudinal isometric tension. During perfusion, resistance to flow was recorded, providing a measure of circular muscle tone. Acetylcholine caused atropine-sensitive increases in tension and resistance to flow. Norepinephrine also produced increases in tension and resistance and these effects were prevented by the α-blocker, phenoxybenzamine. The response of the circular muscle to norepinephrine was greater than that of the longitudinal muscle; with acetylcholine, the longitudinal muscle was most sensitive. Prostaglandins E_1 (PGE_1) and PGE_2 both relaxed precontracted urethral preparations, whereas $PGF_{2\alpha}$ contracted the preparations, increasing both flow and longitudinal tension. Histochemical analyses of the same preparations using the Falck–Hillarp technique demonstrated no fluorescence for adrenergic nerves or ganglion cells in any part

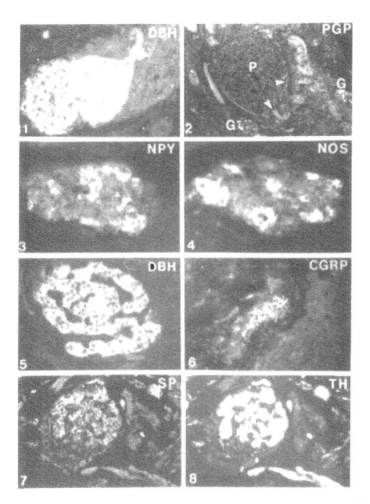

Figure 10   (1) Large paraganglion, intensely immmunopositive for dopamine β-hydroxy-lase (DBH), lies adjacent to unstained primitive autonomic ganglion cells in the adventitia of the bladder neck from a 16-week male fetal specimen; (2) large paraganglion (P) in the adventitia of the bladder wall of a 20-week–male fetal specimen. Several protein gene product 9.5 (PGP)-immunoreactive nerve bundles and two small autonomic ganglia (G) occur in the immediate vicinity, while PGP-immunoreactive nerves (arrowheads) extend into the paraganglion; (3) paraganglion lying lateral to the bladder neck of a 23-week–male fetal specimen. Some of the paraganglion cells are immunoreactive for neuropeptide Y (NPY); (4) paraganglion from the adventitia of the bladder from a 23-week–male fetal specimen in which numerous paraganglion cells are immunoreactive for nitric oxide synthase (NOS); (5) paraganglia in the wall of the bladder from a 7-week–male fetal specimen. All paraganglion cells are dopamine β-hydroxylase (DBH)-immunoreactive, but were negative for the neuropeptides investigated. Note the prominent vascular supply; (6) small intramuscular paraganglion from the urinary bladder of a 2-year-old postnatal male in whom all the cells display calcitonin gene-related peptide (CGRP) immunoreactivity; (7) intramuscular paraganglion from the urinary bladder of a 3-year-old postnatal male in which all the paraganglion cells are immunoreactive for substance P (SP); (8) intramuscular paraganglion from the urinary bladder of a 3-year-old postnatal male in which all the paraganglion cells are immunoreactive for tyrosine hydroxylase (TH) (panels 1, 7, 8: × 150; 2: × 75; 3–6: × 300). (From Ref. 16.)

of the lower urinary tract, in contrast to the findings of von Heyden et al. who used a poly-
clonal antibody to norepinephrine to stain adrenergic nerves in two older fetuses (18).
Whether the differences between these two studies result from the techniques used or the
ages or gender of the fetuses remains to be determined. However, despite the absence of
adrenergic nerves, the presence of functional responsiveness to norepinephrine indicates
that α-adrenergic receptors are present at this early stage in development.

Mitolo–Chieppa and co-workers examined contractile responses of bladder base
strips from human fetuses, aged 3–6 months, to a number of different pharmacological agonists (20). The strips are called sphincter, but the location from which they were removed
and the relative amounts of smooth and striated sphincter are not described. Furthermore,
as neither the gender nor the numbers of fetuses at each age is given, we have no way of
knowing whether responses are representative of more than a single observation. Contractile responses to the muscarinic agonist, bethanechol, were reduced with increasing duration of gestation from 4 to 6 months, suggesting a progressive decline in muscarinic receptor density in the sphincter with increasing gestational age. Contractile responses of
sphincter to α_1-adrenergic stimulation could not be demonstrated in fetuses younger than 6
months, in contrast to the findings of Andersson et al., who showed both an increase in
spontaneous activity and in basal tone after norepinephrine administration in fetuses aged
4–5½ months (19). Developmental changes in autonomic responsiveness have been
demonstrated in rabbit bladder base (21). In this preparation, adrenergic innervation is
sparse at birth and increases with development. Contractile responses to α-adrenergic agonists are absent at birth and increase with increasing age, paralleling development of α-
adrenoceptors. Cholinergic innervation of the rabbit bladder base is dense at birth, and undergoes little change with increasing age. Responses to muscarinic stimulation are
unchanged during development, and muscarinic receptor densities are maximal at birth.
Therefore, although many of these studies do not specifically focus on the external urethral
sphincter, the overall consensus seems to be that cholinergic stimulation has minimal effects on urethral resistance.

VI. IN VIVO PHARMACOLOGY

Because of the inherent difficulties associated with the preparation, little information is
available on in vivo physiology or pharmacology of the fetal external urethral sphincter. In
a series of experiments, Kogan and co-workers monitored responses of the lower urinary
tract of sheep fetuses at varying stages of gestation. Indirect evaluation of urethral sphincter function was made during urodynamic studies in which bladder filling was done through
an urachal catheter. Systemic infusion of the nitric oxide synthase (NOS) inhibitor, N^{ω}-
nitro-L-arginine (L-NNA), into 120-day–gestation fetuses (term 145 days) caused the development of frequent ineffective bladder contractions, yet increased bladder capacity and
postvoid residuals (22). The finding of increased contractions, but poor emptying, suggests
that blockade of nitric oxide synthesis caused a failure of urethral relaxation. After reversal
of the nitric oxide synthase inhibition by infusion of L-arginine, dribbling incontinence occurred, suggesting to the authors that nitric oxide produced from the L-arginine, caused excessive sphincteric relaxation. These observations correlate with data from mature animals
that demonstrate that most NOS is found in the region of the bladder base and urethra (Fig.
11; see color insert). Taken together, these findings suggest that nitric oxide may play an
important role in late gestation sphincteric function.

VII. CONCLUSIONS

When reviewing the literature, one can clearly document the development of the various portions of the urinary sphincter. Histological studies are reasonably complete, but there are major gaps in our understanding of the functional development of the sphincter. Furthermore, there are gender differences that may have significant neonatal consequences that remain to be fully documented.

REFERENCES

1. Bourdelat D, Barbet JP, Butler–Browne GS. Fetal development of the urethral sphincter. Eur J Pediatr Surg 1992; 2:35–38.
2. Tichy M. The morphogenesis of human sphincter urethrae muscle. Anat Embryol 1989; 180: 577–582.
3. Matsuno T, Tokunaka S, Koyanagi T. Muscular development in the urinary tract. J Urol 1984; 132:148–152.
4. Oelrich TM. The striated urogenital sphincter muscle in the female. Anat Record 1983; 205: 223–232.
5. Dröes JTPM, Van Ulden BM, Donker PJ, Landsmeer JWF. [Proceedings]: Studies of the urethral musculature in the human fetus, newborn and adult. Urol Int 1974; 29:231–234.
6. Kokoua A, Homsy Y, Lavigne JF, Williot P, Corcos J, Laberge I, Michaud J. Maturation of the external urinary sphincter: a comparative histotopographic study in humans. J Urol 1993; 150:617–622.
7. Gosling JA, Dixon JS, Humpherson JR. Functional Anatomy of the Urinary Tract. Baltimore: University Park Press, 1982.
8. de Leval J, Chantraine A, Penders L. Le sphincter strié de l'urétre. Première partie: rappel des connaissances sur le sphincter strié de l'urètre. J Urol (Paris) 1984; 90:439–454.
9. Oehich TM. The urethral sphincter muscle in the male. Am J Anat 1980; 158:229–246.
10. Borirakchanyavat S, Baskin LS, Kogan BA, Cunha GR. Smooth and striated muscle development in the intrinsic urethral sphincter. J Urol 1997; 158:1119–1122.
11. Patapoutian A, Wold BJ, Wagner RA. Evidence for developmentally programmed transdifferentiation in mouse esophageal muscle. Science 1995; 270:1818–1821.
12. Woodcock–Mitchell J, Mitchell JJ, Low RB, Kieny M, Sengel P, Rubbia L, Skalli O, Jackson B, Gabbiani G. alpha-Smooth muscle actin is transiently expressed in embryonic rat cardiac and skeletal muscles. Differentiation 1988; 39:161–166.
13. Gilpin SA, Gosling JA. Smooth muscle in the wall of the developing human urinary bladder and urethra. J Anat 1967; 137:503–512.
14. Olszewski VJ, Antoszewska M. Anatomical consideration on innervation of external urethral sphincter. Anat Anz Jena 1988; 166:239–244.
15. Shafik A, Doss S. Surgical anatomy of the somatic terminal innervation to the anal and urethral sphincters: role in anal and urethral surgery. J Urol 1999; 161:85–89.
16. Dixon JS, Jen PYP, Gosling JA. A double-label immunohistochemical study of intramural ganglia from the human male urinary bladder neck. J Anat 1997; 190:125–134.
17. Dixon JS, Jen PYP, Gosling JA. Immunohistochemical characteristics of human paraganglion cells and sensory corpuscles associated with the urinary bladder. A developmental study in the male fetus, neonate and infant. J Anat 1998; 192:407–415.
18. von Heyden B, Jordan U, Hertle L. Neurotransmitters in the human urethral sphincter in the absence of voiding dysfunction. Urol Res 1998; 26:299–310.
19. Andersson K-E, Persson CGA, Alm P, Kullander S, Ulmsten U. Effects of acetylcholine, noradrenaline and prostaglandins on the isolated, perfused human fetal urethra. Acta Physiol Scand 1978; 104:394–401.

20. Mitolo–Chieppa D, Schönauer S, Grasso G, Cicinelli E, Carretú MR. Ontogenesis of autonomic receptors in detrusor muscle and bladder sphincter of human fetus. Urology 1983; 21:599–603.
21. Levin RM, Malkowicz SB, Jacobowitz D, Wein AJ. The ontogeny of the autonomic innervation and contractile response of the rabbit urinary bladder. J Pharmacol Exp Ther 1981; 219:250–257.
22. Mevorach RA, Bogaert GA, Kogan BA. Role of nitric oxide in fetal lower urinary tract function. J Urol 1994; 152:510–514.

2

Functional Anatomy of the Bladder and Urethra in Females

FRANÇOIS HAAB, PHILIPPE SEBE, FABRICE MONDET, and CALIN CIOFU

Saint Antoine University and Tenon Hospital, Paris, France

I. INTRODUCTION

Urinary incontinence in women results from a complex interaction between the bladder, urethra, and pelvic floor. Understanding the functional aspects of the bladder and urethra is necessary to appreciate the pathophysiology of stress urinary incontinence (SUI) and to evaluate its various treatment modalities.

This chapter will focus on the different anatomical structures involved in continence in women and will discuss the functional organization of the pelvis at rest, during stress, and voluntary retention.

II. DESCRIPTIVE ANATOMY

A. The Intrinsic Continence Mechanism

The female urethra is 4 cm long, with a diameter of 6 mm. It begins at the internal vesical orifice, extending downward and forward behind the symphysis pubis, embedding in the anterior vaginal wall, and terminating at the external urethral meatus.

The intrinsic urethral closure continence mechanism relies on the mucosal sealing effect of the urethra, a competent bladder neck, and a functional urethral sphincter (1). Each component contributes approximately one-third of urethral closing pressure at rest (2).

The urethral mucosa is surrounded by a rich, spongy, estrogen-dependent submucosal vascular plexus that is encased in fibroelastic and muscular tissue. Slight compression applied by the surrounding smooth rhabdo sphincters on this layer can result in an excel-

15

lent seal for continence. Estrogens enhance proliferation and maturation of the urethral epithelium and increase vascular pulsations in the urethral wall (3).

According to McGuire and Woodside (4), closure of the bladder neck and proximal urethra is essential to maintain continence, and is even more important than the external sphincteric mechanism. However, the role of the bladder neck in maintaining continence is still controversial. Gosling (5) suggested that the orientation of the smooth-muscle fibers at the bladder neck acts on contraction to open, rather than close the bladder neck. Versi et al. (6) demonstrated that 50% of continent women have an open bladder neck during coughing exercises. Furthermore, using transvaginal ultrasound, Chapple et al. (7) found that 21% of young nulliparous asymptomatic women have an open bladder neck at rest. Finally, recent reports on female orthotopic bladder replacement without preservation of the bladder neck have highlighted the role of the midurethra in maintaining continence (8).

The outer layer of the urethra is formed by the striated sphincter muscle that is present along 80% of the total anatomical urethral length. As seen in magnetic resonance imaging (MRI), the sphincter has its largest diameter in the middle part of the urethra (9). Classically, the urethral striated sphincter muscle is innervated by myelinated somatic fibers, from the S_2 and S_3 levels, which are carried within the pudendal nerves. However, there has been considerable controversy over whether these fibers are purely somatically innervated or if there is a mixture of somatically and autonomically innervated fibers. Evidence suggests that innervation of the urethral sphincter is very complex (10).

The striated urogenital sphincter has two distinct portions: an upper sphincteric portion, which is arranged circularly around the urethra corresponds to the rhabdosphincter classically described in the literature; and a lower portion comprising an arch-like pair of muscular bands (Fig. 1) (11).

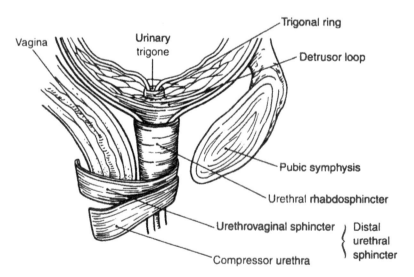

Figure 1 Architectural organization of the striated urethral sphincter. Location of its three components: the urethral rhabdosphincter, the compressor urethra, and the urethrovaginal sphincter. (From Ref. 11.)

1. The Urethral Rhabdosphincter

The fibers of the urethral rhabdosphincter surround the urethral lumen from approximately 20 to 60% of its length. The striated urethral muscle completely surrounds the urethra, although the posterior portion between the urethra and the vagina is relatively thin. Fibers in the posterior plane do not constitute a complete ring, and the gap between the two ends of the rhabdosphincter is bridged by the trigonal plate which completes the ring (11). Therefore, a defect in the muscular ring does not impair contraction because the trigonal plate functions as a tendon, bridging the gap between the muscle on its two ends.

These findings have been reinforced by recent anatomical work on the evolution of the striated sphincter in females with aging (12). The authors have identified that the dorsal wall of the urethral sphincter is present in young females, but its muscular tissue is progressively replaced by fibrotic tissue with aging. The same authors also found a decrease in the number and density of urethral striated muscle fibers with aging, but no decrease in individual fiber size (12). Therefore, aging is characterized at the level of the striated sphincter by a loss of contractile tissue owing to a loss of muscle fibers, rather than by atrophy of the remaining muscle cells. However, although the urethral sphincter plays an important role in continence, little is known about the length and attachment of the endings of its fibers, nor how they are innervated. Circular fibers without tendons have been described (5,13,14), but fibers are also seen attached to connective tissue in the ventral and dorsal parts of the urethra and running along the lateral part (15). The latter observation suggests the existence of two symmetrical muscles. This hypothesis is supported by the presence of two pudendal nerves innervating the rhabdosphincter (16).

Experimental work done in rats has defined and characterized more precisely the functional anatomy and innervation of the striated urethral muscle. These studies have demonstrated that muscle fibers are disposed symmetrically around the urethral lumen, from a ventral to a dorsal insertion into the connective tissue of the urethral wall (Fig. 2A, B) (17). Left and right fibers cross the sagittal plane to overlap (see Fig. 2C). In all cases, the ventral and dorsal insertions of a single fiber are not at the same level of the muscle. On muscle cross sections, the fibers display a cross section near their insertion with the greater part of their length being oriented longitudinally parallel to the urethral lumen (see Fig. 2D). The rhabdosphincter fibers are not inserted in the osteocartilaginous element of the skeleton; therefore, the rhabdosphincter is a nonskeletal striated muscle in which the fibers are inserted directly in the connective tissue of the urethral wall (17).

The orientation of the fibers both transversally and longitudinally suggests that the rhabdosphincter works by nipping the dorsal and ventral walls of the urethra toward each other while simultaneously sliding them one from the other. Staining of the neuromuscular junction reveals a single end plate located at the midpart of each fiber. End plates are always located in contiguous fibers. They are not distributed randomly. In female rats, this lateral disposition of the myofibers is not homogeneous all along the rhabdosphincter: the proximal third contains twofold more end plates than the distal third (17).

2. The Distal Urethral Sphincter

The second portion of the striated urogenital sphincter is at the level of the distal third of the urethra, lying approximately along 60–80% of its length. These striated fibers are not circular in orientation, but consist of two bands that cover the ventral surface of the urethra (11). One of these bands, called the compressor urethra, originates in the perineal membrane. The other band, known as the urethrovaginal sphincter muscle, originates in the vaginal wall.

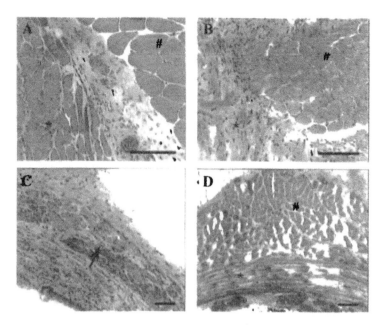

Figure 2   Organization of myofibers in the rat rhabdosphincter: (A) the rhabdosphincter
(*) and the levator ani (#) are separated by connective tissue. Note the respective size of the
muscle fibers; (B) myoconnective junction at the ventral raphe of the rhabdosphincter (*,
connective tissue; #, rhabdosphincter myofibers); (C) crossing of the left and right fascicles
of myofibers at the ventral level, separated by a slight band of connective tissue (arrow) in
females; (D) anterolateral level of the right rhabdosphincter: the saggital lateral fascicle of
myofibers (*) is adjacent to the longitudinal anterior fascicle, showing cross-sectioned fibers
(#). Bars: 20 μm.

B.   The Extrinsic Continence Mechanism

1.   Supportive Structures

The structures involved in urethral and bladder neck support are the arcus tendineus fascia
pelvis, the endopelvic fascia, the pelvic diaphragm, the pubourethral ligaments, and the anterior vaginal wall.

   The endopelvic fascia is the first layer of the pelvic floor. It connects the upper vagina,
cervix, and uterus to the pelvic side walls (Fig. 3). The structure of this fascia varies in different areas of the pelvis, and different ligaments have been identified: the pubourethral ligaments, the urethropelvic ligaments, and the uterosacral ligaments, which are at the level of
the cervix and uterus. All these ligaments are vertical in orientation; therefore, they suspend
the organs from above.

   The region of the external urethral meatus is closely attached to the anterior surface
of the symphysis pubis. This attachment is mainly due to the pubourethral ligaments which
extend between the urethra and the pelvic surface of the pubic bone (18). These ligaments
have a pyramidal form, with a narrow apical bony attachment and a broad urethral attachment. Zaccharin (18) described the pubourethral ligaments as the suspensory mechanism
of the female urethra. This anatomical entity limits excessive urethral mobility in the normal female subject and maintains a close relation between the urethra and the bony con-
tours of the pubic bone and the suprapubic arch.

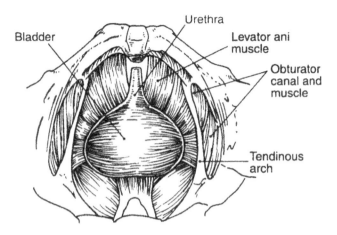

Figure 3 Abdominal view of the pelvic floor with the levator muscle attached laterally to the tendinous arc. (From Ref. 19.)

The arcus tendineus fascia pelvis is a fibrous band that is attached ventrally to the pubic bone and dorsally to the ischial spine (see Fig. 3). This tendinous arc provides lateral attachment to the pelvic floor muscles and ligaments (19).

The pelvic diaphragm represents the muscular component of urethral support and constitutes two different muscles: the levator ani muscle (pubococcygeus and iliococcygeus) and the coccygeus muscle (see Fig. 3). The function of these muscles is to pull the rectum, the vagina, and the urethra anteriorly against the pubic bone to compress their lumen. The pubovaginalis portion, which is the most anterior part of the levator ani, is critical to support the urethra and represents the main muscular component of urethral support.

The perineal body represents dorsal fusion of the three muscles of the perineum: the bulbospongeosus, the ischiocavernosus, and the superficial transverse perinei. Some fibers of the external anal sphincter are also attached at the perineal body. This muscular structure gives stability to the pelvic organs, but does not seem to interfere significantly in continence.

2. The Anterior Vaginal Wall

The anterior vaginal wall and urethra are highly fused by loose areolar tissue so that the vaginal wall conforms to the shape of the periurethral fascia and follows its contour. In the normal female, the vaginal wall ascends laterally and superiorly. The vagina attaches very loosely to the urethropelvic ligaments as it anchors to the lateral pelvic floor, thereby giving the characteristic H-shape of the vaginal lumen in cross-sectional imaging.

The anterior vaginal wall plays an important role in continence mechanisms by supporting the urethra and bladder base. Excessive relaxation of the wall may result in urethral hypermobility and bladder descent.

The anterior vaginal wall is constituted of three different layers: an inner mucosa, a middle connective tissue, and an external muscular layer, including both circular and longitudinal smooth muscle cells. Fu et al. (20) reported that spontaneous contractile activity was increased by prostaglandin F_2 and that norepinephrime augmented muscle tone and induced contractions. According to these preliminary findings, the vaginal wall could be considered not only a passive backboard, but also it clearly has an active role in urethral support.

III. FUNCTIONAL ANATOMY

A. Urinary Continence at Rest

Continence at rest depends on bladder neck closure, urethral sphincter muscle tonic activity, and the urethral mucosa (21).

The fibers within the urethral sphincter are primarily slow-twitch fibers capable of maintaining constant tonic activity. Therefore, the urethral sphincter muscle is well suited to maintain constant tone within the urethral lumen, while retaining the ability to contract when additional occlusive force is needed. The urethral closure pressure measured during static urethral profilometry may represent this permanent intraurethral tone along with the mucosal seal effect. The levator ani muscles also have a constant tone that helps support pelvic structures, including the urethra, by the pubovaginalis portion.

B. Voluntary Continence During Storage

When the bladder is full and when the patient has to postpone urination, additional urethral closure can be elicited through somatic innervation. In this situation, continence relies on active muscle contraction, rather than on pelvic support (21).

Contraction of the striated urogenital sphincter muscle closes the urethral lumen in its upper portion, and the compressor urethra and urethrovaginal muscle sphincter could compress the ventral wall of the distal third of the urethra. Fibers of the striated muscles involved in this process are mainly fast-twitch fibers.

Furthermore, when voluntary continence is needed, active contraction of the pelvic floor may enhance urethral support but, more importantly, contraction of the pelvic floor tends to inhibit any detrusor contraction (22).

C. Continence During Stress

The striated urogenital sphincter by itself is not capable of assuring continence when there is a sudden increase in intra-abdominal pressure. Therefore, the transmission of abdominal pressure to the urethra is almost certainly a primary factor in maintaining continence during stress. This pressure transmission between the abdominal cavity and the urethra is dependent on three factors: urethral support, muscle synergies, and finally, urethral compliance.

1. Urethral Support

The "Hammock" Theory.   The tissue that supports the urethra constitutes a sling ("hammock") under the urethra in its upper and midportions (23). This sling is composed of a segment of the anterior vaginal wall that is attached to the muscles of the pelvic floor (levator ani muscles principally) and to the arcus tendineus fascia pelvis. The levator ani muscles not only help support the visceral structures at rest because of their constant tone, but they act as a backup to the endopelvic fascia, probably serving as the principal support during suddenly increased intra-abdominal pressure. The connection of the urethra to the arcus tendineus assists levator support and limits downward descent of the vesical neck when the levator muscles are relaxed or overcome.

Since support of the bladder neck and proximal urethra is both muscular and ligamentous, proper intrapelvic support requires and active component of muscular contraction during stress, along with the firm strength of the ligaments and vaginal wall. When both active or passive supports are altered, the urethra and bladder base are no longer well supported, resulting in defective transmission of intra-abdominal pressure to the urethra. This type of incontinence is commonly described as type II SUI (24). However, the mechanism responsible for urinary incontinence has not been fully elucidated, since some women are continent despite clinical evidence of urethral hypermobility (1).

The "Intregal Theory."   In 1990, Petros and Ulmsten (25,26) introduced the "integral theory" of female urinary incontinence which states that stress and urge symptoms both arise from the same anatomical defect: a lax vagina. The authors proposed three closure mechanisms (Fig. 4): 1) contraction of the anterior pubococcygeus muscle closes the urethra, and contraction of the periurethral striated muscle provides a watertight seal for the bladder; 2) the bladder neck is closed off by being elongated backward and downwards against an immobilized proximal urethra by stretching of the underlying vagina; 3) a voluntary closure mechanism is mediated by the pelvic floor muscles which, on command, pull the vaginal hammock forward.

Therefore, preservation of continence necessitates adequate functioning of the pubourethral ligament, the suburethral vaginal hammock and the pubococcygeus muscles. Tension in the pubourethral ligament is essential for a correct interplay between the muscles and the vaginal hammock (Fig. 5). The pubourethral ligament acts on an insertion point for horizontal force at the level of the midurethra.

Based on this theory, Ulmsten et al. (27) introduced the tension-free vaginal tape (TVT) technique which reinforces the pubourethal ligament and the suburethral vaginal

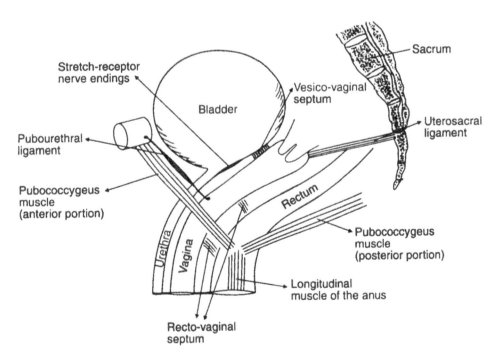

Figure 4   Bladder neck closure mechanism: the anterior and posterior portions of the pubococcygeus muscle contract, creating a semirigid plate. By the contraction of the longitudinal muscle of the anus, the midsection of the plate is pulled downward, "kinking" the bladder base at the internal orifice of the immobilized urethra. The urethra is immobilized by forward contraction of the anterior portion of the pubococcygeus muscle, which pulls against the pubourethral ligament.

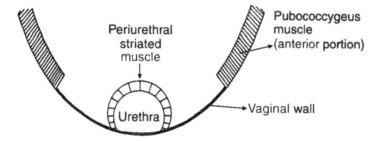

Figure 5 Urethral closure mechanism: contraction of the anterior portion of the pubococ-cygeus muscle closes the urethra. Contraction of the periurethral striated muscle provides a watertight seal.

hammock. The principle of the TVT procedure consists of two parts: an artificial pub-ourethral neoligament is created by the insertion of polyester tape in the position of the natural ligament, and the suburethral hammock is tightened.

2. Muscular Synergies

During stress, various muscle synchronisms or reflexes help maintain continence. First, there is synchrony between the rectus abdominis muscle and the pelvic floor. The posterior portion of the levator ani has constant tone, as mentioned previously, but also contracts further at the time of rectus abdominis contraction during the Valsalva maneuver to maintain a proper vaginal axis (21).

It has been clearly demonstrated that an increase in intraurethral pressure precedes the increase in abdominal pressure by 250 msec, and the pressure rise in the urethra frequently exceeds the increase in intra-abdominal pressure (28). Therefore, there is probably a contraction of the urethral striated muscle in addition to the supportive role of passive compression. Furthermore, the greatest increase in urethral pressure occurs in the distal urethra, rather than in the proximal urethra. This is due to the compressor urethra and ure-throvaginal sphincter muscles that can actively raise intraurethral pressure during stress, and especially when the patient coughs.

From a therapeutic point of view, physiotherapy could help restore continence in two different ways. First, it could reinforce the pelvic floor muscles or the striated urethra sphincter, using either pelvic floor exercises or electrostimulation. Second, physiotherapy could restore muscular synergies between the abdominal wall and pelvic floor by biofeed-back techniques that are relevant to enhance the training of agonistic (levator ani) and antagonistic (rectus abdominis) muscles.

Finally, as mentioned previously, female patients may have lost reflex contraction of the levator ani during a sudden increase in abdominal pressure. One goal of rehabilitation is to relearn this reflex.

3. Urethral Compliance

Urethral compliance or softness is critical for urinary continence during stress (29). When the urethra is rigid, for example, owing to scar tissue after surgery or to pelvic radiation, the various continence mechanisms previously described are not able to compress the urethra and to close the urethral lumen. This situation is commonly known as intrinsic sphincteric deficiency (ISD). However, there is no objective test to quantify urethral wall compliance.

Table 1 Mechanisms of Stress Urinary Incontinence[a]

1. Urethral hypermobility
    Weak muscular support
    Loss of local reflex loop between synergistic muscles
    Ligamentous weakness
    Pathology of connective tissue
2. Urethral insufficiency
    loss of compliance (i.e., pipe stem urethra): mechanical ISD
    Hypotonic urethra (neurogenic ISD)
    Estrogen deficiency

[a]Urinary continence in females results from a complex interaction between urethral support and urethral ability to close. Urethral hypermobility and urethral insufficiency may be associated and should be evaluated to decide the best therapeutic option.

As we have seen before, the definition of ISD is larger than "pipe stem urethra" and probably involves situations during which active reflexes have been damaged by neurological problems.

IV. CONCLUSION

Knowledge of the functional anatomy of continence in females has improved dramatically in the past 10 years. This has helped clinicians to achieve a better understanding of the pathophysiology of stress incontinence and, therefore, to provide a rationale for the use of anti-incontinence procedures.

The objective of surgery is to restore continence without creating outlet obstruction. These procedures could be classified according to their goals: to restore proper urethral support (i.e., bladder neck suspension, vaginal wall sling, pubovaginal sling) or to increase intraurethral pressure (i.e., periurethral injections, artificial urinary sphincter).

A better understanding of the functional anatomy of continence is essential to decide which type of procedure is indicated for each patient. There is certainly no clear separation between type II (hypermobility) and type III (ISD) SUI, for both types may have the same origin (Table 1). For example, neurological pathologies can generate urethral hypermobility by a weak muscular component of urethral support, but can also generate ISD by a defect in active contraction of the urethral wall. For these reasons, we have proposed a pure descriptive classification of SUI which addresses the various components of urethral continence.

REFERENCES

1. Haab F, Zimmern PE, Leach GE. Female stress urinary incontinence due to intrinsic sphincteric deficiency: recognition and management. J Urol 1996; 156:3–17.
2. Rud T, Andersson KE, Asmussen M, Hunting A, Ulmsten U. Factors maintaining intraurethral pressure in women. Invest Urol 1980; 17:343–347.
3. Elia G, Bergman A. Estrogen effects on the urethra: beneficial effects in women with genuine stress incontinence. Obstet Gynecol Surv 1993; 48:509–517.
4. McGuire EJ, Woodside JR. Diagnostic advantages of fluoroscopic monitoring during urodynamic evaluation. J Urol 1981; 125:830–834.

5. Gosling JA. The structure of the female lower urinary tract and pelvic floor. Urol Clin North Am 1985; 12:207–214.

6. Versi E, Cardozo LD, Studd JW. Distal urethral compensatory mechanisms in women with an incompetent bladder neck who remain continent and the effect of menopause. Neurourol Urodynam 1990; 9:579–590.

7. Chapple CR, Helm CW, Blease S, Milroy EJG, Rickards D, Osborne JL. Asymptomatic bladder neck incompetence in nulliparous female. Br J Urol 1989; 64:357–359.

8. Hautman RE, Paiss T, De Petriconi R. The ileal neobladder in women: 9 years of experience with 18 patients. J Urol 1996; 155:76–81.

9. Gosling J, Alm P, Bartsch G, Brubaker L, Creed K, Delmas V, Norton P, Smet P, Mauroy B. Gross anatomy of the lower urinary tract. In: Abrams P, Khoury S, Wein A, eds. Proceedings of the 1st International Consultation on Urinary Incontinence. 1999:23–56.

10. Junemann KP, Schmidt RA, Melch H, Tanagho EA. Neuroanatomy and the clinical significance of the external urethral sphincter. Urol Int 1987; 42:132–136.

11. De Lancey JOL. Structural aspects of the extrinsic continence mechanism. Obstet Gynecol 1988; 72:296–301.

12. Peruchini D, LeLancey JO, Patane L. The number and diameter of striated muscle fibers in the female urethra. Neurourol Urodynam 1997; 16:405–407.

13. Sant GR. The anatomy of the external striated urethral sphincter. Paraplegia 1972; 10:153–156.

14. Oerlich TM. The striated urogenital sphincter in the female. Anat Rec 1983; 205–223.

15. Oerlich. TM. The striated urethral sphincter muscle in the male. Am J Anat 1980; 158–229.

16. Tanagho EA, Schmidt RA, De Araujo CG. Urinary striated sphincter: what is its nerve supply? Urology 1982; 415–417.

17. Mondet F, Haab F, Thibault PH, Sebille A. Histomorphometry and innervation of striated fibers in rat rhabdosphincter muscle. J Urol 1999. In press.

18. Zaccharin RF. The suspensory mechanism of the female urethra. J Anat 1963; 97:423–427.

19. De Lancey JOL. Anatomy and physiology of continence. Clin Obstet Gyncol 1990; 33:298–307.

20. Fu X, Siltberg, Johnson P, Ulmsten U. Viscoelastic properties and muscular function of the human anterior vaginal wall. Int Urogynecol J 1995; 6:229.

21. Leach GE, Haab F. Female pelvic anatomy for the modern day urologist. Contemp Urol 1998; 8:42.

22. Mahony DT, Laferte RO, Blais DJ. Integral storage and voiding reflexes. Neurophysiologic concept of continence and micturition. Urology 1977; 9:95–106.

23. De Lancey JOL. Structural support of the urethra as it relates to stress urinary incontinence: the hammock hypothesis. Am J Obstet Gynecol 1994; 170:1713–1720.

24. Blaivas JG, Olsson CA. Stress incontinence: classification and surgical approach. J Urol 1988; 139:727–731.

25. Petros P, Ulmsten U. An integral theory of female urinary incontinence: experimental and clinical considerations. Acta Obstet Gynecol Scand 1990; 153:7–31.

26. Petros P. The intravaginal slingplasty operation, a minimally invasive technique for cure of urinary incontinence in the female. Aust NZ J Obstet Gynecol 1996; 36:453–461.

27. Ulmsten U, Henriksson L, Johnson P, Varhos G. An ambulatory surgical procedure under local anesthesia for treatment of female urinary incontinence. Int Urogynecol J 1996; 7:81–86.

27. Constantinou CE, Govan DE. Spatial distribution and timing of transmitted and reflexy generated urethra pressures in healthy women. J Urol 1982; 127:964–969.

28. Zinner NR, Sterling AM, Ritter RC. Role of inner urethral softness in urinary continence. Urology 1980; 16:115–117.

3

The Male Striated Urethral Sphincter

ROBERT P. MYERS

Mayo Graduate School of Medicine and Mayo Clinic, Rochester, Minnesota

I. INTRODUCTION

The male striated urethral sphincter (external sphincter) is just one component in a mélange of intricate musculature that composes the pelvic floor and receives innervation primarily from sacral nerve roots. Accurate medical illustration of this part of the human male has always been problematic. Among the numerous offerings available in the literature to understand the complexity of this region, Hinman's *Atlas of Urosurgical Anatomy* (1) is particularly forthcoming in clarifying how pelvic floor structures, including the external sphincter, grossly relate to one another.

II. HISTORY

In 1729, Lorenzo Terraneo (2), an Italian anatomist, unambiguously illustrated what has become known synonymously as the external striated urethral sphincter, external urethral sphincter, external sphincter, or rhabdosphincter (Fig. 1). In his text about periurethral glands, Terraneo related that Galen (130–201 AD) called this muscle "sphincter, or strictor." Vesalius (1514–1564) used "sphincter of the bladder." Later, Riolan (1577–1657), the French anatomist, described it as "sphincter vesicae externus" [as did Henle (3), father of the urogenital diaphragm, in 1866].

In 1836, Müller (4) produced the earliest, most detailed description of the "musculus constrictor urethrae membranaceae." His original copper plates illustrated the external sphincter with superb detail (Fig. 2). Importantly, he depicted the sphincter as a tubular structure around the membranous urethra from the apex of the prostate to the penile bulb. There is no suggestion in his work of any urogenital diaphragm.

Major confusion over the disposition of the external sphincter can be traced to Henle in 1866 (3), who coined the term "diaphragma urogenitale," or urogenital diaphragm. Early

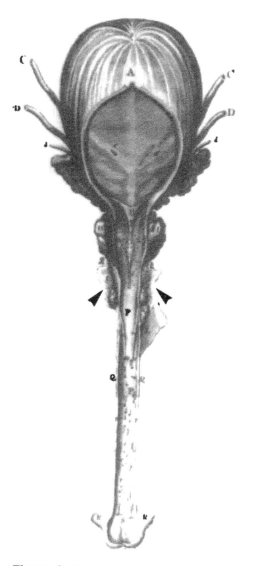

Figure 1 External sphincter (arrowheads): Note embedded bulbourethral glands within distal sphincter. A, bladder; H, prostate; P, urethra; R, glans penis (arrowheads were added). (From Ref. 2.)

in his work, in Figure 285, he showed cylindrical disposition of the external sphincter around the membranous urethra jutting a short distance beyond the apex of the prostate (Fig. 3). The urethra, though, was transected at a level commensurate with the inferior fascia of the pelvic diaphragm, thereby allowing an estimated proximal half to two-third segment of the external sphincter to remain attached to the prostate. He named this proximal segment "sphincter vesicae externus." This then left approximately a half to a third of the sphincter and membranous urethra isolated distal to the inferior fascia of the pelvic diaphragm. He renamed the isolated distal portion of the external sphincter the deep trans-

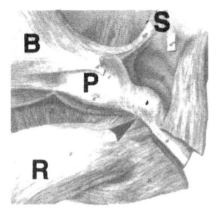

Figure 2 External sphincter (arrowhead) as a vertical tubular structure around the urethra distal to the prostate (P): B, bladder; R, rectum; S, symphysis (arrowhead and capital letters were added). (From Ref. 4.)

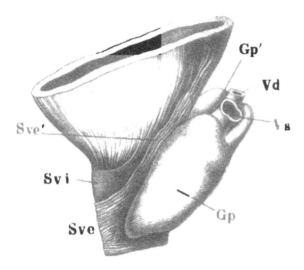

Figure 3 External sphincter as sphincter vesicae externus (Sve): Note transection of urethra close to apex of prostate (Gp). (From Ref. 3.)

verse perinei. Thus, he confusingly divided the external sphincter into two segments with different names.

The inferior fascia of the pelvic diaphragm became the superior fascia, and the perineal membrane became the inferior fascia of a urogenital diaphragm. All of the muscle between the superior and inferior fasciae of the urogenital diaphragm was deep transverse perinei, even the external sphincter. The myth of a muscle sandwich (5) was created. Henle's Figure 392 of the urogenital diaphragm was taken in a coronal plane posterior to the urethra. No urethra was shown penetrating his diaphragm (Fig. 4). The addition of a urethra to a transverse muscle sandwich was the error of subsequent illustrators (Fig. 5). Furthermore,

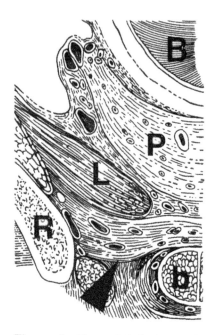

Figure 4 Urogenital diaphragm (arrowhead): Note that no urethra is pictured between prostate (P) and bulb (b). B, bladder; L, levator ani; R, ischiopubic ramus. (Arrowhead and capital letters were added.) (From Ref. 3.)

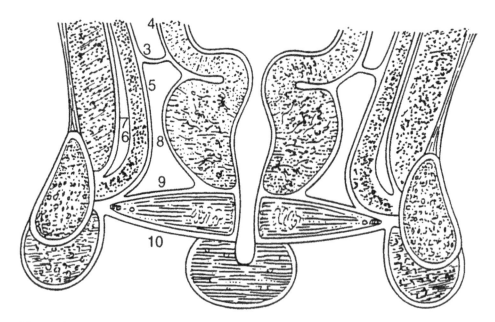

Figure 5 Urogenital diaphragm with urethra erroneously added to same coronal plane as bulbourethral glands. (From Ref. 11.)

illustrators incorrectly added the superior fascia of a urogenital diaphragm as a fascia inferior and separate from a more superiorly situated inferior fascia of the pelvic diaphragm. Henle's concept of a urogenital diaphragm was therefore falsely interpreted and illustrated.

One of the most influential illustrators of the late 20th century was the artist and physician-by-training Frank Netter, whose 1954 atlas (6) continued in color illustration the error of a urogenital diaphragm in both the coronal and the sagittal planes. His work was completed in collaboration with Samuel Vest, one of the most prominent urologists of the mid-20th century. A black-and-white rendition of the coronal illustration appeared for the first time in Lich and Howerton's anatomy chapter in the 2nd edition of Campbell's *Urology* in 1963 (7). The coronal illustration reappeared in both the 3rd edition in 1970 (8) and the 4th edition in 1978 (9). In 1989, Netter's *Atlas of Human Anatomy* (10) carried Plate 361, identical with the 1954 figure with all of the aforementioned error. (The error was captured as early as 1895 in the Basel *Nomina Anatomica;* (11)) For more than 35 years, Netter's coronal illustration of the urogenital diaphragm became the foundation for copies by commercial artists and the advertisers who solicited their work. The urogenital diaphragm as captured so dramatically by Netter mesmerized urological surgeons despite attempts in the literature (12–14) and at a national meeting (5) to dispel the falsehood. Professional journal articles have appeared repeatedly showing the urogenital diaphragm concept in illustration. The illustration of the urogenital diaphragm by Netter (Fig. 6; see color insert) so profoundly influenced urological residents that minds became inured. Recently, a new corruption has evolved in the sagittal plane that combines artistically a pelvic and urogenital diaphragm into a continuous convex entity from coccyx to pubis with the portion anterior to the urethra called the urogenital diaphragm and the portion posterior to the urethra called the pelvic diaphragm (15). This was conceived despite the fact that the pelvic diaphragm and urogenital diaphragm have never been considered the same entity.

Magnetic resonance imaging (MRI) (16) reveals no support for the concept of a urogenital diaphragm, in agreement with Oelrich (13). (Oelrich confirmed Müller (4), who stated, "the membranous part of the urethra does not bore through an aponeurosis . . . [it] goes only through its own constrictor and sinks into the upper surface of the bulb.") There is no structure in coronal MRI that even remotely resembles Netter's urogenital diaphragm (16–18). (Fig. 7). Furthermore, the vertical, tubular MRI configuration is readily confirmed both by gross dissection of fresh cadaveric material (Fig. 8) and by transrectal ultrasonography (Fig. 9).

The major problem of the misinterpretations and the mistaken concept of a urogenital diaphragm has been that it has affected the way surgeons have thought about and approached operations involving the membranous urethra and what Turner Warwick (19) so elegantly called the distal sphincter mechanism. The urogenital diaphragm became synonymous with and, in some illustrations, was labeled the external sphincter. The external sphincter took on the disposition of a flat, horizontal muscle attached bilaterally to the ischiopubic rami, with the prostate perched on top like a plum sitting on a shelf. The idea that the external sphincter was a vertical, tubular structure was lost. Sadly, for those operating with the concept of a urogenital diaphragm in mind, there has been the prospect of an avoidable, significant incidence of urinary incontinence in such operations as radical prostatectomy for localized cancer.

From a historical standpoint, the picture has come full circle from Müller. On a promising note, since Netter's death, the revised 2nd edition of his atlas (20) finally eliminated, after 43 years, a coronal image urogenital diaphragm. A more accurate anatomy proved by

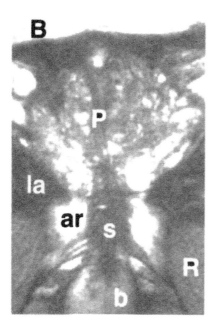

Figure 7 Coronal endorectal coil magnetic resonance imaging scan of external sphincter (s): External sphincter is a vertical tubular structure from prostate (P) to bulb (b) flanked by the fibrofatty anterior recess (ar) of each ischioanal fossa. B, bladder; la, levator ani; R, ischiopubic ramus.

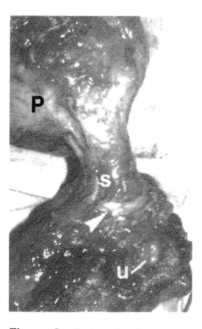

Figure 8 Cadaveric dissection shows external sphincter (s) enveloping membranous urethra between prostate (P) and transverse ligament of perineum (arrowhead) that is situated above bulb and bulbous urethra (u).

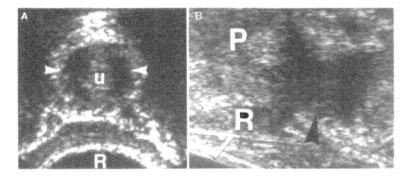

Figure 9   Transrectal ultrasonography: (A) axial image—arrowheads denote hypoechoic external sphincter around urethra (u); (B) sagittal image—hourglass-shaped external sphincter (arrowhead) splays anteriorly over prostate (P) and distally toward bulb; R, rectum (in A and B).

MRI (16) is illustrated. Müller correctly defined and described the extent of the external sphincter as a vertical, tubular structure. [Müller's work (4), in part, appears to have been stimulated by the work of Wilson (21), who, in 1809, described the periurethral muscle that came to be known as Wilson's muscle. Müller was the first to point out that Wilson's muscle was not the true external sphincter, but an artifact in dissecting out as separate muscle the most anteromedial levator ani when investing the urogenital or anterior levator hiatus. Despite Müller's correct analysis in 1836, a misunderstanding of Wilson's muscle as equivalent to the external sphincter is still carried in *Dorland's Medical Dictionary*, 28th edition, published in 1994; (22)].

III. TERMINOLOGY

The external sphincter surrounds what is called the membranous urethra [pars membranaceae, NA (23), pars intermedia, TA (24)]. The membranous urethra extends from the apex of the prostate to the corpus spongiosum of the penis. There is nothing membranous about it, and the name is a misnomer. Membranous urethra is common parlance, but is inaccurate relative to either composition or anatomical placement. The term "membranous" does not appear to be related to the neighboring perineal membrane (16). Because the term membranous urethra is an obvious misnomer, it seems natural to reach for new, more accurate nomenclature. Obvious problems with the term "membranous" led the Federative Committee on Anatomical Terminology in 1998 to recommend "intermediate urethra" (24), for want of a better term. This segment of urethra is unique in that it is the only segment that has intrinsic sphincteric capacity, as opposed to any other segment of the male urethra. It is on this basis that the recommendation was made to change the name from "membranous urethra" to "sphincteric urethra" (16).

Young (25) applied the term sphincteric urethra to the entire posterior urethra. His definition included the vesical neck or preprostatic sphincter as well as the external sphincter and the intrinsic smooth-muscle and elastic tissue sphincter associated with the membranous urethra. To use the term sphincteric urethra for the membranous urethra, one has to accept the sphincteric capability above the verumontanum (supracollicular sphincter) as being vesical in origin (Henle's sphincter vesicae internus) and the infracollicular urethra

as the true urethral sphincteric urethra. Furthermore, one has to accept that the prostatic urethra is defined only by urethra within the prostate, and this is quite variable, depending on
how the prostate grows in an external and quite varied way to encompass the urethra. If
there is an anterior or posterior prostate apical notch (14), the length of the prostatic urethra
will differ if measured anteriorly or posteriorly. Usually it is shorter anteriorly than posteriorly.

Herein, membranous urethra is used only because it is common parlance. Sphincteric
urethra would be preferable and superior to intermediate urethra because it has functional
connotation of immense importance. The membranous urethra with its external sphincter is
part of what is known as the posterior urethra in the male, which also includes the prostatic urethra. The posterior urethra refers to the urethra above the corpus spongiosum and the
perineal membrane. The anterior urethra then refers to the urethra once it has entered the
superior surface of the bulb of the penis into the so-called spongy urethra (pars spongiosa,
NA) that includes both the bulbar urethra and the pendulous urethra, which is distal to the
penoscrotal angle.

Although the infracollicular sphincteric urethra is the true sphincteric urethra, the
supracollicular urethra is a smooth-muscle sphincter associated with the vesical neck, a
sphincter under α-adrenergic neural control, and not a true urethral sphincter. As mentioned, Henle (3) used sphincter vesicae internus, or internal vesical sphincter. The vesical
neck sphincter is not to be confused with the infracollicular internal sphincter, the smooth-
muscle or intrinsic sphincter of the urethral wall (sometimes referred to as the lissosphinc-
ter). Internal sphincter as used herein refers to the smooth-muscle–elastic tissue sphincter,
distal to the verumontanum, that is primary relative to urinary continence; the external
sphincter is secondary (see later discussion).

IV. DEVELOPMENT AND MATURATION

The precise configuration of the external sphincter at any age of life, from the neonate to
the 90-year-old, cannot be understood in the male without an appreciation of the processes
of maturation of the normal prostate and, in middle age, of benign prostatic hyperplasia
(BPH). Both processes alter the disposition of what would otherwise be essentially a female
external sphincter without interruption. The adult female external sphincter is, on average,
approximately 3 cm long and the male sphincter, based on MRI, on average, 2 cm (range,
1.5–2.4 cm) (16). The variable length of the membranous urethra and, thus, the external
sphincter, is readily appreciated with retrograde urethrography (Fig. 10). In the normal
male prostate without BPH, the 1-cm difference from that in the female is due to the displacement anteriorly or the absorption of the anterosuperior striated sphincter fibers into the
fibromuscular stroma (26) of the prostate. When BPH is present, the same absorption occurs, but the length of the anterior fibromuscular stroma in the sagittal plane is variably increased. Thus, a portion of the sphincter becomes prostatic, forming the basis for several
studies of the striated muscle of the prostate and prostatic urethra (27–29).

Development of the external sphincter from the fetus into adulthood was described in
detail by Oelrich (13) in 1980. He examined the fetus at crown–rump heights of 60, 94, 115,
and 245 mm and at term. Then, he traced maturation at 4 years, at puberty, and in young
adult men, aged 21 and 25. He did not formally examine older men in the age range associated with BPH. As he showed so brilliantly, the muscle primordium appears before the
prostate. As the prostate expands within the primordial muscle, it entraps some of the superior sphincter into its anterior stroma. The circumferential disposition of fibers is dis-

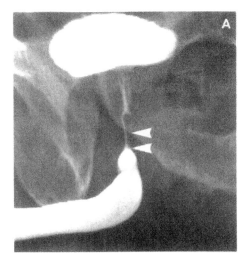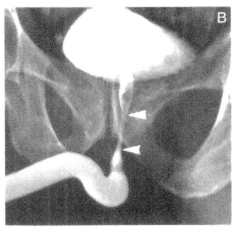

Figure 10 Variable length of membranous urethra and external sphincter in retrograde urethrography: (A) 1 cm; (B) 2.5 cm (arrowheads measure from most distal verumontanum to beginning of bulbous urethra).

rupted so that transverse histological sections show the striated muscle layered out over the anterior surface of the prostate as well as embedded in the stroma. Only distal to the apex of the prostate and around the membranous urethra did Oelrich find the muscle to be sphincteric or circumferential.

When one examines histological sections from the neonate and infant male external sphincter, there is a prominent circumferential distribution of striated fibers around the urethra (30,31). Only a hint of decreased concentration of striated fibers in the posterior midline is present. With increasing age and the development of the adult prostate, the posterior midline becomes progressively devoid of striated sphincter fibers. The posterior midline becomes increasingly fibrotic (31). The result is a posterior midline raphe in continuity with the perineal body. This is not to say that histological sections will not show some striated sphincter fibers in the posterior midline, but the neonatal circumferentiality is lost. The prominent fascia on the posterior surface of the prostate and seminal vesicles known as Denonvilliers' (rectoprostatic and seminal vesicular) fascia is in direct continuity with the midline raphe; hence, with the perineal body. Thus, with advancing age and maturational change, an important alteration takes place in the external sphincter. There is a progressive loss of fibers in the posterior midline so that the disposition of fibers is found, on histological transverse or axial section, to be more of a horseshoe configuration (32). Because the bulk of the fibers are distributed more anterolaterally, the picture changes histologically from true sphincter with a virtually equal circumferential contraction in the neonatal male to more of an anterior compressor in the adult male. Fibers in the posterolateral aspect of the urethra are relatively sparse. This is apparent not only histologically in transverse or axial sections (14,16,31,33), but also in endorectal coil MRI, which demonstrates the external sphincter in exquisite detail (34).

Oelrich dispelled the concept of Henle's urogenital diaphragm, which he never found. Following Müller, he confirmed the unambiguous, tubular, vertical nature of the external sphincter with illustrations showing the extent and disposition of sphincter fibers from the bladder neck to the corpus spongiosum. He found the fascia surrounding the sphincter to be a vertical, tubular sheath and not a pair of transverse planes implicit in a superior and inferior fascia of a urogenital diaphragm. He emphasized that muscle bundles associated with the sphincter were bounded laterally by the pudendal neurovascular pedicles and not the ischiopubic rami, as is so often falsely illustrated.

Oelrich's work did not adequately address the appearance in middle age of BPH. It is evident, however, to someone who performs radical prostatectomy that prostates vary in size, shape, and apical configuration with the onset of BPH. BPH transforms the prostate from a gland with an essentially nonlobar homogeneous stroma and parenchyma to a gland with readily identifiable adenomatous lobes. This phenomenon includes both left and right lateral lobes, symmetrical or asymmetrical, and a median lobe in the floor of the prostatic urethra at the vesical neck, which is often subtrigonal. The lobes vary in degrees of development, and any of the lobes may be absent. Rarely, there is an anterior lobe. Each of these lobes has characteristic adenomatous hyperplasia. The adenomatous lobes develop as a periurethral glandular outbudding. In most cases, as the lobes expand, the normal, relatively homogeneous prostate is compressed posterolaterally outward. With pronounced growth of adenoma, the normal prostate becomes only a thin posterolateral compressed rim around the central BPH. Despite its ubiquity in middle-aged and elderly men, BPH is considered an abnormal condition, and its presence may alter the disposition of the external sphincter at the apex of the prostate. This has important ramifications for proper urethral transection in the course of radical prostatectomy.

The adenomatous prostate may grow to impinge above on the bladder, including its pubovesical (puboprostatic) ligaments, below on the sphincter at the prostate apex, laterally on the levator ani, and backward on the rectum. The pubovesical ligaments may have the illusion of being puboprostatic ligaments, which is their official name, in contrast with women, who unambiguously have pubovesical ligaments. Relative to the sphincter and radical retropubic prostatectomy, growth of the prostate distally does one of three things: (1) the prostate grows to overlap the urethra distal to the veru but not the sphincter; (2) the prostate grows to overlap both the urethra and sphincter distal to the veru; and (3) the prostate grows with no overlap of either urethra or sphincter distal to the veru (Fig. 11). These findings are apparent to one who dissects the apex of the prostate in the course of radical prostatectomy, but these variations have not been formally confirmed in precise coronal histological study. However, one variation, the overlap of the sphincter, has been confirmed in coronal section (35).

Recognizing the variations of the sphincter at the apex is important for optimizing the point of urethral transection and preserving urinary continence. With BPH, distal expansion and growth of the prostate apex around the urethra may be toroidal, circumferentially engulfing the membranous urethra and sphincter. It may grow on either side of the urethra to create an apical notch configuration, or it may produce a combined apical and posterior notch configuration. Alternatively, it may grow asymmetrically with distal expansion on one side, but no growth on the other side. All of the variations constitute some form of BPH overlap of the membranous (sphincteric) urethra.

V. NERVE SUPPLY

The neuroanatomy of the external sphincter has been the subject of continuous controversy and several recent elegant investigations (36–38). Studies support at least dual innervation, both perineal and pelvic (38). The concept of triple innervation (39), which includes auto-

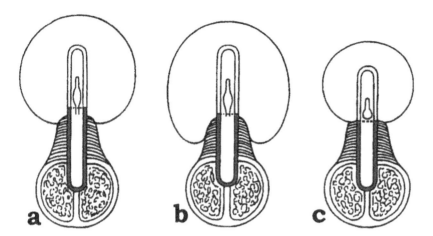

Figure 11   Three configurations of the membranous urethra and external sphincter encountered in radical retropubic prostatectomy: Correct point of urethral transection to ensure postoperative urinary control is at point urethral wall is shaded black at distal verumontanum: (a) Most common, with short intraprostatic urethral cuff; (b) less common, with overlap of sphincter by prostate; (c) Uncommon, with verumontanum at most distal prostatic apex. Urethral crest absent.

nomic as well as dual somatic innervation, has been supported by histochemistry (40) and electron microscopy (41). The idea of autonomic innervation of striated muscle runs counter to the entire rest of the human body; therefore, the concept has its skeptics. (However, the striated muscle fibers of the external sphincter are uniquely different in size and composition, according to electron microscopy; (29))

When the sacral nerve roots are traced as they exit the sacral foramina of S2, S3, and S4, they form a plexus situated along the pelvic sidewall (38). From this plexus, the pelvic nerve courses superficially on the levator ani with branches headed for the apex of the prostate and the external sphincter. In its termination, the pelvic nerve sends branches to both the external sphincter and the levator ani. The pudendal nerve, also formed from the same sacral roots, sends branches that enter the external sphincter from the perineum. The pudendal nerve has a dual supply to the external sphincter, which comprises a superior pelvic surface component and a direct perineal component. Variation of the nerve supply is remarkable (36). Narayan and co-workers (37) found that part of the innervation of the external sphincter originates from special branches that accompany the dorsal nerve of the penis and enter the anterolateral aspect of the sphincter. They suggested possible sensory, as opposed to motor, function for these special branches.

VI. THE SPHINCTER AND MICTURITION

The external sphincter is secondary for urinary continence. It is the internal sphincter, the urethral smooth-muscle wall with its elastic tissue, that is the primary sphincter. If the bladder neck or supracollicular sphincter is not functional, then integrity of the internal sphincter is essential for urinary control. Krahn and Morales (42) demonstrated that the external sphincter is nonessential because pudendal nerve blockade after prostatectomy does not result in urinary incontinence. Recently, Ficazzola and Nitti (43) found that incontinence after radical prostatectomy was associated with deficiency of the internal sphincter in most patients. After prostatectomy, transurethral or radical, the vesical neck sphincter cannot function to provide any degree of continence. Preservation of the distal sphincter mechanism becomes paramount.

The physiology of micturition is so complex that only its basic sequence in ideal circumstances is described (44); that is, a uniform complete emptying of a normal-capacity bladder. Hinman et al. (45) cautioned that interpretation of voiding changes is subject to the state of the bladder, which is variable over time and from situation to situation. It is well known that fear and anxiety, physical activity, ambient temperature, and auditory stimuli, such as running water, all may affect the urge to urinate at different degrees of bladder filling under normal conditions. Sometimes the bladder empties in one continuous stream; sometimes, in a series of interruptions. Under disease conditions of inflammation and obstruction to urinary outflow, voiding becomes increasingly complicated. Inflammation introduces a component of urgency and frequency at less than full capacity. Obstructive diseases, such as BPH, that produce prolonged outflow resistance induce work hypertrophy of the bladder wall with resultant urodynamic abnormality (46). BPH with sufficient increase in outflow resistance leads to detrusor trabeculation with the formation of cellules and diverticula. The result may profoundly affect bladder mechanics and the resultant stream. Hyporeflexia and prolonged residual urine may replace hyperreflexia. Bladder decompensation may occur without a period of hyperreflexia in the face of obstruction. The external sphincter then must function under various events and with individual variation. It is difficult enough to try to assess the normal neurophysiological events of micturition, let alone what is happening in less than ideal circumstances or in the presence of disease.

A. Normal Voiding

With emphasis on the neurophysiological events under normal conditions, Yoshimura and de Groat (44) described voluntary voiding in its simplest form. The pelvic floor and striated urethral sphincter muscles relax as the initial event. The detrusor muscle contracts, and the bladder neck opens. Urine does not flow unless there is reflex inhibition of urethral wall smooth muscle and the external sphincter. Micturition is mediated by activity of autonomic (parasympathetic and sympathetic) and somatic (pudendal) nerves. The precise neurophysiological sequence of events related to the cessation of voiding or to interrupted voiding both in normal and in diseased states is not described in their review.

B. Loop Mechanism?

In extending the work of Oelrich (13), Strasser and colleagues (47) emphasized the change in the male striated urethral sphincter from a circumferential distribution in the fetus to an omega shape in the adult. Others have confirmed the omega shape (30,48). However, axial sections showing an omega shape occur to a very limited degree. Actually, one can find a range of shapes in the axial plane, generally that of a horseshoe, depending on the level of axial or transverse section (32). Whether the axial section is described as omega or horseshoe in shape, at all levels of the membranous urethra in the adult, there is a distinct predominance of the anterolateral striated sphincter fibers. The change in distribution from more circumferential in the child to more horseshoe-configured in the adult suggests that the sphincter cedes true sphincteric ability and comes to function as more of an anterior loop. Recently, in agreement, Myers et al. (49) suggested that not only does the striated sphincter in the male function as an anterior loop but also the puboperinealis portion of the levator ani functions as a posterior loop. The two loops, then, act on the membranous urethra to allow urine to exit in a reflexly relaxed urethra and to produce closure at the termination of voiding (see later discussion).

C. Active or Passive?

There is debate over whether the external sphincter is active or passive (50). Gil Vernet (51) and Burnett and Mostwin (52) supported an active role. Gil Vernet (51) noted the "brusque and violent" closure of the external sphincter in reference to what Gosling et al. (53) termed the quick-stop phenomenon. Burnett and Mostwin illustrated an active mechanism with their schematic of conceptualized function. In the relaxed state, the mass of external sphincter descends with the membranous urethra to a position partially below the pubic arch as the bladder neck and prostatic urethra open. On contraction, the entire mass of sphincter elevates the membranous urethra to a position above the pubic arch and partly anterior to the prostate as the prostatic urethra and bladder neck close tightly.

Several studies (29,53,54) have addressed the physiological capabilities of the external sphincter's striated fibers, which are of much smaller caliber with different tonic capacity compared with ordinary skeletal muscle. Gosling et al. (53) found that the external sphincter fibers were 100% slow-twitch; that is, they would function passively to assist in urethral closure in the absence of urination. Recently, Elbadawi et al. (29) confirmed a predominantly slow-twitch characterization of the external sphincter fibers associated with the prostatic capsule, which can be taken as a reflection of activity of fibers distal to the prostate apex. Only Schrøder and Reske–Nielsen (54) provided controversy by showing a roughly 50:50 slow-twitch–fast-twitch composition. The weight of evidence (two of three studies) supports slow-twitch dominance and, therefore, primarily passive function, but obviously the slow-twitch–fast-twitch controversy needs to be readdressed by new study.

Both transverse histological sections of the membranous urethra and axial images from endorectal coil MRI make it very dubious that the external sphincter could be capable of "brusque and violent" contraction, as described by Gil Vernet (51). Such contraction, however, could clearly reside in the levator ani, particularly in its anteromedial component, the puboperinealis. At the lateral aspects of the urethra, the puboperineales are medial components of the puboanalis (16) (puborectalis, NA, TA) sling that courses posteriorly beneath the anococcygeal ligament. But as medial components, the puboperineales head diagonally downward, anterior to the anorectal flexure, destined for insertion into the perineal body and fusion with the bulbospongiosus and deep portion of the external anal sphincter, as substantiated by MRI (16,49).

The puboperineales, with their attachments to the perineal body, form a powerful loop under voluntary control posterior to the urethra. When the levator ani contracts, this posterior loop is positioned to thrust forward against the back of the urethra, carrying it upward and forward toward the pubis. It is not difficult to imagine that the puboperineales or anteromedial levatores ani are primarily responsible for the quick-stop phenomenon. The problem is one of incontrovertible proof from cineradiography and electrophysiological study, which is lacking.

D. Electrical Stimulation

Stimulation studies do not sort out the exact function of the external sphincter as opposed to the levator ani. Both must stay reflexly relaxed to allow urine to flow freely. Electromyography with use of a perineal cutaneously applied electrode can give only a gross estimate of the function of the perineal and pelvic floor musculature. Studies involving the subcutaneous placement of an electrode are difficult from the standpoint of positioning the electrode accurately. When the external sphincter is said to be stimulated from a posteriorly placed electrode, the electrode tip could be in nonexternal sphincter striated muscle. These muscles include puboperinealis, deep portion of the external anal sphincter, and bulbospongiosus, all present in complex interdigitation anterior to the anorectal angle and at the perineal body. The low-amplitude signal said to be characteristic of the external sphincter has been identified equally with the deep portion of the external anal sphincter (55). Differentiation between the external sphincter and pelvic floor striated muscle, such as the puborectalis (NA, TA), is possible by using an intraurethral electrode and an intraluminal rectal electrode, but it involves two challenging electrode placements (56). Fine-tuning to discriminate between external sphincter and puboperinealis still appears elusive.

VII. SURGICAL CONSIDERATIONS

The less the tissues related to the distal sphincter mechanism, including the external sphincter, are disturbed, the more likely patients will be continent of urine after operations such as radical prostatectomy and cystoprostatectomy with formation of a neobladder anastomosed to the transected membranous urethra. Failure to understand the tubular nature of the external sphincter is one problem. Another is to recognize its variability relative to the apex of the prostate and to transect the urethra with sufficient length and neural innervation to ensure continence.

A. Protection of the External Sphincter

Membranous urethral length varies. When the urethra is very short to begin with, transection too far distal from the prostate apex leaves too little length to expect normal continent coaptation of the urethral lumen. When the membranous urethra is long, there is more latitude in the point of transection. Optimally, one can think of the need to preserve the entire infracollicular sphincteric urethra, which is the goal of urologists performing transurethral resection of the prostate. Transurethral resectionists know that any resection distal to the verumontanum (veru) carries a substantial risk for postoperative urinary incontinence. Turner Warwick (19) illustrated some two-thirds of the sphincter mechanism within the apex of the prostate and one-third distal to the apex. From personal experience performing radical prostatectomy, I would say that it is more realistic to talk about up to one-third of the sphincter mechanism associated with or contained within the apex of the prostate. That is, routine transverse transections of the urethra at the apex or at any point distal to the apex will translate into a finite risk of urinary incontinence because of deliberate sphincter sacrifice. From the standpoint of full sphincter preservation, urethral transection flush with the apex is perfectly acceptable only when the veru is situated at the most distal aspect of the prostatic urethra. This anatomical variant (see Figs. 9A and 10C) can be confirmed either by preoperative retrograde urethrography or endoscopy.

B. Injury

Surgical damage to the external sphincter is a very real issue during the dissection necessary to complete a radical prostatectomy. This includes disruption of the nerves supplying the sphincter from (1) retraction of the levator ani or (2) improperly securing the preprostatic or ventral vascular complex (dorsal vein complex of the penis) (16).

Achievement of postoperative urinary control quickly after radical retropubic prostatectomy includes minimal disruption of the point of attachment of the pubovesical ligaments. (These ligaments are generally called puboprostatic, but are really pubovesical; (16,57). This maneuver preserves the pubourethral fascial support of the membranous (sphincteric) urethra. Because the dorsal vein complex of the penis (ventral vascular complex with respect to the urethra and prostate) is closely adherent to the external sphincter anterolaterally, sutures to secure the plexus in the process of hemostasis should not be placed more distally than the prostatourethral junction or they may injure the sphincter.

In radical perineal prostatectomy (perineal operation), it is customary to provide bilateral anterolateral retraction of the inverted perineal U-shaped incision. The blades of the retractors, handheld or fixed, come to rest against the superficial transverse perineal muscles and the posterior edge of the perineal membrane. Pressure on the pudendal nerve supply to the sphincter that comes in medially from each pudendal neurovascular bundle cannot be avoided. As the prostate is mobilized and the levator sling is retracted laterally, deeper retraction also may affect the nerve supply that comes into the upper portion of the external sphincter through the intrapelvic surface of the levator ani. Handheld retraction that is not constant may be less injurious to the nerves than constant fixed retraction.

Colston (58), a master of the perineal operation, warned many years ago about the insult that multiple simple sutures could inflict on the sphincter and urethra. A ring of fibrosis could easily be produced and a finite portion of the membranous urethra would be defunctionalized. More sutures translate into a more watertight anastomosis after excellent mucosa-to-mucosa approximation, but the drawback is more fibrosis. Fewer sutures provide poorer approximation and the risk of scar formation from local urinary leakage. (Generally, four to six sutures are ideal, with a goal of approximation, not strangulation, of the tissue during the tie-down.)

In an attempt to take pressure off the anastomosis and the external sphincter and urethra and to provide strength, Vest (59) introduced the use of a posterior suture, from the bladder to the midline perineum, tied internally. Subsequently, a modified Vest anastomosis was described by Chute (60) for radical retropubic prostatectomy (the retropubic operation). This involved placing sutures at the 3- and 9-o'clock positions at the reconstructed (plicated) bladder neck and bringing these sutures externally out onto the perineal skin with straight needles. These retention sutures were tied temporarily over a gauze roll (bolster) on the perineal surface. The advantages of this technique are that it avoids the placement of any sutures into the external sphincter and provides results in terms of achievement of urinary control at least as good as the use of simple sutures (61,62). Furthermore, it is technically much simpler in most hands. The downside has been the significant incidence of vesical neck contracture of 10–20%. This type of anastomosis is not watertight, and pooling of urine posteriorly is not uncommon, as demonstrated by retrograde cystography early in the postoperative period. Another downside is that if the perineal sutures are tied too tightly over the sponge or rolled gauze on the perineal surface, the external sphincter becomes squashed with possible ischemic damage and critical decrease in functional urethral length. The right amount of tension on the retention sutures at the time of the tie-down to the perineum is very important. Too much tension produces ischemia and shortens the membranous urethral length, with an obvious threat to urinary continence. Innovation to improve the Vest anastomosis has been introduced recently, and the incidence of vesicourethral anastomotic stricture has been cut to 7.7%, with better mucosa-to-mucosa approximation (63).

The goal in radical prostatectomy is not to disturb the distal continence mechanism. There is some conflicting evidence that neurovascular preservation to protect erectile function may result in improved urinary continence (64). The improved results may have been due to more careful apical dissection and transection of the urethra with more functional length preserved. When the technique of apical dissection was kept constant, neurovascular preservation had no effect on the time to or ultimate success of achieving pad-free urinary control (34,62).

REFERENCES

1. Hinman F Jr. Atlas of Urosurgical Anatomy. Philadelphia: WB Saunders, 1993.
2. Terraneo L. De Glandulis Universum et Speciatim ad Urethram Virilem Novis. Lugduni Batavorum: Haak & Luchtmans, 1729:77–78.
3. Henle J. Handbuch der systematischen Anatomie des Menschen. Vol 2. Braunschweig: F Vieweg & Sons, 1866.
4. Müller J. Über die organischen Nerven der erectilen männlichen Geschlectsorgane des Menschen und der Säugethiere. [Concerning the Autonomic Nerves of the Male Erectile Genital Organs of Man and Mammals.] Berlin: F Dümmler, 1836.
5. Colapinto V. The anatomy of the distal urethral sphincters and the myth of the urogenital "sandwich." J Urol 1984; 131:164A.
6. Netter FH. The CIBA Collection of Medical Illustrations. Vol. 2, Sec. 2. Summit, NJ: CIBA Pharmaceutical Products, 1954: plate 3, p 11; plate 13, p 21.
7. Lich R Jr, Howerton LW. Anatomy and surgical approach to the urogenital tract in the male. In: Campbell, MF, ed. Urology. Vol 1. 2nd ed. Philadelphia: WB Saunders, 1963:23.
8. Lich R Jr, Howerton LW. Anatomy and surgical approach to the urogenital tract in the male. In: Campbell MF, Harrison JH, eds. Urology. 3rd ed. Vol. 1. Philadelphia: WB Saunders, 1970:20.
9. Lich R Jr, Howerton LW, Amin M. Anatomy and surgical approach to the urogenital tract in the male. In: Harrison JH, Gittes RF, Perlmutter AD, Stamey TA, Walsh PC, eds. Campbell's Urology. 4th ed. Vol. 1. Philadelphia: WB Saunders 1978:17.
10. Netter FH. Atlas of Human Anatomy. Summit, NJ: CIBA-GEIGY Corp, 1989: sect. 5, plate 361.
11. His W. Die anatomische Nomenclatur. Nomina anatomica, Verzeichniss der von der anatomischen Gesellschaft auf ihrer IX. Versammlung in Basel angenommenen Namen. Leipzig: Verlag Von Veit, 1895.
12. Elliot JS. Postoperative urinary incontinence, a revised concept of the external sphincter. J Urol 1954; 71:49–57.
13. Oelrich TM. The urethral sphincter muscle in the male. Am J Anat 1980; 158:229–246.
14. Myers RP, Goellner JR, Cahill DR. Prostate shape, external striated urethral sphincter and radical prostatectomy: the apical dissection. J Urol 1987; 138:543–550.
15. Siede BL. Surgical rounds anatomical chart: prostate gland. Surg Rounds 1998; 21:143.
16. Myers RP, Cahill DR, Devine RM, King BF. Anatomy of radical prostatectomy as defined by magnetic resonance imaging. J Urol 1998; 159:2148–2158.
17. Stormont TJ, Cahill DR, King BF, Myers RP. Fascias of the male external genitalia and perineum. Clin Anat 1994; 7:115–124.
18. Myers RP. An anatomic approach to the pelvis in the male. In: Crawford D, Das S, eds. Current Genitourinary Cancer Surgery. 2nd ed. Baltimore: Williams & Wilkins, 1997:155–169.
19. Turner Warwick R. The sphincter mechanisms: their relation to prostatic enlargement and its treatment. In: Hinman F Jr, ed. Benign Prostatic Hypertrophy. New York: Springer-Verlag, 1983:809–828.
20. Netter FH, Dalley AF II, eds. Atlas of Human Anatomy. 2nd ed. East Hanover, NJ: Novartis, 1997.
21. Wilson JA. Description of two muscles surrounding the membranous part of the urethra. Med Chir Soc Trans 1809; 1:175–180.
22. Dorland's Illustrated Medical Dictionary. 28th ed. Philadelphia: WB Saunders, 1994.
23. International Anatomical Nomenclature Committee: Nomina Anatomica, 6th ed. New York: Churchill Livingstone, 1989.

24. Federative Committee on Anatomical Terminology: Terminologia Anatomica: International Anatomical Terminology. Stuttgart: Thieme, 1998.

25. Young BW. Lower Urinary Tract Obstruction in Childhood. Philadelphia: Lea & Febiger, 1972.

26. McNeal JE. The prostate and prostatic urethra: a morphologic synthesis. J Urol 1972; 107: 1008–1016.

27. Manley CB Jr. The striated muscle of the prostate. J Urol 1996; 95:234–240.

28. Haines RW. The striped compressor of the prostatic urethra. Br J Urol 1969; 41:481–493.

29. Elbadawi A, Mathews R, Light JK, Wheeler TM. Immunohistochemical and ultrastructural study of rhabdosphincter component of the prostatic capsule. J Urol 1997; 158:1819–1828.

30. Kokoua A, Homsy Y, Lavigne JF, Williot P, Corcos J, Laberge I, Michaud J. Maturation of the external urinary sphincter: a comparative histotopographic study in humans. J Urol 1993; 150: 617–622.

31. Myers RP. Practical pelvic anatomy pertinent to radical retropubic prostatectomy. AUA Update Ser 1994; 13:26–31.

32. Myers RP. Male urethral sphincteric anatomy and radical prostatectomy. Urol Clin North Am 1991; 18:211–227.

33. Myers RP. Radical prostatectomy: pertinent surgical anatomy. Atlas Urol Clin North Am 1994; 22:1–18.

34. Myers RP. Anatomy and physiology of the external urethral sphincter: implications for preservation of continence after radical prostatectomy. In: Schröder FH, ed. Recent Advances in Prostate Cancer and BPH. New York: Parthenon, 1997:81–86.

35. Blacklock NJ. Surgical anatomy of the prostate. In: Williams DI, Chisholm, GD, eds. Scientific Foundations of Urology. Vol 2. London: William Heinemann Medical Books, 1976:113–125.

36. Zvara P, Carrier S, Kour NW, Tanagho EA. The detailed neuroanatomy of the human striated urethral sphincter. Br J Urol 1994; 74:182–187.

37. Narayan P, Konety B, Aslam K, Aboseif S, Blumenfeld W, Tanagho E. Neuroanatomy of the external urethral sphincter: implications for urinary continence preservation during radical prostate surgery. J Urol 1995; 153:337–341.

38. Hollabaugh RS Jr, Dmochowski RR, Steiner MS. Neuroanatomy of the male rhabdosphincter. Urology 1997; 49:426–434.

39. Donker PJ, Dröes JTPM, Van Ulden BM. Anatomy of the musculature and innervation of the bladder and the urethra. In: Williams DI, Chisholm GD, eds. Scientific Foundations of Urology. Vol 2. London: William Heinemann Medical Books, 1976:32–39.

40. Elbadawi A, Schenk EA. A new theory of the innervation of bladder musculature. 2. Innervation of the vesicourethral junction and external urethral sphincter. J Urol 1974; 111:613–615.

41. Kumagai A, Koyanagi T, Takahashi Y. The innervation of the external urethral sphincter; an ultrastructural study in male human subjects. Urol Res 1987; 15:39–43.

42. Krahn HP, Morales PA. The effect of pudendal nerve anesthesia on urinary continence after prostatectomy. J Urol 1965; 94:282–285.

43. Ficazzola MA, Nitti VW. The etiology of post-radical prostatectomy incontinence and correlation of symptoms with urodynamic findings. J Urol 1998; 160:1317–1320.

44. Yoshimura N, de Groat WC. Neural control of the lower urinary tract. Int J Urol 1997; 4:111–125.

45. Hinman F Jr, Miller GM, Nickel, E, Miller ER. Vesical physiology demonstrated by cineradiography and serial roentgenography: preliminary report. Radiology 1954; 62:713–719.

46. Turner Warwick R, Whiteside CG, Arnold EP, Bates CP, Worth PH Milroy EG, Webster JR, Weir J. A urodynamic view of prostatic obstruction and the results of prostatectomy. Br J Urol 1973; 45:631–645.

47. Strasser H, Klima G, Poise S, Horninger W, Bartsch G. Anatomy and innervation of the rhabdosphincter of the male urethra. Prostate 1996; 28:24–31.

48. Tanagho EA. Anatomy of the lower urinary tract. In: Walsh PC, Gittes RF, Permutter AD, Stamey TA, eds. Campbell's Urology vol. 1. 5th ed. Edited by Philadelphia: WB Sauders, 1986:46.

49. Myers RP, Cahill DR, Kay PA, Camp JJ, Devine RM, Engen DE. Puboperineales: muscular boundaries of the male urogenital hiatus in 3D from magnetic resonance imaging. J Urol 2000; 164:1412–1415.

50. Junemann, KP, Schmidt RA, Melchior H, Tanagho EA. Neuroanatomy and clinical significance of the external urethral sphincter. Urol Int. 1987; 42:132–136.

51. Gil Vernet S. Morphology and Function of Vesico-Prostato-Urethral Musculature. Treviso: Canova, 1968.

52. Burnett AL, Mostwin JL. In situ anatomical study of the male urethral sphincteric complex: relevance to continence preservation following major pelvic surgery. J Urol 1998; 160:1301–1306.

53. Gosling JA, Dixon JS, Critchley HO, Thompson SA. A comparative study of the human external sphincter and periurethral levator ani muscles. Br J Urol 1981; 53:35–41.

54. Schrøder HD, Reske–Nielsen E. Fiber types in the striated urethral and anal sphincters. Acta Neuropathol (Berl) 1983; 60:278–282.

55. Neill ME, Swash M. Increased motor unit fibre density in the external anal sphincter muscle in ano-rectal incontinence: a single fibre EMG study. J Neurol Neurosurg Psychiatry 1980; 43: 343–347.

56. Snooks SJ, Swash M. The innervation of the muscles of continence. Ann R Coll Surg Engl 1986; 68:45–49.

57. Delmas V, Benoit G, Gillot C, Hureau J. Anatomical basis of the surgical approach to the membranous urethra. Anat Clin 1984; 6:69–78.

58. Colston JAC. Perineal prostatectomy. In: Campbell MF, ed. Urology. Vol 3. 2nd ed. Philadelphia: WB Saunders, 1963:2605.

59. Vest SA. Radical perineal prostatectomy, modification of closure. Surg Gynecol Obstet 1940; 70:935–937.

60. Chute R. Radical retropubic prostatectomy for cancer. J Urol 1954; 71:347–372.

61. Igel TC, Barrett DM, Rife CC. Comparison of techniques for vesicourethral anastomosis: simple direct versus modified Vest traction sutures. Urology 1988; 31:474–477.

62. Myers RP. Radical retropubic prostatectomy—balance between preserving urinary continence and achievement of negative margins. Eur Urol 1995; 27 (suppl 2): 32–33.

63. Igel TC, Wehle, MJ. Vesicourethral reconstruction in radical retropubic prostatectomy: an alternative technique. J Urol 1999; 161:844–846.

64. O'Donnell PD, Finan BF. Continence following nerve-sparing radical prostatectomy. J Urol 1989; 142:1227–1228.

4

Physiology of the Smooth Muscles of the Bladder and Urethra

WILLIAM H. TURNER

Addenbrooke's Hospital, Cambridge, England

I. INTRODUCTION

Most of what is known of smooth-muscle function generally comes from study of smooth muscle from other tissues, particularly vascular smooth muscle, and this may be related to research-funding priorities. Many excellent reviews of detailed aspects of smooth-muscle function in general have been produced recently (1–9), and we know much about the membranes of smooth-muscle cells, how they are excited, either electrically or by ligand binding to membrane receptors, how the membrane signal is transduced to the contractile apparatus by second-messenger systems, and how contractile protein function is regulated.

The smooth muscles of the bladder and urethra play a critical part in the normal function of the lower urinary tract, and it is becoming increasingly apparent that smooth-muscle abnormalities play a major role in the pathophysiology of functional lower urinary tract disorders (10). We remain, however, far from a full understanding of how the lower urinary tract works as a whole, functional entity, but since the mid 1980s, there has been a steady increase in study of the smooth muscle of the lower urinary tract, and this has been translated into a broad base of knowledge on many aspects of lower urinary tract smooth-muscle function. The rapid pace at which lower urinary tract smooth-muscle study has moved has been partly due to the development of new techniques in experimental physiology. This presents clinicians with major difficulties in maintaining an up-to-date understanding of how smooth muscle is studied. Therefore, as well as reviewing the present state of knowledge of smooth-muscle physiology in general, and then focusing on what is known about the specific details of detrusor and urethral smooth-muscle physiology, this chapter will outline methods of study of smooth muscle.

II.   METHODS OF STUDY

The classic techniques have included in vitro study of smooth-muscle strip preparations and in vivo studies using pharmacological manipulation of smooth muscles. Techniques in use at present will be considered as those using whole tissues, those using single cells, and molecular techniques.

A.   Whole Tissues

1.   Muscle Tension Studies

Many of the early studies in the recent era of interest in lower urinary tract smooth-muscle physiology were muscle-strip tension studies. A small strip of smooth muscle is dissected free and tied in place, connected to a force transducer, while suspended in an organ bath (Fig. 1). This allows force generation to be measured while the tissue is bathed in physio-

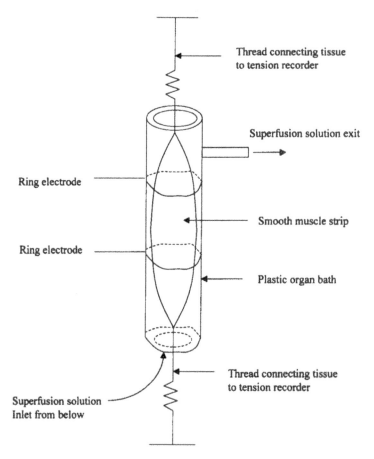

Figure 1   A strip of smooth muscle is suspended between ties, connected to a force transducer. It lies in a small organ bath, superfused by oxygenated, warmed physiological solution, to which drugs can be added. The intrinsic nerves of the strip can be stimulated by the ring electrodes.

COLOR PLATES

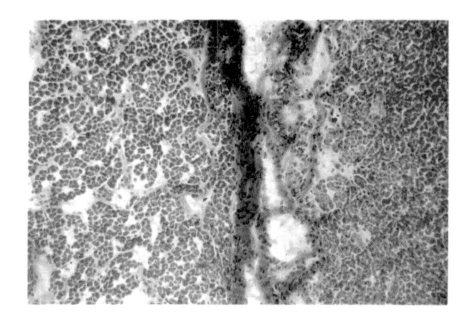

**connective
tissue septum**

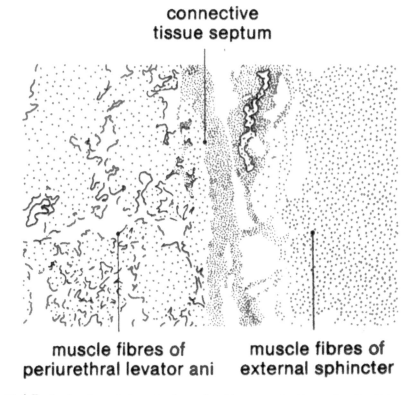

**muscle fibres of
periurethral levator ani**   **muscle fibres of
external sphincter**

Figure 1.5   Section through the striated muscle of the external sphincter (small cells) separated
by a connective tissue septum from the periurethral striated muscle of the levator ani (larger cells):
infant (Masson's trichrome stain). (From Ref. 7.)

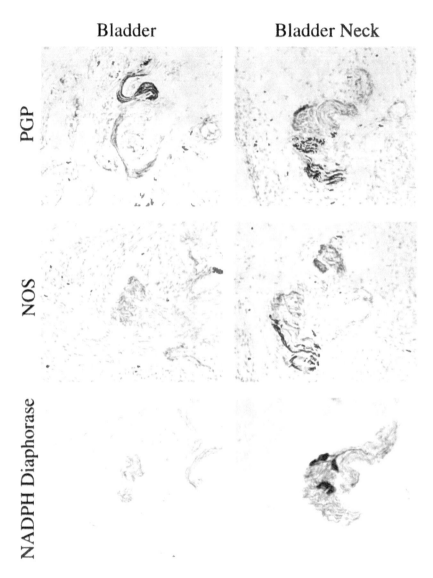

Figure 1.11 Nitric oxide synthase (NOS) immunoreactivity in bladder base and urethra from sheep showing increased staining for NO-containing nerves in bladder neck: (left panel) bladder; (right panel) bladder neck; (top row) PGP immunoreactivity; (center row) NOS immunoreactivity; (bottom row) NADPH diaphorase staining (x 200).

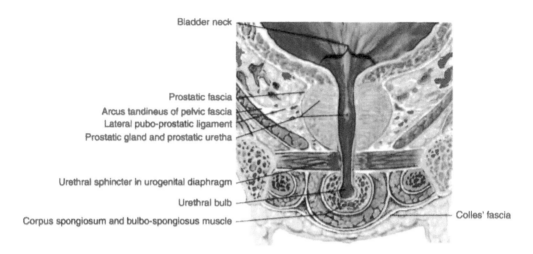

Figure 3.6 Urogenital diaphragm according to Netter.

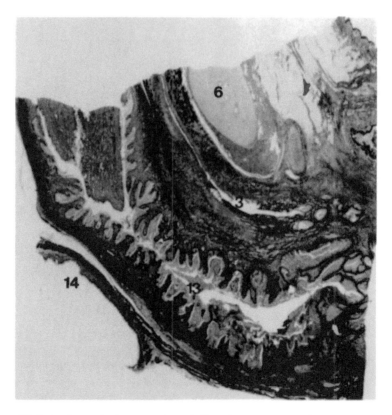

Figure 12.1 Median sagittal section of pelvic floor demonstrates urethra (3) and musculature (7). Pubic symphysis (6), vagina (13), and rectum (14) are also seen. (Courtesy of Dr. K. Colleselli.)

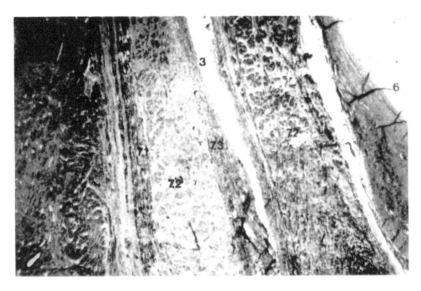

Figure 12.2 Close-up view of cranial two-thirds of female urethra (3). Three layers of smooth muscle—outer (7.1), middle (7.2), and inner (7.3)—are seen. (Courtesy of Dr. K. Colleselli.)

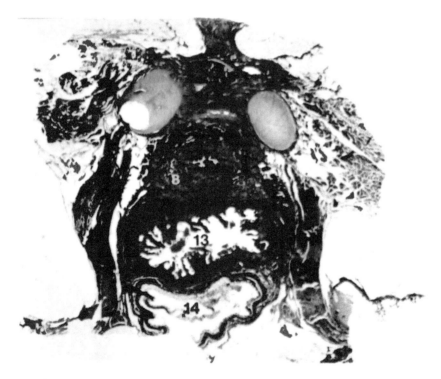

Figure 12.3 Transverse section of female pelvic floor shows omega-shaped rhabdosphincter (8) in caudal third of urethra. Vagina (13) and rectum (14) are also seen. (Courtesy of Dr. K. Colleselli.)

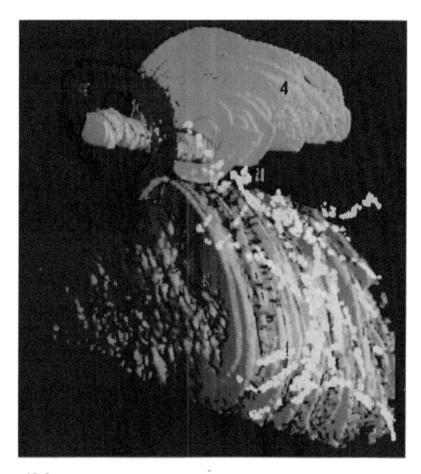

Figure 12.4 Computer 3-D reconstruction of the female pelvic floor shows omega-shaped rhab-dosphincter (8, red); nerve supply (11, yellow) and bladder (4, green), and vagina (13, gray) are also seen. (Courtesy of Dr. K. Colleselli.)

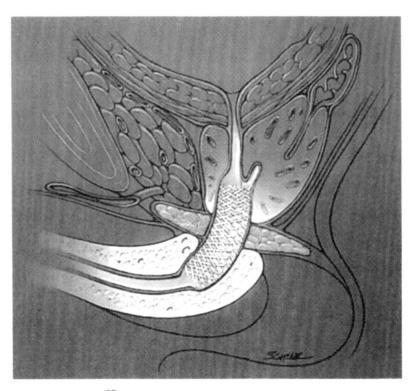

Figure 38.2 Full deployment of the prosthesis after release: The proper position is from the midveru montanum, below the ejaculatory ducts, to the proximal bulbous urethra at least 5 mm beyond the membranous urethra.

logical solution, to which drugs can be added. Electrodes can be either used to stimulate the muscle strip directly, or more usefully, the intrinsic nerves of the preparation (11,12). This allows the effects on contractile function of drugs or changes in the perfusing solution to be assessed. This technique has contributed a huge amount of data on lower urinary tract smooth muscle.

2. Electrical Conduction Properties of Smooth Muscle

A variety of techniques have been used to examine the electrical properties of specimens of smooth-muscle tissue. These include microelectrode techniques that involve the use of very fine glass microelectrodes, that can be filled with physiological solutions, and used to pierce tissue or single cells (Fig. 2) (13,14). The electrode can record electrical potentials that arise in the tissue, it can be used to inject current, or it can record the effects of stimulating the intrinsic nerves of the tissue. This technique depends on factors such as a relative lack of connective tissue for ease of penetration by the electrode, and a lack of movement of the tissue, so that electrode displacement does not occur. Microelectrode studies allow the direct measurement of membrane potentials and estimation of smooth-muscle cell membrane resistance.

The sucrose-gap techniques involve the electrical compartmentalization of a strip of tissue by partly surrounding it with a nonconducting solution (sucrose) (15). Force of contraction and electrical response of the tissue strip can be measured, allowing the two to be correlated (Fig. 3). Similar principles have been used recently to examine the electrical resistance properties of detrusor muscle specimens (16).

3. Flux Studies

Tissues can be incubated in solutions that have been labeled with radioisotopes, allowing the isotopes to be incorporated into the tissues and the rate of efflux to be determined, giving information on the behavior of membrane ion channels (Fig. 4). This technique has been employed particularly in the study of potassium channels (K^+ channels), using potassium or rubidium isotopes (17,18). The use of rubidium depends on the assumption that K^+ channels are equally permeant to K^+ and Rb^+ ions, which is an approximation. Loading

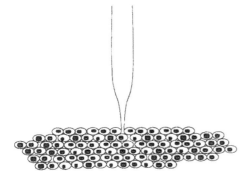

Figure 2 A small piece of smooth muscle, containing thousands of cells, is impaled by a fine glass microelectrode filled with solution, allowing potentials to be recorded and current to be injected.

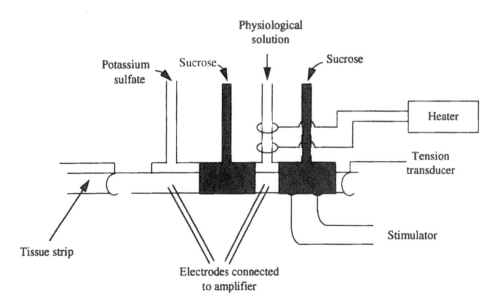

Figure 3   In the double sucrose-gap technique, a tissue strip is held in a partitioned organ bath, and connected to a tension recorder. It is impaled with a microelectrode, to allow recording and current injection. The bath is partitioned to allow recording of potential difference between the depolarized section of tissue (in contact with potassium sulfate), and the section in contact with physiological solution, thus stimulating normal transmembrane potential.

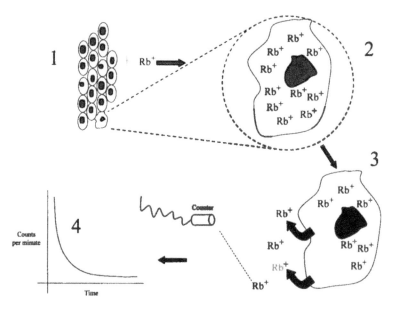

Figure 4   Panel 1 shows isotope added to a tissue preparation. Panel 2 shows isotope taken up by the tissue. Panel 3 shows the rate of efflux of isotope being recorded, and displayed in panel 4, versus time.

cells with these ions may also alter the cell's membrane potential, hence, its channel function, so the results require careful interpretation.

4. Receptor Density Studies

The use of radiolabeled ligands that bind tightly to receptors allows estimation of receptor density in tissue homogenates (19). This requires the use of ligands that bind in a specific manner to a given receptor, and this may not always be true. Information on the localization of the receptors has to be derived from other techniques, such as immunohistochemistry.

B. Single Cells

1. Patch Clamp

The introduction of the patch clamp technique has revolutionized the study of cellular physiology, by allowing membrane currents and ion channels to be studied directly (20). The technique involves the dispersal and isolation of single cells from a tissue and the impalement of a single cell by a glass microelectrode (Fig. 5). The method has been adapted so that either whole cells are studied, or patches of cell membrane in isolation. By varying the nature of the physiological solution bathing the cell, or within the electrode, or both, and by altering the potential at which the electrode holds the cell, current flow into or out of the preparation can be studied. As with microelectrode studies, there may be problems with the preparation of single cell suspensions of the required cells, and this has somewhat limited the use of the technique. Patch clamping also cannot assess the effects of intrinsic innervation or cell-to-cell coupling.

2. Intracellular Calcium Studies

The development of fluorescent calcium indicators, such as Fura 2, has enabled experimental measurement of $[Ca^{2+}]_i$. Cells are loaded with the dye, and when $[Ca^{2+}]_i$ rises in response to some experimental manipulation, light is emitted and can be measured as an index of the change in $[Ca^{2+}]_i$ (Fig. 6). The development of refined techniques of laser-scanning confocal microscopy, used with voltage clamp techniques and calcium indicators, has enabled the precise localization of changes in $[Ca^{2+}]_i$ to particular cellular compartments (1).

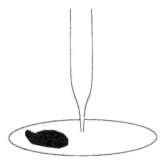

Figure 5 In the patch clamp technique, a single cell has been isolated, and is impaled with a fine glass microelectrode, which can be used to record potential or current flow, or to inject current.

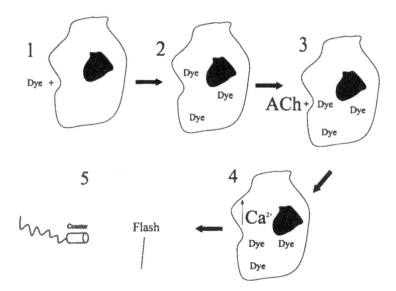

Figure 6 Intracellular calcium release can be recorded using a fluorescent dye, such as Fura-2: Panels 1 and 2 show dye added to the tissue, and then taken up. In panel 3, agonist is added, causing the rise in intracellular calcium shown in panel 4. The rise in intracellular calcium causes release of light by the dye, and this is being recorded in panel 5.

3. Cell Culture

Cell culture has been used for many years in cancer biology in particular. The use of cell culture to develop colonies of isolated smooth-muscle cells has advanced recently, and has been used quite widely (Fig. 7) (21). This allows the study of homogeneous cell populations and the control over many aspects of experimental design. The use of novel experimental designs with cultured cells has allowed study of the effect on smooth-muscle cells of for example, stretch (22,23). It clearly, however, precludes the cellular interactions that occur in living tissue, and this is a limitation of the technique.

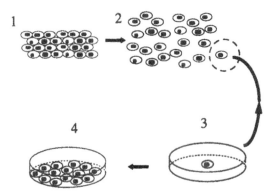

Figure 7 Panels 1 and 2 show dispersal of a tissue preparation into single cells. In panel 3, a cell is taken to a culture dish containing an appropriate culture medium. Panel 4 shows clonal expansion of the cell into a colony of daughter cells.

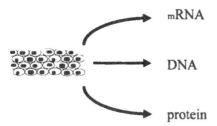

mRNA

DNA

protein

Figure 8   Blotting techniques allow the identification of mRNA, DNA, and protein from tissues.

C. Molecular Techniques

Any more than the briefest outline of the use of these techniques is clearly outside the scope of this chapter. However, with the explosion of molecular techniques used in cell biology and oncology research (24), their use has been adopted to good effect by those studying smooth muscle. Blotting techniques (Fig. 8), to identify mRNA, DNA, and protein products; reverse transcription polymerase chain reaction (RT-PCR) to amplify minute amounts of mRNA (Fig. 9); and gene-cloning techniques, all have been used (Fig. 10). The power of these techniques has been combined with the power of techniques such as patch clamping, to allow the molecular basis of smooth-muscle function to be rapidly further uncovered (25,26).

III.   SMOOTH MUSCLE PHYSIOLOGY

A.   Membrane Properties and Potentials

1.   Membrane Potential

Smooth-muscle cells generally have a resting membrane potential (difference between the inside and the outside) of between –35 and –70 mV relative to the reference electrode, measured either with microelectrodes or, in single cells, by the patch clamp technique (7). A smooth-muscle cell's membrane potential depends on the membrane's ionic permeability and the transmembrane ionic concentration gradients: for each ion, there is a membrane potential (equilibrium potential) that balances the tendency of the ion to move down its con-

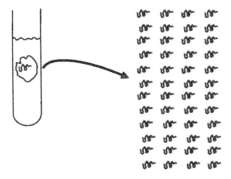

Figure 9   The reverse transcription polymerase chain reaction allows minute amounts of DNA to be amplified enormously.

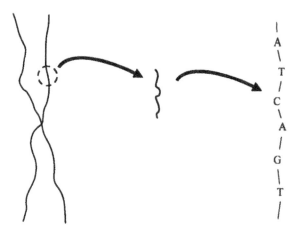

Figure 10 Cloning and sequencing techniques allow the genetic code of DNA and RNA to be identified, allowing the creation of sequences that are exact copies of genes and RNA.

centration gradient (27). This potential is usually close to that of the most permeant ion, generally K⁺ (27). The membrane potential is a consequence of the physical properties of the membrane, its resistance to current flow, and its capacitance (28).

2. Passive Membrane Properties and Cell Coupling

In many tissues (e.g., myometrium or gut), smooth-muscle cells are well coupled electrically, so that electrical activity spreads readily between cells through gap junctions, (29,30)—intimate intercellular connections characterized by the presence of proteins of the connexin family (Fig. 11) (31,32). As well as coupling cells mechanically, gap junctions allow spread of current between cells by the passage of ions through the channels within them. The molecular and electrical properties of connexins have been well defined (7).

    The passive electrical properties of nerve and smooth-muscle cell membranes have been described in mathematical models by analogy to underwater cables (28). The two major parameters of passive electrical properties that are studied are tissue-specific con-

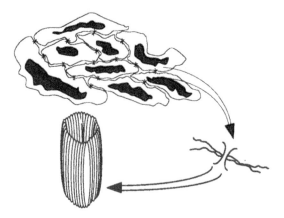

Figure 11 Smooth-muscle cells of many tissues are connected by gap junctions, which are cylindrical pores consisting of copies of specific protein complexes, connexins.

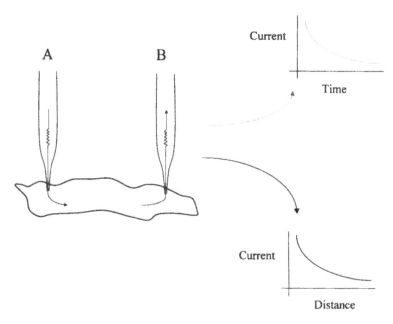

Figure 12   Current is injected into the tissue strip by microelectrode A, and microelectrode B records current. By moving microelectrode B, and by varying the injected current, the decay in current with time and distance can be derived.

stants, called the *space constant* and the *time constant*. These are derived from analysis of the spread of injections of subexcitation threshold current using microelectrodes (Fig. 12). The space constant (λ) is an index of the decay of the injected current with distance, whereas the time constant (τ) describes the decay of current spread with time. Large values of λ indicate good intercellular coupling; for example, as found in pregnant myometrium or cardiac muscle, and large values of τ indicate resistance to membrane charging. Estimation of cable properties has been used as an index of the degree of gap junction distribution in tissues, although molecular techniques now provide an alternative means of investigating this more directly, by looking for connexin mRNA or by immunohistochemistry.

3.   Action Potentials

Some smooth muscles develop spontaneous depolarizations (action potentials), which may propagate among neighboring cells, and are similar in type to nerve action potentials (Fig. 13). Action potentials can be investigated using the microelectrode, patch clamp, or sucrose-gap techniques, and arise from the flow of cations across the cell membrane. Depolarization is due to a rapid inward current, and the cell repolarizes (often with a brief hyperpolarization—"overshoot"), caused by an outward current. Whereas in nerve the inward current is carried by Na^+ ions, in smooth muscle the inward current is a Ca^{2+} current.

   Some smooth muscles develop pacemaker potentials, which are slow depolarizations that trigger a spike (action potential) (7). Slow waves may also occur, and are slow oscillations in membrane potential, which may or may not trigger a spike, and may be due to compound activity in a group of cells, perhaps stimulated by pacemaker cells, such as the interstitial cells of Cajal in the gut (7).

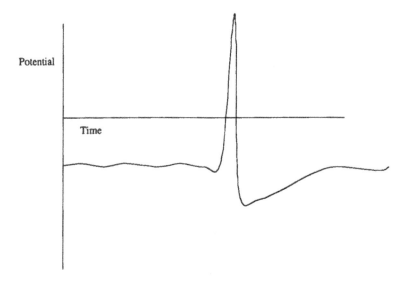

Figure 13 When an action potential occurs, there is a rapid depolarization, followed by hyperpolarization, with a small aftershoot, before the cell's potential returns to resting potential.

4. Spontaneous Activity

Smooth muscles may show spontaneous electrical activity, either action potentials or slow waves as described in the foregoing, or either excitatory junction potentials (EJPs) or inhibitory junction potentials (IJPs). Investigation of EJPs and IJPs using either microelectrodes or sucrose-gap techniques has shown that these represent spontaneous release of single or multiple quanta of neurotransmitter from the smooth muscle's innervation. EJPs may produce sufficient depolarization to reach the threshold for an action potential, which will then evoke a contraction of the smooth-muscle cell. Whether each suprathreshold EJP results in propagated electrical activity and associated contraction, depends largely on the degree of coupling of the smooth muscle in question. When the excitatory innervation of the smooth muscle is activated, there will be massive transmitter release, far beyond the level of EJPs, and smooth-muscle cell membrane receptors will be activated. This may or may not lead to action potentials, depending on the neurotransmitter released. In less well-coupled tissues, it is common to find that the rate of EJPs is much greater than the level of spontaneous mechanical activity, because the spontaneously evoked EJPs cannot propagate sufficiently through the tissues for contractions to occur.

B. Receptors

Transmitters released by nerves activate smooth muscle by binding to specific membrane-bound receptors with two possible main actions: either direct modification of ionic permeability and, hence, membrane potential (ionotropic action), or synthesis of second messengers by a G protein and enzymes such as phospholipase C (PLC) or adenylate or guanylate cyclase (metabotropic action). The second messengers produce phosphorylation of cellular proteins, and they may also regulate ion channels (Fig. 14).

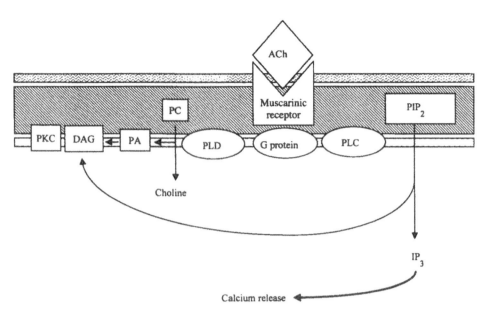

Figure 14 The muscarinic receptor sits in the trilaminar cell membrane. When acetylcholine (ACh) binds to it, a sequence follows whereby the receptor and G protein activate phophsolipase C (PLC) and phophsolipase D (PLD), stimulating synthesis of diacylglycerol (DAG) by phosphatidylcholine (PC) and phosphatidic acid (PA), and synthesis of inositol trisphosphate (IP_3) from phospatidylinositol bisphosphate (PIP_2). DAG then activates protein kinase C (PKC).

The best-studied smooth-muscle cell membrane ligand receptors are adrenoceptors in tissues with adrenergic excitatory innervation, such as the smooth muscle of vascular tissues or the vas deferens. Adrenoceptors are classified as α-adrenoceptors and β-adrenoceptors, with further subclassification of α-adrenoceptors into α_1-(α_{1A-D} and α_{1L}) and α_2-(α_{2A-C}) adrenoceptors, and β-adrenoceptors into β_{1-3} (7). The receptors found in the lower urinary tract also include muscarinic acetylcholine receptors and purinergic receptors. Muscarinic receptors are classified on pharmacological (M_{1-4}) and molecular (m1–5) grounds, with no pharmacological correlate of the m5 subtype yet being identified (6). Purinoceptors have been classified as either P_1 or P_2, with P_1 being further subclassified into A_1 and A_{2A-2B}, and P_2 being further subclassified into P_{2t}, P_{2u}, P_{2x-z} (7). The purinoceptor gene family has been cloned.

C. Ion Channels

1. Sodium Ion Channels

A family of Na^+ channels has been cloned, and they have been characterized pharmacologically, using Na^+ channel antagonists, such as tetrodotoxin (TTX). Although many smooth muscles express Na^+ channels, in contrast to their essential role in mediating the inward current of the upstroke of the nerve action potential, the role of Na^+ channels in smooth-muscle physiology remains to be clarified (7).

2. Potassium Ion Channels

It is now recognized that quite a number of types of K^+ channels exist, with different phys-iological properties (4). Many of them are expressed in smooth-muscle cell membranes, and serve different functions. The genes for many of these channels have been cloned in re-cent years, allowing some clarification of the relation between them. There are two main groups, the classic voltage-sensitive K^+ channels (Kv), and the inward rectifying channels (Kir), which conduct inward K^+ current much more readily than outward K^+ current (7). The voltage-gated channels include the *Shaker, Shab, Shaw,* and *Shal* genetic families, and in functional terms comprise delayed rectifer and transient K^+ channels: this group in-cludes Ca^{2+}-activated K^+ channels (SK, BK, maxi-K^+ channels). The inward rectifying K^+ channels include K_{ATP} channels, which have sufonylurea receptors and are sensitive to the action of glibenclamide.

Inward rectifying K^+ channels probably contribute to vascular smooth-muscle cell resting membrane potential, and this is strongly regulated by the open or closed state of K^+ channels, because the cell's high impedance means that few K^+ channels are open at rest. The opening or closing of a small number of such channels, therefore, has a significant in-fluence on membrane potential and, consequently, on contraction in vascular smooth mus-cle (4). K_{ATP} channels are not dependent on membrane potential, but link the metabolic state of cells to their K^+ permeability. They are closed by intracellular ATP, although this may regulate channel function by producing a low background probability of the channel being in the open (conducting) state, and other factors such as a possible direct effect of hy-poxia, and several protein kinases, then regulate the channel's activity (4). K^+ channel-opening drugs, such as cromakalim, levcromakalim, pinacidil, and nicorandil, probably ac-tivate K^+ channels by reducing their sensitivity to inhibition by ATP, and this action is promoted by magnesium salts of nucleoside diphosphates (4). Acetylcholine can inhibit K_{ATP} channels through a muscarinic mechanism (33).

3. Calcium Ion Channels

Smooth-muscle cells may contain several types of membrane channels, specific or nonse-lective, which allow the influx of Ca^{2+}. However, the main channels through which Ca^{2+} en-ters many smooth-muscle cells are voltage-operated Ca^{2+} channels (1).

Voltage-operated Ca^{2+} channels are classified according to the currents that they per-mit to flow: L-type (long lasting), T-type (transient), or N-type (neither L nor T) (7). Smooth-muscle cell membranes contain L-type Ca^+ channels, and these are sensitive to di-hydropyridine drugs, such as nifedipine. L-type Ca^{2+} channels permit high ion flux rates, but do so in only one of three possible channel states (open state). Membrane potential strongly regulates the open probability of L-type Ca^{2+} channels. The high unitary current of L-type Ca^{2+} channels means that with just a few channels in the open state $[Ca^{2+}]_i$ can rise rapidly, leading to contraction. In many nonspiking smooth-muscle cells, therefore, at resting membrane potentials, the probability of open state is low, and this serves to regulate $[Ca^{2+}]_i$. Many of the genes that control voltage-operated Ca^{2+} channel expression have been cloned, and the molecular structure of the channels is being established (1).

4. Nonselective Cation Channels

Nonselective cation channels include ionotropic channels, such as P_{2x} channels, and metabotropic channels, such as muscarinic receptor-activated cation channels.

P_{2x} channels permit Ca^{2+} flux following binding of ATP. At least seven members of the P_{2x} gene family have been cloned. Activation of P_{2x} receptors leads to membrane depolarization and calcium influx, although Ca^{2+} may carry only 10% of the nonselective cation current (1). The degree to which P_{2x} receptor activation contributes to physiological excitation–contraction coupling in many smooth muscles remains unclear.

In many smooth muscles, acetylcholine activates a depolarizing, nonselective cation current, which may be biphasic, with a Ca^{2+}-activated inward chloride current, followed by a sustained nonselective cation current. Muscarinic currents follow the stimulation of a G–protein-linked membrane receptor, and are strongly facilitated by an increase in $[Ca^{2+}]_i$. There is evidence that physiological activation of this current involves M_2 receptor-mediated second-messenger channel gating, and M_3 receptor-mediated release of Ca^{2+} from intracellular stores (1).

5. Chloride Channels

Intracellular Cl^- concentration is typically 40–50 mM, with a calculated Cl^- equilibrium potential of –35 to –20 mV, indicating an active transport system which contributes to the accumulation of Cl^- in smooth-muscle cells, in addition to passive movement of Cl^- through Cl^- channels (7). Patch clamp studies have shown Ca^{2+}-dependent Cl^- currents in smooth muscle. The genes for Cl^- channel expression have been cloned, and the channels sequenced. Cl^- channels may regulate cell volume and membrane excitability in smooth muscles (7).

D. Second-Messenger Systems

Signal transduction from the smooth-muscle cell membrane is initially mediated either by changes in membrane potential and Ca^{2+} influx directly (ionotropic), or by membrane proteins, the G proteins (metabotropic) (8). G proteins form a vast family of related proteins, each comprising several subunits, and part of the diversity of behavior of smooth muscles may relate to the diversity of G proteins.

Muscarinic receptors (M_1, M_3, and M_5) may link to the $G_{q/11}$ family and cause phospholipase C activation and synthesis of diacylglycerol (DAG) and IP_3, or they may (M_2 and M_4) couple with the $G_{i/o}$ family and induce a rise or fall in K^+ channel activity and a fall in Ca^{2+} channel activity, as well as a fall in cAMP levels. Among α-adrenoceptors, α_1-adrenoceptors (α_{1A}, α_{1B}, and α_{1D}) couple with $G_{q/11}$, whereas β-adrenoceptors (β_{1-3}) are linked to G_s (activation of adenylate cyclase) (7).

E. Calcium

The signal for activation of smooth-muscle cell contractile proteins is a sufficient rise in cytosolic Ca^{2+} concentration, which triggers the formation of a Ca^{2+}–calmodulin complex. As well as entering the cytosol through voltage-operated Ca^{2+} channels or through nonselective cation channels in the cell membrane, Ca^{2+} can also be released from stores within the sarcoplasmic reticulum (SR; Fig. 15). This so-called Ca^{2+}-induced Ca^{2+} release (CICR) occurs through the activation of calcium-release channels (nonselective cation channels) on the sarcoplasmic reticulum (SR) membrane, either when IP_3 receptors are activated by IP_3 following muscarinic receptor activation, or by Ca^{2+} binding to ryanodine receptors (RYR).

IP_3 receptors and ryanodine receptors share substantial sequence homology and similar protein structure (1). Calcium flux is probably 20-fold greater through ryanodine receptors than through IP_3 receptors. IP_3 receptors are strongly regulated by $[Ca^{2+}]_i$, with a marked increase in channel opening as $[Ca^{2+}]_i$ rises, followed by a reduction in activity at higher Ca^{2+} levels (1). CICR occurs when cytosolic Ca^{2+} levels rise, leading to increased probability of ryanodine receptor open state, and hence release of Ca^{2+} from the SR. The

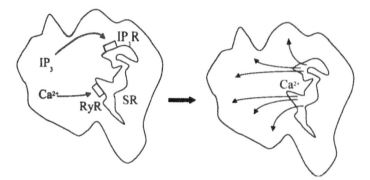

Figure 15 The sarcoplasmic reticulum (SR) contains receptors for ryanodine and for IP_3. If these are bound by calcium or IP_3, respectively, release of calcium from the SR is triggered.

rise in $[Ca^{2+}]_i$ with CICR in smooth muscle may activate not only myosin light-chain kinase (MLCK) and, thereby, lead to contraction, but also may promote activation of membrane-bound Ca^{2+}-activated channels, such as K^+ channels, which can cause membrane hyperpolarization, tending to decrease $[Ca^{2+}]_i$. The net effect would depend on the degree of MLCK activation and membrane hyperpolarization. The activation of Ca^{2+}-activated K^+ channels may also serve to protect the cell from excessive accumulation of calcium, which could be detrimental by activating Ca^{2+}-dependent enzymes, such as proteases and lipases, that could damage the cell.

When multiple ryanodine receptors are activated in the SR, a transient rise in $[Ca^{2+}]_i$ occurs. This has been detected with laser-scanning confocal microscopy and fluorescent calcium indicators; these events have been termed calcium sparks. When sparks occur in the subsarcolemmal space, they may lead to activation of Ca^{2+}-activated K^+ channels (BK channels), leading to outward currents known as spontaneous transient outward currents (STOCs) (2). Further detailed discussion of the regulation of $[Ca^{2+}]_i$ is given by Horowitz and colleagues (3).

F. Contractile Proteins

The contractile elements of smooth muscle are the thick filaments (myosin) and thin filaments (actin, tropomyosin, and caldesmon). Intermediate filaments, mainly desmin, serve as part of the cytoskeleton, maintaining cell shape, and distributing forces (5).

1. Thick and Thin Filaments

Myosin comprises two heavy chains (MHC), which contain the ATP hydrolytic sites and actin-binding sites, and two of each of the two types of light-chain (LC_{17} and LC_{20}). Phosphorylation of LC_{20} leads to ATPase activity in the globular head of the myosin molecule. This is required for cross-bridge cycling between myosin and actin, whereby the filaments slide over each other, leading to smooth-muscle contraction.

2. Myosin Regulation

Myosin light-chain kinase is a specific phosphorylator of LC_{20}. It contains a catalytic domain, a calmodulin (CaM)-binding domain, and actin-binding site, substrate-binding sites, and sites for phosphorylation by various kinases (3). It is primarily regulated by the

Ca^{2+}–CaM complex, but its affinity for CaM can be reduced if it is phosphorylated. This can be accomplished by several kinases. Phosphorylation of LC_{20} leads to not only ATPase activity, but also facilitates the formation of filaments from myosin monomers. The action of MLCK is countered by myosin light-chain phosphatase, which is usually bound tightly to myosin. Its activity is regulated, possibly by arachidonic acid or by protein kinase C.

3. Protein Kinase C

Protein kinase C (PKC) is a family of kinases with diverse roles in cell biology. A variety of agonists induce a sustained rise in (DAG) levels, and DAG is a known physiological activator of PKC. The PKC inhibitors also block agonist-induced contraction, but not KCl-induced contraction (due to depolarization). Therefore, PKC is believed to play an important role in the regulation of sustained smooth-muscle contraction. Related to the PKC activation pathway may be other proteins, such as mitogen-activated protein kinase, caldesmon, small GTP-binding proteins, calponin, and others (3).

4. Thin-Filament Regulation

Some smooth muscles can maintain tone at low levels of LC_{20} phosphorylation: this implies regulation of contraction by the thin filaments. Caldesmon binds to actin and myosin, and can cross-link them, promoting the in vitro assembly of LC_{20} dephosphorylated myosin. This may have a physiological role. Caldesmon also inhibits actomyosin ATPase activity. Calponin is another possible thin-filament regulatory protein, which also inhibits actomyosin ATPase activity.

IV. DETRUSOR PHYSIOLOGY

During filling over a large range of bladder volumes in the guinea pig, the bladder wall thinned, smooth-muscle bundles stretched, and individual smooth-muscle cells stretched by up to fourfold (34). Smooth muscles often respond to stretch by contracting (35), but contraction does not occur during normal filling. The detrusor maintains tone during filling and, thereby, a minimum surface area/volume ratio, allowing efficient pressure generation when a contraction is eventually required. The ability to maintain tone without a contraction despite considerable stretch, probably arises partly from the electrical properties of the bladder, regardless of extrinsic innervation (36). The frequent spontaneous action potentials will produce localized contractile activity, tending to maintain tone in the organ as a whole and to allow adjustment to the increase in volume (37), but poor electrical coupling will prevent synchronous mass contraction of the entire bladder.

The human bladder can normally be emptied at will from a large range of volumes, and the detrusor contraction which brings this about must be sustained until the bladder is empty (38). This requires that contraction be maintained as the bladder volume decreases; therefore, muscle fibers become less stretched. This fiber shortening would normally reduce contractility in smooth muscles. The length–tension characteristics of guinea pig detrusor smooth-muscle cells indicate that, unusually for smooth muscle, force generation remains reasonably constant over a remarkably large change in cell length, remaining nearly maximal at filling volumes of 25–75% of the bladder capacity, in keeping with the functional requirement (34).

A. Passive Membrane Properties

With use of microelectrodes and patch clamp techniques, recordings of detrusor cell membrane potentials have been made a number of times. Values of –40 to –45 mV in the guinea pig and –60 mV in the human have been recorded (13,28,39). Measurement of current spread in guinea pig detrusor, using microelectrodes and with an oil chamber, suggested that many cells were coupled to their close neighbors, but that the tissue as a whole was poorly coupled (13,16).

B. Spontaneous Activity

Spontaneous contractile activity can be recorded in detrusor strips from all species, including humans, although the number of strips showing activity and the frequency of the contractions varies considerably among species (14,40,41). It seems probable, but not certain, that electrical activity in the form of action potentials underlies the contractile activity in all species, but for technical reasons microelectrode recordings from intact smooth-muscle strips have been successfully undertaken only on detrusor from small mammals such as the guinea pig (13,15,42,43), rabbit (44), and rat (45), and combined electrical and mechanical recording has only rarely been performed (43,44,46,47). In these animals, spontaneous action potentials occur continuously. The spontaneous activity (both electrical and mechanical) in isolated strips in all species can be shown to be myogenic, because it is not abolished by receptor antagonists, or by blockade of neuronal activity with tetrodotoxin. Spontaneous actions potentials have also been recorded with patch electrodes in single human detrusor myocytes (48).

   An unusual feature of the spontaneous mechanical activity in normal detrusor strips is the lack of fused tetanic contractions. The individual contractions normally rise from and fall back to a baseline of nearly zero tension, and in many preparations, individual contractions vary in size. Furthermore, in detrusor smooth muscle, action potential frequency recorded from single cells in a strip may greatly exceed that of the spontaneous contractions normally seen. In contrast, in intestinal smooth muscle, each action potential in one cell produces a small increase in tension in the whole strip, and above a critical frequency, the contractions fuse into a tetanus (49). The lack of tetanic contractions in detrusor strips suggests that there is relatively poor electrical coupling between smooth-muscle cells, so spontaneous electrical activity spreads ineffectively among them. Experimental measurements of tissue impedance in the guinea pig support this, showing higher tissue impedance in the detrusor than in other smooth muscles (16,50). Dual microelectrode impalements of cells in guinea pig detrusor show that electrical coupling between cells that are more than 40 μm apart axially occurs only rarely (13). Furthermore, although double sucrose-gap recordings can be made in some small mammal detrusor strips, the electrical activity is not often resolved into clear spikes, and in the normal pig detrusor the technique does not work, probably because of insufficient electrical coupling (18,43). This poor coupling is consistent with the lack of gap junctions in detrusor smooth muscle (51,52). From a functional point of view, these features match well with the requirements that adjustments in the length of the smooth muscles can take place without the activity spreading to produce synchronous activation of the whole bladder wall.

C. Excitatory Innervation

There is a dense excitatory innervation of the detrusor in humans and animals (53,54). In the human, every smooth-muscle cell is probably within at most 200 nm of a nerve fiber (52), and the ratio of axons to detrusor cells in several animal species is 1:1 (53). This could permit virtually synchronous activation of the detrusor, either by direct nerve stimulation of each cell or, more likely, by very widespread nerve stimulation and limited spread of action potentials enabled by the detrusor's meagre electrical coupling. In most species there is dual excitation of the detrusor by release of acetylcholine (ACh) and adenosine triphosphate (ATP), but there is little evidence of separate cholinergic and purinergic innervation; the two neurotransmitters are thought to be coreleased (36,55). Recent evidence supported release of ATP from the excitatory innervation of the rat, and subsequent P_{2x} purinoceptor-mediated contraction (56). Human detrusor excitatory neurotransmission, however, is probably purely cholinergic (40,57–59), although the smooth muscles do respond to bath-applied ATP, and it is probable that ATP is released from the motor nerves. The lack of an effective purinergic innervation could be due to a lack of postsynaptic purinoceptors (60).

Acetylcholine activates detrusor cell membranes through muscarinic receptors. In small mammals it causes little depolarization of the membrane (43,45,61), although it may cause a delayed increase in action potential frequency. Muscarinic receptor stimulation raises intracellular IP_3 levels, implicating release of intracellular stored Ca^{2+} in the initiation of contraction (62,63). In cultured human detrusor smooth-muscle cells, muscarinic receptor activation raises $[Ca^{2+}]$ (64). Activation of P_{2x} purinoceptors by ATP, on the other hand, markedly depolarizes the cells, and causes a large increase in action potential frequency (43,65).

Stimulation of the intrinsic nerves results in depolarizing junction potentials in small mammals (13,43,45,66,67) and in the pig (43). In the guinea pig, these excitatory junction potentials were caused by release of ATP from the motor nerve supply. Under normal circumstances these junction potentials trigger action potentials, but in the presence of L-type Ca^{2+} channel blockers, the junction potentials can be recorded in isolation. They are unaffected by muscarinic receptor blockade, but are abolished by desensitization (43) or blockade (67) of the P_{2x} purinoceptor. No records have been made of the electrophysiological effects of intrinsic nerve stimulation in the human, but the evidence would suggest that excitatory junction potentials may be small or absent in the normal detrusor.

Selective antagonist studies with cultured human detrusor cells suggest that the functionally important muscarinic receptors are of the M_3 subtype (64) and that after their stimulation, desensitization of the resulting IP_3 response occurs (68), potentially representing a further cellular mechanism for regulation of detrusor contraction. However, evidence is accumulating that both M_1 and M_2 receptor subtypes may modulate contractility. In the rat, there appear to be prejunctional muscarinic receptors, M_1 being facilitatory, whereas M_2 are inhibitory (69).

D. Ion Channels

The actions of channel-blocking drugs on the spontaneous mechanical and electrical behavior of detrusor strips can give some indication of the ion channels of functional importance. In detrusor strips from most animals studied, L-type Ca^{2+} channel blockers reduce spontaneous mechanical activity, and K^+ channel-blocking drugs increase it. Action potentials recorded from guinea pig bladder are blocked by L-type Ca^{2+} channel blockers (14). The depolarization phase, which is usually faster than the rising phase and is followed by an after-hyperpolarization (42), is affected in various ways by different K^+ channel-blocking drugs, some blocking after-hyperpolarization, some slowing depolarization, and some doing both (70). Potassium channel blockers also have variable effects on the membrane potential.

The evidence thus suggests that the upstroke of the spike is produced by current flowing through L-type Ca^{2+} channels, and that the tissue contains several types of K^+ channel that may be involved both in determining the membrane potential and in action potential depolarization (71). This has been confirmed by patch clamp studies on isolated detrusor myocytes, particularly from the guinea pig (72–75) and rat (76), and more recently, in cells from human detrusor (48,77,78).

The L-type Ca^{2+} channels in guinea pig bladder are inactivated by a rise in intracellular free Ca^{2+} ions (74), but also show the unusual property of being switched into a long open state by depolarization, and having two open states, features that may have important implications for contractile function (79,80). Currents characteristic of those flowing through several types of K^+ channel have been identified in detrusor myocytes, including voltage-sensitive delayed rectifier current (72), current through Ca^{2+}-activated maxi-K^+ channels (81–84), and glibenclamide-sensitive K^+ channels (75,85). In the rat, an inwardly rectifying current, apparently carried by both Na^+ and K^+ ions has been demonstrated (86). An unusual feature of the electrical activity of the guinea pig bladder is the sensitivity of the action potential frequency to depolarization. Significant increases in frequency can occur in response to very small changes in membrane potential (14,87). It is not yet known what the pacemaker mechanisms are, although recent studies have demonstrated the presence of specialized cells in the detrusor wall, that are reminiscent of the pacemaking interstitial cells of Cajal in the gut (88), and it has been suggested that small conductance Ca^{2+}-activated K^+ channels may regulate pacemaker function in the guinea pig (89). It has been proposed that K^+ channel openers (KCO) may be useful in the treatment of detrusor instability (90). A recent KCO has been shown to activate both glibenclamide-sensitive K^+ channels and Ca^{2+}-activated maxi-K^+ channels (91,92), and to reduce bladder overactivity when given intravesically to obstructed rats (93). Detrusor cells possess stretch-activated nonselective cation channels, and stretch will thus tend to depolarize the cells. However the channels have some permeability to Ca^{2+} ions, and their activation thus results in secondary activation of the Ca^{2+}-activated K^+ channels, which will modulate the response to stretch (94–96). This means that strips of smooth muscle will respond with a rapid depolarization and increase in action potential frequency and force if the stretch is applied rapidly, but the response is transient, and the tension soon falls back toward baseline. Slowly applied stretch does not activate this contractile response, presumably because K^+ channel activation keeps up with opening of the stretch-activated channels, preventing the depolarization. The potential for modulating "mechanogated" ion channels has recently been reviewed (97).

E. Pharmacomechanical and Electromechanical Coupling

Smooth-muscle contraction in the bladder, as in other smooth muscles, is triggered by a rise in intracellular calcium concentration, leading to binding of Ca^{2+} to calmodulin, activation of myosin light-chain kinase, and phosphorylation of the regulatory light chains of the myosin heads, leading to cross-bridge cycling. The initiation of contraction of the detrusor has been reviewed recently (98). Studies in human and guinea pig detrusor suggest that the Ca^{2+} source may be extracellular or intracellular Ca^{2+} stores (27,47,99). Bladder smooth-muscle stores possess both ryanodine receptors (activated by a rapid rise in free-calcium concentration) and IP_3 receptors (activated by IP_3 produced as a result of agonist-stimulated phosphoinositide breakdown). Intracellular calcium release from the sarcoplasmic reticulum can be triggered experimentally through activation of ryanodine receptors with caffeine (100), or through the IP_3 mechanism following activation of muscarinic receptors

(62,63). The link between contraction and its stimulus can occur with or without cell membrane depolarization (electromechanical coupling and pharmacomechanical coupling, respectively (101). Both forms of coupling can occur separately or together, and both can use extracellular or intracellular calcium sources (102). The relative importance of electromechanical and pharmacomechanical coupling, and of intracellular or extracellular Ca^{2+} sources in contraction of the human detrusor are unclear (102,103). The L-type Ca^{2+} channels can access the extracellular Ca^{2+} source either through action potentials, or possibly through continuous Ca^{2+} leakage in the window of membrane potentials at which there is low-level, continuous channel activity (104).

Action potentials will result in transient rapid increases in intracellular Ca^{2+}, and this is thought to be an adequate stimulus for release from the stores by ryanodine receptors. How much of the contraction initiated by action potentials is due to store release and how much by the Ca^{2+} carrying the inward current is presently unclear. Activation of receptors can also access both stores: P_{2x} purinoceptors are nonselective cation channels, and these let in Ca^{2+} ions, as well as depolarizing the membrane and activating the L-type Ca^{2+} channels. Again the rapid rise in intracellular Ca^{2+} could release Ca^{2+} from the stores by ryanodine receptors. Recently, mRNA from ryanodine receptors has been isolated from cultured human detrusor cells, and CICR has been demonstrated from these cells (25) and previously in the guinea pig detrusor (100). Muscarinic receptor activation, although not causing much depolarization, can also cause a small Ca^{2+} entry by activating nonselective cation channels through G proteins (105), and also stimulate Ca^{2+} entry through L-type Ca^{2+} channels by the increase in spike frequency that occurs. The increase in IP_3 that is also stimulated will release Ca^{2+} from the stores. Recent studies of detrusor cell calcium handling have shown that in the guinea-pig, the SR can buffer Ca^{2+} influx (106).

A rise in intracellular Ca^{2+} from whatever source can modulate ion channel function (e.g., inactivate L-type Ca^{2+} channels, activate various K^+ channels, and modulate ryanodine and IP_3 receptor store Ca^{2+} channels). The Ca^{2+} stores in the bladder are relatively labile: they can be readily depleted in Ca^{2+}-free solution, and very rapidly filled from the extracellular source (47). Just which mechanisms are involved in this exchange between stored and extracellular Ca^{2+} is unclear, although the stores can accumulate Ca^{2+} by a CaATPase. Furthermore, acidosis, either extracellular or intracellular, can also modify Ca^{2+} channel activity (107–109).

F. Detrusor Smooth-Muscle Relaxation

Normal bladder compliance requires that the bladder stretches without contracting en masse during filling. This suggests a balance between factors that mediate contraction and those that mediate relaxation. There has been long-standing debate about whether this arose primarily through neurogenic or myogenic mechanisms. Although it remains unclear, some recent data are of interest.

Molecular techniques and muscle strip studies have shown that human detrusor contains β_3-adrenoceptors that can mediate relaxation of agonist-induced contraction (110, 111). Studies in the rat have suggested the presence of an unidentified relaxant factor released by muscarinic receptor activation (112), and the urothelium of isolated pig bladder releases a potent relaxant factor of unidentifiable nature (113). In the marmoset bladder, there appear to be two ATP receptors, a P_{2x} purinoceptor, mediating contraction, whereas a P_{2y} purinoceptor promotes relaxation (114). Finally, stretch of cultured rat detrusor cells stimulated the release of parathyroid hormone-related protein, which was able to oppose carbachol-induced detrusor contraction (22). Any, all, or none of these observations could be involved in the mediation of normal bladder compliance.

V.   URETHRAL PHYSIOLOGY

Much less work has been done on the smooth muscle of the urethra than on the detrusor, although this balance is being rapidly redressed. Whereas the detrusor smooth muscle seems to act as just two units (the body and the base), there is more regional variation in urethral smooth muscle behavior (115), and urethral function is clearly different in males. The in vivo behavior of the urethra has been recently reviewed (116), but remains enigmatic, with no generally accepted view on how the skeletal muscle, smooth muscle, lamina propria, and urothelium bring about continence at rest or under stress. For the smooth muscle in particular, the roles of the circular and longitudinal layers remain unclear, although the circular smooth muscle seems disposed in the manner typical of a muscular sphincter. Experimental studies on the effects of hypoxia and blood flow on urethral pressure generation have been recently reported (117,118).

A.   Innervation

An α-adrenoceptor-mediated contraction in response to norepinephrine, inhibited by isoproterenol or terbutaline by β-adrenoceptors occurs in human urethral smooth muscle (119). There was low sensitivity to acetylcholine, but the resulting contraction was mediated by muscarinic receptors (119). Prostaglandins could increase or decrease both longitudinal and circular smooth-muscle layer tension by nonadrenergic, noncholinergic (NANC) mechanisms (120). At low resting tone, nerve-mediated α-adrenergic contractions occurred, whereas at high tone after norepinephrine pretreatment, nerve-mediated NANC relaxations occurred (121). These differed from relaxations induced with prostaglandin E_2, isoproterenol, ATP, or Vasoactive intestinal peptide (VIP) and the transmitter was not identified (121). This was viewed as in vitro evidence for a mechanism of the urethral relaxation that precedes a detrusor contraction when voiding occurs. Recently, it was suggested that NANC relaxations in urethral smooth muscle in humans are mediated by nitric oxide (122).

Nerve-mediated contractions and relaxations occur in pig urethral smooth muscle, depending on the stimulation parameters (123,124). The contraction is mainly atropine-sensitive and, therefore, cholinergic (115,123,124). The relaxation is at least partly nitrergic (123,125), although another NANC transmitter may also be involved (115). Prostaglandin synthesis inhibition increased tension and spontaneous activity in pig urethral smooth muscle: the opposite effects were produced by both E series prostaglandins and VIP (126,127). Serotonin (5-hydroxy tryptamine; 5-HT) produced substantial relaxations, partly inhibited by specific 5-HT receptor antagonists, although these had no effect on nerve-mediated relaxations, suggesting that 5-HT probably has no physiological role in urethral smooth-muscle relaxation (128). NANC nerve-mediated contractions have been demonstrated in the rabbit, but no muscarinic receptor-mediated contraction occurred (129).

In the rabbit, activation of α_2-adrenoceptors and of muscarinic receptors could inhibit both the release of norepinephrine from adrenergic nerve terminals (130) and the release of acetylcholine from cholinergic nerve terminals (131). This was interpreted as negative-feedback control of norepinephrine and acetylcholine release, indicating that the cholinergic innervation and adrenergic innervation to the urethra could regulate one another. VIP slightly inhibited the contraction induced by norepinephrine, but had no consistent effect on nerve-mediated responses, suggesting that VIP probably did not regulate neurotransmission (132). Recent work showed the presence of heme oxygenase (which produces carbon monoxide) in the smooth muscle of the pig urethra, and that carbon monoxide relaxed urethral smooth-muscle preparations by a mechanism independent of K^+ channels (133). Relaxation of bladder smooth muscle with carbon monoxide was not seen. In the rabbit, nitric oxide was released by nitrergic nerves and caused urethral smooth-muscle relaxation, and inhibited release of norepinephrine from adrenergic nerves (134). In proximal urethra from the female dog, capsaicin produced relaxation in strips precontracted with norepinephrine (135). This was inhibited by L-nitroarginine methyl ester (L-NAME), and by prolonged cold storage, and was thought to be due to the effect of capsaicin on primary afferent nerves (135).

Pig urethral smooth muscle generates considerable myogenic tone, consistent with the ability to maintain continuous sphincter pressure: neither atropine or guanethidine affect this, suggesting that it does not depend on tonic cholinergic or adrenergic innervation (123). Spontaneous tone generation in vitro was greatest from strips of proximal urethral smooth muscle and less in strips from the distal urethra (115).

B. Membrane Properties and Potentials

The resting membrane potential in proximal urethral smooth-muscle cells is −39 mV and −50.6 mV in the male rabbit (measured with microelectrodes) (136,137); −36 mV in the female pig (measured with patch clamp electrodes) (138); −36 mV in sheep of either sex (measured with patch clamp electrodes) (139); and −50.8 mV in female guinea pigs (measured with microelectrodes) (140). In microelectrode studies of the smooth muscle of the proximal urethra of the male rabbit, spontaneous hyperpolarizations and depolarizations occurred in a minority of cells (136). Depolarization and contraction occurred in the double sucrose-gap experiments, and this was contributed to by release of ATP, norepinephrine, and acetylcholine, and large hyperpolarizations occurred which were only partly blocked by nitric oxide synthase inhibitors, suggesting two inhibitory neurotransmitters (136). The implied presence of excitatory and inhibitory innervation differs from the detrusor, which seems to have only direct excitatory innervation (136).

C. Ion Channels

Urethral smooth muscle seems to be unique in responding to depolarization with high K^+ solutions by relaxation, rather than the contraction that invariably occurs with other smooth muscles (141). Levcromakalim produced relaxation of strips of proximal urethral smooth muscle from the female pig, it caused hyperpolarization and an outward K^+ current, both of which were blocked by glibenclamide (138). Metabolic inhibition, stimulated by cyanide, activated the same K^+ channel (138), suggesting involvement of this channel under conditions of hypoxia. This channel was further investigated and was inhibited by intracellular ATP, but reactivated, after running down, by nucleoside diphosphates (142). The channel was felt to differ from the ATP-sensitive channel in the guinea pig bladder, because of different conductance and reactivation properties. Magnesium was thought to contribute to the intracellular regulation of the channel (142). Although differences were seen between this K^+ channel and that in the detrusor, it was felt that KCOs considered for use in detrusor instability should also be assessed for their effect on urethral function, because of the possibility that the therapeutic benefit of inhibiting detrusor instability might be offset by a reduction in urethral closure pressure. The effects of the KCO nicorandil were also studied on proximal urethra of the pig, and two independent mechanisms of nicorandil-induced relaxation were postulated, suggesting too that KCOs might well have unexpected, and possibly adverse clinical effects on the urethra (143).

In urethral smooth muscle of the sheep, guinea pig, and rabbit, L-type Ca^{2+} channels and Ca^{2+}-dependent Cl^- currents seem to act together to produce contraction (137,139, 140). Calcium currents seemed to be responsible for the upstroke of the action potential, whereas the chloride current could have a possible pacemaker function. Ca^{2+}-dependent Cl^- currents resulted from spontaneous release of Ca^{2+} from intracellular stores, and led to spontaneous transient depolarizations. These depolarizations then activated L-type Ca^{2+} channels and resulted in so-called slow waves, depolarizations that probably cause contraction.

VI. CONCLUSION

Skeletal muscle is excited through a single mechanism that involves release of acetylcholine from nerve terminals and the activation of nicotinic receptors. This causes release into the cytosol of Ca^{2+} from the sarcoplasmic reticulum (SR) of the skeletal muscle cell by a single type of SR calcium channel, the ryanodine receptor. In contrast, the excitation of the contractile apparatus of smooth-muscle cells by a rise in intracellular calcium concentration $[Ca^{2+}]_i$, comes about in diverse ways, depending on the smooth muscle in question. Kotlikoff and colleagues have pointed out that redundancy exists at every level of activation of smooth-muscle excitation–contraction coupling (1). The diverse functional requirements of smooth muscles seem to be met by the provision of many possible means of initiating contraction, and this allows many more layers of possible regulation than is probably the case for skeletal muscle. This makes smooth-muscle physiology fascinating, but inherently complex.

Research performed since the mid-1980s has told us a great deal more about the physiology of the detrusor, and to a lesser extent, the urethra, significantly increasing our knowledge base compared with what we knew then (27). Nonetheless, we still are far from understanding how the vast number of pieces of the jigsaw gathered so far fit together. Continued application of the techniques of traditional physiology, pharmacology, and anatomy, coupled with molecular biological methods, seems certain however to bring us toward a clear view of the function of the lower urinary tract.

REFERENCES

1. Kotlikoff MI, Herrera G, Nelson MT. Calcium permeant ion channels in smooth muscle. Rev Physiol Biochem Pharmacol 1999; 134:147–199.
2. Bolton TB, Imaizumi Y. Spontaneous transient outward currents in smooth muscle cells. Cell Calcium 1996; 20:141–152.
3. Horowitz A, Menice CB, Laporte R. Morgan KG. Mechanisms of smooth muscle contraction. Physiol Rev 1996; 76:967–1003.
4. Quayle JM, Nelson MT, Standen NB. ATP-sensitive and inwardly rectifying potassium channels in smooth muscle. Physiol Rev 1997; 77:1165–1232.
5. Zimmem PE, Lin VK McConnell JD. Smooth-muscle physiology. Urol Clin North Am 1996; 23:211–219.
6. Eglen RM, Hegde SS, Watson N, Muscarinic receptor subtypes and smooth muscle function. Pharmacol Rev 1996; 48:531–565.
7. Kuriyama H, Kitamura K, Itoh T, Inoue R. Physiological features of visceral smooth muscle cells, with special reference to receptors and ion channels. Physiol Rev 1998; 78:811–920.

8. Somlyo AP, Wu X, Walker LA, Somlyo AV. Pharmacomechanical coupling: the role of calcium, G-proteins, kinases and phosphatases. Rev Physiol Biochem Pharmacol 1999; 134:201–234.

9. Taggart MJ, Wray S. Hypoxia and smooth muscle function: key regulatory events during metabolic stress. J Physiol (Lond) 1998; 509:315–325.

10. Turner WH, Brading AF. Smooth muscle of the bladder in the normal and the diseased state: pathophysiology, diagnosis and treatment. Pharmacol Ther 1997; 75:77–110.

11. Levin RM, Haugaard N, Hypolite JA, Wein AJ, Buttyan, R. Metabolic factors influencing lower urinary tract function. Exp Physiol 1999; 84:171–194.

12. Brading AF, Sibley GNA. A superfusion apparatus to study field stimulation of smooth muscle from mammalian urinary bladder. J Physiol 1983; 334:11.

13. Bramich NJ, Brading AF. Electrical properties of smooth muscle in the guinea-pig urinary bladder. J Physiol (Lond) 1996; 492:185–198.

14. Mostwin JL. The action potential of guinea pig bladder smooth muscle. J Urol 1986; 135: 1299–1303.

15. Mostwin JL. Electrical membrane events underlying contraction of guinea-pig bladder muscle. Neurourol Urodynam 1988; 6:429–437.

16. Fry CH, Cooklin M, Birns J, Mundy AR. Measurement of intercellular electrical coupling in guinea-pig detrusor smooth muscle. J Urol 1999; 161:660–664.

17. Foster CD, Fujii K, Kingdon J, Brading AF. The effect of cromakalim on the smooth muscle of the guinea-pig urinary bladder. Br J Pharmacol 1989; 97:281–291.

18. Foster CD, Speakman MJ, Fujii K, Brading AF. The effects of cromakalim on the detrusor muscle of human and pig urinary bladder. Br J Urol 1989; 63:284–294.

19. Somogyi GT, de Groat WC. Function, signal transduction mechanisms and plasticity of presynaptic muscarinic receptors in the urinary bladder. Life Sci 1999; 64:411–418.

20. Neher E, Sakmann B. The patch clamp technique. Sci Am 1992; 266:28–35.

21. Harriss DR. Smooth muscle cell culture: a new approach to the study of human detrusor physiology and pathophysiology. Br J Urol 1995; 75(suppl 1):18–26.

22. Steers WD, Broder SR, Persson K, Bruns DE, Ferguson JE, Bruns ME, Tuttle JB. Mechanical stretch increases secretion of parathyroid hormone-related protein by cultured bladder smooth muscle cells. J Urol 1998; 160:908–912.

23. Park JM, Borer JG, Freeman MR, Peters CA. Stretch activates heparin-binding EGF-like growth factor expression in bladder smooth muscle cells. Am J Physiol 1998; 275:C1247–C1254.

24. Watson JD, Gilman M, Witkowski J, Zoller M. Recombinant DNA. New York: Scientific American Books, 1992.

25. Chambers P, Neal DE, Gillespie JI. Ryanodine receptors in human bladder smooth muscle. Exp Physiol 1999; 84:41–46.

26. Davies AM, Jones WD, Eardley I, Beech DJ. Voltage gated potassium channels in detrusor muscle. Neurourol Urodynam 1999; 18:347–348.

27. Brading AF. Physiology of the bladder smooth muscle. In: Torrens M, Morrison JFB, eds. The Physiology of the Lower Urinary Tract. Berlin: Springer-Verlag, 1987:161–191.

28. Mostwin JL, Karim NS, van Koeveringe G. Electrical properties of obstructed guinea pig bladder. Adv Exp Med Biol 1995; 385:21–28.

29. Bortoff A, Sillin LF. Changes in intercellular electrical coupling of smooth muscle accompanying atrophy and hypertrophy. Am J Physiol 1986; 250:C292–C298.

30. Garfield RE, Thilander G, Blennerhassett MG, Sakai N. Are gap junctions necessary for cell-to-cell coupling of smooth muscle? an update. Can J Physiol Pharmacol 1992; 70:481–490.

31. Campos de Carvalho AC, Roy C, Moreno AP, Melman A, Hertzberg EL, Christ GJ, Spray DC. Gap junctions formed of connexin 43 are found between smooth muscle cells of human corpus cavernosum. J Urol 1993; 149:1568–1575.

32. Dermietzel R, Hwang TK, Spray DS. The gap junction family: structure, function and chemistry. Anat Embryol (Berl) 1990; 182:517–528.

33. Bonev AD, Nelson MT. Muscarinic inhibition of ATP-sensitive K^+ channels by protein kinase C in urinary bladder smooth muscle. Am J Physiol 1993; 265:C1723–C1728.

34. Uvelius B, Gabella G. Relation between cell length and force production in urinary bladder smooth muscle. Acta Physiol Scand 1980; 110:357–365.

35. Ruegg JC. Smooth muscle tone. Physiol Rev 1971; 51:201–248.

36. Brading AF. Physiology of the urinary tract smooth muscle. In: Webster GD, Kirby RS, King LR, Goldwasser B, eds. Reconstructive Urology. Boston: Blackwell Scientific, 1993:15.

37. Stewart CC. Mammalian smooth muscle. The cat's bladder. Am J Physiol 1990; 4:185.

38. Morrison JF. The physiological mechanisms involved in bladder emptying. Scand J Urol Nephrol Suppl. 1997; 184:15–18.

39. Fry CH, Wu C, Sui GP. Electrophysiological properties of the bladder. Int Urogynecol J Pelvic Floor Dysfunct 1998; 9:291–298.

40. Sibley GNA. A comparison of spontaneous and nerve-mediated activity in bladder muscle from man, pig and rabbit. J Physiol (Lond) 1984; 354:431–443.

41. Brading AF, Williams JH. Contractile responses of smooth muscle strips from rat and guinea-pig urinary bladder to transmural stimulation: effects of atropine and a,b-methylene ATP. Br J Pharmacol 1990; 99:493–498.

42. Creed KE. Membrane properties of the smooth muscle membrane of the guinea-pig urinary bladder. Pflugers Arch 1971; 326:115–126.

43. Fujii K. Evidence for adenosine triphosphate as an excitatory transmitter in guinea-pig, rabbit and pig urinary bladder. J Physiol (Lond) 1988; 404:39–52.

44. Creed KE, Ishikawa S, Ito Y. Electrical and mechanical activity recorded from rabbit urinary bladder in response to nerve stimulation. J Physiol (Lond) 1983; 338:149–164.

45. Hashitani H, Suzuki H. Electrical and mechanical responses produced by nerve stimulation in detrusor smooth muscle of the guinea pig. Eur J Pharmacol 1995; 284:177–183.

46. Hoyle CH, Bumstock G. Atropine-resistant excitatory junction potentials in rabbit bladder are blocked by alpha, beta-methylene ATP. Eur J Pharmacol 1985; 114:239–240.

47. Mostwin JL. Receptor operated intracellular calcium stores in the smooth muscle of the guinea pig bladder. J Urol 1985; 133:900–905.

48. Montgomery BS, Fry CH. The action potential and net membrane currents in isolated human detrusor smooth muscle cells. J Urol 1992; 147:176–184.

49. Bülbring E. The correlation between membrane potential, spike discharge and tension in smooth muscle. J Physiol (Lond) 1955; 128:200.

50. Parekh AB, Brading AF, Tomita T. Studies of longitudinal tissue impedance in various smooth muscles. Prog Clin Biol Res 1990; 327:375–378.

51. Gabella G, Uvelius B. Urinary bladder of rat: fine structure of normal and hypertrophic musculature. Cell Tissue Res 1990; 262:67–79.

52. Daniel EE, Cowan W, Daniel VP. Structural bases for neural and myogenic control of human detrusor muscle. Can J Physiol Pharmacol 1983; 61:1247–1273.

53. Elbadawi A, Schenk EA. Dual innervation of the mammalian urinary bladder. A histochemical study of the distribution of cholinergic and adrenergic nerves. Am J Anat 1966; 119:405–427.

54. Klück P. The autonomic innervation of the human urinary bladder, bladder neck and urethra: a histochemical study. Anat Rec 1980; 198:439–447.

55. Hoyes AD, Barber P, Martin BG. Comparative ultrastructure of the nerves innervating the muscle of the body of the bladder. Cell Tissue Res 1975; 164:133–144.

56. Tong YC, Hung YC, Shinozuka K, Kunitomo M, Cheng JT. Evidence of adenosine 5′-triphosphate release from nerve and P_{2x}-purinoceptor mediated contraction during electrical stimulation of rat urinary bladder smooth muscle. J Urol 1997; 158:1973–1977.

57. Sjögren C, Andersson KE, Husted S, Mattiasson A, Moller–Madsen B. Atropine resistance of transmurally stimulated isolated human bladder muscle. J Urol 1982; 128:1368–1371.

58. Kinder RB, Mundy AR. Atropine blockade of nerve-mediated stimulation of the human detrusor. Br J Urol 1985; 57:418–421.

59. Chen TF, Doyle PT, Ferguson DR. Inhibition in the human urinary bladder by gamma-amino-butyric acid. Br J Urol 1994; 73:250–255.

60. Inoue R, Brading AF. Human, pig and guinea-pig bladder smooth muscle cells generate similar inward currents in response to purinoceptor activation. Br J Pharmacol 1991; 103:1840–1841.

61. Callahan SM, Creed KE. Electrical and mechanical activity of the isolated lower urinary tract of the guinea-pig. Br J Pharmacol 1981; 74:353–358.

62. Noronha–Blob L, Lowe V, Patton A, Canning B, Costello D, Kinnier WJ. Muscarinic receptors: relationships among phosphoinositide breakdown, adenylate cyclase inhibition, in vitro detrusor muscle contractions and in vivo cystometrogram studies in guinea pig bladder. J Pharmacol Exp Ther 1989; 249:843–851.

63. Iacovou JW, Hill SJ, Birmingham AT. Agonist-induced contraction and accumulation of inositol phosphates in the guinea-pig detrusor: evidence that muscarinic and purinergic receptors raise intracellular calcium by different mechanisms. J Urol 1990; 144:775–779.

64. Harriss DR, Marsh KA, Birmingham AT, Hill SJ. Expression of muscarinic M_3-receptors coupled to inositol phospholipid hydrolysis in human detrusor cultured smooth muscle cells. J Urol 1995; 154:1241–1245.

65. Inoue R, Brading AF. The properties of the ATP-induced depolarization and current in single cells isolated from the guinea-pig urinary bladder. Br J Pharmacol 1990; 100:619–625.

66. Brading AF, Mostwin JL. Electrical and mechanical responses of guinea-pig bladder muscle to nerve stimulation. Br J Pharmacol 1989; 98:1083–1090.

67. Creed KE, Callahan SM, Ito Y. Excitatory neurotransmission in the mammalian bladder and the effect of suramin. Br J Urol 1994; 74:736–743.

68. Marsh KA, Harriss DR, Hill SJ. Desensitisation of muscarinic receptor-coupled inositol phospholipid hydrolysis in human detrusor cultured smooth muscle cells. J Urol 1996; 155:1439–1443.

69. Braverman AS, Kohn IJ, Luthin GR, Ruggieri MR. Prejunctional M_1 facilitory and M_2 inhibitory muscarinic receptors mediate rat bladder contractility. Am J Physiol 1998; 274:R517–523.

70. Fujii K, Foster CD, Brading AF, Parekh AB. Potassium channel blockers and the effects of cromakalim on the smooth muscle of the guinea-pig bladder. Br J Pharmacol 1990; 99:779–785.

71. Brading AF, Turner WH. Potassium channels and their modulation in urogenital smooth muscles. In: Evans JM, Hamilton TC, Longham SD, Stemp G, eds. Potassium Channels and Their Modulators: From Synthesis to Clinical Experience. London: Taylor & Francis, 1996:335.

72. Klöckner U, Isenberg G. Action potentials and net membrane currents of isolated smooth muscle cells (urinary bladder of the guinea-pig). Pflugers Arch 1985; 405:329–339.

73. Isenberg G, Klöckner U. Calcium currents of smooth muscle cells isolated from the urinary bladder of the guinea-pig: inactivation, conductance and selectivity is controlled by micromolar amounts of [Ca]. J Physiol (Lond) 1985; 258:60P.

74. Nakayama S. Effects of excitatory neurotransmitters on Ca_{21} channel current in smooth muscle cells isolated from guinea-pig urinary bladder. Br J Pharmacol 1993; 110:317–325.

75. Bonev AD, Nelson MT. ATP-sensitive potassium channels in smooth muscle cells from guinea pig urinary bladder. Am J Physiol 1993; 264:C1190–C1200.

76. Edwards G, Henshaw M, Miller M, Weston AH. Comparison of the effects of several potassium-channel openers on rat bladder and rat portal vein in vitro. Br J Pharmacol 1991; 102:679–680.

77. Gallegos CR, Fry CH. Alterations to the electrophysiology of isolated human detrusor smooth muscle cells in bladder disease. J Urol 1994; 151:754–758.

78. Wammack R, Jahnel U, Nawrath H, Hohenfellner R. Mechanical and electrophysiological effects of cromakalim on the human urinary bladder. Eur Urol 1994; 26:176–181.

79. Nakayama S, Brading AF. Evidence for multiple open states of the Ca^{2+} channels in smooth muscle cells isolated from the guinea-pig detrusor. J Physiol (Lond) 1993; 471:87–105.

80. Nakayama S, Brading AF. Long Ca^{2+} channel opening induced by large depolarization and Bay K 8644 in smooth muscle cells isolated from guinea-pig detrusor. Br J Pharmacol 1996; 119:716–720.

81. Trivedi S, Potter–Lee L, Li JH, Yasay GD, Russell K, Ohnmacht CJ, Empfield JR, Trainor DA, Kau ST. Calcium dependent K-channels in guinea pig and human urinary bladder. Biochem Biophys Res Commun 1995; 213:404–409.

82. Cotton KD, Hollywood MA, Thornbury KD, McHale NG. Effect of purinergic blockers on outward current in isolated smooth muscle cells of the sheep bladder. Am J Physiol 1996; 270: C969–C973.

83. Hirano M, Imaizumi Y, Muraki K, Yamada A, Watanabe M. Effects of ruthenium red on membrane ionic currents in urinary bladder smooth muscle cells of the guinea-pig. Pflugers Arch 1998; 435:645–653.

84. Hollywood MA, Cotton KD, McHale NG, Thornbury KD. Enhancement of Ca^{2+}-dependent outward current in sheep bladder myocytes by Evans blue dye. Pflugers Arch 1998; 435:631–638.

85. Trivedi S, Stetz S, Levin R, Li J, Kau S. Effect of cromakalim and pinacidil on ^{86}Rb efflux from guinea pig urinary bladder smooth muscle. Pharmacology 1994; 49:159–166.

86. Green ME, Edwards G, Kirkup AJ, Miller M, Weston AH. Pharmacological characterization of the inwardly-rectifying current in the smooth muscle cells of the rat bladder. Br J Pharmacol 1996; 119:1509–1518.

87. Fujii K. Electrophysiological evidence that adenosine triphosphate (ATP) is a cotransmitter with acetylcholine (ACh) in isolated guinea-pig, rabbit and pig urinary bladder. J Physiol (Lond) 1987; 394:26P.

88. Smet PJ, Jonavicius J, Marshall VR, de Vente J. Distribution of nitric oxide synthase-immunoreactive nerves and identification of the cellular targets of nitric oxide in guinea-pig and human urinary bladder by CGMP immunohistochemistry. Neuroscience 1996; 71:337–348.

89. Zografos P, Li JH, Kau ST. Comparison of the in vitro effects of K^+ channel modulators on detrusor and portal vein strips from guinea pigs. Pharmacology 1992; 45:216–230.

90. Brading AF, Turner WH. The unstable bladder: towards a common mechanism. Br J Urol 1994; 73:3–8.

91. Heppner TJ, Bonev A, Li JH, Kau ST, Nelson MT. Zeneca ZD6169 activates ATP-sensitive K^+ channels in the urinary bladder of the guinea pig. Pharmacology 1996; 53:170–179.

92. Hu S, Kim HS. Modulation of ATP-sensitive and large-conductance Ca^{++}-activated K^+ channels by Zeneca ZD6169 in guinea pig bladder smooth muscle cells. J Pharmacol Exp Ther 1997; 280:38–45.

93. Pandita RK, Andersson KE. Effects of intravesical administration of the K^+ channel opener, ZD6169, in conscious rats with and without bladder outflow obstruction. J Urol 1999; 162:943–948.

94. Wellner MC, Isenberg G. Properties of stretch-activated channels in myocytes from the guinea-pig urinary bladder. J Physiol (Lond) 1993; 466:213–227.

95. Wellner MC, Isenberg G. Stretch effects on whole-cell currents of guinea-pig urinary bladder myocytes. J Physiol (Lond) 1994; 480:439–448.

96. Wellner MC, Isenberg G. CAMP accelerates the decay of stretch-activated inward currents in guinea-pig urinary bladder myocytes. J Physiol (Lond) 1995; 482:141–156.

97. Hamill OP, McBride DW Jr. The pharmacology of mechanogated membrane ion channels. Pharmacol Rev 1996; 48:231–252.

98. Fry CH, Wu C. Initiation of contraction in detrusor smooth muscle. Scand J Urol Nephrol Suppl 1997; 184:7–14.

99. Maggi CA, Giuliani S, Patacchini R, Turini D, Barbanti G, Giachetti A, Meli A. Multiple sources of calcium for contraction of the human urinary bladder muscle. Br J Pharmacol 1989; 98:1021–1031.

100. Ganitkevich VY, Isenberg G. Depolarization-mediated intracellular calcium transients in isolated smooth muscle cells of guinea-pig urinary bladder. J Physiol (Lond) 1991; 435:187–205.
101. Somlyo AP. Excitation–contraction coupling and the ultrastructure of smooth muscle. Circ Res 1985; 57:497–507.
102. Andersson KE. Bladder function. In: Webster DG, Kirby RS, King LR, Goldwasser B, eds. Boston: Blackwell Scientific, 1993:27.
103. Andersson KE. Pharmacology of lower urinary tract smooth muscles and penile erectile tissues. Pharmacol Rev 1993; 45:253.
104. Nakayama S, Brading AF. Possible contribution of long open state to noninactivating Ca^{2+} current in detrusor cells. Am J Physiol 1995; 269:C48–C54.
105. Inoue R. Purinergic receptor-operated currents recorded from single isolated cells of guinea-pig urinary bladder. J Physiol (Lond) 1990; 424:22P.
106. Yoshikawa A, van Breemen C, Isenberg G. Buffering of plasmalemmal Ca^{2+} current by sarcoplasmic reticulum of guinea pig urinary bladder myocytes. Am J Physiol 1996; 271:C833–C841.
107. Thomas PJ, Fry CH. The effects of cellular hypoxia on contraction and extracellular ion accumulation in isolated human detrusor smooth muscle. J Urol 1996; 155:726–731.
108. Wu C, Kentish JC, Fry CH. Effect of pH on myofilament Ca(2+)-sensitivity in alpha-toxin penneabilized guinea pig detrusor muscle. J Urol 1995; 154:1921–1924.
109. Wu C, Fry CH. The effects of extracellular and intracellular pH on intracellular Ca^{2+} regulation in guinea-pig detrusor smooth muscle. J Physiol (Lond) 1998; 508:131–143.
110. Takeda, M, Obara K, Mizusawa T, Tomita Y, Arai K, Tsutsui T, Hatano A, Takahashi K, Nomura S. Evidence for P_3-adrenoceptor subtypes in relaxation of the human urinary bladder detrusor: analysis by molecular biological and pharmacological methods. J Pharmacol Exp Ther 1999; 288:1367–1373.
111. Igawa Y, Yamazaki Y, Takeda H, Hayakawa K, Akahane M, Ajisawa Y, Yoneyama T, Nishizawa O, Andersson KE. Functional and molecular biological evidence for a possible β3-adrenoceptor in the human detrusor muscle. Br J Pharmacol 1999; 126:819–825.
112. Fovaeus M, Fujiwara M, Hogestatt ED, Persson K, Andersson KE. A non-nitrergic smooth muscle relaxant factor released from rat urinary bladder by muscarinic receptor stimulation. J Urol 1999; 161:649–653.
113. Hawthorn M, Chapple C, Cock M, Chess–Williams R. Urothelium-derived relaxant factor in the pig bladder. Eur Urol 1999; 35:95.
114. McMurray G, Dass N, Brading AF. Purinoceptor subtypes mediating contraction and relaxation of marmoset urinary bladder smooth muscle. Br J Pharmacol 1998; 123:1579–1586.
115. Bridgewater M, Davies JR, Brading AF. Regional variations in the neural control of the female pig urethra. Br J Urol 1995; 76:730–740.
116. Brading AF. The physiology of the mammalian urinary outflow tract. Exp Physiol 1999; 84:215–221.
117. Greenland JE, Dass N, Brading AF. Intrinsic urethral closure mechanisms in the female pig. Scand J Urol Nephrol Suppl 1996; 179:75–80.
118. Greenland JE, Brading AF. The in vivo and in vitro effects of hypoxia on pig urethral smooth muscle. Br J Urol 1997; 79:525–531.
119. Ek A, Alm P, Andersson KE, Persson CG. Adrenergic and cholinergic nerves of the human urethra and urinary bladder. A histochemical study. Acta Physiol Scand 1977; 99:345–352.
120. Andersson KE, Ek A, Persson CG. Effects of prostaglandins on the isolated human bladder and urethra. Acta Physiol Scand 1977; 100:165–171.
121. Andersson KE, Mattiasson A, Sjögren C. Electrically induced relaxation of the noradrenaline contracted isolated urethra from rabbit and man. J Urol 1983; 129:210–214.
122. Ehrén I, Iversen H, Jansson O, Adolfsson J, Wiklund NP. Localization of nitric oxide synthase activity in the human lower urinary tract and its correlation with neuroeffector responses. Urology 1994; 44:683–687.

123. Bridgewater M, MacNeil HF, Brading AF. Regulation of tone in pig urethral smooth muscle. J Urol 1993; 150:223–228.

124. Klarskov P, Gerstenberg TC, Ramirez D, Hald T. Non-cholinergic, non-adrenergic nerve mediated relaxation of trigone, bladder neck and urethral smooth muscle in vitro. J Urol 1983; 129:848–850.

125. Persson K, Andersson KE. Nitric oxide and relaxation of pig lower urinary tract. Br J Pharmacol 1992; 106:416–422.

126. Klarskov P, Gerstenberg T, Ramirez D, Christensen P, Hald T. Prostaglandin type E activity dominates in urinary tract smooth muscle in vitro. J Urol 1983; 129:1071–1074.

127. Klarskov P, Gerstenberg T, Hald T. Vasoactive intestinal polypeptide influence on lower urinary tract smooth muscle from human and pig. J Urol 1984; 131:1000–1004.

128. Klarskov P, Horby–Petersen J. Influence of serotonin on lower urinary tract smooth muscle in vitro. Br J Urol 1986; 58:507–513.

129. Mattiasson A, Andersson KE, Sjögren C. Adrenergic and non-adrenergic contraction of isolated urethral muscle from rabbit and man. J Urol 1985; 133:298–303.

130. Mattiasson A, Andersson KE, Sjögren C. Adrenoceptors and cholinoceptors controlling noradrenaline release from adrenergic nerves in the urethra of rabbit and man. J Urol 1984; 131:1190–1195.

131. Mattiasson A, Andersson KE, Sjögren C. Inhibitory muscarinic receptors and α-adrenoceptors on cholinergic axon terminals in the urethra of rabbit and man. Neurourol Urodynam 1988; 6:449–456.

132. Sjögren C, Andersson KE, Mattiasson A. Effects of vasoactive intestinal polypeptide on isolated urethral and urinary bladder smooth muscle from rabbit and man. J Urol 1985; 133:136–140.

133. Werkström V, Ny L, Persson K, Andersson KE. Carbon monoxide-induced relaxation and distribution of haem oxygenase isoenzymes in the pig urethra and lower oesophagogastric junction. Br J Pharmacol 1997; 120:312–318.

134. Yoshida M, Akaike T, Inadome A, Takahashi W, Seshita H, Yono M, Goto S, Maeda H, Ueda S. The possible effect of nitric oxide on relaxation and noradrenaline release in the isolated rabbit urethra. Eur J Pharmacol 1998; 357:213–219.

135. Nishizawa S, Igawa Y, Okada N, Ohhashi T. Capsaicin-induced nitric-oxide-dependent relaxation in isolated dog urethra. Eur J Pharmacol 1997; 335:211–219.

136. Creed KE, Oike M, Ito Y. The electrical properties and responses to nerve stimulation of the proximal urethra of the male rabbit. Br J Urol 1997; 79:543–553.

137. Hashitani H, Van Helden DF, Suzuki H. Properties of spontaneous depolarizations in circular smooth muscle cells of rabbit urethra. Br J Pharmacol 1996; 118:1627–1632.

138. Teramoto N, Brading AF. Activation by levcromakalim and metabolic inhibition of glibenclamide-sensitive K channels in smooth muscle cells of pig proximal urethra. Br J Pharmacol 1996; 118:635–642.

139. Cotton KD, Hollywood MA, McHale NG, Thornbury KD. Ca^{2+} current and Ca(2+)-activated chloride current in isolated smooth muscle cells of the sheep urethra. J Physiol (Lond) 1997; 505:121–131.

140. Hashitani H, Edwards FR. Spontaneous and neurally activated depolarizations in smooth muscle cells of the guinea-pig urethra. J Physiol (Lond) 1999; 514:459–470.

141. Brading AF, Chen HI. High potassium solution induces relaxation in the isolated pig urethra. J Physiol (Lond) 1990; 430:118P.

142. Teramoto N, McMurray G, Brading AF. Effects of levcromakalim and nucleoside diphosphates on glibenclamide-sensitive K^+ channels in pig urethral myocytes. Br J Pharmacol 1997; 120:1229–1240.

143. Teramoto N, Brading AF. Nicorandil activates glibenclamide-sensitive K^+ channels in smooth muscle cells of pig proximal urethra. J Pharmacol Exp Ther 1997; 280:483–491.

5

Physiology of the Striated Muscles of the Pelvic Floor

JOHN F. B. MORRISON

United Arab Emirates University, Al Ain, United Arab Emirates

I. INTRODUCTION

This chapter is concerned with the physiological control of pelvic floor muscles and other striated muscles functionally associated with the pelvic diaphragm. The functions of this group of muscles differ between humans and primates, which use the upright posture, and animals that use four limbs to move around. The effects of gravity, the weight of abdominal contents, respiratory movements of the diaphragm and abdominal wall muscles, particularly during coughing and straining, cause greater stress to be borne by the pelvic diaphragm when the upright posture is attained. Nevertheless, many of the basic physiological mechanisms are found in a range of species, which makes analysis of detailed mechanisms of control rather easier than it would be if we had to rely only on human studies.

There has been a mushrooming of basic and applied knowledge in this field, in the last 20 years, that has been marked by a number of reviews and books on the subject (1–5). The striated muscles to be considered are specialized in function, and they form groups of muscle on opposite sides of the body, which are subject to functional coordination that allows them to work together as a functional group. Within this overall concept there remain areas of muscle that are specialized for different tasks—the puborectalis or the fibers of levator ani that loop behind the urethra are examples—and one of the clear conclusions of the last decade or so has been that subdivisions of the muscle of the pelvic floor exhibit some functional differences. There are clear differences, for example, between the urethral sphincter, the associated paraurethral muscles, and the muscle fibers of the major part of levator ani. These differences extend to the histological and biochemical properties of the muscle fibers, the pattern and source of innervation, the reflex behavior, and the role in voluntary control of the lower urinary tract.

II. MORPHOLOGY

A. Anatomy and Histochemistry

The tissues that contribute to the continence mechanisms within the urethra consist of connective tissue, skeletal muscle external to the urethra, and smooth muscle and skeletal muscle within the urethra. The contribution of the pelvic floor to continence arises mainly from skeletal muscle, its tendons, and its fascial attachments. The connective tissue (fasciae) forms a framework against which muscles exert their action and, in addition, provides residual support for the urethra when the muscles of the pelvic floor are relaxed. The main muscle involved in these processes is the levator ani. In the human female, the paraurethral tissues are joined with muscle fibers of the most medial portion of the levator ani in the region of the proximal urethra. At this site, the medial fibers of levator ani are inserted into the anterior vaginal wall and provide an arching mechanism that can constrict the urethra (6); a similar arrangement occurs in female rats (7). It has also been suggested that the medial fibers of the levator ani muscle have a specific role in controlling the vesical neck position and in urinary continence mechanisms (8). The role of the levator ani appears to be to support the proximal urethra and to pull the bladder neck in an anterior direction, such that the lumen is constricted between arching fibers and connective tissue of the levator ani and a connective tissue band (endopelvic fascia) anteriorly. When the levator ani relaxes, the bladder neck can descend, and the lumen can open because the external compression is reduced; at this stage support is provided by the connective tissue of the arcus tendineus fasciae (6,9). Brief spinal anesthesia has been used to block nervous impulses to the pelvic floor and disrupt this active muscular mechanism that supports the bladder neck in healthy continent women (10). A significant loss of support was demonstrable during spinal anesthesia, indicating that activity originating in the spinal cord and pelvic floor muscles was a major factor responsible for support of the bladder neck.

The external urethral sphincter consists of circular striated muscle concentrated over about 40% of the length of the urethra (from 20 to 60% of its length in humans). In the rat the distribution of striated muscle in the urethra is similar, but there is also a mass of muscle that forms an arch at the perineal membrane that can compress the urethra from above in the lower third (11).

B. Types of Striated Muscle and Their Distribution in the Pelvic Floor

Striated muscle fibers can be divided into different types, depending on their speed of contraction and their susceptibility to fatigue. The earliest descriptions of slowly contracting 'red' and fast-contracting 'white' muscle were made in 1874 (12), and were superceded by a recognition, a century later, that the fast group can be divided into two subgroups: fast-fatiguable (FF), and fast fatigue-resistant (FFR) (13). The slow units tend to produce small forces, and are resistant to fatigue. The fast units usually develop much larger forces: those that produce the greatest force have larger diameter fibers and are fatiguable, whereas fast fibers that have a more moderate twitch tension have smaller fibers and are resistant to fatigue. There are also histochemical differences between the different fiber types, and the dominance of oxidative enzymes in slow-twitch fibers and the lack of these in fast-fatiguable fibers is one important histological correlate. The slow-twitch muscle fibers that have high levels of oxidative enzymes are sometimes referred to as type I, and they also receive a rich blood supply. Types IIA and IIB have less ATPase reactivity, have larger diameters, and the capillary supply in IIB, fast-fatiguable fibers is sparse.

C. The Striated Muscle of the Pelvic Floor and Associated Structures

The periurethral fibers of the levator ani contain both type I and larger, type II (fast-twitch) fibers, which suggests that the pelvic floor is more concerned with rapid responses, such as voluntary squeeze (14); in contrast, the striated fibers of the external urethral sphincter consist of type I (slow-twitch) fibers, which are generally associated with the generation of tone (Table 1). Studies of the contractile properties and the actomyosin ATPase levels of the guinea pig external urethral sphincter concluded that the majority of the muscle fibers were of the fast variety (15); the distinction between FF and FFR was not made, but the results indicated close correlation between muscle fiber actomyosin ATPase content and the nature of the mechanical responses.

Biochemical analysis on the myosin chains in different muscles has indicated that the muscle of the rabbit external urethral sphincter has a type of myosin more closely associated with fast red muscles than slow white ones (16,17): the relative proportions of muscle fibers were estimated to be 88% fast type and 12% slow type. The ratio of fast to slow myosins in female external urinary sphincter (EUS) was different from that in male EUS; in addition, there was a suggestion of a selective decrease in the volume of type 2 (fast) muscle fibers or conversion of type 2 to type 1 (slow) muscle fibers with age and multiparity (18,19). In male rabbits, the urethral striated muscle appeared to have mainly fast myosin, but slow myosin occurred in higher amounts in the proximal region and tended to decrease toward the distal end (20,21). In studies of the human external sphincter, the same group found a wide range of muscle properties, and concluded that there is a great diversity in the proportions of fast and slow myosin molecules in different males, and the reasons were unclear. This diversity was also present in females, and was not related to age (22,23). The diversity of these results makes interpretation difficult, and the conclusion

Table 1 Properties of Periurethral Muscle Fibers

	Mechanical properties	Oxidative enzymes	Blood supply	Neuronal conduction velocity	Localized to
Type I	Slow-twitch; maintenance of tone	High	High	Low	External urinary sphincter pelvic floor
Type IIA	Fast-twitch fibers that maintain a high twitch tension during repetitive stimulation (fatigue-resistant)	Intermediate	Intermediate	Intermediate	Pelvic floor
Type IIB	Fast-twitch fibers that cannot maintain a high twitch tension during repetitive stimulation (fatiguable)	Low	Low	High	Certain limb muscles

drawn from mean results may not significantly alter the views expressed in the more traditional view.

The foregoing results indicate that there is a gradation in the properties of striated muscles in the pelvic floor and associated structures, and structures that are specialized for production of tone usually contain mostly slow twitch fibers. These smaller-diameter muscle fibers are innervated by smaller-diameter α-motoneurons, which also conduct more slowly than those that innervate the fast, striated muscle fibers.

II. INNERVATION OF THE PELVIC FLOOR MUSCULATURE

A. Motor Nerves

It is universally accepted that the pudendal nerve innervates many of the striated muscles of the pelvic floor and associated structures. These muscles include the external anal and urethral sphincters, bulbocavernosus, and ischiocavernosus, reflecting a functional role in all the major tracts that pass through the pelvis. It is, therefore, not surprising that there are interrelations between the control of the lower urinary tract (1,2), the gastrointestinal tract, and the reproductive organs (24) at the level of the pelvic diaphragm.

Although the striated muscle of the external urethral sphincter appears to be innervated mainly by the pudendal nerve, there is also evidence of a minor innervation that reaches the muscle by a pathway traversing the pelvis or using the pelvic nerve (25–29). This appears to be true in the rat, dog, and human, although some authors believe that the pelvic pathway is absent in the dog (30). The innervation of the distal urethra by the pudendal nerve appears to be essentially unilateral (31), which is surprising, given that the same arrangement does not apply to the external anal sphincter; in contrast the innervation of the pelvic floor is essentially ipsilateral (32). Some of the innervation of the urethral sphincter, probably sensory in nature, arises from branches of the dorsal nerve of the penis (33). The role of the pudendal innervation of the striated muscles in generating resistance to urethral dilation has been studied, and the conclusion was made that the pudendal nerve was of major importance in maintaining urethral resistance to dilation in healthy human females (34). It has been generally assumed that the innervation of striated muscle in this region is akin to that found in other parts of the somatic musculature. However, it has been found recently that the enzyme nitric oxide (NO) synthase, which generates the neuromodulator nitric oxide, is present in urethral striated muscle (35). Nitrergic nerve fibers were found on the striated urethral sphincter and nitric oxide synthase was also present in the sarcolemma of about half the striated muscle. These results indicate a possible role for NO in the regulation of urethral pressure; some authors have provided evidence that nitric oxide may be involved in the control of the urethral outlet, but have pointed to an action on smooth, rather than on striated muscle (36). It is of interest that nitrergic fibers are also present in the pelvic nerve and that many of these innervate the penis (37,38).

Pudendal motoneurons are smaller in diameter than many somatic neurons, in keeping with the size of the muscle fibers they innervate. The origin of these neurons within the spinal cord is separate from the main somatic motoneurons and also separate from the autonomic cell column, in a group of cells known as Onuf's nucleus (39,40). These neurons have different anatomical characteristics relative to their afferent inputs (41,42). This distinctive group of cells exhibits sexual dimorphism, and testosterone binds to some of these neurons (43), particularly those associated with the bulbocavernosus and ischiocavernosus.

The neurons that innervate the urethra are distinct from those innervating the ischiocavernosus or the external anal sphincter.

The pudendal nerve efferents regulate the activity of skeletal muscle in the external urethral and anal sphincters and in the pelvic floor, and have some properties in common that distinguish them from other somatic motoneurons. Not only are the conduction velocities less (44), but there are few synaptic contacts on their surface (45), which possibly reflects the lack of muscle spindle afferents in urethral muscle, and the lack of type Ia afferent input to these motoneurons (46). There were relatively few monosynaptic inputs from primary afferents in sphincteric motoneurons (45,47). In addition, Renshaw cell inhibition and crossed disynaptic inhibition are absent (45,48).

B. Subgroups of Pudendal Motoneurons Innervating the Pelvic Floor and Associated Muscles

The morphology of the dendritic arborizations of pudendal motoneurons innervating the urethral and anal sphincters of the cat differs in significant ways, reflecting the different terminations of afferent inputs that are associated with the differing functions of these muscles (49). Electrophysiological studies on these neurons (44–51) indicate that those innervating the external urethral sphincter differ in some ways from those innervating the external anal sphincter, but that many of the properties are not dissimilar. The two groups of pudendal motoneurons both belong to the more slowly conducting α-motoneurons that normally innervate slow-twitch muscle fibers, and are tonically active or easily recruited; both also showed hyperpolarizations. Among the differences are the observation that the external urethral sphincter neurons display a greater degree of baseline subthreshold conductances, such as might be caused by anomalous rectification. The responses of these neurons during micturition have been studied (52) using intracellular recordings during micturition, and it was noted that the degree of hyperpolarization of EUS motoneurons was much greater than in motoneurons innervating the external anal sphincter, indicating that there is considerable independence of control of the two sphincters by central nervous pathways.

The role of the pudendal nerve in micturition in humans has been studied by observing the effects of local anesthesia of these nerves (53). The rate of urine flow during voluntary micturition fell to about 50% of the control values. Pudendal nerve degeneration during childbirth has been offered as a reason for denervation of both the anal and the urethral sphincter in women (54–56). In contrast, electromyographic (EMG) studies on the urethral sphincter have shown that in some women who experience urinary retention there is an altered activity of the EUS, which was described as bizarre repetitive discharges (56–58).

C. Tonic Activity of the Pelvic Floor and Urethral Sphincter

The tonic activity in the periurethral skeletal muscle is one of the characteristics of this tissue and is dependent on connections with the spinal cord. The origin of this activity appeared to be almost entirely dependent on a pathway through the pelvic ganglia, as section of the pelvic nerve trunks at this site abolished resting (EMG) activity in most rats (59). Following bilateral pelvic nerve transection, however, reflex activity in this muscle group could be elicited by distension of the anal canal, vaginal stimulation, or pinch of the perineal skin; the afferent and efferent pathways for these evoked effects thus appear to be the pudendal nerve. These results support the view that there is a pelvic nerve pathway to the striated muscles surrounding the urethra, and that branches of the pudendal nerve also excite some of these muscle fibers, and produce phasic responses in response to sudden afferent stimuli. About one-third of the intraurethral pressure at rest is attributable to the striated muscles that influence urethral tone, including those of the pelvic floor (60).

III. REFLEX CONTROL OF THE PELVIC FLOOR

One of the special features of the pelvic floor muscles is that their reaction to stimuli of various sorts can be altered completely by the state of the bladder: if the bladder is relaxed and filling slowly, then one response may occur in studies of the pelvic floor; if the bladder is full and contracting, the behavior of the pelvic floor may be completely different. This is well documented for studies of the bladder and may also be true of the rectum. Reflex control will be considered under the following headings: 1) reflex effects of somatic stimulation on pelvic floor musculature, and 2) effects of visceral stimulation on the pelvic floor.

A. Reflex Effects of Somatic Stimuli on Pelvic Floor Musculature

Studies of the reflex activation of pudendal efferents that innervate the pelvic floor and external anal sphincter in cats have shown that the pudendal motoneurons are excited by segmental stimulation of cutaneous afferents, and that these responses are inhibited during micturition contractions and during distension of the bladder and colon (53,61,62). First, there appears to be no monosynaptic reflex influences on the pelvic floor. Second, excitation of pudendal motoneurons could be elicited by stimulation of afferents in the pudendal and superficial perineal nerves. Third, relaxation of the external anal sphincter and possible the pelvic floor muscles could be achieved by stimulation of some muscle nerves in the hindlimb. Interestingly, in humans, inhibition of the pelvic floor muscles occurs in certain postures, and leg support facilitated this relaxation (63,64). Fourth, presynaptic inhibition of afferents that excite pudendal motoneurons could be demonstrated during micturition. Hence, one component of micturition is a reduction in the amount of transmitter released by afferent terminals in the sacral cord. The disynaptic, trisynaptic, and oligosynaptic pathways responsible for these reflexes utilize sacral interneurons and act both ipsilaterally and contralaterally (47,65).

Sexual reflexes have been reviewed by McKenna and Marson (24). In male and female rats, mechanical stimulation of the urethra elicits a complex urethrogenital reflex that included activation of all of the perineal muscles and clonic activity in some. These authors concluded that this reflex is a coordinated pattern of reflex activity involving the somatic, sympathetic, and parasympathetic systems innervating sexual organs, and is organized by a central motor pattern generator within the spinal cord. The sensory stimulus that elicits activity in this group of pelvic floor muscles is urethral stimulation, and in their experiments these authors found that raising the pressure in the urethra to 60 mmHg followed by a sudden release of pressure was the most effective stimulus.

Painful stimuli in the perineal area have a marked influence on the activity of periurethral striated muscle (59), causing a large increase in EMG activity; cooling the perineal skin caused a smaller increase in activity. These authors (66) have also reported rhythmical oscillation in EMG activity, related to sexual activity in rats. Reference is made later to the influence of afferents from the male genital tract on periurethral muscle function. Finally, acupuncture-like stimulation of somatic structures excites or inhibits the EMG activity of periurethral muscle in rats (67).

In humans, the nerves innervating the pelvic floor are tonically active and generate pelvic floor activity that supports the bladder neck. Anatomical work (4,9) indicating a role of the pelvic floor musculature in continence is supported by functional studies (10) that concluded that a muscular mechanism, the activity of which was dependent on the central nervous system, is responsible for supporting the bladder neck region. Reflex events have been described mainly in paraplegic humans, but in normal healthy women there is evidence for many of the somatic reflexes described in the foregoing. For example, light touch of the perineal area is known to cause reflex contraction of the pelvic floor muscles and external anal sphincter, and is been used as a clinical test of segmental nerves to this region. A more investigative approach was used (68) to study the effects of straining: a straining reflex in which a raised intra-abdominal pressure was accompanied by contraction of the external urethral sphincter in normal adults was found. The response appears to be essentially a protective reflex that causes a rapid response of the sphincter during straining with a rapid onset; slow straining did not induce this response.

Bo and Talseth (69) compared the effects of voluntary pelvic floor muscle contraction and vaginal electrical stimulation on urethral pressure, and found that voluntary pelvic floor muscle contractions increase urethral pressure significantly more than vaginal electrical stimulation does, which also causes pain or discomfort, and is essentially unreliable in producing the desired contractions (70).

1. Responses to Somatic Movements or to Changes in Posture

Contraction or relaxation of the pelvic floor can also occur in response to stimuli that can be considered to alter the pattern of afferent input into the lumbosacral segments of the spinal cord. One consequence of convergence of such afferent inputs from different sources on the activity of pelvic floor and sphincteric muscles is the potential role of afferent impulses from muscles or joints as an adjunct in bladder training. Another type of somatic interactions is coactivation—the degree of synergism and antagonism—between different muscle groups that follow stimulation of the corticospinal tracts (72–74). EMG recordings have been used to analyze postural influences on pelvic floor muscles in girls (63,64); relaxation of the pelvic floor muscles could be improved by appropriate positioning and support of the lower limbs (Table 2). This group also concluded that urodynamic investigations, urobiofeedback training, and the design of pelvic floor exercises for girls could be enhanced by attention to these details (75).

Pelvic floor exercises have been designed that made use of coactivation patterns in synergistic muscles (76); these authors recorded EMG activity from the striated muscle of the urethra and the pelvic floor during relaxation and contraction of the pelvic floor, the Valsalva maneuver, coughing, hip adduction, gluteal contraction, backward tilting of the pelvis, and situps (see Table 2). These authors showed that the urethra contracts concomitantly with the pelvic floor muscles, and during hip adduction and gluteal muscle contraction, but not during contraction of the abdominal muscles.

B. Reflex Effects on the Pelvic Floor Arising from the Urethra and Lower Urinary Tract

Experiments have been performed on cats, showing that forcing fluid along the urethra always augmented the activity of the external urethral sphincter, except when the bladder was stretched passively or was actively contracting (77). These authors believed that this was a sort of guarding reflex that helped maintain continence. Much of the older literature on cats

Table 2 Coactivation Patterns of Different Pelvic Floor and Other Muscles During
Postural Movements or Cortical Stimulation

	Pelvic floor contraction	External urethral sphincter contraction	External anal sphincter contraction	Contraction of other muscles
Valsalva	+	+	+	—
Hip adduction	+	+	—	—
Gluteal muscle contraction	+	+	—	—
Contraction of abdominal muscles	+	—	—	—
Cortical stimulation		+	+	—
Cortical stimulation and voluntary contraction of the EAS	—	—	Facilitation	Facilitation in rectus abdominis and tibialis anterior
Leg support	—	—	—	—
Bladder contraction	—	—	—	—

Source: Refs. 71–73.

indicates that relaxation of the pelvic floor accompanies a rise in bladder pressure or a micturition contraction. Such reciprocal relations have also been demonstrated in the human (1).

More recently, several groups of workers have studied the EMG from periurethral muscle by using fine-wire electrodes directly inserted into the region of the urethral sphincter in anesthetized animals. Morrison et al. (59) observed the effects of cystometry on the EMG activity of the paraurethral muscle–external urinary sphincter complex in the rat. Slow cystometry caused some elevation of intravesical pressure, and culminated in a micturition contraction. During the period of distension, periurethral EMG activity increased gradually and accelerated markedly during the bladder contraction. There was a small increase in pelvic nerve activity recorded on the surface of the bladder during slow distension, and there was a substantial increase just before, or at the start, of a micturition contraction and preceded the increase in EMG activity in periurethral muscles. During the period when the bladder pressure was rising most rapidly, the EMG activity showed an alternating oscillatory pattern in on–off bursting activity. Similar behavior has been reported in several species, including the rat, cat, and dog (78–83).

This oscillatory bursting activity appears to contradict the idea of reciprocity between the parasympathetic drive to the bladder and the somatic drive to the periurethral muscle, because the overall EMG activity in the sphincter was large during the period of elevated bladder pressure. To a certain extent this oscillatory behavior was dependent on the anesthetic used and the physiological condition of these animals: it occurred only when the physiological state was excellent. However, there was an indication that reciprocal activity did exist in these preparations; during the period when the bladder pressure was rising rapidly, there not only was a pattern of on–off oscillatory activity in the periurethral muscle, but there was also a similar pattern in the pelvic nerve supply to the bladder. However, when the EMG activity to the sphincter was "on" the pelvic nerve activity to the bladder was "off." Thus, there was also clear evidence of alternating reciprocal activity between the pelvic nerve discharge to the bladder and the EMG activity of the periurethral muscles.

These periods of high rates of synchronous firing in the periurethral EMG alternating with electrical silence were repeated on several occasions during the rising phase of micturition contraction, particularly during the most rapid rise in intravesical pressure. This oscillatory behavior was never seen in spinal animals, and some authors believe that it is generated by supraspinal mechanisms (84).

C. Reflex Effects on the Pelvic Floor Arising from Other Pelvic Organs

In the rat and cat, colonic distension suppresses both bladder motility and periurethral muscle EMG activity (59,85–88), and stimulation of anogenital afferents in rats caused a prolonged increase in the volume of the bladder at the time of micturition (89). In humans, the same stimulus causes inhibition of the detrusor (90). This is partly due to sensory activity in the pudendal and the pelvic nerves (85,87,91). Vaginal stimulation is also known to suppress bladder motility in cats, and is dependent on the pelvic nerve supply (1,92). Little has been reported, however, concerning the possible interactions between the accessory male reproductive organs and the bladder and periurethral muscle. Morrison et al. (59) showed that that micturition contractions may be inhibited by injection of very small volumes of fluid into the vas deferens, and that this inhibition was accompanied by a marked contraction of the urethral sphincter.

Micturition has a major inhibitory influence on the pelvic floor activity in humans. Relaxation of the external anal sphincter occurs at the start of the rise in bladder pressure, and precedes the start of urine flow (93). It is thought to occur concomitantly with the relaxation of the pelvic floor that allows descent of the bladder (94). The inhibition extends not only to a depression of tonic activity at rest, but causes a reduction in the excitability of pudendal motoneurons involved in reflex functions (95). Similar changes occur during defecation and rectal distension (96), whereas an increase in EMG activity accompanies stimulation of the penile nerve (97). EMG activity has been recorded from the striated muscle of the membranous urethra in humans during ejaculation (98). Before the start of ejaculation there is a contraction of the pelvic floor muscles, and this is followed by a rhythmical bursting activity at 15–20 times per second during a period of some 25 sec.

IV. ROLE OF CENTRAL PATHWAYS IN THE CONTROL OF THE PELVIC FLOOR MUSCULATURE

A. Anatomy

The central nervous control over the pelvic floor muscles and associated sphincters depends on important descending pathways from regions of the brain stem (particularly the pons and medulla) and the hypothalamus. The dorsolateral pons contains two regions that either excite or inhibit tonic activity in the pelvic floor muscles. These regions are close to Barrington's micturition center (99,100). In view of the participation of the pelvic floor in a variety of physiological events, including coughing, vomiting, micturition, defecation, and parturition, it is interesting that these projections to pudendal motoneurons originated in the ipsilateral paraventricular nucleus of the hypothalamus (which also contains oxytocin), and nuclei in the brain stem including the ipsilateral caudal pontine lateral reticular formation, and the contralateral caudal nucelus retroambiguus. These paths descend through the spinal cord in the ipsilateral anterior and contralateral white matter and terminate on Onuf's nucleus motoneurons (101). In the rat, similar pathways have been described that originate in the dorsolateral pontine tegmentum and synapse directly on pudendal motoneurons innervating the external sphincters (102). In this species as well, neurons adjacent to the Barrington micturition center send axons to synapse on pudendal motoneurons, but the projection is predominantly contralateral. The projection is fairly specific for pudendal motoneurons innervating the urethral sphincter, but not those supplying the anal sphincter.

B. Functional Studies

Electrophysiological confirmation of these connections in the cat was provided by Fedirchuk and Shefchyk (52) who stimulated the pontine micturition center directly and showed inhibition of the neurons in Onuf's nucleus. Others (103) had performed an electrophysiological study on this region of the cat brain and had concluded that this region helped cause sphincter relaxation during micturition by means of descending connections with the pudendal motoneurons.

   Descending inhibitory and excitatory pathways from the medulla that act on urethral motoneurons and influence the activity of some of these pathways on bladder motility and sphincteric reflexes, originate in the raphe nuclei and nucleus gigantocellularis reticularis and are predominantly inhibitory in action (45,104,105). In humans, Hansen (73) described the spinal influences on pelvic floor muscles, which he considered to have a significant influence on bladder function. Voluntary influences on the pelvic floor, anal sphincter, urethral sphincter, and bulbocavernosus muscles of humans can be studied by transcranial cortical stimulation using either high voltages or short-duration magnetic pulses (72–74,106). Descending pathways from the cortex are activated by these stimuli and impinge on the cell bodies of pudendal motoneurons in the sacral cord. A small stimulus to the cortex causes a short burst of activity in leg muscles, but in the anal sphincter the response is prolonged, even though the latency of the response is short; sometimes the electrical response of the pudendal motor units lasted 1–2 sec. The response of the external urethral sphincter was similar, whereas that of the bulbocavernosus displayed some differences. Voluntary contraction of the external anal sphincter could cause facilitation of the response to cortical stimulation in various other muscles, such as tibialis anterior. In humans, it had been believed that pelvic floor muscles increase their activity during bladder filling. The methodology employed by Hansen (73) indicated that the excitability of pudendal motoneurons could be either increased or decreased by bladder filling: initially, when bladder volume is low, there appears to be some inhibition of pudendal motoneurons, but when the bladder is full, the motoneurons are facilitated. This facilitation may be voluntary, as a consequence of sensory information from the bladder.

   The excitability of some somatic reflex arcs that excite pudendal motoneurons has been studied during micturition in humans (95) and parallels the results obtained in cats (62,105).

V. REFLEX CONTROL OF THE PELVIC
FLOOR FOLLOWING SPINAL INJURY

Dubrovsky et al. (32) studied the spinal control of pelvic floor muscles in cats. Stimulation of the third sacral ventral root indicated that this segment of the spinal cord innervated the levator ani. Reflex activation of this muscle, unlike the external sphincter, was largely unilateral in nature, and tactile stimulation of the skin innervated by sacral segments cause mainly ipsilateral responses from the pelvic floor. After spinalization, in the early phase of spinal shock, the striated muscle of the pelvic floor becomes hyperreflexic, at a time when detrusor reflexes were absent (107). Balanced bladder function was achieved not long after the end of the period of spinal shock, and detrusor–sphincter dyssynergia was usually absent in this species. More recently, Sasaki et al. (108) described detrusor–sphincteric dyssynergia in about 50% of chronic spinal cats: there was a marked difference between the reflex responses of sphincters that exhibited tonic activity, and those that did not. Rhythmic detrusor contractions were present in all of the spinal animals, and in half of them there was a reciprocal relation between the detruson activity and sphincteric EMG. In the other 50%, detrusor hyperreflexia was present. When the bladder was empty, brushing the perineal skin caused an increase in EUS activity, similar to that seen in normal animals. However, this type of stimulation caused detrusor contractions in spinal animals, the opposite of what occurs in animals with a normal intact neuroaxis. Noxious cutaneous stimulation caused changes similar to those seen in intact animals, but the effects were greater and of longer duration. However, when the bladder was filled, and rhythmic detrusor contractions were present, tactile stimulation caused EUS activity and bladder contractions, and noxious stimulation resulted in an immediate contraction of the bladder, followed by some depression of ongoing rhythmic contractions. The effects on the sphincter depended on whether a normal reciprocal relation between bladder and sphincteric activity existed, or whether dyssynergia was present; when the latter was present it was accompanied by an increased level of ongoing EMG activity. If dyssynergic existed, a prolonged increase in EUS activity was found during innocuous brushing or noxious stimulation of perineal skin, but was not inhibited during micturition contractions. Reflex responses of the sphincter induced by electrical stimulation of afferents in the pudendal nerve were inhibited in spinal animals with a normal synergic relation between the bladder and urethra, but in dyssynergia, relaxation of the sphincter during and inhibition of pudendal nerve reflex responses at high bladder pressures was absent.

It has been known for over 50 years that somatic events influence the bladder of paraplegic patients (109), and recently there is increasing evidence for a role of viscero- or somatic convergence in the control of the human pelvic floor. In experimental studies for the last 30 years, scientists have reported that the motor pathway to the external sphincters and pelvic floor is subject to control from events in viscera and the segmental innervation of somatic structures.

During the phase of spinal shock following spinal cord injury, bladder filling was found to be accompanied by an increased urethral resistance in the bladder neck region, not associated with an increased EMG activity of the pelvic floor (110). The authors concluded that this is associated with smooth-muscle activity, because the EMG activity of the pelvic floor and urethral and anal sphincters was reduced during this phase. Areflexia was also frequently present. In some patients with spinal cord injuries, bladder contraction and distension of the rectum resulted in inhibition of EMG activity in the external urethral and anal sphincters, whereas in the levator ani, there was sometimes an initial excitation of the muscle (111).

VI. CONCLUSIONS

This short review has attempted to focus on the innervation, function, and reflex activity of pelvic floor muscles, and the mechanisms of central control in animals and humans.

The various muscles that act as functional groupings consist of mainly slow-twitch and fast-fatigue–resistant striated muscle fibers. The majority of these are controlled by the pudendal nerve pathway, originating in Onuf's nucleus in the sacral cord. Different muscles behave differently depending on the required activity in the urinary, reproductive, or gastrointestinal tracts. There is some degree of overlap in the way different components of the pelvic floor function in these circumstances, as well as reflex pathways involving somatic afferents innervating skin and muscle of the region, and visceral afferents from the three main visceral systems that enter the sacral cord.

The pelvic floor has a major role to play in supporting the bladder, and tonic activity in this muscle can be supplemented by postural or other reflex activity. The central control of these muscles overlaps to some extent with others, and cortical stimulation, exercises, and reflex activation all indicate that there may be a considerable degree of coactivation of muscles. Certain maneuvers also relax elements of the pelvic floor.

From the point of view of the control of the lower urinary tract, micturition is accompanied by opening of the bladder neck and relaxation of the pelvic floor muscles. Some specialized muscle fibers contribute to urethral closure and these periurethral fibers, and during bladder filling these muscle fibers may contract: it is unclear to what extent this is a reflex or a voluntary response in humans, but it can also be seen in anesthetized animals.

Several areas in the brain stem around the region described as Barrington's micturition center connect with Onuf's nucleus, and there are various studies that show that this region of the brain exerts a coordinated control over the lower urinary tract and pelvic floor.

The pelvic floor is subject to excitatory and inhibitory controls from the skin innervated by the sacral segments, from the pelvic viscera, and from the brain stem. These influences are found commonly in reports in the human and animal literature, and suggest that there are groups of muscle fibers within the pelvis that are subjected to control as a functional unit in resisting the stresses that might lead to incontinence.

REFERENCES

1. Torrens M, Morrison JFB. The Physiology of the Lower Urinary Tract. London: Springer-Verlag, 1987:355.
2. Bock G, Whelan J, eds. Neurobiology of Incontinence. CIBA Found Symp. 1990; 151:334.
3. de Groat WC, Downie JW, Levin RM, Long Lin AT, Morrison JFB, Nishizawa O, Steers WD, Thof KB. Basic neurophysiology and neuropharmacology. In: Abrams P, Khoury S, Wein A, eds. Incontinence. Health Publication Ltd. 1999:105–154.
4. Jordan D. The central control of autonomic function. In: Burnstock G, ed. The Autonomic Nervous System. vol. 2. Amsterdam: Overseas Publishers Association, and Harwood Academic Publishers, 1997.
5. Morrison JFB. Central nervous control of the bladder. In: Jordan D, ed. Central Nervous Control of Autonomic Function. vol 2. Amsterdam: Overseas Publishers Association, and Harwood Academic Publishers, 1997:129–150.
6. DeLancey JO. Functional anatomy of the female lower urinary tract and pelvic floor. Ciba Found Symp 1990; 151:57–69.
7. Russell B, Baumann M, Heidkamp MC, Svanborg A. Morphometry of the aging female rat urethra. Int Urogynecol J Pelvic Floor Dysfunct 1996; 7:30–36.
8. DeLancey JO, Starr RA. Histology of the connection between the vagina and levator ani muscles. Implications for urinary tract function. J Reprod Med 1990; 35:765–771.
9. DeLancey JO. The pathophysiology of stress urinary incontinence in women and its implications for surgical treatment. World J Urol 1997; 15:268–274.
10. Haeusler G, Sam C, Chiari A, Tempfer C, Hanzal E, Koelbl H. Effect of spinal anaesthesia on the lower urinary tract in continent women. Br J Obstet Gynaecol 1998; 105:103–106.
11. Andersson PO, Malmgren A, Uvelius B. Functional responses of different muscle types of the female rat urethra in vitro. Acta Physiol Scand 1990; 140:365–372.
12. Ranvier L. De quelques faits relatifs à l'histologie et à la physiologie des muscles striés. Arch Physiol Norm Pathol 1874; 1:5–18.

13. Burke RE. Motor units: anatomy, physiology and functional organisation. In: Brookhart JM, Mountcastle VB, eds. Handbook of Physiology, Sec 1. The Nervous System. Vol. 2, Part 1. Americal Physiological Society, 1981:345–422.

14. Gosling JA, Dixon JS, Critchley HO, Thompson SA. A comparative study of the human external sphincter and periurethral levator ani muscles. Br J Urol 1981; 53:35–41.

15. Whitmore I, Gosling JA, Gilpin SA. A comparison between the physiological and histochemical characterisation of urethral striated muscle in the guinea pig. Pflugers Arch 1984; 400: 40–43.

16. Tokunaka S, Murakami U, Ohashi K, Okamura K, Yachiku S. Electrophoretic and ultrastructural analysis of the rabbit's striated external urethral sphincter. J Urol 1984; 132:1040–1043.

17. Tokunaka S, Murakami U, Okamura K, Miyata M, Yachiku S. The fiber type of the rabbits' striated external urethral sphincter: electrophoretic analysis of myosin. J Urol 1986; 135:427–430.

18. Tokunaka S, Fujii H, Okamura K, Miyata M, Yachiku S. Biochemical analysis of the external urethral sphincter of female rabbits. Nippon Hinyokika Gakkai Zasshi Jpn J Urol 1992; 83: 493–497.

19. Tokunaka S, Fujii H, Hashimoto H, Yachiku S. Proportions of fiber types in the external urethral sphincter of young nulliparous and old multiparous rabbits. Urol Res 1993; 21:121–124.

20. Fujii H, Tokunaka S, Okamura K, Miyata M, Kaneko S, Yachiku S. Biochemical analysis of the external striated urethral sphincter of male rabbits. Difference in the proportions of muscle fiber types in the male rabbit external urethral sphincter by axial subdivisional study. Nippon Hinyokika Gakkai Zasshi Jpn J Urol 1994; 85:1534–1542.

21. Fujii H, Tokunaka S, Yachiku S. Effects of chronic low-frequency electrical stimulation on the external urethral sphincter of male rabbits—electrophoretic analyses of myosin light and heavy chain isoforms. Nippon Hinyokika Gakkai Zasshi Jpn J Urol 1995; 86:1240–1248.

22. Tokunaka S, Okamura K, Fujii H, Yachiku S. The proportions of fiber types in human external urethral sphincter: electrophoretic analysis of myosin. Urol Res 1990; 18:341–344.

23. Okamura K, Tokunaka S, Yachiku S. Histochemical study of human external urethral sphincter. Nippon Hinyokika Gakkai Zasshi Jpn J Urol 1991; 82:1487–1493.

24. McKenna KE, Marson L. Spinal and brainstem control of sexual function. In: Jordan D, ed. Central Nervous Control of Autonomic Function. Amsterdam: Overseas Publishers Association BV and Harwood Academic Publishers, 1997:151–187.

25. Morita T, Nishizawa O, Noto H, Tsuchida S. Pelvic nerve innervation of the external sphincter of urethra as suggested by urodynamic and horse-radish peroxidase studies. J Urol 1984; 131:591–595.

26. De Leval J, Chantraine A, Penders L. The striated sphincter of the urethra. 1: Recall of knowledge on the striated sphincter of the urethra. J Urol 1984; 90:439–454.

27. Zvara P, Carrier S, Kour NW, Tanagho EA. The detailed neuroanatomy of the human striated urethral sphincter. Br J Urol 1994; 74:182–187.

28. Borirakchanyavat S, Aboseif SR, Carroll PR, Tanagho EA, Lue TF. Continence mechanism of the isolated female urethra: an anatomical study of the intrapelvic somatic nerves. J Urol 1997; 158:822–826.

29. Hollabaugh RS Jr, Dmochowski RR, Steiner MS. Neuroanatomy of the male rhabdosphincter. Urology 1997; 49:426–434.

30. Creed KE, Van Der Werf BA, Kaye KW. Innervation of the striated muscle of the membranous urethra of the male dog. J Urol 1998; 159:1712–1716.

31. Morita T, Kizu N, Kondo S, Dohkita S, Tsuchida S. Ipsilaterality of motor innervation of canine urethral sphincter. Urol Int 1988; 43:149–156.

32. Dubrovsky B, Martinez–Gomez M, Pacheco P. Spinal control of pelvic floor muscles. Exp Neurol 1985; 88:277–287.

33. Narayan P, Konety B, Aslam K, Aboseif S, Blumenfeld W, Tanagho E. Neuroanatomy of the external urethral sphincter: implications for urinary continence preservation during radical prostate surgery. J Urol 1995; 153:337–341.

34. Thind P, Lose G, Colstrup H, Andersson KE. The urethral resistance to rapid dilation: an analysis of the effect of autonomic receptor stimulation and blockade and of pudendal nerve blockade in healthy females. Scand J Urol Nephrol 1995; 29:83–91.

35. Ho KM, McMurray G, Brading AF, Noble JG, Ny L, Andersson KE. Nitric oxide synthase in the heterogeneous population of intramural striated muscle fibres of the human membranous urethral sphincter. J Urol 1998; 159:1091–1096.

36. Bennett BC, Kruse MN, Roppolo JR, Flood HD, Fraser M, de Groat WC. Neural control of urethral outlet activity in vivo: role of nitric oxide. J Urol 1995; 153:2004–2009.

37. Ding YQ, Wang YQ, Qin BZ, Li JS. The major pelvic ganglion is the main source of nitric oxide synthase-containing nerve fibers in penile erectile tissue of the rat. Neurosci Lett 1993; 164:187–189.

38. Vanhatalo S, Soinila S. Direct nitric oxide-containing innervation from the rat spinal cord to the penis. Neurosci Lett 1995; 199:45–48.

39. Ueyama T, Mizuno N, Nomura S, Konishi A, Itoh K, Arakawa H. Central distribution of afferent and efferent components of the pudendal nerve in cat. J Comp Neurol 1984; 222:38–46.

40. Thor KB, Morgan C, Nadelhaft I, Houston M, de Groat WC. Organization of afferent and efferent pathways in the pudendal nerve of the female cat. J Comp Neurol 1989; 288:263–279.

41. Schroder HD. Onuf's nucleus X: a morphological study of a human spinal nucleus. Anat Embryol 1981; 162:443–453.

42. Gibson SJ, Polak JM, Katagiri T, Su H, Weller RO, Brownell DB, Hughes JT, Kikuyama S, Ball J. A comparison of the distributions of eight peptides in spinal cord from normal controls and cases of motor neurone disease with special reference to Onuf's nucleus. Brain Res 1988; 474:255–278.

43. Breedlove SM, Arnold AP. Hormone accumulation in a sexually dimorphic motor nucleus of the rat spinal cord. Science 1980; 210:564–566.

44. Sasaki M. Membrane properties of external urethral and external anal sphincter motoneurones in the cat. J Physiol (Lond) 1991; 440:345–366.

45. Mackel R. Segmental and descending control of the external urethral and anal sphincters in the cat. J Physiol (Lond) 1979; 294:105–122.

46. Jankowska E, Riddell JS. A relay for input from group II muscle afferents in sacral segments of the cat spinal cord. J Physiol (Lond) 1993; 465:561–580.

47. Fedirchuk B, Hochman S, Shefchyk SJ. An intracellular study of perineal and hindlimb afferent inputs onto sphincter motoneurons in the decerebrate cat. Exp Brain Res 1992; 89:511–516.

48. Jankowska E, Padel Y, Zarzecki P. Crossed disynaptic inhibition of sacral motoneurones. J Physiol (Lond) 1978; 285:425–444.

49. Beattie MS, Li Q, Leedy MG, Bresnahan JC. Motoneurons innervating the external anal and urethral sphincters of the female cat have different patterns of dendritic arborization. Neurosci Lett 1990; 111:69–74.

50. Sasaki M. Morphological analysis of external urethral and external anal sphincter motoneurones of cat. J Comp Neurol 1994; 349:269–287.

51. Hochman S, Fedirchuk B, Shefchyk SJ. Membrane electrical properties of external urethral and external anal sphincter somatic motoneurons in the decerebrate cat. Neurosci Lett 1991; 127:87–90.

52. Fedirchuk B, Shefchyk SJ. Membrane potential changes in sphincter motoneurons during micturition in the decerebrate cat. J Neurosci 1993; 13:3090–3094.

53. Brindley GS, Rushton DN, Craggs MD. The pressure exerted by the external sphincter of the urethra when its motor nerve fibres are stimulated electrically. Br J Urol 1974; 46:453–462.

54. Womack NR, Morrison JF, Williams NS. The role of pelvic floor denervation in the etiology of idiopathic faecal incontinence. Br J Surg 1986; 73:404–407.

55. Deindl FM, Vodusek DB, Hesse U, Schussler B. Pelvic floor activity patterns: comparison of nulliparous continent and parous urinary stress incontinent women. A kinesiological EMG study. Br J Urol 1994; 73:413–417.

56. Fowler CJ, Kirby RS, Harrison MJ, Milroy EJ, Turner–Warwick R. Individual motor unit analysis in the diagnosis of disorders of urethral sphincter innervation. J Neurol Neurosurg Psychiatry 1984; 47:637–641.

57. Fowler CJ, Kirby RS, Harrison MJ. Decelerating burst and complex repetitive discharges in the striated muscle of the urethral sphincter, associated with urinary retention in women. J Neurol Neurosurg Psychiatry 1985; 48:1004–1009.

58. Stein R. Possible significance of the urethral paramyotonic outbursts for micturition reflex activation. Scand J Urol Nephrol 1995; 175(suppl):55–56.

59. Morrison JFB, Sato A, Sato Y, Yamanishi T. The influence of afferent inputs from skin and viscera on the activity of the bladder and the skeletal muscle surrounding the urethra in the rat. Neurosci Res 1995; 23:195–205.

60. Rud T, Andersson KE, Asmussen M, Hunting A, Ulmsten U. Factors maintaining the intra-urethral pressure in women. Invest Urol 1980; 17:343–347.

61. McMahon SB, Morrison JFB, Spillane K. An electrophysiological study of somatic and visceral convergence in the reflex control of the external sphincters. J Physiol 1982; 328:379–387.

62. Fedirchuk B, Downie JW, Shefchyk SJ. Reduction of perineal evoked excitatory postsynaptic potentials in cat lumbar and sacral motoneurons during micturition. J Neurosci 1994; 14:6153–6159.

63. Wennergren H, Larsson LE, Sandstedt P. Surface electromyography of pelvic floor muscles in healthy children. Methodological study. Scand J Caring Sci 1989; 3:63–69.

64. Wennergren HM, Oberg BE, Sandstedt P. The importance of leg support for relaxation of the pelvic floor muscles. A surface electromyograph study in healthy girls. Scand J Urol Nephrol 1991; 25:205–213.

65. McMahon SB, Morrison JFB. Two groups of spinal interneurones that respond to stimulation of the abdominal viscera of the cat. J Physiol (Lond) 1982; 322, 21–34.

66. McKenna KE, Knight KC, Mayers R. Modulation by peripheral serotonin of the threshold for sexual reflexes in female rats. Pharmacol Biochem Behav 1991; 40:151–156.

67. Morrison JFB, Sato A, Sato Y, Suzuki A. Long-lasting facilitation and depression of peri-urethral skeletal muscle following acupuncture-like stimulation in anaesthetised rats. Neurosci Res 1995; 23:159–169.

68. Shafik A. Straining urethral reflex: description of a reflex and its clinical significance. Preliminary report. Acta Anat (Basel) 1991; 140:104–107.

69. Bo K, Talseth T. Change in urethral pressure during voluntary pelvic floor muscle contraction and vaginal electrical stimulation [see comments]. Int Urogynecol J Pelvic Floor Dysfunct 1997; 8:3–6.

70. Bo K, Maanum M. Does vaginal electrical stimulation cause pelvic floor muscle contraction? A pilot study. Scand J Urol Nephrol Suppl 1996; 179:39–45.

71. Bo K. Functional aspects of the striated muscles within and around the female urethra. Scand J Urol Nephrol 1995; 175:27–35.

72. Eardley I, Nagendran K, Kirby RS, Fowler CJ. A new technique for assessing the efferent innervation of the human striated urethral sphincter. J Urol 1990; 144:948–951.

73. Hansen M. Spinal Influences on the pelvic floor muscles. Scand J Urol Nephrol Suppl 1995; 175: 37–39.

74. Eardley I, Quinn NP, Fowler CJ, Kirby RS, Parkhouse HF, Marsden CD, Bannister R. The value of urethral sphincter electromyography in the differential diagnosis of parkinsonism. Br J Urol 1989; 64:360–362.

75. Wennergren H, Oberg B. Pelvic floor exercises for children: a method of treating dysfunctional voiding. Br J Urol 1995; 76:9–15.

76. Bo K, Stien R. Needle EMG registration of striated urethral wall and pelvic floor muscle activity patterns during cough, Valsalva, abdominal, hip adductor, and gluteal muscle contractions in nulliparous healthy females. Neurourol Urodynam 1994; 13:35–41.

77. Garry RC, Roberts TD, Todd JK. Reflexes involving the external urethral sphincter in the cat. J Physiol 1959; 149:653–665.

78. Satoh S. Experimental study on the micturition mechanism—the role of the pudendal nerve on the dynamics of micturition in the decerebrated dog. Jpn J Urol 1984; 75:1572–1582.

79. Nishizawa O, Satoh S, Tsukada T, Fukuda T, Moriya I, Tsuchida S. Role of striated urethral sphincter on the voiding cycle in the decerebrated dog. Jpn J Smooth Muscle Res 1984; 20: 413–417.

80. Conte B, Maggi CA, Parlani M, Lopez G, Manzini S, Giachetti A. Simultaneous recording of vesical and urethral pressure in urethane-anesthetized rats: effect of neuromuscular blocking agents on the activity of the external urethral sphincter. J Pharmacol Methods 1991; 26:161–171.

81. Kruse MN, Belton AL, de Groat WC. Changes in bladder and external urethral sphincter function after spinal cord injury in the rat. Am J Physiol 1993; 264:R1157–R1163.

82. Shimoda N, Takakusaki K, Nishizawa O, Tsuchida S, Mori S. The changes in the activity of pudendal motoneurons in relation to reflex micturition evoked in decerebrate cats. Neurosci Lett 1992; 135:175–178.

83. Sackman JE, Sims MH. Electromyographic evaluation of the external urethral sphincter during cystometry in male cats. Am J Vet Res 1990; 51:1237–1241.

84. Kakizaki H, Fraser MO, de Groat WC. Reflex pathways controlling urethral striated and smooth muscle function in the male rat. Am J Physiol 1997; 272:R1647–R1656.

85. de Groat WC. Inhibition and excitation of scarl parasympathetic neurons by visceral and cutaneous stimuli in the cat. Brain Res 1971; 33:399–503.

86. McMahon SB, Morrison JFB. Factors that determine the excitability of parasympathetic reflexes to the cat bladder. J Physiol (Lond) 1982; 322:35–43.

87. Floyd K, McMahon SB, Morrison JFB. Inhibitory interactions between colonic and vesical afferents in the micturition reflex of the cat. J Physiol (Lond) 1982; 322:45–52.

88. Conte B, Maggi CA, Meli A. Vesico-inhibitory responses and capsaicin sensitive afferents in rats. Naunyn Schmiedebergs Arch Pharmacol 1989; 339:178–183.

89. Jiang CH, Lindstrom S. Prolonged increase in micturition threshold volume by anogenital afferent stimulation in the rat. Br J Urol 1998; 82:398–403.

90. Kock NG, Pompeius R. Inhibition of vesical motor activity induced by anal stimulation. Acta Chir Scand 1963; 126:244–250.

91. de Groat WC, Ryall RW. Reflexes to the sacral parasympathetic neurones concerned with micturition in the cat. J Physiol 1969; 200:87–108.

92. Morrison JFB. The neural control of the bladder. In: Bloom SR, Polak JM, Lindenlaub E, eds. Systemic Role of Regulatory Peptides. Symposia Medica Hoechst 1982; 18:381–396.

93. Scott FB, Quesada EM, Cardus D. Studies on the dynamics of micturition: observations on healthy men. J Urol 1964; 92:455–463.

94. Tanagho EA. The anatomy and physiology of micturition. Clin Obstet Gynaecol 1978; 5:3–26.

95. Dyro FM, Yalla SV. Refractoriness of urethral striated sphincter during voiding: studies with afferent pudendal reflex arc stimulation in male subjects. J Urol 1986; 135:732–736.

96. Shafik A. Dilatation and closing anal reflexes. Description and clinical significance of new reflexes: preliminary report. Acta Anat (Basel) 1971; 142:293–298.

97. Shafik A. The peno-motor reflex: study of the response of the puborectalis and levator ani muscles to glans penis stimulation. Int J Impot Res 1995; 7:239–246.

98. Kollberg S, Petersen I, Steiner I. Preliminary results of an electromyographic study of ejaculation. Acta Chir Scand 1962; 123:478–483.

99. Holstege G, Griffiths D, de Wall H, Dalm E. Anatomical and physiological observations on supraspinal control of bladder and urethral sphincter muscles in the cat. J Comp Neurol 1986; 250:449–461.

100. Holstege G, Tan J. Supraspinal control of motoneurons innervating the striated muscles of the pelvic floor including urethral and anal sphincters in the cat. Brain 1987; 110:1323–1344.

101. Kohama T. Neuroanatomical studies on pontine urine storage facilitatory areas in the cat brain. Part II. Output neuronal structures from the nucleus locus subcoeruleus and the nucleus reticularis pontis oralis. Nippon Hinyokika Gakkai Zasshi Jpn J Urol 1992; 83:1478–1483.

102. Ding YQ, Takada M, Tokuno H, Mizuno N. Direct projections from the dorsolateral pontine tegmentum to pudendal motoneurons innervating the external urethral sphincter muscle in the rat. J Comp Neurol 1995; 357:318–330.

103. Kruse MN, Mallory BS, Noto H, Roppolo JR, de Groat WC. Properties of the descending limb of the spinobulbospinal micturition reflex pathway in the cat. Brain Res 1991; 556:6–12.

104. McMahon SB, Spillane K. Brain stem influences on the parasympathetic supply to the urinary bladder of the cat. Brain Res 1982; 234:237–249.

105. McMahon SB, Morrison JF, Spillane K. An electrophysiological study of somatic and visceral convergence in the reflex control of the external sphincters. J Physiol 1982; 328:379–387.

106. Ertekin C, Hansen MV, Larsson LE, Sjodahl R. Examination of the descending pathway to the external anal sphincter and pelvic floor muscles by transcranial cortical stimulation. Electroencephalogr Clin Neurophysiol 1990; 75:500–510.

107. van Gool JD, Schmidt RA, Tanagho EA. Development of reflex activity of detrusor and striated sphincter muscles in experimental paraplegia. Urol Int 1978; 33:293–303.

108. Sasaki M, Morrison JFB, Sato Y, Sato A. Effect of mechanical stimulation pf the skin on the external urethral sphincter muscles in anaesthetised cats. Jpn J Physiol 1994; 44:575–590.

109. Guttmann L. Spinal Cord Injuries. Oxford: Blackwell, 1976:731.

110. Rossier AB, Fam BA, Dibenedetto M, Sarkarati M. Urodynamics in spinal shock patients. J Urol 1979; 122:783–787.

111. Rodriquez AA, Awad E. Detrusor muscle and sphincteric response to anorectal stimulation in spinal cord injury. Arch Phys Med Rehabil 1979; 60:269–272.

6

The Neural Control of Micturition and Urinary Continence

BERTIL F. M. BLOK

Academic Medical Center, University of Amsterdam, Amsterdam, The Netherlands

GERT HOLSTEGE

Groningen University Medical School, Groningen, The Netherlands

I. INTRODUCTION

Micturition and urinary continence depend on coordinated actions between the smooth (detrusor) muscle of the bladder and the striated external urethral sphincter (EUS), which closes the bladder. During urine storage, the detrusor muscle is relaxed and the EUS tonically contracted. This activation pattern is reversed when micturition occurs: the EUS relaxes and the bladder contracts, resulting in expulsion of the stored urine.

Motoneurons of both the bladder and the EUS are located in the sacral spinal cord. However, coordination between these two motoneuronal cell groups in adult animals does not occur in the spinal cord but, rather, in the pontine tegmentum of the caudal brain stem. This region sends fibers to the sacral cord, and their interruption, for example, in patients with thoracic transection of the spinal cord, results in dyssynergic micturition. In such patients, bladder contraction is accompanied by simultaneous EUS contraction. In this condition, to expel urine through the tonically closed urethral sphincter, the bladder has to exert extremely high intravesical pressures. The result is a thickened bladder wall with a smaller bladder capacity, the so-called overflow bladder. Patients with brain lesions rostral to the pons never show bladder–sphincter dyssynergia. However, they may suffer from urge incontinence (i.e., hyperactivity of the bladder and an inability to delay voiding). Apparently, cell groups in the pons coordinate micturition as such, but regions rostral to the pons play a role in the beginning of the micturition act.

89

II. DESCENDING AND EFFERENT (MOTOR) SYSTEMS

A. Motoneurons Innervating the External Urethral Sphincter and Urinary Bladder

The striated EUS, which forms part of the pelvic floor musculature, is innervated by the pudendal nerve. Its motoneurons are located in the so-called nucleus of Onuf, which was first described in 1899 by Onufrowicz (1) as group X in the ventral horn of the human spinal cord, extending from the caudal S1 to the rostral S3 segments. In the cat, motoneurons of the EUS are located in the ventrolateral part of nucleus of Onuf, in the ventral horn, at the S1–S2 level of the spinal cord (2). The dorsomedial part of Onuf's nucleus is occupied by motoneurons innervating the external anal sphincter (EAS). The same situation exists in the hamster, dog, monkey, and human, where motoneurons of the EAS and EUS are also located in the nucleus of Onuf (1,3–5; Fig. 1). In the rat, however, the motoneurons of the EAS and EUS are located in two separate nuclei, the dorsolateral and dorsomedial nucleus, respectively, at L5–L6 (6,7). Remarkably, motoneurons of the EAS in the domestic pig (8) and the Mongolian gerbil (9) are not located in the ventral horn, but in the gray matter just dorsolateral to the central canal, which, in other animals, contains interneurons partly involved in normal micturition.

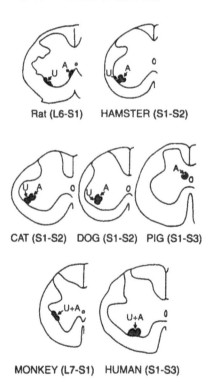

Rat (L6-S1)   HAMSTER (S1-S2)

CAT (S1-S2)   DOG (S1-S2)   PIG (S1-S3)

MONKEY (L7-S1)   HUMAN (S1-S3)

Figure 1 Schematic drawing of the location of the nucleus of Onuf in various mammals: Note that the motoneurons in the rat innervating the external urethral (U) and anal (A) sphincters are located at different sites in the ventral horn, whereas in the hamster, cat, dog, monkey, and humans, they are present in the same nucleus. In the pig, anal sphincter motoneurons are not located in the ventral horn, but are dorsolateral from the central canal.

The smooth detrusor muscle of the bladder is innervated by parasympathetic fibers. Parasympathetic preganglionic motoneurons reside in the sacral intermediolateral (IML) cell group. In cats, these parasympathetic preganglionic motoneurons are located in the S1–S3 segments (10), and in humans, in S2–S4 (11). Their axons reach the bladder through the pelvic nerve and terminate on parasympathetic ganglion cells in the pelvic plexus of the bladder wall. Parasympathetic postganglionic fibers convey the main excitatory output to the bladder muscle fibers. Sympathetic fibers innervating the bladder and urethra are thought to play an important role in promoting continence during the storage phase (12). Human sympathetic preganglionic motoneurons are located in the IML of the rostral lumbar (L1–L4) cord and send their axons to sympathetic ganglion cells in the sympathetic chain and major pelvic ganglia (11). Sympathetic postganglionic fibers run through the pelvic and hypogastric nerves, and have excitatory effects on the smooth musculature of the urethra and bladder base.

B. Brain Stem–Spinal Cord Pathways Coordinate Bladder and Sphincter Motoneurons

In young kittens, the sacral cord in itself is capable of producing a micturition reflex, but needs to be evoked by the mother licking the kittens' perineum (13). This behavior stops after approximately 4 weeks postpartum, following which the supraspinal centers play an essential role.

From the work of Barrington (14), it is known that a crucial structure of the micturition reflex is located in the dorsolateral pontine tegmentum, because bilateral lesions in this area in the cat result in urinary retention. In cats, two different pontine projection systems have been identified (15,16) (Fig. 2). A group of neurons in the medial part of the dorsolateral pons projects to the sacral IML cell column (see also Ref. 17) containing parasympathetic bladder motoneurons. Neurons in the lateral part of the dorsolateral pons specifically project to the nucleus of Onuf. The medial cell group is called the M-region (M = medial), pontine micturition center (PMC) or Barrington's nucleus, and the lateral cell group is known as the L-region (L = lateral) or pontine continence center (PCC). Ultrastructurally, the PMC projection to parasympathetic preganglionic motoneurons of the bladder is monosynaptic and excitatory (18).

In accordance with these findings, electrical and chemical stimulation in the PMC of the cat produces a steep rise in intravesical pressure (16,19), and it also elicits an immediate and sharp decrease in urethral pressure and pelvic floor electromyograms (EMGs). This inhibitory effect is not caused by a direct PMC projection to the nucleus of Onuf, as such a projection does not exist (15,16), and the PMC does not project to the L-region (20). In all likelihood, the PMC projection to interneurons in the sacral intermediomedial (IMM) cell column (15–17) may play a crucial role. PMC fibers terminate in the IMM in the majority of inhibitory γ-aminobutyric acid (GABA) interneurons (21). Retrograde tracing studies using the pseudorabies virus have shown that this area contains interneurons projecting to the nucleus of Onuf (22), and electrical stimulation in the IMM cell column results in inhibition of the EUS by GABAergic interneurons in the IMM (23).

Bilateral lesions of the PMC in the cat cause total urinary retention, leading to depressed detrusor activity and increased bladder capacity (16,24). Stimulation of the L-region elicits strong excitation of the pelvic floor musculature and an increase in urethral pressure (16). Bilateral lesions in the L-region give rise to an inability to store urine; bladder capac-

Descending (motor) pathways

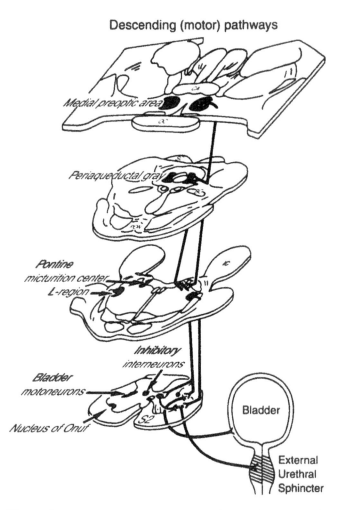

Figure 2 Schematic overview of the spinal and supraspinal structures involved in the descending and efferent control of micturition. The solid lines represent excitatory projections; the line from the sacral inhibitory interneurons to the nucleus of Onuf represents an inhibitory pathway. The nature of the descending pathway from the medial preoptic area is unknown; all other pathways are excitatory. Pathways are indicated on one side only. BC, brachium conjunctivum; CA, anterior commissure; IC, inferior colliculus; OC, optic chiasm; PON, pontine nuclei; SC, superior colliculus; S2, second sacral segment.

ity is reduced, and urine is expelled prematurely by excessive detrusor activity accompanied by urethral relaxation. Outside the episodes of detrusor activity, urethral pressure is not depressed below normal values. These observations suggest that during the filling phase, the L-region has a continuous excitatory effect on the nucleus of Onuf, resulting in contraction of the pelvic floor, including the EUS. Recently, positron emission tomography (PET) studies in healthy men and women have provided evidence of a PMC and a L-region in humans (25,26). About half of the subgroup of right-handed male and female volunteers were able to micturate during scanning. In this subgroup, increased regional blood flow during mic-

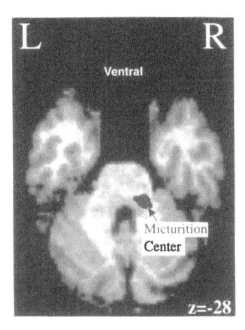

Figure 3 Horizontal section showing significantly increased blood flow with PET in the dorsal pons during micturition in female volunteers. Z, −28 refers to the coordinates in millimeters relative to the intercommissural plane. L, left side; R, right side of the brain.

turition was observed in the dorsomedial part of the pons close to the fourth ventricle (Fig. 3). The location of this area in humans is similar to that of the PMC described in the cat. The other half of the volunteers were not able to micturate during scanning, although they had a full bladder and tried to urinate. In this group, there was activation in the ventrolateral, but not in the dorsomedial pons, as predicted on the basis of the location of the L-region in cats (Fig. 4). Apparently, the volunteers in this nonsuccessful micturition subgroup involuntarily contracted their urethral sphincter and, thus, withheld their urine.

III. ASCENDING AND AFFERENT (SENSORY) SYSTEMS

A. Peripheral Afferent Nerves

Most afferent fibers from the bladder enter the sacral cord by the pelvic nerve. The peripheral fibers of dorsal root ganglia neurons of the pelvic nerve are in contact with bladder wall mechanoreceptors. The proximal fibers enter Lissauer's tract and terminate mainly in Rexed's (27) laminae I, V, VII, and X of the lumbosacral spinal cord at segments L4–S2 (28). The majority of these afferents are thin myelinated and unmyelinated axons, and their conduction velocities are in the Aδ and C-fiber range, respectively (29). Most Aδ fibers originate from slowly adapting mechanoreceptors in the bladder wall, as excitation of these fibers results in activation of the micturition reflex. In all likelihood, Aδ fibers are the peripheral afferent fibers for this reflex (30), for nonmyelinated C-fibers in the pelvic nerve do not respond to distention and contraction of the urinary bladder (31).

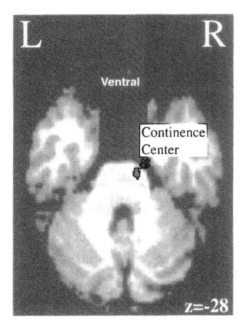

Figure 4 Horizontal section showing significant activity in the ventral pons (presumably the human L-region) when female volunteers tried to micturate, but did not succeed. See Figure 3 for details.

B. Spinal Cord–Brain Stem Pathways Involved in the Micturition Reflex

Obviously, bladder-filling information from sensory neurons in the sacral cord must finally reach the PMC to empty the bladder at an appropriate time. However, we have demonstrated in the cat that the lumbosacral cord does not project to PMC neurons (32). This raises the question about how bladder-filling information is relayed to the PMC. Because the micturition reflex is not abolished by precollicular decerebration (33), lumbosacral projections to forebrain areas, such as the thalamus and hypothalamus, are not essential for this reflex. However, the very strong projections from the lumbosacral cord to the lateral and dorsal parts of the mesencephalic periaqueductal gray (PAG) probably play a much more important role (32) (Fig. 5). The lateral PAG is the only caudal brain stem structure known to project specifically to the PMC (34). The PAG has also been implicated in the control of micturition in humans, because in the previously discussed PET study, the blood flow in this region was significantly increased during micturition (25,26).

IV. FOREBRAIN INVOLVEMENT IN THE CONTROL OF MICTURITION

Although the forebrain is not essential for the micturition reflex, clinical observations suggest that it is important for the beginning of micturition (35). In the cat, stimulation of forebrain structures, such as the anterior cingulate gyrus, preoptic area of the hypothalamus, amygdala, bed nucleus of the stria terminalis, and septal nuclei, elicits bladder contractions (36,37). Although most of these regions are part of the so-called emotional motor system and send fibers to the brain stem (see Ref. 38 for review), only the hypothalamic preoptic area projects specifically to the PMC (39). Our PET study (25) suggests that this might also

Ascending (sensory) pathways

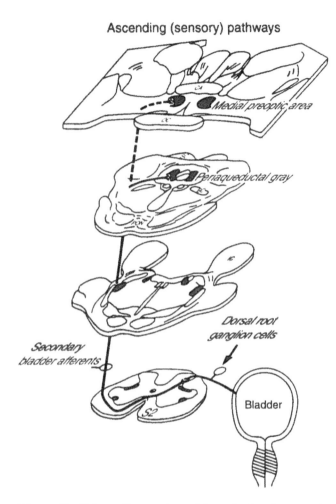

Figure 5 Schematic overview of the spinal and supraspinal structures involved in afferent information concerning bladder filling. Pathways are indicated on one side only. The dotted line represents the sacrohypothalamic pathway, which is not crucial for the micturition reflex. For abbreviations, see Figure 2.

be true in humans, because the hypothalamus, including the preoptic area, shows increased blood flow during micturition. Direct projection of the preoptic area to the PMC is the pathway through which the emotional motor system controls the PMC and, thus, determines whether micturition can take place (see also Ref. 40). The emotional motor system not only gives a "safe signal" to the PMC to start micturition, but also uses micturition in relation to sexual behavior and territorial marking.

V.   THE CEREBRAL CORTEX

A.   Emotional (Involuntary) Control

Our human PET scan results (25,26) point to two cortical areas involved in both micturition and contraction of the pelvic floor. The right dorsolateral prefrontal cortex is active when micturition occurs and also when micturition is involuntarily inhibited. Blood flow in the right anterior cingulate gyrus is significantly decreased during voluntary withholding of urine. In all likelihood, the prefrontal cortex and the anterior cingulate gyrus are not specifically involved in micturition control, but rather, in more general mechanisms, such as attention, intention to perform a task, and response selection (41). The urge incontinence after forebrain lesions including the anterior cingulate gyrus (42) may be due to an attention deficit that interferes with the patient's ability to recognize a filled bladder. A striking observation of these PET studies (25,26) on micturition was that the control areas were predominantly on the right side of the brain and brain stem (cerebral cortex and pons), which corresponds with investigations reporting that urge incontinence is correlated with lesions in the right hemisphere (43).

B. Somatic (Voluntary) Control

In a recent PET study (44) of the brain areas involved in voluntary contraction of the pelvic floor musculature, female volunteers were asked to contract their anal sphincter. The results showed that the superomedial precentral gyrus, which is part of the primary motor cortex, controls voluntary contraction of the pelvic floor (Fig. 6). Furthermore, activation was found in the medial cerebellum, supplementary motor cortex, and thalamus. No activation was detected in the prefrontal cortex.

VI. CONCLUSIONS

The organization of neural control of the urinary bladder and EUS is very similar in cats and humans. Sensory information concerning bladder filling is relayed, by the pelvic nerve and dorsal root ganglion cells, to the sacral cord, where second-order sensory neurons convey it to the caudal PAG. When the amount of urine in the bladder makes voiding desirable,

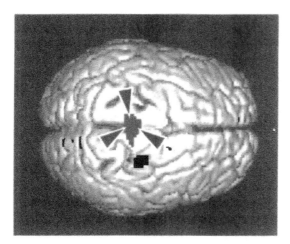

Figure 6 Superior view of the cerebral cortex showing significantly increased blood flow in the superomedial part of the primary motor cortex (indicated by arrowheads) during voluntary contraction of the pelvic floor. The increased blood flow in the more lateral part (not indicated) of the primary motor cortex corresponds with the area controlling the abdominal musculature.

PAG neurons activate neurons in the PMC, which, through the long descending fibers to bladder motoneurons in the sacral cord, produces micturition. Micturition takes place only when the situation is safe, which is assessed by limbic cortical structures. When the situation is considered safe, the prefrontal cortex may send a go signal to the preoptic area of the hypothalamus, from where it is relayed to the PMC, and the PAG may determine the beginning of micturition. In all other situations the L-region is active and produces tonic contraction of the pelvic floor, including the EUS.

REFERENCES

1. Onufrowicz B. Notes on the arrangement and function of the cell groups in the sacral region of the spinal cord. J Nerv Mental Dis 1899; 26:498–504.
2. Sato M, Mizuno N, Konishi A. Localization of motoneurons innervating perineal muscles: a HRP study in cat. Brain Res 1978; 140:149–154.
3. Kuzuhara S, Kanazawa I, Nakanishi T. Topographical localization of the Onuf's nuclear neurons innervating the rectal and vesical striated sphincter muscles: a retrograde fluorescent double labeling in cat and dog. Neurosci Lett 1980; 16:125–130.
4. Roppolo JR, Nadelhaft I, De Groat WC. The organization of pudendal motoneurons and primary afferent projections in the spinal cord of the rhesus monkey revealed by horseradish peroxidase. J Comp Neurol 1985; 234:475–488.
5. Gerrits PO, Sie JAML, Holstege G. Motoneuronal location of external urethral and anal sphincters: a single and double labeling study in the male and female golden hamster. Neurosci Lett 1997; 226:191–194.
6. Schrøder HD. Organization of the motoneurons innervating the pelvic muscles of the rat. J Comp Neurol 1980; 192:567–587.
7. Jordan CL, Breedlove SM, Arnold AP. Sexual dimorphism and the influence of neonatal androgen in the dorsolateral motor nucleus of the rat lumbar spinal cord. Brain Res 1982; 249:309–314.
8. Blok BFM, Roukema G, Geerdes B, Holstege G. Location of external anal sphincter motoneurons in the sacral cord of the female domestic pig. Neurosci Lett 1996; 216:203–206.
9. Ulibarri C, Popper P, Micevych PE. Motoneurons dorsolateral to the central canal innervate perineal muscles in the Mongolian gerbil. J Comp Neurol 1995; 356:225–237.
10. Morgan C, Nadelhaft I, De Groat WC. Location of bladder preganglionic neurons within the sacral parasympathetic nucleus of the cat. Neurosci Lett 1979; 14:189–194.
11. Pick J. The Autonomic Nervous System: Morphological, Comparative, Clinical and Surgical Aspects. Philadelphia: Lippincott, 1970.
12. Vaughan CW, Satchell PM. Role of sympathetic innervation in the feline continence process under natural filling conditions. J Neurophysiol 1992; 68:1842–1849.
13. De Groat WC, Nadelhaft I, Milne RJ, Booth AM, Morgan C, Thor K. Organization of the sacral parasympathetic reflex pathways to the urinary bladder and large intestine. J Auton Nerv Syst 1981; 3:135–160.
14. Barrington FJF. The effect of lesions of the hind- and mid-brain on micturition in the cat. Q J Exp Physiol Cogn Med 1925; 15:81–102.
15. Holstege G, Kuypers HGJM, Boer RC. Anatomical evidence for direct brain stem projections to the somatic motoneuronal cell groups and autonomic preganglionic cell groups in cat spinal cord. Brain Res 1979; 171:329–333.
16. Holstege G, Griffiths D, De Wall H, Dalm E. Anatomical and physiological observations on supraspinal control of bladder and urethral sphincter muscles in the cat. J Comp Neurol 1986; 250:449–461.
17. Loewy AD, Saper CB, Baker RP. Descending projections from the pontine micturition center. Brain Res 1979; 172:533–538.

18. Blok BFM, Holstege G. Ultrastructural evidence for a direct pathway from the pontine mic-
     turition center to the parasympathetic preganglionic motoneurons of the bladder of the cat. Neu-
     rosci Lett 1997; 222:195–198.
19. Mallory BS, Roppolo JR, De Groat WC. Pharmacological modulation of the pontine micturi-
     tion center. Brain Res 1991; 546:310–320.
20. Blok BFM, Holstege G. Two pontine micturition centers in the cat are not interconnected di-
     rectly: implications for the central organization of micturition. J Comp Neurol 1999; 403:209–
     218.
21. Blok BFM, De Weerd H, Holstege G. The pontine micturition center projects to sacral cord
     GABA immunoreactive neurons in the cat. Neurosci Lett 1997; 233:109–112.
22. Nadelhaft I, Vera PL. Neurons in the rat brain and spinal cord labeled after pseudorabies virus
     injected into the external urethral sphincter. J Comp Neurol 1996; 375:502–517.
23. Blok BFM, van Maarseveen JTPW, Holstege G. Electrical stimulation of the sacral dorsal gray
     commissure evokes relaxation of the external urethral sphincter in the cat. Neurosci Lett 1998;
     249:68–70.
24. Griffiths D, Holstege G, Dalm E, De Wall H. Control and coordination of bladder and urethral
     function in the brain stem of the cat. Neurourol Urodynam 1990; 9:63–82.
25. Blok BFM, Willemsen ATM, Holstege G. A PET study on the brain control of micturition in
     humans. Brain 1997; 120:111–121.
26. Blok BFM, Sturms LM, Holstege G. Brain activation during micturition in women. Brain 1998;
     121:2033–2042.
27. Rexed B. A cytoarchitectonic atlas of the spinal cord in the cat. J Comp Neurol 1954; 100:
     297–380.
28. Morgan C, Nadelhaft I, De Groat WC. The distribution of visceral primary afferents from the
     pelvic nerve to Lissauer's tract and the spinal gray matter and its relationship to the sacral
     parasympathetic nucleus. J Comp Neurol 1981; 201:415–440.
29. Hulsebosch CE, Coggeshall RE. An analysis of the axon populations in the nerves to the pelvic
     viscera in the rat. J Comp Neurol 1982; 211:1–10.
30. De Groat WC, Booth AM, Milne RJ, Roppolo JR. Parasympathetic preganglionic neurons in
     the sacral spinal cord. J Auton Nerv Syst 1982; 5:23–43.
31. Jänig W, Morrison JF. Functional properties of spinal visceral afferents supplying abdominal
     and pelvic organs, with special emphasis on visceral nociception. Prog Brain Res 1986;
     67:87–114.
32. Blok BFM, De Weerd H, Holstege G. Ultrastructural evidence for the paucity of projections
     from the lumbosacral cord to the pondine micturition center or M-region in the cat. A new con-
     cept for the organization of the micturition reflex with the periaqueductal gray as central relay.
     J Comp Neurol 1995; 359:300–309.
33. Tang PC, Ruch TC. Localization of brain stem and diencephalic areas controlling the micturi-
     tion reflex. J Comp Neurol 1956; 106:213–245.
34. Blok BFM, Holstege G. Direct projections from the periaqueductal gray to the pontine mic-
     turition center (M-region). An anterograde and retrograde tracing study in the cat. Neurosci Lett
     1994; 166:93–96.
35. Blaivas JG. The neurophysiology of micturition: a clinical study of 550 patients. J Urol 1982;
     127:958–963.
36. Gjone R, Setekleiv J. Excitatory and inhibitory bladder responses to stimulation of the cerebral
     cortex in the cat. Acta Physiol Scand 1963; 59:337–348.
37. Gjone R. Excitatory and inhibitory bladder responses to stimulation of "limbic," diencephalic
     and mesencephalic structures in the cat. Acta Physiol Scand 1966; 66:91–102.
38. Holstege G. Descending motor pathways and the spinal motor system: Limbic and non-limbic
     components. Prog Brain Res 1996; 107:307–421.
39. Holstege G. Some anatomical observations on the projections from the hypothalamus to brain-
     stem and spinal cord: an HRP and autoradiographic tracing study in the cat. J Comp Neurol
     1987; 260:98–126.

40. Blok BFM, Holstege G. The neuronal control of micturition and its relation to the emotional motor system. Prog Brain Res 1996; 107:113–126.

41. Pardo JV, Pardo PJ, Janer KW, Raichle ME. The anterior cingulate cortex mediates processing selection in the Stroop attentional conflict paradigm. Proc Natl Acad Sci USA 1990; 87:256–259.

42. Andrew J, Nathan PW. Lesions of the anterior frontal lobes and disturbances of micturition and defaecation. Brain 1964; 87:233–262.

43. Kuroiwa Y, Tohgi H, Ono S, Itoh M. Frequency and urgency of micturition in hemiplegic patients: relationship to hemisphere laterality of lesions. J Neurol 1987; 234:100–102.

44. Blok BFM, Sturms LM, Holstege G. A PET study on cortical and subcortical control of pelvic floor musculature in women. J Comp Neurol 1997; 389:535–544.

7

The Pelvic Floor:
Lessons from Our Past

RICHARD A. SCHMIDT

University of Colorado Medical School and Rose Hospital, Denver, Colorado

I. INTRODUCTION

The basic goal of all research is to build on an existing understanding of why the body is designed to function in a specific way. This is essential to understanding why the body begins to fail (i.e., prone to cancer, choking, myositis, tendenitis, voiding dysfunction, or other). However, there are times when we encounter a roadblock in our attempts to understand problems. In situations such as this an insight of how to proceed can be gleaned by reflection on the past (1,2). Through a better appreciation of the body design, we can develop better directional concepts as to therapy.

The pelvic floor is clearly becoming an ever-increasing focal point of pelvic medicine, especially in the arena of urogynecology, female urology, and male prostatism. Much discussion goes on concerning its role in health and disease. The following reflection is offered from the direction of what evolution might teach us about the pelvic floor. Perhaps, through a greater awareness of developmental pressures, a better appreciation of nature's intended purpose for the pelvic muscles, and the risk that come with failure to achieve desirable functional endpoints, can be achieved.

This approach to medical science is referred to as Evolutionary Biology. It seeks answers to problems or diseases through study of the evolutionary paths of development. This is a distinctly different, yet complementary, approach from modern medicine, which seeks answers to disease processes through study of anatomy and physiology of the existing organism. When this latter approach is unsuccessful the study of evolutionary roots can often provide understanding that will open new directions of research along more traditional lines. Our various body functions evolved because of environmental pressures that were different from those that evolved our present-day physiology.

II. EVOLUTIONARY TRADE-OFFS

The biology of evolution follows certain rules (3). Time was required for natural selection to occur and there was clearly a trade-off between the benefits and consequences. A highly successful gene mutation might allow a bird or animal to be more competitive in one food niche, but less so in another. Here, as with most of our evolved adaptions, advantages clearly outweigh any disadvantages. However natural selection was not always perfect in its results. There are examples of less successful attempts by nature to preserve the gene pool. The sickle cell gene appeared as a protection against malaria. Although one copy may have conferred immunity to malaria, two copies of the gene can lead to an early death and terrible suffering. Cystic fibrosis and typhoid are other examples of less than perfect attempts to protect humans from environmental risks. The natural selection of benefits, against any downside trade-off, were intended for the good of species survival and as an ultimate advantage for successful passage of the gene pool. The end result was a compromise, the best solution possible, but always attached with attendant risks.

III. HERITAGE LEGACY

Another rule of evolutionary biology is that there is no turning back. We must live with our heritage. Our respiratory passage may expose us to death with each swallow. However, evolutionary forces had no other option. We evolved with a heritage to the lung fish, which had an air hole on the top of its head. As the airway shrank back there was no choice but to link it with the swallowing mechanism. Along similar lines, we have evolved muscles of certain strength, bones of a certain size, and organs with only so much redundancy. These we cannot change because evolution generally involves compromise of available solutions—how much of a certain function is necessary, how much redundancy can be allowed without sacrificing efficiency? There is never too much nor too little.

Nature has provided the human body with just the right amount of behavior needed for survival. This formula drove the design of each and every cell or organ in our bodies. The design had one purpose, to assure passage of the gene pool, and preference was given to the more advantaged designs. These trends hold true for the nervous system. Mature adult reflexes that govern automated body functions did not eliminate the immature precursor reflexes of our predecessors. Instead, evolution provided for suppression or inhibition of these reflexes with maturing of the nervous system. Sherrington (4) first ascribed the role of keeping lower central nervous system (CNS) levels in check to our hierarchical nervous system, similar to the sheriff controlling an unruly mob. If this higher center control is lost, for whatever reason, primitive reflex behavior can emerge. The anatomist A. Gonzalez described precursor reflexes as being relegated to the background where they remain dormant, but subject to reactivation with appropriate stimuli. Thus, the overwhelming response to neural stress, whether it is physical, emotional, or behavioral, is an upregulation of neural metabolism and signaling, with the emergence of hypersensitivity and spasticity.

IV. NEURAL EFFICIENCY

A third observation of nature's design, is neural efficiency. Successful solutions are applied throughout the body. Some examples would include the flexion–extension muscle collaboration in upper and lower limbs, the use of similar neurotransmitters throughout all levels of the CNS, memoried striated muscle tone (e.g., massater, paraspinal, and pelvic floor), and the provision for a striated muscle gate for the visceral systems of respiration and continence. The latter is of special interest because of the intricate relation with the pelvic visceral organs. The pelvic floor, although composed of many separate muscle partitions (5), is designed to function as a unit in regulating pelvic visceral organ behavior. Any breakdown in the unit, for example, separation of the levator bellows-like (S3,4) actions, from the sphincter clamp-like actions (S2—pudendal), or abuses in range of motion usage (e.g., excessive holding) of either group, can only lead to a breakdown in behavior of the various pelvic organ systems. However, unlike other striated muscle groups in the body, the pelvic floor dysfunction will impinge on both the striated and smooth-muscle organs of the pelvis.

V. PENALTIES

A fourth observation of evolution is that penalties exist on either side of evolved solutions (Fig. 1). Too much or too little of a trait decreased competitiveness either because of inefficiency of function or disease, or both (1). This was part of natures selection of the strongest and fittest to assure survival of a species. For example, larger internal organs would necessitate a redesign of the body cavities, sacrifice of agility, and yet not provide greater survival. Smaller organs would compromise endurance. Bigger bones would exact a heavy price of energy expenditure through having to carry all the extra weight. Larger muscles would encumber the long-distance hunter lifestyle of early humans. Lean and mean has always been the formula for success. We have adequate muscle strength for our needs. If demand increases, muscle strength and resistance to fatigue improves. If demand

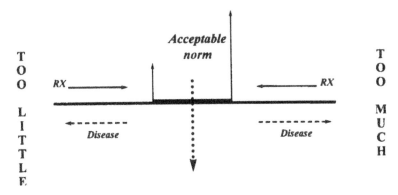

Figure 1 Diagrammatic representation of the evolutionary design: There is an ideal norm that maximizes efficiency of performance. For the pelvic floor, there should be a midrange sphincter tension, with a volitionally directed wide excursion of tone on either side of the midrange. This would be considered the ideal pelvic floor dynamic. It is the "gold standard" for efficiency of function with a minimum of risk. The more inefficient the excursion, the greater the risk of consequences. Treatment should always seek to restore behavior back toward the ideal for which it was designed. This is essential for successful therapy.

goes down, there is a rapid loss of muscle to conserve energy. The additional argument would be that bigger, stronger muscles would not be in the interest of encouraging cleverness to solve problems.

VI. THE PSYCHOLOGICAL ROOTS OF TOILETING

Prior to 1800 few people lived in congested environments of a city. By the mid-1800s the number was still low, roughly fewer than 30%. The circumstances of voiding and defecation changed dramatically in the latter half of the century. The industrial revolution brought more than inventions and financial wealth. Cultural adaptions began to reshape our physiology and disease risk (6). Early man died from infections, starvation, trauma, and predation. As psychological stress became more a part of every day life, people began to die from stress-related disease: heart disease, cancer, and autoimmune disease. By 1900 voiding in crowded environments was only starting to become an issue. Today numerous studies have pointed out the preference of spaced traffic flow through the urinal (7). Privacy remains a primary concern with our basic faculties, yet it is difficult to find. Our heritage for millions of years was to use open space for toileting needs. Then, within a relatively short time span of a few decades, a psychological adaptation was necessitated for the circumstances of toileting. The shy bladder syndrome represents the disadvantages that comes with higher-center regulation of voiding (7). Too much of a good thing can be a bad thing.

Our body physiology has had to readapt the basic response to stress (8). We have inherited a stress response from our evolutionary roots. In our beginnings, our bodies were designed to handle the stress of the chance occasional threat; for example, the encounter with a predator. Muscles tighten, Blood pressure and pulse rise, glucose stores are mobilized, and fat stores are broken down to increase triglycerides. In the interests of preserving the gene pool, the response was set on a hair-trigger. However, today we are prone to activate this stress response with every traffic jam or phone call. The continued elevation of stress hormones, corticotropin (ACTH), cortisone and cortisol, epinephrine, and norepinephrine, exact a price on tissues over time. Chronically elevated triglycerides, glucose, and autoimmune responses have obvious consequences in diseases that make up the common afflictions of today. These include damage to our heart and arteries, autoimmune diseases, suggested links to cancer, and a multitude of lower urinary tract syndromes tied to pelvic floor overuse or misuse. A response designed to protect us from random danger has now become one of our greatest risks to health. It is no wonder that the professional athlete is now trained to deal with both the physical and the mental aspects of his trade. An important corollary of being able to control the psychology aspects of stress is that memoried muscle behavior is less prone to distortion. Performance improves and injury risk declines. Our bodies do not do well with chronic stress. This is evidenced in the host of known stress syndromes as well as recent MRI evidence of actual shrinkage of important brain stem nuclei (e.g., the hypothalamus and amygdala).

A. Cultural Hurdles

Many parents still view discipline as a way to manage the eneuretic, encopretic child. Tradition has taught, and many parents still believe, that toilet training should take place by the third year of life, or roughly parallel to anatomical development of the myelin sheath. This teaching ignores the fact that voiding requires a higher center direction, a degree of control that is dependent on a level of psychological and intellectual maturity, or between ages 8 and 10 years. The stress associated with unrealistic expections for voiding control can result in distorted behavior of the striated sphincter. Eventually, with sufficient repetition, the distortion becomes the norm. Problems, as with any abnormal muscle behavior, may not become apparent for years, possibly decades. Expectations for normal toileting, in all circumstances, before "the age of reason" are simply naive. There can be great risk in pushing the envelope of continence control in children.

The circumstantial stresses placed on the micturition control center are many and varied (7). Single bathrooms in large families, outhouses, public troughs for voiding, deadlines that cut into void time, cultural inhibitions, or to a refusal to sit down to void. These situations lead to an exaggeration of the holding reflex, eventually leading to memoried distortions in sphincter tone. This is the downside of a protective reflex, initially designed for a different purpose.

B. Why a Sphincter

There are three basic needs for a sphincter. Each has an evolutionary purpose.

1. Continence

This primordial need extends to virtually all species. For land mammals there was an obvious benefit from the cleanliness this capability provided. Survival would not be helped by having continuous ooze of waste that would stain fur or skin. The associated odors would make an animal easy feed for a predator. In addition, skin breakdown and infections would undoubtedly risk illness and premature death. None of this would be in the interest of survival of the species, as transfer of the better gene pool would be constantly under pressure. The process of natural selection would clearly benefit those with control of their bowel and bladder.

It is consistent with the pressures of survival that the patterns of evacuation would vary among ecological niches. Fish and birds do not need a great deal of storage time. A degree of continence is required for health reasons, but predation risk is less tied to olfactory function than for land mammals.

2. Reproduction

The safe delivery of sperm requires a reliable delivery method. This would seem to be a priority of Mother Nature in its evolutionary design. Many mammals rely on the sphincter for an ejaculatory push of sperm along the urethral tube for safe deposition in the female. This evolutionary design is shared liberally across species. For land quadripeds this same mechanism overlaps with micturition, as part of the reproductive design.

3. Convenience

Voiding at convenient intervals has links to both the need for survival and reproduction. Reflex voiding could be a problem for an animal trying to outrun a predator, or the hunter closely stalking a prey. Territorial marking became essential for selective passage of the better gene pool from the more dominant or fit male animals. A consciously directed passage of urine was required that could be turned on and off at will. It is a process that continues to assure survival of the more advantaged gene pool. Most importantly, it required a link to higher neural regulatory centers. In turn, the timing of voids became, of necessity, inextricably linked to the conscious mind. This evolutionary role must be dealt with in humans in modern-day life. Micturition in land animals evolved to be consciously directed.

However, too little direction leads to reflex voiding (the unstable bladder), whereas too much control equates to retention and hesitant voiding. However, without this conscious control, reflex voiding would be the norm, as in fish and birds. This would not make sense from an evolutionary prospectus for land mammals.

VII. CONTINENCE AND POSTURE EVOLUTION FROM FISH TO FROG TO ERECT POSTURE

Dogs, a well-studied laboratory resource, have only a minimal degree of active sphincter closure. Being quadriped, and having a bladder that tips down from the symphysis, they do not have much need for an active high-pressure sphincter. Continence requirements necessitate only a low-pressure, more-passive sphincter tone. There is no need for the degree of memoried tone characteristic of biped humans. Gravity faciltiates continence in the quadriped, but works against continence in the human.

The pelvic diaphragm forms a vertical wall in the quadriped-tailed animal and is neurologically linked to muscle involved in movement of the tail (9). Indeed, stimulation of the S2 root in a quadriped (equivalent with S3 in the human) vigorously contracts the tail as well as the sphincter and bladder. However, unlike the biped human, there is no lifting of the rectum or compression of the prostate. In humans the pelvic floor muscles have evolved to serve needs that are entirely different from those of the quadriped. These added muscles have a lifting (bellows) action when stimulated. This lifting capability of pelvic floor serves multiple functions: 1) provides support for the abdominal organs, 2) contributes to active and passive bowel and bladder continence, 3) participates in ejaculation functions, and 4) provides structural support for the true sphincters. The levator muscle became a separate neurological unit from those that originally composed the pelvic floor. The levator remained linked to the motor innervation of the bladder, with minimal ties to the feet. S3 stimulation contracts the visceral organs, the levator, and the large toe. The original pelvic floor, or true sphincters, separated from the motor outflow from the cord to the viscera, but remained closely tied to the motor innervation of the feet. (S2 stimulation in the human will contract the sphincters and the foot but not the pelvic viscera.) However, the central reflex ties remain, at both the brain stem and lumbosacral cord, linking the sphincters, the feet, and the pelvic viscera (10–12).

The greatly expanded role of the pelvic floor muscles in the human contributed to a change in the structural anatomy of the pelvic bones—evident in the formation of the ischial spines and a widening of the sacral ala (9). The spines result from the medial pull of muscles inserted directly or indirectly onto the sacral spinous ligament. All this results in a stable pelvic girdle facilitating ambulation. The absence of pelvic floor innervation in spina bifida and sacral agenesis leaves a wider sacral outlet and absence of spines.

An additional need for the close central neurological ties between the pelvic muscles and the muscles of ambulation was the need for continence with movement. Increases in abdominal pressure occur in both the quadripeds and bipeds—anger, territorial battles, coughs, sneezes, and so on. The evolutionary need for reflex regulation of sphincter tone to avoid random soiling of the perineum seems clear. Animals required this reflex mechanism for continence, as do humans.

The neuroregulation of sphincter behavior evolved to fit each and every requirement. There is never too much or too little. Quadripeds do not need to spend energy maintaining sphincter pressures on the level of humans. However, reflex protection against leakage during territorial battles was a necessity. Human requirements are different, and this led to a redesign of the system.

A. Muscle Memory

As humans evolved to the biped state there was a need to transfer force from the lower extremities to the vertebral spine. This need evolved the design of the pelvis and the pelvic floor muscles. The design of the pelvic bones in humans incorporates an efficient transfer of force from the lower extremities. More importantly, it intimately tied the lower extremities to the pelvic muscles. Movements of the lower limbs require a fulcrum point achievable only through stabilization of the pelvis. Innervation of the feet is linked to the same dermatome (13) as the bladder in much the same way that extensor muscles are linked to flexor muscles. This would seem to satisfy nature's need for efficiency in essential cooperation of movement and broad-based application of successful formulas.

Muscle memory is important for reasons of posture control, sphincter control, and learning of various survival skills (e.g., walking, running, and defensive postures). The more efficient muscle memory systems were passed ultimately on, as are the more successful gene pools, to obvious advantages in speed, food production, and defense. Today these memoried behaviors remain essential in our daily travels and duties. However, the advantage of efficient muscle control remains, and it becomes obvious in competitive arenas such as sports. Better performance follows better-conditioned movement. More importantly, the wear-and-tear–type injury risk is decreased, and recovery from these types of injuries is more complete when muscle movement is associated with conditioned muscle.

B. Gating Distractions and Overuse Syndromes

The afferent feedback to the spinal cord at the lumbosacral level is 90–98% concerned with control of the lower extremities—ambulating: walking, running, posture regulation, and such. Only 2–10% is concerned with regulation of the pelvic floor. Much of this afferent activity is concerned with the unconscious regulation of automated behavior. The conscious element requires a practiced effort. This effort must be ongoing or higher-center representation for these activities can shrink dramatically (13). Eventually subconscious reflex behavior will escape the conscious regulation of the higher centers. It will then either shut down completely, as with a squinted eye, or revert to a more vestigial state of activity (nociception owing to upregulated spinal circuits). The shift in neural regulation has been evidenced in functional magnetic resonance imaging (MRI) and positron emission tomography (PET) scan studies that show expanded or contracted CNS activity that directly mirrored the limb or hand usage (13,14). Similarly, in functional MRI studies of the brain stem micturition centers show voiding or holding efforts, but absence of any change without contraction or relaxation in the lower urinary tract. The changes can be permanent and associated with decline in tissue integrity.

These phenomena can be referred to as negative-gating because there are negative consequences to tissues linked to this lack of CNS conscious regulation.

VIII. DISCUSSION

There is one very important lesson to be drawn from this discussion of our evolutionary roots. Placing excessive demands on the body design leads to deterioration. The examples are everywhere—fatty food and atherosclerosis, inefficiencies in locomotion lead to tendentitis, excess sugar intake leads to diabetes, and so on. These same principles apply to the muscle-overuse syndromes that represent one of the most common afflictions of modern medicine.

If muscles are used inefficiently anywhere, there are negative inflammatory consequences, with eventual deterioration in integrity of the tissue. Initially, terms used are tendonitis, housemaid's knee, back pain, muscle strain, torticollis, surgeon's neck, writer's cramp, carpel tunnel, osteoarthritis, and so on. Repair mechanisms are switched on within the CNS to manage the strain placed on tissue. This involves upregulation in the production of peptides, growth factors, and cytokines to repair and rebuild damaged or stressed tissues. The problem is that if the behavioral stress is repetitive, the upregulation becomes permanent, and the processes become destructive to tissue. Given the unique responsibility of the pelvic floor sphincters to regulate the excitability of the visceral organs, dysfunction of the pelvic floor will have destructive cascade effects on the integrity of the pelvic viscera. Therefore, regardless of the presenting symptoms, there should always be an assessment of function of the pelvic floor muscles in every patient. If dysfunction is identified, then functional restorative efforts should be part of the therapeutic plan (Fig. 2).

IX. SUMMARY

The body is constantly regulating activity toward a certain norm. Variance too far from the norm triggers repair circuits within the CNS. These are very delicate pathways prone to becoming unstable. The reasons for this lie in our evolutionary heritage. The CNS is uniquely designed to respond to environmental stress. It was and is the means by which we evolved. There is, however, an unfortunate downside to our ability to adapt to our environment. Stress, whether from our surrounding environment or lifestyle behaviors, triggers neuronal survival mechanisms that were designed to be fail-safe. They cannot be circumvented. Presently there is no longer evidence of the kind of environmental stress that caused adaptation to our physical makeup, but we still carry the mechanisms attached to those evolutionary roots. Now we are more likely to suffer consequences from these pathways than we are to see change in our physical makeup. This risk comes from everyday stress and the biological hair-triggers that set off primitive reflex activity within the core basal levels of our nervous system. Hence, it is not surprising that treatment is so difficult. Medications, while useful, are pathway-limited in efficacy and side effects. On the bright side, modulation-based therapies are promising, for they follow nicely the evolutionary rules. For just as higher CNS centers suppress and selectively regulate primitive neural reflex activity, so too will neurostimulation. The other hope on the horizon is the human genome project. Unmasking our genetic past may unravel the secrets of fail-safe response mechanisms of our nervous system (15). The therapies of the future will most certainly evolve along lines that are in keeping with our evolutionary heritage. The most promising avenues of development involve selective modulation of the CNS, such as target-specific drug delivery (e.g., neurotoxins), neurostimulation, or gene manipulation. Treatments along these lines will open up exciting new avenues of management for the dysfunctional pelvic floor.

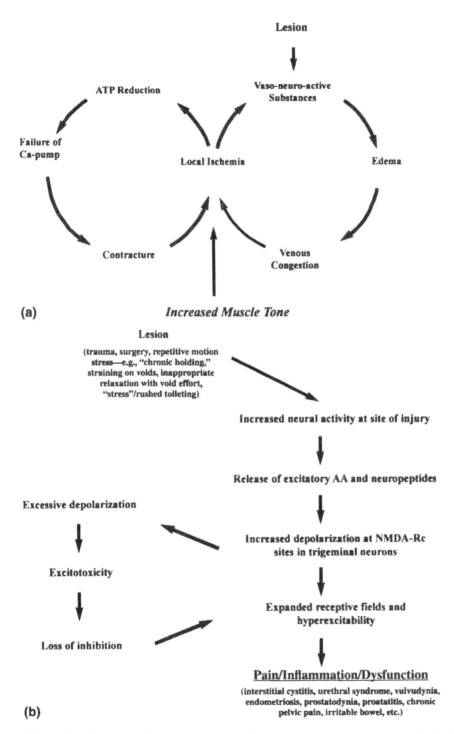

Figure 2 Diagrammatic representation of sequence of events that underlie the inflammatory response in tissue in repetitive use syndromes: (a) various cycles triggered by muscle overuse syndromes; (b) consequences of tissue injury or behavioral stress. (From Ref. 16.)

REFERENCES

1. Nesse RM, Williams GC. Evolution and the origins of disease. Sci Am 1998; 279:86–93.
2. Ruse M. The origin of life: philosophical perspectives. J Theor Biol 1997; 187:473–482.
3. McCormack K. Fail safe mechanisms that perpetuate neuropathic pain. International Association for the Study of Pain. Clinical Updates V, VII (3), 1999.
4. Sherrington CS. The Integrative Action of the Nervous System. London: Churchill Livingstone, 1947.
5. Dubrovsky B, Filipini D. Neurobiological aspects of the pelvic floor muscles involved in defecation. Neurosci Behav Rev 1990; 14:157–168.
6. Sapolsky R. How the other half heals. Discov Mag 1998; April:46–52.
7. Hinman F Jr. Voiding Habits of Man and Beast. Vacaville, CA: Vespasian Press, 1999.
8. Adler J. How stress attacks you. Newsweek June 14, 1999:56–63.
9. Abitol MM. Evolution of the ischial spine and of the pelvic floor in the Hominoidea. Am J Anthropol 1988; 75:53–67.
10. Zermann D, Ishigooka M, Doggweiler R, Schmidt RA. Central autonomic innervation of the lower urinary tract—a neuroanaomic study. World J Urol 1998; 16:417–422.
11. Zermann D, Ishigooka M, Doggweiler R, Schmidt RA. Neurological insights into etiology of genito-urinary pain in men. J Urol 1999; 161:903–908.
12. Vanderhorst VG, Holstege G. Organization of lumbosacral motoneuronal cell groups innervating hindlimb, pelvic floor, and axial muscles in the cat. J Comp Neurol 1997; 382:46–76.
13. Kandel ER, Schwartz JH, Jessell TM. Language, learning and memory. In: Essentials of Neural Science and Behavior, Sec. IX. Appleton & Lange, 1995.
14. Blok BF, Sturms LM, Holstege G. Brain activation during micturition in women. Brain 1998; 121:2033–2042.
15. Woolf CJ, Mannion RJ. Neuropathic pain: aetiology, symptoms, mechanisms, and management [review]. Lancet 1999; 353:1959–1964.
16. Pain Forum. 1997; 6:158.

8

The Role of Connective Tissue at the Level of the Pelvic Floor

ATSUO KONDO

Komaki Shimin Hospital, Komaki, Japan

MOMOKAZU GOTOH

Nagoya University School of Medicine, Nagoya City, Japan

I. INTRODUCTION

The pelvic floor has to resist gravitational forces, and in this, the levator ani muscles and the fasciae play essential roles. Although the levator ani muscles and the bony structure provide space to accommodate pelvic viscerae, the fasciae glue the muscles, bone, and intrapelvic organs together, giving them mechanical strength. Histochemical and neurophysiological studies have provided evidence of partial denervation of the pelvic floor muscle and the striated urethral sphincter, which may be responsible for urinary and fecal incontinence as well as prolapse of the pelvic organs (1).

Stress urinary incontinence is a multifactorial disease observed preponderantly in females in their 30s and older. The overall affliction rates are 30% for females and 5% for males who are otherwise healthy and reside in their own homes. Prevalence definitely increases with age (2). Anatomical and histological investigations suggest that the proximal urethra and bladder neck are secured onto the endopelvic fascia that covers the anterior vaginal wall, and this supporting shelf is firmly connected to the arcus tendineus fasciae pelvis (the white line) at the lateral wall of the levator ani muscles. The urethra, with its inner longitudinal and outer circular smooth muscle, is not fixed directly to the lateral wall by any means. At the proximal urethra and bladder neck, pubovesical muscles arise from the detrusor muscle and connect with the white line. In the same area, pubourethral ligaments connect the vagina and periurethral tissues to the side of the levator ani muscles and run under the urethra. Although the striated urethral sphincter wraps around the smooth muscle of the urethral wall from the 20th to the 60th percentile, the concentric muscular structure is incomplete on the vaginal surface in some aged persons. In the distal portion, two bands of striated muscle (formerly known as the deep transverse muscle of the perineum) begin at the upper portion of the lower third of the urethra and arch over it: the urethrovaginal sphincter encircles both the vagina and urethra, with compressor urethrae passing out laterally and inserting into the urogenital diaphragm near the pubic rami (3).

Recent studies indicate that, in addition to these anatomical and functional disorders, defective biochemical composition of collagen may play a significant role in rendering women incontinent. Ulmsten et al. (5), who investigated connective tissues extensively by biochemical methods (4), proposed a new hypothesis to account for stress incontinence, and devised a minimally invasive sling operation to correct this pathology. Recent meta-analysis of surgery for stress incontinence has clearly demonstrated that long-term surgical results are better in those whose operation was retropubic suspension or sling surgery than in those treated with vaginal needle suspension or anterior vaginal wall repair (6,7). To improve surgical success rates, the most appropriate surgical technique has to be chosen, depending on the type of stress incontinence (8) as well as anatomical and histological defects in the paraurethral tissues. It is suggested that some incontinent women really suffer from hereditary disorders of connective tissues in terms of qualitative, quantitative, or biomechanical properties (4,9,10). If these anomalies are really correlated with the development of stress incontinence in women, analyses of the tissue sampled from the pubocervical fascia or the abdominal rectus fascia may eventually indicate early surgical intervention; for instance, without wasting time and money on those whose collagen is found to be defective.

We review here the clinical significance and evidence relating to the fascial sphincteric complex that plays a key role in maintaining urinary continence, but we do not claim to be complete in all aspects. We have subdivided this chapter into four main investigative techniques (i.e., anatomy and histology, magnetic resonance imaging [MRI], biochemistry, and biomechanical studies).

II. ANATOMY AND HISTOLOGY

The intrinsic continence mechanism is composed of submucosal sealing effects, with smooth-muscle tone, a competent bladder neck, and the striated external sphincter. Urethral resistance comprising the urethral mucosa and submucosal vasculature provides coaptation and compression on the urethral lumen. In the proximal urethra, the anterior vaginal wall is firmly attached to the arcus tendineus fasciae pelvis (the white line), which is a band of dense connective tissue suspended between the back of the lower edge of the pubis and the ischial spine. The anterior vaginal wall provides a hammock-like layer on which the bladder and urethra rest.

The extrinsic continence mechanism comprises the levator ani muscles and the deep transverse muscle of the perineum. The former promptly compress the urethra in response to voluntary or involuntary elevation of intra-abdominal pressure, with huge power in the anterosuperior direction. With detrusor instability, however, which is characterized by slow contraction of the smooth muscle lasting several seconds, with peak pressure of more than 100 cmH$_2$O, simple mechanical power is often demanded. Boys squeeze the penis to obstruct the urethral lumen, and girls firmly cross their legs or push the perineum down on the edge of a chair or on the ankle (11).

A. Endopelvic Paravaginal Defect

The concept of a paravaginal defect is rather unique in that defective connection of the vaginal wall with the white line is responsible for causing cystocele, with or without stress incontinence. Richardson et al. (12) reported the case of a woman who suffered from cystourethrocele with eversion of the right superior sulcus of the vagina. The fact that manual support of this everted area alone simply eradicated the pathology led him to first believe the presence of a specific defect or tear of the paravaginal connection from the white line (12). Of 93 patients with symptomatic anterior pelvic relaxation, 60 who were deemed to have lateral defects underwent paravaginal repair through an abdominal incision. Excellent results were obtained in 92% of the cases 20 months later. Shull and Baden (13) employed Richardson's technique in 149 consecutive patients with stress incontinence and reported cures in 97% of them; blood transfusion was required in 6 patients, and postoperative catheter use lasted 4 days. In 1990, Richardson (14) schematically depicted how to repair paravaginal defects and obtained satisfactory results in 95% of cases. This operation is not indicated for those suffering from stress incontinence, but is designed to correct cystourethrocele caused by a paravaginal defect, when stress incontinence may or may not also be present.

B. Slow- and Fast-Twitch Fibers

Contraction of the pelvic diaphragm pushes the vagina anteriorly against the posterior surface of the urethra and obstructs the urethral lumen. The striated urethral sphincter that comprises slow-twitch fibers (type 1) is fatigue-resistant and contracts, maintaining urethral tone over a prolonged period with less energy expenditure. On the other hand, the pubococcygeus muscle (a part of the levator ani muscles) is composed 24–33% fast-twitch fibers (type 2) (15). The latter are recruited during stress conditions, contracting forcefully and rapidly for a short time. To cough, to strain abdominally, or to voluntarily interrupt the urinary stream, type 2 fibers have to be called into play. Consequently, patients should be taught pelvic floor exercises involving two modes of muscle contraction to recruit motor units of both fiber types, one to slowly contract to maximal strength in 3 sec and to hold it for the next 5 sec, and the other to exert rapid and maximal contractions for 1–2 sec. These contractions are to be repeated 40–50 times a day (16). However, in some women, nerve supply to the pelvic muscles is compromised, and their musculature is torn or detached from the white line. Because these women will not be relieved by practicing pelvic floor exercises, they should be triaged into other forms of treatments that will increase the success rates of physiotherapy (17). Support of the urethra at rest comes from both its attachment to the arcus tendineus fasciae pelvis and the resting tone of the pelvic diaphragm muscles. Relaxation of the muscles allows the bladder neck to descend and facilitates opening (18).

C. The Pubourethral Ligaments and the Pubovesical Muscles

The posterior pubourethral ligaments were studied by Wilson and his associates (19) using light and electron microscopy, as well as neurohistochemistry. Specimens were obtained from ten continent women and nine genuine stress incontinence patients during Burch colposuspension procedures. Their findings did not differ between the two groups. The ligaments were composed of smooth-muscle bundles and a matrix of dense connective elements. There was no evidence of any striated muscles or elastic tissue. They confirmed the presence of acetylcholinesterase-positive (presumptive by cholinergic) nerve fibers by a histochemical technique. The characteristics of the smooth muscle and cholinergic nerve terminal regions were also identified by electron microscopy. The authors claimed that any disorders of these ligaments are unlikely to become an etiological factor in genuine stress incontinence.

In 1989, DeLancey (20) defined the pubourethral ligaments and pubovesical muscles through elaborate studies on histological sections from fresh and preserved cadavers. He reported that the pubovesical muscles lie anterior to the urethra and anterior and superior to the paraurethral vascular plexus. The muscles are an extension of the detrusor muscle and its adventitia, and they attach to the pubic bone and arcus tendineus fasciae pelvis. They contract to facilitate opening the bladder neck but are unable to support the urethra. Delicate and easily torn, they are digitally lifted upward, showing a plexus of blood vessels between the muscles above and the urethral supports (i.e., pubourethral ligament below Figs. 1 and 2). The pubourethral ligament runs underneath the urethra and vascular plexus bilaterally and supports the urethra.

The pubocervical fascia in the precervical area was investigated histologically by Mäkinen et al. (21) in ten women with uterine prolapse in comparison with ten women who underwent hysterectomy for uterine fibroids. They found that the pubocervical fascia with

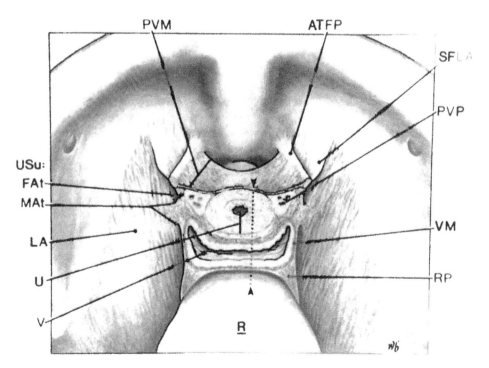

Figure 1   Schematic axial section of the proximal urethra and vagina: The paravascular plexus (PVP) is located between the pubovesical muscles above and the pubourethral ligaments (the urethral support) below. PVM, pubovesical muscles; USu, urethral supports or pubourethral ligaments; FAt, fascial attachment; MAt, muscular attachment; LA, levator ani muscles; U, urethra; V, vagina; ATFP, arcus tendineus fasciae pelvis; SFLA, superior fascia of levator ani; PVP, paraurethral vascular plexus; VM, vaginal wall muscularis; RP, rectal pillar; R, rectum. (From Ref. 20.)

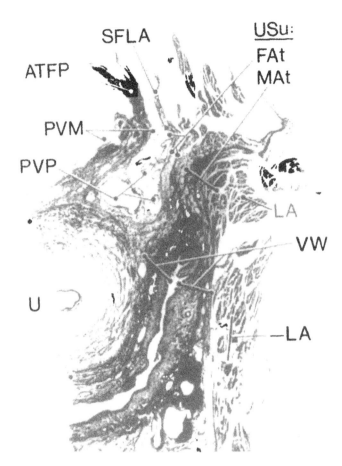

Figure 2   Axial section of paraurethral tissues: The paravesical vascular plexus (PVP) is sandwiched by the pubovesical muscles (PVM) and the pubourethral ligaments (urethral supports; USu). The PVM are attached to the ATFP, and USu runs underneath the urethra. Abbreviations are the same as in Figure 1. (From Ref. 20.)

a decreased number of fibroblasts and increased collagen fibers is correlated with laxity of the connective tissue and uterine prolapse (p < 0.05).

D. The Male Sphincteric Complex

The male pelvis obtained from fresh cadavers was investigated by Burnett and Mostwin (22). The structure of the male urethral sphincteric complex includes the cylindrical rhabdosphincter surrounding the prostatomembranous urethra and a fascial framework. The histological appearance of the rhabdosphincter at its dorsal aspect suggests a suburethral musculofascial plate. Rhabdosphincteric muscle fibers are oriented in vertical and ventrolateral directions, with attachments to the subpubic fascia and the medial fascia of the levator ani. The complex consists of musculofascial structures that provide key areas of attachment, suggesting suspensory and stabilization functions. Myers (23) stressed that the length of the membranous urethra is a vital portion for urinary continence following radical prostatectomy and is variable on retrograde urethrograms with a mean of 1.96 cm (1.2–5.0 cm). He described the membranous urethra as a continence package comprising several soft-tissue elements to provide coaptation of the urethral lumen. Steiner (24) reported that the male urethral suspensory mechanism is composed of the anterior, intermediate, and posterior pubourethral ligaments. Attachment of these ligaments forms a support sling from the pubic arch. Careful handling of these anatomical structures is essential to preserve both potency and urinary continence.

III. MAGNETIC RESONANCE IMAGING

Conventional anatomy studies use tissues and organs obtained from cadavers. Because the pelvic floor plays an important role in retaining urinary and fecal continence, its functions need to be investigated: not in cadavers, but in living subjects. With the recent advent of magnetic resonance imaging (MRI), which is a simple and noninvasive technique, several characteristics of the musculature and connective tissue are under intense investigation, with gratifying outcomes. Because soft tissues are not well visualized on T1-weighted sequences, fast spin-echo T2-weighted sequences are used in most studies. There are, however, a few disadvantages of MRI for evaluating continence mechanisms: it is expensive, imaging time is rather long, and patients cannot keep contracting or straining their muscles for this period of time while their position is not erect but supine. Figure 3 illustrates a 36-year-old continent women by axial section. The thick urethrovesical and vaginorectal fasciae are clearly visible.

A. Studies on Living Subjects

Klutke and his associates (25) studied 45 women with stress incontinence, 5 normal controls, and 1 female cadaver without a history of incontinence, correlating findings on the paraurethral and bladder neck area with data obtained by MRI (0.3-tesla permanent magnet,

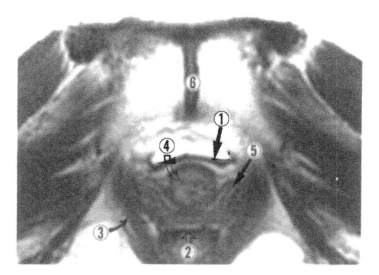

Figure 3 Axial section from continent women (T2-weighted spin-echo sequence, GE Signa Horizon). Note the thick urethrovesical fascia (1) covering the urethra (4), the vaginorectal fascia (2), the levator ani muscle (3), the vagina (5), and the symphysis pubis (6).

T2-weighted spin-echo sequence). It was recognized that the bladder neck and the proximal urethra were supported by a so-called urethropelvic ligament, originating from the levator ani at the lateral pelvic sidewall (the arcus tendineus fasciae pelvis, or the white line). A case of paravaginal defect (Fig. 4) was demonstrated. Their finding of a urethropelvic ligament was, however, later challenged by Kirschner–Hermanns et al. (26) and Aronson et al. (27), who could not locate the ligament in a similar MRI study. Histological investigations suggest that the ligament is consistent with a complex of pubovesical muscles and pubourethral ligaments (20).

Yang et al. (28) evaluated 26 patients, with either pelvic prolapse or stress incontinence, and 16 controls by dynamic fast MRI. The pelvis was evaluated relaxed and under maximal strain. They found MRI useful in diagnosing prolapse involving the anterior (cystocele), middle (vaginal prolapse, uterine prolapse, and enterocele), and posterior (rectocele) compartments. A woman with rectocele demonstrated replacement of her Denonvilliers' fascia by fat (Fig. 5).

Sugimura et al. (29) identified a low-intensity signal in the outer muscular layer, which was thickest in the middle third, a high-intensity signal in the submucosal layer, and a low-intensity ring in the mucosal plate. The posterior pubourethral ligaments were observed unilaterally or bilaterally in 80% of subjects. It was suggested that gadopentetate dimeglumine injection would enhance the target-like view of the urethral lumen on T1-weighted images (30).

Kirschner–Hermanns et al. (26) found that the urethra was not directly connected to the levator ani muscles, for which sharp dorsal angulation in control subjects was lost in 65% of patients, and the muscles themselves were damaged or degenerated in 45% of these patients because of episiotomy, surgical injury, or trauma during childbirth.

Christensen et al. (31,32) investigated 17 physiotherapists by MRI, subtracting images of the pelvic floor muscles in submaximal contraction from those at rest. Using sophisticated computer programs, they beautifully depicted for the first time, the extent of changes in normal pelvic floor displacement during physiotherapy. In sagittal scans, for instance, they recorded anterosuperior movement of the levator ani muscles and the entire

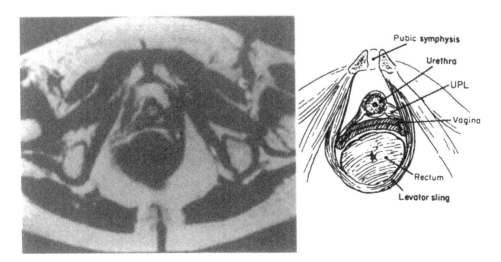

Figure 4 A patient with stress incontinence shows bladder neck descent and a paravaginal defect of the right side in an axial section. UPL, urethropelvic ligaments. (From Ref. 25.)

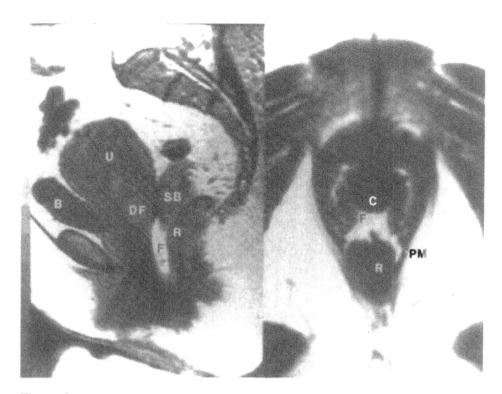

Figure 5   A defect in Denonvilliers' fascia (the rectovaginal septum) is replaced by fat in (left) sagittal and (right) axial images: U, uterus; B, bladder; DF, degenerating fibroid; SB, small bowel; F, fat; R, rectum; C, cervix; PM, puborectal muscle. (From Ref. 28.)

bladder, with narrowing of the retropubic space owing to anterior motion of the urethra (Fig. 6). In short, pelvic floor exercises augmented the contractile force of the levator ani muscles.

Aronson et al. (27) were successful in visualizing the posterior pubourethral ligaments and paravaginal attachments (Fig. 7) in patients with continence, which, however, were distorted and defective in those with urinary incontinence. Because of paravaginal detachment at the arcus tendineus fasciae pelvis, the space of Retzius tended to be enlarged in incontinent subjects.

Tunn et al. (33) found one difference in the thickness of the levator muscles, urethral diameter, distance from the symphysis to the urethra, or the thickness of the anterior vaginal wall between continent and incontinent women, but the concave configuration of the anterior vaginal wall was significantly lost in most patients with stress incontinence or genital prolapse.

B.   Studies on Cadavers

Strohbehn et al. (34) assimilated MRI data on the levator ani muscles of two female cadavers into anatomical sections of the same cadavers and correlated the images with MRI of ten living patients. The levator ani muscles have traditionally been subdivided into the iliococcygeus and pubococcygeus muscles. By MRI analysis, they found that the pubococcygeus muscle actually comprises a few muscles that form a sling behind the rectum, the

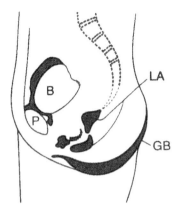

Figure 6 Black portions indicate movement distances observed by subtracted MRI in a sagittal scan: The levator ani muscle (LA) made a dominant movement, whereas the bladder (B) and gluteal muscles moved moderately. The retropubic space was narrowed because of urethral displacement: P, pubis; GB, gluteal border. (From Ref. 31.)

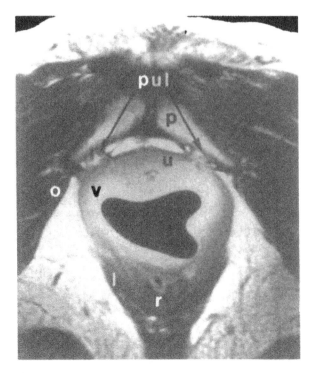

Figure 7 An axial T1-weighted image assisted by an endoluminal coil in a continent woman. The posterior pubourethral ligament connects the vagina to the posterior pubic bone. Pul, posterior pubourethral ligaments; p, pubic bone; u, urethra; o, obturator internus muscle; v, vagina; l, levator ani muscle; r, rectum. (From Ref. 27.)

vagina, and the anus in the intersphincteric groove. They subsequently proposed use of the term *puboviscceral muscle,* which was first coined by Lawson (35), instead of the pubococcygeus muscle.

Strohbehn et al. (36) studied the urethra and bladder neck removed en block from 13 female cadavers. The distinct layers of the cadaveric urethra were best recognized on proton density and T2-weighted images. At the midurethra, the mucosa was seen as a bright ring, the submucosa as a dark ring, the longitudinal and circular smooth muscle as a bright outer ring, and the striated urogenital sphincter muscle as a dark outer ring. These observations confirm the previous report of Sugimura et al. (29).

IV. BIOCHEMISTRY

The etiology of stress incontinence is multifactorial, stemming from bladder neck incompetence, traumatized muscles, torn fasciae, a denervated musculature, obesity, surgical interventions, menopause, aging, and genetic defects in connective tissue. Recent developments in biochemical, bioassay, histochemical, and immunochemical technologies during the past 10–15 years have revealed that several genetically distinct forms of collagen are involved in stress incontinence (37). Collagen, a major protein, accounts for 30% of all body protein. The fundamental unit, the collagen molecule (tropocollagen), is a long 300×1.5-nm rod, with a molecular weight of 285,000. It is involved in maintaining urinary continence in endopelvic fasciae overlying organs and in pelvic floor muscles (see Figs. 3, 4, and 7). The structural unit, the fibril, forms a collagen framework that is rather inextensible, but of high tensile strength. In certain cases, the mechanical properties of collagen change in (in the cervix after parturition) and play an important role in physiological conditions (38).

On the basis of the biochemical composition of their chains, several collagens are recognized. Type I is considered to be supportive collagen and is found in abundance in tissue where mechanical support is required, such as in tendons, bones, ligaments, cornea, and the dentine. Type III collagen, on the other hand, occurs in tissues in which less rigidity is required (e.g., the vascular system and the intestine). A reduction in type I over III in women with stress incontinence means that less supportive collagen is present around the urethra and pelvic floor. The major biological change that occurs is proline hydroxylation in the α-position, providing collagen with its characteristic high hydroxyproline concentration (14%). Lysine oxidation is the extracellular modification that results in cross-linkages between α-chains of adjacent molecules and is the basis of the structural stability of collagen. Cross-linkage is a major contributor to its tensile strength, and types I, III, IV, and V are the predominant components in the ligaments and periurethral structures (39). Fibroblasts are key producers of extracellular matrix proteoglycans. Three small proteoglycans have been identified: decorin, biglycan, and fibromodulin.

Elastin is the major component of elastic fibers, which form a network that contributes to the elasticity of tissue. Fibronectin is a multifunctional molecule that can bind to collagen, heparin, and specific receptors of various cell types. Hyaluronan is a large non-sulfated glycosaminoglycan that aggregates the core protein of vesican and water molecules. Integrin comprises glycoproteins that connect the cell surface to the extracellular matrix. Falconer's (40) schematic illustration of the fibrous connective tissue components appears in Figure 8. Changes in their biochemical and biomechanical characteristics are dependent on age (41), hormonal milieu (42), neuromuscular disease (43), denervation (44), and mechanical strain (45).

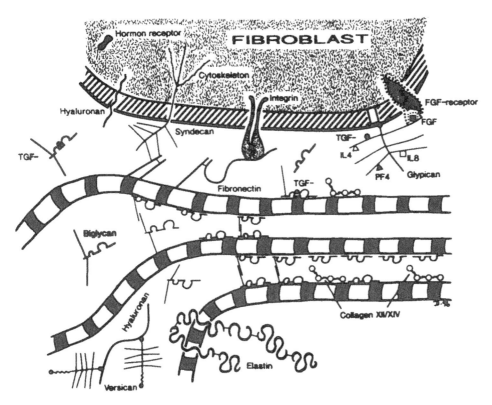

Figure 8   Schematic illustration of fibrous connective tissue components: three large lines with a zebra pattern stand for collagen fibrils. (From Ref. 40.)

Murakumo et al. (46) investigated the three-dimensional arrangement of collagen and elastin fibers in the bladder with chemical digestion methods and scanning electron microscopy. They demonstrated that the serosal layer of the bladder consisted of wavy collagen bundles piled up in sheets intercalated by clusters of adipose cells, but elastin fibers were sparse throughout the bladder wall.

Chang et al. (45) localized collagen type III fibers with an immunohistochemical technique and showed that detrusor accommodation to gradual urine accumulation was maintained mainly by changing the form of collagen type III. They distended the bovine bladder from 0, to 25 or 100% of maximum capacity and, with epifluorescence microscopy, observed that the coiled type III fibers connecting the muscle bundles orthogonally changed their arrangements to extended, longer and taut forms that were oriented parallel to the lumen (Fig. 9).

A.   Collagen Defects

In 1987, Ulmsten et al. (4) measured collagen content of the skin and ligament rotundum in continent controls and incontinent patients. Collagen concentration in both tissues was significantly decreased in those with stress incontinence compared with the continent controls, but its extractability was not different between the two groups (Table 1). They hypothesized that women suffering from stress incontinence may have defective biochemical composition of their connective tissues.

Empty or Partially
Distended Bladder
(top-bottom conformation)

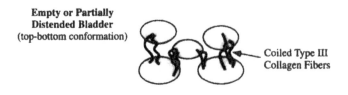

Coiled Type III
Collagen Fibers

Completely Distended
Bladder
(side-side conformation)

Uncoiled Type III
Collagen Fibers

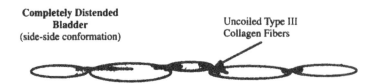

Figure 9   Relation between the detrusor muscle arrangement and the shapes of type III collagen fibers. In the contracted bladder, coiled type III collagen fibers connect the muscle bundles orthogonally, whereas in the full bladder they become extended, taut, and uncoiled. (From Ref. 45.)

Brincat et al. (42) correlated the amount of collagen in the skin with the presence or absence of sex hormone. Skin collagen concentration, quantified biochemically, was 221 $\mu g/mm^2$ in the group treated with sex hormone implants and 164 $\mu g/mm^2$ in the untreated group without implants (p < 0.001). In the untreated group, a decrease of collagen was significantly correlated with menopausal age, but not with chronological age (p < 0.001). Skin thickness, measured radiologically, was also significantly different, being 30% thicker in those with implants than in untreated women (p < 0.001).

Versi et al. (47) investigated correlations between collagen concentration in the skin, skin thickness of the forearm, and several parameters of urethral pressure profile in a group of 50 postmenopausal women who were urodynamically normal, with a mean age of 51. A majority of urethral pressure parameters were significantly correlated with collagen concentration (149 $\mu g/mm^2$), but not with skin thickness (0.82 mm). They concluded that estrogen may have beneficial effects on sphincteric function.

Sayer et al. (48) studied 60 women with stress incontinence in terms of collagen concentration in the pubocervical fascia, abdominal striae, and innervated smooth muscle (electromyography; EMG). An incontinent group without bladder neck prolapse (group A)

Table 1   Collagen Content ($\mu g/mg$ w wt) and Extractability (%) of Collagen[a]

	Group A		Group B	
	Skin (n = 6)	Lig rotundum (n = 7)	Skin (n = 8)	Lig rotundum (n = 3)
Total collagen	30.9	11.6	17.6**	8.4*
Extractability in acetic acid	1.8	1.0	1.4	1.7
Extractability in pepsin	26.2	49.7	34.4	50.4

**p < 0.01 *p < 0.05.
[a]Group A (seven continent women) and group B (eight incontinent women). Collagen content was significantly decreased in incontinent women compared with the control.
Source: Ref. 4.

Table 2 Three Parameters Were Compared Between Group A
(Stress Incontinence Without Bladder Neck Prolapse) and Group B
(Stress Incontinence with Bladder Neck Prolapse)

	Group A	Group B
Abdominal striae	32%	92%
Smooth-muscle denervation	54%	17%
Collagen content	9.3 (µg/g)	9.4 (µg/g)

Source: Ref. 48.

was characterized by greater denervation of the smooth-muscle bundles, whereas the incontinent group with severe bladder neck prolapse (group B) had a greater incidence of abdominal striae. The amount of collagen was the same in the two groups (Table 2). They postulated that there were actually two groups of incontinent women, one suffering from a weakened sphincter owing to damaged neuromuscular components, and the other with defective connective tissue, manifested by abdominal striae, leading to compromised sphincter function and bladder neck prolapse.

Rechberger et al. (49) quantified collagen concentration and estrogen receptors in vesicovaginal fascia harvested from 11 incontinent patients and 5 continent controls. Those with stress incontinence were characterized by less collagen (13.9 µg/mg wet weight) and more estrogen receptors (49.4 fmol/mg protein) than the control group, which might be explained by the stimulatory effects of estrogen on procollagenase gene expression. This observation is consistent with the previous report by Ulmsten et al. (4).

Falconer and his associates (50) from Sweden have been investigating the relation between collagen and stress incontinence. In 1994, they cultured fibroblasts from skin biopsies of incontinent patients and continent controls. Cultures from incontinent patients produced 30% less collagen than those from the controls, but general protein synthesis was similar in the two groups. These results suggest that women with stress incontinence have altered connective tissue metabolism, and reduced collagen production weakens their paraurethral support system. In 1996, they studied the characteristics of collagen taken from the paraurethral connective tissue of six incontinent patients before and 2 years after intravaginal slingplasty (51). Although collagen concentration was unchanged during this time, its metabolism in terms of solubility by pepsin digestion increased from 41 to 66%, which is consistent with less collagen cross-linking. It is known that aging augments the amount of stable cross-linking which, in turn, decreases protein turnover and makes tissues stiffer. The increase in solubility implies that slingplasty helped the paraurethral tissue to become more compliant and the urethral lumen to close promptly. In 1998, they compared the ultrastructure and metabolism of paraurethral connective tissue in stress urinary incontinent and control women (52). They found that collagen concentration was almost 30% greater (17.9 vs. 13.5 µg/mg wet weight) with a significantly larger collagen fibril diameter (76 vs. 58 nm) in the incontinent group (40) (Fig. 10), that mRNA expressions for collagen I and III were twice as high, and that the ratio of proteoglycans over collagen was significantly lower when compared with that of the controls (0.10 vs. 0.15). Notably, the increased collagen concentration they reported in incontinent women contradicted their own article published in 1994, which they now suspect may reflect different reactions from different portions of the body (Falconer, personal communication, 1999).

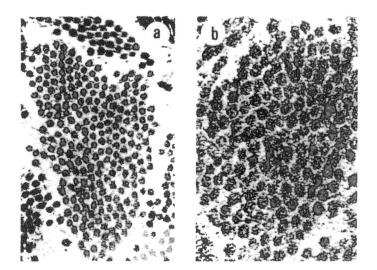

Figure 10 The diameter of collagen fibrils of paraurethral connective tissue, observed by electron microscopy, was (a) 58 nm in the control group and (b) 76 nm in the stress incontinent group (p < 0.0005). (From Ref. 40.)

B. Type I to Type III Collagen Ratio

Norton et al. (53) investigated collagen type I/III ratios in three groups of age-matched women: 8 with genital prolapse, 6 with stress incontinence, and 15 controls. Vaginal skin was obtained from the vaginal apex for this purpose (normal ratio: 6:1–7:1). A reduced type I/III ratio implies that less supportive collagen is available. The ratio was normal in those with stress incontinence (6.7:1) and in the controls (6.3:1.0), but abnormal in genital prolapse (3.4:1). They hypothesized that some patients with a reduced ratio may be predisposed to genital prolapse and that a normal ratio in women with stress incontinence is indicative of a multifactorial pathophysiology.

Bergman et al. (54) studied type III collagen in the perineal skin, uterosacral ligaments, and round ligaments of the uterus among three groups comprising, respectively, six patients with pelvic prolapse and stress incontinence, four controls, and four subjects with pelvic prolapse only. The total amount of collagen in these three groups did not differ, but the collagen type III ratio of the three tissues was significantly lower in the first compared with the other two groups (Table 3). Conversely, group 1 had more type I collagen, which is not in agreement with the report of Norton et al. (53).

Table 3 Percentage of Type III Collagen Among Three Groups[a]

	Group 1 ($n = 6$)	Group 2 ($n = 4$)	Group 3 ($n = 4$)
Skin (%)	21*	29	27
Uterosacral ligament (%)	17*	21	26
Round ligament (%)	17*	22	21

*$p < 0.05$.
[a]Group 1 comprising those with pelvic relaxation and stress incontinence, group 2 control women, and group 3 those with pelvic relaxation without stress incontinence.
Source: Ref. 54.

Table 4 Comparison of Tissue Collagen Content in Two Groups[a] of Women

	Incontinent nulliparous ($n = 36$)	Continent nulliparous ($n = 25$)	P value
Age	38 (13–49)	25 (16–50)	
Collagen content	29% (14–53)	39.7% (20–54)	<0.0001
Type I/III ratio	65:35	71:29	0.0008

[a]Patient group comprises 36 incontinent nulliparous women and 25 continent nulliparous women.
Source: Ref. 9.

Keane et al. (9) recruited 36 premenopausal nulliparous women with stress incontinence and 25 nulliparous controls to exclude contributory factors produced by pregnancy and childbearing. Tissue biopsy of the periurethral vagina revealed that less collagen was present in the patient group, that the ratio of type I to type III collagen was altered, that the proportion of type I was lower in those with stress incontinence, and that mature cross-linked collagen, which accounts for the rigidity and strength of tissues, was also reduced (Table 4). These authors clearly demonstrated that defective collagen in connective tissue was one of the causes of stress incontinence in a select group of patients not compromised by childbirth.

C. Is Urinary Incontinence Hereditary?

Mushkat et al. (55) attempted to answer a conventional question: "Is urinary incontinence hereditary?" They evaluated 780 first-degree relatives (mothers, sisters, and children) of 259 women suffering from stress incontinence in comparison with 474 first-degree relatives of 165 continent women. The overall prevalence rate was 20.3% in the former and 7.8% in the latter, the difference being statistically significant (Table 5). The answer to the question is "yes" in that some genetic factors must be involved in initiating stress incontinence among the first-degree relatives of incontinent women.

V. BIOMECHANICAL STUDY

Collagenous tissues have a structural function in the organism (i.e., they support load and respond to stress). One of the features of collagenous tissues is the periodicity of light optical dimensions, ranging from a few microns to a few tenths of a millimeter. The waveform describing this periodicity is best approximated as a regular-repeating crimp, the function

Table 5 Familial Prevalence of Stress Incontinence[a]

	Study group	Control group	p value
Mothers	71/203 (35.0%)	19/140 (13.6%)	<0.005
Sisters	73/367 (19.9%)	15/229 (6.6%)	<0.005
Daughters	14/210 (6.7%)	3/105 (2.9%)	>0.05
Total	158/780 (20.3%)	37/474 (7.8%)	<0.0001

[a]Study group originated in 259 incontinent patients and control group of 165 continent women.
Source: Ref. 55.

of which is consistent with that of a linear shock-absorbing mechanism by the creation of a compliant toe region in the force-elongation diagram (56). Cross-link formation has been demonstrated during normal maturation, and the effects of aging on the morphological properties of collagenous tissues have been recently investigated. Hamlin and Kohn (41) reported that collagen samples obtained from the diaphragms of male accident victims became progressively more resistant to collagenase digestion with increasing age. This was represented by a linear relation between age and the logarithm of time required to digest 50% of the collagen. Yamauchi and his associates (57) appropriately demonstrated that an abundance of cross-linked collagen is related to chronological aging in bovine and human skin. Quantification of the cross-link showed that it increased rapidly from birth through maturation, and subsequently was gradually augmented. Using ligaments of rabbit hind limbs, Amiel et al. (58) observed that aging was an important factor in reducing collagen concentration and its synthesis rates. Aging increased nonreducible cross-linkage with maturation in 36-month-old rabbits compared with 2-month-old controls.

A few articles have described the biomechanical characteristics of connective tissue, which is vital in maintaining urinary continence. Changes in the biomechanical properties of collagen during pregnancy are responsible for occasional urinary incontinence, which is well documented. Incontinence appearing in many women during this period will be overcome after childbearing. In a few women, however, incontinence does not subside and is sometimes aggravated, especially when hereditary collagen deficiency is involved (4,9).

A. Mechanical Strength of the Fascia and Joint Mobility

In 1976, Minns and Tinckler (59) biomechanically investigated the fascia transversalis obtained during herniorrhaphy from patients and compared the results with those of postmortem specimens taken from the same region. Fascia from hernia patients showed lower ultimate tensile strength compared with the controls, but the strain at rupture was practically the same. These data are in general agreement with those of Landon et al. (10), who studied the effects of pregnancy on the strength of rectus fascia, 35-mm long and 7-mm wide, in vitro. The tissue was sampled from 24 pregnant women and 92 nonpregnant controls. Ultimate tensile strength was weaker and strain (percentage extension) at failure was higher in the pregnant women compared with the controls ($p < 0.0001$) (Fig. 11). Pregnancy altered the mechanical properties of the fascia, favoring more distensible, gradual, and safe fetal growth without disturbing the intrauterine milieu. There is a notable analogy between hernia and pregnancy in terms of biomechanical strength in both clinical settings.

The relation of joint mobility to pelvic prolapse was first studied by Marshman et al. (60), who found that patients with rectal prolapse showed significantly increased extensibility of the fifth finger (81 degrees) compared with the controls (68 degrees) ($p < 0.001$). Subsequently, Norton et al. (61) looked for a correlation between joint hypermobility and genitourinary prolapse or stress incontinence in 107 women. They discovered that patients with joint hypermobility had a significantly higher incidence of cystocele, rectocele, and uterine or vault prolapse, implying that genetic deficits in connective tissue are responsible for pelvic laxity, but not for stress incontinence.

Landon et al. (62) investigated in vitro tensile strength of the rectus fascia obtained from 14 women with stress incontinence and 25 continent controls. They loaded the specimens on a test system with force and length measurements. There was no significant difference among any of the parameters they investigated (Table 6), indicating no variance in the basic biomechanical properties of the fascia from the two groups. Their conclusion is inconsistent with our in vivo results.

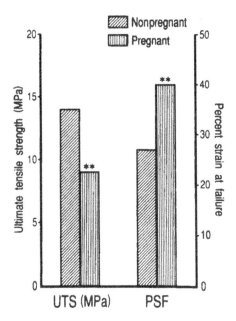

Figure 11 Ultimate tensile strength (UTS) was lower, and the percentage strain at failure (PSF) was higher in pregnant women compared with nonpregnant women (** p < 0.0001). (From Ref. 10.)

That we noted a fragile anterior vaginal wall in some incontinent women when a long needle was used for penetration during the Stamey procedure motivated us to undertake an in vivo study (63). Twenty-six women with stress incontinence and 21 continent controls who underwent transabdominal hysterectomy for myoma uterii were recruited. A Stamey needle was connected to a digital force gauge and pushed downward into the rectus fascia, then into the pubocervical fascia bilaterally (Fig. 12). The force required for penetration (shear strength of the tissue) was read. The shear strength of both the rectus fascia and the pubocervical fascia was lower in the patient group than in the controls (p < 0.01) (Table 7). Shear strength of the vaginal wall was not correlated with aging, irrespective of the continence status. Consequently, our data indicate that some women suffering from stress incontinence may have hereditary disorders of the biomechanical properties of connective

Table 6 Biomechanical Properties of the Rectus Fascia In Vitro[a]

	Incontinent women (n = 14)	Continent women (n = 25)
UTS (n/mm^2)[b]	19.51	17.66
Strain (%)	29.73	27.06
Young modulus	1.079	1.196
Stress at 10% strain (n/mm^2)	6.03	6.45
Energy for failure	0.118	0.92

[a]There was no significant difference in any parameters between the groups.
[b]UTS; ultimate tensile strength.
Source: Ref. 62.

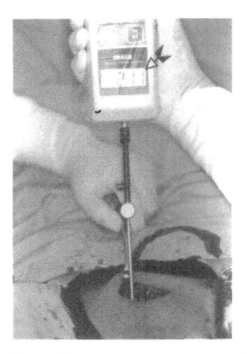

Figure 12   Stamey needle connected to a digital force gauge: a force of 2.11 kg, indicated by an arrow, was necessary to penetrate the right pubocervical fascia in vivo.

tissues, and these weak connective tissues may be responsible for lax support of the urethra and the vagina at the time of a sudden increase in intra-abdominal pressure.

VI.   SUMMARY AND CONCLUSION

Endopelvic paravaginal defect is a rather new concept, but any stress incontinence without this pathology should not be treated by ligating the vaginal fascia to the white line. Two modes of muscle contractions are of importance for training pelvic floor muscles (i.e., gradual and maximum contractions for slow-twitch fibers, and fast, maximum contractions for fast-twitch fibers, respectively). Good practice of pelvic floor exercises is consistent with strong, repeated contractions of the levator ani muscles which shifts the vagina, urethra, and bladder to an anterosuperior direction. Pubourethral ligaments run underneath the urethra and support it together with a hammock-like bed of the anterior vaginal wall. MRI can iden-

Table 7   Shear Strength (kg) of Two Fasciae Measured In Vivo Revealed Statistically Significant Difference Between a Patient Group and a Control Group

	Patient group[a] ($n = 26$)	Control group[a] ($n = 21$)
Pubocervical fascia, left	2.81 (0.81)**	3.74 (0.87)
right	2.87 (0.75)**	3.62 (0.87)
Rectus fascia, left	2.48 (0.99)**	3.20 (0.86)
right	2.36 (0.80)**	3.26 (0.82)

[a]Values in parentheses stand for standard deviation. **$p < 0.01$.

tify the characteristics of the musculature and the connective tissue without exposing the subject to ionizing radiation.

Women who suffer from stress incontinence in general are characterized by decreased collagen concentration in connective tissues and a lower ratio of type I over type III collagen compared with that of normal controls. Pregnancy alters the mechanical properties of the rectus fascia, making it more distensible. Hypermobility of the fifth finger is correlated with a high incidence of cystocele, rectocele, and uterine prolapse, but not stress incontinence. Epidemiology has confirmed that stress urinary incontinence is a hereditary disease in some women. Shear strength of the rectus fascia and the pubocervical fascia is significantly weaker in those with stress incontinence.

In conclusion, stress incontinence is a multifactorial disease brought about by menopause, aging, denervation, traumatized levator ani muscles, hypermobility of the bladder neck, and intrinsic sphincter deficiency. As we have seen in this chapter, we should be aware that genetic deficiencies in connective tissues have been definitely involved in initiating stress incontinence or pelvic relaxation in some patients, but further biochemical and genetic investigations are warranted.

REFERENCES

1. Smith ARB. Role of connective tissues and muscle in pelvic floor dysfunction. Curr Opin Obstet Gynecol 1994; 6:317–319.
2. Kondo A, Saito M, Yamada Y, Kato T, Hasegawa S, Kato K. Prevalence of hand-washing incontinence in healthy subjects in relation to stress and urge incontinence. Neurourol Urodynam 1992; 11:519–523.
3. DeLancey JOL. Correlative study of paraurethral anatomy. Obstet Gynecol 1986; 68:91–97.
4. Ulmsten U, Ekman G, Giertz G, Malmström A. Different biochemical composition of connective tissue in continent and stress incontinent women. Acta Obstet Gynecol Scand 1987; 66:455–457.
5. Petros PEP, Ulmsten U. An integral theory of female urinary incontinence. Acta Obstet Gynecol Scand Suppl 1990; 153:7–31.
6. Jarvis GJ. Surgery for genuine stress incontinence. Br J Obstet Gynaecol 1994; 101:371–374.
7. Leach GE, Dmochowski RR, Apell RA, Blaivas JG, Hadley HR, Luber KM, Mostwin JL, O'Donnel PD, Roehrborn CG. Female stress urinary incontinence Clinical Guidelines Panel Summary Report on surgical management of female stress urinary incontinence. J Urol 1997; 158:875–880.
8. McGuire EJ. Urodynamic findings in patients after failure of stress incontinence operation. Prog Clin Biol Res 1981; 78:351–360.
9. Keane DP, Sims TJ, Abrams P, Bailey AJ. Analysis of collagen status in premenopausal nulliparous women with genuine stress incontinence. Br J Obstet Gynaecol 1997; 104:994–998.
10. Landon CR, Crofts CE, Smith ARB, Trowbridge EA. Mechanical properties of fascia during pregnancy: a possible factor in the development of stress incontinence of urine. Contemp Rev Obstet Gynaecol 1990; 2:40–46.
11. Kondo A, Kato K, Takita T, Otani T. Holding postures characteristic of unstable bladder. J Urol 1985; 134:702–704.
12. Richardson AC, Lyons JB, Williams NL. A new look at pelvic relaxation. Am J Obstet Gynecol 1976; 126:568–573.
13. Shull BL, Baden WF. A six-year experience with paravaginal defect repair for stress urinary incontinence. Am J Obstet Gynecol 1989; 160:1432–1440.
14. Richardson AC. How to correct prolapse paravaginally. Contemp OB/GYN 1990; 35:100–114.
15. Gilpin SA, Gosling JA, Smith ARB, Warrell DW. The pathogenesis of genitourinary prolapse and stress incontinence of urine. A histological and histochemical study. Br J Obstet Gynaecol 1989; 96:15–23.

16. Kondo A, Yamada Y, Morishige R, Niijima R. An intensive programme for pelvic floor muscle exercises: short- and long-term effects on those with stress urinary incontinence. Acta Urol Jpn 1996; 42:853–859.

17. DeLancey JOL. The pathophysiology of stress urinary incontinence in women and its implications for surgical treatment. World J Urol 1997; 15:268–274.

18. DeLancey JOL. Functional anatomy of the female lower urinary tract and pelvic floor. Ciba Found Symp 1990; 151:57–76.

19. Wilson PD, Dixon JS, Brown ADG, Gosling JA. Posterior pubo-urethral ligaments in normal and genuine incontinent women. J Urol 1983; 130:802–805.

20. DeLancey JOL. Pubovesical ligament: a separate structure from the urethral supports ("pubo-urethral ligaments"). Neurourol Urodynam 1989; 8:53–61.

21. Mäkinen, J, Söderström K–O, Kiiholma P, Hirvonen T. Histological changes in the vaginal connective tissue of patients with and without uterine prolapse. Arch Gynecol 1986; 239:17–20.

22. Burnett AL, Mostwin JL. In situ anatomical study of the male urethral sphincteric complex: relevance to continence preservation following major pelvic surgery. J Urol 1998; 160:1301–1306.

23. Myers RP. Male urethral sphincteric anatomy and radical prostatectomy. Urol Clin North Am 1991; 18:211–227.

24. Steiner MS. The puboprostatic ligament and the male urethral suspensory mechanism: an anatomic study. Urology 1994; 44:530–534.

25. Klutke C, Golomb J, Barbaric Z, Raz S. The anatomy of stress incontinence: magnetic resonance imaging of the female bladder neck and urethra. J Urol 1990; 143:563–566.

26. Kirshner–Hermanns R, Wein B, Niehaus S, Schaefer W, Jakse G. The contribution of magnetic resonance imaging of the pelvic floor to the understanding of urinary incontinence. Br J Urol 1993; 72:715–718.

27. Aronson MP, Bates SM, Jacoby AF, Chelmow D, Sant GR. Periurethral and paravaginal anatomy: Endovaginal magnetic resonance imaging study. Am J Obstet Gynecol 1995; 173:1702–1710.

28. Yang A, Mostwin JL, Rosenshein NB, Zerhouni EA. Pelvic floor descent in women: Dynamic evaluation with fast MRI and cinematic display. Radiology 1991; 179:25–33.

29. Sugimura K, Yoshikawa K, Okizuka H, Kaji Y, Ishida T. Normal female urethra and paraurethral structure: evaluation with MRI. Nippon Acta Radiol (Tokyo) 1991; 51:901–905.

30. Hricak H, Secaf E, Buckley DW, Brown JJ, Tanagho EA, McAninch JW. Female urethra: MR imaging. Radiology 1991; 178:527–535.

31. Christensen LL, Djurhuus JC, Lewis MT, Dev P, Chase RA, Constantinou PS, Constantinou CE. MRI of voluntary pelvic floor contractions in healthy female volunteers. Int Urogynecol J 1995; 6:138–152.

32. Christensen LL, Djurhuus JC, Constantinou CE. Imaging of pelvic floor contractions using MRI. Neurourol Urodynam 1995; 14:209–216.

33. Tunn R, Paris S, Fischer W, Hamm B, Kuchinke J. Static magnetic resonance imaging of the pelvic floor muscle morphology in women with stress urinary incontinence and pelvic prolapse. Neurourol Urodynam 1998; 17:579–589.

34. Strohbehn K, Ellis JH, Strohbehn JA, DeLancy JOL. Magnetic resonance imaging of the levator ani with anatomic correlation. Obstet Gynecol 1996; 87:277–285.

35. Lawson JON. Pelvic anatomy. 1. Pelvic floor muscles. Ann R Coll Surg Engl 1974; 54:244–252.

36. Strohbehn K, Quint LE, Prince MR, Wojno KJ, DeLancy JOL. Magnetic resonance imaging anatomy of the female urethra: a direct histologic comparison. Obstet Gynecol 1996; 88:750–756.

37. Macarak EJ, Howard PS, Lally ET. Production and characterization of a monoclonal antibody to human type III collagen. J Histochem Cytochem 1986; 34:1003–1011.

38. Harkness RD. Biological functions of collagen. Biol Rev 1961; 36:399–463.

39. Morley R, Cumming J, Weller R. Morphology and neuropathology of the pelvic floor in patients with stress incontinence. Int Urogynecol J 1996; 7:3–12.

40. Falconer C. Stress urinary incontinence in women; pathophysiological aspects. PhD dissertation, Stockholm, 1997.
41. Hamlin CR, Kohn RR. Evidence for progressive, age-related structural changes in post-mature human collagen. Biochim Biophys Acta 1971; 236:458–467.
42. Brincat M, Moniz CJ, Studd JWW, Dabby A, Magos A, Emburey G, Versi E. Long-term effects of the menopause and sex hormones on skin thickness. Br J Obstet Gynaecol 1985; 92:256–259.
43. Stepens HR, Duance VC, Dunn MJ, Bailey AJ, Dubowitz V. Collagen types in neuromuscular diseases. J Neurol Sci 1982; 53:45–62.
44. Salonen V, Lehto M, Kalimo H, Penttinen R, Aro H. Changes in intramuscular collagen and fibronectine in denervation atrophy. Muscle Nerve 1985; 8:125–131.
45. Chang SL, Howard PS, Koo HP, Macarak EJ. Role of type III collagen in bladder filling. Neurourol Urodynam 1998; 17:135–145.
46. Murakumo M, Ushiki T, Abe K, Matsumura K, Shinno Y, Koyanagi T. Three-dimensional arrangement of collagen and elastin fibers in the human urinary bladder: a scanning electron microscopic study. J Urol 1995; 154:251–256.
47. Versi E, Cardozo L, Brincat M, Cooper D, Montgomery J, Studd J. Correlation of urethral physiology and skin collagen in postmenopausal women. Br J Obstet Gynaecol 1988; 95:147–52.
48. Sayer TR, Dixon JS, Hosker GL, Warrell DW. A study of paraurethral connective tissue in women with stress incontinence of urine. Neurourol Urodynam 1990; 9:319–320.
49. Rechberger T, Donica H, Baranowski W, Jakowicki J. Female urinary stress incontinence in terms of connective tissue biochemistry. Eur J Obstet Gynecol Reprod Biol 1993; 49:187–191.
50. Falconer C, Ekman G, Malmström A, Ulmsten U. Decreased collagen synthesis in stress-incontinent women. Obstet Gynecol 1994; 84:583–586.
51. Falconer C, Ekman–Ordeberg G, Malmström A, Ulmsten U. Clinical outcome and changes in connective tissue metabolism after intravaginal slingplasty in stress incontinence women. Int Urogynecol J 1996; 7:133–137.
52. Falconer C, Blomgren B, Johansson O, Ulmsten U, Malmström A, Westergren–Thorsson G, Ekman–Ordeberg G. Different organization of collagen fibril in stress-incontinence women of fertile age. Acta Obstet Gynecol Scand 1998; 77:87–94.
53. Norton P, Boyd C, Deak S. Collagen synthesis in women with genital prolapse or stress urinary incontinence. Neurourol Urodynam 1992; 11:300–301.
54. Bergman A, Elia G, Cheung D, Perelman N, Nimni ME. Biochemical composition of collagen in continent and stress urinary incontinence women. Gynecol Obstet Invest 1994; 37:48–51.
55. Mushkat Y, Bukovsky L, Langer R. Female urinary stress incontinence—does it have familial prevalence? Am J Obstet Gynecol 1996; 174:617–619.
56. Gathercole LJ, Keller A. Crimp morphology in the fibre-forming collagens. Matrix 1991; 11:214–234.
57. Yamauchi M, Woodley DT, Mechanic GL. Aging and cross-linking of skin collagen. Biochem Biophys Res Commun 1988; 152:898–903.
58. Amiel D, Kuiper SD, Wallace CD, Harwood FL, VandeBerg JS. Age-related properties of medial collateral ligament and anterior cruciate ligament: a morphologic and collagen maturation study in the rabbit. J Gerontol 1991; 46:B159–165.
59. Minns RJ, Tinckler LF. Structural and mechanical aspects of prosthetic herniorrhaphy. J Biomech 1976; 9:435–438.
60. Marshman D, Percy J, Fielding L, Delbridge L. Rectal prolapse: relationship with joint mobility. Aust NZ J Surg 1987; 57:827–829.
61. Norton P, Baker J, Shaarp H, Warenski J. Genitourinary prolapse: relationship with joint mobility. Neurourol Urodynam 1990; 9:321–322.
62. Landon CR, Smith ARB, Crofts CE, Trowbridge A. Biomechanical properties of connective tissue in women with stress incontinence of urine. Neurourol Urodynam 1989; 8:369–370.
63. Kondo A, Narushima M, Yoshikawa Y, Hayashi H. Pelvic fascia strength in women with stress urinary incontinence in comparison with those who are continent. Neurourol Urodynam 1994; 13:507–513.

9

The Pelvic Floor in Infancy and Childhood

PATRICK H. McKENNA

Southern Illinois University School of Medicine, Springfield, Illinois

C. D. ANTHONY HERNDON

University of Connecticut, Farmington, Connecticut

I. INTRODUCTION

The underlying causes, methods of evaluation, and treatment differ greatly for children with pelvic floor dysfunction when compared with those of adults. Unlike adults the main issue with the pediatric sphincter and pelvic floor is lack of relaxation with voiding and defecation. This can lead to life-threatening complications that are exceedingly rare in adults. Only in unusual cases, in whom severe neurological abnormalities lead to denervation, or congenital anatomical abnormalities are present, is the flaccid sphincter and pelvic floor the underlying cause of stool and bowel incontinence in children.

Pediatric patients have a higher probability of an underlying congenital abnormality as the cause of pelvic floor dysfunction. The methods used to evaluate children are far more complex because there is often less cooperation, there are equipment size issues, and methodology must be changed with the decreasing patient size. Unlike adults, history, particularly in infants, plays a much smaller role in the differential diagnosis. Methods of treatment are hindered by lack of available medications approved for use in children, low attention span with behavioral techniques, and added difficulty because of patient size and future growth that complicates surgical options.

The object of this chapter will be to review the current state of knowledge of the unique aspects of the pediatric external sphincter and pelvic floor. It will include a review of the most recent theories that form the basis for current treatment options for both congenital and acquired problems with the pediatric external sphincter and pelvic floor.

II. DEVELOPMENTAL ANATOMY

There are specific striated sphincteric muscles identified in both pediatric boys and girls. The innervation of these muscles arise from branches of the pudendal nerve that follows the course of the pudendal vessels through the perineum. There appears to be some differences in the development of these mechanisms between the sexes, and these muscles do not function entirely independently from the pelvic floor musculature and anal sphincteric mechanism that all share innervation from branches of the pudendal nerve. This explains why there is often associated bowel problems with urethral sphincter dysfunction (1–4).

Evidence is building that sphincter development in the fetus may predispose to early fetal bladder outlet obstruction and may be responsible for high-grade reflux, which is seen predominantly in male infants who do not have bladder outlet obstruction by the time of birth (5–10).

In adolescents and adults, the sphincter is intrinsic to the urethral wall and closely applied to the smooth muscle at the level of the membranous urethra in the male and midurethra in the female (11). The sphincter is described as being omega-shaped in adolescents and adults (12) (Fig. 1). A ring-shaped sphincter has been seen in early adolescence, but this is most often noted before age 1 (Fig. 2). The development of the urorectal septum, Cowper's glands, and the perineal body in the male may account for the transition from ring-shaped to omega-shaped. The development of the urogenital septum in the female may be responsible for the transition. The thick ring-shaped configuration is most often seen in the male infants and may explain initial high voiding pressures seen predominately in male newborns (7), and the propensity for male infants to have high-grade vesicoureteral reflux at birth that has a high spontaneous resolution rate (10).

III. CONGENITAL ABNORMALITIES

In pediatrics, there is a higher probability than in adults that an underlying congenital abnormality can account for anatomical and neurological problems. This can affect the function of the sphincteric mechanism and pelvic floor. A complete history and physical examination can identify most of the congenital problems. Occasionally, appropriate screening studies are required to correctly categorize the patients.

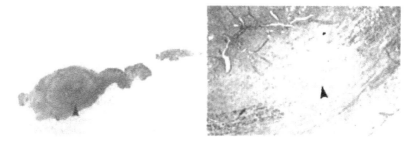

Figure 1   The sphincter is omega-shaped with posterior deficiency in 14-month-old female subject. (Arrowheads show posterior deficiency of rhabdosphincter.) (From Ref. 7.)

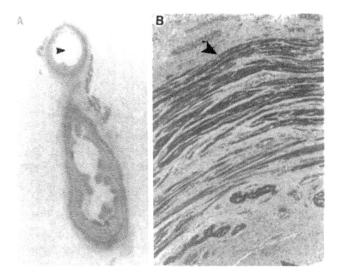

Figure 2   The sphincter is a complete ring-shaped muscle in a 3-month-old male subject (small arrowhead in A). Portion of urethral wall shows concentric striated fibers (large arrowhead in B). (From Ref. 7.)

A. Myelodysplasia

In the past this was the most common form of neurogenic bladder dysfunction in children, but its incidence has been steadily decreasing because of early detection in the antenatal period, resulting in termination of the pregnancy (13), and folic acid treatment, which markedly decreases the likelihood of developing spinal defects (14–16). There is a slight increase in the incidence of myelodysplasia if other family members also have this disorder (17).

In cases of open myelomeningocele (Fig. 3), it is readily identifiable at birth. The neurological effect cannot be determined by the level of the lesion because some nerve roots may be left intact, an Arnold–Chiari malformation can affect the brain stem and pontine center, and often the tethering of the spinal cord along with different growth rates of the vertebral bodies can affect the final neurological deficit (18). Likewise, immediately

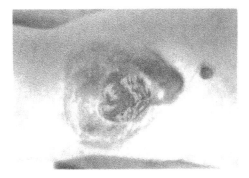

Figure 3   Patient with posterior open sacral level myelomeningocele. (Courtesy of Dr. Patrick McKenna.)

after birth and during infancy and early childhood, there is often a changing pattern seen in the urodynamics of these patients (19–21). It is impossible to make broad generalizations about the patients, but in cases with high thoracic lesions, patients may have an intact sacral reflex arc. Patients with lesions at S1 and below can have normal bladder function, but upper or lower motor lesions involving the bladder and or pelvic floor are also seen. Complete urological evaluations of these infants, including renal ultrasound and voiding cystourethrogram; a full urodynamic assessment is required because it is predictive of future deterioration (19,22–25). Clear evidence exists that starting prophylactic treatment in situations for whom there is high risk for deterioration (uninhibited bladder contraction in association with sphincter dyssynergy) is beneficial in decreasing the likelihood of upper-tract and bladder deterioration (26–28). Management usually involves initiation of clean, intermittent catheterization (CIC) and an anticholinergic medication. The dynamic nature of this disease requires routine surveillance throughout the patient's life, but particularly during periods of rapid linear growth (26,29).

B. Lipomeningocele

The lipomeningocele abnormality is more difficult to identify on physical examination. It is important to have a high level of suspicion and to carefully examine the lower spine because the vast majority of children that have these lesions have an identifiable superficial lesion. The changes occur because of an intradural lipoma. This lesion results in a broad spectrum of disease and presentation (30). Typically during early childhood there are few outward physical abnormalities, and only with complete urodynamic assessment is the effect on the bladder identified (31). The most common urodynamic findings are consistent with an upper motor neuron lesion. Sphincter dyssynergy is less often identified in this group. In older children in whom the diagnosis has not been made earlier, there are often lower extremity neurological changes noted (32). The urodynamic changes in the older group are mixed between detrusor hyperreflexia and detrusor areflexia. The best method to identify these lesions are by magnetic resonance imaging (MRI) and complete urodynamic assessment (33).

C. Sacral Agenesis

The sacral agenesis lesion is even more difficult to identify on physical examination, and often the patients present at an older age when they fail to become continent (34,35). Loss of the lower vertebral bodies can be easily seen on lateral lower plain film of the spine or on a MRI study. Klauber felt that palpation of the coccyx could identify absent vertebral bodies, but radiological confirmation is the best method (36). The patients appear to develop a stable neurological lesion that does not progress with growth and is urodynamically varied (37). Patients may have no sign of denervation, hyperreflexia, areflexia, intact sphincter function, sphincter dyssynergy, and some have absent control over the sphincter (38). A high level of suspicion, radiological confirmation, and complete urodynamics characterizes treatment (34). Specific intervention is based on the identified findings (35).

D. Tethered Cord

Isolated tethered cord is the most difficult lesion to identify in its early stages (21,39,40). It is most commonly seen in patients who have had previous surgery for myelodysplasia and lipomeningocele, but there is a small group of patients who can have isolated tethering of the spinal cord (41,42). Khoury has identified a group of patients with severe bladder dysfunction and refractory incontinence who had occult spinal dysraphism, many without radiographic evidence of a low conus, but improvement after surgical division of the filum and others question the significance of spina bifida occulta with negative MRI findings (43–45). He suggests that the static nature of the MRI may miss a functional tethering that can be identified only with movement. The changes seen in patients with myelodysplasia occur more commonly with growth and are most often characterized by development of un-inhibited contractions and worsening lower extremity bony abnormalities (46–49). These patients are best managed by routine surveillance urodynamics and neurosurgical evalua-tion when significant pattern changes on urodynamics are noted (50).

E. Cerebral Palsy

Cerebral palsy develops most commonly from a serious medical event in the premature in-fant (51). The initiating event is usually infection or anoxia that results in a variable non-progressive brain lesion and varying degrees of muscular disability. Continence is often de-layed in these patients, but ultimately, even with severe disability, most patients gain reasonable continence. Evaluation with urodynamics and invasive studies should be post-poned until the child has reached a level of mental maturity in which continence is expected or development of a urinary tract infection or constipation indicates needed intervention (52). As expected with a disease from variable causes and severity, Decter showed a vari-able urodynamic pattern (53). The primary lesion is an upper motor lesion characterized by uninhibited bladder contractions (54). The mainstay of treatment of these patients is with anticholinergic medication and occasionally clean intermittent catheterization (55).

F. Spinal Cord Injury

Children younger than 16 years of age account for less than 5% of all spinal cord injuries (56). Spinal cord tumors are also rare, but when encountered, can result in injury and neu-rological effects on the sphincter. When spinal injury does occur, the initial effect on the bladder is often urinary retention from spinal shock. The initial management is placement of a Foley catheter followed by institution of clean intermittent catheterization (57). If nor-mal bladder function does not return, full urodynamic assessment is usually postponed for up to 3 months postinjury so the acute spinal changes become stabilized. The most com-mon long-term urodynamic finding in cord trauma is evidence of an upper motor neuron le-sion and sphincter dyssynergia. Institution of anticholinergics, with or without clean inter-mittent catheterization, is the main long-term treatment. Routine screening of the upper tracts with ultrasound and surveillance urodynamics should also be instituted (58).

G. Bladder Exstrophy

Classical exstrophy is a rare lesion characterized by exstrophic bladder, abdominal wall de-fect, epispadias, pelvic diastasis, vesicoureteral reflux, and bilateral inguinal hernias (Fig. 4). The method of reconstruction is based on a staged strategy (59). The first stage involv-ing abdominal wall closure and usually pelvic osteotomy. The epispadias is reconstructed in the next stage, and finally the bladder neck continence mechanism and reflux is corrected in the final phase. Recently, Mitchell has advocated combining the first two stages into one operation soon after birth (60).

Exstrophy reconstruction has led to a greater understanding of sphincter and pelvic floor anatomy and function. Patients with improved pelvic floor reconstruction after os-teotomy have better continence rates (61–63). This is felt to better approximate the pelvic

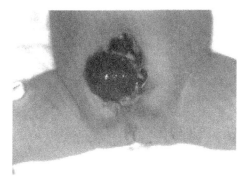

Figure 4 Patient with classic bladder exstrophy. (Courtesy of Dr. Patrick McKenna.)

floor muscle. In addition, the close relation between bladder size and continence has been clearly established. In situations for which capacity is inadequate, bladder augmentation, bladder neck closure, and an alternative site for catheterization is indicated (64).

H. Bilateral Single System Ectopic Ureters

Bilateral single system ectopic ureters is an extremely rare congenital abnormality in girls that results in a combination of problems leading to incontinence and difficult reconstruction (65,66). When both ureters attach ectopically past the bladder neck there is obstruction and dilation of the ureters associated with a high likelihood of renal injury (Fig. 5). It is believed that dilation of the ureter through the bladder neck destroys or prevents normal sphincter muscle development. In addition, the urine bypasses the bladder during development, which results in a small-capacity bladder. Incontinence develops in all cases and the small bladder capacity and lack of muscle at the bladder neck complicate reconstruction. Standard

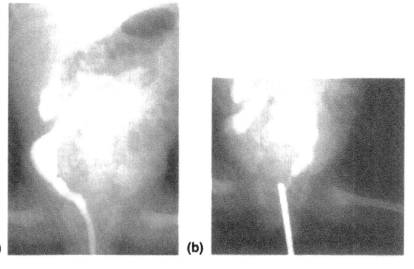

(a)   (b)

Figure 5 (a) Retrograde pyelogram demonstrating ectopic right ureter. (b) Retrograde pyelogram demonstrating ectopic left ureter. (Courtesy of Dr. Patrick McKenna.)

Young–Dee–Leadbetter's bladder neck reconstruction fails because of the lack of bladder neck muscle and inadequate bladder capacity. Bladder augmentation, bladder neck closure, and an alternative site for catheterization, using the Mitroffanoff principle is a proved method of reconstruction (67). Recently, the Pippi Salle bladder neck reconstruction with bladder augmentation has also been successfully used for this rare abnormality (65).

I. Posterior Urethral Valves

Posterior urethral valves remains the most common cause of bladder outlet obstruction in the newborn period. Currently, it is almost always identified antenatally (Fig. 6). The antenatal identification has resulted in an opportunity to intervene during pregnancy in severe cases and accomplish early evaluation and treatment before infection after birth. Whether this advantage will result in better patient outcomes is yet to be determined. The type I posterior urethral valve, described by Young et al. (68), is the most common type of valve identified. It radiates from the posterior edge of the verumontanum to the membranous urethra. Modern endoscopic equipment makes primary valve ablation the most frequent form of treatment (69,70). Valve patients have a wide spectrum of disease. In the less severe forms it may not present until the patient is much older (71). The late presentation of incontinence and recurrent urinary tract infections in older male patients may represent the late presentation, which is why a voiding cystourethrogram should be obtained in male patients with development of these symptoms. When patients with known valve disease develop incontinence later in life, it is almost always secondary to bladder dysfunction, rather than to injury to the bladder neck or sphincter from a previous valve ablation (72–74). It is crucial to

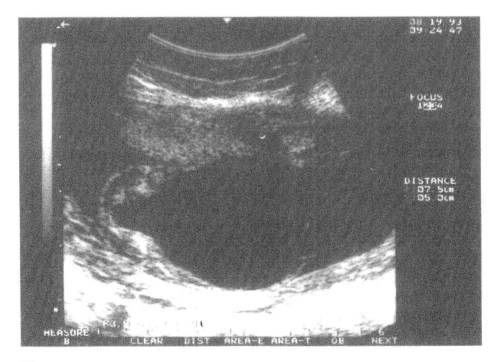

Figure 6 Antenatal ultrasound in third trimester demonstrating classic "keyhole" abnormality indicative of PUV. (Courtesy of Dr. Patrick McKenna.)

follow patients with severe valve disease through adolescence because there is the possibility of bladder decompensation that may result in upper tract injury. When the nadir creatinine falls below 0.8 mg/dL after treatment of severe valve disease, it is unlikely those patients will develop renal failure at a later date. The exception is patients who are lost to follow-up and have later unsuspected bladder dysfunction and new renal injury from high-pressure reflux and infection (75).

When bladder injury is severe and patients develop a valve bladder with incontinence and upper tract deterioration, clean intermittent catheterization and anticholinergic medication is required (76,77). Patients with severe valve disease are one of the most difficult subgroups of patients to train to do clean intermittent catheterization because they have full sensation and a high bladder neck that makes CIC more difficult. When medical therapy fails, bladder augmentation is indicated. In severe cases of posterior urethral valves the body often sacrifices one upper tract system to protect the remaining system. This phenomenon has come to be known as the vesicoureteral reflux dysplasia syndrome (VRDS) (78). Physicians have made use of this phenomenon by resisting the urge to remove the dilated ureter and nonfunctioning kidney until it is certain that it is not needed for an autoaugmentation of the bladder. Ureter has been shown to be the best bladder augmentation tissue (79,80).

J. Anal Rectal Malformations

Anal rectal malformations represent rare congenital lesions of the cloaca. These malformations are important lesions in relation to the urethral sphincter and pelvic floor because of the often associated neurological abnormalities leading to a neurogenic bladder. There is also a high incidence of other congenital genitourinary abnormalities associated with these malformations. There have been multiple classification systems, but none have been widely used. From a urological prospective the simple distinction of "high," "intermediate," or "low" anal rectal lesions is probably sufficient. Low lesions being ones that occur inferior to the levator muscles. High lesions occur superior to the levator muscles and intermediate ones occur in between (Fig. 7). From a clinical point of view, most intermediate lesions are

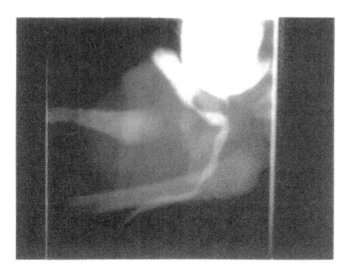

Figure 7 Patient with high level imperforate anus and communicating urethrorectal fistula. (Courtesy of Dr. Michael Bourque.)

treated similar to high lesions. The surgical correction of these malformations is most often by a technique repopularized by de Vries and Pena using the posterior sagittal approach (81). Associated urological abnormalities occur in up to 20% of patients with low lesions and up to 60% of patients with high lesions (46,82). The most common findings are vesicoureteral reflux, neurogenic bladder, renal agenesis, renal dysplasia, and cryptorchidism. It is not surprising that there is a high incidence of neurogenic bladder because of the likely association of vertebral abnormalities with anal rectal malformations. They occur in as many as 50% of the patients (46). The main anatomical finding in patients with vertebral abnormalities is a tethered cord. Only recently has this association been identified and its associated high incidence of neurogenic bladder and dysfunctional pelvic floor. Patients with anal rectal malformations should be screened urodynamically, especially if they have high lesions or spinal abnormalities.

IV. PATIENT EVALUATION

A. History

The urodynamic assessment of the pediatric or neonatal patient should commence with an in-depth history focusing on areas that may indicate an occult underlying pathological lesion. The antenatal period, past surgical history, neurological history, including the presence of spinal cord lesion, developmental history, and urinary and bowel history, all should be assessed during the initial patient evaluation. Antenatally, genitourinary abnormalities, specifically hydronephrosis, an enlarged bladder, or an open spinal cord defect should be investigated. Past surgical history may include detethering procedures, ventriculoperitoneal shunts, and urinary or bowel diversions. The neurological history should include a global assessment of motor and sensory function by assessing gait, coordination, and muscle strength. An evaluation of developmental milestones, such as urinary and bowel control, ambulation, present education level, sexual history, functional needs such as a wheelchair or braces, should be obtained. The urinary history should assess the onset of urinary control, technique used to facilitate bowel emptying, urinary frequency, presence of nocturnal or diurnal enuresis, stress urinary incontinence, weakness of urinary stream, urgency, hematuria, dysuria, a history of urinary infections, and the presence and grade of vesicoureteral reflux, hydronephrosis, and posterior urethral valves. The classic Vincent's curtsey may be elicited, which is a maneuver employed by children to prevent urinary incontinence by compressing the perineum with their heel while performing a curtsey maneuver (Fig. 8) (83). Catharization schedule, size of catheters, amount with each catheterization, person who catheterizes (parent or child), and presence of any aberrations from normal routine should be investigated in children who manage their bladder with clean intermittent catheterization. When specifically dealing with a child with a spinal dysraphism, questions should be directed at change in urinary symptoms and occurrence of urinary tract infection, which may indicate the presence of cord retethering and accompanying lower tract changes that place the upper tract at risk for renal deterioration. The medical history should document dosage and frequency of medications. A bowel history should assess the normal bowel pattern; the bowel regimen used to maintain bowel pattern, including stool softeners, laxatives, or enemas; the presence and frequency of encopresis and fecal incontinence; and the date of last anometric study if indicated. A nursing assessment sheet with the aforementioned questions should be completed at the initiation of an urodynamic assessment with any child (84,85) (Fig. 9).

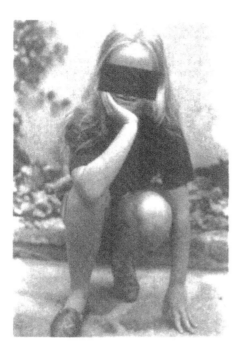

Figure 8   Patient demonstrating Vincent's curtsey maneuver with heel compressing perineum to prevent incontinence. (From Ref. 84.)

B.   Physical Examination

Similar to the history, the physical examination should focus on areas that may reveal occult underlying pathology. The neurological assessment of the child should include two-point discrimination of all extremities, assessment of gross motor strength in both upper and lower extremities, deep tendon reflexes (specifically the Achilles tendon [S1–S2]) and bulbocavernosal reflex (S2–S4). The bulbocavernosal reflex is performed by stimulation of the sacral afferents through pinching the glans penis or clitoris or gentle manipulation of an indwelling Foley catheter while placing a finger at the anal sphincter to assess its contraction. The reflex may be absent in neurologically intact individuals, and the usefulness of the test is optimized with a positive reflex, indicating an intact sacral arc. The abdominal examination should investigate for the presence of a mass, which may represent a full bladder, or other masses indicative of upper tract urinary obstruction. The back, specifically, the sacral region should be assessed for the presence of a dimple, hair patch, or underlying lipoma, suggestive of an occult spinal dysraphism (86).

C.   Urodynamics and Videourodynamics

Urodynamics in the pediatric population is quite different from that of the adult population because of the level of maturity of the patient population. The child is typically extremely anxious; thus, the evaluation should be performed in a warm, quiet setting. Empiric anxiolytics should be avoided because they may masquerade an abnormality. Urodynamics is a diagnostic modality used by the urologist to identify pathology of the lower urinary tract during urinary storage or voiding. Although multiple factors may contribute to voiding dysfunction, preservation of renal function is the foremost goal in managing the neurogenic

Urology Nursing History

I. Background Information

Mother's Name: _____   Child lives with:_____
Father's Name: _____   Informant: _____

Comments family/social situation/stressors:

II. Pregnancy & Delivery History

Problems during pregnancy? (Bleeding, rash, diabetes, injury, elevated blood pressure, infection, etc.):

Medications taken during pregnancy: _____
Drug/Alcohol use during pregnancy? yes ☐, no ☐
Birth Weight: lb.   oz, Weeks gestation:_____ Delivered by C-section: ☐   Vaginally: ☐

III. Health History

Current Medications & dosage:

Allergies: Reaction:

Previous Hospitalizations/Surgeries:

History of:
Seizures ☐ (Type _____ Frequency _____ . Date last seizure _____)
Diabetes ☐, Myelo/lipomeningocele ☐ (Level_____), Tethered cord ☐ Hydrocephalus ☐,
CP ☐, SCI ☐ (Level _____), Autonomic dysreflexia, ☐, TBI ☐, ADD ☐, Poor weight gain ☐,
Failure to thrive ☐, Pulmonary problems ☐ (describe:_____),
Cardiac problems ☐ (describe: _____)
(Name of Cardiologist/Pulmonologist_____)
OTHER:_____
_____

Family History of: Myelomeningocele ☐, Urinary tract surgery ☐, UTIs ☐,
Bowel/Bladder problems ☐ (describe_____)
OTHER: _____
_____

IV. Developmental History

Present grade in school _____, Special needs classes: yes ☐, no ☐, first walked at age _____
Uses: crutches ☐, braces ☐, wheelchair ☐. menses started ☐, LMP _____,
sexually active ☐
Notes:

MB
9/96

Figure 9 Urological nursing-screening medical history sheet used at Connecticut Children's Medical Center. (Courtesy of Dr. Patrick McKenna.)

bladder. The urodynamic assessment involves a filling and voiding assessment with simultaneous electromyographic recording of urinary sphincter, with or without videofluoroscopy.

1. Cystometrogram

During the filling phase, the cystometrogram (CMG) measures the bladder pressure during filling (Fig. 10). The filling rate in children is quite different from that of adults and is dependent on patient age. The filling phase of urodynamics measures the sensory component

V. Urinary & Bowel History

History of: Frequent urination ☐, Infrequent urination ☐ (# of voids/day _____),

Night time incontinence ☐ (frequency_____)

Daytime incontinence ☐ (frequency_____)

Awakening at night to urinate ☐ (frequency _____)

Wetting with increased activity ☐, with laughing ☐, with coughing/sneezing ☐,

Dribbling urine ☐, Urgency ☐, Trouble starting urination ☐, Intermittent stream ☐, weak stream ☐,

bloody urine ☐, painful urination ☐ (describe _____) UTIs ☐ (Last one _____),

Reflux ☐ (grade _____, L/R/B), Hydronephrosis ☐ (grade _____ L/R/B),

Posterior urethral valves ☐

OTHER:

_____

_____

_____

Cath schedule _____, consistent ☐ inconstant ☐ Type & size of cath _____

Who performs catheterization? Parent(s) ☐ Child ☐ Other ☐ _____

Wet between catheterizations? yes ☐ no ☐ (describe frequency/amount_____

_____)

If wet between caths, was there ever a time of complete dryness? yes ☐, no ☐. (When? _____)

Problems with catheterization? _____

Wears: Diaper day & night ☐, night only ☐, day only ☐ "Pull up" day & night ☐, night only ☐, day

only ☐ Sanitary napkin day & night ☐, night only ☐, day only ☐ Incontinence pads day & night ☐,

night only ☐, day only ☐ Primarily due to Bowel incontinence ☐ Bladder incontinence ☐, Both ☐

Toilet trained?: yes ☐ no ☐ never attempted ☐

Age toilet training completed for bladder _____   Age toilet training completed for bowel _____

If incontinent now, ever a period of complete control? yes ☐ no ☐ (When?_____)

Normal bowel pattern: _____

Bowel program? yes ☐, no ☐ Describe:_____

_____

History of : Staining/soiling of underpants with stool ☐ (frequency _____)

Incontinence of stool ☐ (frequency _____), constipation ☐, diarrhea ☐,

use of suppositories ☐, enemas ☐, stool softeners ☐, laxatives ☐, other ☐ (type _____)

special diet ☐ (type _____)

Last urodynamics study _____   Last manometric study _____

VI. Homecare

Copy of homecare instructions given to _____. Reviewed by _____

Caregiver verbalizes an understanding of instructions☐   Released to home with _____

NOTES:

Figure 9 continued

of voiding cycle. Decreased bladder capacity may be due to urgency and likewise increased bladder compliance results from sensory denervation such as diabetes or tabes dorsalis. In the neonate, a 5-Fr feeding tube and warm normal saline infused at a rate of 5 mL/min is appropriate, in a young child a 7-Fr catheter and 10 mL/min is fairly standard, and in older children a 10-Fr catheter and 20 mL/min is routine. The estimated bladder capacity can be determined by the formula initially introduced by Koff: Age + 2 × 30 = bladder capacity in ounces (87). Another formula to determine the correct rate is to instill 10% of the estimated bladder capacity per minute (88). Houle evaluated 923 pediatric urodynamic evaluations and derived a formula to measure minimal total bladder capacity, which is 16(age) + 70 mL (89,90). It is extremely important to commence the study with the patient and family's full

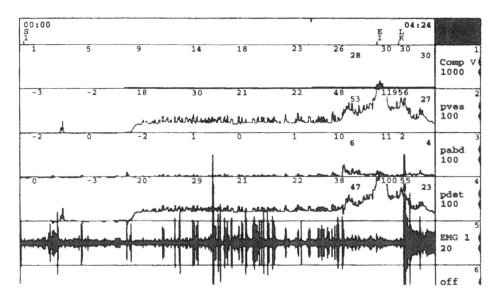

Figure 10   Filling phase of urodynamic assessment with detrusor, vesical, and abdominal pressure profile. (Courtesy of Dr. Patrick McKenna.)

understanding of the urodynamic setup and exactly what the urodynamic information will provide in the care of their child. The examining room should be a warm and quiet place.

The formal cystometrogram consist of four phases: The first phase involves a rapid increase in bladder pressure. The second phase consists of rapid filling at a static bladder pressure. The third phase involves a second increase in bladder pressure. The fourth phase involves the initiation of voluntary voiding (91). A dual lumen catheter is used to measure bladder pressure and a triple lumen catheter can measure the functional urethral length as well. With the addition of a rectal balloon catheter, abdominal pressure can be inferred and used to calculate detrusor pressure. The detrusor pressure is a crucial component of the urodynamic evaluation in managing a child with a neurogenic bladder. The detrusor pressure is the product of vesicle pressure—abdominal pressure. In addition to the abdominal, vesicle, and detrusor pressure, several variables can be used to identify underlying voiding dysfunction abnormalities.

The bladder compliance is measured by observing the change in bladder pressure as bladder volume increases. Normal compliance should be less than 10 cmH$_2$O during the tonus phase (second) of bladder filling (92). Conditions associated with decreased compliance place the upper tracts at risk for deterioration. In the presence of a functional urethral sphincter, elevated detrusor pressure is transmitted directly to the upper tracts. Factors that lead to decreased bladder compliance include fibrosis, detrusor hypertrophy, or neuroplasitic changes secondary dysfunctional pelvic floor syndrome (93). In cases of spinal shock or autonomic neurogenic bladder, increased bladder compliance, combined with decreased urine flow, creates a functional obstructive pattern on urodynamic evaluations (91).

The presence of bladder contractions, may be initiated or uninhibited. An initiated bladder contraction may occur with straining or coughing. Alternatively, with decreased bladder compliance uninhibited bladder contractions occur in response to elevated detrusor pressure. The uninhibited contractions may overcome urethral pressure and produce clinical urinary incontinence.

2. Leak Point Pressure

The leak point pressure is used to monitor the risk of upper tract deterioration and urinary continence. The *detrusor leak point pressure* (DLPP) is defined as the amount of detrusor pressure required to cause urinary leakage. McGuire eloquently demonstrated that detrusor leak point pressures greater than 40 cmH$_2$O place the upper tracts at significant risk of deterioration (22). The Valsalva leak point pressure (VLPP) is used to identify anatomical stress urinary incontinence. The VLPP records the amount of abdominal pressure required to produce urinary leakage. A VLPP of 90 cmH$_2$O indicates anatomical stress incontinence and a VLPP of less than 60 cmH$_2$O indicates intrinsic sphincter deficiency. The VLPP normally should be infinite, that is abdominal straining should not generate urinary leakage (94). The VLPP is used to develop a continence program for patients with spinal dysraphisms.

3. Electromyography

Electromyography (EMG) can be used to assess voiding dysfunction and monitor the potential risk of upper tract deterioration. Electromyography of the external sphincter can be performed accurately with external patch electrodes (95). The motor end plate action potential of the external sphincter is recorded by the EMG electrodes; it is first initiated in the anterior horn of the spinal cord (96). The postsynaptic sympathetic receptor is adrenergic, and the neurotransmitter is norepinephrine (91,97). The activity of the pelvic floor and external sphincter are recorded with perineal electrodes placed at the 3- and 9-o'clock positions on the perineum. Additionally, abdominal patch, perineal (male) and paraurethral (female) can be used to record pelvic floor activity (98–100). Normally, the EMG activity should increase steadily with bladder filling and on initiation of voiding, a silence of EMG activity should occur (99,101). Abnormalities of sphincter activity in children with spinal cord lesions have been described by McGuire and include three types of detrusor sphincter dyssynergia (DSD): type I involves the onset of increased EMG activity with the initiation of voiding; type II involves intermittent inappropriate contraction of the external sphincter during voiding, which causes a reflex inhibition of detrusor contraction; type III involves inappropriate relaxation of sphincteric activity during bladder filling which results in incontinence (102). Pseudodyssynergia reveals a similar EMG finding and occurs with neurologically intact patients who demonstrate an increase in pelvic floor activity with voiding.

4. Urethral Pressure Profile

The primary focus of this chapter is the urethral sphincter, and its functional length is measured by the urethral pressure profilometry (UPP) (Fig. 11). First described in 1969, the total resistance is measured by the pressure required to maintain flow through the side lumen of a catheter placed in the urethra. The UPP is performed with the bladder empty and, therefore, is a static UPP. Some feel that the intraurethral resistance is dynamic, and changes with bladder capacity and compliance, and that the static UPP fails to take these factors into consideration. The total resistance is the sum of several factors, including the smooth and skeletal muscle composing the urethral sphincter, as well as the elastic properties of the connective tissue of the urethral lumen (103). Nonetheless, the static UPP is procedure of choice to measure functional urethral length. Three techniques are available to record this information; perfusion urethral pressure profile, balloon catheter technique, and the catheter tip transducer (103).

The perfusion urethral pressure profile is performed by placing a triple-lumen catheter into the bladder and infusing saline at 2 mL/min as the catheter is withdrawn at 2 mm/sec (104). The catheter's side lumen records the pressure required to maintain flow intra-

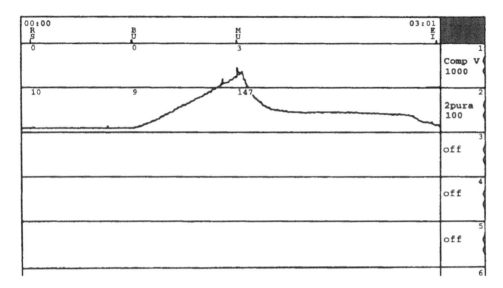

Figure 11 Urethral pressure profile demonstrating a maximal urethral pressure of 147 cmH₂O. (Courtesy of Dr. Patrick McKenna.)

urethrally. The recorded pressure is mapped over the length of urethra and defines the functional urethral length. The International Continence Society developed standard nomenclature; the maximal urethral pressure, maximum urethral closing pressure (maximum urethral pressure—bladder pressure), and the functional urethral length. The female maximal urethral pressure is in the midurethra and the male maximal urethral pressure is at the level of the membranous urethra (91). Additionally, a UPP can be performed with CO_2 but requires 150 mL/min to record an accurate study. The balloon catheter system is less popular technique, but employs a closed system consisting of plastic balloons along the side of the catheter that record urethral pressure. The system is technically demanding and requires frequent calibration. Finally, the catheter tip transducer system relies on transducers that are mounted on the end of the catheter. Simultaneous vesical and urethral pressure can be recorded in addition to a voiding urethral pressure. The transducer system is expensive.

5. Videourodynamics

Videourodynamics add a dynamic component to the urethral profilometry and may identify pathological factors amenable to treatment (105,106). With the addition of fluoroscopy to the urodynamic assessment, genuine stress incontinence, with hypermobility, can be differentiated from intrinsic sphincter deficiency. In the pediatric population, dilation of the proximal urethra, coupled with increased EMG activity during detrusor contractions indicative of detrusor sphincter dyssynergia, can be seen during the fluoroscopic assessment of voiding (107). In addition, lower tract pathology such as vesicoureteral reflux can be documented. Although infrequently used in patients with dysfunctional voiding, some authors advocate its use (108). The voiding phase of the urodynamic assessment commences with a decrease in EMG-recorded activity, indicating relaxation of the external sphincter (109). The child should be allowed to void in a quiet warm environment devoid of excessive external stimuli. Abnormalities of voiding are either secondary to an abnormal bladder or to an abnormal outlet (increased pelvic floor activity versus anatomical obstruction) (103). Normal voiding pressures for boys are 55–80 cmH₂O and for girls 30–65 cmH₂O (101).

The simultaneous measurement of the detrusor and abdominal pressures in context of the urine flow should isolate the pathology to one of these two areas. For example, decreased flow with increased abdominal pressure and increased detrusor pressure with decreased compliance indicate bladder outlet obstruction. The information gained from EMG electrodes will isolate the pathology to increased pelvic floor activity versus an anatomical obstruction. In addition, a patient with DSD may display detrusor hyperreflexia with uninhibited detrusor contractions during the filling phase of the urodynamic assessment. An example of bladder pathology is demonstrated by a low flow, increased detrusor compliance with a low detrusor pressure, increased abdominal pressure, and silent EMG activity. This clinical picture is similar to the patient with a sensory neurogenic bladder secondary to diabetes.

6. Indications for Urodynamic Studies

In the pediatric population, the indications for formal urodynamics include patients with spinal dysraphisms (58), spinal cord injury patients (56), cerebral palsy patients with voiding dysfunction (54,110), patients with sacral agenesis, imperforate anus patients, patients with suspicious voiding history, infants with urinary tract infections (111–113), and in select refractory cases, diurnal enuresis (114).

Allen and Bright first identified a dyssynergic voiding pattern in children with symptoms of dysfunctional voiding and felt that this may represent a transitional phase of voiding (115). Bauer utilized urodynamics to classify children with dysfunctional voiding into four distinct groups: small-capacity hypertonic bladder, detrusor hyperreflexia, lazy bladder syndrome, and Hinman's syndrome (nonneurogenic neurogenic bladder). In these neurologically intact individuals he performed formal urodynamics in an effort to develop a treatment plan based on the interaction of the bladder and external sphincter. The usefulness of urodynamics resides in its ability to monitor the bladder response to medical therapy (111). Likewise, Mayo and Burns further defined a population with pure detrusor instability who benefit from anticholinergic therapy in the absence of dysfunctional voiding (116). Recent studies involving patients with voiding dysfunction indicate that most of these patients can be managed successfully without a formal urodynamic assessment (93).

Urodynamics are a standard means to assess the risk of upper tract deterioration in patients with spinal cord dysraphism, the most common cause of neurogenic bladder in children. In managing newborns with neurogenic bladders secondary to myelomeningocele, Bauer has identified three distinctive voiding patterns that occur as a result of combined bladder and external sphincter interaction: synergic, dyssynergic with and without detrusor hypertonicity, and complete denervation (19).

A review of urodynamics in the patient with the neurogenic bladder should be performed in the context of assessing the possibility of cord tethering, the risk of upper tract deterioration, and the development of a continence program. The first manifestation of spinal cord retethering may be the sudden onset of detrusor sphincter dyssynergia (19,117, 118). An assessment of upper tract deterioration is made through a critical review of the urodynamic assessment. If the CMG reveals a compliant bladder, then the upper tracts are protected. If the CMG reveals a noncompliant bladder with uninhibited contractions and the UPP reveals an elevated urethral pressure greater than detrusor pressure, then upper tracts are at risk for deterioration. Children with spinal dysraphisms are at risk of excoriation of skin from long-term incontinence. The VLPP coupled with the UPP can identify the presence of stress incontinence, define the urethral anatomy and facilitate a treatment program.

D. Other Diagnostic Tools

Scintigraphic evaluation of urine flow has been evaluated in one center and may have a future role as a means of assessing voiding dysfunction (119).

1. Uroflow–EMG

The measurement of the urine flow curve combined with EMG activity of the pelvic floor provides a valuable diagnostic tool for the urologist. To assure a valid study, the patient should void with a full bladder and is instructed to try and let the pelvic floor muscles relax as they try to urinate (120). After completion of urination, a bladder scan is performed to assess the postvoid residual urine volume. Normally, the postvoid residual volume in children is less than 5 mL. The uroflow curve varies with sex and age, but in general, a bell-shaped curve exist for most boys and girls (121). In children with voiding dysfunction, a noninvasive assessment of bladder function can be recorded with a uroflow–surface EMG with measurement of postvoid residual urine by a bladder scan (95). Patients with a history suggestive of dysfunctional voiding should be screened properly to rule out anatomical abnormalities with a voiding cystourethrogram (VCUG) and renal ultrasound. Findings on VCUG suggestive of dysfunctional voiding include pelvic floor muscle contraction during voiding, which produces the classic spinning top deformity, the presence of vesicoureteral reflux, as well as constipation (4,93). In addition, a screening uroflow should be performed to document the presence of suspected pseudodyssynergia. The setup for a uroflow involves the measurement of a flow curve with simultaneous recording of pelvic floor activity. EMG patches are placed on the perineum a technique described by Maziels (122). Four main uroflow–EMG patterns have been identified in children with dysfunctional pelvic floor syndrome (Fig. 12): flattened flow pattern, increased pelvic floor activity, increased postvoid residual; a flattered flow pattern, increased pelvic floor activity, and decreased postvoid residual; a staccato flow pattern, increased pelvic floor activity and increase postvoid residual; and a staccato flow pattern, increased pelvic floor activity and decreased postvoid residual. In a population of patients with voiding dysfunction, only a few patients demonstrated the classic staccato flow pattern (93). In addition to a screening tool, the uroflow can be used to document improvement during rehabilitation of the pelvic floor in children with dysfunctional voiding (93,122,123). The abnormal flow pattern produced by children with dysfunctional voiding may represent a transitional period of voiding control (115).

2. Bowel Manometrics

A clear association exists between constipation, voiding dysfunction, and vesicoureteral reflux (3,4). The urologist may work in concert with other specialist in evaluation of the bowel and should be familiar with bowel manometrics. An assessment of bowel manometrics, specifically anorectal manometrics, may be indicated to formulate an appropriate treatment program for patients with chronic constipation and voiding dysfunction. Anorectal manometrics have been used to evaluate the anal sphincter in children with chronic constipation and has identified paradoxical contraction of the external anal sphincter and a dilated low-tonicity rectal vault as two main abnormalities that may represent the pathogenesis of chronic constipation and encopresis (124,125). Although used to evaluate many children with chronic constipation, little evidence exist to correlate subjective symptoms and objective findings of the manometrics. However, the identification of a population of children who contract the anal sphincter during defecation appears to correlate with increasing subjective symptoms of constipation (126). Similar to patients with dysfunctional voiding, this

Flow Report

Q max: 25 mL/sec   T to Max: 6 sec   T Flow: 17 sec   Volume 286 mL
Q ave: 17 mL/sec   T Void: 17 sec   PVR: .44 mL

Position: . . . . . .   Pattern: continuous   Conclusion: . . . .

Comments:

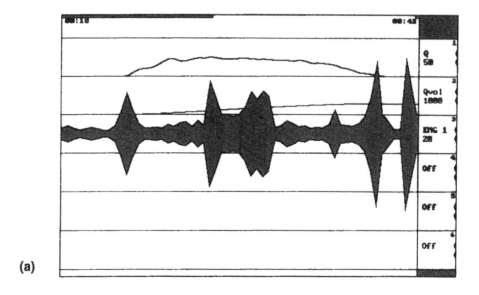

(a)

Flow Report

Q max: 27 mL/sec   T to Max: 4 sec   T Flow: 11 sec   Volume 172 mL
Q ave: 16 mL/sec   T Void: 11 sec   PVR: 0 mL

Position: sitting   Pattern: continuous   Conclusion: . . . .

Comments:

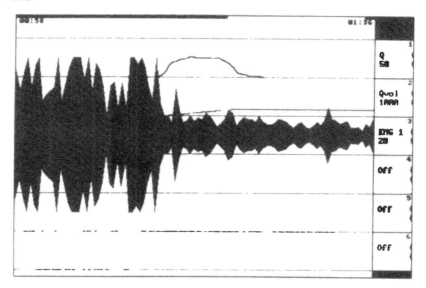

(b)

Figure 12 (a) Uroflow-EMG demonstrating flattened flow pattern, increased pelvic floor activity and increased postvoid residual. (b) Uroflow-EMG demonstrating flattened flow pattern, increased pelvic floor activity and no postvoid residual. (c) Uroflow-EMG demonstrating staccato flow pattern, increased pelvic floor activity, and increased postvoid residual. (d) Uroflow-EMG demonstrating staccato flow pattern, increased pelvic floor activity, and no postvoid residual. (Courtesy of Dr. Patrick McKenna.)

Flow Report

Q max:	21 mL/sec	T to Max: 40 sec	T Flow:	37 sec	Volume	291 mL
Q ave:	8 mL/sec		T Void:	44 sec	PVR:	191 mL

Position: sitting   Pattern: intermittent   Conclusion: . . . .

Comments:

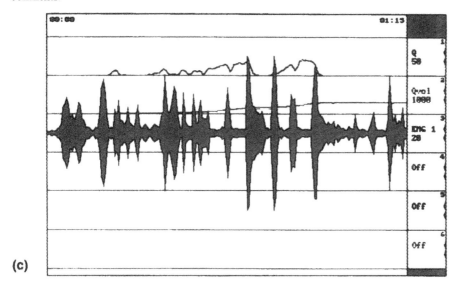

(c)

Flow Report

Q max:	12 mL/sec	T to Max: 3 sec	T Flow:	12 sec	Volume	75 mL
Q ave:	6 mL/sec		T Void:	12 sec	PVR:	7 mL

Position: sitting   Pattern: continuous   Conclusion: . . . .

Comments:

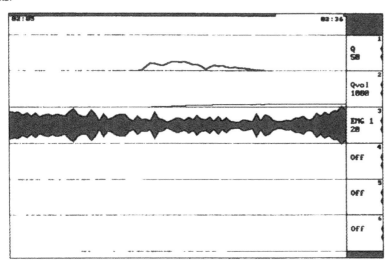

(d)

Figure 12 continued

cohort of patients may benefit from pelvic floor rehabilitation directed at identification and relaxation of the pelvic floor (127).

The manometric device is a hydraulic infusion system with three infusion ports spaced at 6, 7, and 9 cm from the tip of the tube. The pressure of each port is calibrated against a mercury column. The catheter is inserted into the anus until all three ports are inserted. The patient is asked to defecate, and the catheter and rectal and anal sphincter pressure are recorded. In addition, an assessment of rectal vault capacity is recorded by inflation of the proximal port with up to 250 cc of air (126).

V. DYSFUNCTIONAL VOIDING, URINARY TRACT INFECTIONS, AND VESICOURETERAL REFLUX

Several authors have demonstrated the association between diurnal enuresis, urinary urgency, urinary frequency, constipation, urinary tract infections, and vesicoureteral reflux (1,4,26,43,115,128–130,132,134). Currently, several theories exist to explain this association. Bauer initially focused his evaluation and subsequent medical treatment of these patients based on his interpretation of the urodynamic findings (111). A decrease in the incidence of breakthrough urinary tract infections and increased resolution of vesicoureteral reflux has been demonstrated with a urodynamic-directed medical program (128). The increased intravesical pressure, created by the functional obstruction, that develops from contraction of the pelvic floor (external sphincter) with voiding creates increased filling pressures that may result in the development of vesicoureteral reflux (130). The classic spinning top deformity will be present in a significant number of patients as well (Fig. 13). Recently, dysfunctional bowel evacuation and subsequent fecal retention has been described to be the key component in the pathogenesis of dysfunctional voiding and may have a significant influence on the natural history of children with vesicoureteral reflux when treated appropriately (4). Unfortunately, there is no literature to support the pathophysiological association between fecal retention, dysfunctional voiding, vesicoureteral reflux, and the development

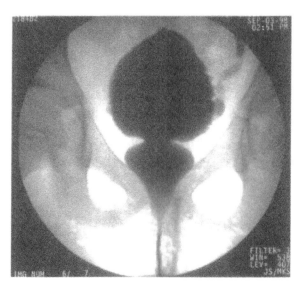

Figure 13 Spinning top deformity and grade 2 vesicoureteral reflux demonstrating on voiding cystourethrogram. (Courtesy of Dr. Patrick McKenna.)

of urinary tract infections. A new theory, developed by McKenna, formulates that neural plastic changes are created by long-standing pelvic floor dysfunction. Three abnormal patterns exist, the most common being chronic pelvic floor dysfunction that results in paradoxical sphincter contraction with voiding. Pelvic floor laxity exists in a minority of pediatric patients but is fairly common in the geriatric population. Finally, inappropriate stimulation of the guarding reflex results in inhibition of appropriate detrussor contractions in a third population of patients. This neuroplasticity causes collateral affects on other organs, such as the bladder and bowel, through an unidentified neurotrophic factor, perhaps nerve growth factor. This theory more clearly explains the symptoms of bowel and bladder that patients with dysfunctional voiding commonly manifest (93).

The development of urinary tract infections is a common presentation for children with dysfunctional voiding. Bacteria gain access to bladder through an ascending route from fecal contamination of the perineum. Host and bacterial factors predispose to recurrent infections. A majority of children with dysfunctional voiding have been described to carry an elevated postvoid residual urine volume (93). These findings are contrary to the common practice of indiscriminate use of anticholinergic therapy for children with dysfunctional voiding (133). The host resistance factors include the bladder's ability to wash out pathogens with each void. Therefore, patients should be instructed to stay well hydrated, void with a strong stream, and void to completion. The bacterial factors include specific *Escherichia coli* which manifest fibrae that enable its attachment to bladder mucosa (136). Treatment plans should incorporate programs that relax the pelvic floor and not the bladder, which will allow efficient synergistic voiding.

A.   Nonneurogenic Neurogenic Bladder

Hinman's syndrome, as it is more commonly known, probably represents the severest form of external sphincter and pelvic floor dysfunction (67,137–141). The most common presentation includes patients with a symptom complex including nocturnal enuresis, diurnal enuresis, constipation, encopresis, urinary tract infection, and upper urinary tract dilation (Fig. 14). Thought initially to be an acquired illness of older children in socially stressed situations, more recently it has been identified in early infancy (67). This has brought into question whether it truly represents an acquired abnormality. The syndrome primarily affects males, and its diagnosis is based on excluding other anatomical causes, such as posterior urethral valves and a tethered cord.

Hinman, for whom the syndrome is named, emphasized the psychological factors associated with the syndrome; however, other reports have not found these factors in even the majority of patients (138,142). The theoretical cause for the sphincter and pelvic floor dysfunction has been thought to be the result of uninhibited bladder contraction associated with chronic conscious contraction of the sphincter to block incontinence (140). Although accepted by multiple authors, this theory fails to completely account for the associated bowel dysfunction seen in most patients and the cases that have been identified in infancy for which continence is not an issue. Urodynamic evaluation of the older patients with this syndrome has shown a mixed picture with some controversy. Most patients have evidence of sphincter contraction associated with increase bladder pressure that appears to be an uninhibited contraction (115,143–146). Hanna noted that it appeared the sphincter contraction may actually occur before the bladder pressure elevation, and speculated that the bladder pressure rise may be the result of sphincter contraction, rather than the sphincter contraction as the result of an uninhibited bladder contraction (147).

Treatment of nonneurogenic neurogenic bladder has centered on a combination of

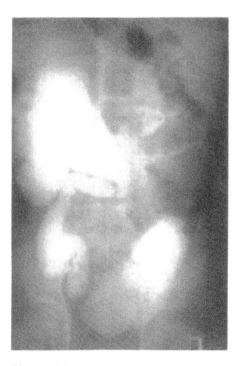

Figure 14 Voiding cystourethrogram demonstrating bilateral grade 5 vesicoureteral reflux and a neurogenic bladder in a patient with Hinmann's syndrome. (Courtesy of Dr. Patrick McKenna.)

voiding retraining, biofeedback, anticholinergic medications, hypnosis, psychotherapy, management of constipation, antibiotics, and clean intermittent catheterization (Masek 1985). Surgical intervention on the bladder neck has proved ineffective and is seldom indicated. Correction of the voiding dysfunction is indicated before surgical correction of associated problems, such as reflux.

B. Constipation and Encopresis

The association of urinary tract infections, dysfunctional voiding, abnormalities of the upper urinary tract, and constipation is a recognized entity (1,135,148–151). Recently, Koff has proposed that correction of constipation may have a dramatic effect on the natural history of children with dysfunctional voiding and vesicoureteral reflux (4). The underlying etiology of constipation in children is most commonly voluntary functional fecal retention; in a subset of patients paradoxical contraction of the external sphincter with defecation occurs and produces fecal retention. This form of functional constipation likely coexists with dysfunctional voiding in patients who are typically evaluated in the urological community and likely results from dysfunctional pelvic floor syndrome (93). Several observations have been made in children with chronic constipation, including hypertrophy of the external and internal sphincters (152) and an alteration in the sensory afferent loop from the rectum (153).

1.   Definition of Constipation

A single definition of constipation does not exist; however, aberrations of stool frequency, consistency, and size, all are components that occur with its diagnosis. An agreed-on normal defecation schedule in infants is four stools per day during the first week, which decreases to about two stools a day at 2 days of age, and decreases furthermore to about one stool per day at 4 days of age (154–157). Further definitions include the passage of firm stools that may produce significant discomfort (158). Encopresis is an accepted term used to describe fecal soiling and the passage of liquid-like stools, which commonly occurs in association with constipation and a result of fecal impaction after the age of 4 years (159,160).

2. Evaluation

The normal defecation process involves a complex synergistic relations between the rectum, the anus, internal sphincter reflex relaxation, and volitional control of the external sphincter (161). The involuntary and voluntary reflexes respond to either luminal pressure sensors in the rectum and stimulation of anoderm receptors in the anus (162). Up to 30% of initial evaluations by the pediatric gastroenterologist will be for constipation or encopresis and involves an imbalance of the variables involved in the normal defecation (158–160,163).

The evaluation of constipation or encopresis should be performed in context of an outline of functional or organic etiological factors. The organic factors include neurological (occult spinal dysraphism, spinal cord trauma), endocrinological (hypothyroidism, hypercalcemia, hypokalemia, diabetes), pharmacological (codeine, lead poisoning, psychotrophics, laxative abuse), and congenital (Hirschbrung's, anal stenosis, anterior anus placement) (164). The functional factors include fecal retention syndrome, prolonged use of diapers, the grunting baby syndrome, and infant dyschesia (158).

The diagnostic modalities employed in the evaluation of abnormalities of defecation are directed at presenting symptoms at initial evaluation. The history should evaluate the size, frequency, and consistency of bowel movements. The age of toilet training, hydration, and fiber intake assessment, medications, and family history should be recorded. The physical examination may reveal a palpable mass to the left of the rectus muscle or, in infants, occupying the suprapubic space. The remainder of the examination is similar to those previously described earlier in this chapter for urodynamic assessment.

After an appropriate history and physical examination, the use of specific diagnostic modalities may facilitate a definitive diagnosis. The diagnosis of Hirschbrung's disease is suspected by failure to pass meconium within the first 24 hr of birth and, when located distally, can be suggestive by barium enema. With the addition of fluoroscopy, an assessment of colonic and rectal mobility can be performed. The colonic transit time utilizes radiopaque markers to evaluate gastrointestinal motility. Normally, 80% of pellets are evacuated within 5 days and 100% within 7 days (165). Anorectal manometry is used to evaluate the coordinated activity between the rectum, anus, and the sphincters. In children with chronic constipation, significant abnormalities in rectal compliance and function, and coordination of sphincteric activity during defecation (Fig. 15) are present (166–168). A catheter with a inflatable balloon is placed in the rectum to measure compliance and motility and two balloons are held at the level of the sphincter to evaluate the internal sphincter rectosphincteric relaxation reflex and the inflation reflex in both the internal and external sphincter (169). Other functional disorders of defecation present with varied anometric findings. The use of electromyography during defecation is employed to confirm suspected inappropriate contraction of external sphincter with defecation. Another indication for anometric evaluation includes chronic constipation persisting into adolescence (170). Hirschbrung's disease demonstrates inappropriate failure to manifest a rectosphincteric relaxation with rectal distention. In addition, other anorectal malformations may be identified with manometrics (171). Colonic manometry is used to differentiate functional fecal retention

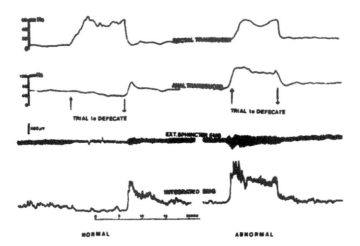

Figure 15 Tracings depict pressure changes in rectum and anal canal, and EMG changes from EAS during trial to defecate. Duration of defecation trial is indicated by arrows. Normal defecation consists of increased rectal (intra-abdominal) pressure, decreased anal pressure, and decreased direct and integrated EMG activity. Abnormal defecation dynamics consists of increased rectal (intra-abdominal) pressure, anal pressure, and direct and integrated EMG activity. (From Ref. 181.)

from organic constipation (162). Some authors feel that the diagnosis should not involve the use of invasive manometrics (172).

3. Therapy

A therapeutic program designed for constipation and encopresis in children involves patient and family education, an initial regimen tailored to relieve fecal impaction, and a maintenance protocol to maintain adequate bowel elimination for hard-core, chronic constipation. Less severe cases of constipation in children is addressed with a dietary regimen consisting of a high-fiber low-fat diet and refractory cases managed with stool softeners (e.g., senna preparations; Senokot) and in severe cases laxatives (158–160,162,163,172). Children who present with encopresis typically have associated fecal impaction and a long-standing history of constipation that should be addressed with treatment.

Pediatric gastroenterologists prefer to evacuate fecal retention or disimpaction with the use of mineral oil, enemas, magnesium citrate, or polyethylene glycol. The dosage of mineral oil is 30 mL/yr of age, up to 8 oz. administered twice daily for 3 consecutive days (173). Encopresis usually completely resolves with adequate disimpaction. After successful disimpaction, a maintenance regimen should be instituted that prevents the reaccumulation of hard stool by combining medical and behavioral therapy. In terms of medical therapy, nightly mineral oil (15 mL/yr of age up to 60 mL), laxatives, high-fiber diet, milk of magnesia or lactose may be instituted. Behavioral therapy involves strict adherence to a high-fiber diet and monitoring the consistency and frequency of defections and attempting to defecate after each meal by sitting from 5 to 15 min in hopes of benefiting from the gastrocolic reflex. Multiple trials have demonstrated success with a combined medical and behavioral program for preventing the recurrence of fecal retention (173,174). After a successful period of maintenance therapy, laxatives are weaned off, and the condition is managed with a high-fiber dietary regimen (158,162,175). A subpopulation of children, with constipation and encopresis and paradoxical contraction of anal sphincters with defecation, will benefit from biofeedback therapy (176–180). Although successful in centers, some studies provide evidence that biofeedback may not be superior to a strict medical and behavioral regimen (181–185). Refractory cases of chronic constipation, who are unresponsive to standard medical and behavioral therapy, should be considered for rectal biopsy to rule out neuroenteric disorders.

The surgical management of constipation involves mainly the treatment of Hirschsprung's disease (186). Failure to pass meconium within the first 24 hr occurs in 95% of patients with this disease. The remaining 5% present later in life with constipation and encopresis. After an appropriate rectal biopsy confirms the absence of ganglion cells in Auerbach's and Meissner's plexus, a surgical procedure is performed in an effort to relieve the functional colonic obstruction and provide an anatomically correct means for evacuation of stool. Primarily two main procedures, the Duhamel and the Soave, have evolved into the two most commonly used pull-through procedures today (187,188).

C. Nocturnal Enuresis

Nocturnal enuresis is the most common form of pediatric incontinence, affecting up to 15% of children at age 5; 5% at age 10; and 1% at age 15 (189). It is more common in males, most patients have had nocturnal enuresis since birth, and only a small percentage have associated daytime accidents. The causes of nocturnal enuresis appear to be multifactoral. Much work has been performed in an attempt to identify a unifying underlying cause, but it appears that most children are physically and psychologically normal (190). Extensive urodynamic studies have identified that bladder instability is present in a wide range of patients (191–193). Studies by Norgaard showed that uninhibited contractions induced by bladder filling during sleep were as likely to awaken the patient as to cause incontinence (194). Bladder instability and sphincter dysfunction do not play a major role in the pathophysiology. The cause of nocturnal enuresis appears to be a functionally insufficient bladder capacity. There are multiple potential etiological factors that could be at work (195,196). For most patients identifying these factors provide little help in treatment. Potential etiological factors include the following:

Sleep disorders
Maturational lag
Developmental delay
Psychological factors
Genetic factors
Stress
Underlying urological disease
Abnormal antidiuretic hormone secretion

In evaluating patients it is important to identify patients who have a higher probability of underlying urological problems that need more extensive evaluation. Patients with a history of urinary tract infections, daytime incontinence, or clear physical or neurological abnormalities on physical examination should undergo a complete evaluation with renal ultrasound and voiding cystourethrogram to exclude treatable urological problems. Recently, Yeung has identified a higher incidence of underlying urological, anatomical, and urodynamic abnormalities in older patients that are refractory to treatment (197,279). The recommended treatment for most of children with nocturnal enuresis without underlying urological abnormalities is outlined in Table 1.

Table 1 Recommended Treatments for Nocturnal Enuresis

1. Conservative treatments
    Restrict fluids in the evening
    Completely empty bladder before going to sleep
    Awaken the patient during the night to empty bladder
2. Medical treatment
    Desmopressin (DDAVP)
    Imipramine (Tofranil)
3. Behavioral treatment
    Alarm system
    Vibratory system

In the adolescent population, treatment does result in improvement in behavioral problems (198).

VI. THEORETICAL CAUSES OF SPHINCTER AND PELVIC FLOOR DYSFUNCTION

Unlike the adult situation, most problems with the sphincter and pelvic floor in children result from overactivity and lack of relaxation during voiding, in contrast with the adult population in whom the mechanism may be that the sphincter and pelvic muscle is too relaxed or damaged. The exceptions to this occur with severe congenital abnormalities (i.e., exstrophy, bilateral ectopic ureters in females), rare neurological disorders, or trauma. The causes of sphincter dysfunction that result because of congenital or acquired abnormalities and neurological disorders are easily understood. The muscle is either undeveloped, destroyed, or the innervation is affected. These disorders are managed by complete urodynamic assessment, specific surgical approaches, medication, and often clean intermittent catheterization.

The cause of sphincter and pelvic floor dysfunction in the patient who has no underlying neurological, acquired, or congenital abnormality is less well understood. The classic theory holds that the sphincter dyssynergia results as a response to an uninhibited bladder contraction. The uninhibited contraction resulting in a forced sphincter contraction to prevent spontaneous loss of urine (Fig. 16). Historically, most of the emphasis has been placed on a complete invasive urodynamic study that concentrates on the full evaluation of the bladder during filling (26,111,115,123,196,199).

Bauer in his unstable bladder article outlined a series of bladder categories he identified in children with voiding dysfunction, without obvious neurological disease (111). He coined the commonly referred to terms: hypertonic bladder, hyperreflexic bladder, lazy bladder, nonneurogenic neurogenic bladder. The hypertonic bladder being of small capacity, with sustained uncontrolled detrusor contraction, normal sphincter activity with bladder filling, and incomplete relaxation of the external sphincter in some patients during voiding; the recommended treatment of anticholinergics and antibiotics was not effective in preventing recurrent UTIs, nor in stopping incontinence. The hyperreflexic bladders have uninhibited contractions, appropriate sphincter reactivity on voiding, and complete sphincter relaxation; anticholinergics alone were helpful in preventing incontinence in most of these patients, but were unhelpful in preventing urinary tract infections. The lazy bladder is characterized by absent bladder contraction at high volumes, voiding with Valsalva ma-

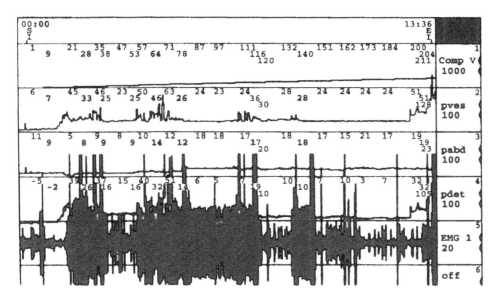

Figure 16 Multiple uninhibited bladder contractions during filling phase of urodynamic assessment in a patient with a neurogenic bladder. (Courtesy of Dr. Patrick McKenna.)

neuver, and complete relaxation during voiding; there was a 77% improvement in a small group of patients with a change in voiding habits, bethanechol, and intermittent catheterization. The nonneurogenic bladder group had the same findings and approach as described by Hinman; treatment was directed at the social pressures (140). Van Gool's review also identified four patterns, but he concentrated more on urine flow and sphincter dysfunction. Unlike Bauer's findings, van Gool implicated abnormal sphincter dysfunction in the majority of patients he studied. He showed that recurrent urinary tract infections, vesicoureteral reflux, and abnormal sphincter function strongly correlated. He also felt that the lazy bladder syndrome represented a decompensation of a dysfunctional voider and not a primary unique voiding pattern (200,201).

As early as the late 1970s Koff and Lapides identified the strong correlation between dysfunctional voiding, urinary tract infections, and vesicoureteral reflux (144). They documented that the most common finding was sphincter contraction, in combination with uninhibited contractions. Koff later showed that by treating patients with voiding dysfunction and reflux with anticholinergics; he could decrease the rate of infection and increase the spontaneous resolution rate of reflux (128). However, what he and others did not emphasize at the time was that his initial program also concentrated on treating constipation, which was probably the main reason he had such good results in decreasing urinary tract infections. In 1998 Koff published his concept of "dysfunctional elimination syndromes" (4). He noted that the association of constipation with incontinence problems had been identified since the early 1950s, but largely disregarded as important by urologists (202). He did not offer a pathophysiological explanation why the bowel and bladder problems occur together so often in cases of voiding dysfunction.

The classic theory that bladder dysfunction is at the root of voiding dysfunction, by long-standing conscious contraction of the sphincter to prevent incontinence, fails to explain many of the findings that have been reported over the last 25 years: findings of non-

neurogenic neurogenic bladder in infants (67); that there is a high association of constipation and stooling dysfunction; and that some centers have had difficulty in eliminating recurrent urinary tract infections when their treatment is directed solely at the bladder function (111,133).

We recently proposed a new theory, called the neural plastic theory, that suggests the
pelvic floor is the common denominator when dysfunctional elimination syndromes are
identified (93). Three types of dysfunction are proposed; chronic dysfunctional contraction
of the pelvic floor (the most common); chronic pelvic floor laxity, which is rare in pediatric
patients; and the inappropriate stimulation of the guarding reflex that results in the inhibition of appropriate bladder contractions. Rather than concentrating solely on the external
sphincter, we have advocated evaluating the entire pelvic floor. Rather than directing treatment at the bladder dysfunction, we have managed children with medical therapy directed
solely at the bladder, the pelvic floor, and the bowel. With this approach, without anticholinergics, we have been successful in curing or significantly improving voiding symptoms in close to 90% of the children studied, and associated bowel problems in close to
100% of the children. The approach involves increasing fluids, timed voiding with voiding
tricks, aggressively addressing constipation, screening for pelvic floor dysfunction, and
using computer games to retrain and correct pelvic floor dysfunction. We, too, have found
that there is a high association between voiding dysfunction, constipation, recurrent urinary
tract infections, and reflux, especially in girls. By employing our system, we have seen a
precipitous drop in surgical intervention for reflux mainly because the recurrent urinary
tract infection rate is so low. It appears that the underlying cause of reflux in most female
patients is secondary, rather then primary, reflux as once thought.

We proposed that, with the most common type, chronic dysfunctional contraction of
the pelvic floor that is present since before birth sets up a collateral neural plastic effect on
the bladder, resulting in a variable pattern of bladder dysfunction. Several authors have
shown that stimulating or denervating peripheral muscles can have a direct effect on bladder function (203–211). So, it is possible that chronic pelvic floor contraction may have a
similar but negative effect on the bladder. Steers has proposed a theory of how this may occur
in bladder neck obstruction secondary to benign prostatic hypertrophy (BPH) (212–215).
The pathway involves stimulation of nerve growth factor (NGF) which, in turn, stimulates
increase neuron size and subsequently bladder muscle hypertrophy. Furthermore, he has
speculated that increased NGF creates a functional plasticity in the spinal reflex as well as
potentiates hyperactive voiding in a rat model (216,217). Afferent pathway changes may
contribute to the variety of changes seen in bladder outlet obstruction (97). The obstruction
of the pediatric bladder and bowel could be initiated by pelvic floor dysfunction and then set
up changes similar to those Steers has identified in bladder neck obstruction from BPH.

We are moving closer to understanding the pathophysiology of voiding dysfunction,
and it is clearly more complicated then the classic theory that bladder dysfunction alone is
its cause.

VII. THERAPY FOR DYSFUNCTIONAL PELVIC FLOOR SYNDROME

Various management strategies have developed over the last 20 years to manage children
with dysfunctional voiding symptoms. In addition, several theories have developed in an attempt to bring together the symptoms of dysfunctional voiding, constipation, and associated upper urinary tract changes. The therapeutic strategies have been directed at the underlying etiology of these symptoms and include medical therapy, behavioral therapy,
electrical stimulation, and surgical intervention (218).

Medical therapy is used to inhibit detrusor contractions and to facilitate urinary storage and bladder emptying. In treating children with dysfunctional voiding without a neurological lesion, Bauer felt that the underlying pathology consistent in all children with dysfunctional voiding was an abnormal bladder. He based his therapy on the urodynamic assessment of the bladder. Medical therapy consisting mainly of anticholinergics, and tricyclic antidepressants were instituted and children were followed with serial urodynamics, but this method achieved only moderate success (219). Recently, Snodgrass has advocated a similar strategy in the management of children with dysfunctional voiding and vesicoureteral reflux. The disadvantage of this approach is that the desired effect of the anticholinergic medication relaxes the bladder, but also adversely affects colonic motility (133). Propantheline (Pro-Banthine) has also been successfully used to relax the bladder (220).

Medication used to inhibit detrusor instability as well as facilitate urinary storage includes anticholinergics, tricyclic antidepressants, and β-adrenergic agonists. Available anticholinergics include oxybutynin chloride (Ditropan XL) and tolterodine. The mechanism of action involves inhibition of the muscarinic cholinergic postganglionic parasympathetic innervation to the bladder in addition to a mild analgesic effect (221). Side effects associated with oxybutynin are secondary to the antimuscarinic effects and include dry mucus membranes and constipation. Oxybutynin XL is delivered in a steady-rate fashion that reduces its side effects through the elimination of the peaks and troughs historically associated with oxybutynin chloride (222). Tolterodine reportedly manifest fewer side effects because of its specificity for the M_3 cholinergic receptor, in addition to calcium antagonistic properties (223). The anticholinergic action inhibits detrusor contractions and should be used with caution because of the inherent risk of urinary retention and constipation. In addition, others have demonstrated effective treatment programs for dysfunctional voiding with pharmacological treatment (224,225).

In addition to patients with voiding dysfunction, the population of children with neurogenic bladders secondary to posterior urethral valves, myelomeningocele, cerebral palsy, and multiple sclerosis are managed with anticholinergics. In this population, the medication is used primarily to facilitate urinary storage and maintain a low detrusor pressure in an effort to prevent upper tract changes and subsequent renal deterioration (22). With pharmacological urinary retention, clean intermittent catheterization (CIC) is an effective modality to provide bladder emptying. The routine use of CIC has revolutionized the management of children with severe neurogenic bladders by significantly altering the need for surgical intervention. This treatment has turned poorly compliant bladders into compliant reservoirs drained by a catheter, through the prevention of increasing in detrusor pressure and development of detrusor sphincter dyssynergia (226). In addition to the anticholinergics, the use of tricyclic antidepressants, including imipramine and doxapin, appear to benefit patients with neurogenic bladders because of their unique combined properties of both anticholinergic–antimuscarinic activity, which relaxes the bladder, and α-adrenergic activity, which tightens the bladder neck by affecting the α_1-receptors primarily located in the urinary sphincter (220,227). Imipramine use in children has fallen out of favor because of the known risk of cardiac arrhythmia's in addition to the side effects of abdominal cramping, nausea, lethargy, and headache (228). In the presence of intrinsic sphincter deficiency, the α-adrenergic agonist, pseudoephedrine (30 mg q 4–6 hr) or phenylpropanolamine (25 mg q 4 hr), can be used to increase urethral closure pressure to maintain continence in patients receiving CIC and maximal antispasmodics.

Pelvic floor muscle rehabilitation or biofeedback utilized for the management of dysfunctional voiding facilitates the identification and subsequent rehabilitation of the pelvic floor, including the urinary sphincter, in an attempt to achieve a synergistic voiding pattern.

Biofeedback is defined as a modality used to provide instantaneous output about a given system or treatment regimen (229). Initially introduced by Sugar and Firlit, biofeedback for the management of dysfunctional voiding has been extremely successful in many institutions (93,122,230–247). Kegel is credited for introducing pelvic floor rehabilitation as a means to improve urinary symptoms (248). Biofeedback therapy is quite different in the pediatric population because its success relies directly on patient motivation that may be poor in young children. To address this lack of interest some institutions depend on inpatient treatment programs (201,244,249) and the use of invasive urodynamics as an initial means to assess bladder function (230,232–234,240,242,243,245,246). For biofeedback to be successful, the participant must be highly motivated. McKenna and Herndon have integrated interactive computer games with standard biofeedback based on noninvasive initial uroflow–surface EMG as a means to identify and engage children with dysfunctional voiding (Fig. 17). Biofeedback has proved to be an effective modality to manage children with dysfunctional voiding by correcting the paradoxical contraction of the urinary sphincter and pelvic floor with voiding. In addition, McKenna and Herndon have demonstrated significant cure rates in patients with constipation and encopresis, presenting with dysfunctional voiding, with biofeedback to suggest that their common etiology lies in a dysfunctional sphincteric mechanism or pelvic floor (93).

Although used with success in the adult population, electrical stimulation for the treatment of voiding symptoms has a limited role in the treatment of the pediatric population. Trsinar and Kralj reported on 73 girls with dysfunctional voiding and bladder instability managed successfully with maximal electrical stimulation through an anal plug. Others have demonstrated similar results (250–252). Electrical stimulation of the anal sphincter travels along the afferent pudendal nerve fibers and inhibits uninhibited bladder contractions. Several theories exist to describe the effect of electrical stimulation, which include a downregulation of cholinergic detrusor receptors and reactivation of functional detrusor units (253).

The surgical management of urinary incontinence secondary to anatomical urinary sphincter abnormalities includes several reconstructive procedures. The decision for surgical intervention should be made after all conservative approaches, including maximal anticholinergic therapy and α-adrenergic therapy, when appropriate, have been exhausted. A

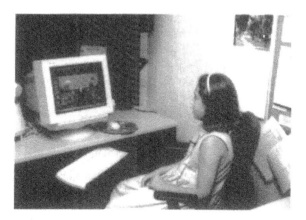

Figure 17   Patient with dysfunctional pelvic floor syndrome playing a computer-integrated biofeedback baseball game. (Courtesy of Dr. Patrick McKenna.)

detailed outline of available procedures and their indications is covered elsewhere in this text. The endoscopic management of intrinsic sphincter deficiency involves the injection of a bulking agent into the proximal bladder neck in an effort to increase urethral closure pressure (254,255). The two approaches include transurethral or intraurethral injection. Initially, several agents were available for injection includes Teflon, spheres, and autologous fat. Recently, the U.S. Food and Drug Administration (FDA) approved the use of bovine collagen, which is now used in most centers with acceptable continence rates (254–257). Another option for intrinsic sphincter deficiency is the pubovaginal sling that creates a compressive force on the urethra that may provide urinary continence for patients. It is usually more successful in female patients than male patients with a fixed bladder neck and prostate (258–261). The Young–Dees–Leadbetter bladder neck reconstruction achieves the same effect by employing the proximal bladder neck and tubularizing it into a functional urethra (262–264). The Kroop onlay and Pippi Salle utilize the principle of gaining functional urethral length by isolating an anterior vesical flap (265,266). In males, the placement of an artificial urinary sphincter should be considered when all available options have been exhausted (267–269). An alternative approach to severe urinary incontinence is ligation of the bladder neck and alternative site for catheterization. Several procedures that use this principle include the appendicovesicostomy (270,271), ileonipple conduit (272), ileal reservoir (273), cecoileal pouch(Mainz)(274), Indiana pouch (275), Penn pouch (276), gastric reservoir (277), and ureterosigmoidostomy (278). Finally, in patients with detrusor sphincter deficiency an external sphincterotomy provides a decrease in urethral closure pressure and facilitates bladder emptying.

VIII. SUMMARY

The pediatric approach to sphincteric and pelvic floor dysfunction differs greatly from that of the adult population because of the higher probability of an underlying anatomical or neurological abnormality. A complete history and physical examination and appropriate screening studies can identify these patients. Whether there is an underlying problem or the child has voiding dysfunction many options are available for treatment. It is becoming very clear that the pelvic floor is important in many instances and that most cases of dysfunctional voiding are also associated with dysfunctional stool elimination. A management strategy directed at the pelvic floor rehabilitation can correct both problems.

ACKNOWLEDGMENT

We want to thank Ms. Barbara Corcoran for her help in completing this manuscript.

REFERENCES

1. O'Regan S, Yazbeck S, Schick E. Constipation, bladder instability, urinary tract infection syndrome. Clin Nephrol 1985; 23:152–154.
2. O'Regan S, Schick E, Hamburger B, Yazbeck S. Constipation associated with vesicoureteral reflux. Urology 1986; 28:394–396.
3. O'Regan S, Yazbeck S, Hamburger B, Schick E. Constipation: a commonly unrecognized cause of enuresis. Am J Dis Child 1986; 140:260–261.
4. Koff SA, Wagner TT, Jayanthi VR. The relationship among dysfunctional elimination syndromes, primary vesicoureteral reflux and urinary tract infections in children. J Urol 1998; 160:1019–1022.

5. Yeung CK, Dhillon HK, Duffy PG, Ransley PG. Vesicoureteral reflux in infants with prenatally diagnosed hydronephrosis. Presented to the Section on Urology, American Academy of Pediatrics, New Orleans, LA, 1991: 111; abtr. 83.

6. Sillén U, Hjälmås K, Aili M, Bjure J, Hanson E, Hansson S. Pronounced detrusor hypercontractility in infants with gross bilateral reflux. J Urol 1992; 148:598–599.

7. Kokoua A, Homsy Y, Lavigne J, Williot P, Corcos J, Laberge L, Michaud J. Maturation of the external urinary sphincter: a comparative histotopographic study in humans. J Urol 1993; 150: 617–622.

8. Yeung CK, Godley ML, Ho CK, Ransley PG, Duffy PG, Chen CN, Li AK. Some new insights into bladder function in infancy. Br J Urol 1995; 76:235–240.

9. Yeung CK, Godley ML, Duffy PG, Ransley PG. Natural filling cystometry in infants and children. Br J Urol 1995; 75:531–537.

10. Herndon CDA, McKenna PH, Kolon TF, Gonzalez E, Baker L, Docimo SG. A multi-center outcomes analysis of neonatal reflux patients presenting with antenatal hydronephrosis. J Urol 1999; 162:1203–1208.

11. Stephens, FD. Congenital Malformations of the Urinary Tract. New York: Praeger, 1983: 84–85.

12. Tanagho EA. Anatomy of the lower urinary tract. In: Campbell's Urology, 1986; 1:46–60.

13. Cromie WJ, Lee K, Houde K, Holmes L. Implications of the decrease in major genitourinary malformations in the United States, 1972–1974. Am Acad Pediatr Annu Meet, San Francisco, CA, 1998: abstr 106.

14. Stein SC, Feldman JG, Freidlander M, Klein RJ. Is myelomeningocele a disappearing disease? Pediatrics 1982; 69:511–514.

15. MMW Morb Mortal Wkly Rep. Use of folic acid for prevention of spina bifida and other neural tube defects—1983–1991. 1991;40:513–516.

16. Lewis DP, Van Dyke DC, Stumbo PJ, Berg MJ. Drug and environmental factors associated with adverse pregnancy outcomes. Part II: Improvement with folic acid. Ann Pharmacother 1998; 32:947–961.

17. Scarff TB, Fronczak S. Myelomeningocele: a review and update. Rehabil Lit 1981; 42:143–146.

18. Lais A, Kasabian NG, Dyro FM, Scott RM, Kelly MD, Bauer SB. Neurosurgical implications of continuous neuro-urological surveillance of children with myelodysplasia. J Urol 1993; 150:1879–1883.

19. Bauer SB, Hallet M, Khoshbin S, Lebowitz RL, Winston KR, Gibson S, Colodny AH, Retik AB. The predictive value of urodynamic evaluation in the newborn with myelodysplasia. JAMA 1984; 650:652.

20. Roach MB, Switters DM, Stone AR. The changing urodynamic pattern in infants with myelomeningocele. J Urol 1993; 150:944–947.

21. Sillén U, Hansson E, Hermansson G, Hjälmås K, Jacobsson B, Jodal U. Development of the urodynamic pattern in infants with myelomeningocele. Br J Urol 1996; 78:596–601.

22. McGuire EJ, Woodside JR, Borden TA, Weiss RM. Prognostic value of urodynamic testing in myelodysplasia patients. J Urol 1981; 126:205–209.

23. van Gool JD, Kuijten RH, Donckerwolcke RA, Kramer PP. Detrusor–sphincter dyssynergia in children with myelomeningocele: a prospective study. Z Kinderchir 1982; 37:148.

24. Dator DP, Hatchett L, Dyro FM, Sheffier JM, Bauer SB. Urodynamic dysfunction in walking myelodysplastic children. J Urol 1992; 148:362–365.

25. Andros GJ, Hatch DA, Walter JS, Wheeler JS, Schlehahn L, Damaser MS. Home bladder pressure monitoring in children with myelomeningocele. J Urol 1998; 160:518–521.

26. Bauer SB. [Editorial] The challenge of the expanding role of urodynamic studies in the treatment of children with neurological and functional disabilities. J Urol 1998; 160:527–528.

27. Perez LM, Khoury J, Webster GD. The value of urodynamic studies in infants less than one year old with congenital spinal dysraphism. J Urol 1992; 148:584–587.

28. Wu HY, Baskin LS, Kogan BA. Neurogenic bladder dysfunction due to myelomeningocele: neonatal versus childhood treatment. J Urol 1997; 157:2295–2297.

29. Bauer SB, Lais A, Scott RM. Continuous urodynamic surveillance of babies with myelodysplasia: implications for further neurosurgery. Eur J Pediatr Surg 1992; 2(suppl):35–36.

30. Foster LS, Kogan BA, Cogan PH, Edwards MSB. Bladder function in patients with lipomyelomeningocele. J Urol 1990; 143:984–986.

31. Atala A, Bauer SB, Dyro FM, Sheffner J, Shillito J, Sathi S, Scott RM. Bladder functional changes resulting from lipomeningocele repair. J Urol 1992; 148:592–594.

32. Bruce DA, Schut L. Spinal lipomas in infancy and childhood. Child Brain 1979; 5:192–203.

33. Colak A, Pollack IF, Albright AL. Recurrent tethering: a common long-term problem after lipomyelomeningocele repair. Pediatr Neurosurg 1998; 29:184–190.

34. Guzman L, Bauer SB, Hallet M, Khoshbin S, Colodny AH, Retik AB. The evaluation and management of children with sacral agenesis. Urology 1983; 23:506–510.

35. Gotoh T, Shinno Y, Kobayashi S, Watarai Y, Koyanagi T. Diagnosis and management of sacral agenesis. Eur Urol 1991; 20:287–292.

36. White RI, Klauber GT. Sacral agenesis. Analysis of 22 cases. Urology 1976; 8:521–525.

37. Koff SA, DeRidder PA. Patterns of neurogenic bladder dysfunction in sacral agenesis. J Urol 1977; 118:87–89.

38. Borrelli M, Bruschini H, Nahas WC, Figueiredo JA, Prado MJ, Spinola R, Walligora M, Freire GC, de Goes GM. Sacral agenesis: why is it so frequently misdiagnosed? Urology 1985; 26: 351–355.

39. Palmer LS, Richards I, Kaplan WE. Subclinical changes in bladder function in children presenting with nonurological symptoms of the tethered cord syndrome. J Urol 1998; 159:231–234.

40. Giddens JL, Radomski SB, Hirshberg ED, Hassouna M, Fehlings M. Urodynamic findings in adults with the tethered cord syndrome. J Urol 1999; 161:1249–1254.

41. Flanigan RC, Russell DP, Walsh JW. Urologic aspects of tethered cord. Urology 1989; 33: 80–82.

42. Shurtleff DB, Duguay S, Duguay G, Moskowitz D, Weinberger E, Roberts T, Loeser J. Epidemiology of tethered cord with meningomyelocele. Eur J Pediatr Surg 1997; (suppl 1):7–11.

43. Khoury AE, Hendrick EB, McLorie GA, Kulkarni A, Churchill B. Occult spinal dysraphism: clinical and urodynamic outcome after diversion of the filum terminate. J Urol 1990; 144: 426–429.

44. Ritchey ML, Sinha A, DiPietro MA, Huang C, Flood H, Bloom DA. Significance of spina bifida occulta in children with diurnal enuresis. J Urol 1994; 152:815–818.

45. Pippi Salle JL, Capolicchio G, Houle A, Vemet O, Jednak R, O'Gorman AM, Montes JL, Fanner J. Magnetic resonance imaging in children with voiding dysfunction: is it indicated? J Urol 1998; 160:1080–1083.

46. McLorie GA, Sheldon CA, Fleisher M, Churchill BM. The genitourinary system in patients with imperforate anus. J Pediatr Surg 1987; 22:1100–1104.

47. Flanigan RF, Russell DP, Walsh JW. Urologic aspects of tethered cord. Urology 1989; 33: 80–82.

48. Fone PD, Vapnek JM, Litwiler SE, Couillard DR, McDonald CM, Boggan JE, Stone AR. Urodynamic findings in the tethered spinal cord syndrome: does surgical release improve bladder function? J Urol 1997; 157:604–609.

49. Satar N, Bauer SB, Shefner J, Kelly MD, Darbey MM. The effects of delayed diagnosis and treatment in patients with an occult spinal dysraphism. J Urol 1995; 154:754–758.

50. Kaplan WE, McLone DG, Richards I. The urologic manifestations of the tethered spinal cord. J Urol 1988; 140:1285–1288.

51. Naeye RL, Peters EC, Bartholomew M, Landis R. Origins of cerebral palsy. Am J Dis Child 1989; 143:1154–1161.

52. Brodak PP, Sherz HC, Packer MG, Kaplan GW. Is urinary screening necessary for patients with cerebral palsy? J Urol 1994; 152:1586–1587.

53. Decter RM, Bauer SB, Khoshbin S, Dyro FM, Krarup C, Colodny AH, Retik AB. Urodynamic assessment of children with cerebral palsy. J Urol 1987; 138:1110–1112.

54. Mayo ME. Lower urinary tract dysfunction in cerebral palsy. J Urol 1992; 147:419–420.

55. Murphy KP, Molnar GE, Lankasky K. Medical and functional status of adults with cerebral palsy. Dev Med Child Neurol 1995; 37:1075–1084.

56. Chao R, Mayo ME. Long-term urodynamic follow-up in pediatric spinal cord injury. Paraplegia 1994; 32:806–809.

57. Barkin M, Dolfin D, Herschorn S, Bharatwal N, Comisarow R. The urologic care of the spinal cord injury patient. J Urol 1983; 129:335–339.

58. Decter RM, Bauer SB. Urologic management of spinal cord injury in children. Urol Clin North Am 1993; 20:475–483.

59. Gearhart JP, Jeffs RD. State of the art reconstructive surgery for bladder exstrophy at the Johns Hopkins Hospital. Am J Dis Child 1989; 143:1475–1478.

60. Grady RW, Carr MC, Mitchell ME. Complete primary closure of bladder exstrophy. Epispadias and bladder exstrophy repair. Urol Clin North Am 1999; 26:95–109.

61. McKenna PH, Khoury AE, McLorie GA, Churchill BM, Wedge JH. Anterior diagonal mid-innominate osteotomy. Dialog Pediatr Urol 1993; 16:1.

62. McKenna PH. A functional classification of ectopic ureteroceles based on renal unit jeopardy. Dialog Pediatr Urol 1993; 16:9.

63. McKenna PH, Khoury AE, McLorie GA, Churchill BM, Babyn PB, Wedge JH. Iliac osteotomy: model to compare options in bladder and cloacal exstrophy reconstruction. J Urol 1994; 151:182–186 [discussion 186–187].

64. Gearhart JP, Jeffs RD. Augmentation cystoplasty in the failed exstrophy reconstruction. J Urol 1988; 139:790–793.

65. Herndon CDA, Ferrer FA, McKenna PH. A complex urologic problem demonstrates how far pediatric urology has progressed. In: Crombie D, ed. CT Medicine. 1999; 63:707–711.

66. Jayanthi VR, Churchill BM, Khoury AE, McLorie GA. Bilateral single ureteral ectopia: difficulty attaining continence using standard bladder neck repair. J Urol 1997; 158:1933–1936.

67. Jayanthi VR, Khoury AE, McLorie GA, Agarwal SK. The nonneurogenic neurogenic bladder of early infancy. J Urol 1997; 158:1281–1285.

68. Young HH, Frontz WA, Baldwin JC. Congenital obstruction of the posterior urethra. J Urol 1919; 3:289.

69. Kim YH, Horowitz M, Combs A, Nitti VW, Libretti D, Glassberg KI. Comparative urodynamic findings after primary valve ablation, vesicostomy or proximal diversion. J Urol 1996; 156:673–676.

70. Kim YH, Horowitz M, Combs AJ, Nitti VW, Libretti D, Borer J, Glassberg KI. Management of posterior urethral valves on the basis of urodynamic findings. J Urol 1997; 158:1011–1016.

71. Pieretti RV. The mild end of the clinical spectrum of posterior urethral valves. J Pediatr Surg 1993; 28:701–706.

72. Peters CA, Bauer SB. Evaluation and management of urinary incontinence after surgery for posterior urethral valves. Urol Clin North Am 1990; 17:379–387.

73. Holmdahl G, Sillén U, Hanson E, Hermansson G, Hjälmås K. Bladder dysfunction in boys with posterior urethral valves before and after puberty. J Urol 1996; 155:694–698.

74. Holmdahl G, Sillén U, Bertilsson M, Hermansson G, Hjälmås K. Natural filling cystometry in small boys with posterior urethral valves: unstable valve bladders become stable during sleep. J Urol 1997; 158:1017–1021.

75. Merguerian PA, McLorie GA, McKenna PH, Khoury AE, Churchill BM. Radiographic and serologic correlates of azotemia in patients with posterior urethral valves. J Urol 1992; 148:1 499–1503.

76. Kaefer M, Keating MA, Adams MC, Rink RC. Posterior urethral valves, pressure pop-offs and bladder function. J Urol 1995; 154:708–711.

77. Holmdahl G, Sillén U, Bachelard M, Hansson E, Hermansson G, Hjämås K. The changing uro-dynamic pattern in valve bladders during infancy. J Urol 1995; 153:463–467.
78. Reinberg Y, McKenna PH. Nephrectomy combined with lower abdominal extraperitoneal ureteral bladder augmentation in the treatment of children with the vesicoureteral reflux dysplasia syndrome. J Urol 1995; 153:177–179.
79. Churchill BM, Aliabadi H, Landau EH, McLorie GA, Steckler RE, McKenna PH, Khoury AE. Ureteral bladder augmentation. J Urol 1993; 150:716–720.
80. McKenna PH, Bauer MB. Bladder augmentation with ureter. Dialog Pediatr Urol 1995; 18:1.
81. de Vries PA, Friedland GW. The staged sequential development of the anus and rectum in human embryos and fetuses. J Pediatr Surg 1974; 9:755–769.
82. Levitt MA, Patel M, Rodriguez G, Gaylin DS, Pena A. The tethered spinal cord in patients with anorectal malformations. J Pediatr Surg 1997; 32:462–468.
83. Robson WLM, Leung AKC, Mathers MS. Kegel exercises and squatting behavior. J Pediatr Edit Corresp 7/1994:169–170.
84. Himsl KK, Hurwitz RS. Pediatric urinary incontinence. Urol Clin North Am 1991; 18:283–293.
85. Bloom DA, Park JM, Koo HP. Comments on pediatric elimination dysfunctions: the Whorf hypothesis, the elimination interview, the guarding reflex and nocturnal enuresis. Eur Urol 1998; 33(suppl 3):20–24.
86. Maizels M, Gandhi, Keating B, Rosenbaum D. Diagnosis and treatment for children who cannot control urination. Curr Prob Pediatr 1993; 402–450.
87. Koff SA. Estimating bladder capacity in children. Urology 1983; 21:248.
88. Wan J, Greenfield SP. Pediatric urodynamics. In: Blaivas JG, Chancellor M, eds. Atlas of Urodynamics. Baltimore: Williams & Wilkins, 1996:251–270.
89. Houle AM, Gilmour RF, Churchill BM, Gaumond M, Bissonnette B. What volume can a child normally store in the bladder at a safe pressure? J Urol 1993; 149:561–564.
90. Mattsson SH. Voiding frequency, volumes and intervals in healthy school children. Scand J Urol Nephrol 1994; 28:1–11.
91. Barrett DM, Wein AJ. Voiding dysfunction: diagnosis, classification and management. Adult Pediatr Urol 1987; 1:863–962.
92. Gilmour RF, Churchill BM, Steckler RE, Houle AM, Khoury AE, McLorie GA. A new technique for dynamic analysis of bladder compliance. J Urol 1993; 150:1200–1203.
93. McKenna PH, Herndon CDA, Connery S, Ferrer FA. Pelvic floor muscle retraining for pediatric voiding dysfunction using interactive computer games. J Urol 1999; 162:1056–1062.
94. Wan J, McGuire EJ, Bloom DA, Ritchey ML. Stress leak point pressure: a diagnostic tool for incontinent children. J Urol 1993; 150:700–702.
95. Maizels M, Firlit CF. Pediatric urodynamics: a clinical comparison of surface versus needle pelvic floor/external sphincter electromyography. J Urol 1979; 122:518–522.
96. Diokno AC, Koff SA, Anderson W. Combined cystometry and perineal electromyography in the diagnosis and treatment of neurogenic urinary incontinence. J Urol 1976; 115:161–163.
97. Chai TC, Gemalmaz H, Andersson KE, Tuttle JB, Steers WD. Persistently increased voiding frequency despite relief of bladder outlet obstruction. J Urol 1999; 161:1689–1693.
98. Diokno AC, Koff SA, Bender LF. Periurethral striated muscle activity in neurogenic bladder dysfunction. J Urol 1974; 112:743–749.
99. Blaivas JG, Labib KB, Bauer SB, Retik AB. A new approach to electromyography of the external urethral sphincter. J Urol 1977; 117:773–777.
100. Koff SA, Kass EJ. Abdominal wall electromyography: a noninvasive technique to improve pediatric urodynamic accuracy. J Urol 1982; 127:736–739.
101. Blaivas JG, Labib KB, Bauer B, Retik AB. Changing concepts in the urodynamic evaluation of children. J Urol 1977; 117:778–781.
102. McGuire EJ. Electromyographic evaluation of sphincteric function and dysfunction. Urol Clin North Am 1979; 6:121–124.
103. Wein AJ, VanArsdalen KN. Nonsurgical management of neuropathic voiding dysfunction. Semin Urol 1985; 3:216–237.

104. Yalla SV, Sharma GURK, Barsamian EM. Micturitional static urethral pressure profile method of recording urethral pressure profiles during voiding and implications. J Urol 1980; 124:649–656.

105. Bachelard M, Sillén U, Hansson S, Hermansson G, Jodal U, Jacobsson B. Urodynamic pattern in infants with urinary tract infection. J Urol 1998; 160:522–526.

106. Porter T, Weerasinghe N, Malone PS. Modification of therapy based on videourodynamics in neurologically normal children: Southampton 1988–1993. Br J Urol 1995; 76:779–782.

107. Glazier DB, Murphy DP, Fleisher MH, Cummings YB, Barone JG. Evaluation of the utility of video-urodynamics in children with urinary tract infection and voiding dysfunction. Br J Urol 1997; 80:806–808.

108. Weerasinghe N, Malone PS. The value of videourodynamics in the investigation of neurologically normal children who wet. J Urol 1993; 73:539–542.

109. Passerini–Glazel G, Cisternino A, Camuffo MC, Ferrarese P, Aragona F, Artibani W. Video-urodynamic studies of minor voiding dysfunctions in children: an overview of 13 years' experience. Scand J Urol Nephrol 1992; 141:70–86.

110. Reid CJ, Borzyskowski M. Lower urinary tract dysfunction in cerebral palsy. Arch Dis Child 1993; 68:739–742.

111. Bauer SB, Retik AB, Colodny AH, Hallett M, Khoshbin S, Dyro FM. The unstable bladder of childhood. Urol Clin North Am 1980; 7:321–336.

112. Williams MA, Noe HN, Smith RA. The importance of urinary tract infection in the evaluation of the incontinent child. J Urol 1994; 151:188–190.

113. Batista JE, Bauer SB, Shefner JM, Kelly MD, Darbey MD, Siroky NM. Urodynamic findings in children with spinal cord ischemia. J Urol 1995; 154:1183–1187.

114. Medel R, Ruarte AC, Castera R, Podesta MI. Primary enuresis: a urodynamic evaluation. Br J Urol 1998; 81 (suppl 3):50–52.

115. Allen TD, Bright TC III. Urodynamic patterns in children with dysfunctional voiding problems. J Urol 1978; 119:247–249.

116. Mayo ME, Burns MW. Urodynamic studies in children who wet. Br J Urol 1990; 65:641–645.

117. Blaivas JG, Sinha HP, Zayed AAH, Labib KB. Detrusor–external sphincter dyssynergia. J Urol 1981; 125:542–544.

118. Blaivas JG, Sinha HP, Zayed AAH, Labib KB. Detrusor–external sphincter dyssynergia: a detailed electromyographic study. J Urol 1981; 125:545–548.

119. van der Vis-Melsen MJE, Baert RJM, Rajnherc JR, Groen JM, Bemelmans LNMJ, DeNef JJEM. Scintigraphic assessment of lower urinary tract function in children with and without outflow tract obstruction. J Urol 1989; 64:263–269.

120. Jorgensen JB, Jensen KM. Uroflowmetry. Urol Clin North Am 1996; 23:237–242.

121. Segura CG. Urine flow in childhood: a study of flow chart parameters based on 1,361 uroflowmetry tests. J Urol 1997; 157:1426–1428.

122. Maizels M, King LR, Firlit CF. Urodynamic biofeedback: a new approach to treat vesical sphincter dyssynergia. J Urol 1979; 122:205–209.

123. van Gool JD, Hjälmås K, Tamminen–Mobius T, Olbing H. Historical clues to the complex of dysfunctional voiding, urinary tract infection and vesicoureteral reflux. The International Reflux Study in Children. J Urol 1992; 148:1699–1702.

124. Meunier P, Marechal JM, de Beaujeu MJ. Rectoanal pressures and rectal sensitivity studies in chronic childhood constipation. Gastroenterology 1979; 77:330–336.

125. Di Lorenzo C, Flores AF, Reddy SN, Hyman PE. Use of colonic manometry to differentiate causes of intractable constipation in children. J Pediatr 1992; 120:690–695.

126. Borowitz SM, Sutphen J, Ling W, Cox DJ. Lack of correlation of anorectal manometry with symptoms of chronic childhood constipation and encopresis. Dis Colon Rectum 1996; 39:400–405.

127. Keren S, Wagner Y, Heldenberg D, Golan M. Studies of manometric abnormalities of the rectoanal region during defecation in constipated and soiling children: modification through biofeedback therapy. Am J Gastroenterol 1988; 83:827–831.

128. Koff SA, Murtagh DS. The uninhibited bladder in children: effect of treatment on recurrence of urinary infection and on vesicoureteral reflux resolution. J Urol 1983; 130:1138–1141.

129. Allen TD. Commentary: voiding dysfunction and reflux. J Urol 1992; 148:1706–1707.

130. Koff SA. Relationship between dysfunctional voiding and reflux. J Urol 1992; 148:1703–1705.

131. Chandra M, Maddix H, McVicar M. Transient urodynamic dysfunction of infancy: relationship to urinary tract infections and vesicoureteral reflux. J Urol 1996; 155:673–677.

132. Bomalaski MD, Bloom DA. Urodynamics and massive vesicoureteral reflux. J Urol 1997; 158:1236–1238.

133. Snodgrass W. The impact of treated dysfunctional voiding on the nonsurgical management of vesicoureteral reflux. J Urol 1998; 160:1823–1825.

134. Yeung CK, Godley MI, Dhillon HK, Duffy PG, Ransley PG. Urodynamic patterns in infants with normal lower urinary tracts or primary vesicoureteral reflux. Br J Urol 1998; 81:461–467.

135. Dohil R, Roberts E, Jones KV, Jenkins HR. Constipation and reversible urinary tract abnormalities. Arch Dis Child 1994; 70:56–57.

136. Svanborg–Eden C, Hanson LA, Jodal U, Lindberg U, Akerlund AS. Variable adherence to normal human urinary tract epithelial cells of *Escherichia coli* strains associated with various forms of urinary tract infection. Lancet 1976; 2:490–492.

137. Beer E. Chronic retention of urine in children. JAMA 65:1709, 1915.

138. Allen TD. The non-neurogenic neurogenic bladder. J Urol 1977; 117:232–238.

139. Hinman F, Baumann FW. Vesical and ureteral damage from voiding dysfunction in boys without necrologic or obstructive disease. J Urol 1973; 109:727–730.

140. Hinman F Jr. Nonneurogenic neurogenic bladder (the Hinman syndrome)—15 years later. J Urol 1986; 136:769–777.

141. Johnson JF III, Hedden RJ, Piccolello ML, Wacksman J. Distention of the posterior urethra: association with nonneurogenic neurogenic bladder (Hinman syndrome). Radiology 1992; 185:113–117.

142. Williams DI, Taylor JS. A rare congenital uropathy: vesicourethral dysfunction with upper tract anomalies. Br J Urol 1969; 41:307–313.

143. Firlit CF, Smey P, King LR. Micturition urodynamic flow studies in children. J Urol 1978; 119:250–253.

144. Koff SA, Lapides J, Piazza DH. Association of urinary tract infection and reflux with uninhibited bladder contractions and voluntary sphincteric obstruction. J Urol 1979; 122:373–376.

145. Koff SA. Bladder–sphincter dysfunction in childhood. Urology 1982; 19:457–461.

146. McGuire EJ, Savastano JA. Urodynamic studies in enuresis and the nonneurogenic neurogenic bladder. J Urol 1984; 132:299–302.

147. Hanna MK, Di Scipio W, Suh KK, Kogan SJ, Levitt SB, Donner K. Urodynamics in children, part II. The pseudoneurogenic bladder. J Urol 1981; 125:534–537.

148. Herbetko J, Hyde I. Urinary tract delation in constipated children. Br J Radiol 1990; 63:855–857.

148a. Masek, 1985.

149. Blethyn AJ, Jenkins HR, Roberts R, Jones KV, Verrier–Jones K. Radiological evidence of constipation in urinary tract infection. Arch Dis Child 1995; 73:534–535.

150. Dierks SM, Colberg JW. Urinary retention in a child secondary to Hirschsprung's disease. Br J Urol 1997; 79:806.

151. Loening–Baucke V. Urinary incontinence and urinary tract infection and their resolution with treatment of chronic constipation of childhood. Pediatrics 1997; 100:228–232.

152. Hosie GP, Spitz L. Idiopathic constipation in childhood is associated with thickening of the internal anal sphincter. J Pediatr Surg 1997; 32:1041–1044.

153. Loening–Baucke VA, Yamada T. Is the afferent pathway from the rectum impaired in children with chronic constipation and encopresis? Gastroenterology 1995; 109:397–403.

154. Colon AR, Jacob LJ. Defecation pattern in American infants and children. Clin Pediatr 1977; 16:999–1000.

155. Lemon AN, Booke OG. Frequency and weights of normal stools in infancy. Arch Dis Child 1979; 54:719–722.
156. Weaver LT, Steiner H. The bowel habits of young children. Arch Dis Child 1984; 59:649–652.
157. Potts MJ, Sesney J. Infant constipation: maternal knowledge and beliefs. Clin Pediatr 1992: 143–148.
158. Lewis LG, Rudolph CD. Practical approach to defecation disorders in children. Pediatr Ann 1997; 26:260–268.
159. Loening–Baucke V. Constipation in children. Curr Sci 1994; 556–561.
160. Loening–Baucke V. Management of chronic constipation in infants and toddlers. Am Fam Physician 1994; 397–406.
161. Young RJ. Pediatric constipation. Gastroenterol Nurs 1996; 88–95.
162. Seth R, Heyman M. Management of constipation and encopresis in infants and children. Gastroenterol Clin North Am 1994; 23:621–636.
163. Loening–Baucke V. Functional constipation. Semin Pediatr Surg 1995; 4:26–34.
164. Hyman PE, Fleisher DR. A classification of disorders of defecation in infants and children. Semin Gastrointest Dis 1994; 5:20–23.
165. Eastwood HDH. Bowel transit studies in the elderly: radiopaque markers in the investigation of constipation. Gerontol Clin 1972; 14:154–159.
166. Loening–Baucke VA, Cruikshank BM. Abnormal defecation dynamics in chronically constipated children with encopresis. J Pediatr 1986; 108:562–566.
167. Kaya IS, Dilmen U, Ceyhan M, Saglain R. Rectal and anal pressure profile in constipated children. Lancet 1988; 1:1198–1199.
168. Sutphen J, Borowitz S, Ling W, Cox DJ, Kovatchev B. Anorectal manometric examination in encopretic-constipated children. Dis Colon Rectum 1997; 40:1051–1055.
169. Schuster MM, Hookman P, Hendreix TR Mendeloff AI. Simultaneous manometric recording of internal and external anal sphincteric reflexes. Bull Johns Hopkins Hosp 1965; 116:79–88.
170. Rex DK, Fitzgerald JF, Goulet RJ. Chronic constipation with encopresis persisting beyond 15 years of age. Dis Colon Rectum 1992; 35:242–244.
171. Rintala RJ, Lindahl H. Is normal bowel function possible after repair of intermediate and high anorectal malformations? J Pediatr Surg 1995; 30:491–494.
172. Beach RC. Management of childhood constipation. Lancet 1996; 348:766–767.
173. Gleghorn EE, Rudoph C, Heyman MB. No-enema therapy for idiopathic constipation and encopresis. Clin Pediatr 1991; 30:669–672.
174. Nolan T, Debelle G, Oberklaid F, Coffey C. Randomized trial of laxatives in treatment of childhood encopresis. Lancet 1991; 338:523–527.
175. Katz C, Drongowski A, Coran AG. Long-term management of chronic constipation in children. J Pediatr Surg 1987; 22:976–978.
176. Dahl J, Lindquist BL, Tysk C, Leissner P, Philipson L, Järnerot G. Behavioral medicine treatment in chronic constipation with paradoxical anal sphincter contraction. Dis Colon Rectum 1991; 34:769–776.
177. Benninga MA, Büller, Taminiau JA. Biofeedback training in chronic constipation. Arch Dis Child 1993; 68:126–129.
178. Cox DJ, Sutphen J, Borowitz S, Dickens MN, Singles J, Whitehead WE. Simple electromyographic biofeedback treatment for chronic pediatric constipation/encopresis: preliminary report. Biofeedback Self Regul 1994; 19:41–50.
179. Berquist WE. Biofeedback therapy for anorectal disorders in children. Semin Pediatr Surg 1995; 4:48–53.
180. van der Plas RN, Benninga MA, Taminiau JAJM, Btiller HA. Treatment of defecation problems in children: the role of education, demystification and toilet training. Eur J Pediatr 1997; 156:689–692.
181. Loening–Baucke VA. Modulation of abnormal defecation dynamics by biofeedback treatment in chronically constipated children with encopresis. J Pediatr 1990; 116:214–222.

182. Loening–Baucke V. Persistence of chronic constipation in children after biofeedback treatment. Dig Dis Sci 1991; 36:153–160.
183. Loening–Baucke V. Biofeedback treatment for chronic constipation and encopresis in childhood: long-term outcome. Pediatrics 1995; 96:105–110.
184. Loening–Baucke V. Biofeedback training in children with functional constipation. Dig Dis Sci 1996; 41:65–71.
185. Loening–Baucke V. Constipation and biofeedback in children. Dig Dis Sci 1996; 41:1653–1657.
186. Simpson BB, Ryan DP, Schnitzer JJ, Flores A, Doody DP. Surgical evaluation and management of refractory constipation in older children. J Pediatr Surg 1996; 31:1040–1042.
187. Soave F. Hirschsprung's disease: a new surgical technique. Arch Dis Child 1964; 39:116–124.
188. Duhamel B. A new operation for the treatment of Hirschsprung's disease. Arch Dis Child 1960; 35:38–39.
189. Forsythe WI, Redmond A. Enuresis and spontaneous cure rate: study of 1129 enuretics. Arch Dis Child 1974; 49:259–263.
190. Byrd RS, Weitzman M, Lanphear NE, Auinger P. Bed-wetting in US children: epidemiology and related behavior problems. Pediatrics 1996; 98:414–419.
191. Mahony DT, Laferte RO, Blais DJ. Studies on enuresis: IX. Evidence of a mild form of compensated detrusor hyperreflexia in enuretic children. J Urol 1981; 126:520–523.
192. Nørgaard JP. Urodynamics in enuretics. II. A pressure–flow study. Neurourol Urodynam 1989; 8:213–217.
193. Nørgaard JP. Urodynamics in enuretics. I. Reservoir function. Neurourol Urodynam 1989; 8:199–211.
194. Nørgaard JP, Ritting S, Djurhuus J. Nocturnal enuresis: an approach to treatment based on pathogenesis. J Pediatr 1989; 114:705–710.
195. Rushton HG. Evaluation of the enuretic child. Clini Pediatr (Phila) 1993; spec ed:14–18.
196. Rushton HG. Wetting and functional voiding disorders. Urol Clin North Am 1995; 22:75–93.
197. Moore KH, Richmond DH, Parys BT. Sex distribution of adult idiopathic detrusor instability in relation to childhood bedwetting. Br J Urol 1991; 68:479–482.
198. Fergusson DM, Horwood LJ. Nocturnal enuresis and behavioral problems in adolescence: a 15-year longitudinal study. Pediatrics 1994; 94:662–668.
199. Bloom DA, Faerber G, Bomalaski MD. Urinary incontinence in girls. Evaluation, treatment, and its place in the standard model of voiding dysfunctions in children. Urol Clin North Am 1995; 22:521–538.
200. van Gool JD, De Jonge GA. Urge syndrome and urge incontinence. Arch Dis Child 1989; 64:1629–1634.
201. van Gool JD, Vijverberg MAW, de Jong TPVM. Functional daytime incontinence: clinical and urodynamic assessment. Scand J Urol Nephrol 1992; 141:58–69.
202. Swenson O. A new concept in the pathology of megaloureters. Surgery 1952; 32:367.
203. Pape KE, Kirsch SE. Technology-assisted self-care in the treatment of spastic diplegia. The diplegia child evaluation and management. AAP Orthop Surg 1991; 19:241–251.
204. Pape KE, Kirsch SE, Galil A, Boulton JE, White MA, Chipman M. Neuromuscular approach to the motor deficit of cerebral palsy: a pilot study. J Pediatr Orthop 1993; 13:628–633.
205. Pape KE. Therapeutic electrical stimulation: the past, the present, the future. Neuro-Dev Treat Assoc Prog Motion 1996:1–7.
206. Pape KE. Therapeutic electrical stimulation (TES) for the treatment of disuse muscle atrophy in cerebral palsy. Pediatr Phys Ther 1997:110–112.
207. Martínez–Piñeiro L, Dahiya R, Nunes LL, Tanagho EA, Schmidt RA. Pelvic plexus denervation in rats causes morphologic and functional changes of the prostate. J Urol 1993; 150:215–218.
208. Schurch B, Rodic B, Jeanmonod D. Posterior sacral rhizotomy and intradural anterior sacral

root stimulation for treatment of the spastic bladder in spinal cord injured patients. J Urol 1997; 157:610–614.

209. Steinbok P, Reiner A, Kestle JRW. Therapeutic electrical stimulation following selective posterior rhizotomy in children with spastic diplegic cerebral palsy: a randomized clinical trial. Dev Med Child Neurol 1997; 39:515–520.

210. Houle AM, Vernet O, Jednak R, Pippi Salle JL, Fanner JP. Bladder function before and after selective dorsal rhizotomy in children with cerebral palsy. J Urol 1998; 160:1088–1091.

211. Beck S. Use of sensory level electrical stimulation in the physical therapy management of a child with cerebral palsy. Pediatr Phys Ther 1997; 137–138.

212. Steers WD, Ciambotti J, Erdman S, de Groat WC. Morphological plasticity in efferent pathways to urinary bladder of the rat following urethral obstruction. J Neurosci 1990; 10:1943–1951.

213. Steers WD, Ciambotti J, Etzel B, Erdman S, de Groat WC. Alterations in afferent pathways from the urinary bladder of the rat in response to partial urethral obstruction. J Comp Neurol 1991; 310:401–410.

214. Steers WD, Creedon DJ, Tuttle JB. Immunity to nerve growth factor prevents afferent plasticity following urinary bladder hypertrophy. J Urol 1996; 155:379–385.

215. Steers WD, Kolbeck S, Creedon D, Tuttle JB. Nerve growth factor in the urinary bladder of the adult regulates neuronal form and function. J Clin Invest 1991; 88:1709–1715.

216. Clemow DB, Spitsbergen JM, McCarty R, Steers WD, Tuttle JB. Arterial nerve growth factor (NGF) MRNA, protein, and vascular smooth muscle cell NGF secretion in hypertensive and hyperactive rats. Exp Cell Res 1998; 244:196–205.

217. Clemow DB, Steers WD, McCarty R, Tuttle JB. Altered regulation of bladder nerve growth factor and neurally mediated hyperactive voiding. Am J Physiol 1998; 275:R1279–1286.

218. Edens JL, Surwit RS. In support of behavioral treatment for day wetting in children. Urol 1995; 45:905–908.

219. Hellström A, Hjälmås K, Jodal U. Terodiline in the treatment of children with unstable bladders. Br J Urol 1989; 63:358–362.

220. Diokno AC, Hyndman CW, Hardy DA, Lapides J. Comparison of action of imipramine (Tofranil) and propantheline (ProBanthine) on depressor contraction. J Urol 1972; 107:42–43.

221. Diokno AC, Lapides J. Oxybutynin: a new drug with analgesic and anticholinergic properties. J Urol 1972; 108:307–309.

222. Wein AJ. Pathophysiology and categorization of voiding dysfunction. In: Walsh PC, Retik AB, Vaughan ED Jr, Wein AJ, eds. Campbell's Urology. 7th ed. Philadelphia: Saunders, 1998:917–926.

223. Abrams P. Terodiline in clinical practice. Urology 1990; 36(suppl 4):50–57.

224. Smey P, Firlit CF, King LR. Voiding pattern abnormalities in normal children: results of pharmacologic manipulation. J Urol 1978; 120:574–577.

225. Smey P, King LR, Firlit CF. Dysfunctional voiding in children secondary to internal sphincter dyssynergia: treatment with phenoxybenzamine. Urol Clin North Am 1980; 7:337–347.

226. Lapides J, Diokno AC, Silber S, Lowe BS. Clean, intermittent self-catheterization in the treatment of urinary tract disease. J Urol 1972; 107:458–461.

227. Cole AT, Fried FA. Favorable experiences with imipramine in the treatment of neurogenic bladder. J Urol 1972; 107:44–45.

228. Tingelstad JB. The cardiotoxicity of the tricyclics. J Am Acad Child Adolesc Psychiatry 1991; 30:845–846.

229. Orne MT. The efficacy of biofeedback therapy. Annu Rev Med 1979; 30:489–503.

230. Cardozo LD, Abrams PD, Stanton SL, Feneley RCL. Idiopathic bladder instability treated by biofeedback. Br J Urol 1978; 50:521–523.

231. Cardozo LD, Stanton SL. Biofeedback: a 5-year review. Br J Urol 1984; 56:220.

232. Wear JB Jr, Wear RB, Cleeland C. Biofeedback in urology using urodynamics: preliminary observations. J Urol 1979; 121:464–468.

233. Hellström A, Hjälmås K, Jodal U. Rehabilitation of the dysfunctional bladder in children: method and 3-year follow-up. J Urol 1987; 138:847–849.

234. Jerkins GR, Noe HN, Vaughn WR, Roberts E. Biofeedback training for children with bladder sphincter incoordination. J Urol 1987; 138:1113–1115.

235. Wennergren HM, Öberg BE, Sandstedt P. The importance of leg support for relaxation of the pelvic floor muscles. Scand J Urol Nephrol 1991; 25:205–213.

236. Philips HC, Fenster HN, Samsom D. An effective treatment for functional urinary incoordination. Behav Med 1992; 15:45–63.

237. van Gool JD, Vijverberg MAW, Messer AP, Elzinga–Plomp A, de Jong TPVM. Functional daytime incontinence: non-pharmacological treatment. Scand J Urol Nephrol 1992; 141(suppl): 93–105.

238. Kjølseth D, Knudsen LM, Madsen B, Norgaard JP, Djurhuus JC. Urodynamic biofeedback training for children with bladder–sphincter dyscoordination during voiding. Neurol Urodynam 1993; 12:211–221.

239. Schneider MS, King LR, Surwit RS. Kegel exercises and childhood incontinence: a new role for an old treatment. J Pediatr 1994; 124:91–92.

240. Kjølseth D, Madsen B, Knudsen LM, Norgaard JP, Djurhuus JC. Biofeedback treatment of children and adults with idiopathic detrusor instability. Scand J Urol Nephrol 1994; 28:243–247.

241. Stein M, Discippio W, Davia M, Taub H. Biofeedback for the treatment of stress and urge incontinence. J Urol 1995; 153:641–643.

242. Wennergren H, Öberg B. Pelvic floor exercises for children: a method of treating dysfunctional voiding (Published erratum in Br J Urol 1995; 76:815). Br J Urol 1995; 76:9–15.

243. Hoebeke P, Vande Walle J, Theunis M, De Paepe H, Oosterlinck W, Renson C. Outpatient pelvic-floor therapy in girls with daytime incontinence and dysfunctional voiding. Urology 1996; 48:923–927.

244. Vijverberg MAW, Elzinga–Plomp A, Messer AP, Van Gool JD, de Jong TPVM. Bladder rehabilitation, the effect of a cognitive training program on urge incontinence. Eur Urol 1997; 31: 68–72.

245. Combs AJ, Glassberg AD, Gerdes D, Horowitz M. Biofeedback therapy for children with dysfunctional voiding. Urology 1998; 52:312–315.

246. De Paepe H, Hoebeke P, Renson C, et al. Pelvic-floor therapy in girls with recurrent urinary tract infections and dysfunctional voiding. Br J Urol 1998; 81(suppl 3):109–113.

247. Hoekx L, Wyndaele J, Vermandel A. The role of bladder biofeedback in the treatment of children with refractory nocturnal enuresis associated with idiopathic detrusor instability and small bladder capacity. J Urol 1998; 160:858–860.

248. Kegel AH. The physiologic treatment of poor tone and function of the genital muscles and of urinary stress incontinence. West J Surg Obstet Gynacol 1949; 527–535.

249. Sugar EC, Firlit CF. Urodynamic biofeedback: a new therapeutic approach for childhood incontinence. infection (vesical voluntary sphincter dyssynergia). J Urol 1982; 128:1253–1258.

250. Trsinar B, Plevnk S, Vracnik P, Drobnic J. Maximal electrical stimulation for enuresis. Proceedings International Continence Society 4th Meeting, Inssbruck 1984:495–496.

251. Plevkik S, Janez J, Vrtacnik P, Trsinar B, Vodusek DB. Short-term electrical stimulation. Home treatment for urinary incontinence. World J Urol 1986; 4:24–26.

252. Trsinar B, Kralj B. Maximal electrical stimulation in children with unstable bladder and nocturnal enuresis and/or daytime incontinence: a controlled study. Neurol Urodynam 1996; 15: 133–142.

253. Janez J, Plevnik S, Korosec L, Stanovnik L, Vrtacnik P. Changes in depressor receptor activity after electric pelvic floor stimulation. Proceedings International Continence Society 11th Meeting 1981:22–23.

254. Perez LM, Smith EA, Parrott TS, Broecker BH, Massad CA, Woodard JR. Submucosal bladder neck injection of bovine dermal collagen for stress urinary incontinence in the pediatric population. J Urol 1996; 156:633–636.

255. Chernoff A, Horowitz M, Combs A, Libretti D, Nitti V, Glassberg KI. Periurethral collagen injection for the treatment of urinary incontinence in children. J Urol 1997; 157:2303–2305.

256. Leonard MP, Decter A, Mix LW, Johnson HW, Coleman GU. Treatment of urinary incontinence in children by endoscopically directed bladder neck injection of collagen. J Urol 1996; 156:637–641.

257. Sundaram CP, Reinberg Y, Aliabadi HA. Failure to obtain durable results with collagen implantation in children with urinary incontinence. J Urol 1997; 157:2306–2307.

258. McGuire IJ, Wang CC, Usitalo H, Savastano J. Modified pubovaginal sling in girls with myelodysplasia. J Urol 1986; 135:94–96.

259. Bauer SB, Peters CA, Colodny AH, Mandell J, Retik AB. The use of rectus fascia to manage urinary incontinence. J Urol 1989; 142:516–521.

260. Gormley EA, Bloom DA, McGuire EJ, Fitchey ML. Pubovaginal slings for the management of urinary incontinence in female adolescents. J Urol 1994; 152:822–825.

261. Kurzrock EA, Lowe P, Hardy BE. Bladder wall pedicle wraparound sling for neurogenic urinary incontinence in children. J Urol 1996; 155:305–308.

262. Young HH. An operation for the cure of incontinence of urine. Surg Gynecol Obstet 1919; 28:84.

263. Leadbetter GW Jr. Surgical correction for total urinary incontinence. J Urol 1964; 91:261.

264. Dees JE. Congenital epispadias with incontinence. J Urol 1949; 62:513.

265. Kropp KA, Angwafo FF. Urethral lengthening and reimplantation for neurogenic incontinence in children. J Urol 1986; 135:533.

266. Pippi Salle JL, De Fraga JCS, Amarant A, Silveira ML, Lambertz M, Schmidt M, Rosito NC. Urethral lengthening with anterior bladder wall flap for urinary incontinence: a new approach. J Urol 1994; 152:803–806.

267. Barrett DM, Furlow WL. The management of severe urinary incontinence in patients with myelodysplasia by implantation of the AS791/792 urinary sphincter device. J Urol 1982; 128: 484–486.

268. Light JK, Hawila M, Scott FB. Treatment of urinary incontinence in children: the artificial sphincter vs. other methods. J Urol 1983; 130:518–521.

269. Bosco PJ, Bauer SB, Colodny AH, Mandell J, Retik AB. The long-term results of artificial urinary sphincters in children. J Urol 1991; 146:396–399.

270. Mitrofanoff P. Cystométrie continente trans-appendiculaire dans le traitement des vessies neurologiques. Chir Pediatr 1980; 21:297–305.

271. Woodhouse CRJ, Malone PR, Cumming J, Reilly TM. The Mitrofanoff principle for continent urinary diversion. Br J Urol 1989; 63:53–57.

272. Benchekroun A. The ileocecal continent bladder. In: King L, Stone AR, Webster GD, eds. Bladder Reconstruction and Continent Urinary Diversion. Chicago: Year Book Medical Publishers 1987:324–336.

273. Kock NG, Nilson AE, Nilsson LO, Norlen LJ, Philipson BM. Urinary diversion via a continent ileal reservoir: clinical results in 12 patients. J Urol 1982; 128:469–475.

274. Thuroff JW, Alken P, Reidmiller H, Engelmann U, Jacobi GH, Hohenfellner R. The Mainz pouch (mixed augmentation ileum and cecum) for bladder augmentation and continent diversion. J Urol 1986; 136:17–26.

275. Rowland RG, Mitchell ME, Birhle R, Kahnoski RJ, Piser JE. Indiana continent urinary reservoir. J Urol 1987; 137:1136–1139.

276. Duckett JW, Snyder HM. Use of the Mitrofanoff principle in urinary reconstruction. World J Urol 1985; 3:191–193.

277. Carr MC, Mitchell ME. Continent gastric pouch. World J Urol 1996; 14:112–116.

278. Ambrose SS. Ureterosigmoidostomy. In Glenn JF, ed. Urologic Surgery. 3rd ed. Philadelphia: JB Lippincott, 1983.

279. Yeung CK, Chiu HN. Bladder dysfunction in children with refractory monosymptomatic primary nocturnal enuresis. Am Acad Pediatr Annu Meet. San Francisco, CA, 1998: abstr 25.

10

The Aging Pelvic Floor

CARA TANNENBAUM

McGill University Health Centre, Montreal, Quebec, Canada

LOUISE PERRIN

McGill University, Montreal, Quebec, Canada

GEORGE A. KUCHEL

University of Connecticut Center on Aging and University of Connecticut Health Center, Farmington, Connecticut

I. DEMOGRAPHIC ISSUES

In recent years there has been an unprecedented expansion in the numbers of persons reaching advanced age (1). These changes have been most dramatic in industrialized western countries, yet increasing evidence points to the fact that many other countries in Asia and Africa, particularly Japan, will be facing similar and perhaps even more striking demographic challenges in future decades (1). Nevertheless, to date, this phenomenon has been most dramatic and best documented in North America and the countries of Western Europe (1). For example, in 1975, people aged 75 and older represented only 5–6% of the North American population. In contrast, today the percentage has increased to 7% and is expected to increase to 15–18% by the year 2050 (1). It is projected that by the year 2050, the elderly will constitute 23% of the U.S. population (2). European projections are even higher, with a prediction that 25% of the overall European and 35% of the Italian population will be elderly in 2050 (1).

In addition to the overall foregoing changes, several additional trends involving our older citizens merit consideration. Individuals who are 85 years and older (the oldest old) constitute the most rapidly growing demographic group in western countries (3). These individuals now constitute approximately 10% of all North American seniors, but this proportion is expected to increase more than 160% by the year 2041. In fact, according to

World Bank estimates, the number of centenarians is expected to double every decade, with the expectation that there will be 2.2 million people in the world over 100-years old in 2050 (1,3). Another trend is the increasing "feminization" of the older population, as women continue to benefit from a substantial survival advantage, as compared with men. For example, a 65-year-old woman living in North America has a 50% chance of reaching age 85, and at that age she will outnumber her male counterparts by a ratio of approximately 2.6:1 (2,3).

Although the issue of growing old often evokes rather common stereotypical reactions among both the general public, as well as health care providers, most evidence points to increasing, rather than decreasing, interindividual heterogeneity as we grow old (4). The issue of "compression of morbidity" continues to be debated, because it is not clear whether disability rates have, on average, changed to a lesser or greater extent than have mortality rates (5). At the same time, although there may have been some recent changes in disability rates (6), actual numbers of older individuals who survive into old age with minimal or no functional deficits continue to increase, as do the numbers of frail and disabled elderly.

The influence of all these demographic changes on the practice profiles of health professionals dealing with problems related to the pelvic floor will be complex. Not only will most health care providers be seeing much larger numbers of older and elderly individuals, but these patients' general health status, burden of comorbid diseases, and overall level of functional independence will vary tremendously. Clearly, in the next few decades, age-related biological degenerative processes involving the genitourinary tract will be among the most important challenges facing physicians and other health care professionals dealing with pelvic floor and urogynecological pathology. Care of such patients will often require highly specialized and targeted clinical expertise. At the same time, optimum care of the older patient usually necessitates a more global approach, one that extends beyond the pelvic floor and beyond the actual presenting complaint. This truism is particularly so in the case of older individuals who are more "frail" or disabled. In addition to considering the contribution played by specific disease processes, the role of normal aging cannot be neglected even in healthy older individuals. Normal aging can influence the presentation of individual clinical symptoms, as well as their effect on quality of life (7). Moreover, specific physiological changes associated with normal aging may influence such important factors as fluid balance, blood pressure regulation, the effectiveness of standard anesthetic regimens, as well as metabolism and risk–benefit profiles of many categories of medications (7).

II. "NORMAL" AGING OF THE PELVIC FLOOR
   AND ASSOCIATED STRUCTURES

The term *urogenital aging* has been used in recent years to define the normal physiological changes that occur in the female lower genitourinary tract with age, which then predispose to a complex of symptoms involving the lower urinary tract, the genital tract, and the pelvic floor (8,9). A variety of symptoms referable to the pelvic floor and associated structures may be influenced by urogenital aging. These include urinary incontinence, fecal incontinence and other bowel symptoms, sexual dysfunction, as well as urogenital atrophy and prolapse in the female (8,9).

Complicating the foregoing approach is that, in contrast to many other organ systems, our current state of knowledge of urogenital aging does not allow us to clearly delineate between changes that result from normative aging and those that are due to the presence of disease processes that are common in older women. For example, many studies of vaginal cytology performed in older and elderly women, who are not receiving any hormonal replacement therapy (HRT), have shown the presence of highly variable cytological profiles (10–12). Although considered as a part of urogenital aging, only a minority of elderly women not receiving HRT develop clinical and cytological evidence of atrophic vaginitis (8–12). Moreover, this condition usually requires treatment because it is commonly associated with bothersome symptoms, including vaginismus and dysparunia, while also being a major risk factor for such problems as recurrent urinary tract infections (8,9,12). Thus, although advanced age and lower estrogen both appear to be risk factors, atrophic vaginitis and its associated sequelae can hardly be considered normal.

Even though ovarian estrogen production generally ceases within a few years of the menopause, serum estrogen levels are still detectable in nearly all elderly women, even if they are not receiving any HRT (13). In addition, nearly two-thirds of these women exhibit evidence of variable degrees of estrogenic stimulation on vaginal cytology (10,14). Both the serum (13) and cytological indices (14) of endogenous estrogens vary greatly in elderly women and correlate with body weight and body mass index. Based on these considerations, as well as the presence of aromatase enzyme activity in adipose tissues, it has been proposed that most "residual" estrogens in elderly women are derived from the adipose tissue conversion of adrenally derived androstenedione into low-potency estrone (13). However, there has also been a growing awareness of the presence and potential importance of compounds with nonnegligible estrogenic properties in the form of dietary isoflavones, as well as various "carrier" compounds commonly present in topical creams.

The lack of a clear understanding of what constitutes urogenital and pelvic aging, combined with ongoing demographic imperatives, present the investigator with unique challenges, as well as opportunities. Future research efforts in this area will need to more carefully consider the recruitment and characterization of aged subjects, particularly in terms of excluding confounding disease and considering nutritional and lifestyle factors that can influence aging. Levels of "residual" estrogens cannot be neglected when evaluating urogenital aging because these previously neglected hormones clearly have physiological effects on bone turnover and risk of fractures (15), as well as the maturation of vaginal cells (14). Moreover, there is a growing need to consider, whenever possible, the inclusion of a prospective study design, as a strong reliance on cross-sectional methodology can confound gerontological studies (16). Finally, there is an urgent need to develop appropriate animal and in vitro models, bringing the full potential of biomedical translational research into this field.

III. PREVALENCE OF SYMPTOMS RELATED TO THE PELVIC FLOOR

Review of the literature demonstrates a great variability in the prevalence of genitourinary symptoms in older women. This variability appears to be due to differences in populations being studied, variations in research design, as well as varying definitions. In one typical European survey the prevalence of symptoms caused, at least in part, by changes associated with aging of the urogenital structures, was estimated to be between 25 and 40% (9,17).

Urinary incontinence alone has been reported to occur in 15–35% of individuals 60 years and older living in the community, and in more than one-half of those living in long-term care facilities (18). Older women are particularly vulnerable, with a prevalence more than twice as high in older women than men (18). With these considerations in mind, it becomes worthwhile to examine the specific urodynamic, anatomical, biochemical, and pharmacological changes that occur in the pelvic floor as a function of age to better understand the resulting pathological processes in general and dysfunction of the urinary sphincter in particular.

IV. URODYNAMIC CHANGES WITH AGING

Intuitively, the effects of normal aging on the human urethra and the pelvic floor should be reflected by variations in urodynamic measurements in elderly subjects. Changes in levator ani muscle strength and tone, as well as intrinsic urethral factors involving autonomic innervation, mucosal coaptation, striated and smooth muscles changes in the urethral wall, vascular congestion of the submucosal venous plexus, and elasticity of the urethral wall itself, often lumped under the heading of "urogenital atrophy," should lead to subtle differences in the normative urodynamics of elderly individuals compared with their younger counterparts. Unfortunately, there are no gold standard longitudinal studies examining intraindividual changes in urodynamic parameters over time. This consideration is also true for urethral pressure profilometry (UPP), which has much potential for the study of normal changes seen in urethral integrity and dynamic function as part of the aging pelvic floor in both men and women. In spite of the potential limitations of cross-sectional studies, we will examine available data on aging urodynamic function in the elderly. In view of significant anatomical and physiological differences between older men and women, as well as the effects of prostatic enlargement and estrogenic insufficiency, respectively, these two groups will be considered separately.

A. Urodynamic Changes in the Aging Male

The natural history of sphincter function changes in elderly men was examined most extensively by Hammerer et al. (19) by analyzing urodynamic studies utilizing UPP in 257 men 44–88 year of age. They found that sphincter length decreased with age from 24.3 to 14.8 mm, that maximal urethral pressure decreased from 88.7 to 55 cmH_2O and that maximal urethral pressure during voluntary contraction decreased from 221.4 to 166.3 cmH_2O. No morphometric correlation was obtained, which could have clarified whether the observed decrease in maximal urethral closure pressure was caused by decreased activity of the periurethral striated musculature, smooth-muscle activity, or organic narrowing of the urethral lumen owing to enlarged glandular tissue. Another a confounding variable is that localized prostatic cancer, benign prostatic hyperplasia (BPH), and superficial bladder cancer were not excluded in this study. Because all these conditions, as well as prostatic volume, tend to increase with patient age, it is not entirely surprising that among the elderly individuals included in this study, none were completely free of these conditions. Thus, it is unclear whether these data reflect changes of normal aging or concomitant lower urinary tract disease. Whereas, histological evidence of BPH is present nearly universally among elderly men, significant prostatic enlargement results in only about half of affected individuals (20). We cannot, therefore, extrapolate these findings to all healthy elderly men, although the trend toward decreased urethral resistance is supported theoretically by some of the anatomical changes that are seen with normal aging. No studies of the changes with age in urethral compliance have been reported in men.

Studies of uroflowmetry in men all document a decrease in urine flow with age (21–23). Unfortunately, examination of the various reports demonstrates a tremendous variability between different studies. Moreover, intraindividual variability, attributed to varying studies, contexts and measurement surroundings, have also been reported. As a result of these difficulties, uroflowmetry often does not provide a clear distinction between normal, unobstructed, and obstructed voiding.

There are currently no universally accepted nomograms for decremental increments in urine flow in men with normal aging. However, it has been proposed that, with a minimum void of 200 mL, a minimally acceptable maximum urine flow rate should be 21 mL/sec for men aged 14–45, 12 mL/sec for those aged 46–65, and 9 mL/sec for those aged 66–80 (24). Although based on clinical experience, these recommendations have not been validated in large longitudinal studies. Moreover, is it unclear whether the decline in maximal flow is due to decreased bladder contractility, effects of luminal obstruction, decreased urethral resistance or, most likely, a combination of the three.

Postvoid residual urine volumes (PVR) have generally been assumed to increase with age (25), although a clear-cut normative cutoff value for unobstructed men has not been established. The prevalence, median, and range of residual urine in elderly men in the community was documented by Bonde et al. (26) using nonrepeated sonographic measurement in 92 randomly selected 75-year-old men with a prevoid volume of 150 mL. One man had 1502 mL of residual urine, and the remaining 91 men had PVR measurements in the range of 10–400 mL, with 75% of men having PVRs greater than 50 mL. Correlation with lower urinary tract symptoms was not reported. Resnick et al. (27) measured PVRs using repeated urinary catheterization in 17 institutionalized incontinent elderly men; however, the high prevalence of impaired detrusor contractility in this population makes it difficult to extrapolate the findings to the general-aging population.

B. Urodynamic Changes in the Aging Female

In studies of continent women, UPP has demonstrated that the maximal urethral pressure, maximal urethral closure pressure, and functional urethral length decrease with age, especially beyond the age of 60 (28). Abrams et al. (29) reported a decline in maximal urethral pressure to 65 cmH$_2$O in women older than age 64 in whom no pathological abnormality had been found. These findings have been ascribed to reduced urethral vascularity, a decrease in α-adrenergic receptors, and soft tissue atrophy—all presumably occurring secondary to low levels of circulating estrogens found in postmenopausal women. Results from detailed morphometric studies of age changes in the various tissue components of the normal human urethra have demonstrated a decrease in the relative volume of striated muscle in the urethra with increasing age and a decrease in the volume fraction of blood vessels, lending support to this hypothesis (30,31). An increase in the connective tissue component of the female urethra with age has also been observed, although no changes in the smooth-muscle category have been reported (30). Susset et al. (32) examined changes in the compliance of the female urethra with age and found that compliance also decreased significantly, perhaps as a result of the aforementioned increased connective tissue content. None of the women studied in Susset's analysis were truly normal, however, as all presented with lower urinary tract symptoms, so these results must be interpreted with caution.

Some studies of uroflowmetry in women fail to demonstrate an age effect (33–34), whereas others do (35). All studies were subject to potential bias due to the presence of lower urinary tract symptoms, degree of straining and volume, and method of measurement. Abrams et al. (24) reported a minimum acceptable maximum urine flow of 10 mL/sec in women with normal urinary tract function, aged 66–80, with a voided volume of 200 mL or more, compared to 18 mL/sec in women aged 14–45 and 15 mL/sec for women aged 46–65. As discussed in the foregoing, these stated criteria for uroflowmetry "normalcy" are based on clinical experience and need to be validated by large longitudinal studies.

The influence of age on PVR in women was evaluated most extensively by Brocklehurst et al. (37), who found that 88% of the women studied without prior incontinence or left cerebral hemispheric lesions had residual volumes of less than 100 mL, with a median of 50 mL. Bonde et al. (26) confirmed a median PVR measurement of 45 mL in 48 75-year-old community-dwelling women, with a range of 0–180 mL. As is true with men, it is difficult to discern the effects of normal aging on PVR from the influence of the silent phenomenon of impaired detrusor contractility, which appears to increase in incidence with age (27).

V. SUMMARY

Increasing numbers of individuals are reaching advanced age. Symptoms related to the pelvic floor are common in late life and can have a major influence on the quality of life of older women and men. As a result, the health professional dealing with pelvic floor dysfunction will need to be increasingly familiar with the care of older and elderly individuals. Considerable evidence points to unique clinical needs of older patients. Future research into the aging pelvic floor is needed to develop a better understanding of the effect of aging and of specific disease processes on the pelvic floor.

REFERENCES

1. United Nations Department of Economic and Social Affairs Population Division. World population prospects: the 1996 revision. New York: United Nations, 1997.
2. Day JC. Bureau of the Census. Current Population Reports. Population Projections of the United States by Age, Sex, Race, and Hispanic Origin: 1993 to 2050. Washington DC: Government Printing Office, 1993:P25–1104.
3. Suzman RM, Willis DP, Manton KG. The Oldest Old. New York: Oxford University Press, 1992.
4. Rowe JW, Kahn RL. Human aging: usual and successful. Science 1987; 237:143–149.
5. Fries JF. Physical activity, the compression of morbidity, and the health of the elderly. J R Soc Med 1996; 89:64–68.
6. Manton KG, Corder L, Stallard E. Chronic disability trends in elderly United States populations: 1982–1994. Proc Natl Acad Sci USA 1997; 94:2593–2598.
7. Katzman R, Rowe JW. Principles of Geriatric Neurology. Philadelphia: FA Davis, 1992.
8. Lovatsis D, Drutz HP. The role of estrogen in female urinary incontinence and urogenital aging: a review. Ostomy Wound Manage 1998; 44:48–53.
9. Bachmann G. Urogenital ageing: an old problem newly recognized. Maturitas 1995; 22(suppl): S1–S5.
10. Meisels A. The menopause: a cytohormonal study. Acta Cytol 1966; 10:49–55.
11. Wied GL, Bibbo M. Hormonal cytology. In: Bibbo M, ed. Comprehensive Cytopathology. Philadelphia: WB Saunders, 1991:85–114.
12. Bergh PA. Vaginal changes with aging. In: Breen JL, ed. The Gynecologist and the Older Patient. Rockville, MD: Aspen Publishers, 1988:299–311.
13. Judd HL, Fournet N. Changes of ovarian hormonal function with aging. Exp Gerontol 1994; 29:285–298.
14. Morse AR, Hutton JD, Jacobs HS, Murray MA, James VH. Relation between the karyopyknotic index and plasma oestrogen concentrations after the menopause. Br J Obstet Gynaecol 1979; 86:981–983.
15. Cummings SR, Browner WS, Bauer D, Stone K, Ensrud K, Jamal S, Ettinger B. Study Osteoporotic Fractures Research Group. Endogenous hormones and the risk of hip and vertebral fractures among older women. N Engl J Med 1998; 339:733–738.
16. Bleich HL, Boro ES, Rowe JW. Clinical research on aging: strategies and directions. N Engl J Med 1977; 297:1332–1336.
17. Pan-European study on the prevalence of urogenital aging and its perceived impact on "quality of life." Med Radar Int 1995:project No. 94069.
18. Fantl JA, Newman DK, Colling J, et al. Clinical Practice Guideline. Quick Reference Guide for

Clinicians, No. 2, 1996 Update. Rockville, MD: U.S. Department of Health and Human Services, Public Health Service, Agency for Health Care Policy and Research. AHCPR Pub. 96-0686, March 1996.

19. Hammerer P, Michl U, Meyer–Moldenhauer WH, Huland H. Urethral closure pressure changes with age in men. J Urol 1996; 156:1741–1743.

20. Isaacs JT, Coffey DS. Etiology and disease process of benign prostatic hyperplasia. Prostate Suppl 1989; 2:33–50.

21. Frimodt-Moller C. A urodynamic study of micturition in healthy men and women. Dan Med Bull 1974; 21:41–48.

22. Drach GW, Layton TN, Binard WJ. Male peak urinary flow rate: relationships to volume voided and age. J Urol 1979; 122:210–214.

23. Drach GW, Layton T, Bottacini MR. A method of adjustment of male peak urinary flow rate for varying age and volume voided. J Urol 1982; 128:960–962.

24. Abrams P, Feneley R, Torrens M. Urodynamics. New York: Springer-Verlag, 1983:35.

25. Resnick NM. Geriatric incontinence. Urol Clin North Am 1996; 23:55–74.

26. Bonde HV, Sejr T, Erdmann L, Meyhoff HH, Lendorf A, Rosenkilde P, Bodker A, Nielsen MB. Residual urine in 75-year-old men and women. A normative population study. Scand J Urol Nephrol 1996; 30:89–91.

27. Resnick NM, Yalla SV, Laurino E. The pathophysiology of urinary incontinence among institutionalized elderly persons. N Engl J Med 1989; 320:1–7.

28. Rud T. Urethral pressure profile in continent women from childhood to old age. Acta Obstet Gynecol Scand 1980; 59:331–335.

29. Abrams P, Fenelay R, Torrens M. Urodynamics. New York: Springer-Verlag, 1983:56.

30. Carlile A, Davies I, Rigby A, Broclehurst JC. Age changes in the human female urethra: a morphometric study. J Urol 1988; 139:532–535.

31. Huisman AB. Aspects on the anatomy of the female urethra with special relation to urinary continence. Contrib Gynecol Obstet 1983; 10:1–31.

32. Susset JG, Ghoniem GM, Regnier CH. Abnormal urethral compliance in females: diagnosis, results and treatment. Preliminary study. J Urol 1983; 129:1063–1065.

33. Griffiths DJ. Urodynamic assessment of bladder function. Br J Urol 1977; 49:29–36.

34. Drach GW, Ignatoff J, Layton T. Peak urinary flow rate: observations in female subjects and comparison to male subjects. J Urol 1979; 122:215–219.

35. Fanti JA, Smith PJ, Schneider V, Hurt WG, Dunn LJ. Fluid weight uroflowmetry in women. Am J Obstet Gynecol 1983; 145:1017–1024.

36. Backman KA. Urinary flow during micturition in normal women. Acta Chir Scand 1965; 130:357–370.

37. Brocklehurst JC, Dillane JB. Studies of the female bladder in old age. 1. Cystometrograms in nonincontinent women. Gerontol Clin 1966; 8:285–305.

11

Epidemiology of the Dysfunctional Urinary Sphincter

ANDREW K. CHUNG, KENNETH M. PETERS, and ANANIAS C. DIOKNO

William Beaumont Hospital, Royal Oak, Michigan

I. COMPONENTS OF THE URINARY SPHINCTER

The urinary sphincter comprises an internal component, predominantly made up of smooth muscle, and an external component of striated muscle fibers (rhabdosphincter). The musculature of the bladder is complex and has a plexiform organization without recognizable arrangement into discrete layers. As the muscle bundles approach the ureteral orifices and bladder neck, however, they become organized into three distinct layers: an inner longitudinal layer, a middle circular layer, and an outer longitudinal layer. It is controversial whether these extend into the urethra. Tanagho (1), Woodburne (2), Elbadawi (3), and Hutch and Rambo (4) state that the longitudinal muscle of the bladder base extends into the proximal urethra as its inner longitudinal layer. However, others maintain that all muscle bundles of the detrusor end at the urethral orifice (5–7). Although the vesical neck does not have an anatomical sphincter, the circular fibers of the deep detrusor musculature may provide a functional sphincter. The abundance of elastic tissue in the submucosa and the tone of the urethral muscles also contribute to the sphincter-like properties of this area (8). It may act as a mechanism for urinary continence and may also prevent retrograde ejaculation (9). An analogous sphincter is not present in females.

The male sphincter mechanism has been described by Turner–Warwick as two continence zones located in the posterior urethra: a proximal zone and a distal urethral zone. The proximal zone involves the bladder neck and the preprostatic sphincter. The distal urethral zone extends from the verumontanum, traverses the prostatic apex, and ends at the perineal membrane. Both of these zones are important, as surgery that preserves at least one mechanism maintains urinary continence. The proximal urethral continence mechanism is under involuntary control, whereas the external distal sphincter mechanism is under voluntary control.

Sphincteric resistance may be implied in a measure called functional urethral length. This refers to the length of the posterior urethra which is capable of exerting pressure that exceeds intravesical pressure without a detrusor contraction. Radical retropubic prostatectomy shortens functional urethral length, and preservation of the more distal sphincter helps reduce the incidence of postprostatectomy incontinence.

One can also view the entire posterior urethra (from the bladder neck to the distal end of the membranous urethra) as a single continence mechanism. The vesicourethral junction, prostatic urethra, and membranous urethra would then be considered the intrinsic or internal sphincter, and the periurethral striated muscle surrounding the internal sphincter considered to be the external sphincter. The intrinsic sphincter is involuntary, and the periurethral striated muscle, which is heavily concentrated at the region of the membranous urethra, is voluntary. Continence may be dependent on a variety of factors, including urethral wall tension, caliber of the urethral lumen, and functional length of the urethra (10,11). The striated muscles surrounding the urethra augment the internal sphincter during strenuous activity, but are not essential for continence during nonstrenuous activities. The external sphincter is important for voluntary termination of micturition.

The female continence mechanism is different from its male counterpart. A physiological internal sphincter is not present. The main sphincter activity is found in the proximal three-fourths of the urethra. At this site, especially the midurethra, the vascular plexus is most abundant, and the smooth and striated muscles are best developed.

To be continent, the urethra must seal properly, urethral pressure must be higher than bladder pressure, and the bladder must be under control. Urethral compression and inner urethral folding are thought to contribute to urethral sealing. The inner epithelial surface is richly folded to allow complete apposition of the mucosa. There is a network of veins, elastic tissue, and collagen fibers that form a spongy layer that fills the urethral folds (12). The urethral venous plexus has been theorized to contribute to the urethral high-pressure zone and is considered to be an auxiliary closure mechanism (13). This theory is based on the findings of Enhorning (13) in which vascular pulsation, especially at the urethral high-pressure zone, affected urethral profilometry. These findings have been confirmed by others (14,15).

The urethral-sealing effect has been noted to decrease with increasing age. Hormonal factors have been implicated, for an atrophic mucosa seen in menopausal women can lead to decreased urethral sealing. With aging, muscle tone likewise diminishes, thereby increasing the risk of incontinence.

The anatomy of the urethral smooth muscles has been well studied. It consists of a thick inner longitudinal layer and a thin outer circular layer. Because the outer circular layer is thin, its exact role in the urethral closure mechanism is unclear. Evidence shows that the urethral smooth muscles play an important role, as manifested by a 35–65% drop in urethral pressure when the drug phentolamine is given intravenously (16–18).

The striated urethral muscle is also an important component of the urethral closure mechanism. It is composed of muscles of the urogenital diaphragm, which is a continuous fan of skeletal muscle oriented transversely and covers the anterior surface of the urethra and distal vagina. Striated urethral muscle fibers surround the entire urethra in the region of the bladder neck and proximal third of the urethra. They incompletely surround the urethra, beginning at the middle third, with some fibers encircling both the urethra and vagina to insert posteriorly at the rectovaginal septum.

Multiple etiologies can cause dysfunction in either or both the striated sphincter and smooth-muscle sphincter. Dysfunction of the urinary sphincter can be divided into three classifications: incompetent urinary sphincter, hypertonic urinary sphincter, and dyssynergic urinary sphincter.

II. INCOMPETENT URINARY SPHINCTER

The incompetent urinary sphincter comprises a large component of sphincteric dysfunction. However, the exact prevalence is unknown. An incompetent urinary sphincter may result in *stress urinary incontinence* (SUI), which is defined as an involuntary loss of urine when intravesical pressure exceeds maximum urethral pressure (19). Valsalva maneuvers, such as coughing, sneezing, straining, or physical activity, lead to urinary incontinence. Stress incontinence may be secondary to pelvic muscle relaxation or intrinsic sphincter deficiency (ISD).

Stress incontinence affects 15–60% of women (20,21) and rarely touches men. Studies have demonstrated that 50% of young nulliparous nursing students and 25% of nulliparous varsity athletes have some component of stress incontinence (22,23). Pregnancy increases the likelihood of developing SUI. The Medical Epidemiologic and Social Aspects of Aging Study interviewed 1145 women 60 years or older and found a 37.6% prevalence of urinary incontinence (24). Of these, 26.7% complained of pure stress incontinence, and 55.3%, of both stress and urge (mixed) incontinence. Thus, 64% of incontinent women older than the age of 60 had a component of stress incontinence from either pelvic floor relaxation or ISD.

ISD is unlikely to occur de novo. Its incidence in patients with stress incontinence and no previous operative therapy has been reported to be only 6–9% (25,26). In men, the most common cause of stress incontinence resulting from ISD is prostate surgery. Radical prostatectomy culminates in SUI in 2.5–87% of men (27–31). On the basis of urodynamic studies, sphincteric damage is the sole factor behind postradical prostatectomy incontinence in 5–62% of men (32–39). The incidence of incontinence after transurethral resection of the prostate is approximately 1% (40–42), although sphincteric damage is not the sole cause of incontinence in all these cases. Other surgeries can lead to an incompetent urinary sphincter owing to damaged pelvic and pudendal nerves. Motor parasympathetic denervation after abdominoperineal resection (APR) was first reported to be close to 60% (43,44). More recent studies have demonstrated the rate to be 7.5–12% (45,46). Although urinary retention is more common after APR, urinary incontinence has been noted to be 9–17% (47). Radical hysterectomy produces postoperative incontinence rates of 4–27% (48). Incontinence is directly related to the extent of dissection of the pelvic plexus as it travels around and over the upper third of the vagina on its way to the bladder and urethra. The proportion of incontinence elicited solely by sphincteric damage is unknown in these cases.

An incompetent urethral sphincter can be caused by inherited syndromes, such as myelodysplasia and Shy–Drager syndrome. The incidence of myelodysplasia is 1:1000 live births. The incidence doubles when more than one family member has a neurospinal dysraphism (49). The typical myelodysplastic patient shows an areflexic bladder with an open bladder neck. Urodynamically, 69% of myelodysplastic patients have some evidence of striated sphincter denervation, whereas only 15% have true detrusor–sphincter dyssynergia (DSD) (50). Shy–Drager syndrome is a progressive disease causing cell loss and gliosis in the cerebellum, substantia nigra, globus pallidus, caudate, putamen, inferior olives, interomediolateral columns of the spinal cord and Onuf's nucleus (51,52). The disease occurs predominantly in middle age. Initial urological findings are urgency, frequency, and urge incontinence. Cystourethrography and videourodynamics generally reveal an open bladder neck and evidence of striated sphincter denervation on motor unit electromyography (EMG). Striated sphincter abnormalities make prostate surgery hazardous in men and predispose women to sphincteric incontinence.

III. HYPERTONIC URINARY SPHINCTER

The hypertonic urinary sphincter occurs primarily after anti-incontinence procedures. The true incidence of iatrogenic obstruction after anti-incontinence procedures is unknown, but has been estimated to be between 2.5 and 24% (53–57). Transient urinary retention has been reported in up to 41% of patients, whereas prolonged urinary retention is seen in less than 5% (58).

Primary bladder neck obstruction is defined as the inability of the bladder neck to open properly in the presence of a normal detrusor contraction. It was originally described in a male by Marion in 1933 (59). On endoscopy, there is no visible lesion, and this traditionally was a diagnosis of exclusion. With the use of videourodynamic testing, the diagnosis of primary bladder neck obstruction can be made accurately. Primary bladder neck obstruction in women is very rare (60–62).

Another rare cause of the hypertonic sphincter is external sphincter spasticity owing to increased tone of the pelvic floor–external sphincter complex in women (63,64). The syndrome may result from introital or vaginal infections, urethritis, Skene's gland abscesses, anorectal disease, or adnexal disease.

IV. DYSSYNERGIC SPHINCTER

A DSD results from a suprasacral spinal cord lesion causing a detrusor contraction against a closed external sphincter that may lead to damage of the upper urinary tract. Supraspinal cord injury has an annual incidence exceeding 10,000, and its prevalence is estimated to be over 200,000 (65,66). More than 50% of those with suprasacral spinal cord lesions are between 16 and 35 years old, and more than 80% are male (66,67). Lesions between the sacral spinal cord and the area of sympathetic outflow result in detrusor hyperreflexia, absent sensation below the level of the lesion, smooth sphincter synergia, and striated sphincter dyssynergia. Lesions above the spinal cord level of T7 and T8 may lead to in smooth sphincter dyssynergia as well. The level of the clinical neurological disorder often does not correlate with expected vesicourethral function; thus, management of the urinary tract must be based on urodynamic findings (68,69).

Multiple sclerosis is a very common cause of DSD. The prevalence of multiple sclerosis is between 6:100,000 and 122:100,000 individuals (70). It affects young and middle-aged adults, with an increased incidence in women, urban dwellers, and inhabitants of temperate climates (71,72). The demyelinating process most commonly involves the posterior and lateral columns of the cervical spinal cord (73,74). DSD occurs in 12–66% of patients with multiple sclerosis. A recent metanalysis of 22 studies put the frequency of DSD in multiple sclerosis patients at 25% (75).

Nonneurogenic–neurogenic bladder (Hinman's syndrome) is a learned behavior resulting in active contraction of the striated sphincter during voiding. This leads in urgency, urge or stress incontinence, intermittent urination associated with straining, recurrent urinary tract infections, and profound changes to the urinary tract. Hydroureteronephrosis, vesicoureteral reflux, and grossly trabeculated, large-capacity bladder are often seen. The prevalence of this disorder is unknown.

There are a variety of disorders that cause urinary tract dysfunction, but ordinarily with smooth and striated sphincter synergia. These include cerebrovascular accident (CVA), for which EMG studies show that true detrusor–external sphincter dyssynergia is rare, but a voluntary contraction of the external sphincter during an involuntary detrusor contraction (pseudodyssynergia) may occur (68). The majority of patients have detrusor hyperreflexia with synergic voiding (76–79).

Likewise, most patients with cerebral palsy have detrusor hyperreflexia with synergic voiding. In patients younger than 20 years of age, however, 25% exhibit striated sphincter dyssynergia (80). As they age, though, it appears that sphincter dysfunction is attributable to problems relaxing the pelvic floor and not true striated sphincter dyssynergia (81).

Sporadic involuntary activity in the striated sphincter during involuntary bladder contractions may be detected in as many as 60% of patients with Parkinson's disease. However, this does not cause obstruction, and thus is not true dyssynergia (82,83). Perineal EMG reveals a delayed relaxation of the external sphincter during bladder contraction in 25–60% of parkinsonian patients (84,85), but again, true striated sphincter dyssynergia does not occur.

Herniated disk disease may also cause voiding dysfunction, which is most commonly seen when the lesions occur at the T12–L1, L4–L5, or L5–S1 interspaces (86). T12–L1 (conus medullaris) disease impairs the thoracolumbar sympathetic nuclei and associated sympathetic pathways subserving vesicourethral function. They may impair smooth muscle function at the bladder neck and proximal portions of the urethra, resulting in SUI (87). L4–L5 and L5–S1 disease impairs the parasympathetic pelvic nerve and the pudendal nerve, and may cause detrusor denervation, ISD, and denervation of the external urethral sphincter (88,89).

V. CONCLUSION

The urinary sphincter is generally thought to have a voluntary (striated) sphincter and an involuntary (smooth) sphincter. The location of the well-developed striated muscle in the male is primarily in the membranous urethra, whereas in the female it is in the midurethra and poorly developed. The smooth muscle is located in the proximal three-fourths of the urethra in women, whereas the position is primarily at the bladder neck and prostatic urethra in men.

There are multiple etiologies of sphincteric dysfunction. These may be divided into the incompetent urinary sphincter, hypertonic urinary sphincter, and dyssynergic urinary sphincter. The incompetent urinary sphincter usually manifests as stress urinary incontinence, and affects as many as 60% of women. Many disorders may cause sphincteric incompetence, and includes postsurgical changes, radiation, myelodysplasia, and the Shy–Drager syndrome, among others. A hypertonic sphincter may be caused by postsurgical changes, primary bladder neck obstruction (Marion's syndrome) or increased tone of the pelvic floor–external sphincter complex. A dyssynergic sphincter may result from spinal cord injuries, multiple sclerosis, and neurogenic bladder, among others. Various other disorders may also cause dyssynergia in a few cases. The key to any urological treatment plan is urodynamic testing when the diagnosis is in doubt.

REFERENCES

1. Tanagho EA. The ureterovesical junction: anatomy and physiology. In: Chishold GD, Williams DJ, eds. Scientific Foundations of Urology. Chicago: Year Book, 1982:295–404.
2. Woodburne RT. Anatomy of the bladder outlet. J Urol 1968; 100:474–487.

3. Elbadawi A. Functional pathology of urinary bladder muscularis: the new frontier in diagnostic uropathology. Semin Diagn Pathol 1993; 10:314–354.
4. Hutch JA, Rambo ON Jr. A new theory of the anatomy of the internal urinary sphincter and the physiology of micturition. III. Anatomy of the urethra. J Urol 1967; 97:696–704.
5. Dorschner W, Stolzenburg J–U, Leutert G. A new theory of micturition and urinary continence based on histomorphological studies. I. The musculus detrusor vesicae: occlusive function or support of micturition? Urol Int 1994; 52:61–64.
6. Gilpin SA, Gosling JA. Smooth muscle in the wall of the developing human bladder and urethra. J Anat 1983; 137:503–512.
7. Gosling JA. Anatomy. In: Stanton SL, ed. Clinical Gynecologic Urology. St Louis: Mosby, 1984:3–12.
8. De Groat WC. Anatomy and physiology of the lower urinary tract. Urol Clin North Am 1993; 20:383–401.
9. Dorschner W, Stolzenburg JU, Dieterich F. A new theory of micturition and urinary continence based on histomorphological studies. 2. The musculus sphincter vesicae: continence or sexual function? Urol Int 1994; 52:154–158.
10. Lapides J. Structure and function of the internal vesical sphincter. J Urol 1958; 50:341–353.
11. Staskin DR, Zimmem PE, Hadley HR, Raz S. The pathophysiology of stress incontinence. Urol Clin North Am 1985; 12:271–278.
12. Zinner NR, Sterling AM, Ritter RC. Role of inner urethral softness in urinary continence. Urology 1980; 16:115–117.
13. Enhoming G. Simultaneous recording of intravesical and intraurethral pressure. Acta Chir Scand Suppl 1961; 276:1–6.
14. Raz S, Caine M, Ziegler M. The vascular component in the production of intraurethral pressure. J Urol 1972; 108:93–96.
15. Rud T, Andersson KE, Asmussen M, Hunting A, Ulmsten U. Factors maintaining the intraurethral pressure in women. Invest Urol 1980; 17:343–347.
16. Donker PJ, Ivanovici F, Noach EL. Analysis of urethral pressure profile by means of electromyography and administration of drug. Br J Urol 1972; 44:180–193.
17. Mattiasson A, Andersson KE, Sjogren C. Adrenoceptors and cholinoceptors controlling noradrenaline release from the adrenergic nerves in the urethra of rabbit and man. J Urol 1984; 131:1190–1195.
18. Nordling J. alpha-Blockers and urethral pressure in neurological patients. Urol Int 1978; 33:304–309.
19. Bates G, Bradley WE, Glen E, et al. First report on the standardization of lower urinary tract function: procedures related to the evaluation of urine storage: cystometry, urodynamics. Br J Urol 48:39–42, 1976.
20. Foldspang A, Mommsen S. Adult female urinary incontinence and childhood bedwetting. J Urol 1994; 152:85–88.
21. Burgio KL, Matthews KA, Engel BT. Prevalence, incidence and correlates of urinary incontinence in healthy, middle-aged women. J Urol 1991; 146:1255–1259.
22. Wolin LH. Stress incontinence in young, healthy nulliparous female subjects. J Urol 1969; 101:545–549.
23. Nygaard IE, Thompson FL, Svengalis SL, Albright JP. Urinary incontinence in elite nulliparous athletes. Obstet Gynecol 1994; 84:183–187.
24. Diokno AC, Brock BM, Brown MB, Herzog AR. Prevalence of urinary incontinence and other urological symptoms in the noninstitutionalized elderly. J Urol 1986; 136:1022–1025.
25. McGuire EJ. Adult female urology. In: Yalla SV, McGuire EJ, Elbadawi A, Blaivas JG, eds. Neurourology and Urodynamics: Principles and Practice, New York: Macmillan, 1988.
26. McGuire EJ. Urodynamic findings in patients after failure of stress incontinence operations. In: Zinner NR, Sterling AM, eds. Female Incontinence. New York: Alan R Liss, 1980.
27. Nanninga JE, O'Connor VJ Jr. Suprapubic and retropubic prostatectomy. In: Walsh PC, Gittes

RF, Perlmutter AD, Stamey TA, eds. Campbell's Urology. 5th ed. Philadelphia: WB, Saunders, 1986.

28. Rudy DC, Woodside JR, Crawford ED. Urodynamic evaluation of incontinence in patients undergoing modified Campbell radical retropubic prostatectomy: a prospective study. J Urol 1984; 132:708–712.

29. Walsh PC, Jewett HJ. Radical surgery for prostatic cancer. Cancer 1980; 45:1906–1911.

30. Leach GE, Yun SK. Post-prostatectomy incontinence, part I. The urodynamic findings in 107 men. Neurourol Urodynam 1992; 11:91–97.

31. Fowler FJ Jr, Barry MJ, Lu–Yao G, Roman A, Wasson J, Wennberg JE. Patient-reported complications and follow-up treatment after radical prostatectomy, The National Medicare Experience: 1988–1990 (updated June 1993). Urology 1993; 42:622–629.

32. Fitzpatrick JM, Gardiner RA, Worth PHL. The evaluation of 68 patients with postprostatectomy incontinence, Br J Urol 1979; 51:552–555.

33. Khan Z, Mieza M, Starer P, Singh VK. Post-prostatectomy incontinence. A urodynamic and fluoroscopic point of view. Urology 1991; 38:483–488.

34. Leach GE, Yip CM, Donovan BJ. Post-prostatectomy incontinence: the influence of bladder dysfunction, J Urol 1987; 138:574–578.

35. Chao R, Mayo ME. Incontinence after radical prostatectomy: detrusor or sphincter causes. J Urol 1995; 154:16–18.

36. Mayo ME, Ansell JS. Urodynamic assessment of incontinence after prostatectomy. J Urol 1979; 122:60–61.

37. Yalla SV, Karsh L, Kearney G, Fraser L, Finn D, DeFelippo N, Dyro FM. Post prostatectomy urinary incontinence: urodynamic assessment. Neurourol Urodynam 1982; 1:77–87.

38. Goluboff ET, Chang DT, Olsson CA, Kaplan SA. Urodynamics and the etiology of post-prostatectomy urinary incontinence: the initial Columbia experience. J Urol 1995; 153:1034–1037.

39. Leach GE, Trockman B, Wong A, et al. Post prostatectomy incontinence: 10 year experience with 215 men. J Urol (in press).

40. Habib NA, Luck RJ. Results of transurethral resection of the benign prostate. Br J Surg 1983; 70:218–219.

41. Meyhoff HH, Nordling J. Long term results of transurethral and transvesical prostatectomy. A randomized study. Scand J Urol Nephrol 1986; 20:27–33.

42. Mebust WK, Holtgrewe HL. Current status of transurethral prostatectomy: a review of the AUA National Cooperative Study. World J Urol 1989; 6:194.

43. Tank ES, Ernst CB, Woolson ST, Lapides J. Urinary tract complications of anorectal surgery. Am J Surg 1972; 123:118–122.

44. Fowler JW, Bremner DN, Moffat LE. The incidence and consequences of damage to the parasympathetic nerve supply to the bladder after abdominoperineal resection of the rectum for carcinoma. Br J Urol 1978; 50:95–98.

45. Kinn, AC, Ohman U. Bladder and sexual function after surgery for rectal cancer. Dis Colon Rectum 1986; 29:43–48.

46. Chang PL, Fan HA. Urodynamic studies before and/or after abdominoperineal resection of the rectum for carcinoma. J Urol 1983; 130:948–951.

47. Petrelli NJ, Nagel S, Rodriguez–Bigas M, Piedmonte M, Herrera L. Morbidity and mortality following abdominoperineal resection for rectal adenocarcinoma. Am Surg 1993; 59:400–404.

48. Manzl J, Marberger F, Hetzel H, Klammer J, Geir W, Dapunt O. Funktionelle Storungen des unteren Hamtraktes nach Radikaloperationen des Kollumkarzinoms. Geburtshilfe Frauenheilkd 1981; 41:145–150.

49. Scarff TB, Fronczak S. Myelomeningocele: a review and update. Rehabil Lit 1981; 42:143–146.

50. Webster GD, el-Mahrouky A, Stone AR, Zakrzewski C. The urological evaluation and management of patients with myelodysplasia. Br J Urol 1986; 58:261–265.

51. Shy M, Drager GA. A neurologic syndrome association with orthostatic hypotension, Arch Neurol 1960; 2:511.

52. Salinas JM, Berger Y, De La Rocha RE, Blaivas JG. Urological evaluation in the Shy Drager syndrome. J Urol 1985; 135:741–743.

53. Juma S, Sdrales L. Etiology of urinary retention after bladder neck suspension J Urol 1993; 149:401A.

54. Zimmern PE, Hadley HR, Leach GE, Raz S. Female urethral obstruction after Marshall–Marchetti–Krantz operation. J Urol 1987; 138:517–520.

55. McDuffie RW Jr, Litin RB, Blundon KE. Urethrovesical suspension (Marshall–Marchetti–Krantz operation). Experience with 204 cases. Am J Surg 1981; 141:297–298.

56. Spencer JR, O'Conor VJ Jr. Comparison of procedures for stress urinary incontinence, AUA Update Series, vol 6, lesson 28. Baltimore: American Urological Association, 1987.

57. McGuire EJ, Lytton B. Pubovaginal sling procedure for stress incontinence. J Urol 1978; 119:82–84.

58. Raz S. Complications of vaginal surgery. In: Raz S, ed. Atlas of Transvaginal Surgery. Philadelphia: WB Saunders, 1992.

59. Marion G. Surgery of the neck of the bladder. Br J Urol 1933; 5:351.

60. Massey JA, Abrams PH. Obstructed voiding in the female. Br J Urol 1988; 61:36–39.

61. Farrar DJ, Osbome JL, Stephenson TP, Whitesise CG, Weir J, Berry J, Milroy EJ, Warwick RT. A urodynamic view of bladder outflow obstruction in the female: factors influencing the results of treatment. Br J Urol 1975; 47:815–822.

62. Diokno AC, Hollander JB, Bennett CJ. Bladder neck obstruction in women: a real entity. J Urol 1984; 132:294–298.

63. Raz S, Smith RB. External sphincter spasticity syndrome in female patients. J Urol 1976; 115:443–446.

64. Webster JR. Combined video/pressure–flow cystourethography in female patients with voiding disturbances. Urology 1975; 5:209–215.

65. Guttman L. Spinal Cord Injuries: Comprehensive Management and Research. Oxford: Blackwell Scientific, 1973; 628.

66. Ditunno JF Jr, Formal CS. Chronic spinal cord injury. N Engl J Med 1994; 330:550–556.

67. Le CT, Price M. Survival from spinal cord injury J Chronic Dis 1982; 35:487–492.

68. Blaivas JG. The neurophysiology of micturition: a clinical study of 550 patients. J Urol 1982; 127:958–963.

69. Kaplan SA, Chancellor MB, Blaivas JG. Bladder and sphincter behavior in patients with spinal cord lesions. J Urol 1991; 146:113–117.

70. Poser CM. The epidemiology of multiple sclerosis: a general overview. Ann Neurol 1994; 36:S180–S193.

71. Goldstein I, Siroky MB, Sax DS, Krane RJ. Neurourologic abnormalities in multiple sclerosis. J Urol 1982; 128:541–545.

72. Miller H, Simpson CA, Yeates WK. Bladder dysfunction in multiple sclerosis. Br Med J 1965; 1:1265.

73. Fog T. Topographic distribution of plaques in the spinal cord in multiple sclerosis. Arch Neurol Psychiatry 1950; 63:382–414.

74. Oppenheimer DR. The cervical cord in multiple sclerosis. Neuropathol Appl Neurobiol 1978; 4:151–162.

75. Litwiller SE, Frohman EM, Zimmern PE. Multiple sclerosis and the urologist. J Urol 1999; 161:743–757.

76. Arunabh MB, Badlani G. Urologic problems in cerebrovascular accidents. Probl Urol 1993; 7:41–53.

77. Tsuchida S, Noto H, Yamaguchi O, Itoh M. Urodynamic studies on hemiplegic patients after cerebrovascular accidents. Urology 1983; 21:315–318.

78. Motola JA, Mascarenas B, Badlani G. Cerebrovascular accidents: urodynamic and neuroanatomical findings. J Urol 1988; 139:512A.

79. Badlani GH, Sanjeev V, Motola JA. Detrusor behavior in patients with dominant hemispheric strokes. Neurourol Urodynam 1991; 10:119–123.

80. Reid CJD, Borzykowski M. Lower urinary tract dysfunction in cerebral palsy. Arch Dis Child 1993; 68:739–742.

81. Mayo ME. Lower urinary tract dysfunction in cerebral palsy. J Urol 1992; 147:419–420.

82. Sotolongo JR, Chancellor M. Parkinson's disease. Probl Urol 1993; 7:54–67.

83. Berger Y, Salinas J, Blaivas J. Urodynamic differentiation of Parkinson's disease and the Shy–Drager syndrome. Neurourol Urodynam 1990; 9:117–121.

84. Pavlakis AJ, Siroky MB, Goldstein I, Krane RJ. Neurourologic findings in Parkinson's disease. J Urol 1983; 129:80–83.

85. Berger Y, Blaivas JG, De La Rocha ER, Salinas JM. Urodynamic findings in Parkinson's disease. J Urol 1987; 138:836–838.

86. Rosomoff HL, Johnston JD, Gallo AE, et al. Cystometry in the evaluation of nerve compression in lumbar spine disorders. Surg Gynecol Obstet 1963; 117:263.

87. McGuire EJ. Urodynamic evaluation after abdominal perineal resection and lumbar intervertebral disk herniation. Urology 1975; 6:63–70.

88. Appell RA, et al. Assessment of vesico-urethral dysfunction in lumbar spine disorders. In: Sundin T, Mattiasson A, eds. Proceedings Eleventh Annual Meeting of the International Incontinence Society, Trelleborg, Sweden, 1981, Skogs.

89. Andersen JT, Bradley WE. Neurogenic bladder dysfunction in protruded lumbar disc and after laminectomy. Urology 1976; 8:94–96.

12

Pathophysiology of the Incompetent Urinary Sphincter

FIROUZ DANESHGARI

University of Colorado Health Sciences Center, Denver, Colorado

PHILIPPE E. ZIMMERN

The University of Texas Southwestern Medical Center at Dallas, Dallas, Texas

I. INTRODUCTION

The *urinary sphincter* is a term applied to the structures in the urethra that contribute to the function of opening and closing of the urethra. Anatomically, several structures have been identified that participate in the "sphincter" function of the urethra. Although the focus of this chapter is not on the detailed description of these structures, their mention is needed to allow the discussion on the pathophysiological causes of *sphincteric failure*.

The participating structures in the urethral continence mechanism follow:

A. Smooth-Muscle Fibers

Several studies have demonstrated the presence of two or three layers of smooth-muscle fibers in the urethral wall. In the proximal two-thirds of the urethra, three smooth-muscle layers are identified that form an outer, middle, and inner layer (Fig. 1; see color insert). The inner layer appears to be in continuation with bladder neck fibers. The middle layer contains the thickest layer of muscle fibers (Fig. 2; see color insert). The autonomic nerve fibers that supply the urethral smooth musculature arise from the pelvic plexus, which contains sympathetic and parasympathetic fibers. The sympathetic fibers reach the pelvic plexus through the superior hypogastric plexus, which is located ventral to the common iliac arteries. The parasympathetic fibers originate from the sacral segments of the splanchnic nerves.

Several studies have investigated the functional role of the smooth (1–3) and striated muscles (4) of the urethra. Several investigators have shown that in patients with both natural or pharmacological paralysis or surgical interruption of the striated muscle, urinary continence is maintained by the smooth muscles of the proximal urethra (5–7). Moreover, stimulation of the smooth musculature of the urethra through the autonomic pelvic plexus results in an increase in urethral closure pressure throughout the urethra which, in itself, can maintain urinary continence (3).

B. Striated Muscle Fibers

Striated muscle fibers have been identified in the distal one-third of the urethra (8). These fibers are more prominent on the ventral than on the dorsal surface, making the appearance of the Greek letter "omega." Recent studies show that the omega-shaped rhabdosphincter is present from the beginning of life (Figs. 3 and 4; see color insert) (8). This is in contrast with previous findings suggesting a nearly ring-shaped configuration, which becomes omega-like during the first year of life (9). The innervation of these fibers is through the pudendal nerve, which courses alongside the internal pudendal vessels on the lateral aspect of the ischiorectal fossa inside the pudendal canal. Branches of the inferior rectal nerves, perineal nerves, and dorsal nerve of the clitoris branch off in the region of the pelvic floor. Several thin branches of the pudendal nerve run to the rhabdosphincter, lie under the levator ani muscle fibers, and enter the distal urethra on its lateral aspect.

C. Vascular Component

Although no specific "sphincteric" function has been assigned to the thick vascular component of the urethra, several investigators (2,5) have clearly demonstrated that interruption of the circulation to the "vascular bed" of the urethra leads to a drop in urethral pressure that is essential for the continence mechanism. From these studies, it is clear that the presence and the quality of the rich vascular network of the urethra plays a "washer"-like effect in, at least, the passive control of continence. Some investigators have attributed 30% of the continence mechanisms to this structure (5,10,11). Figure 5 demonstrates the cystoscopic appearance of a urethra in which most of the vascular washer was destroyed, except for a

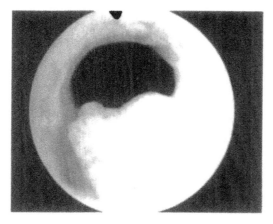

Figure 5   A cystoscopic view of the urethra shows the soft tissue "washer" is destroyed except between 5- and 7-o'clock.

bridge of tissue between 5- and 7-o'clock. The destruction of the vascular tissue in this patient had occurred after transurethral injection of Teflon.

D. Pelvic Floor Structures and Vaginal Wall

Several layers of striated muscle and fascia support the pelvic viscera in both men and women. These layers have been named the *pelvic diaphragm* or *urogenital diaphragm*. The most important part of these structures is the levator ani muscle. The levator ani muscle is often divided into three components: the pubococcygeus, iliococcygeus, and ischiococcygeus muscles, according to their origin from the pelvic side wall (12). The literature is replete with various descriptions of the pelvic diaphragm and of its role in the support of the bladder, bladder neck, and urethra. In fact the urethra and bladder neck lie on a supportive layer that is composed of endopelvic fascia and anterior vaginal wall. The structural stability of this supportive layer seems to derive from its lateral attachments to the arcus tendineus fascia pelvic and levator ani muscles (13,14). DeLancey has compared this supportive relation to a "hammock." This hammock-like structure provides a compressive force for the urethral closure during increase in intra-abdominal pressure with cough and sneeze (15). Gosling et al. have reported that the pelvic floor musculature has an important role in urinary continence, providing an additional occlusive force on the urethral wall (16,17). Petros and Ulmsten have recently introduced the "integral" theory of female urinary incontinence (18). By describing three closure mechanisms, these authors propose that stress and urge incontinence may both derive from the same anatomical defect, a lax vagina. Altered collagen or elastin in the vaginal connective tissue or its ligamentous supports may cause this laxity.

Whether these components of the continence mechanism act independently or as a part of one sphincteric mechanism is debatable. The authors favor the concept of "one sphincter, multiple components." Given these concepts, the pathophysiological causes of sphincteric failure are discussed herein.

II. CLASSIFICATION

The causes, and thus the classification, of sphincteric failure can be divided into two main categories: neurogenic and nonneurogenic. Although many causes in the nonneurogenic group could easily have a neurological etiology, such as pelvic trauma or extensive pelvic surgery, the neurogenic term is generally applied to disturbances of the "central control mechanisms." The central control mechanisms include the cortical portion of the frontal lobe of the brain, the pons micturition center, and the thoracic and lumbar spinal cord segments. Diseases and pathological conditions affecting any of these centers would lead to disturbances in the function of the lower urinary tract organs, including the continence mechanism. Myelodysplastic disease and spinal cord injuries are among the more prevalent causes in the younger population, and lesions of the central nervous system, such as cerebrovascular accidents and Parkinson's disease, are more common among the older population. Although the central lesions rarely result in an isolated sphincteric failure, they commonly disturb the function of the bladder and parts of the lower urinary tract system.

The term *nonneurogenic* is generally applied to other causes, which may or may not involve the innervation of the lower urinary tract or continence mechanisms. Such causes include trauma (childbirth trauma, pelvic fracture, pelvic surgeries), radiation, previous anti-incontinence surgery, and changes related to aging or menopause. In the following section, each of these causes is discussed.

A.   Neurogenic Causes of Impaired Urinary Sphincter

Various classifications of neurogenic causes of voiding dysfunction that include an impaired urinary sphincter, have been proposed over the last several decades (19). Despite attempts to simplify the complex relation between the central control mechanisms and the resulting lower urinary tract symptoms, most of these classifications have fallen out of favor. The most recent classification, proposed by Wein, is the International Continence Society's classification (20,21). By ICS's classification, the urethral sphincter can be normal, over-active–obstructed, or incompetent. An overactive urethra contracts involuntarily against the detrusor contraction (dyssynergia), or fails to relax during attempted micturition. An incompetent urethra will result in incontinence. This could occur during an increase in intra-abdominal pressure (stress), during a rise in detrusor pressure (urge), or be related to a continuous failure to close, which will lead to unaware incontinence. Failure of the urethra to promptly close or open in response to detrusor contraction has been termed *urethral instability* and is a recognized cause of urinary incontinence (22).

Because the contraction and relaxation of the layers of the smooth muscle, and also the smooth-muscle component of the urethral vascular bed, are under sympathetic control: any damage to this inflow may cause paralysis of the smooth-muscle component. In contrast, damage to the somatic or pudendal nerve inflow may lead to malfunction of the rhabdosphincter.

B.   Nonneurogenic Causes of Impaired Urinary Sphincter

1.   Trauma

A variety of pelvic traumas could impose substantial damage to the urinary sphincter. Pelvic fracture, extensive pelvic surgery, and traumatic vaginal delivery are among the most common causes. Combination of urinary and anal sphincter damage can coexist. The occurrence of sphincteric damage is often associated with damage to the pudendal nerve terminal, which can last several weeks (23) (Figs. 6 and 7). The incidence of urinary sphincter damage during obstetrical anal sphincter injury reached 50% in some series (24).

2.   Prostatectomy

All versions of radical prostatectomies, either open simple, radical, or transurethral carry a risk of urinary incontinence. Urinary incontinence after simple or radical prostatectomy may or may not fit into the categories of causes of urinary sphincter failure. However, its inclusion may be warranted in this chapter because the possible cause of urinary incontinence after prostatectomy is either removal or severe damage of the smooth-muscle and vascular components of the continence mechanism or ISD (25). Despite a poor definition of incontinence, a recent survey by the American College of Surgeons (26), reported for 1990 and 1993, respectively, complete control or only occasional urinary incontinence requiring no pads in 81.3 and 79.8% of patients after radical retropubic prostatectomy (RRP). Interestingly, a nerve-sparing technique may be associated with more use of absorbent pads at 3 and 12 months following treatment (27). In general, the prevalence and severity of incontinence after RRP improve over time, with a long-term incidence remaining near 8% (28,29).

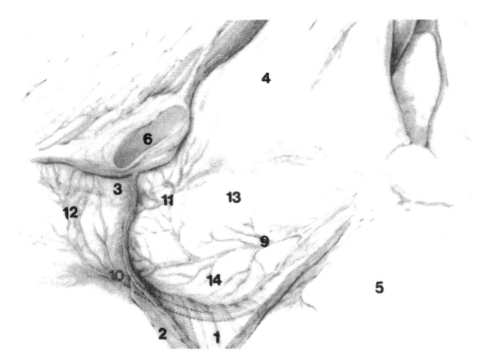

Figure 6   Schematic of lateral view of female pelvic floor dissection showing autonomic nerve supply to urethra (3), bladder (4), and vagina (13): (1) levator ani muscle; (2) obturator internus muscle; (5) ischial spine; (6) symphysis pubic; (9) pelvic plexus; (10) pudendal nerve; (11) fibers of pelvic plexus; (12) fibers of pudendal nerve. (Courtesy of Dr. K. Colleselli.)

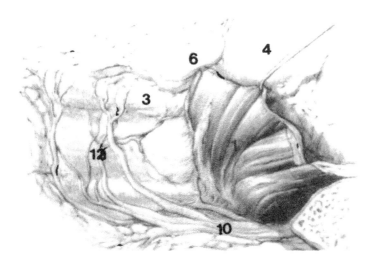

Figure 7   Schematic and close-up of lateral view of female pelvic floor dissection showing branches emerging from pudendal nerve (10) course to caudal third of urethra (3). (1) levator ani muscle; (6) pubic symphysis; (10) pudendal nerve; (12) fibers of pudendal nerve. (Courtesy of Dr. K. Colleselli.)

3. Radiation

Radiation therapy is used in the treatment of a variety of carcinomas in both men and women, including prostate cancer in men and advanced cervical cancer in women. Treatment of uncommon causes such as vaginal rhabdomyosarcoma of infancy can also lead to urinary sphincteric failure later in life (30).

The incidence of urinary incontinence after radiation therapy for prostate cancer appears to be similar to that of radical prostatectomy (31). It is suspected that the damage to the urinary sphincter takes place at the level of the mucosal seal of the sphincter, as well as at the level of the sphincter's innervation (32).

C. Anti-incontinence Surgery

Previous anti-incontinence surgery is becoming an increasing cause of urinary sphincter failure. Indeed the incidence of urethral sphincteric failure increases after each anti-incontinence surgery. In reviewing the causes of urinary incontinence in 648 patients, urethral sphincteric failure was seen in 28% of patients after one previous anti-incontinence surgery (33). This incidence increased to 75% in patients after a secondary operation. In addition, in comparing the causes of stress incontinence in women with no prior history of anti-incontinence surgery with those who had prior surgery, a threefold increase in the incidence of type III incontinence or intrinsic sphincteric deficiency (ISD) was noted (33). Whether urethral sphincteric failure occurs because the patient has this condition originally or as a result of the operative procedure is hard to judge. Recent anatomical and histochemical studies of the lower urinary tract point to a rich neurovascular supply in the urethra and the bladder neck areas most exposed during anti-incontinence procedures. In a recent review of the literature of 35 series of patients who had undergone surgical treatments for ISD, from 1977 to 1997, we found no group of patients without risk factors who had primary ISD (Table 1) (34). This is in contrast to a 13% rate of ISD reported by McGuire in patients with no prior anti-incontinence surgery (33). This difference may be because McGuire's study did not consider vaginal delivery and menopause as risk factors for ISD.

D. Menopause and Aging

Video urodynamic studies of women older than 70 years who presented with new-onset stress urinary incontinence suggested that incontinence was related to poor urethral function, rather than urethral hypermobility (32). On the other hand, estrogen deficiency in postmenopausal women is thought to be responsible for atrophic urethral mucosal changes (35).

Table 1 Causes of Intrinsic Sphincteric Deficiency (ISD) in 1471 Patients Who Underwent Treatment for ISD

Cause	No. of patients
Previous anti-incontinence surgery	1363
Prior pelvic or urethra surgery or trauma	18
Neurogenic causes	45
Radiation changes	12
Others:	33
(Senile atrophic changes, steroid therapy, severe COPD)	
Primary ISD (no risk factor)	0

Although the incidental relation between an incompetent sphincter and menopause may suggest that estrogen deficiency could be an important contributing factor in compromising urethral function (36), most studies do not support the contention that bladder neck integrity is estrogen-dependent, or is age-dependent (37).

III. SUMMARY

The contributing elements to the function of the urinary sphincter are smooth-muscle fibers, striated muscle fibers, rhabdosphincter, and the rich vascular plexus of the urethra. Failure of the urinary sphincter can result from damage to any of these structures. Stress urinary incontinence will occur when such damage overwhelms the continence threshold of the sphincter. The pathophysiological causes can be divided into neurogenic and nonneurogenic. The neurogenic causes mostly interrupt the central control mechanism of the urinary sphincter. Most nonneurogenic causes damage the elements of the peripheral control mechanism. A more refined understanding of the pathophysiological mechanisms resulting in urethral sphincteric failure would assist the clinicians in properly selecting the best therapeutic modality for their incontinent patients.

REFERENCES

1. Kleeman FJ. The physiology of the internal urinary sphincter. J Urol 1970; 104:549–554.
2. Raz S, Caine M, Zeigler M. The vascular component in the production of intraurethral pressure. J Urol 1972; 108:93–96.
3. Tanagho EA, Meyers FH, Smith DR. Urethral resistance: its components and implications. I. Smooth muscle component. Invest Urol 1969; 7:136–149.
4. Tanagho EA, Meyers FH, Smith DR. Urethral resistance: its components and implications. 11. Striated muscle component. Invest Urol 1969; 7:195–205.
5. Donker PJ, Ivanovici F, Noach EL. Analyses of the urethral pressure profile by means of electromyography and the administration of drugs. Br J Urol 1972; 44:180–193.
6. Lapides J. Stress incontinence. J Urol 1961; 85:291–294.
7. McGuire EJ. The effects of sacral denervation on bladder and urethral function. Surg Gynecol Obstet 1977; 144:343–346.
8. Colleselli K, Stenzl A, Eder R, Strasser H, Poisel S, Bartsch G. The female urethral sphincter: a morphological and topographical study. J Urol 1998; 160:49–54.
9. Kokoua A, Homsy Y, Lavigne JF, Williot P, Corcos J, Laberge I, Michaud J. Maturation of the external urinary sphincter: a comparative histotopographic study in humans. J Urol 1993; 150:617–622.
10. Raz S, Caine M, Zeigler M. The vascular component in the production of intraurethral pressure. J Urol 1972; 108:93–96.
11. Rud T, Andersson KE, Asmussen M, Hunting A, Ulmsten U. Factors maintaining the intraurethral pressure in women. Invest Urol 1980; 17:343–347.
12. Thiede HA. Prevalence of pelvic floor dysfunction in women. Conference on Pelvic Floor Dysfunction—An Initiative for Curriculum Enhancement in Residency Education. Chicago: American Board of Obstetrics and Gynecology, 1992.
13. DeLancey JO. Correlative study of paraurethral anatomy. Obstet Gynecol 1986; 68:91–97.
14. DeLancey JO. Anatomy and physiology of urinary continence. Clin Obstet Gynecol 1990; 33:298–307.
15. DeLancey JO. Structural support of the urethra as it relates to stress urinary incontinence. The hammock hypothesis. Am J Obstet Gynecol 1994; 170:1713–1723.
16. Gosling JA, Dixon JS, Critchley HO, Thompson SA. A comparative study of the human external sphincter and periurethral levator ani muscles. Br J Urol 1981; 53:35–41.

17. Gosling JA, Dixon JS, Lendon RG. The autonomic innervation of the human male and female bladder neck and proximal urethra. J Urol 1977; 118:302–305.
18. Petros PE, Ulmsten UI. An integral theory of female urinary incontinence. Experimental and clinical considerations. Acta Obstet Gynecol Scand 1990; 153:7–31.
19. Steers WD, Barrett DM, Wein AJ. Voiding dysfuction: diagnosis, classification, and management. In: Gillenwater JY, Grayhack JT, Howards SS, Duckett JW, eds. Adult and Pediatric Urology. 3rd ed. St Louis: Mosby-Year Book, 1996:1220–1327.
20. International Continence Society Standardisation Committee. Fourth report on the standardisation of terminology of lower urinary tract function. Br J Urol 1981; 53:333–335.
21. Wein AJ. Classification of neurogenic voiding dysfunction. J Urol 1981; 125:605–609.
22. McGuire EJ. Reflex urethral instability. Br J Urol 1978; 50:200–204.
23. Snooks SJ, Swash M. Abnormalities of the innervation of the urethral striated sphincter musculature in incontinence. Br J Urol 1984; 56:401–405.
24. Tetzschner T, Sorensen M, Lose G, Christiansen J. Anal and urinary incontinence in women with anal sphincter rupture. Br J Obstet Gynaecol 1996; 103:1034–1040.
25. Ficazzola MA, Nitti VW. The etiology of post-radical prostatectomy incontinence and correlation of symptoms with urodynamic findings. J Urol 1998; 160:1317–1320.
26. Mettlin CJ, Murphy GP, Sylvester J, McKee RF, Morrow M, Winchester DP. Results of hospital cancer registry surveys by the American College of Surgeons: outcomes of prostate cancer treatment by radical prostatectomy. Cancer 1997; 80:1875–1881.
27. Talcott JA, Rieker P, Propert KJ, Clark JA, Wishnow Ki, Loughlin KR, Richie JP, Kantoff PW. Patient-reported impotence and incontinence after nerve-sparing radical prostatectomy. J Natl Cancer Inst 1997; 89:1117–1123.
28. Goluboff ET, Saidi JA, Mazer S, Bagiella E, Heitjan DF, Benson MC, Olsson CA. Urinary continence after radical prostatectomy: the Columbia experience. J Urol 1998; 159:1276–1280.
29. Leandri P, Rossignol G, Gautier JR, Ramon J. Radical retropubic prostatectomy: morbidity and quality of life. Experience with 620 consecutive cases. J Urol 1992; 147:883–887.
30. Lagro–Janssen AL, Debruyne FM, van Weel C. Value of the patient's case history in diagnosing urinary incontinence in general practice. Br J Urol 1991; 67:569–572.
31. Uhle CA, Blakey EE. Post-prostatectomy urinary incontinence: experience with a group of diverse surgical techniques. J Urol 1960; 83:454–457.
32. Horbach NS, Ostergard DR. Predicting intrinsic urethral sphincter dysfunction in women with stress urinary incontinence. Obstet Gynecol 1994; 84:188–192.
33. McGuire EJ. Urodynamic findings in patients after failure of stress incontinence operations. Prog Clin Biol Res 1981; 78:351–360.
34. Daneshgari F, Zimmern PE. Does ISD exist in women in absence of risk factors? 77th Annual Meeting of South Central Section of American Urological Association, Cancun, Mexico. 1998: abstr 92.
35. Staskin D, Zimmern PE, Hadley R, Raz S. The pathophysiology of stress incontinence. Urol Clin North Am 1985; 12:271–278.
37. Elia G, Bergman A. Estrogen effects on the urethra: beneficial effects in women with genuine stress incontinence. Obstet Gynecol Surv 1993; 48:509–517.
38. Versi E, Cardozo L, Studd J. Distal urethral compensatory mechanisms in women with an incompetent bladder neck who remain continent, and the effect of the menopause. Neurol Urodynam 1990; 9:579–590.

13

Pathophysiology of the Hypertonic Sphincter or Hyperpathic Urethra

DIRK-HENRIK ZERMANN

University Hospital, Friedrich-Schiller-University, Jena, Germany

MANABU ISHIGOOKA

Yamagata University School of Medicine, Yamagata, Japan

RICHARD A. SCHMIDT

University of Colorado Medical School and Rose Hospital, Denver, Colorado

I. INTRODUCTION

In general, lower urinary tract dysfunction may be attributable to any disease process or injury that affects the neural reflexes governing urine storage or release (1–5). Many clinical conditions affecting the lower urinary tract (LUT) are poorly understood. The underlying cause of LUT dysfunction can be very difficult to discover, given the complexity of the central and peripheral neural system, and that pathophysiological changes at one site in the nervous system or in a target organ may induce changes in another site.

One of these disorders is the *hypertonic sphincter* or *hyperpathic urethra*. In contrast, the hypotonic urethra is relatively well investigated, and much research work in the past has provided insights into the epidemiology, clinical course, diagnosis, and treatment options for this problem (6).

Before going into detail concerning clinical approaches to management of the hypertonic sphincter, we will discuss recent developments in basic and behavioral neurourology.

II. SCIENTIFIC BACKGROUND

A. Principles of Learning: Toilet-Training Risks

Acquiring LUT control is a gradual evolutionary process. Traditional teaching implies that voiding control is asserted automatically, usually by age 3. However, it is also a learned process, very much linked to the complex processing of environmental information fed into the brain. Although there is overall basic organization to the brain and central nervous system (CNS), it is also true that within this gross organization, the degree of dendritic interconnectivity is greatly influenced by the afferent information carried to the brain circuitry. All repeated experiences, even the most basic routines, such as toileting behavior, generate changes in our nervous systems (7–15). Changes in the type and competitive nature of the sensory inputs can have a profound influence on overall neural interconnectivity. Even a few minutes a day for several days a week can produce major changes in the control of somatosensory regulatory areas of the brain. This is especially true during childhood when the brain is much more plastic and moldable. Adjustments in the way in which information is handled and processed go on throughout life, but much more slowly as the nervous system ages.

Plasticity, or CNS adaptation to varying sensory inputs, slows considerably according to variable learning deadlines. For voiding, this probably occurs in late childhood, between the ages of 8 and 10. Sophisticated body functions, such as toileting, require a degree of psychological maturity for proper regulation. Children have difficulty relating bladder fullness feelings to a timeframe for voiding. As a result, they tend to be retentive, reluctant to break away from "play" for routine voids, except for those last minute, strong impending urges. It is, therefore, not unusual for children to get "caught" in a car ride, in school, at a playground, in a department store, or at a sports event, as they cannot judge time until access to a toilet. Unfortunately, there remains this adult parenteral tendency to scold the child if there is a wetting accident, a behavior that potentially aggravates, rather than helps, the development of micturition control.

Because of learning deadline principles, a child with repetitive retentive tendencies, dating from early childhood, is prone to evolve a permanent regulatory circuitry that will favor persistence of this type of behavior throughout life. This retentive behavior is readily reinforced by pressures that result from our deadline-orientated society. Tension in the home, overbearing parents pushing their children to be toilet trained, intolerance of parents toward bedwetting, a daycare center that demands that the child be toilet trained before entry, examinations in school, grant and contract applications, the stresses of venture capitalism, family economic strains, corporate takeovers, long meetings, nurses in long surgical cases, public toilet inaccessibility, excessive exercise routines, local traumas from instrumentation, previous surgical interventions or delivery, psychological distress, and so on, all are potential contributors to fixed alterations in pelvic floor physiology (6). Behavioral stress is a basic risk to any muscle system in the body. Any muscle action, if sufficiently repetitive, and sufficiently noxious, along with time and age, could eventually couple to precipitate a breakdown in the functional and anatomical integrity of tissue.

Relevant concepts have emerged from myofascial pain research. Changes in central processing, expansion of receptor fields within the CNS and even cell death have been experimentally induced by noxious inputs to the spinal cord (16). The actual mechanisms that allow for overfacilitated and permissive communication within the CNS are unclear. In all probability, however, they would be along the lines of flawed inhibitory gating observed in neuropathic spastic states (i.e., the spastic urethral sphincter–hyperpathic urethra).

It is especially important to appreciate that incorrect conditioning of these reflexes during the time the nervous system is maturing, could result in voiding dysfunctions ranging from incontinence to retention. Symptoms may be in evolution for years, even decades before they become incapacitating. Therefore, prevention of dysfunctional voiding or urogenital pain syndromes should begin by addressing the toileting habits of children. This is not only logical, but also critically important to the long-term management of the "overactive" or hyperpathic sphincter.

Inappropriate, nociceptive somatic afferent bombardment of delicate central regulatory micturition circuits could, over time, be extremely harmful to the integrity of central pelvic organ regulation. Any persistent cascade of abnormal neural events could trigger a breakdown of the normal inhibitory gating within these CNS centers. Chronic LUT dysfunction is maintained by permanently upregulated sacral reflex arcs, and a variety of dysfunctional and autonomic symptoms could logically follow.

This hypothesis is supported by the consistent improvement rates reported for modulation-based therapies. Most (i.e., biofeedback programs, timed voids, and such) address pelvic floor dysfunction by focusing on achieving direct improvements in dynamic behavior. Others attempt to modulate sacral reflex arc excitability with medications, acupuncture, and neurostimulation (17).

B. Pelvic Floor and Perineal Sensation

Anatomically, the pelvic floor encompasses two functional layers. The deeper layer is composed of the levator and its various components. This is a hammock-like structure attached to the pelvic brim (18–20). It slings across the pelvic outlet supporting the internal pelvic organs. Contraction of the levator occurs with stimulation of the third and fourth sacral nerves. The pelvic organs are then lifted upward and anterior toward the pubis. With this movement, there is actual physical compression of the proximal urethra or bladder neck. With voluntary tightening and relaxation efforts, the perineum should move with a bellows-like action. There should be a visible deepening and flattening of the buttock crease.

The second functional layer to the pelvis is composed of all of the muscles below the levator: the transversus peronealis, the ischeo- and bulbocavernosus muscles, the urethral sphincter, and the superficial anal sphincter. These muscles are innervated by the pudendal nerve, which is derived primarily from S2. Stimulation of the pudendal nerve produces anteroposterior squeezing, or clamp-like activity, consistent with the anteroposterior orientation of muscle fibers.

These two motions, the bellows and the clamp, are distinctly different from a functional perspective. Normally, the two actions blend together, with the bellows response being much more evident and easy to appreciate. In voiding dysfunction, these movements become fractionated or dyssynergic relative to each other and to the bladder.

The integrity of the S2, S3, and S4 nerves can be judged to a great degree by physical examination. All perineal skin sensation is derived from the S2 (pudendal) nerve. There is no significant skin sensation sourced from either the S3 or the S4 nerves. Skin sensation will be impaired unilaterally or bilaterally with deficits in the S2 nerves (Fig. 1). Although loss of perineal skin sensation often reflects a loss of urethral sphincter integrity, the presence of normal perineal skin sensation does not guarantee sphincter integrity or vice versa.

The presence of two distinct anatomical and functional layers to the pelvic floor is important clinically. Deficits in the S3 or S4 nerves should not be associated with significant incontinence, loss of perineal skin sensation, or sphincter tone. These are mainly motor

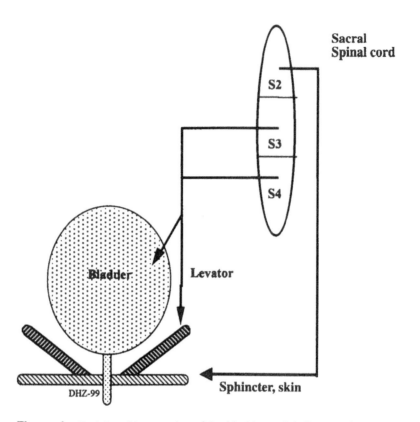

Figure 1   Peripheral innervation of the bladder, pelvic floor, and perineal skin.

nerves, and neuropathies at these levels are expressed primarily as motor deficits of bladder and levator support. Hypersensitivity of the bladder is often mirrored by hypersensitivity of the levator.

The urethal and superficial anal sphincter muscles (S2) have an important integrated role in reflex regulation of micturition. Loss of pudendal afferent input to the micturition center can significantly dampen the detrusor reflex. Conversely, enhanced input to the cord, by C fiber pudendal afferents, can augment the detrusor reflex. Suppression of the detrusor reflex can result from either excess supraspinal inhibition (e.g., the shy voider), or by increased inhibitory input into the micturition center (e.g., a voluntary hold). These examples include common chronic anxiety states, with upregulated tension in the sphincters, or a complete loss of the volitional ability to physically identify and relax the pelvic floor and sphincter with the void effort. As both are noxious, either behavioral pathway, over time, can result in a permanent loss of higher center inhibition with emergence of urethral instability and incontinence. Admittedly, this logic is as yet unproved, but it is consistent with the established neurophysiological principles of windup and hyperalgesia that result from enhanced noxious afferent input in the CNS (21–22).

Functional as well as pathological events in the periphery can bring about changes in the behavior of the pelvic viscera, with consequent anatomical changes over time. The presumed mediator of such changes is peptide release from nerve endings secondary to metabolic stress within the nerves. The result is enhanced production, peripheral transport, and then release of inflammatory or neural-sensitizing peptides into tissue. Most of the behavioral problems involving the LUT are associated with inadequate pelvic floor control.

Thus, rectal examination is the key to diagnosing and managing many of these conditions (i.e., urge incontinence, urge-frequency syndromes, recurrent urinary tract infections, chronic urinary retention, pelvic pain syndromes, prostatitis) (23–25). It is very important to manage the overall pelvic floor dyscoordination stemming from lack of conscious voluntary control. Too often the focus of rectal examination is on anatomical findings. Although overt pathology is important to identify, behavioral dysfunction contributing to anatomical findings should be quantified (26).

Finally, the clinician should be aware of the neurological link between the feet and the pelvis. The anatomy of the feet, and overall excitability of lower extremity reflexes, can give an indication of problems in the sacral segments of the cord. High arches or hammertoes imply loss of S2, caused by a disproportionate tone in the dorsiflexors of the foot versus the plantar flexors. Loss of sensation along the outer part of the foot can imply selective deficits of S2, but in reality, there is usually a more general loss of the distal half of the foot.

C. General CNS Aspects

Regulation of the LUT by the CNS (i.e., the bladder, urethral sphincter, and levator muscle) is directly linked to the brain stem. Proper function is dependent on information processing in a number of brain stem nuclei (27–32) (Table 1). Logically, any pathology in these regions could have tremendous influence on the functional integrity of the LUT. Also, a dysfunctional LUT could have a tremendous effect on information processing in various brain stem nuclei.

The paraventricular nucleus of the hypothalamus is a well-known site for regulation

Table 1 Pseudorabies Virus Studies on the Central Neuroanatomical Pathways Involved in Innervation of the Pelvic Area

Mapped structure	Spinal representation	Major brain stem representation	Ref.
Bladder	L6–S1	PMC, RO, NGC, LC, A_5, PVN	30
Bladder trigone	Th12–L2 L6–S2	Cortex, PMC, LC, PVN, PAG, RM, VML	31
Perineal muscles (IC, BS)	T13–L2 L6–S1	PMC, RP, VML, A_5, LC, PVN	27
External urethral sphincter	L6–S1	PMC, RM, A_5, A_7, LC, PAG	28
Prostate gland	T13–L2 S1–S2	PMC, PAG, RM, A_5, LC, PVN	32
Urethra	L6–S1	PMC, RN, LC, PVN	29

Abbreviations: A_5, A_5 noradrenergic cell group; A_7, A_7 noradrenergic cell group; LC, locus caeruleus; NGC, nucleus gigantocellularis; PAG, periaquaductal gray; PMC, pontine micturition center; PVN, paraventricular nucleus of the hypothalamus; RM, raphe magnus; RN, red nucleus; RO, raphe obscurus; RP, raphe pallidus; VML, ventrolateral medulla; IC, m. ischiocavernosus; BS, m. bulbospongiosus.

of the autonomic nervous system (33). It contains many putative peptides, and there are important projections from this area to the hypophysis, the spinal control centers for the pelvic floor (Onuf's nucleus), the parasympathetic motor nucleus, and the intermediolateral cell column (sympathetic motor nucleus) as well as the dorsal horns (lamina I and lamina X) (Figs. 2–4). These connections can tie pelvic physiology to hormonal regulation of the hypophysis, allowing potential linkage between dysmenorrhea symptoms (e.g., oxytocin-mediated cramps) and LUT dysfunction in patients.

Another important brain stem–sphincter linkage occurs through the dorsal pontine reticular formation (DPRF). The DPRF gives projections to the nucleus retroambiguus which, in turn, projects heavily to both the abdominal muscles and the pelvic floor muscles (Table 2). Discomforts in the upper abdomen can, therefore, be associated with, or stem from, spastic dysfunction of the pelvic muscles.

Physiological studies in animals and positron-emission tomography (PET) imaging in humans have identified two important regions in the brain stem: (1) the medial part of the dorsal pontine tegmentum (M-region), which results in sphincter relaxation and detrusor contraction when stimulated; and (2) the lateral part of the pontine tegmental field (L-region), which leads to sphincter contraction and detrusor inhibition when stimulated (34,35).

From these areas of the brain stem there are norepinephrine projections throughout the length of the spinal cord, including the parasympathetic motor nucleus, the intermediolateral nucleus, and Onuf's nucleus (34,36,37). They have a general excitatory influence. α-Adrenergic blockers, because of their lipophilic properties, can cross the blood–brain barrier, and downregulate the excitability of these noradrenergic pathways that modulate pelvic floor excitability. Similarly, the nucleus pallidus and the ventromedullary reticular formation have strong projections to somatic and autonomic motoneurons throughout the cord. Many of these projections are serotonergic, but contain substance P (SP) and leu-enkephalin. They have a facilitatory role. New serotonergic blockers may have a therapeutic effect in modulating LUT dysfunction.

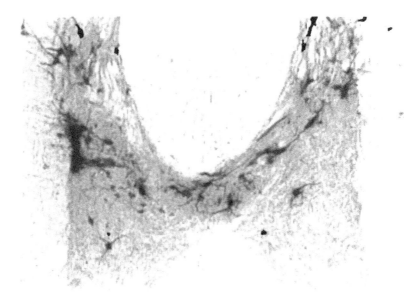

Figure 2   Spinal cord (Th 12) after injection of pseudorabiesvirus (PRV) into the urinary bladder (trigone). Note strong labeling of the intermediolateral cell column.

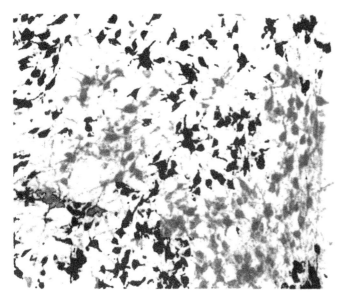

Figure 3 Labeling of the hypothalamus (nucleus periventricularis) after PRV injection into the urinary bladder (trigone).

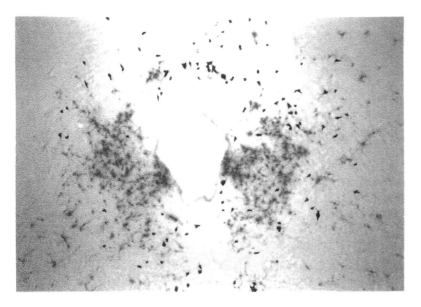

Figure 4 Labeling of the periaquaductal gray after PRV injection into the urinary bladder (trigone).

Given the extensive neurological linkage between the brain stem and the LUT, the integrity of CNS peptide pools could be reflected in the activity or behavior of the bladder, the urethra or the pelvic floor, or same combination thereof (Table 3). It is difficult to imagine the LUT as being normal in the face of brain stem neuropathology. It is also difficult to consider these same brain stem nuclei, with profound regulatory influence over continence and micturition, as being metabolically normal in the presence of a significantly dysfunc-

Table 2 Hypothalamic Regions Involved in Lower Urinary Tract Control

Lateral area		Medial area
Parabrachial		Rostral raphe N.
Subcaeruleus		Edinger Westphal N.
Locus caeruleus		Dorsal substantia nigra
	Periaquaductal gray	
	Interpeduncular N.	
	Nucleus retroambiguus	

tional LUT. In the future, functional imaging of the brain may provide insight into the integrity of these various nuclei and how they are affected in patients with "ideopathic" LUT dysfunction.

D. Peripheral Muscle: Peripheral and CNS Pathophysiology

A primary difficulty noted in patients with chronic urinary retention and pelvic pain syndromes is the inability to voluntarily relax their perineums on command. As many of these patients, not uncommonly, describe bladder difficulties in childhood, there may very well be a progressive drift with time toward memorized high-pressure activity within the striated pelvic muscles.

Noxious sensory information is relayed to the CNS from the pelvic floor striated muscles by thin myelinated Aδ fibers (group III) or unmyelinated C fibers (group IV). This information is then filtered and modulated within the CNS before any muscle activity can occur. The release of neuropeptides mediates all CNS events (38,39). They are, therefore, the important link between sensations experienced by patients and consequent activity in muscle. They are also potentially important therapeutic pathways for drug therapy.

Similar peptides influence both sensory and muscular events. For example, dorsal root ganglion cells, which project to muscle tissue, contain SP, calcitonin gene-related peptide (CGRP), and somatostatin (40,41). These neuropetides are not only effective in connection with pain, but also influence motor fiber tonicity. CGRP coexists with acetylcholine (ACh) in a subpopulation of motoneurons and enhances the contraction of skeletal muscle (42). Furthermore, CGRP can increase spontaneous ACh release (43) and ACh synthesis at the neuromuscular junction (44). Neuropeptides are released from both spinal terminals within the CNS and receptive endings in the peripheral target (i.e., muscle) (45). In this

Table 3 Central Peptide Pools Linked to CNS Centers
Regulating Lower Urinary Tract Function

Paraventricular peptide pool
    Vasopressin, oxytocin, substance P
    Somatostatin, dopamine, neurotensin
    Glucagon, renin
    Corticotropin-releasing factor
    Met- and leu-enkephalin
Nucleus Onuf peptides (for sphincter control)
    Somatostatin, neuropeptide Y, serotonin
    Substance P (from paraventricular nucleus, dorsal and ventral roots)
    Met- and leu-enkephalin

way, CGRP and SP influence the biochemical environment of both central and peripheral receptors from which they are released (46).

It is known that SP release from nociceptive peripheral nerve endings can cause neural inflammation (47). The microcirculation within the muscle can be changed by the vasodilating actions of CGRP (48) and by the increased vascular permeability effects of SP and neurokinins A and B (49). Thus, a whole chain of events in peripheral muscle (21), once triggered, can contribute to the development of deleterious muscle pathophysiology. Any underlying primary muscle dysfunction will not only be supported, but will also be aggravated.

A continued stream of nociceptive information associated with repetitive dysfunctional behavior of the pelvic floor muscles, especially if memorized and chronic, puts those CNS circuits involved in a state of metabolic stress. Architectural and communicative changes can subsequently occur within the CNS. Motor neurons can have increased numbers of dendritic buttons and receive enhanced afferent input from a variety of competing sources. Cross talk, convergence, and windup can occur within the dorsal root laminations as well as at other levels within the CNS. The progressive chaos in sensory processing will eventually result in the emergence of irritative voiding symptoms and dyssynergic void efforts.

Afferents from both viscera and pelvic striated muscle enter the cord primarily within laminas I and V (50–52). Skin afferents enter the cord in laminas II–IV (53). Cross-communication and excitation, within or between lamina, would explain the cutaneous and visceral hypersensitivity (pelvic pain) found with pelvic floor striated muscle dysfunction. The mechanisms would be based on afferent–afferent interactions within the cord, convergence projection, dichotomized sensory C fibers, or aberrant sympathetic reflex activity (54,55).

Sensitization, windup, and expansion of receptive fields are classic response properties of the CNS to nociceptive input (56–60). Symptoms of urethral allodynia, referred pain, frequency, and urgency are consistent with these CNS events, as are the signs of sphincter hyperalgesia (local pain), pelvic floor tenderness and rigidity of movement, and dyssynergic voiding (Fig. 5). Any breakdown in the pathway (i.e., loss of gated regulation), that assures coordinated CNS regulation of pelvic floor behavior, only reinforces pathophysiological behavior. A vicious cycle of pain and dysfunction, involving organs within a dermatome, and an expanded receptive field then result.

Recently, we determined the distribution of spinal nociceptive neurons, which receive afferent inputs from the bladder, the prostate, and the urethral sphincter. The c-*fos*-immunoreactive cells within the spinal cord were evaluated in response to chemical irritation of these three organs. Through this study, it was found that c-*fos*-positive cells were most evident in the dorsal commissure and spinal parasympathetic nuclei regions for stimulation of all three organs. A significant overlap in spinal c-*fos* expression following irritation of three separate LUT segments was established. The experiments suggest a close linkage in central nociceptive processing from these organs. Chronic nociceptive input leads to expansion of receptive fields in dorsal horn neurons in the spinal cord (57). This expansion of receptive fields would include activation of a greater number of neurons than would be activated normally (61). These phenomena, along with the demonstrated convergence of afferent input to the cord, strongly favor viewing chronic nociceptive inputs from one pelvic organ as being capable of adversely affecting the integrity, functional or morphological, of other pelvic organs. For example, afferent inputs from an inflamed prostate, or a dysfunctionally irritated sphincter (hypertonic sphincter), could adversely influence spinal regulatory circuits of micturition through neurogenically mediated inflammation mechanism (54,55).

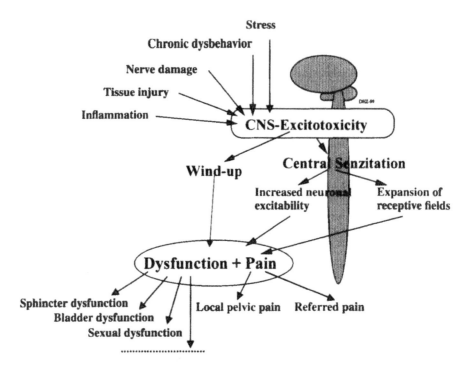

Figure 5 Neurobiological background of chronic pelvic pain and dysfunction in the pelvic area.

III. CLINICAL APPROACH: DIAGNOSTICS, CLASSIFICATION GUIDELINES, AND TREATMENT

A. History and Clinical Examination

At a first visit in a neurourology clinic, before "hypertonic urethra," is diagnosed, patients usually complain about a variety of symptoms. However, this is only one point that makes the diagnosis of a hypertonic urethra really difficult. Patients report frequency, urgency, suprapubic, perineal, or deep pelvic pain; they complain about slow urinary stream, the necessity of double voiding, and recurrent urinary tract infections. Some patients, mostly women, are in chronic urinary retention.

After carefully recording the patient's history (Table 4), objectivation of the reported symptoms is mandatory. This includes a micturition diary of at least 14 days. The patient is asked to note emptying parameters (time, volume, leakage, pad change) as well as fluid intake data (time, volume). Comments on pain, autonomic signs (headache, sweating, tachycardia, palpitation, on other), and defecation are requested.

The history recorded should include at least those data shown in Table 4.

B. Physical Examination

Pelvic floor and digital rectal examinations are the main focus. Initially, the clinician should observe voluntary attempts to tighten and relax the perineum. This is done with the patient

Table 4 Recorded Data for Basic History

Current symptoms?
    Since when? development over the last time? change in last time?
    Pain?
        Where?, character?, intensity (using visual analog scale 0–10), Change over time?
    Micturition?
        Any problems?, double voiding?, infections?, burning?, inability to void?
    Defecation?
        Frequency, consistency
    Sexual life?
        Dysfunction?, emotional problems?, *female:* vaginism?
Childhood
    prolonged bedwetting?, excessive exercises to achieve early urinary continence?, punishment
    for bedwetting?, retentive voiding habits (i.e., low micturition frequency?), sexual abuse (fe-
    male)?
Adolescence
    Female: painful menses?, frequent urinary tract infections?
    Male: urinary tract infections
Adulthood
    Female: childbirths?, vaginal delivery?, pelvic surgery?, infections?, voiding habits over time,
    profession, personal satisfaction
    Male: voiding habits, profession, social life

in the lithotomy position, or stooped over, with arms on an examination table. A visual assessment is then carried out.

With a "hold" effort, contraction and relaxation of the pelvic floor muscles should be clearly evident. There should be an instantaneous, unhesitating identity with the rectal muscles. The movement should be effortless and free of extraneous muscular activity (i.e., abdominal tightening, Valsalva, pelvic tilt, or other). The "bellows"-like movement of the levator should be repeatable with consistency, and the contraction should be sustainable for 2–3 sec before relaxation is permitted. Often, the effort is flawed dynamically, with contraction–relaxation inconsistencies, or frank tightness or weakness is evident.

Subsequently, the buttocks should be slightly separated, and the anal skin observed for "clamp-like" wrinkling with the hold effort. Occasionally, one may see fibrillations in the superficial anal muscle fibers. Alternatively, an easier way to check on voluntary recruitment of the pudendal innervated perineal muscles is to observe contraction of the base of the penis during hold and relaxation. Shortening of the ischiocavernosus muscles should pull the penis (clitoris) toward the pubic bone.

Poor identity with the pelvic muscles, or inconsistencies in recruitment, reflect inefficiencies in neural regulation of the sphincter.

Digital rectal examination is then performed, both for anatomical aberrations and functional behavior. The following should be assessed and quantified mentally:

1. Tonus of the deep and superficial and sphincter muscles: Is sphincter tone normal, weak, or high?
2. Evidence of hypersensitivity: Is there tenderness of the levator posterolaterally? Is there tenderness of the prostate apex, base, or external sphincter?

3. Motor identity: Can the patient contract on the examining finger? Is the movement repetitively consistent? Is there a distinct contraction as well as relaxation above and below the basal tone? Is the levator edge distinct or mushy? Is there movement in both the levator and pudendal sphincter components?

The clinician should learn to recognize degrees of inefficiency that affect the behavior of the pelvic floor between, as well as during, voids. Patients with "shy bladders," "recurrent urinary tract infections," or a "frequency issue" often have high-pressure, tender, and inefficient pelvic floor muscles and muscular dynamics.

This examination should follow a careful clinical examination of the patient (Table 5). For this part, the patient can be examined standing, sitting, or in the lateral decubitus position. A systematic assessment of pelvic floor sensation, anal tone, strength of the lower limbs and feet, and the lability of reflexes involving the bulbocavernosus, anal, knee, and ankle muscles should be carried out.

Table 5 Suggested Scheme for Clinical Evaluation of the Pelvic Area

Clinical assessment of pelvic floor and sphincter	
Asymmetry of gluteal–thigh creases:	
none (0), some (1+), major (2+)	2
Symmetry of greater trochanters (pelvic tilt):	
none (0), some (1+), major (2+)	2
Total	4
Visual assessment	
Bellows (levator)	
Gluteal cleft: deep (2+), flat (2+), moderate (0)	2
Hold: definitive (0), some (1+), none (2+)	2
Relaxation: complete (0), some (1+), none (2+)	2
Repetitious: consistency on three tries; identical movement (0), some (1+), none (2+)	2
Penile retraction (sphincter)	
Hold: definitive (0), some (1+), none (2+)	2
Relaxation: complete (0), some (1+), none (2+)	2
Repetitious: consistency on three tries; identical movement (0), some (1+), none (2+)	2
Visual total	14
Voluntary contraction assessment (digital rectal examination)	
Levator (bellows)	
Resting tone: none (0), moderate/normal (1+), increased (2+)	2
Hold: definitive (0), some (1+), none (2+)	2
Relaxation: complete (0), some (1+), none (2+)	2
Repetitious: consistency on three tries; identical movement (0), close (1+), none (2+)	2
Rectal (levator) sensation: no pain (0), some discomfort (1+), very painful (2+)	2
Anal sphincter (clamp)	
Resting tone: moderate, normal (0), increased, weakened (1+), tight, none (2+)	2
Hold: definitive (0), some, flutter, or premature release (1+), none (2+)	2
Relaxation: complete (0), some (1+), none (2+)	2
Repetitious: consistency 3 tries; identical movement (0), some (1+), none (2+)	2
Perianal skin sensation: normal (0), increased, decreased (1+), hyperaesthetic, numb (2+)	
Total examination points	20
Total possible score	38

When completed, this examination should provide useful insight into the functional integrity of the sacral nerve roots controlling bladder and sphincter behavior. Reflex excitability should be an important focus of the examination. Brisk lower extremity reflexes are often a good indication of a hyperexciteable pelvic floor.

C. Urodynamics

Urodynamic studies are meant to include all techniques used to provide objective documentation of LUT functional integrity (6,62). Traditionally, urodynamic testing includes a cystometrogram, urethral pressure profile (UPP), urinary flow rate, and documentation of residual urine. Additional tests include leak point pressure and various neurological tests: EMG monitoring of the pelvic floor, pudendal motor term latencies, and evoked potential studies. Radiologic tests include videomonitoring of the bladder during filling and emptying (videourodynamics). The most meaningful assessment is achievable by recordings of LUT behavior.

1. Cystometry

Just what is normal bladder function? There is good urodynamic evidence that the adult bladder should be able to hold 400–500 mL without much more than a sense of fullness.

As with low urinary volumes, storage above 500 mL is considered abnormal and quite possibly a sign of a hypertonic sphincter. There is a range, and the greater the departure from the ideal norm, the greater the neuromuscular abnormality of the bladder, the greater the risk of complications, and the greater the difficulty to be expected in correcting the problem.

Void diaries are very helpful, but can be misleading. A void frequency of four to six times per day may be normal with a 24-hr output of 2 L (500 mL/void), but abnormal with a 24-hr output of 800 mL (200 mL/void). Smaller-volume voids reflect such abnormalities of the bladder wall as instability, hyperreflexia, hypersensitivity, or poor compliance.

A cystometrogram is obtained with the patient lying down and a filling rate of 20 mL/min. The cool temperature of the filling fluid, or standing the patient, is provocative of the void reflex. Contraction and voiding should occur as a voluntary event with filling near the ideal range. Otherwise, the test should be considered a departure from an idealized norm.

2. Recording of Urethral Sphincter Activity

The value of UPP recording, lies not so much in the absolute pressure reading, but in documentation of the degree of facilitation or inhibition that may exist within CNS regulatory circuits. UPP is recorded with the bladder filled to roughly 25–75% of suspected capacity, for there are different micturition gates operational at different fill volumes. Sensitivity to the presence of the catheter is noted (hypersensitive urethras are most often associated with labile activity and with irritative voiding symptoms). Each time the profile is repeated, changes in urethral tone, reflex excitability of the pelvic floor striated muscles, and any triggering of an unstable bladder contraction are noted. The real value of UPP is achieved only when the data are collected and viewed with a dynamic perspective. Static pressure readings have limited value as, for example, may be true with pure intrinsic sphincter weakness (63–65).

Dynamic recording is able to show sphincter overactivity and spasticity (Fig. 6).

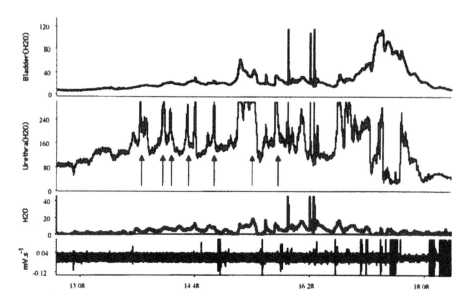

Figure 6 Storage failure: spastic urethral sphincter behavior during bladder filling phase (see arrows).

3. Urethral Reflexes and Continence

It has been reported that the striated sphincter contributes more than 50% of closure tone to the bladder outlet (66). The remainder results from smooth-muscle tone and the fibroelastic components of the urethra. Although this may be a quantitative measure, it does not imply that 50% of continence comes from the smooth muscle of the urethra. Patients with weak sphincters can present with retention, and patients with high-pressure sphincters can present with incontinence. Although urethral closure pressures do generally correlate with symptoms, there are common discrepancies. An aberrance in behavior and excitability is usually more evident in dynamic sphincter recordings.

4. Dynamic Behavior: Importance

Basal tone is provided to the sphincter via the CNS regulatory pathways. During periods of stress, the sphincter mechanism must compensate, through reflex contraction, for the immediate rise in intra-abdominal pressure. Animal studies (67–70) have shown that passive increases in intra-abdominal pressure are reflected equally within the bladder and the bladder neck, but are lost progressively in the more distal urethra. Conversely, abrupt intra-abdominal pressure change (e.g., coughing) evokes a brisk rise in external sphincter closure that is not seen at the level of the bladder neck or within the bladder.

These studies have demonstrated that continence during acute stress (e.g., coughing) is preserved by the efficiency of urethral striated sphincter closure. Thus, a passive, slow pressure rise can be partially balanced by the bladder neck and urethral smooth muscle, but it is the modulating and protective neuroreflex regulation of the striated sphincter that maintains continence. Hence, assessment of the integrity of these reflexes is important in evaluating urethral competence.

5. Urethral Sphincter Activity Assessment

The bladder is filled while bladder and urethral pressures are monitored simultaneously. Spontaneous fluctuations in urethral sphincter activity are indicators of instability and flawed CNS reflex regulation. During filling of the bladder, the perineum is carefully observed for spontaneous muscle activity, the degree of activity triggered by coughing, straining, or movement of the catheter in the urethra. The ability to voluntarily recruit pelvic floor muscle activity (i.e., the levator) is visually assessed, whereas the urethral sphincter contraction is recorded urodynamically. Also, the patient's ability to "strain" and "hold" is observed to assess concepts of proper voluntary coordination of the pelvic floor with voiding and continence. The perineum should move down with a strain and up with a hold, respectively. The cough reflex, or the bulbocavernosus reflex, is recorded on the urethral channel.

6. Voiding Behavior

There are four stages of voiding behavior, which can potentially be involved in lower urinary tract pathophysiology (Table 6; Figs. 7 and 8).

7. The Hypertonic Sphincter–Hyperpathic Urethra: A Classification

What constitutes a dyssnergic sphincter? Is it lack of relaxation? Is it hypersensitivity? Are tonicity and reflex excitability both factors in dyssnergia? The answers to these questions are not really addressed by the terms overactive or hypertonic sphincter. Perhaps, it is time to revisit the old terminology, as it can frequently be overly subjective and nonquantitative. If there is little accuracy in the terms used to describe a condition, it is very difficult to associate prognosis with the treatments generally available.

The term *hypertonic sphincter* is intended to describe a sphincter that has a higher than normal sustained pressure in the resting state. However, although there are case examples that might fit this definition, the behavior cannot be reliably assigned as a trait of any one particular diagnosis, as, for example, can the term cogwheel rigidity reliably de-

Table 6 Four States of Voiding Behavior

1. Fill phase (normally very stable pressures 60–80 cmH$_2$O)
   Pathology High sphincter pressure (>80)
   Hypersensitivity
   Clonic or hyperreflexic dynamic
   Spasms (pain) versus spontaneous relaxations (leakage episodes)
2. Transition phase (normally smooth)
   Pathology Nonrelaxation
   Hesitant/delayed relaxation
   Precipitous relaxation
   Aborted relaxation
   Rising sphincter pressures
3. Void phase (normally coordinated)
   Pathology Partial relaxations
   Intermittency of sphincter relaxation
4. Recovery stage (normally smooth)
   Pathology Intermittency (dribbling)

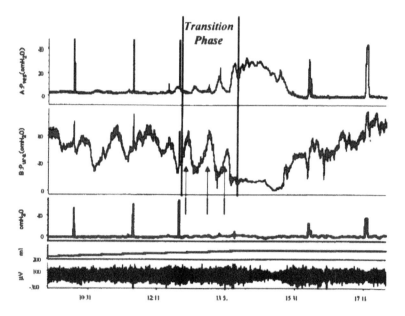

Figure 7 Transition failure: unable to initiate voiding properly, owing to spastic urethral sphincter activity during transition phase.

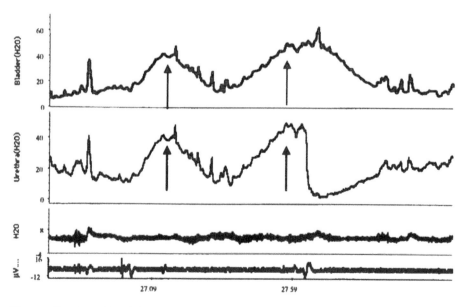

Figure 8 Micturition failure: increase of bladder pressure is paralleled by an increase of urethral pressure.

scribe the muscle tone of parkinsonism. Instead, the hypertonic sphincter is only one behavioral component of what could be better termed the *hyperpathic urethra*. This latter term would better incorporate the three implied aspects of sphincter dysfunction:

1. Hypertonicity (T)
2. Hyperreflexia (R)
3. Hypersensitivity (S)

As the term is accurately descriptive, it can be inclusive of both nonneurogenic as well as neurogenic LUT disorders. It can be objectively quantitative when used to summarize urodynamic findings, or subjectively quantitative when used to describe physical findings.

As an example, the sphincter could be described as being any one of the following subtypes: (1) hyperpathic—TRS; (2) hyperpathic—TR; (3) hyperpathic—RS; (4) hyperpathic—S; (5) hyperpathic—R; (6) hyperpathic—TS; (7) hyperpathic—T; or other. Each example denotes a particular type of hyperpathic behavior of the urinary sphincter.

One could then subcategorize each category into quantifiable degrees of severity [i.e., none (0), mild (1), moderate (2), or severe (3)]. Hence, two variations could be as follows: (1) hyperpathic—$T_1R_3S_3$, to describe the *dysfunctional prostatodynia sphincter*—mildly hypertonic (T_1), severely hyperreflexic (R_3), and severely hypersensitive (S_3); or (2) hyperpathic—$T_2R_0S_0$, to describe a parkinsonian patient with a moderate degree of sphincter hypertonicity, no hyperreflexic activity, and no hypersensitivity.

The scheme may appear unwieldy at first. However, it is logical, easy to write, and far more descriptively accurate than the alternatives employed today. To complete this logic and extend the classification scheme to include the hypopathic urethra, minus numbers for sphincter tonicity could be used. Thus, the cauda equina sphincter would be described as T_{-1} or T_{-2}, depending on pressure. The R and S components would remain as zeros. Thus, the cauda equina patient, with a 1000-mL bladder, absent sensation, and a sphincter closure pressure of less than 30 cmH$_2$O becomes a $T_{-2}R_0S_0$ sphincter dysfunction.

The rationale behind this classification is simply to have better accuracy in the stated diagnosis and, consequently, to evolve therapeutic regimens that would best address each of the different clinical presentations.

There are no recommended normal values for urethral closure pressure. However, clinical experience would suggest normal resting urethral closure pressures in the following range:

Women: 60–70 cmH$_2$O
Men: 60–80 cmH$_2$O

Consequently, female urethral closure pressure of more than 70 cmH$_2$O, and male urethral closure pressure greater than 80 cmH$_2$O, would be considered an hypertonic urethra (or hyperpathic—T). Often, nonneuropathic patients with these high sphincter pressures have additional hypersensitivity problems in the urethral sphincter and bladder neck areas. Any degree of noxious discomfort caused by movement of the urodynamic catheter while performing UPP would constitute hypersensitivity. Neurometer measurements would be better at assessing sensitivity, but are expensive. Therefore, for the present, the term should be based on clinical testing as it is carried out in most clinics today. Reflex contractions to movement of the urodynamic catheter of more than 5 cmH$_2$O would represent a state of significant hyperreflexia.

IV. CONCLUSION: AN ALTERNATIVE URODYNAMIC PHILOSOPHY

The CNS is composed of a delicately balanced (i.e., gated) circuitry, with a built-in predisposition toward instability. Tissue or nerve injury or chronic behavioral dysfunction can trigger a release of excitotoxic transmitters. These, in turn, can create prolonged changes in central neural circuitry, with resultant permanent change in the way in which nociceptive sensory information is processed (71).

Given the association between pelvic neuromuscle integrity and "overcontinence," urethral sphincter failure can be viewed, apart from iatrogenic factors, as being a myofascial degenerative condition linked to an acute or chronic neurogenic compromise. The association of a hypertonic sphincter with CNS pathology is easy to understand. However, by far, the majority of LUT symptoms—overcontinence and pelvic pain syndromes remain unexplained by existing theories.

Chronic misuse of the striated muscles, regardless of body location, whether through lifestyle or habit, is capable of triggering aberrant plasticity changes within the CNS. This concept of LUT failure over time should be considered when there is an obvious disconnection of conscious CNS modulation of pelvic floor behavior, and there is no explainable cause of the symptoms. This is a neurological perspective of the problem and requires a more behavioral-based neurodiagnostic evaluation. The approach is consistent with the present shift in emphasis of care toward modulation-based treatments. The goal is to "wind down" CNS excitability first and foremost, before moving to surgical-based treatments. The preventative approach should result in marked improvement of patient care and satisfaction. Educating patients about the risks of stress, hurried voids, or retentive tendencies should be part of every routine physical. By initiating treatment and prophylaxis programs early in life, the problems of the elderly could be greatly diminished.

REFERENCES

1. Floman Y, Wiesel SW, Rothman RH. Cauda equina syndrome presenting as a herniated lumbar disk. Clin Orthop Rel Res 1980; 147:234–237.
2. Borges PM, Hackler RH. The urologic status of the Vietnam war paraplegic: A 15-year prospective follow-up. J Urol 1982; 127:710–711.
3. Andersen JT. Disturbances of bladder and urethral function in Parkinson's disease. Int Urol Nephrol 1985; 17:836–838.
4. Pavlakis AJ, Siroky MB, Goldstein I, Krane RJ. Neurourologic findings in Parkinson's disease. J Urol 1983; 129:80–83.
5. Blaivas JG. Management of bladder dysfunction in multiple sclerosis. Neurology 1980; 30: 12–18.
6. Schmidt RA, Zermann DH, Doggweiler R. Urinary incontinence update: old traditions and new concepts. Adv Intern Med 1999; 44:19–57.
7. Hawkins RD, Kandel ER, Siegelbaum SA. Learning to modulate transmitter release: themes and variations in synaptic plasticity. Annu Rev Neurosci 1993; 16:625–665.
8. Kandel ER. Genes, nerve cells, and the remembrance of things past. J Neuropsychiatry 1989; 1:103–125.
9. Sasaki K, Gemba H. Plasticity of cortical function related to voluntary movement, motor learning and compensation following brain dysfunction. Acta Neurochir 1987; 41(suppl):18–28.
10. Dickinson A. Contemporary Animal Learning Theory. Cambridge, UK: Cambridge University Press, 1980.
11. Tulving E, Schacter DL. Priming and human memory system. Science 1990; 247:301–306.

12. Bailey CH, Bartsch D, Kandel ER. Toward a molecular definition of long-term memory storage. Proc Natl Acad Sci USA 1996; 93:13445–13452.

13. Plunkett K, Karmiloff–Smith A, Bates E, Elman JL, Johnson MH. Connectionism and developmental psychology. J Child Psychol Psychiatry 1997; 38:53–80.

14. Cohen NJ, Poldrack RA, Eichenbaum H. Memory for items and memory for relations in the procedural/declarative memory framework. Memory 1997; 5:131–178.

15. Domjan M, Burkhard B. The Principles of Learning and Behavior. 2nd ed. Monterey, CA: Brooks & Cole, 1986.

16. McMahon SB, Wall PD. Receptive fields of rat lamina 1 projection cells move to incorporate a nearby region of injury. Pain 1984; 19:235–247.

17. Food and Drug Administration (FDA) Gastroenterology and Urology Device Panel, Rockville, MD. Aug 6, 1997.

18. DeLancey JO. The anatomy of the pelvic floor. Curr Opin Obstet Gynecol 1994; 6:313–316.

19. DeLancey JO. Functional anatomy of the female lower urinary tract and the pelvic floor. Ciba Found Symp 1990; 151:57–69.

20. Matzel KE, Schmidt RA, Tanagho EA. Neuroanatomy of the striated muscular anal continence mechanism. Implications for the use of neurostimulation. Dis Colon Rectum 1990; 33:666–673.

21. Mendell LM, Wall PD. Responses of dorsal horn cells to peripheral cutaneous unmyelinated fibers. Nature 1965; 206:97–99.

22. Pockett S. Spinal cord synaptic plasticity and chronic pain. Anesth Analg 1995; 80:173–179.

23. Schmidt RA, Pelvic pain. Probl Urol 1989; 3:270–281.

24. Hellstrom WJG, Schmidt RA, Lue TF, Tanagho EA. Neuromuscular dysfunction in nonbacterial prostatitis. Urology 1987; 30:183–188.

25. Zermann DH, Ishigooka M, Doggweiler R, Schmidt RA. Neuro-urological insights to the etiology of genitourinary pain in men. J Urol 1999; 161:903–908.

26. Zermann DH, Ishigooka M, Wunderlich H, Reichelt O, Schubert J. A study of pelvic floor function pre- and post-radical prostatectomy using clinical neurourological investigations, urodynamics and electromyography. Eur Urol 2000; 37:156–160.

27. Marson L, McKenna KE. CNS cell groups involved in the control of the ischiocavernosus and bulbospongiosus muscles: a transneurological tracing study using pseudorabies virus. J Comp Neurol 1996; 374:161–179.

28. Nadelhaft I, Vera PL. Neurons in the rat brain and the spinal cord labeled after pseudorabies virus injected into the external urethral sphincter. J Comp Neurol 1996; 375:502–517.

29. Vizzard MA, Erickson VL, Card JP, Roppolo JR, de Groat WC. Transneuronal labeling of neurons in the adult rat brainstem and spinal cord after injection of pseudorabies virus into the urethra. J Comp Neurol 1995; 355:629–640.

30. Nadelhaft I, Vera PL, Card JP, Miselis RR. Central nervous system neurons labeled following the injection of pseudorabies virus into the rat urinary bladder. Neurosci Lett 1992; 143:271–274.

31. Zermann DH, Ishigooka M, Doggweiler R, Schmidt RA. Central autonomic innervation of the lower urinary tract—a neuroanatomical study. World J Urol 1998; 16:417–422.

32. Zermann DH, Ishigooka M, Ebersberger A, Schubert J, Schmidt RA. Spinal and supraspinal neurons labeled after pseudorabies virus injected into the prostate gland. Soc Neurosci Abstr 1999; 25(part 1):104.

33. Benarroch EE. The central autonomic network: functional organization, dysfunction and perspective. Mayo Clin Proc 1993; 68:988–1001.

34. Holstege G, Tan J. Supraspinal control of motoneurons innervating the striated muscles of the pelvic floor including urethral and anal sphincters in the cat. Brain 1987; 110:1323–1344.

35. Blok BFM, Willemsen ATM, Holstege G. PET study on brain control of micturition in humans. Brain 1997; 120:111–121.

36. Kruse MN, Noto H, Roppolo JR, de Groat WC. Pontine control of the urinary bladder and external urethral sphincter in the rat. Brain Res 1990; 532:182–190.

37. Blok BFM, Holstege G. Neuronal control of micturition and its relation to the emotional motor system. Prog Brain Res 1996; 107:113–126.

38. Höfkelt T, Johansson O, Ljungdahl A, Lundberg JM, Schultzberg M. Peptidergic neurons. Nature 1980; 284:515–521.

39. Cuello AC. Peptides as neuromodulators in primary sensory neurons. Neuropharmacology 1987; 26:971–979.

40. O'Brien C, Woolf CJ, Fitzgerald M, Lindsay RM, Molander C. Differences in the chemical expression of rat primary afferent neurons which innervate skin, muscle or joint. Neuroscience 1989; 32:493–502.

41. Molander C, Ygge I, Dalsgaard CJ. Substance P, somatostatin-, and calcitonin gene-related peptide-like immunoreactivity and fluoride resistant acid phosphatase-activity in relation to retrogradely labeled cutaneous, muscular and visceral primary sensory neurons in the rat. Neurosci Lett 1987; 74:34–42.

42. Takami K, Kawai Y, Uchida S, Tomyama M, Shiotani Y, Yoshida H, Emson PC, Girgis S, Hillyard CJ, MacIntyre I. Effect of calcitonin gene-related peptide on contraction of striated muscle in the mouse. Neurosci Lett 1985; 60:227–230.

43. Jinnai K, Chihara K, Kanda F, Tada K, Fujita T. Calcitonin gene-related peptide enhances spontaneous acetylcholine release from the rat motor nerve terminal. Neurosci Lett 1989; 103: 64–68.

44. New HV, Mudge AW. Calcitonin gene-related peptide regulates muscle acetylcholine receptors synthesis. Nature 1986; 323:809–811.

45. Kruger L. Morphological correlates of "free" nerve endings—a re-appraisal of thin sensory axon classification. In: Schmidt RF, Schaible HG, Vahle–Hinz C, eds. Fine Afferent Nerve Fibers and Pain. Weinheim: Verlagsgesellschaft, 1987:1–13.

46. Holzer P. Local effector functions of capsaicin-sensitive sensory nerve endings: involvement of tachykinins, calcitonin gene-related peptide and other neuropeptides. Neuroscience 1988; 24: 739–768.

47. Lembeck F, Holzer P. Substance P as neurogenic mediator of antidromic vasodilation and neurogenic plasma extravasation. Naunyn-Schmiedebergs Arch Pharmacol 1979; 310:175–183.

48. Brian SD, Williams TJ, Tippins JR, Morris HR, MacIntyre I. Calcitonin gene-related peptide is a potent vasodilatator. Nature 1985; 313:54–56.

49. Couture R, Kerouac R. Plasma protein extravasation induced by mammalian tachykinins in rat skin: influence of anaesthetic agents and acetylcholine antagonist. Br J Pharmacol 1987; 91: 265–273.

50. Brushart TM, Henry EW, Mesulam MM. Reorganization of muscle afferent projection accompanies peripheral nerve regeneration. Neuroscience 1981; 6:2053–2061.

51. Brushart TM, Mesulam MM. Transganglionic demonstration of central sensory projections from skin and muscle with HRP–lectin conjugates. Neurosci Lett 1980; 17:1–6.

52. Nadelhaft I, Roppolo J, Morgan C, de Groat WC. Parasympathetic preganglionic neurons and visceral primary afferents in monkey sacral spinal cord revealed following application of horseradish peroxidase to pelvic nerve. J Comp Neurol 1983; 216:36–52.

53. Koerber HR, Brown PB. Projections of two hindlimb cutaneous nerves to the cat dorsal horn. J Neurophysiol 1980; 44:259–269.

54. Wesselmann U, Lai J. Mechanism of referred visceral pain: uterine inflammation in the adult virgin rat results in neurgenic plasma extravasation in the skin. Pain 1997; 73:309–317.

55. McMahon SB, Dmitrieva N, Kolzenburg M. Visceral pain. Br J Anaesth 1995; 75:132–144.

56. Coderre TJ, Katz J, Vaccarino AL, Melzack R. Contribution of central neuroplasticity to pathological pain: review of clinical and experimental evidence. Pain 1993; 52:259–285.

57. Hylden JLK, Nahin RL, Traub RJ, Dubner R. Expansion of receptive fields in spinal lamina I projections in rats with unilateral adjuvant-induced inflammation: the contribution of dorsal horn mechanism. Pain 1989; 37:229–243.

58. Calverley RKS, Jones DG. Contributions of dendritic spines and perforated synapses to synaptic plasticity. Brain Res Rev 1990; 15:215–249.
59. Wall PD, Woolf CJ. Muscle but not cutaneous C-afferent input produces prolonged increase in the excitability of the flexion reflex in rat. J Physiol 1984; 356:443–458.
60. Woolf CJ, Wall PD. Relative effectiveness of C primary afferent fibers of different origins in evoking a prolonged facilitation on the flexor reflex in the rat. J Neurosci 1986; 6:1433–1442.
61. Dubner R. Neuronal plasticity and pain following peripheral tissue inflammation or nerve injury. In: Bond MR, Charlton VE, Woolf CJ, eds. Proceedings of the VIth World Congress on Pain. Amsterdam: Elsevier, 1991: 246–276.
62. Abrams P, Blaivas JG, Stanton SL, Andersen JT. The standardisation of terminology of lower urinary tract function. The International Continence Society Committee on Standardisation of Terminology. Scand J Urol Nephrol 1988; 114:5–19.
63. Anderson RS, Shepherd AM, Feneley RC. Microtransducer urethral profile methodology: variations caused by transducer orientation. J Urol 1983; 130:727–728.
64. DeJonge MC, Kornelis JA, van den Berg J. The static urethral closure pressure profile in female incontinence. A comparison between sphincter and detrusor incontinence. Prog Clin Biol Res 1981; 78:231–238.
65. Bruskewitz R, Raz S. Urethral pressure profile using microtip catheter in females. Urology 1979; 14:303–307.
66. Tanagho EA, Schmidt RA, Araujo GG. Urinary striated sphincter: what is the nerve supply? Urology 1982; 20:415–417.
67. Thüroff JW, Bazeed MA, Schmidt RA, Tanagho EA. Mechanism of urinary incontinence: an animal model to study urethral responses to stress conditions. J Urol 1982; 127:1202–1206.
68. Thüroff JW, Schmidt RA, Bazeed MA, Tanagho EA. Chronic stimulation of the sacral roots in dogs. Eur Urol 1983; 9:102–108.
69. Thüroff JW, Casper F, Heidler H. Pelvic floor stress response: reflex contraction with pressure transmission to the urethra. Urol Int 1987; 42:185–189.
70. Heidler H, Casper F, Thüroff JW. Role of striated sphincter muscle in urethral closure under stress conditions: an experimental study. Urology 1987; 42:195–200.
71. Dubner R, Ruda MA. Activity-dependent neuronal plasticity following tissue injury and inflammation. Trends Neurosci 1992; 15:96–103.

14

The Dyssynergic Sphincter

GÉRARD AMARENCO and SAMER SHEIKH ISMAEL

Rothschild Hospital, Paris, France

JEAN MARC SOLER

Bouffard-Vercelli Medical Center, Cerbere, France

I. INTRODUCTION

Normal micturition (1), evoked by a sacral spinal reflex under cortical influences, is characterized by a detrusor contraction associated with complete urethral sphincter relaxation. Thus, the voiding reflex is accomplished with low detrusor pressure and without residual volume.

Detrusor–sphincter dyssynergia is a voiding dysfunction of the emptying phase of micturition. By definition, it is urodynamic, with involuntary contraction of the external urethral sphincter during detrusor contraction (2–5). It constitutes an obstructive phenomenon and can lead to urological complications, such as hydroureteronephrosis and renal failure. Patients with spinal cord injuries are particularly vulnerable. Treatment is always necessary to avoid these complications: intermittent self-catheterization can be proposed in association with anticholinergic drugs, α-adrenergic blockers, antispastic agents, transperineal injections of botulinum toxin, intraurethral stent prosthesis, or sphincterotomy. In some cases, incoordination between the bladder and urethral sphincter is not due to a neurological lesion, but is secondary to a behavioral dysfunction. Pelvic floor rehabilitation is advisable with biofeedback exercises.

II. DEFINITIONS

Detrusor–external sphincter dyssynergia (DESD) is characterized by involuntary contractions of the external urethral sphincter during involuntary detrusor contraction. It is caused by neurological lesions between the brain stem (pontine micturition center) and the sacral spinal cord (sacral micturition center). These include especially traumatic spinal cord injury as well as multiple sclerosis, myelodysplasia, and other forms of transverse myelitis.

DESD was hypothesized to be an abnormal flexor response of the perineal musculature to bladder contraction (6) and was considered an exaggerated continence reflex owing to the loss of supraspinal influences (7).

This incoordination between the detrusor smooth muscle and the external urethral sphincter or the bladder neck induces an obstruction that creates excessive bladder pressures during voiding and residual volume. Thereby, the risk increases for recurrent urinary tract infections, vesicoureteral reflux, hydronephrosis, and pyelonephritis.

III. PHYSIOLOGY

A. Introduction

The storage and periodic elimination of urine are dependent on the activity of two functional units in the lower urinary tract: a reservoir (the bladder) and an outlet consisting of the bladder neck, the urethra, and the striated urethral sphincter. These structures are controlled by autonomic and somatic innervation: sacral parasympathetic (pelvic), thoracolumbar sympathetic (hypogastric), and sacral somatic (pudendal) nerves.

Many reflexes control the storage phase and micturition. Urine storage is dependent on spinal reflexes. The efferent pathways are the somatic nerves (external sphincter contraction) and the sympathetic nerves (internal sphincter contraction, detrusor inhibition, or ganglionic inhibition). Micturition is under the control of spinobulbospinal reflexes, which determine the inhibition of sympathetic activity and the activation of parasympathetic activity (detrusor contraction). The expulsion phase consists of initial relaxation of the urethral sphincter, followed in a few seconds by contraction of the detrusor. Secondary reflexes elicited by urine flow through the urethra facilitate bladder emptying.

B. Anatomy of the Central Nervous System Controlling the Detrusor–Sphincter Synergia

1. Pathways in the Spinal Cord

Parasympathetic preganglionic neurons are located in the intermediolateral gray matter in the sacral segments. Sympathetic preganglionic neurons are located in both medial and lateral sites in the intermediate gray matter of the lumbar spinal cord. Pelvic and pudendal afferent pathways project into the sacral spinal cord. The overlap of bladder and urethral afferents indicates the importance of this region in coordinating bladder and urethral sphincter activity. Ascending sensory pathways terminate in different sites, including the periaqueductal gray and the gracile nucleus. Neurons of the periaqueductal gray nucleus relay information to the pontine micturition center and initiate the micturition reflex.

2. Pathways in the Brain

Many areas are involved in control of the urinary tract: the pontine micturition center (Barrington's nucleus), the locus caeruleus, the periaqueductal gray, the hypothalamus, and the medial frontal cortex.

The cerebrocortical areas concerned with innervation of the periurethral striated sphincter are located on the medial aspect of the sensorimotor cortex. Axons that originate from neurons in this region pass through the internal capsule and cerebral peduncles, then continue in the lateral columns of the spinal cord as corticospinal tracts.

C. Organization of Voiding Reflexes

We do not describe here the different storage reflexes, which are not involved in physiological and pathophysiological mechanisms of urethral sphincter–detrusor synergia. Micturition is achieved by activation of the parasympathetic efferent pathways to the detrusor, and by concomitant inhibition of the somatic pathways to the urethral sphincter. Neurons of the inferior colliculus have an essential role in the parasympathetic component. Pontine micturition center neurons are activated by afferent activity arising from tension receptors in the bladder, and modulated by inhibitory and excitatory influences from the diencephalon and cerebral cortex.

The pontine micturition center plays a very important role in micturition. It coordinates the activity of the bladder and external urethral sphincter. Electrical or chemical stimulation of the pontine micturition center of animals determines suppression of urethral sphincter electromyographic (EMG) activity, firing of sacral preganglionic neurons, and detrusor contraction (8–11). Suprapontine organization controlling micturition is less known. The frontal cortex plays an important role, and lesions of this area remove inhibitory control over the hypothalamic area, which normally provides excitatory input to micturition centers in the brain stem. This modulatory effect of hypothalamic centers on the reflex pathways is probably mediated by direct inputs to both the pontine and sacral micturition centers.

Coordination between detrusor contraction and urethral sphincter relaxation is mediated by different reflexes, or neurological loops (12). Loop 2 (corticospinal reflex) allows an adequate temporal duration of detrusor contraction (and sphincter relaxation) to obtain the complete evacuation of intravesical contents. Loop 3 consists of peripheral detrusor afferent axons and their pathways in the spinal cord that terminate by synapsing on pudendal motor neurons that innervate the urethral sphincter. This loop allows inhibition of pudendal motor efferents by impulses from detrusor afferents. Thus, striated sphincter contraction is possible during the filling phase and its relaxation during the emptying phase of micturition. Dysfunction of this loop determines detrusor sphincter dyssynergia. Loop 4A consists of the suprasacral afferent and efferent innervation of pudendal motor neurons to the striated sphincter. Loop 4B consists of afferent fibers from the striated sphincter that synapse on pudendal motor neurons. Pudendal nerve afferents produce excitatory potentials in these motor neurons. Anomalies of suprasacral control result in abnormal responses of pudendal motor neurons to bladder filling and emptying, and may determine detrusor–sphincter dyssynergia.

1. Different Phases of the Voiding Reflex

Initiation of voiding is the first phase. Tanagho and Miller (13) described the progressive drop in urethral pressure that occurs slightly before a corresponding increase in detrusor pressure. Urethral pressure could remain constant, with detrusor contraction eventually exceeding it. This process is accompanied by the bladder outlet assuming a funneled shape. This funneling begins before any modification of detrusor pressure. Intraurethral pressure decreases for 3 sec before the detrusor begins to contract. The drop in urethral pressure is due to relaxation of the striated muscle, which is confirmed by EMG studies (diminution of EMG activity as soon as the premicturition phase starts). Bladder neck opening may be passive, as a result of pelvic floor relaxation. Torrens (14) demonstrated that stimulation of the sacral nerves produces a reduction in urethral pressure that is independent of any afferent activity and bladder contraction. This response is blocked by β-$_2$adrenergic antagonists.

Ghoneim et al. (15) showed that bladder distension produces an additional drop in urethral resistance to flow after striated function has been abolished by succinylcholine. Continuation of voiding is the second phase. It depends on pure automatic activity. The afferent input from tension receptors in the bladder, and the presence of urine in the posterior urethra, control the voiding reflex. Indeed, the passage of urine through the urethra may reinforce and facilitate complete bladder emptying.

Thus, concomitant lowering of resistance of the smooth and striated sphincter, associated with coordinated detrusor contraction, determines complete and easy micturition.

IV. PATHOPHYSIOLOGICAL MECHANISMS

Blaivas et al. (4,5) identified three types of DESD. Type 1 is defined by a concomitant increase in both detrusor pressure and sphincter EMG activity, but at the peak of detrusor contraction, the sphincter suddenly relaxes and unobstructed voiding occurs. Type 2 DESD is characterized by sporadic contractions of the external urethral sphincter throughout detrusor contraction (clonic sphincter contractions). In type 3 DESD, there is a crescendo–decrescendo pattern of sphincter contraction that results in urethral obstruction throughout detrusor contraction (sustained sphincter contraction).

Detrusor–internal sphincter dyssynergia is a failure of the smooth muscle of the bladder neck and proximal urethra to relax during detrusor contraction.

A. Pathophysiological Result of Dyssynergia

Bladder–sphincter dyssynergia may have an indirect effect on spinal reflex pathways and reflex mechanisms. Tonic activity of the urethral sphincter can determine morphological changes in bladder afferent neurons. Anatomical tracing studies in chronic spinal rats have revealed that afferent neurons innervating the bladder are markedly increased in size and associated with sprouting of afferent axons in the bladder to innervate the larger target tissue.

Outlet obstruction induces hypertrophy of bladder afferent and efferent neurons, accompanied by increased levels of nerve growth factor in the bladder as well as expansion of the bladder afferent terminals in the cord and facilitation of the spinal micturition reflex (16). Spinal reflex mechanisms are thus affected by the changes in organ functions that occur following spinal injury (17).

V. CLINICAL FEATURES, ETIOLOGIES, AND COMPLICATIONS

A. Clinical Features

Incoordination between the bladder and urethra during voiding produces a weak stream or urinary retention. Urinary flow can be low during the entire voiding (*tonic dyssynergia*) or can be irregularly interrupted by perineal muscle spasms (*clonic dyssynergia*). The symptoms are often variable, and can be influenced by general fatigue, subject position, bladder repletion, concomitant anorectal dysfunction, urinary tract infection, urinary lithiasis, orthopedic complications and, generally, by any factor inducing increased spasticity.

B. Etiologies

The main cause of detrusor–sphincter dyssynergia is a CNS lesion located between the brain stem micturition center and the sacral spinal cord. It may be confused with a failure of urethral relaxation owing to local urethral causes, such as inflammation or edema, or to psychogenic causes.

DESD is one of the major urodynamic arguments for a neurogenic bladder, and its presence demonstrates an upper motor neuron lesion. However, persistence of the bulbocavernosus reflex during voiding is a more sensitive, although slightly less specific, sign of upper motor neuron bladder dysfunction than detrusor–sphincter dyssynergia (18).

1. Neurological Lesions

DESD is seen in 70–100% of patients with suprasacral cord lesions following spinal cord injury (19). Autonomic dysreflexia is often associated with DESD, and a high correlation exists between the magnitude of the blood pressure response, the level of injury, and the severity of detrusor–sphincter dyssynergia (20). Other nontraumatic spinal cord injuries, such as cervical myelopathy, may elicit DESD (21).

In rare cases, DESD can be observed without spinal cord diseases. Although normal coordinated micturition (spincteric relaxation followed by detrusor contraction) is essentially dependent on no interruption of the neurological connection between the brain stem and sacral spinal cord, an intact brain stem is probably also necessary. Thus, in acute hemispheric stroke, detrusor–sphincter dyssynergia is not infrequent (noted in 14%), and uninhibited spincter relaxation occurs in 36% of patients (22).

DESD is also very frequent in multiple sclerosis (28–82%) (23). However, in different studies, in comparison with spinal cord injury, few multiple sclerosis patients with detrusor–sphincter dyssynergia had such complications as hydronephrosis or elevated creatine levels (24).

2. Nonneurological Lesions

Clinical manifestations of detrusor–sphincter dyssynergia can be revealed in patients without neurological disease. The symptoms are long voiding duration, hesitancy, intermittent stream, straining to void, recurrent cystitis, enuresis, frequent voiding, pain during voiding, and anal discomfort. Vesicoureteral reflux can be observed. The etiology of detrusor–sphincter dyssynergia in these nonneurological patients should be discussed. Highly frequent, intermittent spasms of the urethra during voiding represent a persistent transitional phase in development of the cerebral control of voiding (25). A search for psychogenic causes and a history of sexual abuse or rigid education may be needed. In these cases, failure of relaxation of the external (striated muscle) urethral sphincter during detrusor contraction results in a micturitional disorder, and perineal EMG demonstrates no evidence of denervation with increased activity during attempts to void.

One of the major problems is the necessity of tracking down a neurological disease when these sorts of symptoms are observed. A history of complaints, physical examination (without pyramidal signs), urodynamic data (absence of phasic contraction, preserved bladder sensation), and the normality of electrophysiological testing (EMG examination of the perineal muscles, the normality of sacral reflex latency, and cortical-evoked responses following pudendal nerve stimulation) are strong arguments against a neurological origin.

When doubt persists, other investigations (brain stem MRI; spinal cord MRI; auditory-, visual- and somesthesic-evoked potentials; cerebrospinal fluid analysis, and such) are necessary to definitely rule out a neurological cause.

Psychometric testing, or even psychiatric consultation, may be helpful in pinpointing psychogenic conditions before beginning a specific psychological treatment.

3. DESD Complications

The association of autonomic dysreflexia and DESD is frequent. DESD is an important risk factor for upper tract deterioration in patients with chronic spinal cord injury (26). Pyelonephritis, hydronephrosis, and renal failure are the main complications. The necessity of treating DESD can induce iatrogenic complications: orthostatic hypotension with α-adrenergic blockers, urethral stenosis with intermittent self-catheterization, urinary incontinence, and retrograde ejaculation with sphincterotomy.

VI. EVALUATION OF DESD

The classic test to recognize DESD is combined cystometry and external sphincter EMG. Meanwhile, DESD can be suggested when flowmetry is possible to investigate interrupted urine flow and residual volume.

Cystometry may be recorded by rectal pressure measurement to analyze abdominal pressure simultaneously with bladder pressure to eliminate artifacts caused by abdominal muscle contraction. Indeed, the diagnosis of DESD requires detrusor contraction. However, many patients are unable to initiate such a contraction, particularly in pronounced DESD.

Furthermore, in moderate DESD, some patients will strain to try to urinate, which causes a simultaneous increase in sphincter activity and bladder and rectal pressure. "Pseudodyssynergia" can be observed in patients with hyperreflexia secondary to a brain stem lesion, and in those who try to inhibit bladder contractions with voluntary contractions of the external sphincter.

Sphincter dyssynergia is diagnosed by increased EMG activity during an involuntary detrusor contraction. Unlike neurologically intact patients, there is no prevoiding decrease in urethral pressure, and external sphincter contraction occurs simultaneously with or immediately after the onset of a detrusor contraction. The dyssynergia can be quantified with a specific EMG technique, such as power spectrum analysis with fast Fourier transformation of the external urethral sphincter (27). DESD is further suggested by high voiding pressure and persistently elevated maximal urethral pressure.

Smooth-sphincter dyssynergia is more difficult to confirm. Videoimaging techniques allow the diagnosis of bladder neck dyssynergia. Fluoroscopic imaging during an involuntary contraction objectifies persistent narrowing of the external sphincter or of the bladder neck.

When micturition is possible, combined uroflow and sphincter EMG (eventually with a single rectal pressure recording) allow DESD screening. This investigation is particularly interesting in evaluating children. Abdominal wall EMG can be used in substitution of rectal pressure recording to eliminate strain pseudodyssynergia.

In fact, a very common and important question is whether dyssynergia can be diagnosed in the absence of a bladder contraction. Despite failure to arrive at a true definition, we can consider that DESD is the sole mechanism of urinary retention in patients with spinal cord injury who have an overactive bladder without cervicourethral organic obstruction (urethral stenosis, prostatic hypertrophy). However, recognition of DESD is not the main problem in management of the neurogenic bladder. The real challenge is not to prove DESD absolutely with urodynamic tests, but to evaluate its consequences, especially high detrusor pressure during storage or micturition, which can determine bladder or renal complications. Urodynamic investigation allows the study of detrusor compliance and the bladder response to anticholinergic treatment. Clinical (micturition chart) or echographic evaluation quantifies residual volume, the source of urinary tract infections and possible renal complications.

For Geirsson and Fall (28), a simple ice water test can replace EMG to prove DESD. This test involves rapid intravesical infusion of 100 mL of sterile ice water during continuous pressure measurement with recording of fluid leakage. In a typical positive test, fluid leaks around the catheter during the peak of detrusor contraction elicited by cold stimulation. A nonleaking positive ice water test with high detrusor pressure may indicate DESD.

REFERENCES

1. Denny–Brown D, Robertson E. On the physiology of micturition. Brain 1933; 56:149–190.
2. Anderson JT, Bradley WE. The syndrome of detrusor–sphincter dyssynergia. J Urol 1976; 116: 493–495.
3. Yalla SV, Blunt KJ, Fam BA, Constantinople NL, Gittes RF. Detrusor–urethral sphincter dyssynergia. J Urol 1977; 118:1026–1029.
4. Blaivas JG, Sinha HP, Zayed AA, Labib KB. Detrusor–external sphincter dyssynergia. J Urol 1981; 125:542–544.
5. Blaivas JG, Sinha HP, Zayed AA, Labib KB. Detrusor–external sphincter dyssynergia: a detailed electromyographic study. J Urol 1981; 125:545–548.
6. Siroky MB, Krane RJ. Neurologic aspects of detrusor–sphincter dyssynergia, with reference to the guarding reflex. J Urol 1982; 127:953–957.
7. Rudy DC, Awad SA, Downie JW. External sphincter dyssynergia: an abnormal continence reflex. J Urol 1988; 140:105–110.
8. de Groat W, Boorth A, Yoshimura N. Neurophysiology of micturition and its modifications in animal models of human disease. In: Maggi CA, ed. The Autonomic Nervous System. Vol. 3. Nervous Control of the Urogenital System. London: Harwood Academic, 1993:227–290.
9. Torrens M, Morrison JFB. The Physiology of the Lower Urinary Tract. Berlin: Springer-Verlag, 1987.
10. Mallory BS, Roppolo JR, de Groat WC. Pharmacological modulation of the pontine micturition center. Brain Res 1991; 546:310–320.
11. Noto H, Roppolo JR, Steers WD, de Groat WC. Electrophysiological analysis of the ascending and descending components of the micturition reflex pathways in the rat. Brain Res 1991; 549: 95–105.
12. Hald T, Bradley W. The Urinary Bladder: Neurology and Dynamics. Baltimore: Williams & Wilkins, 1982:5–36.
13. Tanagho EA, Miller ER. The initiation of voiding. Br J Urol 1970; 42:175–183.
14. Torrens MJ. Urethral sphincteric responses to stimulation of the sacral nerves in the human female. Urol Int 1978; 33:22–26.
15. Ghoneim MA, Fretin JA, Gagnon DJ, Susset JG. The influence of vesical distension on urethral resistance to flow: The expulsion phase. Br J Urol 1975; 47:663–670.
16. Steers WD, Ciambotti J, Etzel B, Erdman S, de Groat WC. Alterations in afferent pathways from the urinary bladder of the rat in response to partial urethral obstruction. J Comp Neurol 1991; 310:401–410.
17. de Groat WC. A neurological basis for the overactive bladder. Urology 1997; 50(suppl. 6A): 36–53.
18. Sethi RK, Bauer SB, Dyro FM, Krarup C. Modulation of the bulbocavernosus reflex during voiding: loss of inhibition in upper motor neuron lesions. Muscle Nerve 1989; 12:892–897.
19. Thomas DG, Smallwood R, Graham D. Urodynamic observations following spinal trauma. Br J Urol 1975; 47:161–175.

20. Perkash I. Autonomic dysreflexia and detrusor–sphincter dyssynergia in spinal cord injury patients. J Spinal Cord Med 1997; 20:365–370.

21. Sakakibara R, Hattori T, Tojo M, Yamanishi T, Yasuda K, Hirayama K. The location of the paths subserving micturition: studies in patients with cervical myelopathy. J Auton Nerv Syst 1995; 55:165–168.

22. Sakakibara R, Hattori T, Yasuda K, Yamanishi T. Micturitional disturbance after acute hemispheric stroke: analysis of the lesion site by CT and NMI. J Neurol Sci 1996; 137:47–56.

23. Amarenco G, Kerdraon J, Denys P. Bladder and sphincter disorders in multiple sclerosis. Clinical, urodynamic and neurophysiological study of 225 cases. Rev Neurol (Paris) 1995; 51:722–730.

24. Sirls LT, Zimmerm PE, Leach GE. Role of limited evaluation and aggressive medical management in multiple sclerosis: a review of 113 patients. J Urol 1994; 151:946–950.

25. Jorgensen TM, Djurhuus JC, Schroder HD. Idiopathic detrusor sphincter dyssynergia in neurologically normal patients with voiding abnormalities. Eur Urol 1982; 8:107–110.

26. Geffidzen RG, Thijssen AM, Dehoux E. Risk factors for upper tract deterioration in chronic spinal cord injury patients. J Urol 1992; 147:416–418.

27. Mizuo T, Suzuki M, Oya K, Kura N, Terao T. Electromyographic study on the external urethral sphincter of male-power spectrum analysis with fast Fourier transformation. Nippon Hinyokika Gakkai Zasshi 1994; 85:632–641.

28. Geirsson G, Fall M. The ice-water test in the diagnosis of detrosor–external sphincter dyssynergia. Scand J Urol Nephrol 1995; 29:457–461.

15

Prolapse and Urethral Sphincteric Dysfunction

SERGE PETER MARINKOVIC, KAVEN BAESSLER,
and STUART L. STANTON

St. George's Hospital Medical School, London, England

Massive vaginal eversion is clearly associated with gross distortion of normal pelvic anatomy, and I believe that this also is often associated with damage to the bladder neck which may produce refractory stress incontinence.

L. Lewis Wall, M.D.

I. INTRODUCTION

In the third millennium there will be 20 million women between the ages of 45 and 65 and another 23 million older than 65 years of age in the United States (1). This alarming number and the cost of these 43 million patients requiring the diagnosis and treatment of genital prolapse (Fig. 1) or urinary incontinence in their lifetime will be staggering. We are experiencing an increase in genital prolapse particularly posthysterectomy vaginal vault prolapse, but most commonly seen are cystourethrocele, uterine descent, and rectocele (2). These patients may present with a protruding vaginal mass, and up to 25% may complain of urinary incontinence, usually stress urinary incontinence (2). Patients may also recognize that as the pelvic prolapse worsens their urinary incontinence becomes less noticeable (2). This cause and effect may be attributable to urethral kinking or urethral compression enhancing the urethral sphincteric continence mechanism (2). There is now a consensus opinion among urogynecologists, gynecologists, and urologists that these two conditions—prolapse and urinary incontinence—often occur concomitantly, so that relaxation of the anterior vaginal wall may lead to urethrovesical hypermobility and genuine stress incontinence (2–4). However, with pelvic relaxation being a global phenomenon, a coexisting cystocele, rectocele, enterocele, uterine descent, or vaginal vault prolapse may be present

231

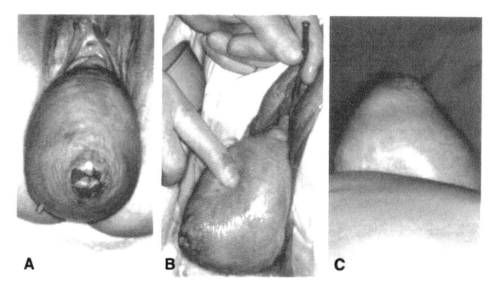

Figure 1 Complete procidentia: (A) sagittale view; (B) lateral view; (C) superior view.

and symptomatic (1–4). It has also been advocated not to treat the three pelvic compartment prolapses in isolation, but to address all defects simultaneously, under ideal circumstances, and under one anesthetic (2,5). The role that each of these three pelvic compartments' prolapse has on urinary sphincteric dysfunction is similar, and its pathophysiology will be the focus of our discussion.

II. GENITAL PROLAPSE: DEFINITION, CLASSIFICATION, AND INCIDENCE

Genital prolapse is the protrusion of a pelvic organ beyond its normal anatomical confines within the vagina. This represents the failure of the fibromuscular supports of the pelvis to maintain normal position (6). The three pelvic compartments are 1) anterior—pertaining to urethral descent (urethrocele) or bladder descent (cystocele); 2) middle—pertaining to uterine descent, vaginal vault descent, or enterocele; 3) posterior—pertaining to the rectum (rectocele). Staging or grading of genital prolapse is not absolute, a multitude of classifications systems abound from the simple to the complex. A commonly used system is to classify prolapse as first degree—descent within the vagina; second degree—descent to the introitus; and third degree—descent beyond the introitus. But this system is too simple and arbitrary and may lack intraobserver accuracy for scientific comparisons.

In 1994, the International Continence Society Committee for Standardization of Terminology adopted a more comprehensive and complex method hoping to improve intra- or interobserver comparisons for genital prolapse (7). With this system the hymen is the reference point for all measurements (in centimeters) of the anterior and posterior vaginal walls. Also included are the length of the genital hiatus, width of the perineal body, and total vaginal length. These nine measurements are formatted onto a three-by-three grid board (8)

anterior wall	anterior wall	cervix or cuff
Aa	Ba	C
genital hiatus	perineal body	total vaginal length
gh	pb	tvl
posterior wall	posterior wall	posterior fornix
Ap	Bp	D

Figure 2 Three-by-three grid for recording quantitative description of pelvic support. (From Ref. 7.)

(Figs. 2 and 3). Once these measurements are recorded, it is possible to grade the severity and extent of the genital prolapse on a scale of 0–4 (Fig. 4). Its is also critically important to relate the conditions of the physical examination (i.e., position of the patient, and position of prolapse with a Valsalva maneuver).

The incidence of genital prolapse is difficult to accurately assess because mild degrees of prolapse may be asymptomatic (6). However, estimates of prolapse have been made and vary with parity, age, and race (6). Fifty percent of parous women may demonstrate some degree of prolapse, but only 10–20% of these patients report symptoms severe enough to warrant further gynecological investigation (9). Symptomatic prolapse is rare in nulliparous women and comprises less than 2% of prolapse patients (10). The incidence of prolapse increases with age (11). Symmonds et al. reviewed 190 women with severe vaginal prolapse, and over 60% of the study population were older than 60 years of age (11). The incidence of genital prolapse is most common among white races 5.4–11% (10,12), and least common amongst African–Americans and Orientals 0.6–2% (10,13). About 50% of women with genuine stress incontinence have significant prolapse of the anterior vaginal wall (14).

A. Cystourethrocele and Cystocele

Anterior vaginal wall prolapse may present with stress incontinence, particularly if there is hypermobility of the urethrovesical junction or a history of prior anti-incontinence procedures. Anti-incontinence procedures may lead to periurethral and bladder neck scarring, thereby, reducing maximum urethral closure pressures. A reduced maximum urethral closure pressure of 20 cmH$_2$O or less may then be evident when urodynamic studies are performed (15). A large cystocele may cause urethral kinking and overflow incontinence (2). This voiding symptom can be addressed by manually reducing the cystocele or placing a

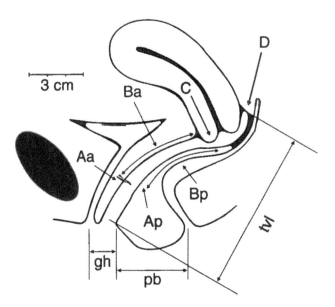

Figure 3 Six sites (points Aa, Ba, C, D, Bp, Ap), genital hiatus (gh), perineal body (pb), and total vaginal length (tvl) used for pelvic organ support quantitation. (From Ref. 7.)

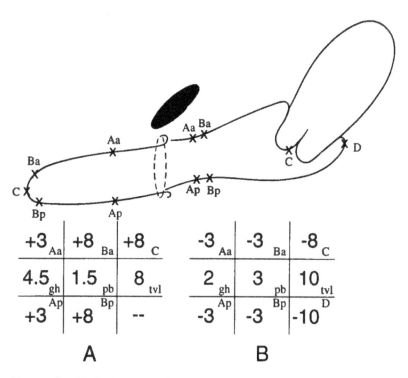

Figure 4 (A) Grid and line diagram of complete vaginal eversion stage; (B) normal support stage O. (From Ref. 7.)

pessary. Determining postvoid residuals with portable ultrasound scanners can identify these patients.

B. Uterine Descent

Uterine descent can cause lower back and sacral discomfort by placing tension on the uterosacral ligaments and accompanying nerves. This discomfort is usually relieved by a ring pessary to support the prolapse or by lying down. Occasionally, there are symptoms of bladder outlet obstruction or urinary retention secondary to uterine descent (16).

C. Enterocele or Vault Prolapse

These may present with only vague symptoms of vaginal discomfort. However, because enteroceles usually occur with other types of prolapse it becomes difficult to discern which symptoms are related. Dehiscence of the vaginal vault presents with acute pain and small bowel may be seen at the vulva, which may then strangulate and become an acute surgical emergency (2).

D. Rectocele

A rectocele can lead to incomplete evacuation of stool from the rectum. Digital reduction may be necessary to help evacuate stool. Patients can also complain of backache or left lower quadrant abdominal pain if constipated. Sometimes a large rectocele or enterocele may mask potential stress urinary incontinence. After reparative surgery, these patients may then complain of stress incontinence.

III. HISTORY AND PHYSICAL EXAMINATION

A thorough history and physical examination is the most valuable tool to assess prolapse and urinary complaints. The history is focused on the type of symptoms, and whether stress incontinence, urgency, urge incontinence, and nocturia are present. Detailed assessment is made on the duration of symptoms and what conditions make the symptoms better or worse. Has the patient received prior medical therapy (oxybutynin, phentolamine) or had surgical therapy (prior anti-incontinence or prolapse surgery)? A careful review of the patient's medication list and over-the-counter medications can provide useful information. α-Adrenergic blockers for hypertension can decrease maximum urethral closure pressure so that stress incontinence may become evident. Sometimes changing the type of antihypertensive (ACE inhibitor or β-adrenergic blocker) medication can resolve this symptom. Constipation is a common complaint and may stimulate bladder μ-receptors leading to bladder hypocontractility while also directly reducing bladder capacity.

The patient is examined in the supine position. The abdominal examination determines if there is a distended bladder, abdominal mass, or painful areas to palpation. The patient is asked to Valsalva to discern whether sphincteric incompetence is present. If with straining or coughing there is a momentary pause before leakage, cough-induced detrusor instability may be present. A complete neurological examination of both sensory and motor function of the lower extremities and perineum should be performed (17). A bulbocavernosal reflex and digital rectal examination help determine function of the S2–S4 sacral nerve arc. The patient is then repositioned to either a lithotomy or left lateral recumbent position. Using a Sims' speculum the posterior vaginal wall is retracted to expose the anterior vaginal wall. The patient is asked to strain or Valsalva to demonstrate a cystourethrocele or cystocele and whether stress incontinence is present. Retracting the bladder neck with the Sims' speculum can determine if the bladder neck is mobile and whether a Burch colposuspension could be used. The posterior vaginal wall is then retracted while the patient is asked to strain or bear down, with a hand placed firmly over her perineum to support it, the presence of a rectocele, enterocele, uterine descent, or vault prolapse is noted. The degree of uterine prolapse is gauged by placing a tenaculum on the lower lip of the cervical os and applying gentle traction. A concomitant digital rectal examination while retracting the anterior vaginal wall may aid in evaluating the grade of rectocele and enterocele. The examination is completed by performing a bimanual pelvic examination to assess the presence and size of the uterus and adnexa. Measurements of the anterior/posterior vaginal wall prolapse are recorded in accordance with the International Continence Society recommendations (7).

A. Diagnostic Testing

Diagnostic testing includes a urine culture and sensitivity, urine cytology, if urgency is evident, a voiding diary, uroflow, multichannel cystometry with or without video, and radiological scanning. Perineal ultrasonography or dynamic pelvic floor fluoroscopy (18) will image the three compartments. Dynamic magnetic resonance imaging (MRI) can image the pelvic floor and provide excellent tissue visualization, but its application to pelvic floor prolapse remains to be evaluated (19–21).

1. Anterior Compartment

Mild or moderate genital prolapse with a grade 1 cystourethrocele or cystocele can often be associated with stress urinary incontinence. However, in striking contrast, women with advanced anterior compartment prolapse (grade 2 or 3) often do not complain of stress incontinence (22). The continence mechanism may be related to an artificial enhancement of the urethral sphincter through urethral kinking or urethral compression (23). Once relieved and the cystourethrocele or cystocele is returned to its normal resting position by a vaginal pessary, a urethral pressure or abdominal pressure transmission ratio of urethra/bladder less than 1 may become evident (22). Occult stress urinary incontinence (stress urinary incontinence associated with genital prolapse) may then become evident because of this pressure dissipation. The pubocervical fascia (endopelvic fascia) attaches to the arcus tendineus fascia pelvis and helps these components of the anterior vaginal wall from a "hammock" for support of the bladder and bladder neck (24,25). Deficiencies in this pelvic support may lead to a cystourethrocele (Fig. 5) or cystocele. Poor abdominal pressure transmission to the urethra with this poor support during sudden increases in intra-abdominal pressure, is believed to be a contributing factor in the genesis of occult stress incontinence (26).

A grade 2 or grade 3 cystocele may cause urethral kinking, urethral compression, pressure dissipation, and bladder outlet obstruction while enhancing maximum urethral closure pressure (22,27,28) (Fig. 6A). However, once the cystocele is reduced to its normal position with a pessary (22,27) or vaginal packing (28) the maximum urethral pressure may be significantly reduced and stress incontinence may become evident. Bergman et al. (22) performed multichannel urodynamics and urethral pressure profiles at rest and with straining in 67 patients with grade 3 cystoceles before and after reduction with a Smith–Hodge pessary. Of the 67 patients, 24 (36%) had an abdominal pressure transmission ratio of urethra/bladder less than 1. Seventeen of these 24 patients demonstrated stress incontinence

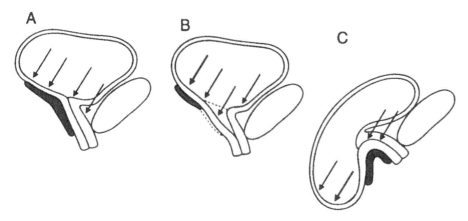

Figure 5 (A) Diagram showing abdominal pressure closing the urethra against the underlying urethral supports; (B) in this diagram the supporting tissues are unstable and do not form a firm layer against which the urethra can be compressed; (C) a cystourethrocele in which the urethra is much lower than normal but has a strong supportive layer that allows urethral compression. (From Ref. 25.)

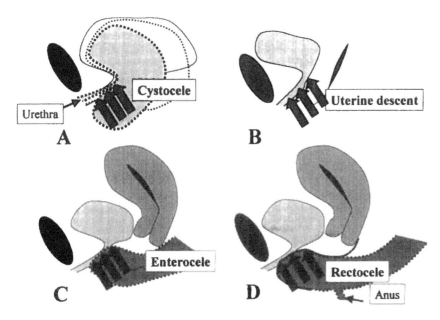

Figure 6 (A) Cystocele; (B) uterine descent; (C) enterocele; (D) rectocele. All causing urethral compression or kinking. This enchances the urethral sphincteric continence mechanism. Reduction of the prolapse during urodynamics minimizes this artifact.

with reduction of the prolapse, and all 24 underwent a modified Pereyra procedure in addition to an anterior repair. After 3–6 months follow-up all 24 patients were continent. Urethral pressure profiles showed all patients with good abdominal pressure transmission on coughing. The remaining 43 patients underwent cystocele repair without bladder back suspension and all were continent. Versi et al. (27), Ghoniem (28), and Romanzi et al. (29) used videourodynamics or urethral pressure profiles to assess patients with grade 2 or grade 3 cystoceles. With pessary reduction, 25–69% of patients demonstrated occult genuine stress incontinence, with 40–50% of these patients demonstrating intrinsic sphincter deficiency by Valsalva leak point pressures or maximum urethral closure pressure of less than 20 cm H_2O. Additionally, Romanzi et al. (29) found that patients with grade 2 or 3 cystoceles have a 52% incidence of detrusor instability (DI), whereas those with grade 1 cystoceles had a 20% incidence. Videourodynamic assessment is expensive, labor intensive, and may be indicated only in patients with multiple prior surgeries for prolapse or incontinence. Whether videourodynamics is necessary to evaluate a pessary possibly producing bladder outlet obstruction during urodynamic assessment is still uncertain. However, these studies do emphasize the importance of urodynamic assessment with prolapse reduction to properly ascertain occult stress incontinence and DI.

2. Middle Compartment

Reduction of uterine or vaginal vault prolapse is associated with a reduction in pressure transmission ratios (30) (PTR < 1) and a significant decrease in maximum urethral closure pressures (23,30,31). The reasons for continence before pessary or barrier placement, or surgical correction, are the same as for cystoceles, namely urethral kinking and compression enhancing the urethral sphincteric mechanism (see Fig. 6B and C). Bump et al. (30) evaluated 11 continent women with grade 3 vaginal vault or uterine descent and found 8 out of 11 women with a PTR less than 0.90 of normal. Their maximum urethral closure pressure significantly declined with a barrier in place from 75 to 45 cmH_2O (p = 0.03). Wall and Hewitt (32) assessed 19 patients with posthysterectomy vaginal vault prolapse using pressure–flow studies before surgical correction. They found their patients had obstructive voiding dynamics characterized by a mean peak flow rate of 11 mL/sec and a detrusor pressure at peak flow of 50 cmH_2O. Forty-seven percent demonstrated occult stress incontinence with barrier placement. Voiding complaints included urgency (79%) and urge incontinence (63%), whereas urodynamically confirmed DI was present in only 16%. Some patients (5–15%) can have urethral sphincteric incompetence following correction of vault prolapse (i.e., sacrocolpopexy or sacrospinous fixation).

3. Posterior Compartment

Myers et al. (33) evaluated 90 patients urodynamically with isolated posterior compartment prolapse. Only patients with reduced grade 3 posterior wall defects had significant decreases in maximum urethral closure pressure, functional urethral length, and increases in leakage volume with a Valsalva maneuver. The largest individual change in maximum urethral closure pressure with a posterior defect retracted was 15 cmH_2O. This may become clinically significant in patients with a maximum urethral closure pressure between 25 and 35 cmH_2O. These patients after barrier reduction may reveal a maximum urethral closure pressure less than 20 cmH_2O or urethral sphincteric deficiency. As with anterior and middle compartment prolapse, a third-degree posterior compartment prolapse may also cause bladder outlet obstruction by urethral compression (see Fig. 6D).

IV. CONCLUSION

Advanced genital prolapse may have a significant clinical effect on urethral sphincteric function. Before prolapse surgery, we should perform a detailed history and physical examination, with urodynamic studies with the prolapse present and reduced. All clinically significant prolapse should be corrected under one anesthetic. Correction of genital prolapse may lead to another prolapse or to urethral sphincter incontinence.

REFERENCES

1. Shull BL. Pelvic organ prolapse: anterior, superior and posterior vaginal segment defects. Am J Obstet Gynecol 1999; 181:6–11.
2. Grody MHT. Urinary incontinence and concomitant prolapse. Clin Obstet Gynecol 1998; 41: 777–785.
3. Jackson SL, Weber AM, Hull TL, Mitchinson AR, Walters NO. Faecal incontinence in women with urinary incontinence and pelvic organ prolapse. Obstet Gynecol 1997; 89:423–427.
4. Seim A, Eriksen BC, Hunskaar S. A study of female urinary incontinence in general practice. Demography, medical history and clinical findings. Scand J Urol Nephrol 1996; 30:465–471.
5. Nichols DH. Surgery for pelvic floor disorders. Surg Clin North Am 1991; 71:927–946.
6. Harris TA, Bent AE. Genital prolapse with and without urinary incontinence. J Reprod Med 1990; 35:792–798.
7. Hall AF, Theofrastous JP, Cundiff GW, Harris RL, Hamilton LF, Swift SE, Bump RC. Interobserver and intraobserver reliability of the proposed International Continence Society, Society of Gynecologic Surgeons, and American Urogynecologic Society pelvic organ prolapse classification system. Am J Obstet Gynecol 1996; 175:1467–1471.
8. Bump RC, Mattiasson A, Bo K, Brubaker LP, Delancey JO, Klarskov P, Shull BL, Smith AR. The standardization of terminology of female pelvic organ prolapse and pelvic floor dysfunction. Am J Obstet Gynecol 1996; 175:10–17.
9. Beck RP. Pelvic relaxational prolapse. In: Kase NG, Weingold AB, eds. Principles and Practice of Clinical Gynecology. New York: John Wiley & Sons, 1983:677–685.
10. Nichols DH, Randall CL. Types of prolapse. In: Nichols DH, Randall CL, eds. Vaginal Surgery. Baltimore: Williams & Wilkins, 1996:107–109.
11. Symmonds BRE, Williams TJ, Lee RA, Webb MJ. Post hysterectomy enterocele and vaginal prolapse. Am J Obstet Gynecol 1981; 140:852–859.
12. Olsen AL, Smith VJ, Bergstrom JO, Colling JC, Clark AL. Epidemiology of surgically managed pelvic organ prolapse and urinary incontinence. Obstet Gynecol 1997; 89:501–506.
13. Heynes OS. Genital prolapse. In: Charlewood GP, ed. Bantu Gynecology. Johannesburg: Witwatersrand University Press, 1956:41–52.
14. Jackson S, Smith P. Fortnightly review: diagnosing and managing genitourinary prolapse. Br Med J 1997; 314:875–880.
15. Stanton SL. Vaginal prolapse. In: Shaw RW, Souter WP, Stanton SL, eds. Gynaecology. New York: Churchill Livingstone, 1997:759–769.
16. Carr LK, Webster GD. Bladder outlet obstruction in women. Urol Clin North Am 1996; 23:385–391.
17. Lind LR, Rosenzweig BA, Bhatia NN. Urologically oriented neurological examination. In: Ostergard DR, Bent AE, eds. Urogynecology and Urodynamics. Theory and Practice. Baltimore: Williams & Wilkins, 1996:101–102.
18. Altringer WE, Saclarides TJ, Dominguez JM, Brubaker LT, Smith CS. Four-contrast defecography:pelvic floor-oscopy. Dis Colon Rectum 1995; 38:695–699.
19. Yang A, Mostwin JL, Rosenshein NB, Zerhouni EA. Pelvic floor descent in women: dynamic evaluation with fast MR imaging and cinematic display. Radiology 1991; 179:25–33.
20. Gufler H, Laubenberger J, DeGregorio G, Dohnicht S, Langer M. Pelvic floor descent: dynamic MIR imaging using a half-Fourier RARE sequence. J Magn Reson Imaging 1999; 9:378–383.
21. Fielding JR, Versi E, Mulkem RV, Lerner MH, Griffiths DJ, Jolesz FA. MR imaging of the female pelvic floor in the supine and upright positions. J Magn Reson Imaging 1996; 6:961–963.
22. Bergman A, Koonings PR, Ballard CA. Predicting postoperative urinary incontinence development in women undergoing operation for genitouninary prolapse. Am J Obstet Gynecol 1988; 158:1171–1175.

23. Richardson DA, Bent AE, Ostergard DR. The effect of uterovaginal prolapse on urethrovesical pressure dynamics. Am J Obstet Gynecol 1983; 146:901–905.

24. DeLancey JO. Structural support of the urethra as it relates to stress urinary incontinence: the hammock hypothesis. Am J Obstet Gynecol 1994; 170:1713–1723.

25. DeLancey JO. The pathophysiology of stress urinary incontinence in women and its implications for surgical treatment. World J Urol 1997; 15:268–274.

26. Enhoming GE. Simultaneous recording of intravesical and intraurethral pressure. A study of urethral closure in normal and stress incontinent women. Acta Clin Scand Suppl 1961; 276: 1–68.

27. Versi E, Lyell DJ, Griffiths DJ. Videourodynamic diagnosis of occult genuine stress incontinence in patients with anterior vaginal wall relaxation. J Soc Gynecol Invest 1998; 5:327–330.

28. Ghoniem GM, Walters F, Lewis V. The value of the vaginal pack test in large cystoceles. J Urol 1994; 152:931–934.

29. Romanzi LJ, Chaikin DC, Blaivas JG. The effect of genital prolapse on voiding. J Urol 1999; 161:581–586.

30. Bump RC, Fantl A, Hurt WG. The mechanism of urinary continence in women with severe uterovaginal prolapse: results of barrier studies. Obstet Gynecol 1988; 72:291–295.

31. Veronikis DK, Nichols DH, Wakamatsu MM. The incidence of low pressure urethra as a function of prolapse reducing technique in patients with massive pelvic organ prolapse (massive descent at all vaginal sites). Am J Obstet Gynecol 1997; 177:1305–1314.

32. Wall LL, Hewitt JK. Urodynamic characteristics of women with complete posthysterectomy vaginal vault prolapse. Urology 1994; 44:336–342.

33. Myers DL, Lasala CA, Hogan JW, Rosenblatt PL. The effect of posterior wall support defects on urodynamics indices in stress urinary incontinence. Obstet Gynecol 1998; 91:710–714.

16

Clinical History

LINE LEBOEUF and ERIK SCHICK

University of Montreal and Maisonneuve–Rosemont Hospital, Montreal, Quebec, Canada

I. GENERAL CONSIDERATIONS

Medical training places great emphasis on the diagnostic value of careful symptom assessment. Such an evaluation forms a major part of any clinical consultation. However, on the whole, most contemporary reports claim few and weak relations between the presence of lower urinary tract symptoms (LUTS) and clinical measures such as urodynamics. Multiple studies have shown that bladder is an unreliable witness; urinary symptoms alone inaccurately reflect the cause of urinary tract dysfunction (1–4). For example, Jarvis et al. (4) compared the results of clinical and urodynamic diagnosis for 100 women presenting with LUTS. There was agreement between subjective and objective data in 68% of the cases of genuine stress incontinence, but only in 51% of cases of detrusor instability. Patients whose symptoms suggest pure stress incontinence will, on the urodynamic study, demonstrate detrusor instability 11–16% of the time (5,6), whereas up to 22% of women with filling symptoms will actually have pure genuine stress incontinence (4). We analyzed the relation between clinical symptoms and urodynamic data in a group of 267 women presenting in a urological clinic with LUTS. Of these 267 patients, 62 (23%) had pure genuine stress incontinence, and 45 had (17%) symptoms of urgency or of urge incontinence on a questionnaire, without a history of stress urinary incontinence (SUI). On subsequent multichannel urodynamic evaluation, among the 62 patients with genuine stress incontinence, 47 (76%) had stable bladders, and 15 (24%) had unstable bladder contractions during the filling phase of the study. In the group of 45 patients with symptoms suggesting bladder instability, but no SUI, only 29 (64%) had urodynamically proved unstable detrusor, and 16 (36%) showed stable bladder (Table 1). In spite of a "typical" history of detrusor instability, in one-third of the patients, no uninhibited contractions could be demonstrated.

Table 1   Incidence of SUI[a] in Urodynamically Stable and Unstable Women

	Urodynamically stable	Urodynamically unstable
Clinically stable (SUI without urge/urge incontinence)	47/62 (76%)	15/62 (24%)
Clinically unstable (Urge/urge incontinence without SUI)	16/45 (36%)	29/45 (64%)

[a]SUI, stress urinary incontinence.

Lagro–Jansson et al. (6) showed that symptoms of stress incontinence, in the absence of symptoms of urge incontinence, had a sensitivity of 78%, specificity of 84%, and a positive-predictive value of 87%. Bergman and Bader (7) evaluated 122 incontinence patients and found that a detailed urinary symptom questionnaire had a positive-predictive value of 80% for genuine stress incontinence, and only 25% for detrusor instability. A few studies have demonstrated that when stress incontinence is the only symptom reported, then genuine stress incontinence is likely to be present in over 90% of cases (8,9). Unfortunately, few patients present with symptoms of stress incontinence alone (10). Symptom complexes have also been used in an attempt to improve diagnostic accuracy, reaching 96% in some conditions (8). In an effort to eliminate the need for urodynamic studies, we retrospectively analyzed a standardized questionnaire and the corresponding multichannel urodynamic studies of 406 women. We found that if a patient has a clinical history of increased voiding frequency, urgency or of urge incontinence, and urgency provoked by the sound of the running water, this patient has a 70% chance of having an unstable bladder on urodynamic study. In other words, the positive-predictive value of this symptom triad is 70%. This can be further improved if, during cystourethroscopy, the bladder wall showed significant (grade ≥ 2) trabeculation. Under these circumstances, the positive-predictive value for detrusor instability increased to 80% (Figs. 1 and 2). This, in several clinical situations, seems to be acceptable level of certitude to initiate noninvasive or not too expensive, mainly pharmacological, treatment.

In recent years, lower urinary tract questionnaires have been developed, some focusing on men with LUTS secondary to benign prostatic hyperplasia (11–13), and others on LUTS in women (14–16). These questionnaires provide a method of measuring symptom

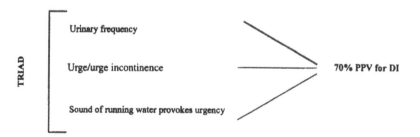

Figure 1   Triad of clinical symptoms suggesting unstable bladder behavior. PPV, positive predictive value; DI, detrusor instability.

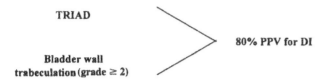

TRIAD

80% PPV for DI

Bladder wall
trabeculation (grade ≥ 2)

Figure 2 Combination of subjective symptoms (see Fig. 1) and cystoscopic findings in predicting unstable bladder. PPV, positive predictive value; DI, detrusor instability.

severity and life quality in a reproducible and valid fashion, as well as allowing an in-depth assessment of specific LUTS (14,17). To be clinically useful though, they require strong psychometric properties and good validity and reliability. Urinary diaries (also known as frequency–volume charts) are also widely used to assess frequency, nocturia, and incontinent episodes (18,19) (see Chap. 18 on diaries). Finally, Wise et al. (20) evaluated the diagnostic accuracy of visual analog scores and found that these did not increase discrimination between women with genuine stress incontinence and those with detrusor instability.

When questioning a patient complaining of urinary symptoms, one should aim to determine the length of time that they have been present and whether the symptom(s) have changed over time. Also, the degree of bother that the symptoms cause and general effect of these on the quality of life should be assessed. In the general inquiry about LUTS, care should be taken to avoid medical jargon and to use a language accessible to the patient, as he or she may be unable to understand or describe them. Effects of the symptoms on sexual practices should be sought, for it is known that LUTS can be associated with significant sexual dysfunction (21). Finally, attention to the patient's body language and verbal cues may provide the physician with an idea of the patient's comprehension as well as treatment preferences.

II. SPECIFIC SYMPTOMS

Lower urinary tract symptoms should be divided into storage and voiding symptoms (Table 2). Whereas in men voiding symptoms are most prevalent, in women, storage symptoms appear more common (22). Many studies have examined the effect of LUTS: those causing

Table 2 Lower Urinary Tract Symptoms

Storage	Voiding
Frequency	Hesitancy
Nocturia	Straining
Urgency	Decreased urinary stream
Incontinence	Intermittency
Stress	Terminal dribble
Urgency	Incomplete emptying
Continuous	Dysuria
Coital	
Overflow	
Enuresis	

the most bother include those associated with storage (so-called irritative or filling symptoms), such as frequency, urgency, nocturia, and incontinence (23,24). Moreover, incontinence reduces social relations and activities, impairs emotional and psychological well-being, and impairs sexual relations (15,21). It is quite clear, however, that there is considerable variability in complaints of deleterious effects of LUTS among patients experiencing them (15).

A. Frequency

Frequency is defined as the number of times a patient voids during waking hours. Studies have estimated normal diurnal frequency to be between four and seven voids per day (18,19,25,26). Abnormal urinary frequency, whether increased or decreased may occur for a number of reasons, including reduced structural or functional bladder capacity, increased bladder capacity or bladder sensation, excessive fluid intake, as well as the ingestion of caffeine, alcohol, and strong citrus juices (27). Urgency and frequency are often linked, as shown by that operative cure of one is usually associated with cure of the other (28). Nevertheless, frequency is not diagnostic for detrusor instability (21), nor for genuine stress incontinence (29), although women with detrusor instability do void more frequently. The actual incidence of voidings can be charted by a patient using a frequency–volume chart that records input and output volumes and allows an objective assessment of urine loss together with episodes of urgency and leakage (see Chap. 18).

B. Nocturia

Nocturnal frequency is arousal from sleep to pass urine (25). It is important to discriminate between that scenario and the one when a person voids because he or she is awake. The number of voids at night changes with age, and there is an increase, on average, of one void per night every decade after the age of 70 years. Changes in sleep pattern in the elderly and nighttime recumbent mobilization of pooled fluid of the lower limbs probably account for the alteration in nocturnal diuresis (26).

C. Urgency

Urgency is a strong and sudden impulse to void that if uncontrolled or unfulfilled, may result in urge incontinence. Urgency on its own seems to be a commonplace symptom; Bungay et al. (30) studied fit women between 30 and 65 years old and found that approximately 20% had urgency. Also, some older women complain of urgency and urge incontinence only when their bladder is full and when they stand up from their bed in the morning. Evidence suggests that this may be a response of the bladder to acute postural changes with or without neurological abnormalities (31).

D. Incontinence

Urinary incontinence is defined as the involuntary loss of urine that is objectively demonstrable and is a social or hygienic problem (32). The prevalence rates of incontinence, as determined by the Agency of Health Care Policy and Research guidelines on incontinence are 1.5–5.0% for men, 10–25% for women aged 15–64 years, and 15–30% for persons older than 60 years. Women are twice likely to experience incontinence than men and, in addition, more than one-half of all those in nursing homes may also be incontinent (15). Loss of urine through channels other than the urethra is extraurethral incontinence (32). A major barrier to gauging the severity of urinary incontinence is that women differ vastly in their perception of the distress and infuence of incontinence on their lives and activities (15).

1. Stress Incontinence

Stress incontinence is the sudden leakage of urine while accomplishing activities that increase intra-abdominal pressure above urethral resistance, such as coughing, lifting, or running. The urine is usually lost in discrete amounts, and there is no associated urgency (31).

2. Urgency Incontinence

Urgency incontinence is the precipitous loss of urine preceding the symptoms of urgency (strong urge to void). The quantity of urine lost can be a few drops just before voiding or it can be a large volume, urine "pouring down both legs" uncontrollably. The sound of running water, changes in temperature, or orgasm can possibly trigger episodes of urge incontinence. Urge incontinence has limited sensitivity of 78% and specificity of 39% in the diagnosis of detrusor instability (3).

3. Continuous Incontinence

Continuous incontinence refers to the involuntary loss of urine at all times and in all positions (25). It is usually seen when there is an ectopic urethra or a urinary fistula, following pelvic surgery, radiotherapy, or malignancy.

4. Coital Incontinence

Urinary incontinence can occur during sexual intercourse either on penetration or during orgasm. Leakage on penetration is more likely to occur in women with urethral sphincter incompetence (21), whereas leakage with orgasm is associated with urgency and is thought to be related to detrusor instability (33).

5. Overflow Incontinence

Often called paradoxical incontinence, it is secondary to chronic urinary retention and high residual urine volumes. The bladder, chronically distended, never empties completely and patients may dribble out small amounts of urine as the bladder overflows. This type of incontinence usually develops over a considerable length of time and patients may be totally unaware of incomplete bladder emptying.

6. Enuresis

Enuresis is urinary loss during sleep. The causes can be abnormal circadian secretion of antidiuretic hormone (34), detrusor instability, abnormal control of the micturition reflex, or abnormal sleep pattern. It is important to differentiate between this complaint and waking with urgency and then leaking before arriving to the toilet.

E. Hesitancy

Urinary hesitancy refers to a delay in the initiation of micturition when the person wished to void. Normally, urination begins within a second after relaxing the urinary sphincter (25), but it may be delayed by the presence of bladder outlet obstruction, detrusor–sphincter dyssynergia, ineffective contraction of the detrusor muscle, or by psychological inhibition of bladder contraction, which occurs in patients who can void only in privacy. The symptom of hesitancy by itself, however, does not discriminate between any of these problems.

F. Straining

Straining refers to the use of the abdominal musculature, which increases the intravesical pressure, to improve bladder emptying.

G. Decreased Urinary Stream

The condition of a decreased urinary stream can be secondary to bladder outlet obstruction, reduced volume of urine, or decreased bladder contractility. However, except for severe degrees of obstruction, most patients are unaware of a change in the force and caliber of their urinary stream (25). As the urine flow rate can be dependent on the urinary volume, the complaint of decreased urinary stream should be assessed with reference to a frequency–volume chart.

H. Intermittency

Intermittency is the involuntary starting or stopping of the urinary stream (25). This is caused by intermittent occlusion of the urinary stream, most commonly by lateral obstructive prostatic lobes, or by a hypertonic urethral striated sphincter (see Chap. 13)

I. Terminal Dribble

Also referred to as postvoid dribbling, this is the terminal release of drops of urine at the end of micturition. This is thought to be secondary to a small amount of residual urine in either the bulbar or prostatic urethra that normally is milked back into the bladder at the end of micturition (25). Postvoid dribbling, by itself, is often an early symptom of urethral obstruction related to benign prostatic hyperplasia.

J. Incomplete Emptying

Incomplete emptying is a sensation that micturition does not completely empty the bladder. It can be caused by fluid remaining in the bladder or by an abnormality of sensation of detrusor instability.

K. Dysuria

Dysuria is painful urination. Pain occurring at the start of urination may indicate urethral pathology, whereas pain occurring at the end of micturition (strangury) as the bladder mucosa closes down is usually of bladder origin. Suprapubic pain may also be associated with pathology outside the bladder, but within the pelvis. Dysuria is often accompanied by frequency and urgency.

III. SPECIFIC HISTORY

A. Gynecological

Close anatomical, physiological, and embryological relations exists between urological and genital tracts. That is the reason why lesion of one of these systems can affect the other (35). The lower urinary tract is estrogen-sensitive and estrogen-dependent (36). The relation of the menstrual cycle and menopause to urethral function is important. Smith has demonstrated the symptomatic and cytological changes associated with postmenopausal estrogen deficiency and the benefits of estrogen therapy. Thus, women should be queried about changes in urinary symptoms during the menstrual cycle.

The majority of patients complaining of urological symptoms have coexisting gynecological pathology (38). Ovarian and uterine enlargement may cause symptoms of frequency and urinary retention if impaction occurs. Endometriosis and pelvic inflammatory disease can involve the bladder, leading to frequency and urgency. Urethral sphincter incompetence can be masked by a vaginal prolapse, rending crucial the identification of the former before the urodynamic tests are undertaken so that it can be reduced to expose any underlying urethral sphincter incompetence (see Chap. 15). Also, over 40% of women with urethral sphincter deficiency will have significant cystoceles (26).

The effect of previous gynecological surgical interventions on the urological system can be important; the urethral sphincter and bladder may have been damaged by scarring, distortion of tissues, or simply by direct alteration of their innervation during intervention.

B. Neurological

The frequent occurrence of bladder disturbances associated with neurological disease makes it imperative that a neurological history and examination be completed. Some of the common neurological diseases that may appear are central intervertebral disk prolapse, peripheral neuropathy associated with diabetes mellitus, cerebrovascular accidents, parkinsonism, multiple sclerosis, on others (39,40). Evidence of neurological disease should be sought, especially questions directed toward past surgery on the spine and in alteration in sensation and motor power in legs or perineum. The latter may be described as altered sensation during sexual intercourse or inability to feel urinary stream during micturition.

C. Medical

Recording of all past major abdominal and pelvic surgery, as well as complications eventually related to them is mandatory. One should aim to inquire particularly about urinary retention that could indicate prolonged overdistention, which can lead to bladder-emptying difficulties caused by detrusor hypotonia (41). Surgery on the large bowel, such as abdominoperineal resection of the rectum and pelvic surgery are of particular importance, for they may result in denervation of the bladder or lesions to the urethra. Urinary tract infection and its treatment should be inquired about, as well as the frequency of episodes and treatments over the past 2 years.

General conditions that have potential to increase abdominal pressure and induce or worsen stress incontinence should be sought. Also, cardiac and renal failure can produce frequency and nocturia. Endocrine disorders, such as diabetes, may lead to frequency secondary to impaired bladder sensation and a hypotonic detrusor. Finally, patients suffering from dementia may not empty their bladders frequently and may not be aware of the need to void.

D. Drug

The current drug regimen is important. Drugs taken for gynecological or urological symptoms and for other conditions should be noted, because many drugs affect the lower urinary tract (e.g., benzodiazepines, diuretics, anticholinergics, sympathicomimetics, or others). It is relevant to confirm the time of administration because a common cause for nocturia is late administration of diuretic therapy. A note should be made about drug allergy and history of alcohol ingestion because the latter produces a diuresis and can alter a person's perception of bladder filling.

IV. CONCLUSION

Finally, history taking can be disappointing, because it does not allow the diagnosis of urinary disorders. Nonetheless, LUTS should be assessed with great care and empathy; they may be unvaluable to provide an assessment of disease severity and quality of life and to serve as a guide in determining further management, as cure can be achieved by directing treatment to relieve the troublesome symptoms.

REFERENCES

1. De La Rosette JJMCH, Witjes WPJ, Schäfer W, Abrams P, Donovan JL, Peters TJ, Millard RJ, Frimond–Møller C, Kalomiris P, the ICS-"BPH" Study Group. Relationships between lower urinary tract symptoms and bladder outlet obstruction: results from the ICS–BPH study. Neurourol Urodynam 1998; 17:99–108.
2. Ezz El Din K, Koch WFRM, De Wildt MJAM, Kiemeney LALM, DeBruyne FMJ, De La Rosette JJMCH. Reliability of the International Prostate Symptom Score in the assessment of patients with lower urinary tract symptoms and/or benign prostatic hyperplasia. J Urol 1996; 155:1959–1964.
3. Sand PK, Ostergard DR. Incontinence history as a predictor of detrusor stability. Obstet Gynecol 1988; 71:257–259.
4. Jarvis GJ, Hall S, Stamp S, Millar DR, Johnson A. An assessment of urodynamic examination in incontinent women. Br J Obstet Gynaecol 1980; 87:893–896.
5. Byrne DJ, Hamilton Stewart PA, Gray BK. The role of urodynamics in female urinary stress incontinence. Br J Urol 1987; 59:228–229.
6. Lagro–Janssen FM, DeBruyne FMJ, Van Weel C. Value of the patient's case history in diagnosing urinary incontinence in general practice. Br J Urol 1991; 67:569–572.
7. Bergman A, Bader K. Reliability of the patient's history in the diagnosis of urinary incontinence. Int J Gynecol Obstet 1990; 32:255–259.
8. Hastie KJ, Moisey CU. Are urodynamics necessary in female patients presenting with stress incontinence? Br J Urol 1989; 63:155–156.
9. Farrar DJ, Whiteside CG, Osborne JL, Turner–Warwick RT. A urodynamic analysis of micturition symptoms in the female. Surg Gynecol Obstet 1975; 141:875–881.
10. Haylen BT, Sutherst JR, Frazer MI. Is the investigation of most stress incontinence really necessary? Br J Urol 1989; 64:147–149.
11. Madsen PO, Iversen P. A point system for selecting operative candidates. In: Hinman F, ed. Benign Prostatic Hypertrophy. New York: Springer-Verlag 1983:763–765.
12. Barry MJ, Fowler FJ, O'Leary MP. The American Urological Association Symptom Index for Benign Prostatic Hyperplasia. J Urol 1992; 148:1549–1557.
13. Donovan JL, Abrams P, Peters TJ, Kay HE, Reynard J, Chapple C, De La Rosette JJMCH, Kondo A. The ICS-"BPH" study: the psychometric validity and reliability of the ICS male questionnaire. Br J Urol 1996; 77:554–562.
14. Jackson S, Donovan J, Brookes S, Eckford S, Swithinbank L, Abrams P. The Bristol Female Lower Urinary Tract Symptoms questionnaire: development and psychometric testing. Br J Urol 1996; 77:805–812.
15. Donovan J, Naughton M, Gotoh M, Corcos J, Jackson S, Kelleher C, Lukacs B, Costa P. Symptom and quality of life assessment. In: Abrams P, Khoury S, Wein A, eds. Proceedings of the First WHO and UICC International Consultation on Incontinence. Monaco; 1998. Plymouth: Health Publication 1999:295–331.

16. Black N, Griffiths J, Pope C. Development of a symptom severity index and a symptom impact index for stress incontinence in women. Neurourol Urodynan 1996; 15:630–640.

17. Moon TD, Hagen L, Heisey DM. Urinary symptomatology in younger men. Urology 1997; 50: 700–703.

18. Larsson G, Victor A. Micturition patterns in a healthy female population, studied with a frequency/volume chart. Scand J Urol Nephrol Suppl 1988; 114:53–57.

19. Larsson G, Abrams P, Victor A. The frequency/volume chart in detrusor instability. Neurourol Urodynam 1991; 10:533–543.

20. Wise BG, Cutner A, Cardozo LD, Kelleher CJ, Burton G, Abbott D. Do detailed symptom questionnaires negate the need for urodynamic investigation? Neurourol Urodynam 1992; 11:353–355.

21. Kelleher CJ, Cardozo LD, Wise BG, Cutner A. The impact of urinary incontinence on sexual function. Neurourol Urodynam 1992; 11:359–360.

22. Abrams P. Lower urinary tract symptoms in women: who to investigate and how? Br J Urol 1997; 80:43–48.

23. Jolleys JV, Donovan JL, Nanchanal K, Peters TJ, Abrams P. Urinary symptoms in the community: how bothersome are they? Br J Urol 1994; 74:551–555.

24. Peters TJ, Donovan JL, Kay HE, Abrams P, De La Rosette JJMCH, Porru D, Thüroff JW, the International Continence Society "Benign Prostatic Hyperplasia" Study Group. The bothersomeness of urinary symptoms. J Urol 1997; 157:885–889.

25. Brendler CB. History, physical examination and urine analysis. In: Walsh PC, Retik AB, Darracott Vaughan E Jr, Wein AJ, eds. Campbell's Urology. Philadelphia: WB Saunders, 1998:131–157.

26. Cardozo L. History and examination. In: Cardozo L, ed. Urogynecology: The King's Approach. Edinburgh: Churchill–Livingstone, 1997:85–99.

27. Theofrastous JP, Swift SE. The clinical evaluation of pelvic floor dysfunction. Obstet Gynecol Clin North Am 1998; 25:783–801.

28. Stanton SL, Williams JE, Ritchie D. The colposuspension operation for urinary incontinence. Br J Obstet Gynecol 1976; 83:890–895.

29. Larsson G, Victor A. The frequency/volume chart in genuine stress incontinent women. Neurourol Urodynam 1992; 11:23–31.

30. Bungay GT, Vessey MP, McPherson CK. Study of symptoms in middle life with special reference to the menopause. Br Med J 1980; 281:181–183.

31. James ED. The behavior of the bladder during physical activity. Br J Urol 1978; 50:387–394.

32. Abrams P, Blaivas JG, Stuart L, Andersen T. The standardization of terminology of lower urinary tract function. Scand J Urol Nephrol Suppl 1988; 114:5–17.

33. Sutherst JR. Sexual dysfunction and urinary incontinence. Br J Obstet Gynecol 1979; 86:387–388.

34. Carter PG, McConnell AA, Abrams P. The significance of atrial natriuretic peptide in nocturnal urinary symptoms in the elderly. Neurourol Urodynam 1992; 11:420–421.

35. Stanton SL. History and physical examination. In: Stanton SL, ed. Clinical Gynecologic Urology. St Louis: CV Mosby, 1984:46–58.

36. Iosif CS, Batra S, Ek A, Ashedt B. Estrogen receptors in the human female lower urinary tract. Am J Obstet Gynecol 1981; 141:817–820.

37. Smith P. Age changes in the female urethra. Br J Urol 1972; 44:667–676.

38. Benson JT. Gynecologic and urodynamic evaluation of women with urinary incontinence. Obstet Gynecol 1985; 66:691–694.

39. Chanceller MB, Blaivas JG. Practical Neuro-urology. Genitourinary Complications in Neurologic Disease. Boston: Butterworth–Heinemann, 1995.

40. Corcos J, Schick E. Les vessies neurogènes de l'adulte. Paris: Masson, 1996.

41. Hinman F. Postoperative overdistension of the bladder. Surg Gynecol Obstet 1976; 142:901–902.

17

Physical Examination

ERIK SCHICK

University of Montreal and Maisonneuve–Rosemont Hospital, Montreal, Quebec, Canada

I. INTRODUCTION

Physical examination of the patient, together with a detailed clinical history, and whenever possible, the voiding diary, are the three cornerstones on which any further evaluation, diagnosis, and therapeutic plan are built. Except for neurourological examination, there are presently no scientific data documenting the parameters of a normal pelvic examination (especially in the female) and, consequently, the components of the examination have not been universally agreed on (1). Furthermore, we often assume that findings on physical examination correlate with lower urinary tract function. This is not necessarily true: For example, no specific physical sign can be found in patients with unstable bladders, even when sophisticated neurological examinations are performed (2). Also, in a recent analysis of 221 female patients, no urethral hypermobility was demonstrated on vaginal examination, yet 122 (55%) claimed urinary stress incontinence in their clinical history. On the other hand, 90% of 233 patients with grade II cystourethrocele reported clinically significant stress urinary incontinence on a questionnaire (3), yet 10% of these patients claimed perfect continence during physical stress (Table 1). These observations by no means imply that physical examination should be neglected but, rather, it should be put in its proper perspective.

A. Children

Physical examination of children with overt neurological lesions, such as neurospinal dysraphism (e.g., spina bifida), cerebral palsy, or traumatic injury to the spine, is obvious and does not require detailed description here. Children with functional voiding disorders (i.e., lazy bladder syndrome, Hinman's syndrome, and such) often appear remarkably normal on physical examination.

Table 1 Relation Between Stress Urinary Incontinence (Obtained from
History) and the Degree of Cystourethrocele Evident on Physical Examination

Grade of cystourethrocele (no. of patients in each category)	SUI on history-taking	No SUI on history-taking
0 (221)	122 (55%)	99 (45%)
I (224)	159 (71%)	65 (29%)
II (233)	209 (90%)	24 (10%)
III (79)	68 (86%)	11 (14%)
IV (10)	8 (80%)	2 (20%)

SUI, stress urinary incontinence.

One should verify, however, that the rectum is empty. Fecalome suggests that chronic constipation can be responsible for urinary tract infection, vesicoureteral reflux, or unstable bladder contractions (4). Digital rectal examination also assesses rectal tone (S3–S5), and the bulbocarvernous reflex (L5–S5). The presence of this reflex indicates that the pudendal nerves are intact, which suggests that the pelvic nerves are also intact at the level of the spinal cord, because the two nerves originate from the same sacral roots (S2–S4). Two clinical entities, however, deserve more detailed comments.

1. Occult Dysraphism

Occult dysraphism is a condition characterized by an abnormality of the spinal column which, unlike classic spina bifida does not result in an open vertebral canal (5). Associated anomalies include intradural lipome, diastematomyelia, and short filum terminale. In more than 80% of these children very discrete skin lesions at the midline portion of the lower back may be detected (6). Lower limb abnormalities are also common, including a high arch in the feet and different muscle size and strength between the two legs. In about 40% of these children, the lower urinary tract is affected (7).

2. Sacral Agenesis

Sacral agenesis is a congenital malformation characterized by the absence of part or all of two or more vertebral bodies. Interestingly, the diagnosis is often made only after failed attempts at bladder training. Sensation is normal, including perianal dermatomes, and lower extremity function is intact (5). Palpation of the coccyx will reveal the absent vertebrae.

B. Male

Physical examination of the male patient can be performed in three steps:

1. Abdomen

Recently, Giovanucci et al. (8) found that abdominal obesity increases the frequency and severity of lower urinary tract symptoms as well as the likelihood of undergoing prostatectomy. Palpation of the lower abdomen focuses on the detection of bladder distension, particularly if the examination is done immediately following urination. If the bladder is palpable, postvoid residual urine should be determined by ultrasound or urethral catheterization.

2. Digital Rectal Examination

As in children, this allows evaluation of rectal tone and detection of the bulbocavernous reflex. This reflex is intact if squeezing the glans penis provokes reflex contraction of the anal sphincter. According to Blaivas et al. (9), 98% of neurologically normal males will have a normal bulbocarvernous reflex at clinical examination. In contrast, only 10 patients out of a group of 34 (34%) with incomplete lower motor lesions had a clinically normal bulbocavernous reflex (9).

This suggests that the absence of the bulbocavernous reflex in the male is an indication of a neurological lesion involving the sacral cord, but its presence does not rule out the possibility of a significant lesion at this level.

Rectal examination also assesses the size, consistency, and tenderness of the prostate. It should be pointed out that prostate size does not correlate with symptom severity or degree of urodynamic obstruction (10,11).

3. Neurological Examination

Neurourological examination is almost identical in the male and the female; accordingly, it is discussed in the following.

C. Female

The physical examination of the female should also focus on three areas:

1. Abdomen

As in males, the main reason for abdominal examination is the detection of a distended or overdistended bladder, in which case postvoid residual urine should be determined by ultrasound or catheterization.

2. Pelvic Examination

Estrogen deficiency is manifested at the level of the vaginal mucosa by a thinned epithelium. The appearance of vaginal secretions may indicate infection, which should be documented by culture.

Bimanual examination permits determination of the size and position of the uterus and the ovaries. Pelvic organ prolapse can be present at the anterior, apical, or posterior segments of the vaginal wall, or simultaneously at two, or even all three segments of the vagina. Anterior vaginal wall descent represents cystourethrocele. Urethrocele alone is almost nonexistent. It is always accompanied by cystocele. On the other hand, cystocele may exist without concomitant urethrocele, especially in patients who have previously undergone a successful urethropexy.

Gynecologists often classify cystourethroceles in three grades, whereas urologists prefer a four-grade classification. For the gynecologist, grade I cystourethrocele represents anterior vaginal wall descent that, with a forceful Valsalva maneuver, still remains within the introitus, whereas the urologist considers slight hypermobility as grade I and moderate hypermobility as grade II cystourethrocele.

In gynecological grade II or urological grade III, the anterior vaginal wall reaches the plane of the vulva, whereas gynecological grade III or urological grade IV represents complete prolapse outside the vulva (Table 2). Baden and Walker (12) proposed a classification in which different grades were established relative to the hymen (Table 3).

Table 2 Widely Used Classification by Urologists and Gynecologists to Describe the Degrees of Cystourethrocele on Physical Examination

Description	Urological classification	Gynecological classification
Slightly hypermobile vaginal wall	Grade I	Grade I
Moderately hypermobile vaginal wall that still remains inside the introitus	Grade II	Grade I
Hypermobility reaches the vulvar plane	Grade III	Grade II
Prolapsus outside the vagina	Grade IV	Grade III

Table 3 Baden–Walker Classification, the So-Called Halfway System, Which Inspired the Classification Proposed by the International Continence Society

Grade	Definition
Grade I	Descent halfway to the hymen
Grade II	Descent to the hymen
Grade III	Descent halfway past the hymen
Grade IV	Complete prolapse outside the vagina

Source: Ref. 11.

None of the classifications of pelvic organ prolapse became widely accepted by the scientific community. Recognizing the problem, the International Continence Society (ICS) put together an international, multidisciplinary terminology standardization committee for the description and classification of pelvic organ prolapse. The report of this committee was published in 1996 (13). For the purpose of this classification, the hymen was chosen as a fixed point, and six sites on the vaginal wall were referenced to this fixed point: two anterior, two posterior, and two apical (cervix or vaginal cuff and the posterior fornix). Furthermore, the genital hiatus (anteroposterior axis of the hymenal ring), the perineal body (distance between the posterior fornix of the vulva and the anal margin), and total vaginal length were measured. Their displacements were defined in centimeters and expressed as negative (above the hymen) or positive (below the hymen), the presented in the form of a three-by-three grid, with the first line describing the anterior vaginal wall; the second line, the dimension of the hymenal ring, the perineal body and the total vaginal length; and the third line, the posterior vaginal wall (Table 4). Studies relative to the validation (reproducibility, reliability) of this classification were presented in 1995 at the ICS Annual Meeting in Sydney, Australia (14,15) and published in more detail in 1996 (16).

Table 4 The Three-by-Three Grid Proposed by the International Continence Society to Characterize Pelvic Organ Prolapse

First line	Point A_a (anterior wall)	Point B_a (anterior wall)	Point C (cervix or cuff)
Second line	Genital hiatus (hymenal ring)	Perineal body	Total vaginal length
Third line	Point A_p (posterior wall)	Point B_p (posterior wall)	Point D (posterior fornix or the Douglas pouch)

Table 5 International Continence Society Classification of Pelvic
Organ Prolapse, Using Data Obtained from the Three-by-Three Grid
of Table 4

Stage	Position of the leading edge of the prolapse in relation to the hymenal ring[a,b]
0	All points are –3 cm; point C or D is at no more than –(X–2) cm
I	Less than –1 cm
II	Between –1 cm and +1 cm
III	Greater than +1 cm but less than +(X–2) cm
IV	At least +(X–2) cm

[a]X, total vaginal length in centimeters.
[b](+) and (–), below or above the hymenal ring, respectively.

Derived from this detailed description, the ICS proposed a staging system based on
the position of the leading edge of the prolapse in relation to the hymenal ring (Table 5).
This allows comparison of well-defined patient populations with the assessment of symptoms in relation to parameters, such as pelvic floor weakness and treatment outcomes. Furthermore, the leading edge of the prolapsus can be specified as being anterior or posterior.

If the classic Sims speculum is not available, vaginal examination can be improved
using one blade of a dismounted, normal speculum (Fig. 1). This allows one to examine
separately the mobility of the anterior and the posterior vaginal wall. For example, a relatively small rectocele can be easily visualized this way (Fig. 2).

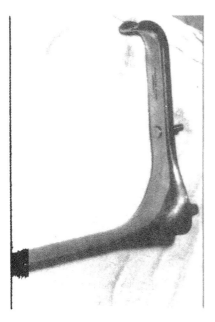

Figure 1 Single blade of a dismounted ordinary vaginal speculum, which allows an easier visualization of the mobility of the anterior and posterior vaginal wall.

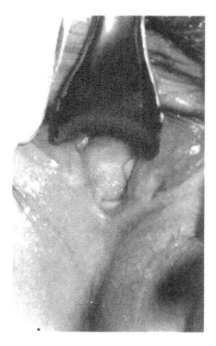

Figure 2   Retracting the anterior vaginal wall with the single blade of a speculum allows one to visualize a relatively small rectocele.

In the case of urethral hypermobility, careful inspection of the anterior vaginal wall can yield some information about its cause.

In the case of central protrusion of the anterior vaginal wall, the normally present mucosal folds of the vagina will be absent, and the mucosa will have a shiny, smooth appearance (Fig. 3). This finding suggests that a defect in the midline of the pubocervical fascia below the trigone and the bladder base is responsible for the central herniation of these structures. Hypermobility of the anterior vaginal wall may also result from uni- or bilateral detachment of the pubocervical ligament and the endopelvic fascia from the arcus tendineous of the obturator. Under these circumstances, the mucosal folds of the vaginal wall will be preserved (Fig. 4).

While asking the patient to contract the perineal muscle, the strength of the pelvic floor musculature should also be tested, especially in the incontinent female. This can be done by simple observation (narrowing of the vaginal introitus, in-drawing of the anus), by palpation, or with a pressure probe (perineometer) in the vaginal or anal canal. Urethral and bladder neck mobility can be quantified using the Q-Tip test (17).

Booney's bladder neck elevation test (18) was originally described as having prognostic value for stress incontinence: If elevation of the bladder neck with the index and middle finger at the anterior vaginal wall eliminated urine leakage during stress, then surgical correction of bladder neck hypermobility was thought likely to cure stress incontinence. However, in our experience as well as that of other investigators (19,20), this test has no prognostic value, for it is always positive, that is, no urine leakage is observed once the bladder neck is elevated, irrespective of the etiology of incontinence. We no longer use the Booney maneuver although we routinely ask patients with a full bladder to cough forcefully during physical examination to visualize urine leakage.

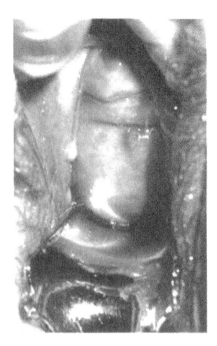

Figure 3 Hypermobility of the anterior vaginal wall, result of the central herniation of the bladder base and the trigone. Note the absence of mucosal folds.

D. Neurourological Examination

During a physical examination, all patients should have at least a simple neurological examination, including 1) assessment of anal tone, 2) its voluntary contraction, 3) clinical evaluation of the bulbocavernous (or clitoridoanal) reflex, and 4) evaluation of perineal sensation.

Blaivas et al. (9) reported that 81% of normal females had a normal clitoridoanal reflex. This implies that in about 20% of neurologically intact females this reflex is absent, which is in contrast to 2% of males. As mentioned earlier, the clinical absence of this reflex necessitates further electrophysiological studies in the male. In females, however, the clitoridoanal reflex may be absent as a consequence of trauma from vaginal childbirth (1).

To verify the anal reflex, light stroking of the perianal skin should provoke visible contraction of the anal sphincter. Alternatively, simple movement of the index finger in the anal canal should provoke perceptible contraction of the sphincter. When a more detailed neurological examination is needed, this is generally done by the neurologist. It should be mentioned that the anal reflex is mediated through S2–S5; the bulbocavernous reflex through S2–S4; the cremasteric reflex in the male through L1–L2; and the abdominal reflexes through T6–L2 (stroking the abdominal skin toward the umbilicus causes the umbilicus to move in the direction of the stimulus) (Table 6).

II. CONCLUSION

The first International Consultation on Incontinence (1), held in Monaco in 1998, made some specific recommendations for the physical examination of different groups of patients: children, females, males, frail elderly, adults, and neurogenic patients. These recommendations, slightly modified, are summarized in Table 7.

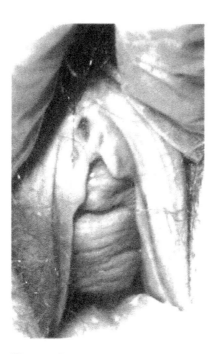

Figure 4 In this patient, the grade II (almost grade III) cystourethrocele is the consequence of a paravaginal defect. The endopelvic fascia and the pubocervical fascia have
been detached from the arcus tendineous of the obturator muscle. The mucosal folds of the
anterior vaginal wall have been conserved, because there is no central rupture of the pubocervical fascia, as in Figure 3.

Table 6 Different Nerve Roots Involved in Some of
the Sensory and Deep Tendon Reflexes Useful in
Neurourological Evaluation

	Type of reflex	Nerve roots involved
Sensory	Abdominal	T6–L2
	Cremasteric	L1–L2
	Bulbocavernous	S2–S4
	Anal	S2–S5
Deep tendon	Quadriceps	L3–L4
	Achilles	L5–S1 or S2

Table 7 Recommendations of the First International Consultation on Incontinence for Physical Examination of Different Groups of Patients (author's modifications are in *italics*)

Children
    Psychomotor development
    Examination of the lower back for spinal abnormality
    Observe voiding
Female
    Abdomen (palpable bladder)
    Pelvic examination
        External genitalia
        Vaginal epithelium
    Bladder neck mobility (*Q-Tip test*)
    Evidence of fistula or diverticulum
    Size of uterus and ovaries
    Support of anterior, apical, and posterior segments of the vagina
    Digital rectal examination
        Sphincter tone
        Clitoridoanal reflex or voluntary contraction
Male
    Abdomen (palpable bladder)
    Lower back
    Digital rectal examination
        Sphincter tone
        Anal reflex or bulbocavernous reflex, or voluntary contraction
        Evaluation of prostate
    Scrotum
    Urethral meatus
    Inguinal area (re: hernia)
Frail elderly
    General systemic examination
    Comorbid conditions (i.e., heart failure)
    Manual dexterity
Neurogenic
    Complete neurological examination
    Observe voiding

REFERENCES

1. Shull BL, Halaska M, Hurt G, Kinn A, Laycock J, Palmtag H, Reilly N, Yang Y, Zubieta R. Physical examination. In: Abrams P, Koury S, Wein A, eds. Incontinence. Plymouth, UK: Health Publication, 1999:335–349.
2. Del Carro U, Riva D, Comi GC, Locatelli T, Magnani G, Levati N, Vigano R, Sambruni I, Canal N. Neurophysiological evaluation in detrusor instability. Neurourol Urodynam 1993; 12:455–462.
3. Schick E. Unpublished data, 1999.
4. O'Regan S, Yazbeck S, Schick E. Constipation, bladder instability and urinary tract infection. Clin Nephrol 1985; 23:152–154.
5. Bauer SB. Pediatric urodynamics: lower tract. In: O'Donnell B, Kuff SA, eds. Pediatric Urology. 3rd ed. Oxford: Butterworth–Heinemann, 1997:125–151.

6. Anderson FM. Occult spinal dysraphism: a series of 73 cases. Pediatrics 1975; 55:826–835.
7. Dubrowitz V, Lorber J, Zachary RB. Lipoma of the caudal equina. Arch Dis Child 1965; 40: 207–213.
8. Giovanucci E, Rimm EB, Chute CG, Kawachi I, Colditz GA, Stamfer MJ, Willett WC. Obesity and benign prostatic hyperplasia. Am J Epidemiol 1994; 140:989–1002.
9. Blaivas JG, Zayed AAH, Labib KB. The bulbocavernous reflex in urology: a prospective study of 299 patients. J Urol 1981; 126:197–199.
10. Simonsen O, Møller–Madsen B, Dorflinger T, Nørgoaard JP, Jørgensen HS, Lundhus E. The significance of age on symptoms and urodynamic and cystoscopic findings in benign prostatic hypertrophy. Urol Res 1987; 15:355–358.
11. Barry MJ, Cockelt ATK, Holdgrowe HL, McConnell JD, Sihelnik SA, Winfiled HN. Relationship of symptoms of prostatism to commonly used physiologic and anatomical measures of the severity of benign prostatic hyperplasia. J Urol 1993; 150:351–358.
12. Baden W, Walker T. Surgical Repair of Vaginal Defects. Philadelphia: JB Lippincott, 1992.
13. Bump R, Mattiasson A, Bø K, Brubaker LP, Delancey JOL, Klarskov P, Schull BL, Smith ARB. The standardization of terminology of female pelvic organ prolapse and pelvic floor dysfunction. Am J Obstet Gynecol 1996; 175:10–17.
14. Athanasiou S, Hill S, Gleeson C, Anders K, Cardozo L. Validation of the ICS proposed pelvic organ prolapse descripting system. Neurourol Urodynam 1995; 14:414–415.
15. Schüssler B, Perschers U. Standardization of terminology of female genital prolapse according to the new ICS criteria: inter-examiner reproducibility. Neurourol Urodynam 1995; 14:437–438.
16. Hall AF, Theofrastous JP, Cundiff GC, Harris RL, Hamilton LF, Swift SE, Bump RC. Inter- and intra-observer reliability of the proposed International Continence Society, Society of Gynecologic Surgeons, and American Uro-gynecologic Society Pelvic Organ Prolapse Classification System. Am J Obstet Gynecol 1996; 175:1467–1471.
17. Crystie CD, Charm LS, Copeland WE. Q-Tip test in stress urinary incontinence. Obstet Gynecol 1971; 38:313–315.
18. Berkeley C, Booney V. A Textbook of Gynecologic surgery. 3rd ed. London: Cassell, 1935.
19. Bhatia NN, Bergman A. Urodynamic appraisal of the Booney test in women with stress urinary incontinence. Obstet Gynecol 1983; 62:696–699.
20. Migliorini GD, Glenning PP. Booney's test—fact or fiction? Br J Obstet Gynaecol 1987; 94: 157–159.

18

The Voiding Diary

MARTINE JOLIVET-TREMBLAY and ERIK SCHICK

*University of Montreal and Maisonneuve–Rosemont Hospital,
Montreal, Quebec, Canada*

I. INTRODUCTION

Lower urinary tract symptoms (LUTS) are common in the general population. It is generally estimated that about 50% of patients who consult a general practitioner have some kind of LUTS, even if they are not the main reason for the consultation. The bladder is unreliable for investigation, as it is difficult to depend solely on subjective symptoms to establish a diagnosis of bladder–urethral dysfunction.

Although frequently overlooked, one of the simplest, objective, and noninvasive tests to evaluate the function of the lower urinary tract (LUT) is the voiding diary. It is completed by patients, and it offers the advantage of assessing the severity of LUTS in their own environment. By filling out the voiding diary, patients become active participants in the diagnostic process.

At first, studies published about voiding diaries concerned only urinary incontinence. Since the end of the 1980s; however, the voiding diary has become a widely accepted tool in the investigation of voiding dysfunctions, including obstructive uropathy, urinary tract infection, and vesicoureteral reflux.

II. TERMINOLOGY

In an effort to standardize the terminology in the literature, Abrams and Klevmark (1) described four different voiding diaries, depending on the type and amount of information contained in each of them (Table 1).

Table 1   Different Types of Voiding Diaries

	Voiding diary		
Frequency chart	Frequency severity chart	Frequency–volume chart	Urinary diary
No. of voidings	No. of voidings	Time of each voiding	Time of each voiding
No. of incontinence episodes	No. of inconti- nence episodes	Volume of each voiding	Volume of each voiding
	+	Time of incontinence episodes	Time of incontinence episodes
	No. of pads used		+
			No. and type of drinks/food
			Activities related to LUTS

A.   Frequency Chart

Only the number of micturitions and the number of incontinence episodes per 24 hr are reg-istered. This is the simplest possible voiding diary. It objectively determines micturition and incontinence frequency. It does not provide information about diuresis, mean voided vol-ume, or the severity of incontinence.

B.   Frequency–Severity Chart

In addition to the number of micturitions and incontinence episodes, this type of diary reg-isters the number of protective pads used or clothing changes, objectively defining the de-gree of severity of incontinence. No effort is made to quantify the amount of urine lost.

C.   Frequency–Volume Chart

This type of voiding diary is probably the most widely used by the urological community. It demands only a minimum effort on the part of the patient and provides maximum infor-mation to the physician. Together with the number and timing of the incontinence episodes and the time when micturition occurred, the amount of urine voided at each micturition is also registered. This determines 24-hr diuresis, the functional capacity of the bladder, the frequency of micturition, and daytime diuresis, compared with nocturnal diuresis. This type of diary does not, however, estimate the amount of fluid intake or its distribution through-out a 24-hr period.

D.   Urinary Diary

This is the most elaborate voiding diary. Together with data obtained from the fre-quency–volume chart, it also contains information on the number and types of beverages and foods taken and activities related to LUTS. This type of chart is too cumbersome to fill out correctly and precisely by the patient in routine clinical practice and is sometimes dif-ficult for the physician to analyze. It is used mainly as a research tool within a given protocol. From the clinical point of view, knowledge of volume ingested is not necessary if diuresis is measured, because these run parallel to each other in normal circumstances.

III. OBJECTIVES OF THE VOIDING DIARY

Incorporation of the voiding diary in the investigation and follow-up of patients with LUTS serves four objectives:

First, it allows an objective measure of the patient's subjective complaints. McCormack et al. (2) studied 88 consecutive patients in whom urinary frequency was evaluated by questionnaire at the first visit. This was compared with the frequency obtained by analyzing the frequency–volume chart filled out by the patient for 7 consecutive days. A wide discrepancy was noted between subjective-estimated frequency and chart-determined frequency.

Second, it may contribute to establishment of the etiology of LUTS. Later in this chapter, we will discuss the application as well as the limitations of the voiding diary as a diagnostic tool.

Third, it encourages the patient to participate actively in the evaluation of his or her LUTS. This allows the physician to evaluate the patient's willingness to follow a therapeutic plan.

Finally, the voiding diary is an invaluable tool in measuring the results of surgery or for following the progress of a medical treatment. Siltberg et al. (3) estimated that the voiding diary provided the best tool for follow-up in the treatment of patients with urge syndrome.

IV. PARAMETERS DERIVED FROM THE VOIDING DIARY

Careful examination of the voiding diary can disclose important information about the frequency of micturition and the number of incontinence episodes. It can also give an estimate of diuresis. The data can be entered into a computer and, by a simple computer program, more precise and detailed analysis can be done.

This computer program, developed in our laboratory, calculates the following parameters: mean voided volume per micturition (mL), frequency (units), diuresis (mL/min), mean interval between micturitions (min), and volume voided during a specified period of the day (mL). All these parameters are calculated separately for daytime and for nighttime. The first daytime voiding is when the person urinates on rising. This voided volume is considered part of nocturnal diuresis and treated as such by the computer program. It is assumed that daytime lasts 16 hr (960 min), and nighttime 8 hr (480 min). Therefore, the amount of urine voided during the day is divided by 960 and during the night (including the first micturition on rising) by 480, to give the day and night diuresis in milliliters per minute. Further analysis produces two more parameters: output/24 hr (mL), which is the total voided volume during a 24-hr period, and the ratio between nighttime and daytime diuresis. In addition, the computer prints out the number of days analyzed, the number of incontinence episodes occurring during this period, and the number of micturitions for which volume was not measured. This last figure is also expressed as a percentage of the total number of voidings during the observation period.

The computer program is designed to automatically correct daytime and nighttime diuresis as well as the total volume voided (output per day, output per night, output per 24 hr) for those urinations when voided volume was not measured. Mean voided volume is calculated from recorded voided volumes. This mean volume is then substituted for each and every unrecorded voiding volume to give the final corrected output. The diuresis ratio (night/day) is derived from this corrected diuresis (4).

To facilitate interpretation of the patient's data, the computer will print out the normal value for each parameter, along with the standard deviation (SD) and the standard normal deviation (Z-value), which is the number of SDs an observation lies away from the mean. A Z-value of 2.00 or more suggests a significant deviation from the mean (5) (Table 2).

We have used this computer program in our urodynamic laboratory for over 15 years, analyzing thousands of frequency–volume charts (Fig. 1).

A. Normal Values

Surprisingly, very few data are available in the literature concerning the normal values of voiding diaries. We consider this an important issue because baseline figures are needed to compare data from patients with different LUTS.

1. Children

Reference values are difficult to obtain in children. Data in the literature are rare. Mattsson (6) studied 206 children, aged 7–15, considered to be asymptomatic. All of them completed a 24-hr frequency–volume chart. They voided two to ten times a day, and 95% of them had a voiding frequency of three to eight. About 10% voided once during the night. Voided volumes varied greatly, the morning voiding being the largest, and the last voiding before bedtime, the smallest. Single voided volume varied between 20 and 800 mL, with total volumes over 24 hr between 325 and 2100 mL.

Table 2 Basic Screen Provided by Computer

No. of days analyzed:
    No. of incontinence episodes
    No. of micturitions without recorded volume: (%)

		Patient's data	Normal	± 1SD	Z-value
Day:	Mean voided volume (mL)		237	67	
	Frequency		5.63	1.26	
	Diuresis (mL/min)		1.11	0.35	
	Corrected diuresis (mL/min)		1.11	0.35	
	Interval between micturitions (min)		222	60	
	Output (mL)		1005	497	
	Corrected output (mL)		1005	497	
Night:	Mean voided volume (mL)		379	132	
	Frequency		0.08	0.16	
	Diuresis (mL/min)		0.84	0.27	
	Corrected diuresis (mL/min)		0.84	0.27	
	Interval between micturitions (min)		454	50	
	Output (mL)		409	130	
	Corrected output (mL)		409	130	
Output/24 hr (mL)			1473	386	
Corrected output/24 hr (mL)			1473	386	
Diuresis ratio (night/day)			0.81	0.30	

SD, standard deviation; Z-value: standard normal deviation (see text).

Day	Time/Volume (day) (in oz or mL)					Time/Volume (night) (in oz or mL)
1						
2						
3						
4						
5						
6						
7						

For details on how to proceed, see reverse side.

Figure 1   Frequency–volume chart to be filled out by patient.

Bloom et al. (7) analyzed the toilet habits of 1192 children without any history of urinary tract infection. They obtained a mean frequency of about four to five micturitions a day. However, the data were obtained by questionnaire, and no frequency–volume chart was filled out.

When using a frequency chart on which urine volume could be measured, but was not mandatory, Wan et al. (8) estimated that voiding frequency for normal children was approximately six times daily (or near once every 3–4 hr). They found the diary particularly useful in infrequent voiding.

Hellström et al. (9), studying the micturition habits of 3556 7-year-old children, found that the frequency of micturition was three to seven times per day among those without symptoms of bladder disturbance and with no previous urinary tract infection.

Esperanca and Gerrard (10) determined urinary frequency in 297 normal children aged 4–14 years. The average frequency for 4-year-olds was 5.3 micturitions, whereas for 12-year-olds it was 4.8 voidings.

Bower et al. (11) constructed nomograms for mean maximum voided volume, mean voided volume, and mean minimum voided volume for specific age groups using data obtained from 322 incontinent children, aged 6–11 years, who completed a 2-day frequency–volume chart. They noted a wide variation of all voided volumes, very much as Mattsson and Lindström did in normal children (12). Because of this, frequency–volume charts alone seem to be an unsuitable screening tool for children.

2. Females

Most of the published data on frequency–volume charts were obtained in women. Several authors (3,4,13–15) established normal values for healthy females. Comparison of these data is given in Table 3.

Only Saito et al. (14), and Kassis and Schick (4) analyzed diurnal and nocturnal data separately. This appears important, because nighttime diuresis may exceed daytime diuresis and be responsible for nocturia, especially in the elderly.

According to Saito et al. (14) an increase in urine volume during the night can be induced by three physiological events, all related to aging: 1) the circadian rhythm of antidiuretic hormone, the renin–angiotensin–aldosterone system or atrial natriuretic hormone secretion may be abnormal (16); 2) the glomerular filtration rate or renal plasma flow may be altered because of a reduction in the concentrating ability of the distal tubules; and, finally, 3) an impaired cardiovascular system may not be able to supply sufficient amounts of blood to the kidneys during waking hours, creating edema of the lower extremities which become immobilized in the supine position. The calculated ratio of night over day diuresis can draw attention to one of these phenomena, which is important to recognize, because its logical consequence, nocturia, has nothing to do with a vesicourethral pathology (such as outflow obstruction, unstable bladder function, and such).

Table 3 Data Obtained from Frequency–Volume Charts of Normal Females

	Boedker et al. (15) ($n = 123$)	Larsson and Victor (13) ($n = 151$)	Siltberg et al. (3) ($n = 151$)	Saito et al.[a] (14) ($n = 20$)	Kassis and Schick (4) ($n = 33$)
Mean voided volume (day) in mL		250 (± 79)	240	179	237 (± 67)
Mean voided volume (night) in mL				230	379 (± 132)
Mean frequency (day)				6.8	5.63 (± 1.26)
Mean frequency (night)	5.7	5.8 (± 1.41)	5.5	0.5	0.08 (± 0.16)
Diuresis in mL/min (day)					1.11 (± 0.35)
Diuresis in mL/min (night)					0.84 (± 0.27)
Excreta in mL (day)				1149	1,005 (± 497)
Excreta in mL (night)				234	409 (± 130)
Diuresis/24 hr in mL	1350	1430 (± 487)	1350	1272	1473 (± 386)
Night diuresis					
Day diuresis					0.81 (± 0.30)
Functional capacity in mL		460 (± 174)	450		

[a]Also includes normal males.

3. Males

No data were found in the literature concerning reference values for frequency–volume charts in males. A study by Saito et al. (14) included males and females, but did not separate them into two subgroups. One reason for this might be the difficulty in defining the clinical characteristics of a normal male. These probably change with age, so that normal parameters should be established for different age groups in males.

B. Duration of the Chart

No clear guidelines can be found in the literature indicating the minimum number of days necessary to maintain a diary to furnish reliable data. Abrams (17) recommends a 7-day chart, Barnick and Cardozo (18) a 5-day chart, Sommer et al. (19) a 3-day chart, and Larsson and Victor (13) a 48-hr chart.

Barnick and Cardozo (18) were the only authors to compare a 5-day chart with a 1-day chart in a group of 150 women attending a urodynamic clinic. They found a significant correlation between the two sets of results with $p < 0.0001$.

Wyman et al. (20) studied a 2-week diary in 55 incontinent women, and compared the first week with the second week. They concluded that a 1-week diary is sufficient to assess the frequency of micturition and incontinence episodes. The 7-day diary can consequently be considered as the gold standard for voiding diaries.

C. The Way We Proceed

At our institution, patients are invited to fill out a 7-day frequency–volume chart, in which diurnal and nocturnal voidings are clearly separated (Fig. 1). The patient is asked to register the time and the volume of each voiding as well as the time of each incontinence episode. When, for some reason, the patient is unable to measure voided volume, he or she notes only the time, and puts an "X" instead of the volume. Volume can be expressed in millileters (mL) or in fluid ounces (fl oz), but should be uniform throughout the chart. The back of the chart (Fig. 2) offers simple instructions on how it should be completed with examples for the patient to consult.

Over 95% of patients fill out the chart correctly. We initially explain the use of the chart to every patient. With time, written instructions prove clear enough to forego verbal explanations. The chart can be sent out by mail even before the patient comes to the office, so that he or she will arrive for his or her first visit with complete frequency–volume information.

D. The Frequency–Volume Chart as a Diagnostic Tool

Several authors have explored the possibility of using the frequency–volume chart as a diagnostic tool.

Larsson et al. (21) analyzed the frequency–volume chart in detrusor instability, compared it with a group of healthy women, and related it to cystometric findings, in an attempt to evaluate the quantitative aspects of motor urgency incontinence. The chart was filled out for 7 days, but only 2-day periods were evaluated. None of the parameters of the frequency–volume chart (frequency of micturition, mean voided volume, largest single voided volume, and variability in voided volumes) were useful in differentiating between motor urgency and normal voiding habits. An adequate correlation was not found between any of the data from the frequency–volume chart and the quantitative cystometry data (first desire

Fill out this voiding calendar precisely for 7 consecutive days.

Turn in your completed calendar when you present yourself for cystoscopy (bladder examination).

To fill in the calendar :

1) Note the time and quantity of your micturition (passing water).

2) If unable to measure the quantity of your micturition (away from home), note only the time when voiding occurred.

3) If you lose urine (wet yourself, incontinent), note the time followed by the letters U.I.

4) Day means when you are awake, night means when you are woken from sleep by the desire to void.

Example:

Day	Time / Volume (day) (oz or mL)		Time / Volume (night) (oz or mL)
1	7:00 AM / 200 mL 10:00 AM / 150 mL 1:30 PM / 320 mL 5:00 PM / X 8:45 PM/U.I.		3:00 AM / 280 mL
	At 5:00 PM you were in a store You lost urine or measurement was impossible. at 8:45 PM.		

Figure 2   Explanations and examples for filling out the chart.

to void, bladder volume at first unstable contraction, bladder capacity, and bladder volume at first leakage). The authors concluded that frequency–volume charts cannot aid in differential diagnosis, but that mean voided volume represents a good measure of the severity of detrusor instability symptoms.

Larsson and Victor (22) compared the frequency–volume charts of 81 genuine stress incontinent patients with those of 151 asymptomatic women. Interestingly, all four parameters (total voided volume, frequency, largest single voided volume, and variability of voided volumes) differed statistically between the two groups; however, because of marked overlapping between the two populations, the frequency–volume chart became an uncertain diagnostic tool.

Fink et al. (23) compared the 24-hr frequency–volume chart in genuine stress incontinent and urge incontinent women. When applying logistic regression to these two groups, the frequency of micturition during nighttime was the parameter that best discriminated between these medical conditions. Mean voided volume (over the 24-hr period) showed the highest differentiating power (p < 0.0001), but the large overlap between populations limited the value of the frequency–volume chart for differential diagnostic purposes.

Recently, Siltberg et al. (3) proposed a nomogram on which the frequency of micturition was plotted against the range of voided volumes. According to these authors, this plot could be used to select the level of certainty (with 10% intervals for the probability) of having motor urgency incontinence–stress incontinence. Tincello and Richmond (24) tested this nomogram in 216 patients. For detrusor instability, it had a maximum sensitivity of 52% and a specificity of 70%. For genuine stress incontinence, the sensitivity and specificity were 66 and 65%, respectively. They concluded that formal cystometric evaluation is necessary in incontinent females, because the nomogram does not provide enough diagnostic information.

These observations are not really surprising. It seems simplistic to attempt characterization of such different complex physiopathological entities as continence and voiding with a single parameter, in this case, the frequency–volume chart. Nonetheless, it remains one of many important elements in our understanding of patient symptomatology.

E. Chart Completion

To be reliable, frequency–volume charts must be filled out correctly. In an effort to verify their accuracy when recorded by patients, Palnaes Hansen and Klarskov (25) studied 18 subjects who noted their fluid intake and voided volumes and collected 24-hr urine samples for three consecutive days. They concluded that self-reported frequency–volume chart data were valid and useful for patients with voiding symptoms.

Barnick and Cardozo (18) studied 106 consecutive patients who received a 5-day frequency–volume chart by mail, to be filled out before their physical examination. Only 40% of them completed the chart correctly for the full 5 days.

Robinson et al. (26) compared two 7-day diaries in 278 incontinent women. The first was completed with minimal instructions, the second after receiving extensive instructions. They concluded that a 7-day diary remained a reliable tool to assess urinary symptoms, even if patients received minimal instructions on filling out the chart.

According to our own experience, more than 95% of patients correctly complete the frequency–volume chart without any special verbal instructions. The fact that we allow patients to use milliliters or fluid ounces for volume measurement is probably helpful, because older people are less familiar with the metric system. Bailey et al. (27) presented results similar to our own, with most patients completing the chart correctly before their first visit.

F. Interpretation of Frequency–Volume Charts

In our department, every frequency–volume chart filled out by a patient is analyzed by the afore described computer program. The most important parameters in the clinical setting are the frequency of micturition (day and night), 24-hr urinary output, the ratio of night diuresis (in mL/sec) to daytime diuresis (in mL/sec), and mean voided volume (day and night).

Table 4 Increased 24-hr Urinary Output (for explanations, see text)

No. of days analyzed: 7
No. of incontinence episodes: 0
No. of micturitions without recorded volume: 0 (0%)

		Patient's data	Normal	± 1SD	Z-value
Day:	Mean voided volume (mL)	143	237	67	(1.41)
	Frequency	17.0	5.63	1.26	9.02
	Diuresis (mL/min)	238	1.11	0.35	3.63
	Corrected diuresis (mL/min)	238	1.11	0.35	3.63
	Interval between micturitions (min)	60	222	60	(2.70)
	Output (mL)	2286	1005	497	2.58
	Corrected output (mL)	2286	1005	497	2.58
Night:	Mean voided volume (mL)	186	379	132	(1.46)
	Frequency	2.14	0.08	0.16	12.89
	Diuresis (mL/min)	122	0.84	0.27	1.41
	Corrected diuresis (mL/min)	122	0.84	0.27	1.41
	Interval between micturitions (min)	153	454	50	(6.03)
	Output (mL)	586	409	130	1.36
	Corrected output (mL)	586	409	130	1.36
Output/24 hr (mL)		2871	1473	386	3.62
Corrected output/24 hr (mL)		2871	1473	386	3.62
Diuresis ratio (night/day)		0.51	0.81	0.30	(0.99)

1. Increased 24-Hour Urinary Output

This is usually seen in patients with unbalanced diabetes or simple potomania. Table 4 illustrates the voiding diary of a 60-year-old diabetic man. His urinary output was almost double the normal volume. Coupled with a decrease in diurnal and nocturnal mean voided volumes, this led to increased urinary frequency, which was his main complaint. It should be noted that nocturia was not the consequence of nocturnal polyuria, because the nocturnal/diurnal diuresis ratio was not increased (0.51). Further investigation was necessary to explain the low mean voided volumes.

2. Increased Frequency

Increased urinary frequency may have several causes. If exclusively diurnal, it is often psychogenic. Table 5 gives an example of an 81-year-old woman presenting a significant rise in diurnal and nocturnal frequency. Her symptom could not be attributed to increased 24-hr urinary output (which was within normal limits), nor to nocturnal polyuria, because the nocturnal/diurnal diuresis ratio was only slightly elevated (1:11) and was not high enough to explain this degree of nocturia (3.43 micturitions). Because of a significant decrease in mean voided volume, she had an increased frequency. Urodynamic studies revealed uninhibited contractions during the filling phase, with a small cystometric capacity, but a normally compliant bladder wall. This confirmed the diagnosis that an unstable bladder was responsible for her decreased mean voided volume.

Another example of increased frequency is presented in Table 6. This 67-year-old man complained of a weak stream, significant nocturia, and voiding every 2 hr during the day. Urinalysis was normal. His frequency–volume chart indicated more severe pollakiuria

Table 5 Increased Frequency (for explanations, see text)

No. of days analyzed: 7
No. of incontinence episodes: 0
No. of micturitions without recorded volume: 0 (0%)

		Patient's data	Normal	± 1SD	Z-value
Day:	Mean voided volume (mL)	143	237	67	(1.41)
	Frequency	15.43	5.63	1.26	9.02
	Diuresis (mL/min)	1.00	1.11	0.35	3.63
	Corrected diuresis (mL/min)	1.00	1.11	0.35	3.63
	Interval between micturitions (min)	143	222	60	(2.70)
	Output (mL)	959	1005	497	2.58
	Corrected output (mL)	959	1005	497	2.58
Night:	Mean voided volume (mL)	195	379	132	(1.46)
	Frequency	3.43	0.08	0.16	12.89
	Diuresis (mL/min)	1.01	0.84	0.27	1.41
	Corrected diuresis (mL/min)	1.01	0.84	0.27	1.41
	Interval between micturitions (min)	177	454	50	(6.03)
	Output (mL)	529	409	130	1.36
	Corrected output (mL)	529	409	130	1.36
Output/24 hr (mL)		1488	1473	386	3.62
Corrected output/24 hr (mL)		1488	1473	386	3.62
Diuresis ratio (night/day)		1.11	0.81	0.30	(0.99)

Table 6 Increased Frequency (for explanations, see text)

No. of days analyzed: 7
No. of incontinence episodes: 0
No. of micturitions without recorded volume: 7 (5.6%)

		Patient's data	Normal	± 1SD	Z-value
Day:	Mean voided volume (mL)	95	237	67	(2.11)
	Frequency	12.17	5.63	1.26	5.19
	Diuresis (mL/min)	1.03	1.11	0.35	(0.24)
	Corrected diuresis (mL/min)	1.11	1.11	0.35	0.00
	Interval between micturitions (min)	93	222	60	(2.15)
	Output (mL)	986	1005	497	(0.04)
	Corrected output (mL)	1065	1005	497	0.12
Night:	Mean voided volume (mL)	217	379	132	(1.23)
	Frequency	5.50	0.08	0.16	33.88
	Diuresis (mL/min)	2.94	0.84	0.27	7.77
	Corrected diuresis (mL/min)	2.94	0.84	0.27	7.77
	Interval between micturitions (min)	74	454	50	(7.60)
	Output (mL)	1410	409	130	7.70
	Corrected output (mL)	1410	409	130	7.70
Output/24 hr (mL)		2396	1473	386	2.39
Corrected output/24 hr (mL)		2475	1473	386	2.60
Diuresis ratio (night/day)		2.86	0.81	0.30	6.84

than that reported by the patient. Increased frequency had several causes in this case: (1) polyuria (2475 mL/24 hr); (2) nocturnal polyuria (night/day diuresis ratio of 2.86); and (3) decreased mean voided volumes (day: 95 mL; night: 217 mL). The increased day time frequency, however, could not be explained by the daily diuresis, which was normal (1065 mL), but rather by decreased diurnal mean voided volume (95 mL). Urodynamic studies later revealed an unstable bladder as the cause of this decreased mean voided volume.

3. Nocturnal Polyuria

Causes of nocturnal polyuria have been described in the foregoing. The frequency–volume chart of a 53-year-old woman showed a significant increase of 24-hr diuresis (2681 mL). This increase, however, was almost exclusively nocturnal (1500 mL), and her night/day ratio was 2.65 (Table 7). Nocturnal frequency was somewhat less than expected, with this major increase in nocturnal diuresis being tempered to some extent by an elevation of mean voided volume during the night (525 mL). This patient showed a stable bladder on urodynamic investigation.

These few examples demonstrate the usefulness of the frequency–volume chart in the routine evaluation of LUTS patients. They also illustrate the value of computer-analyzed reports in extracting maximum information from the patient's voiding charts and demonstrate the need for other techniques, such as urodynamic study, to explain the patient's clinical complaints.

Table 7 Nocturnal Polyuria (for explanations, see text)

No. of days analyzed: 7
No. of incontinence episodes: 7
No. of micturitions without recorded volume: 1 (2.27%)

		Patient's data	Normal	± 1SD	Z-value
Day:	Mean voided volume (mL)	344	237	67	1.60
	Frequency	4.43	5.63	1.26	(0.95)
	Diuresis (mL/min)	1.18	1.11	0.35	0.20
	Corrected diuresis (mL/min)	1.23	1.11	0.35	0.34
	Interval between micturitions (min)	292	222	60	1.17
	Output (mL)	1132	1005	497	0.26
	Corrected output (mL)	1181	1005	497	0.35
Night:	Mean voided volume (mL)	525	379	132	1.11
	Frequency	1.86	0.08	0.16	11.11
	Diuresis (mL/min)	3.13	0.84	0.27	8.47
	Corrected diuresis (mL/min)	3.13	0.84	0.27	8.47
	Interval between micturitions (min)	1.68	454	50	(5.72)
	Output (mL)	1500	409	130	8.39
	Corrected output (mL)	1500	409	130	8.39
Output/24 hr (mL)		2632	1473	386	3.00
Corrected output/24 hr (mL)		2681	1473	386	3.13
Diuresis ratio (night/day)		2.65	0.81	0.30	6.14

V. CONCLUSIONS

This overview of the published literature on voiding diaries as well as our own experience leads us to some conclusions:

Frequency–volume charts are an invaluable and indispensable tool in the investigation of LUTS patients and in understanding their symptoms. Interpretation of the results is greatly simplified by a simple computer program. The commercial unavailability of such software may explain why frequency–volume charts are not more popular.

More research should be done to study voiding diaries in children. Reference values for males are desperately needed:

Although the 7-day diary is currently considered the gold standard, comparative studies are needed to determine the minimum number of days necessary for the frequency–volume chart to be completed and still remain reliable.

The voiding diary is a precious diagnostic tool, but cannot guarantee a precise diagnosis. Because of the complex nature of LUT dysfunction, it has become evident that frequency–volume charts will never replace urodynamic studies.

In addition to their value as a diagnostic tool, frequency–volume charts play an important role in evaluating the success of a surgical intervention (i.e., detrusorectomy for refractory unstable bladder) or during the follow-up of medical therapy.

Urodynamic studies are the gold standard for diagnosing an unstable bladder. Although several attempts have been made to characterize an unstable bladder by number, amplitude, and point of occurrence in relation to bladder volume; urodynamics remains a *qualitative* instrument for diagnostic purposes. Frequency–volume charts provide a *quantitative* measure of unstable bladder behavior, because severity is reflected quantitatively by mean voided volume.

REFERENCES

1. Abrams P, Klevmark B. Frequency–volume charts: an indispensable part of lower urinary tract assessment. Scand J Urol Nephrol Suppl 1996; 179:47–53.
2. McCormack M, Infante–Rivard C, Schick E. Agreement between clinical methods of measurement of urinary frequency and functional bladder capacity. Br J Urol 1992; 69:17–21.
3. Siltberg H, Larsson G, Victor A. Frequency/volume chart: the basic tool for investigating urinary symptoms. Acta Obstet Gynecol Scand 1997; 76(suppl 166):24–27.
4. Kassis A, Schick E. Frequency–volume chart pattern in a healthy female population. Br J Urol 1993; 72:708–710.
5. Duncan RC, Knapp RG, Miller MC III. Introductory Biostatistics for the Health Sciences. New York: John Wiley & Sons, 1977.
6. Mattsson SH. Voiding frequency, volumes and intervals in healthy schoolchildren. Scand J Urol Nephrol 1994; 28:1–11.
7. Bloom DA, Seeley WW, Ritchey ML, McGuire EJ. Toilet habits and continence in children: an opportunity sampling in search of normal parameters. J Urol 1993; 149:1087–1090.
8. Wan J, Kaplinsky R, Greenfield S. Toilet habits of children evaluated for urinary tract infection. J Urol 1995; 154:797–799.
9. Hellström AL, Hanson E, Hansson S, Hjälm$ås K, Judal U. Micturition habits and incontinence in 7-year-old Swedish school entrants. Eur J Pediatr 1990; 149:434–437.
10. Esperanca M, Gerrard JW. Nocturnal enuresis: studies in bladder function in normal children and enuretics. Can Med Ass J 1969; 101:324–327.
11. Bower WF, Moore KH, Adams RD, Shepherd RB. Frequency–volume chart data from incontinent children. Br J Urol 1997; 80:658–662.

12. Mattsson S, Lindström S. Diuresis and voiding pattern in healthy schoolchildren. Br J Urol 1995; 76:783–789.

13. Larsson G, Victor A. Micturition patterns in a healthy female population, studied with a frequency/volume chart. Scand J Urol Nephrol Suppl 1988; 114:53–57.

14. Saito M, Kondo A, Kato T, Yamada Y. Frequency–volume charts: comparison of frequency between elderly and adult patients. Br J Urol 1993; 72:318–341.

15. Boedker A, Lendorf A, H–Nielsen A, Ghahn B. Micturition pattern assessed by the frequency/volume chart in a healthy population of men and women. Neurourol Urodynam 1989; 8:421–422.

16. Matthiesen TB, Rittig S, Norgaard JP, Pedersen EB, Djurhuus JC. Nocturnal polyuria and natriuresis in male patients with nocturia and lower urinary tract symptoms. J Urol 1996; 156:1292–1299.

17. Abrams P. Urodynamics. 2nd ed. London: Springer-Verlag 1997.

18. Barnick C, Cardozo L. Unpublished data quoted by Barnick C. In: Cardozo L, ed. Urogynecology. London: Churchill Livingstone 1997:101–107.

19. Sommer P, Bauer T, Nielsen KK, Kristensen ES, Hermann GG, Steven K, Nordling J. Voiding patterns and prevalence of incontinence in women. A questionnaire survey. Br J Urol 1990; 66:12–15.

20. Wyman JF, Choi SC, Harkins SW, Wilson MS, Fantl JA. The urinary diary in evaluation of incontinent women: a test–retest analysis. Obstet Gynecol 1988; 71:812–817.

21. Larsson G, Abrams P, Victor A. The frequency–volume chart in detrusor instability. Neurourol Urodynam 1991; 10:533–543.

22. Larsson G, Victor A. The frequency–volume chart in genuine stress incontinent women. Neurourol Urodynam 1992; 11:23–31.

23. Fink D, Perucchini D, Schaer GN, Haller U. The role of the frequency–volume chart in the differential diagnosis of female urinary incontinence. Acta Obstet Gynecol Scand 1999; 78:254–257.

24. Tincello DG, Richmond DH. The Larsson frequency/volume chart is not a substitute for cystometry in the investigation of women with urinary incontinence. Int Urogynecol J Pelvic Floor Dysfunct 1998; 9:391–396.

25. Palnaes Hansen C, Klarskov P. The accuracy of the frequency–volume chart: comparison of self-reported and measured volumes. Br J Urol 1998; 81:709–711.

26. Robinson D, McClish DK, Wyman JF, Bump RC, Fantl JA. Comparison between urinary diaries completed with and without intensive patient instructions. Neurourol Urodynam 1996; 15:143–148.

27. Bailey R, Shepherd A, Trike B. How much information can be obtained from frequency–volume charts? Neurourol Urodynam 1990; 9:382–385.

19

Detection and Quantification of Urine Loss: The Pad-Weighing Test

ERIK SCHICK and MARTINE JOLIVET-TREMBLAY

*University of Montreal and Maisonneuve–Rosemont Hospital,
Montreal, Quebec, Canada*

I. INTRODUCTION

Urinary incontinence, defined by the International Continence Society (ICS) as involuntary urine loss, is an hygienic and social problem (1). The magnitude of the condition differs from individual to individual. From the urologist's everyday experience, tolerance toward incontinence is wide-ranging. Some patients cannot accept the loss of a few drops of urine which happens only under certain circumstances, whereas others wear diapers for years before seeking medical advice.

Incontinence is not easy to quantify from patient interviews or clinical examination (2). This is the role of the pad-weighing test. It is the best available instrument to document the amount of urine lost. It does not evaluate, however, the effect that a given degree of incontinence has on the patient's quality of life.

The Urodynamic Society recommended use of the pad-weighing test in the pretreatment evaluation of incontinent patients as well as in their posttreatment evaluation at each follow-up visit (3). However, the society did not specify the type of pad test to be used. On the other hand, the Agency for Health Care Policy and Research of the United States Department of Health and Human Services did not mention the pad test for the identification and evaluation of urinary incontinence (4).

II. DISCRIMINATION BETWEEN CONTINENCE AND INCONTINENCE

Before interpreting pad test results, it is important to know the upper limit of weight gain by the pad in normal continent persons. Perineal pads can absorb perspiration, vaginal discharge, and such, even in a perfectly continent patient.

Several authors have analyzed this question (Table 1). In general, the shorter the test duration is, the lower is the extraurinary weight gain. In the protocol described by Hahn and Fall (5), in which the duration of the exercise program is very short, each and every gram gained by the pad is considered urine lost. Continent patients do not show any pad weight gain. On the other hand, Griffiths et al. (6), investigating elderly people for 10 days, considered urinary incontinence only if pad weight gain exceeded 10 g/24 hr.

Most authors estimate that during the 1-hr test the upper limit of pad weight gain in continent subjects is close to 1 g, whereas during a 24-hr test it is between 4 and 10 g, with a limit of 15 g/24 hr. According to these authors, a weight gain of more than 1 g in a single pad or 8 g/24 hr may be considered significant. It should be remembered, however, that weight gains less than these limits do not exclude incontinence, and additional measures may be necessary to confirm the diagnosis (7).

Nygaard and Zmolek (8) analyzed in detail the reproducibility of three similar exercise protocols, their correlation with voided volume and pyridium staining in 14 continent volunteers. The mean pad weight gain during these three sessions was 3.19 g ($\pm$ 3.16 g), with a range of 0.1–12.4 g. Because of the large variation between subjects, they were unable to establish a clear cutoff value separating continence from incontinence. Adding pyridium did not improve the specificity of the test.

III. TYPES OF PAD TESTS

Pad tests can essentially be divided into two categories: qualitative tests and quantitative tests.

Table 1 Discrimination Between Continence and Incontinence

Length of test	Authors	Suggested value for continence	Comments
No time limit	Hahn and Fall (5)	0 g	—
40 min	Martin et al. (46)	< 2 g	(with 75% of cysto-metric capacity)
1 hr	Kroman–Andersen et al. (37)	≤ 1 g	—
	Sutherst et al. (2)	1 g	—
	Versi and Cardozo (47)	< 0.94 g	—
	Ali et al. (42)	< 0.5	—
2 hr	Walsh and Mills (48)	1.2 g ($\pm$ 1.35 g)/2 hr	
24 hr	Mouritzen et al. (44)	<5 g/24 hr	
	Lose et al. (43)	4 g/24 hr	(max: 8 g)
	Versi et al. (41)	7.13 g ($\pm$ 4.32 g)/24 hr	(95% upper confidence level < 15 g)
	Griffiths et al. (6)	≤ 10 g/24 hr	

A. Qualitative Tests

The qualitative test uses a dye to color urine (e.g., phenazopyridine [Pyridium] 200 mg tid). The patient is asked to wear protective pads and change them regularly during normal daily activities. The amount of staining on the pads is a rough estimate of the severity of incontinence (9). This test is particularly useful to document very small amounts of urine loss (which may seriously bother the patient), or when vaginal discharge cannot be distinguished easily from urinary incontinence.

Another approach has been suggested by Mayne and Hilton (10), who compared the distal urethral electrical conductance test (DUEC) with weighted perineal pads and found that the DUEC was very sensitive in detecting leakage (sensitivity = 97%). Janez et al. reported similar observations (11).

B. Quantitative Tests

One of the earliest attempts to quantify urine loss was, interestingly, made with an electric device, the so-called Urilos system, designed by James et al. (12). It consists of a pad impregnated with a dry electrolyte. The addition of urine changes the capacitance of aluminum strip electrodes in the pad in proportion to the amount of urine, thereby giving an estimate of the urine lost. Stanton et al. (13,14) tested the device extensively. They observed problems with reproducibility in different batches. Among 26 women showing symptoms of urinary incontinence, but with a negative stress test, 9 demonstrated leakage. In another group of 30 patients with symptoms of stress incontinence, one-third had a negative clinical stress test, but presented leakage with the Urilos system. Eadie et al. (15) concluded that the system was useful to verify patient histories, although it was difficult to obtain a quantitative measure of urine loss, especially because errors were observed at volumes greater than 50 mL owing to movement up to 35%. Probably because it did not fulfill its initial promise in reliably quantifying urine loss, the device never gained wide acceptance.

A more practical approach to the quantification of urine loss is to weigh perineal pads after various lengths of time during which patients are invited to perform standardized exercises. This has generated a great amount of literature in which authors tested different time intervals, with or without diverse exercise protocols, in an effort to find the best combination of reproducibility, reliability, and practicality.

1. Children

Very few reports are found in the literature on application of the pad test to the pediatric patient population.

Hellström et al. (16) compared a 2-hr pad test on the ward (with standardized activities and fluid provocation) with a 12-hr pad test done at home. Both tests were comparable in the detection of urine loss (68 and 70%, respectively), but frequency increased in about 10% of patients when fluid provocation was included in the home pad test.

Imada et al. (17) studied 23 incontinent children with a 1-hr pad test, as proposed by the ICS (1), and compared the results with an "interval test," during which the pad was applied between three consecutive voidings and then weighed. They concluded that the interval test reflected the clinical symptoms better than the 1-hr pad test. They recommended the former for the objective assessment of urinary incontinence in children.

2. Adults

Several reports on the pad-weighing test have been published in the literature. They differ mainly in the length of time the pad is used. The short ones last 1 hr (2,18–26) or 2 hr (27), and are usually combined with a standardized exercise or activity program, but there can also be no time limit imposed, only an exercise protocol performed (5,28,29). The longer ones last from 12 hr up to 10 days (6,30–34). Several authors have compared tests of different lengths (29–31) or those done in different environments (35).

Exercise Protocol Without a Fixed Time Schedule. The provocative pad test proposed by Hahn and Fall (5) consisted of a series of exercises, with the bladder being filled to half of its cystometric capacity. The test–retest correlation was good ($r = 0.94$). In control groups of clinically continent females, urine loss during this exercise program was 0 g. The test takes about 20 min to complete. It seems to be particularly adapted to stress-incontinent females. Because urge symptoms appear irregularly and in specific situations of daily life for patients with bladder instability, a test of longer duration, for example 24 hr, is more reliable.

   Mayne and Hilton (28), after filling the bladder with 250 mL of normal saline solution, compared a short pad test program with the 1-hr test in the same patient population. They failed to demonstrate any significant difference between the two methods.

   More recently, Miller et al. (29) proposed an even simpler test, the paper towel test, to quantify urine loss related to stress. During three consecutive deep coughs, the authors calculated the amount of urine lost from the wetted area on a tri-folded paper towel maintained on the perineal region. They found this test simple and its test–retest reliability accurate. They recommended its application for losses less than 10 mL, because the towel saturates with volumes exceeding 15 mL.

The 1-Hour Test. The 1-h pad test is the most extensively studied, since it was chosen by the Standardization Committee of the ICS (1).

   The reproducibility and reliability of this test have been investigated by several authors. Klarskov and Hald (21) found the test to be reproducible and reliable when compared with subjective daytime incontinence. Jorgensen et al. (24) attested to its reproducibility, especially when bladder volume at the start of the test and diuresis during the test were taken into consideration ($r = 0.93$; $p < 0.0001$). When the test was performed with a standardized bladder volume, the test–retest results were even better ($r = 0.97$; $p < 0.001$), even if individual variations up to ± 24 g were observed (25).

   Mayne and Hilton (28) suggested performing the test with 250 mL of fluid in the bladder. Lose et al. (22) filled the bladder up to 50% of its cystometric capacity, whereas Kinn and Larsson (36) preferred 75%.

   The sensitivity of the test (i.e., the proportion of patients with incontinence who have a positive result) varies between 58 and 81%. Its positive predictive value (i.e., the probability of a patient with a positive test being incontinent), which is more relevant to clinical practice, is over 90%. The false-negative rate (i.e., incontinent patients with a negative pad test), however, is quite high (19–56.8%) (Table 2).

   It appears that the 1-hr test proposed by the ICS is not optimal, and its reliability is insufficient (37). It can be improved, however, when bladder volume at the beginning and during the test is known and standardized.

Table 2 Short-Term Pad Test

Authors	Sensitivity (%)	False negative rate (%)	PPV (%)	NPV (%)	Comments
Anand et al. (49)	70	30	92	53	Patients with LUTS
	81	19	91	72	Patients with SUI
Janez et al. (50)	—	39.4	—	—	No fixed bladder volume
Cardozo and Versi (51)	68	32	91	48	No fixed bladder volume
Schüssler et al. (52)	—	56.8	—	—	Fixed bladder volume
Jorgensen et al. (24)	68	32	—	—	—
Jorgensen et al. (53)	58	42	—	—	Fixed bladder volume

PPV, positive predictive value; NPV, negative predictive value; LUTS, lower urinary tract symptoms; SUI, stress urinary incontinence.

The 2-Hour Test.   Some authors have suggested extending the test to 2 hr because they felt that its accuracy might be improved. During this test, the patient is asked to drink a given amount of liquid as quickly as possible at the beginning of the first hour to provoke a constant level of diuresis. The pad test itself starts at the second hr and consists of a fixed exercise protocol.

Richmond et al. (27) studied two groups of incontinent patients who were submitted to the same protocol except that the exercise sequence was varied between groups. They found that the order in which the exercises were performed did not influence the overall identification of incontinent patients. They estimated that the optimum length of the test was 2 hr. Haylen et al. (38) arrived at the same conclusion. Eadie et al. (39), however, comparing the 2-hr pad test with the Urilos system, estimated that the former was not reliable.

The 12-Hour Test.   When medium- or long-term pad tests are considered, it is important to ensure that no significant evaporation takes place between the end of the test and the time the pads are weighed. In the evaporation test, the mean weight loss of the pads, placed in a hermetically sealed plastic bag, is 0.2 g (0.1–0.3 g) after 24 hr, irrespective of the water volume in the pad. Mean weight loss after 48 hr and 6 days is 0.4 g (0.2–0.7 g) and 0.8 g (0.5–1.2 g), respectively (40). No difference in weight after 1 week, and less than 5% change in weight after 8 weeks (with the upper 95% confidence limit of less than 10% loss), were observed by Versi et al. (41).

This test has not been analyzed on its own, but compared with the 1-hr test by Ali et al. (42) who found that the 1-hr pad test on the ward was representative of the degree of urinary loss the patient experienced during normal activity. Consequently, a 12-hr extension was not judged necessary.

The 24-Hour Test.   This test was analyzed extensively on its own by Rasmussen et al. (40) and considered to be reproducible when there is only moderate variation in activity and fluid intake. However, with drastically decreased fluid intake or extreme activity, significant variations in urine leakage can be observed. Lose et al. (43) compared this test with the 1-hr test. Among 31 stress or mixed incontinent women, 58% were classified as incontinent with the 1-hr test and 90% with the 24-hr home test. They concluded that it is practical as a screening tool for incontinence, but its reproducibility is too poor to allow its use in scientific studies.

Recently, Versi et al. (41) analyzed the 24- and 48-hr tests. Test–retest analysis showed a strong correlation with coefficients of 0.90 and 0.94, respectively. The reproducibility of the two time schedules was also good, demonstrating no advantage of a longer 48-hr test compared with the 24-hr schedule.

The same observation was made by Mouritzen et al. (44), who compared the 1-, 24-, and 48-hr tests. They concluded that the 1-hr test underestimated the grade of incontinence and correlated less with clinical parameters than the 24-hr test. On the other hand, the 24-hr test was as informative as the 48-hr test, making it unnecessary to prolong the test over 24 hr. Hence, the 24-hr test was confirmed as the test of choice for the diagnosis and quantification of urinary incontinence.

The 48-Hour Test.   The reproducibility of the 48-hr test seems to be good ($r = 0.90$) and comparable with the 1-hr test. However, there was no correlation between these two tests ($r = 0.10$) according to Victor and Åsbrink (45). Ekelund et al. (33) demonstrated that this test can be successfully administered in the patient's home environment, even among elderly women.

3. The Elderly

The elderly group of patients represents a particular challenge to clinicians attempting to quantify urine loss.

There is a high incidence of severe urge incontinence among these patients. Furthermore, some of them have significant cognitive impairment, making their performance of the test difficult. Finally, a number of these patients are unable to perform any kind of previously determined exercise program.

Griffiths et al. (6,30,31) extensively studied the pad test in geriatric populations. They found that physical examination frequently failed to demonstrate leakage in incontinent patients; the patients' subjective reports and the 1-hr pad-weighing test were too unreliable to be useful. In their experience, the 24-hr pad test stood out as a superior method for demonstrating and assessing incontinence.

Combining this noninvasive test with invasive videourodynamics, they characterized the type of urinary incontinence in 100 elderly patients. They showed that the 24-hr test had adequate reproducibility and high sensitivity (88%) for detecting urine loss, which was predominantly nocturnal in urge incontinence. Its amount depended, however, on the previous evening's fluid intake and on nocturia. This suggested that nocturnal toileting and evening fluid restriction could reduce nocturnal incontinence by a small, but useful, amount in older patients with severe urge incontinence.

O'Donnell et al. (34) described a method that allowed the nursing staff to identify, measure, and record incontinence severity while monitoring multiple patients simultaneously. The method, however, has not been tested for its reproducibility and sensitivity.

IV. CONCLUSION

From the clinician's point of view, the pad-weighing test is useful when the amount of urine loss can be an important element in treatment decisions. It is also helpful whether the sensation of dampness the patient is complaining of is urinary in origin or is secondary to excessive sweating or vaginal discharge. In these circumstances, the 1-hr test, or even a shorter one, is quite adequate. In this eventuality, however, the test should be performed with a known volume in the bladder. This will yield practical, useful information to complete the clinical investigation of the patient.

For scientific and research purposes, the 24-hr pad test should be used because it has good reproducibility, it is easy to perform, it is done in the patient's own environment, and it has a better potential to detect and quantify urine loss in urge incontinence than the 1-hr test. It should also be incorporated, together with other outcome measures, in the follow-up of different treatment modalities.

REFERENCES

1. Abrams P, Blaivas JG, Stanton SL, Andersen JT. The standardization of terminology of lower urinary tract function. Scand J Urol Nephrol Suppl 1988; 114:5–19.
2. Sutherst JR, Brown MC, Richmond D. Analysis of the pattern of urine loss in women with incontinence as measured by weighing perineal pads. Br J Urol 1986; 58:273–278.
3. Blaivas JG, Appell RA, Fantl JA, Leach G, McGuire EJ, Resnick NM, Raz S, Wein AJ. Standards of efficacy for evaluation of treatment outcomes in urinary incontinence: recommendations of the Urodynamic Society. Neurourol Urodynam 1997; 16:145–147.
4. Fantl JA, Newman DK, Colling J, et al. Urinary incontinence in adults: acute and chronic management. Clinical Practice Guideline No. 2, 1996 Update. Rockville, MD: Department of Health and Human Services. Public Health Service, Agency for Health Care Policy and Research. AHCPR Publication 96-0682, March 1996.
5. Hahn I, Fall M. Objective quantification of stress urinary incontinence: a short, reproducible, provocative pad-test. Neurourol Urodynam 1981; 10:475–481.
6. Griffiths DJ, McCracken PN, Harrison GM, Gormley EA. Relationship of fluid intake on voluntary micturition and urinary incontinence in geriatric patients. Neurourol Urodynam 1993; 12:1–7.
7. Siltberg H, Victor A, Larsson G. Pad weighing tests, the best way to quantify urine loss in patients with incontinence. Acta Obstet Gynecol Scand Suppl 1997; 166:28–32.
8. Nygaard I, Zmolek G. Exercise pad testing in continent exercisers: reproducibility and correlation with voided volume, pyridium staining and type of exercise. Neurourol Urodynam 1995; 14:125–129.
9. Iselin CE, Webster GD. Office management of female urinary incontinence. Urol Clin North Am 1998; 25:625–645.
10. Mayne CJ, Hilton P. The distal urethral electric conductance test: standardization of method and clinical reliability. Neurourol Urodynam 1988; 7:55–60.
11. Janez J, Rudi Z, Mihelic M, Vrtacnik P, Vodusek DB, Plevnik S. Ambulatory distal urethral electric conductance testing coupled to a modified pad test. Neurourol Urodynam 1993; 12:324–326.
12. James ED, Flack FC, Caldwell KP, Martin MR. Continuous measurement of urine loss and frequency in incontinent patients. Preliminary report. Br J Urol 1971; 43:233–237.
13. Stanton SL. Urilos: the practical detection of urine loss. Am J Obstet Gynecol 1977; 128:461–463.
14. Robinson H, Stanton SL. Detection of urinary incontinence. Br J Obstet Gynaecol 1981; 88:59–61.
15. Eadie AS, Glen ES, Rowan D. The Urilos recording nappy system. Br J Urol 1983; 55:301–303.
16. Hellström AL, Anderson K, Hjälm$ås K, Jodal U. Pad tests in children with incontinence. Scand J Urol Nephrol 1986; 20:47–50.
17. Imada N, Kawauchi A, Tanaka Y, Watanabe H. The objective assessment of urinary incontinence in children. Br J Urol 1998; 81(suppl 3):107–108.
18. Sutherst J, Brown M, Shawer M. Assessing the severity of urinary incontinence in women by weighing perineal pads. Lancet 1981; 1:1128–1129.

19. Murray A, Price R, Sutherst J, Brown M. Measurement of the quantity of urine lost in women by weighing perineal pads. Proceeding International Continence Society, Leiden, 1982:243–244.

20. Wood P, Murray A, Brown M, Sutherst J. Reproducibility of a one hour urine loss test (pad test). Proceeding International Continence Society, Aachen, 1983; II:515–517.

21. Klarskov P, Hald T. Reproducibility and reliability of urinary incontinence assessment with a 60 min test. Scand J Urol Nephrol 1984; 18:293–298.

22. Lose G, Gammelgaard J, Jorgensen TJ. The one-hour pad-weighing test: reproducibility and the correlation between the test result, the start volume in the bladder and the diuresis. Neurourol Urodynam 1986; 5:17–21.

23. Christensen SJ, Colstrup H, Hertz JB, Lenstrup C, Frimodt–Møller C. Inter- and intra-departmental variations of the perineal pad weighing test. Neurourol Urodynam 1986; 5:23–28.

24. Jorgensen L, Lose G, Andersen JT. One-hour pad-weighing test for objective assessment of female urinary incontinence. Obstet Gynecol 1987; 69:39–42.

25. Lose G, Rosenkilde P, Gammelgaard J, Schroeder T. Pad-weighing test performed with standardized bladder volume. Urology 1988; 32:78–80.

26. Donnellan SM, Duncan HJ, MacGregor RJ, Russell JM. Prospective assessment of incontinence after radical retropubic prostatectomy: Objective and subjective analysis. Urology 1997; 49:225–230.

27. Richmond DH, Sutherst RJ, Brown MC. Quantification of urine loss by weighing perineal pads. Observations on the exercise regimen. Br J Urol 1987; 59:224–227.

28. Mayne CJ, Hilton P. Short pad test: method and comparison with 1-hour test. Neurourol Urodynam 1988; 7:443–445.

29. Miller J, Ashton–Miller JA, Delancey JOL. The quantitative paper towel test for measuring stress related urine loss. Proceedings International Continence Society, Yokohama, 1997:43–44.

30. Griffiths DJ, McCracken PN, Harrison GM. Incontinence in the elderly: objective demonstration and quantitative assessment. Br J Urol 1991; 67:467–471.

31. Griffiths DJ, McCracken PN, Harrison GM, Gormley EA. Characteristics of urinary incontinence in elderly patients studied by 24-hour monitoring and urodynamic testing. Age Aging 1992; 21:195–201.

32. Ryhammer AM, Laurberg S, Djurhuus JC, Hermann AP. No relationship between subjective assessment of urinary incontinence and pad test weight gain in a random population sample of menopausal women. J Urol 1998; 159:800–803.

33. Ekelund P, Bergstrom H, Milsom I, Norlen L, Rignell S. Quantification of urinary incontinence in elderly women with the 48-hour pad test. Arch Gerontol Geriatr 1988; 7:281–287.

34. O'Donnell PD, Finkbeiner AE, Beck C. Urinary incontinence volume measurement in elderly male inpatients. Urology 1990; 35:499–503.

35. Wilson PD, Mason MV, Herbison GP, Sutherst JR. Evaluation of the home pad test for quantifying incontinence. Br J Urol 1989; 64:155–157.

36. Kinn A, Larsson B. Pad test with fixed bladder volume in urinary stress incontinence. Acta Obstet Gynecol Scand 1987; 66:369–372.

37. Kroman–Andersen B, Jakobsen H, Thorup–Andersen J. Pad-weighing tests: a literature survey on test accuracy and reproducibility. Neurourol Urodynam 1989; 8:237–242.

38. Haylen BT, Fraser MI, Sutherst JR. Diuretic response to fluid load in women with urinary incontinence: optimum duration of pad test. Br J Urol 1988; 62:331–333.

39. Eadie AS, Glen ES, Rowan D. Assessment of urinary loss over a two-hour test period: a comparison between Urilos recording nappy system and the weighed perineal pad method. Proc ICSW, Innsbruck, 1984:94–95.

40. Rasmussen A, Mouritzen L, Dalgaard A, Frimond-Møller C. Twenty-four hour pad weighing test: reproducibility and dependency of activity level and fluid intake. Neurourol Urodynam 1994; 13:261–265.

41. Versi E, Orrego G, Hardy E, Seddon G, Smith P, Anand D. Evaluation of the home pad test in the investigation of female urinary incontinence. Br J Obstet Gynaecol 1996; 103:162–167.

42. Ali K, Murray A, Sutherst J, Brown M. Perineal pad weighing test: comparison of one hour ward pad test with twelve hour home pad test. Proceeding International Continence Society, Aachen, 1983; I:380–382.

43. Lose G, Jorgensen L, Thunedborg P. 24-Hour home pad weighing test versus 1-hour ward test in the assessment of mild stress incontinence. Acta Obstet Gynecol Scand 1989; 68:211–215.

44. Mouritzen L, Berild G, Hertz J. Comparison of different methods for quantification of urinary leakage in incontinent women. Neurourol Urodynam 1989; 8:579–587.

45. Victor A, Åsbrink AS. A simple 48-hour test for quantification of urinary incontinence. Proceeding International Continence Society, London, 1985:507–508.

46. Martin A, Halaska M, Voigt R. Our experience with modified pad weighing test. Proceeding International Continence Society, Halifax, 1992:233–234.

47. Versi E, Cardozo L. One hour single pad test as a simple screening procedure. Proceeding International Continence Society, Innsbruck, 1984:92–93.

48. Walsh JB, Mills GL. Measurement of urinary loss in elderly incontinent patients. A simple and accurate method. Lancet 1981; 1:1130–1131.

49. Anand D, Versi E, Cardozo L. The predictive value of the pad test. Proceeding International Continence Society, London, 1985:290–291.

50. Janez J, Plevnik S, Vrtacnik P. Short pad test versus ICS pad test. Proceeding International Continence Society, London, 1985:386–387.

51. Cardozo L, Versi E. The use of a pad test to improve diagnostic accuracy. Proceeding International Continence Society, Boston, 1986:367–369.

52. Schüessler B, Hesse U, Horn J, Lentsch P. Comparison of two clinical methods for quantification of stress urinary incontinence. Proceeding International Continence Society, Boston, 1986: 563–565.

53. Jorgensen L, Lose G, Thunedborg P. Diagnosis of mild stress incontinence in females: 24-hour home pad weighing test versus the 1-hour ward test. Neurourol Urodynam 1987: 6:165–166.

20

Uroflowmetry and Postvoid Residual

JERZY B. GAJEWSKI

Dalhousie University, Halifax, Nova Scotia, Canada

MOSTAFA E. ABDELMAGID

Al-Azhar University, Cairo, Egypt

I. INTRODUCTION

Uroflowmetry is a graphic depiction (curve) of urinary flow through the urethra. The urine flow curve is a velocity plot of voided urine against time. The urine stream is affected by voiding pressure and bladder outlet resistance. Therefore, uroflowmetry evaluates the interaction between urinary bladder contraction strength and bladder outlet resistance. It is a preliminary, noninvasive screening procedure for the investigation of patients with voiding dysfunction, for the assessment of progression of the disease, and for evaluation of the results of treatment. It is a reliable tool to quantify and graphically depict urinary flow. It can also be performed as part of a full urodynamics study.

The first observations on urinary flow were recorded by Guiteras in 1912 (1). Normal stream projection was noted for a distance of 0.91–1.5 m (3–5 ft). Schwartz and Brenner (2) quantified the urine stream by measuring its greatest horizontal distance (i.e., "voiding" or "cast" distance). A decrease to one-half or one-third of previous values was an indication for surgery (3). Some urologists (4) have suggested measuring the height of a vertical stream of urine, the total voiding time, or the time taken to fill a 100-mL container as an estimate of the urine flow rate.

The first urine flowmeter was developed by Rehfisch in 1897 (5). A urine-collecting chamber was connected to Marey's tambour, and flow was plotted on a kymograph (6). Drake (7) and Kaufman (8) invented a uroflowmeter that calculated the weight of voided urine. Von Garrelt (9) applied an electronic pressure transducer to record urine flow. In

1963, Cardus et al. (10) designed the electromagnetic uroflowmeter. Recently, microprocessor technology delivered different types of uroflometers with the capability of computing different flow measurements.

II. TECHNIQUES

Uroflow is best performed in private and in the patient's accustomed position. Patients should be familiar with the apparatus and have clear instructions about how it works. Multiple recording is indicated if any doubt exists about the accuracy of the procedure (4). Comparison of 23 males and 27 females in a hospital setting versus the physician's office showed that male patients voided with a significantly lower Q_{max} in the hospital urodynamic laboratory than in the office: 9.2 versus 14.2 mL/sec (11).

Uroflowmetry should be performed without previous catheterization, especially in men. In women, there seems to be no difference between uroflow recorded without versus with catheterization (12). Uroflow examination should be completed by measurement of postvoid residual (PVR), which can be done by invasive or noninvasive techniques. The invasive technique includes in-and-out catheterization with endoscopy. When catheterization is used for PVR measurements, complete drainage of the bladder should be ensured to account for any urine from ureter reflex or bladder diverticulum (13). The catheter should be slowly withdrawn with intermittent twisting and application of suprapubic pressure.

Noninvasive methods of PVR measurements can utilize lower abdominal ultrasound or radioisotope study. Isotope investigations for PVR measurements were introduced before the era of ultrasound (14) and are now occasionally used in children. Lower abdominal ultrasound is a simple, noninvasive technique, but very expensive. PVR calculations are based on several different volume formulas, employing transverse and longitudinal ultrasound bladder images, with a standard error ranging from 12.9 to 20.0 (15–19). All formulas are equally accurate for assessing PVR (20,21). Portable devices available for PVR measurement are cheaper, but less accurate (22). In 100 measurements, the mean absolute error of the scanner was 52 mL.

III. EQUIPMENT

The uroflowmeter consists of a flow transducer and a recording device that plots the volume of voided urine against time. There are several different types of transducers, and some have only historical significance. Volume transducers are used for fractionated measurement of volume voided in calibrated tubes at fixed intervals (23). Capacitance (dipstick) transducers on two metal plates attached to a plastic stick immersed in samples of urine conduct electricity across the capacitor. Changes in capacitance reflect alterations in voided volume (24). The passage of electrolytes in the urinary stream through a magnetic field induces an electric current (10) that can be measured by an electromagnetic transducer. An air displacement uroflowmeter measures the amount of air displaced from a container in which the urine is collected. The amount of power needed to keep the wire at 82°C (180°F) is proportional to urine flow (25).

The most widely used are weight, pressure, and spin transducers. The weight transducer was invented by Drake (7) and developed further by Kaufman (8). The patient voided into a container suspended on a spring. The increasing weight of the container stretched the spring for kymograph recording. This transducer was not sensitive to a flow rate less than 10 mL/sec or to voided volume less than 150 mL. Von Garrelt (9) placed an electronic pressure transducer at the bottom of a container into which the patient voided, and connected it to a photokymograph. Changes in urine flow were measured by recording its hydrostatic pressure. In a spinning disk transducer, a servomotor spins a plastic disk at a constant speed. The urine falling onto the disk decelerates it and the electrical energy needed by the motor to keep it rotating at constant speed is proportional to the flow rate. This is an accurate and sensitive method that can detect both low flow rate and interrupted flow. However, the response is conditioned by the site of impact of the jet stream on the disk (26). More futuristic designs utilize spectrometry (27), radioisotopes (28), and audiorecording (29).

IV. MEASUREMENTS

Uroflow variables include voided volume (V_{comp}), flow time (TQ), maximum flow rate (Q_{max}), and average flow rate (Q_{ave}). V_{comp} (mL) is the amount of urine recorded during flow measurements; TQ is the time over which measurable flow actually occurs; Q_{max} (mL/sec) is maximum flow recorded at any time; and Q_{ave} (mL/sec) is V_{comp} divided by TQ. According to the International Continence Society (ICS)(30), PVR measurement is the essential part of the uroflow report, which should contain V_{comp}/Q_{max}/PVR. PVR is the volume of urine in the bladder immediately after voiding. Occasionally, it can be expressed as a percentage of bladder capacity.

The uroflow report should also include some specifications for the technique, as recommended by the ICS (30):

1. Patient position (supine, sitting, or standing)
2. Mode of bladder filling
    a. By diuresis—either spontaneous or forced (specify the regimen)
    b. By catheter—transurethral or suprapubic (state the filling rate)
    c. Fluid temperature
3. The measuring equipment
4. A solitary procedure or combined with complete urodynamic study
5. Patient age and sex.

The shape of the uroflow curve, although defined by the Standardization Committee of the ICS (30) as either continuous or intermittent, has limited diagnostic application.

A. The Nomenclature of Continuous Flow

Voided volume (V_{comp}) is the total volume expelled by the urethra.
Q_{max} is the maximum measured value of the flow rate (i.e., peak flow).
Q_{ave} is V_{comp} divided by TQ. It is meaningful only if the flow is continuous and without terminal dribbling.
TQ is the time over which measurable flow actually occurs.
Time to maximum flow (TQ_m) is the elapse time from the onset of flow to maximum flow.

B. The Nomenclature of Intermittent Flow

The same parameters use for continuous flow, except for TQ, can also be used with terminal dribbling

TQ is the time intervals between flow episodes or terminal dribbling are disregarded.
Voided time (T_{100}) is the total duration of micturition, including interruptions.

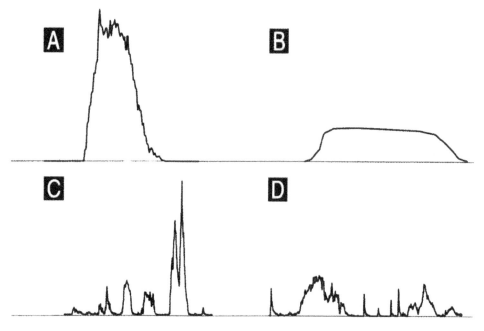

Figure 1 Examples of uroflows: (A) normal flow; (B) urethral stricture; (C) obstruction; (D) voiding with abdominal straining.

V. CLINICAL APPLICATIONS

A. Normal Flow Pattern

A flow curve is normally continuous, bell-shaped, and should rise steeply (Fig. 1). Time to Q_{max} is less than one-third of total time. Q_{ave} should be approximately half of Q_{max} (31). Q_{max} is a good parameter to differentiate between normal and abnormal voiding. However, the lower limit of normal Q_{max} is not well-defined and is still controversial. It depends on age, sex, and V_{comp}. Recommended values for the lower limits of normal Q_{max} in men range between 15 mL/sec (32,33) and 20 mL/sec (8,24,34). In women, it ranges between 12 mL/sec (35) and 20 mL/sec (8). These minimum rates are considered reliable when V_{comp} is 150 mL (9) to 200 mL (24). In children, Q_{max} ranges between 10 mL/sec (age 4–7 years) to 13 mL/sec (up to 14 years) at minimum V_{comp} of 100–150 mL (8,24).

There are practically no upper limits of normal flow. Very high Q_{max} values do not necessarily indicate good detrusor power or normal detrusor–sphincter function. They can be seen in patients with powerful unstable detrusor or following relief of infravesical obstruction (36). We have also observed high Q_{max} values in some patients with stress urinary incontinence.

Urinary flow rates are dependent on voided urine volume in both sexes (7,25). With low voided volume, urine may be expelled before the maximum effect of the bladder can be attained, resulting in low-flow rates (37). In large bladders with an overstretched detrusor muscle, the contractile response can be diminished, eliciting a falsely low Q_{max} (38).

The recommended minimum adequate V_{comp} is 150 mL (8) to 200 mL (38). By increasing V_{comp} more than 200 mL, changes in Q_{max} will be insignificant. The maximum suggested V_{comp} is 450 mL (38,39). The relation between V_{comp} and flow rate is logarithmic. Increased flow is most marked with small volumes (7,40). Because V_{comp} has such an influence on Q_{max}, many authors recommend the use of urine flow nomograms that plot Q_{max} against V_{comp} (28,39,40–42). Nomograms may overcome the necessity of referencing flow rates to a particular V_{comp}. They also allow interpretation of flow rates for volumes as low as 50 mL. Von Garrelt (39) created maximum flow nomograms for normal males. He correlated the results for different age groups from younger than 20 years to older than 60 years. By using the square root of V_{comp}, he developed a volume-independent linear correlation. Backman (41) conducted a similar study on normal women within the same age group. Susset et al. (25) developed a nomogram from a series of 300 curves obtained in 80 normal men and 150 curves obtained in 50 normal women, but without stratification for age. Siroky et al. (43) developed nomograms for both average and maximum flow rates in normal men with ages ranging from 21 to 45 years. They related TQ to initial bladder volume, rather than to V_{comp}. They noted that the use of V_{comp} results in overestimation of the flow rate, which is more significant with low V_{comp} and large residual urine. In comparing a diagnosis of bladder outlet obstruction (BOO) based on pressure–flow studies, the Siroky nomogram showed-false positive results in 22% of patients. The sensitivity and specificity of the nomogram were reported to be 91 and 30%, respectively.

The Bristol nomogram was developed on the basis of 286 voidings in 123 men older than the age of 50 (44). Sensitivity and specificity for the diagnosis of BOO with this nomogram are 54 and 70%, respectively (45). Jorgensen et al. (46) promoted a nomogram for normal men older than 50 years, based on 121 flows from asymptomatic elderly men. They calculated the corrected Q_{max} by dividing the actual Q_{max} by the square root of V_{comp}. This created a linear nomogram for volumes between 50 and 500 mL. Haylen et al. (47) developed a nomogram in centile form from both maximum and average flow rates in relation to both V_{comp} (15–600 mL) and age for males (aged 16–64 years) as well as females (aged 16–63 years). They plotted mean curves for the age group younger than 50 and for those older than 50. Toguri et al. (48) and Szabo and Fegyverneki (49) developed pediatric uroflow nomograms for Q_{ave} and Q_{max} rates based on body surface area, V_{comp} and sex. The overall Q_{ave} for 104 boys was 14 mL/sec and for 96 girls, 16 mL/sec (49).

Urinary flow rate is directly related to the pressure created and maintained within the bladder (32). Differential uroflowmetry has been suggested to distinguish between low-flow rates caused by infravesical obstruction or a weak detrusor, but the technique is not practical and is not widely used (32,50).

In elderly patients, a urinary flow rate of 24 SD below the mean Siroky nomogram has a positive predictive value for obstruction of 0.97 (43). In the same age group, patients with a single normal peak flow rate have a 0.31 probability of uroflow obstruction (51). According to Abrams (52), a maximum flow of less than 10 mL/sec correctly diagnosed an obstruction in 90% of patients with benign prostatic hyperplasia (BPH). Others reported that a Q_{max} less than 15 mL/sec is the cutoff point for predicting a successful outcome (71 vs. 92%) of transurethral resection of the prostate (TURP) (53). PVR has a questionable role as an outcome prognostic factor in patients with bladder outlet obstruction. There is no correlation between PVR and symptoms, prostate volume, and the degree of obstruction (54–56).

Several other factors may influence normal uroflow. The urine flow rate decreases as part of the normal aging process, in both sexes (38,40,41). Von Garrelt (39) noted a reduction of Q_{max} in men of 1 mL/sec for every 10 years of age, and Jorgensen et al. (40), of 4 mL/sec for every 10 years. Haylen et al. (47) found a decline in Q_{max} of 1–1.6 mL/sec per

10 years and an Q_{ave} of 0.6–1 mL/sec per 10 years. In a large Olmsted County study, Girman et al. (57) and Oesterling et al. (42) observed a decrease in Q_{max} of 2 mL/sec per decade of life. Median Q_{max} decreased from 20.3 mL/sec in men 40–44 years old to 11.5 mL/sec in men 75–79 years old. Infants and children have small voided volumes and low-flow rates (8,58,59).

     Differences in urinary flow rates between men and women of comparable ages have been described (24,26,39). Backman (41) reported variances in flow rates between parous and nonparous women, which were not, however, confirmed by Haylen et al. (47). Uroflow measurements antepartum and postpartum showed direct correlation with the V_{comp} and not with the stages of pregnancy (60).

VI. FLOW-RECORDING ARTIFACTS AND PITFALLS

Spikes and artifacts are often seen when the urinary stream moves in relation to the collecting funnel. Tracings show sudden increases and decreases in the flow rate. Several papers have suggested that visual interpretation of the uroflow curve is more accurate than electronic display. Grino et al. (61) observed that, on average, manually read values of Q_{max} were 1.5 mL/sec lower than automatic electronically read values. In 20% of recordings, the difference was 2 mL/sec, and in 9%, 3 mL/sec. Jorgensen et al. (62) obtained similar results with a mean difference of 2.5 mL/sec. In conclusion, the electronic automatic determination of Q_{max} may be misleading and should not replace visual evaluation. New computer-based urodynamic machines incorporate electronic filters for uroflow readings to reduce these artifact errors. The 18-F urethral catheter decreases Q_{max} on average by 0.5 mL/sec during pressure–flow studies (63).

     Significant variability of repeated uroflow recordings has been reported in the same patient (64). Q_{max} readings, corrected for V_{comp} in uroflows 2 weeks apart in the same patient, differed from −14.7 to +13.8 mL/sec. Others found increased Q_{max} values in consecutive voidings and attributed them to the patient's learning effect (65,66). Mean Q_{max} of 164 men with LUTS increased from 9.0 to 14.3 in four consecutive flows (66,67). Similarly, Underberg–Poulsen and Kirkeby (68) noted little diversity in Q_{max} in 459 flows from 13 healthy volunteers (25–40 years of age). Hence, it is preferable to have at least two independent flow rate recordings for the proper interpretation of urinary flow.

     Recording of PVR may not always be accurate. The intraindividual variability of PVR is high and can be influenced by unfamiliar surroundings, an under- or overfilled bladder, and the interval between voidings. PVR variability within 24-hr periods has been reported in men with BPH (69). In elderly patients, within-patient variability may be as high as 128 mL (70).

VII. CONCLUSION

Uroflowmetry is a simple noninvasive urodynamic method. It is widely used as a screening test for patients with voiding dysfunction. Although it is very simple, the results are nonspecific and require cautious interpretation. The flow rate curve is a reproducible method to quantify urinary flow. Urine flow rate is related to bladder pressure, bladder outlet resistance, V_{comp}, as well as residual urine volumes. It is affected by patient age and sex. Therefore, uroflowmetry is not a diagnostic tool, and patients with low or equivocal flow rates should be investigated by a complete pressure–flow study. PVR measurement should be an integral part of uroflowmetry and, if necessary, several measurements should be performed.

As in any urodynamic test, the results of uroflowmetry and PVR alone may be misleading and should always be analyzed in conjunction with the patient's clinical status.

REFERENCES

1. Guiteras R. The diseases of the urinary tract in men and women. In: Urology. New York: D Appleton, 1912:239. Quoted in: Perez LM, Webster GD. The history of urodynamics. Neurourol Urodynam 1992; 11:1–21.
2. Schwartz O, Brenner A. Untersuchungen uber die Physiologie und Pathologie der Blasen-function VIII: Die Dynamik der Blase. Z Urol Chir 1922; 32:32 (quoted in Ref. 21).
3. Smith JC. Urethral resistance to micturition. Br J Urol 1968; 40:125–156.
4. Tanagho EA. Urodynamic studies. In: Tanagho EA, McAnich JW, eds. Smith's General Urology. Connecticut: Appleton & Lang, 1995:514.
5. Rehifisch E. Ueber den Mechanismus des Larnblasenverschlusses und der Harenentleering. Virch Arch 1897; 150:111 (quoted in Ref. 7).
6. Von Garrelt SB. Micturition in the normal male. Acta Chir Scand 1958; 114:197–210.
7. Drake WM. The uroflowmeter: an aid to the study of the lower urinary tract. J Urol 1948; 59:650.
8. Kaufman JI. A new recording uroflowmeter: a simple automatic device for measuring voiding velocity. J Urol 1957; 78–97.
9. Von Garrelt SB. Analysis of micturition. A new method of recording the voiding of the bladder. Acta Chir Scand 1956; 112:326–340.
10. Cardus D, Quesada EM, Scott FB. Use of an electromagnetic flowmeter for urine measurements. J Appl Physiol 1963; 18:845–847.
11. Reid RE, Maliver L, Laor E, Tolia BM, Freed SZ. Office vs. urodynamic flows: is there a difference. Neurourol Urodynam 1986; 5:273–276.
12. Bergman A, Bhatia NN. Uroflowmetry; spontaneus versus instrumented. Am J Obstet Gynecol 1984; 15:788–790.
13. Stoller ML, Millard RJ. The accuracy of catheterized residual urine. J Urol 1989; 141:15–16.
14. Mulrow PJ, Huvos A, Buchanan DL. Measurement of residual urine with I-131-labeled Diodrast. J Lab Clin Med 1961; 57:109–113.
15. Hakenberg OW, Ryall RL, Langlois SL, Marshall VR. The estimation of bladder volume by sonocystography. J Urol 1983; 130:249–251.
16. Poston GJ, Joseph AE, Riddle PR. The accuracy of ultrasound in the measurement of changes in bladder volume. Br J Urol 1983; 55:361–363.
17. Hartnell GG, Kiely EA, Williams G, Gibson, RN. Real-time ultrasound measurement of bladder volume: a comparative study of three methods. Br J Radiol 1987; 60:1063–1065.
18. Rageth JC, Langer K. Ultrasonic assessment of residual urine volume. Urol Res 1982; 10:57–60.
19. Orgaz RE, Gomez AZ, Ramirez CT, Torres JLM. Applications of bladder ultrasonography. I. Bladder content and residual. J Urol 1981; 125:174–176.
20. Griffiths CJ, Murray A, Ramsden PD. Accuracy and repeatibility of bladder volume measurement using ultrasonic imaging. J Urol 1986; 136:808–812.
21. Beacock CJM, Roberts EE, Rees RWM, Buck AC. Ultrasound assessment of residual urine. A quantitive method. Br J Urol 1985; 57:410–413.
22. Ding YY, Sahadevan S, Pang WS, Choo PW. Clinical utility of portable ultrasound scanner in the measurement of residual urine volume. Singapore Med J 1996; 37:365–368.
23. Koontz WW, Rowan GA. A uroflowmetry recording changes in rate each second. Invest Urol 1967; 5:35.
24. Abrams PH, Feneley RCL, Torrens MJ. Urodynamics. Berlin: Springer–Verlag, 1983:28–96.
25. Susset JG, Picker P, Kretz M, Jorest R. Critical evaluation of uroflowmeters and analysis of normal curves. J Urol 1973; 109:874–878.

26. Rowan D, McKenzie AL, McNee SG, Glen ES. A technical and clinical evaluation of the DISA uroflowmeter. Br J Urol 1977; 49:285–291.

27. Zinner NR, Ritter RC, Sterling AM, Harding DC. Drop spectrometer: a non-obstructive, non-interfering instrument for analysing hydrodynamic properties of human urination. J Urol 1969; 101:914–918.

28. Winter CC. Radio-isotope uroflowmetry and bladder residual test. J Urol 1964; 91:103–106.

29. Keitzer WA, Huffman GC. The voiding audiograph: a new voiding test. J Urol 1966; 96:404–410.

30. Abrams P, Blaivas JG, Stanton SL, Andersen JT. Standardisation of terminology of lower urinary tract function. Neurourol Urodynam 1988; 7:403–427.

31. Abrams PH. Urodynamic equipment. In: Mundy AR, Stephenson TP, Wein AJC, eds. Urodynamics: Principles, Practice and Application. New York: Churchill Livingstone, 1984:69–75.

32. Stewart BH. Clinical experience with the uroflowmeter. J Urol 1960; 84:414–419.

33. Holm HH. A uroflowmeter and a method for combined pressure and flow measurement. J Urol 1962; 88:318–321.

34. Drake WM. The uroflowmeter in the study of bladder neck obstruction. JAMA 1954; 156:1079.

35. Massey JA, Abrams PH. Obstructed voiding in the female. Br J Urol 1988; 61:36–39.

36. Stephenson TP, Wein AJ. The interpretation of urodynamics. In: Mundy AR, Stephenson TP, Wein AJ, eds. Urodynamics: Principles, Practice and Application. New York: Churchill Livingstone, 1984:93–115.

37. George NJR. Obstructive and functional abnormalities of the lower tract. In: O'Reilly PH, ed. Obstructive Uropathy. Berlin: Springer–Verlag, 1986:235–275.

38. Drach GW, Layton TN, Binard WJ. Male peak urinary flow rate: relationship to volume voided and age. J Urol 1979; 122:210–214.

39. Von Garrelt B. Intravesical pressure and urinary flow during micturition in normal subjects. Acta Chir Scand 1957; 112:49.

40. Jorgensen JB, Jensen KM, Morgensen P. Longitudinal observations on normal and abnormal voiding in men over the age of 50 years. Br J Urol 1993; 72:413–420.

41. Backman KA. Urinary flow during micturition in normal women. Acta Chir Scand 1965; 130:357.

42. Oesterling JE, Girman CJ, Panser LA, Chute CG, Barrett DM, Guess HA, Lieber MM. Correlation between urinary flow rate, voided volume, and patient age in a community based population. Prog Clin Biol Res 1994; 386:125–139.

43. Siroky MB, Olsson CA, Krane RJ. The flow rate nomogram: I. Development. J Urol 1979; 122:665–668.

44. Kadow C, Howells S, Lewis P, Abrams P. A flow rate nomogram for normal males over the age of 50. Proceedings ICS 15th Annual Meeting, London, 1985:138–139.

45. Lim CS, Reynard J, Abrams P. Flow rate nomograms: their reliability in diagnosing bladder outlet obstruction. Proceedings 24th Annual Meeting ICS, Prague, 1994:74–75.

46. Jorgensen JB, Jensen KME, Bille–Brahe NE, Mogensen P. Uroflowmetry in asymptomatic elderly males. Br J Urol 1986; 58:390–395.

47. Haylen BT, Ashby D, Sutherst JR, Frazer MI, West CR. Maximum and average urine flow rates in normal male and female populations—the Liverpool nomograms. Br J Urol 1989; 64:30–38.

48. Toguri AG, Uchida T, Bee DE. Pediatric uroflow rate nomograms. J Urol 1982; 127:727–731.

49. Szabo L, Fegyverneki S. Maximum and average urine flow rates in normal children—the Miskolc nomograms. Br J Urol 1995; 76:16–20.

50. Shields JR, Daird RA, McDonald DF. Differential uroflowmetry. J Urol 1958; 79:580.

51. Matzkin H, Van der Zwaag R, Chen Y, Patterson LA, Braf Z, Soloway MS. How reliable is a single measurement of urinary flow in the diagnosis of obstruction in benign prostatic hyperplasia? Br J Urol 1993; 72:181–186.

52. Abrams P, Bruskewitz R, de la Rosette J, Griffiths D, Koyanagi T, Nordling J, Park YC, Schafer W, Zimmern P. Pressure–flow studies in BPH. 3rd WHO International Consultation on BPH, Monte Carlo, 1995:299–367.

53. Jensen KM, Jorgensen JB, Mogensen P. Urodynamic in prostatism. I. Prognostic value of uroflowmetry. Scand J Urol Nephrol 1988; 22:109–117.
54. El Din KE, Kiemeney LALM, DeWildt MJAM, Debruyne FMJ, de la Rosette JJMCH. Correlation between uroflowmetry, prostate volume, post void residue and lower urinary tract symptoms as measured by International Prostate Symptom Score. Urology 1996; 48:393–397.
55. Abrams PH, Griffiths DJ. The assessment of prostatic obstruction from urodynamic measurements and from residual urine. Br J Urol 1979; 51:129–134.
56. Barry MJ, Cockett AT, Holtgrewe HL, McConnel JD, Sihelnik SA, Winfield HN. Relationship of symptoms of prostatism to commonly used physiological and anatomical measures of the severity of benign prostatic hyperplasia. J Urol 1993; 150:351–358.
57. Girman CJ, Panser LA, Chute CG, Oesterling JE, Barrett DM, Chen CC, Arrighi HM, Guess HA, Lieber MM. Natural history of prostatism: urinary flow rates in a community-based study. J Urol 1993; 150:887–892.
58. Gierup J. Micturition studies in infants and children. Normal urinary flow. Scand J Urol Nephrol 1970; 4:191–197.
59. Griffiths DJ, Scholtmeijer RJ. Momentum flux measurement in boys. A clinical evaluation. Neurourol Urodynam 1982; 1:173–182.
60. Hong PL, Leong M, Seltzer V. Uroflowmetric observations in pregnancy. Neurourol Urodynam 1988; 7:61–70.
61. Grino PB, Bruskewitz R, Blaivas JG, Siroky MB, Andersen JT, Cook T, Stoner E. Maximum urinary flow rate by uroflowmetry: automatic or visual interpretation. J Urol 1993; 149:339–341.
62. Jorgensen JB, Mortensen T, Hummelmose T, Sjorslev J. Mechanical versus visual evaluation of urinary flow curves and patterns. Urol Int 1993; 51:15–18.
63. Reynard J, Lim CS, Abrams P. Pressure–flow studies in men: the obstructive effect of a urethral catheter. J Urol 1995; 153:453A.
64. Barry MJ, Girman CJ, O'Leary MP, Walker–Corkery ES, Binkowitz BS, Cockett ATK, Guess HA, BPH Treatment Outcomes Study Group. Using repeated measures of symptom score, uroflowmetry and PSA in the clinical management of prostatic disease. J Urol 1995; 153:99–103.
65. Frimodt–Moller C, Hald T. Clinical urodynamics. Methods and results. Scand J Urol Nephrol, 1972; 6(suppl 15):143–145.
66. Reynard J, Lim C–S, Abrams P. The value of multiple free flow studies in men with lower urinary tract symptoms (LUTS). J Urol 1995; 153:397A.
67. Jensen KM, Jorgensen JB, Mogensen P. Reproducibility of uroflowmetry variables in elderly males. Urol Res 1985; 13:237–239.
68. Poulsen EU, Kirkeby HJ. Home-monitoring of uroflow in normal male adolescents relation between flow-curve, voided volume and time of day. Scan J Urol Nephrol Suppl 1988; 114:58–62.
69. Bruskewitz RC, Iversen P, Madsen PO. Value of post-void residual urine determination in evaluation of prostatism. Urology 1982; 20:602–604.
70. Griffiths DJ, Harrison G, Moore K, McCracken P. Variability of post-void residual urine volume in the elderly. Urol Res 1996; 24:23–26.

21

Urethral Pressure Profile

JERZY B. GAJEWSKI

Dalhousie University, Halifax, Nova Scotia, Canada

I. INTRODUCTION

To maintain continence during the storage phase, occlusive pressure of the urethra, generated by active and passive structures of the urethral wall, should exceed bladder pressure (1,2). Resistence in the urethra drops only during the voiding phase, owing to relaxation of the sphincter, allowing flow to commence. The urethral pressure profile (UPP) was mostly used as a urodynamic test in the past to evaluate competence of the urethra.

The first urethral pressure measurements, using a double-lumen catheter, were reported in 1933 by Denny–Brown and Robertson (3). In 1953, Karlson introduced microtransducers to measure bladder and urethral pressures simultaneously (4). Urethral perfusion pressure was introduced by Olanesco and Streja in 1960 (5). Lapides et al. (6) used an intermittent withdrawal technique with a water column, and published elegant diagrams of normal urethral resistance in men and women. Harrison and Constable (7) added a puller, and Gleason (8), a pump, to the method. Since then, several additional modifications and accessories have been incorporated, but the basic system remains unchanged. The International Continence Society (ICS) published recommended terminology and techniques for this test in 1988 (9).

II. TECHNIQUE

Measurements by UPP can be recorded during the storage (filling) phase when the urethra is empty (resting UPP), during coughing or straining (stress UPP), or during the voiding phase (voiding UPP). The latter has not been used widely.

UPP can be measured in the supine, sitting, or standing position. Intraluminal pressure is recorded by a perfusion catheter with side holes, microtip transducer catheter, or balloon catheter. The classic technique of Brown and Wickham utilizes saline perfusion

(10,11) through a double-lumen catheter with side holes (12,13). The recommended saline perfusion rate is between 2 and 10 mL/min to prevent the catheter holes from being occluded by urethral mucosa. The most acceptable curves are achieved by employing a syringe driver, rather than a peristaltic pump. Perfusion with CO_2 is seldom used and requires a much higher perfusion rate (60–150 mL/min) (14). This perfusion technique gives correct readings only if the urethra seals the fluid chamber almost completely at both ends. In such a case, the fluid pressure measured by the catheter corresponds to the true pressure exerted by the urethral wall. If the seal is insufficient, the UPP results may be incorrect (15). The speed of response to pressure changes of the perfusion catheter is about 34 cm/sec at a perfusion rate of 2 mL/min, too slow for the accurate recording of "stress" events (16). Perfusion catheters require precise balancing, with reference being the level of the center of the bladder. Any change in patient (bladder) position during the test may offset accuracy of the readings because of the water column effect. Liquid-perfused catheters are relatively simple and economical; some of them are disposable. They are not suitable for prolonged recordings because of necessary connections to cumbersome equipment. Perfusion itself may trigger urethral reflexes and cause artifacts (17).

The microtip transducer catheter consists of miniature pressure recorders (one or more) localized at its tip and then some distance from it to allow simultaneous pressure monitoring from different locations in the urethra and bladder (18). Some catheters also have a perfusion channel. Compared with liquid-perfused catheters, tip-transducer catheters are not affected by position (height) of the bladder and are balanced at atmospheric pressure. Tip-transducer catheters do not measure intraluminal pressure, but rather, direct pressure of the urethral wall applied on the transducer itself (19). Microtip-transducer catheters allow rapid pressure changes to be recorded with a frequency response of 2000 Hz (20), making them most suitable for assessing stress UPP. They are also very stable during prolonged recordings. However, they are prone to positional artifacts, are expensive, and require sterilization. They are also very sensitive and break easily when bent or sterilized.

The balloon catheter is either connected to an external transducer (2) or contains a modified tip transducer inside the balloon (21,22). The size of the balloon is approximately 5–10 mm. The balloon catheter measures true hydrostatic pressure exerted by the urethral wall. These catheters are more suitable for recording intraluminal pressure in a fixed location of the urethra, rather than performing formal profilometry. The speed of response to pressure changes (125 cmH$_2$O/sec) is better than with perfusion catheters, but slower than tip transducers. During slow, constant withdrawal, balloons can evoke urethral spasm and artifact reading. A major drawback of the balloon catheter is the necessity of frequent calibration and keeping the tubing free of air bubbles (23).

Catheters between 4F and 10F gauge have shown satisfactory results (24,25). Larger and more rigid catheters will overestimate UPP because of the limited elastic property of the urethra. Tip-transducer techniques have the highest reproducibility rate (26–28).

The UPP shows significant dependence on catheter (actually microtransducer or hole) orientation in the urethra (29). It is significantly higher when the transducer or hole is oriented anteriorly (toward the pubis) with a shorter functional urethral length than when it is oriented posteriorly (27,30). Lateral orientation seems to give optimal results (31). These variations in recording are caused mainly by the weight and stiffness of the catheters (32).

During UPP, the catheter is withdrawn constantly and steadily by a mechanical puller. Speed of withdrawal is synchronized and, in new equipment, computerized with the speed of recording to allow measurements at anatomical distances of the urethra. The optimal withdrawal rate suggested is 7 mm/sec (26). In stress UPP, withdrawal speed is low (1 mm/sec) to allow pressure transmission readings from each 2-mm segment of the urethra. In the fixed position test, measurements are usually taken at the point of maximal urethral pressure to record any pressure fluctuation with time. Continuous recording of urethral pressure at one or more points is called dynamic UPP. It is mainly performed for research purposes to discriminate between smooth and striated sphincter activity of the urethra (33). Sometimes, intermittent withdrawal can be used to measure urethral pressure at different locations. In stress UPP, urethral pressure and bladder pressure are measured simultaneously. Repeated coughs or Valsalva maneuvers are exercised to evoke "stress." In the "normal" urethra, there is adequate pressure transmission from the abdomen to the urethra. This test is difficult to standardize, however, because of difficulty in evoking precise abdominal pressure and uncertainty of accuracy in actual pressure transmission (34,35). Although pressure with Valsalva maneuvers is easier to control, the consistency of pressure transmission with coughing is more reliable (36).

Urethral pressure usually rises with increased bladder volume in normal women, but it falls in patients with stress incontinence (11,37). Bladder capacity at half maximal cystometric capacity is technically acceptable. Patient position has an effect. Urethral pressure increases in continent women in the erect position and decreases in women with stress incontinence (38,39).

III. MEASUREMENTS

Relevant measurements relating to resting UPP include maximal urethral pressure (MUP), maximal urethral closure pressure (MUCP), functional urethral length (Fig. 1), and pressure profile (Fig. 2). In stress UPP, important calculations include the pressure transmission ratio (PTR) and pressure transmission profile. *PTR* is defined as a percentage of the increment in urethral pressure versus the increment in bladder pressure, with stress (Fig. 3).

IV. CLINICAL APPLICATIONS

Many factors influence intraurethral pressure, including smooth and striated sphincter activity, tension of the connective tissue and blood flow through the urethra (24,40). Resting

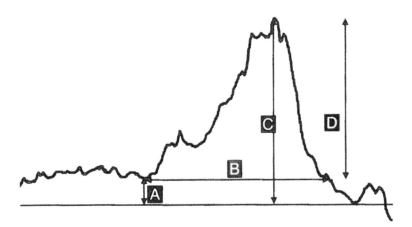

Figure 1 Relevant measures relating to UPP: (A) intravesical pressure; (B) functional profile length; (C) maximum urethral pressure; (D) maximum urethral closure pressure.

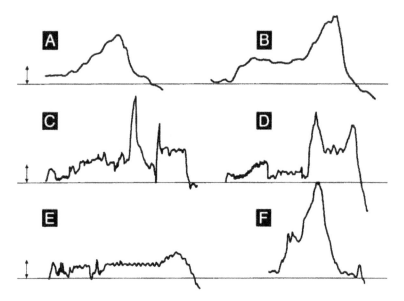

Figure 2   Example of the urethra pressure profiles: (A) female urethral pressure profile (UPP): (B) male UPP; (C) postfascial sling obstruction; (D) meatal obstruction; (E) type III stress urinary incontinence; (F) urethral stenosis.

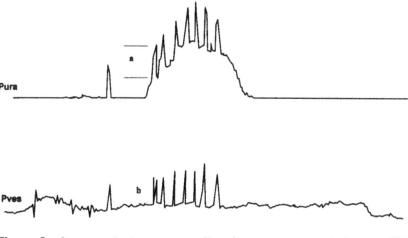

Figure 3   Stress urethral pressure profile. a/b, pressure transmission rate (PTR).

UPP does not necessarily reflect physiological changes that occur during stress. There are no normal values defined for UPP because considerable variations have been reported. Resting MUP declines with age (41). Although MUCP tends to be lower in women with genuine stress incontinence in comparison with healthy subjects, there is significant overlap between the two groups, hampering clinical usefulness of the UPP test (42–45). Also, the severity of stress incontinence correlates more with lower MUCP (46), but this has limited relevance. Because of inter- and intraindividual variations, UPP has limited application as a diagnostic tool (47), but in patients with low preoperative UPP (<20 cmH$_2$O), there is a significantly lower success rate by conventional surgical procedures (48–52). Others (53) have found no significant correlation between low MUCP and conventional surgical failure in patients with mobile urethra. UPP alone, therefore, cannot be a diagnostic tool for intrinsic sphincter deficiency.

In healthy patients, continuous recording of urethral pressure displays variations in MUCP between 10 and 25 cmH$_2$O (54–57). It has been suggested that variation in excess of one-third of MUCP should be considered abnormal (58,59) and defined as unstable urethra (56). The ICS initially clarified unstable urethra as an involuntary fall in urethral pressure in the absence of detrusor activity (60). However, recent revision in ICS standardization recommends further data collection and precise definition (9).

In men, static UPP has been used to assess the length of the prostate as related to possible outlet obstruction (61). There is, however, little correlation between length, size of the prostate, and outlet obstruction. The test was not widely adopted for this reason.

V. SUMMARY

Although widely used in the past, UPP has limited clinical application. UPP evaluation is not necessary for standard investigation of stress incontinence (62–64). The possible clinical value of UPP lies in its extreme low reading, possibly suggesting, but not discriminating, intrinsic sphincter deficiency diagnosis. It may also have some pertinence in research or as a follow-up investigational tool.

REFERENCES

1. Barnes A. The method of evaluating the stress of urinary incontinence. Am J Obstet Gynecol 1940; 40:381.
2. Enhorning G. Simultaneous recording of intravesical and intraurethral pressure. Acta Chirur Scand Suppl 1961; 276:1–68.
3. Denny–Brown D, Robertson EG. On the physiology of micturition. Brain 1948; 56:650.
4. Karlson S. Experimental studies on functioning of the female urinary bladder and urethra. Acta Obstet Gynecol Scand 1953; 32:285–307.
5. Olanesco G, Streja M. La role de la cystosphincerometrie dans l' investigation des troubles de la miction. Acta Urol Belg 1960; 28:77.
6. Lapides J, Ajemian EP, Stewart BH, Breskey BA, Lichtwart JR. Further observations on the kinetics of the urethrovesical sphincter. J Urol 1960; 84:86.
7. Harrison NW, Constable AR. Urethral pressure measurements: a modified technique. Br J Urol 1970; 42:229–233.
8. Gleason DM, Reilly RJ, Bottaccini MR, Pierce MJ. The urethral continence zone and its relation to stress incontinence. J Urol 1974; 112:81–88.
9. Abrams P, Blaivas JG, Stanton SI, Adersen JT. Standardisation of terminology of lower urinary tract function. Neurourol Urodynam 1988; 7:403–427.
10. Abrams PH, Martin S, Griffiths DJ. The measurement and interpretation of urethral pressures obtained by the method of Brown and Whickham. Br J Urol 1978; 50:33–38.
11. Glen ES, Rowan D. Continuous flow cystometry and urethral pressure profile measurement with monitored intravesical pressure: a diagnostic and prognostic investigation. Urol Res 1973; 1: 97–100.
12. Toews HA. Intra-urethral and intra-vesical pressures in normal and stress incontinent women. Obstet Gynecol 1967; 29:613–624.
13. Brown M, Wickham JEA. The urethral pressure profile. Br J Urol 1969; 41:211–217.

14. Raz S, Kaufman JJ. Carbon dioxide urethral pressure profile. J Urol 1976; 115:439–442.
15. Griffiths DJ. Urodynamics: the mechanics and hydrodynamics of the lower urinary tract. Medical Physics Handbook 4. Bristol: Hilger, 1980.
16. Abrams PH, Martin S, Griffiths DJ. The measurement and interpretation of urethral pressure obtained by the method of Brown and Wickham. Br J Urol 1978; 50:33–38.
17. Rossier AB, Fam BA, Dibenedetto M, Sarkarati M. Urodynamics in spinal shock patients. J Urol 1979; 122:783–787.
18. Millar HD, Baker LE. Stable ultraminiature catheter tip pressure transducer. Med Biol Eng 1973; 11:86–89.
19. Hilton P, Stanton S. Urethral pressure measurement by micro-transducer—I: an analysis of variance. In: XIth Annual Meeting of the International Continence Society; Lund, Sweden, 1981: 69.
20. Asmussen M. Urethrocystometry in women [MD]: Lund, Sweden, 1975.
21. Van der Kooi JB, van Wanroy PJA, de Jonge MC, Kornelis JA. Standardization of stress urethral pressure profile measurements with microtransducers. Proceedings 15th Annual Meeting ICS, London, 1985:408–410.
22. Lose G, Colstrup H, Saksager K, Kristensen JK. New probe for measurement of related values of cross-sectional area and pressure in biological tube. Med Biol Eng Comput 1986; 24:488–492.
23. Schmidt RR, Witherow R, Tanago EA. Recording urethral pressure profile: comparison of methods and clinical implications. Urology 1977; 10:390–397.
24. Edwards L, Malvern J. The urethral pressure profile: theoretical considerations and clinical application. Br J Urol 1974; 46:325–335.
25. Harrison N. Urethral pressure profile. Urol Res 1976; 4:95–100.
26. Hilton P. Urethral pressure measurement at rest: an analysis of variance. Neurourol Urodynam 1982; 1:303–311.
27. van Geelen JM, Doesburg WH, Martin CB Jr. Female urethral pressure profile; reproducibility, axal variation and effects of low dose oral contraceptives. J Urol 1984; 131:394–398.
28. Ghonheim M, Rottenbourg J, Fretin J, Susset J. Urethral pressure profile: standardisation of technique and study of reproducibility. Urology 1975; 5:632–637.
29. Hilton P, Stanton S. Urethral pressure measurement by micro-transducer—II: an analysis of rotational variations. In: XI Annual Meeting of the International Continence Society, Lund, Sweden, 1981: 70.
30. Anderson RS, Shepherd AM, Feneley RCL. Microtransducer urethral profile methodology: variations caused by transducer orientation. J Urol 1983; 130:727–728.
31. Teague CT, Merrill DC. Laboratory comparison of urethral profilometry techniques. Urology 1979; 13:221–228.
32. Plevnik S, Janež J, Vrtačnik P, Brown M. Directional differences in urethral pressure recordings: contributions from the stiffness and weight of recording catheter. Neurourol Urodynam 1985; 4:117.–128.
33. Rossier AB, Bushra AF, Lee IY, Sarkarati M. Evans DA. Role of striated and smooth muscle components in the urethral pressure profile in traumatic neurogenic bladder: a neuropharmacological and urodynamic study. Preliminary report. J Urol 1982; 128:529–535.
34. Schick E. Objective assessment of resistance of female urethra to stress. A scale to establish degree of urethral incompetence. Urology 1985; 26:518–526.
35. Cundiff GW, Harriss RI, Theofrastous JP, Bump RC. Pressure transmission ratio reproducibility in stress continent and stress incontinent women. Neururol Urodynam 1997; 16:161–166.
36. Hilton P. Urethral pressure measurement on stress: a comparison of profiles on coughing and straining. Neurourol Urodynam 1983; 2:55–62.
37. Awad SA, Bryniak SR, Lowe PJ, Bruce AW, Twiddy DA. Urethral pressure profile in female stress incontinence. J Urol 1978; 120:475–479.
38. Henriksson L, Ulmsten U, Anderson KE. The effects of changes of posture on the urethral closure pressure in healthy women. Scand J Urol Nephrol 1977; 11:201–206.

39. Henriksson L, Ulmsten U, Anderson KE. The effects of changes in posture on the urethral closure pressure in stress incontinent women. Scand J Urol Nephrol 1977; 11:207–210.
40. Anderson JT, Bradley WE. The urethral closure pressure profile. Br J Urol 1976; 48:341–343.
41. Hammerer P, Michl U, Meyer–Molden Rauer WH, Huland H. Urethral closure pressure changes with age in men. J Urol 1996; 156:1741–1743.
42. Hilton P, Stanton SL. Urethral pressure measurement by micro-transducer: the results in symptom free women and those with genuine stress incontinence. Br J Obstet Gynaecol 1983; 90: 919–933.
43. Henriksson L, Anderson K, Ulmsten U. The urethral pressure profile in continent and stress incontinent women. Scand J Urol Nephrol 1979; 13:5.
44. Meyer S, De Grandi P, Schmidt N, Sanzeni W, Spinosa JP. Urodynamic parameters in patients with slight and severe genuine stress incontinence: is the stress profile useful? Neurourol Urodynam 1994; 13:21–28.
45. Versi E. Discriminant analysis of urethral pressure profilometry data for the diagnosis of genuine stress incontinence. Br J Obstet Gynaecol 1990; 97:251–259.
46. Theofrastous JP, Bump RC, Elser DM, Wyman JF, McClish DK. Correlation of urodynamic measures of urethral resistance with clinical measures of incontinence severity in women with pure genuine stress incontinence. The Continence Program for Women Research Group. Am J Obstet Gynecol 1995; 173:407–412.
47. Swift SE, Rust PF, Ostergard DR. Intrasubject variability of the pressure–transmission ratio in patients with genuine stress incontinence. Int Urogynecol J Pelvic Floor Dysfunct 1996; 7:312–316.
48. Hilton P, Stanton SL. A clinical and urodynamic assessment of the Burch colposuspension in genuine stress incontinence. Int Urogynecol 1996; 7:312–316.
49. Weil A, Reyes H, Bischoff P, Rottenberg RD, Krauer F. Modifications of urethral rest and stress profiles after different types of surgery for urinary stress incontinence. Br J Obstet Gynaecol 1984; 91:46–55.
50. Francis LN, Sand PK, Hamrang K, Ostergard DR. A urodynamic appraisal of success and failure after retropubic urethropexy. J Reprod Med 1987; 32:693–696.
51. Sand PK, Bowen LW, Panganiban R, Ostergard DR. The low pressure urethra as a factor in failed retropubic urthropexy. Obstet Gynecol 1987; 69:399–402.
52. Bowen LW, Sand PK, Ostergard DR, Franti CE. Unsuccessful Burch retropubic urethropexy: a case–controlled urodynamic study. Am J Obstet Gynecol 1989; 160:452–458.
53. Ramon J, Mekras JA, Webster GD. The outcome of transvaginal cystourethropexy in patient with anatomical stress urinary incontinence and outlet weakness. J Urol 1990; 144:106–109.
54. Plevnik S, Janez J. Urethral pressure variations. Urology 1983; 21:207–209.
55. Sorenson S. Urethral pressure variations in healthy and incontinent women. Neurourol Urodynam 1992; 11:549–591.
56. Vereecken RL. Physiological and pathological urethral pressure variations. Urol Int 1996; 57:145–150.
57. Tapp AJ, Cardozo LD, Versi E, Studd JW. The prevalence of variation of resting urethral pressure in women and its association with lower urinary tract function. Br J Urol 1988; 61:314–317.
58. Versi E, Cardozo L. Urethral instability: diagnosis based on variations of the maximum urethral pressure in normal climacteric women. Neurourol Urodynam 1986; 5:535–541.
59. Hilton P. Unstable urethral pressure—toward a more relevant definition. Neurourol Urodynam 1988; 6:411–418.
60. Bates CP, Bradley WE, Glen ES, Melchior H, Rowan D, Sterling AM, Sundin T, Thomas D, Torrens M, Turner–Warwick R, Zinner NR, Hald T. Fourth report on the standardization of terminology of lower urinary tract function. Terminology related to neuromuscular dysfunction of the lower urinary tract. Br J Urol 1981; 53:333–335.
61. Abrams PH. Sphincterometry in the diagnosis of male outflow obstruction. J Urol 1976; 116: 489–492.

62. Blavias JG, Awad SA, Bissada N, Khanna DP, Krane RJ, Wein AJ, Yalla S. Urodynamic procedures: recommendations of the Urodynamic Society I. Procedures that should be available for routine urological practice. Neurourol Urodynam 1982; 1:51–55.
63. Urinary Incontinence Guideline Panel. Urinary incontinence in adults: clinical practice guideline. AHCPR Publication 96-0682. Rockville, MD: Agency for Health Care Policy and Research, Public Health and Human Services, 1996.
64. Report on The Surgical Management of Female Stress Urinary Incontinence. The American Urological Association Female Stress Urinary Incontinence Clinical Guidelines Panel, 1997.

22

Leak Point Pressure

JERZY B. GAJEWSKI

Dalhousie University, Halifax, Nova Scotia, Canada

I. INTRODUCTION

The concept of leak point pressure (LPP), which is the value of detrusor pressure when leakage occurs in the absence of a rise in abdominal pressure, was introduced by McGuire et al. (1) to evaluate the risk of upper tract deterioration in children with myelomeningocele. This test was later adapted to women with stress urinary incontinence (SUI) by using abdominal LPP (ALPP), the value of bladder pressure (P_{ves}) at which leakage occurs in the absence of detrusor contraction (2). If the patient is straining or coughing to provoke leakage, the test is called Valsalva leak point pressure (VLPP) or cough leak point pressure (CLPP), respectively.

II. TECHNIQUE

The patient has to be properly instructed as to how the test will be performed. LPP measurement is usually done during urodynamic testing, after cystometrography with an intraurethral catheter. Some centers recommend recording abdominal pressure with a rectal (3,4) or vaginal catheter (5) to avoid possible interference of the urethral catheter with leakage. Vaginal recording, however, has been shown overall to give significantly lower values than those from the bladder (5). The bladder is filled to 50% (6,7) of cystometric capacity or another constant value set by a particular urodynamic laboratory. The patient is then asked to perform the Valsalva maneuver with a stepwise increase in abdominal pressure. If straining produces no urine leak, the patient is instructed to cough several times with increasing strength (Fig. 1). The lowest bladder or abdominal pressure at which leaks occur is defined as LPP. Some laboratories use visual recording (5,6,8,9), uroflow or videourodynamics (1,10,11), and electric conductance (12–14) to register the presence of leakage. LPP results are reproducible as long as the method of measurement and bladder volumes are kept constant (15,16).

III. CATHETERS

Catheter size significantly affects LPP results (17). Bump et al. (5,18) obtained significantly higher VLPP values with an 8F than with a 3F urethral catheter. Others also reported dependence on caliber (4). VLPP measured by urethral catheter is almost always higher than by rectal catheter, exceeding 20 cmH$_2$O in 50% of cases (19). However, Flood and Liu (20) found that measurements with or without a 10F urethral catheter did not modify VLPP values. A subsequent report from the same group showed that an indwelling 10F urethral catheter is much more likely to affect ALPP measurement in men than in women with intrinsic sphincter deficiency (ISD) (21).

IV. BLADDER VOLUME

Increased bladder volume correlates with decreased VLPP values (22). Theofrastous et al. (7) examined 120 women with genuine SUI, using VLPP measurements at bladder volumes of 100, 200, 300 mL, and maximum cystometric capacity (7). Thirty-three women had leakage starting at a bladder volume of 100 mL; 18 at 200 mL, 19 at 300 mL, and 17 had leakage only at maximum cystometric capacity. They noted that VLPPs at lower volume were significantly higher than at maximum capacity.

Faerber and Vashi (23) compared LPPs determined at 50-mL volume increments, with fluoroscopic criteria of SUI. Women with type I SUI had high LPP which remained high at increasing vesical volumes. Those with type III had low LPP which remained low at increasing vesical volumes. In patients with type II incontinence, initially high LPP decreased significantly at increasing vesical volumes. The optimal bladder volume for LPP testing was 250–300 mL.

Petrou and Kollmorgen (24), however, found no significant difference in VLPP determinations or type of SUI at various bladder volumes (150, 300 mL, and maximal cystometric capacity).

V. POSITION

Examination can be done in a supine, sitting, or standing position. It has been suggested that VLPP in a supine position better assesses ISD (25). Hsu et al. (25) demonstrated that a positive VLPP test is a reliable predictor of IUD, whereas a negative test correlates highly with the absence of IUD. They performed a supine stress test using coughing and Valsalva maneuvers after bladder filling to 200 mL. ISD was diagnosed if ALPP was less than 100 cmH$_2$O. With ALPP measurement, the supine stress test had 93.5% sensitivity, 90.0% specificity, 96.7% positive-predictive value, and 81.8% negative predictive value for detecting ISD diagnosed by videourodynamics. Others also reported a statistically significant relation between low LPP ($\leq$ 60 cmH$_2$O) and a positive supine empty stress test, which had a sensitivity of 79% and a specificity of 62.5% for the detection of low LPP (26).

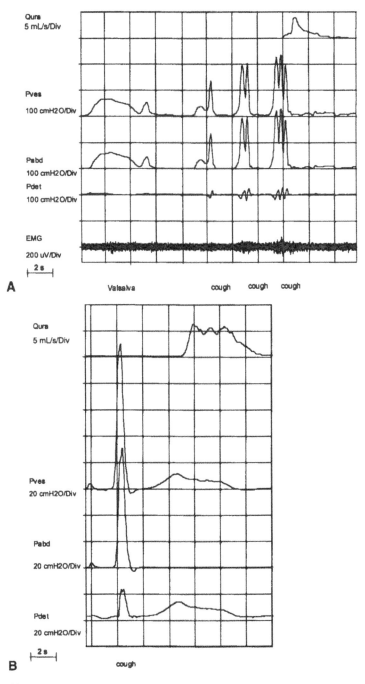

Figure 1 Criteria for positive LPP: (A) positive LPP test; (B) negative LPP test (leak caused by detrusor contraction).

VI. MEASUREMENTS

Several study conditions have to be specified when reporting LPP: the position of the patient, type of LPP, bladder volume in milliliters or percentage of maximal cystometric capacity, location and type of pressure transducer, type of catheter, and provoking maneuvers.

Detrusor LPP is the value of detrusor pressure (P_{det}) at which leakage occurs in the absence of a rise in abdominal pressure. ALPP is the lowest total bladder or abdominal pressure at which urinary leakage occurs during a progressive increase in intra-abdominal pressure by Valsalva maneuvers (VLLP) or coughing (CLPP). LPP can be expressed as an absolute value or as a change in total bladder (vesical) or abdominal pressure from baseline (before straining) to the pressure at which leakage occurs. There is no advantage of one calculation over another.

$$\text{ALPP} = \max P_{ves} \text{ or } \max P_{ves} - \text{base } P_{ves} \text{ at leakage}$$

$$\text{Detrusor LPP} = \max P_{det} \text{ or } \max P_{det} - \text{base } P_{det} \text{ at leakage}$$

VII. CLINICAL APPLICATIONS

A. Neurogenic Bladder

McGuire et al. (27) reported that children with myelomeningocele and with detrusor LPP of more than 40 cmH$_2$O are at increased risk of renal failure (1,22). Pressure of 40 cmH$_2$O or more at normal bladder capacity was significantly more common in patients with (44%) than in those without reflux (20%). In another study, in the areflexic group of patients with myelomeningocele, LPP was useful in assessing incontinence, whereas in the hyperreflexic group, leak point volume (LPV) was more useful. The addition of LPP and LPV during routine urodynamic studies in myelodysplastic patients enhances accurate diagnosis and may select those who will best benefit from bladder augmentation or a procedure to increase outlet resistance (28).

Modification of the LPP test in children with spina bifida was suggested by Combs and Horowitz (29). They measured LPP at leakage and then removed the catheter. Immediately after leakage ceased, the catheter was reinserted and detrusor pressure recorded again. Three groups of children were identified: 1) detrusor LPP greater than 40 and less than 40 cmH$_2$O with the catheter in and out, respectively; 2) detrusor LPP consistently less than 40 cmH$_2$O with the catheter in and out; and 3) detrusor LPP consistently greater than 40 cmH$_2$O with the catheter in and out. There was a 5% incidence of upper tract changes in group 1 and a 40% incidence in group 3. All patients in group 2 had normal upper tracts.

Others (30) also showed that patients with neurogenic bladder owing to spinal cord injury and with bladder LPP higher than 40 cmH$_2$O had a significantly higher incidence of upper tract damage and persisting external detrusor–sphincter dyssynergia.

Detrusor LPP or ALPP has also been applied to evaluating the outcome of different operative procedures, such as sphincterotomy (31), UroLume (32) and Memotherm prosthesis (33), that are performed to reduce bladder outlet obstruction in patients with spinal cord injury.

B. Stress Urinary Incontinence in Women

Conventional urodynamic evaluation of SUI based on maximum urethral closing pressures is less useful than ALPP in detecting ISD. McGuire et al. (2) adopted LPP for investigation of SUI in women and suggested VLPP for the detection of ISD. They demonstrated that almost 80% of women who had VLPP less than 60 cmH$_2$O had type III SUI based on videourodynamics. VLPP values higher than 90 cmH$_2$O usually rule out ISD and are associated with pure urethral hypermobility (2). VLPP results, combined with history, physical examination, and some other urodynamic studies, allow accurate classification of SUI and become a useful tool to the clinician in choosing the most appropriate treatment (34). Others (6,35,36) have also suggested that low ALPP usually indicates ISD.

Swift and Ostergard (37) established that ALPP is superior to maximal urethral closure pressure in evaluating SUI. They suggested a value less than, or equal to, 60 cmH$_2$O to be an appropriate cutoff for screening patients at risk of potential ISD.

Cummings et al. (38) reported low VLPP in 83% of women with severe leakage and previous surgery. They also noted, however, that 47% of patients without predisposing factors also had low VLPP.

Nitti and Combs (36) found some correlation between the subjective degree of incontinence and VLPP values. They evaluated 64 consecutive women with SUI. The subjective degree of SUI was graded as 1, 2, or 3, according to the SEAPI-QMN classification. Statistical analysis demonstrated a significant difference in the number of patients with a VLPP of 90 cmH$_2$O or less, and one of 60 cmH$_2$O, among the three symptom groups. However, others (39) have shown that the severity of SUI symptoms assessed by the Urogenital Distress Inventory (UDI-6) does not correlate with the severity of VLPP. CLPP has been used to measure the dynamics of female urethral function (40). It reportedly increases from 99.9 to 138.9 cmH$_2$O when intravaginal anti-incontinence devices are employed.

C. Urinary Diversion

Leak point pressure was adopted also to evaluate function of the stoma in patients with urinary diversion. In subjects with mean stomal LPP of 7.7 cmH$_2$O (range 5–10), there was no vesicoureteral reflux, calculus formation, hydronephrosis, autonomic dysreflexia, or worsening renal function in follow-up of 12–15 months (41).

VLPP has also been used successfully to assess the continence mechanism of the ileal neobladder (42). Intraoperative stomal LPP measurement of cutaneous continent diversions has helped reduce the revision rate (43). Good long-lasting results have been obtained with intraoperative stomal LPP higher than 80 cmH$_2$O.

D. Incontinence in Men

Ficazzola and Nitti (44) used VLPP to assess sphincteric function after radical prostatectomy (RP). They defined ISD as incontinence associated with increased intra-abdominal pressure and concluded that it was due to ISD in 54 out of 57 men. Others (45) also found post-RP sphincteric damage to be the cause of urinary incontinence in 95% of patients; 69% had VLPP less than 103 cmH$_2$O, with a urethral urodynamic catheter in place. An additional 26% had VLPP less than 150 cmH$_2$O on removal of the catheter. It was concluded that the degree of VLPP is an indication of the severity of sphincteric damage (4,5). Given measurements of maximum urethral pressure and ALPP, Gudziak et al. (46) also suggested that postprostatectomy incontinence owing to sphincter dysfunction results from intrinsic and not extrinsic urethral sphincter deficiency.

VIII. SUMMARY

Leak point pressure testing is useful in evaluating patients with suspected ISD and in monitoring or predicting treatment outcomes. As with any urodynamic test, however, LPP results have to be interpreted in conjunction with the patient's clinical status.

REFERENCES

1. McGuire EJ, Woodside JR, Borden TA, Weiss RM. Prognostic value of urodynamic testing in myelodysplastic children. J Urol 1981; 126:205–209.
2. McGuire EJ, Fitzpatrick CC, Wan J, Bloom D, Sanvordenker J, Ritchey M, Gormley EA. Clinical assessment of urethral sphincter function. J Urol 1993; 150:1452–1454.
3. Miklos JR, Sze EH, Karram MM. A critical appraisal of methods of measuring leakpoint pressures in women with stress incontinence. Obstet Gynecol 1995; 86:349–352.
4. Siltberg H, Larsson G, Victor A. Reproducibility of a new method to determine cough-induced leak point pressure in women with stress urinary incontinence. Int Urogynecol J Pelvic Floor Dysfunct 1996; 7:13–19.
5. Bump RC, Elser DM, Theofrastous JP, McClish DK, the Continence Program for Women Research Group. Valsalva leak point pressures in women with genuine stress incontinence. Reproducibility, effect of catheter caliber, and correlations with other measures of urethral resistance. Am J Obstet Gynecol 1995; 173:551–557.
6. Bump RC, Coates KW, Cundiff GW, Harris RL, Weidner AC. Diagnosing intrinsic sphincteric deficiency—comparing urethral closure pressure, urethral axis, and Valsalva leak point pressures. Am J Obstet Gynecol 1997; 177:303–310.
7. Theofrastous JP, Cundiff GW, Harris RL, Bump RC. The effect of vesical volume on Valsalva leak-point pressures in women with genuine urinary stress incontinence. Obstet Gynecol 1996; 87:711–714.
8. Van Venrooij GE, Blok C, Van Riel MP, Coolsaet BL. Relative urethral leakage pressure versus maximum urethral closure pressure. The reliability of the measurement of urethral competence with the new tube-foil sleeve catheter in patients. J Urol 1985; 134:592–595.
9. Sultana CJ. Urethral closure pressure and leak point pressure in incontinent women. Obstet Gynecol 1995; 86:839–842.
10. McGuire EJ. Urodynamic evaluation of stress incontinence. Urol Clin North Am 1995; 22:551–555.
11. Hernandez RD, Hurwitz RS, Foote JE, Zimmern PE, Leach GE. Nonsurgical management of threatened upper urinary tracts and incontinence in children with myelomeningocele. J Urol 1994; 152:1582–1585.
12. Plevnik S, Vrtacnik P, Janez J. Detection of fluid entry into the urethra by electric impedance measurement: electric fluid bridge test. Clin Phys Physiol Measur 1983; 4:309–313.
13. Plevnik S, Brown M, Sutherst JR, Vrtacnik P. Tracking of fluid in the urethra by simultaneous electric impedance measurement at three sites. Urol Int 1983; 38:29–32.
14. Sutherst J, Brown M. The fluid bridge test for urethral incompetence. A comparison of results in women with incontinence and women with normal urinary control. Acta Obstet Gynecol Scand 1983; 62:271–273.
15. Heritz DM, Blaivas JG. Reliability and specificity of leak point pressure. J Urol 1995; 153:492A.
16. Gormley EA, McGuire EJ. Reproducibility of abdominal leak point pressure in the diagnosis of stress urinary incontinence. J Urol 1994; 151:478A.
17. Decter RM, Harpster L. Pitfalls in determination of leak point pressure. J Urol 1992; 148:588–591.
18. Bump RC, Elser DM, McClish DK. Valsalva leak point pressure in adult women with genuine stress incontinence. Reproducibility, effect of catheter caliber, and correlation with passive urethral pressure profilometry. Neurourol Urodynam 1993; 12:307–308.
19. Payne CK, Raz S, Babiarz JW. The Valsalva leak point pressure in evaluation of stress urinary incontinence. Technical aspects of measurements. J Urol 1994; 151:478A.
20. Flood HD, Liu J. The effect of the urethral catheter on leak point pressure in patients being assessed for urethral reconstruction. Process Urodynamic Society, Las Vegas, April 1995.
21. Flood HD, Alevizatos C, Liu JL. Sex differences in the determination of abdominal leak point pressure in patients with intrinsic sphincter deficiency. J Urol 1996; 156:1737–1740.

22. McGuire EJ, Cespedes RD, O'Connell HE. Leak-point pressures. Urol Clin North Am 1996; 23:253–262.

23. Faerber GJ, Vashi AR. Variations in Valsalva leak point pressure with increasing vesical volume. J Urol 1998; 159:1909–1911.

24. Petrou SP, Kollmorgen TA. Valsalva leak point pressure and bladder volume. Neurourol Urodynam 1998; 17:3–7.

25. Hsu TH, Rackley RR, Appell RA. The supine test: a simple method to detect intrinsic urethral sphincter dysfunction. J Urol 1999; 162:460–463.

26. McLennan MT, Bent AE. Supine empty stress test as a predictor of low Valsalva leak point pressure. Neurourol Urodynam 1998; 17:121–127.

27. Flood HD, Ritchey ML, Bloom DA, Huang C, McGuire EJ. Outcome of reflux in children with myelodysplasia managed by bladder pressure monitoring. J Urol 1994; 152:1574–1577.

28. McCormack M, Pike J, Kiruluta G. Leak point of incontinence. A measure of the interaction between outlet resistance and bladder capacity. J Urol 1993; 150:162–164.

29. Combs AJ, Horowitz M. A new technique for assessing detrusor leak point pressure inpatients with spina bifida. J Urol 1996; 156:757–760.

30. Kim YH, Kattan MW, Boone TB. Bladder leak point pressure: the measure for sphincterotomy success in spinal cord injured patients with external detrusorsphincter dyssynergia. J Urol 1998; 159:493–496.

31. Juma S, Mostafavi M, Joseph A. Sphincterotomy: long-term complications and warning signs. Neurourol Urodynam 1995; 14:33–41.

32. Chancellor MB, Gajewski JB, Ackman CFD, Appell RA, Bennett J, Binard J, Boone TB, Chetner MP, Crewalk JA, Defalco A, Foote J, Green B, Juma S, Jung SY, Linsenmeyer TA, MacMillan R, Mayo M, Ozawa H, Roehrborn CG, Shenot PJ, Stone A, Vazquez A, Killorin W, Rivas DA. Long-term (5 years) follow-up of the North American Multicenter UroLume Trial for the treatment of detrusor–external sphincter dyssynergia. J Urol 1999; 161:1545–1550.

33. Juan Garcia FJ, Salvador S, Montoto A, Lion S, Balvis B, Rodriguez A, Fernandez M, Sanchez J. Intraurethral stent prosthesis in spinal cord injured patients with sphincter dyssynergia. Spinal Cord 1999; 37:54–57.

34. Cespedes RD, Cross CA, McGuire EJ. Selecting the best surgical option for stress urinary incontinence. Medscape Women's Health 1996; 1:3.

35. Haab F, Zimmern PE, Leach GE. Female stress urinary incontinence due to intrinsic sphincteric deficiency: recognition and management. J Urol 1996; 156:3–17.

36. Nitti VW, Combs AJ. Correlation of Valsalva leak point pressure with subjective degree of stress urinary incontinence in women. J Urol 1996; 155:281–285.

37. Swift SE, Ostergard DR. A comparison of stress leak-point pressure and maximal urethral closure pressure in patients with genuine stress incontinence. Obstet Gynecol 1995; 85:704–708.

38. Cummings JM, Boullier JA, Parra RO, Wozniak–Petrofsky J. Leak point pressures in women with urinary stress incontinence—correlation with patient history. J Urol 1997; 157:818–820.

39. Lemack GE, Zimmern PE. Predictability of urodynamic findings based on the Urogenital Distress Inventory-6 questionnaire. Urology 1999; 54:461–466.

40. Siltberg H, Larsson G, Victor A. Cough-induced leak-point pressure—a valid measure for assessing treatment in women with stress incontinence. Acta Obstet Gynecol Scand 1998; 77:1000–1007.

41. Mutchnik SE, Hinson JL, Nickell KG, Boone TB. Ileovesicostomy as an alternative form of bladder management in tetraplegic patients. Urology 1997; 49:353–357.

42. Aboseif SR, Borirakchanyavant S, Lue TF, Carroll PR. Continence mechanism of the ileal neobladder in women: a urodynamic study. World J Urol 1998; 16:400–404.

43. Bissada NK, Marshall L. Leak point pressure use for intraoperative adjustment of the continence mechanism in patients undergoing continent cutaneous urinary diversion. Urology 1998; 52:790–792.

44. Ficazzola MA, Nitti VW. The etiology of post-radical prostatectomy incontinence and correlation of symptoms with urodynamic findings. J Urol 1998; 160:1317–1320.

45. Desautel MG, Kapoor R, Badlani GH. Sphincteric incontinence: the primary cause of post-prostatectomy incontinence in patients with prostate cancer. Neurourol Urodynam 1997; 16: 153–160.
46. Gudziak MR, McGuire EJ, Gormley EA. Urodynamic assessment of urethral sphincter function in post-prostatectomy incontinence. J Urol 1996; 156:1131–1134.

23

Multichannel Urodynamic and Videourodynamic Testing

VICTOR W. NITTI

New York University School of Medicine, New York, New York

YOUNG H. KIM

Brown University School of Medicine, Providence, Rhode Island

I. INTRODUCTION

The lower urinary tract is responsible for the storage and evacuation of urine. Storage should occur at low pressure to assure continence and protection of the kidneys, and evacuation should be voluntary. However, a variety of problems may arise that interfere with these two basic functions. Urodynamics is the dynamic study of the transport, storage, and evacuation of urine by the urinary tract. It comprises several tests that individually or collectively can be used to gain information about lower urinary tract function. It can be an invaluable tool in the evaluation of urinary storage and voiding dysfunction. When several parameters are measured simultaneously, we refer to the collective test as multichannel urodynamics.

Normal lower urinary tract function is dependent on normal anatomy and function of the bladder and the bladder outlet, including the urethra, as well as normal interactions between the two. Abnormalities in any of these may result in various lower urinary tract disorders that are discussed throughout this text. Multichannel urodynamics are critical in detecting abnormal bladder or urethral function as well as disorders in bladder–urethral interactions. Several parameters are measured during storage and emptying, including total vesical pressure, abdominal pressure, subtracted detrusor pressure, urinary flow rate and, in select cases, intraurethral pressure and pelvic floor electromyography (EMG).

Because urodynamics is the clinician's tool to measure lower urinary tract function and diagnose abnormalities it is ideal to have a classification of urodynamic findings that not only differentiates abnormalities, but also helps direct appropriate treatment. The classification system for voiding dysfunction proposed by Wein (1) is extremely useful, for it is based on function (and thus urodynamic findings) of each part of the lower urinary tract and permits planning of treatment options based on these findings. Functionally, lower urinary tract dysfunction can be divided into 1) failure to store urine; 2) failure to empty urine; and 3) failure to store and empty. Each functional abnormality can then be attributed to the bladder, the bladder outlet, or both; for example 1) bladder dysfunction (overactive, underactive); 2) bladder outlet dysfunction (overactive, underactive); or 3) combined dysfunction. Thus, the urodynamic evaluation should help determine if there is bladder or bladder outlet dysfunction (or both) and whether there is a storage or emptying problem. By providing answers to these questions, urodynamic testing can lead to a correct diagnosis and institution of appropriate treatment.

Multichannel urodynamics involves the recording, display, and analysis of several urodynamic parameters simultaneously. Videourodymanics incorporates the simultaneous imaging of the lower urinary tract using fluoroscopy. Typically, total vesical pressure, total abdominal pressure, subtracted detrusor pressure, and urinary flow rate are recorded (Fig. 1). In addition, pelvic floor EMG or urethral pressure may be recorded. To perform multichannel urodynamics, it is necessary to place a catheter into the bladder to fill and measure pressure. This is usually accomplished with a urethral catheter (7–10F) which has two lu-

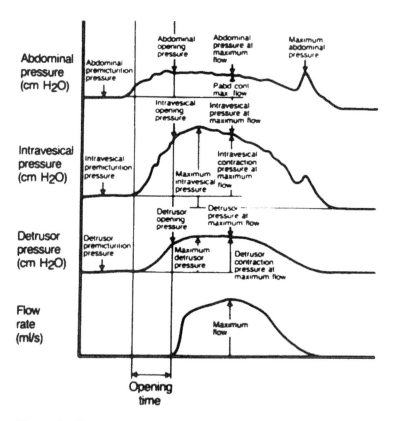

Figure 1 Recommended International Continence terminology for combined pressure(s) and flow recording (multichannel urodynamics). (From Ref. 4.)

mens, one for filling and one for pressure monitoring. A triple-lumen urethral catheter may also be used if one wishes to measure urethral pressure. (A suprapubic catheter may be used if one wishes to avoid urethral catheterization.) A rectal (or vaginal) balloon catheter is used to measure intra-abdominal pressures. A computer is used to subtract intra-abdominal pressure from intravesical pressure to record and display a subtracted detrusor pressure. Pelvic floor EMG can be performed with surface electrodes placed in the perianal area or with needle electrodes placed directly in the anal or urethral sphincter. A full description of the technical aspects of performing a urodynamic study are found elsewhere (2,3).

II. SPECIFIC MEASURES OF STORAGE AND EMPTYING

A. Parameters of Filling and Storage

Normal storage of urine in the bladder requires maintenance of low bladder pressures during bladder filling and storage of a normal capacity of urine. Thus, during filling there should be no bladder contractions or significant rises in pressure until voluntary voiding is initiated. The cystometrogram (CMG) is a measure of the bladder's response to being filled (4). It measures the pressure–volume relation within the bladder and one hopes, mimics normal bladder filling and storage of urine (Fig. 2). The CMG also provides a subjective measure of bladder sensation with the cooperation of the patient. Filling cystometry can evaluate the following parameters:

1. Filling pressure (direct measurement)
2. Sensation (subject measurement dependent on patient cooperation)
3. Presence of involuntary or unstable contractions (direct measurement)
4. Compliance—change in pressure/change in volume (direct measurement)
5. Capacity (direct measurement, but dependent on subjective response of the patient)
6. Control over micturition

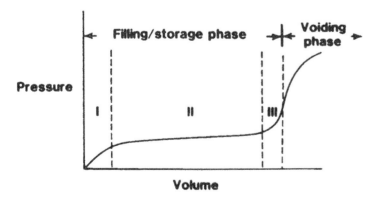

Figure 2 Idealized normal adult cystometrogram: phase I reflects the bladder's initial response to filling; phase II is the tonus limb and reflects bladder pressure during most of the filling phase. As the vesicoelastic properties of the bladder reach their limit, phase III is entered where pressures begin to increase just before phase IV, the voluntary contraction phase. (From Ref. 4.)

Cystometry can be performed as a single-channel study in which the bladder pressure is measured and recorded during filling and storage. However, intravesical pressure that is monitored during cystometric studies is actually the sum of intra-abdominal pressure (P_{abd}) and the pressure generated by the detrusor itself, either through a contraction or wall tension with bladder filling (compliance). The simultaneously recording of P_{abd} and vesical pressure (P_{ves}) during multichannel urodynamics provides a means of calculating the true detrusor pressure (P_{det}) by subtracting abdominal P_{abd} from P_{ves}. The ability to calculate subtracted P_{det} allows one to distinguish between a true rise in detrusor pressure (either through a contraction or loss of compliance) and the effect of increased abdominal pressure (e.g., movement, Valsalva). This is especially important when rises in detrusor pressure are small or when they are accompanied by changes in abdominal pressure (5) (Fig. 3). Another application of abdominal pressure monitoring is its use in assessing the effects of abdominal pressure on the lower urinary tract; specifically, urethral sphincteric function (abdominal leak point pressure). In adults, filling CMG is usually performed at a rate of 30–50

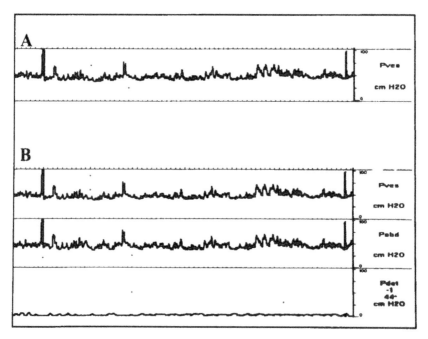

Figure 3 Adding intra-abdominal pressure monitoring gives a better representation of the true detrusor pressure: (A) Total vesical pressure tracing; note the multiple spikes and rises in pressure. Without having simultaneous monitoring of intra-abdominal pressure, it is impossible to tell if these pressure spikes are due to a rise in detrusor or abdominal pressure. (B) This same tracing with intra-abdominal pressure monitoring added. One can clearly see now that the changes in vesical pressure were due to the changes in abdominal pressure. When one looks at the P_{det} curve it is noted to be flat and without any rises in pressure. P_{ves}, total vesical pressure; P_{abd}, total abdominal pressure; P_{det}, subtracted detrusor pressure. (From Ref. 3.)

mL/min using physiological saline or radiographic contrast (for videourodynamics), although faster and slower rates can be used in special circumstances.

1. Sensation

Sensation is a truly subjective parameter; therefore, it requires an alert and attentive patient and clinician. It may be affected by the infusion rate and temperature of the filling solution as well as the level of the patient's distraction. It is difficult to precisely define a hypersensitive or hyposensitive bladder and there are no absolute values for such terms. Even though most urodynamicists would agree that a patient who feels nothing with 1 L in the bladder has a "hyposensitive bladder" and a patient who has a strong urge to void with 50 mL in the bladder has a "hypersensitive bladder," there is a large gray zone in between. Ultimately, sensitivity and functional bladder capacity are best determined through voiding diaries and not by CMG. The true value of the CMG relative to sensation is when a symptom is mimicked and sensation can be correlated, or not correlated, with changes in vesical pressure. There are several subjective parameters that can be recorded during the CMG. It is important to note the exact time at which these occur and whether or not they are associated with changes in P_{ves}. The following list of sensory parameters are defined by the International Continence Society (6):

1. First sensation of bladder filling: This is clearly the most variable of sensory parameters. Many patients will describe a filling sensation almost immediately and then will go on to have an otherwise unremarkable CMG from a sensory perspective.
2. Desire to void:
   a. First desire to void.
   b. Normal desire to void: "The feeling that leads the patient to pass urine at the next convenient moment, but voiding can be delayed if necessary."
   c. Strong desire to void: "Persistent urge to void without the fear of leakage."
3. Urgency: "A strong desire to void accompanied by fear of leakage or fear of pain." Some investigators will use the terms first urge and strong or severe urge.
4. Pain: "The site and character of which should be specified. Pain during bladder filling or micturition is abnormal."

2. Filling Pressure

Normally as the bladder fills, detrusor pressure remains relatively constant and low, usually not exceeding 5–10 cmH$_2$O (see Fig. 2). As the vesicoelastic properties of the bladder reach their limit, there may be a slight rise in pressure, before voluntary contraction takes place. There are two ways that filling pressure may abnormally rise. The first is with an involuntary contraction and the second is as a result of impaired compliance.

Involuntary contractions, also known as uninhibited bladder contractions, often result in an abnormal sensation of urgency or even urinary incontinence (Fig. 4). Involuntary contractions may have a neurological or nonneurological etiology. According to the standards of the International Continence Society (6), when the cause is neurological in origin, involuntary contractions are termed *detrusor hyperreflexia* and when nonneurologicaly they are referred to as *detrusor instability.* Suprapontine lesions, such as cerebrovascular accident, cerebral atrophy, and brain tumor, will result in a loss of inhibitory input to the pontine micturition center, resulting in detrusor hyperreflexia. Suprasacral spinal cord injury

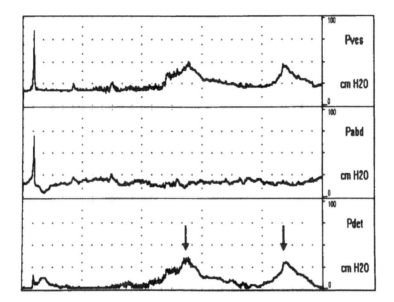

Figure 4   Detrusor instability: This is a CMG of patient with severe urinary frequency and urgency. Note the rises in detrusor pressure during filling (arrows). These are unstable contractions and were accompanied by urges. P_{ves}, total vesical pressure; P_{abd}, total abdominal pressure; P_{det}, subtracted detrusor pressure.

can also lead to impaired supraspinal inhibitory input, resulting in detrusor hyperreflexia (7). Causes of detrusor instability include bladder outlet obstruction, bladder mucosal irritants, urinary tract infection, bladder cancer, bladder stones and foreign bodies, and estrogen deficiency in women. Recently, the normal aging process has been associated with detrusor instability (8). In either case, whether instability or hyperreflexia, involuntary contractions may result as a response to abnormal urethral function (i.e., anatomical or functional obstruction).

The International Continence Society originally defined an *involuntary contraction* as a contraction of at least 15 cmH$_2$O (6). However, it is now generally accepted that a rise in detrusor pressure that is accompanied by an urge may be considered an involuntary contraction (i.e., detrusor instability or hyperreflexia). Instability and hyperreflexia may look identical on CMG. The terms instability and hyperreflexia are strictly defined by the patient's neurological status and not the CMG appearance of the involuntary contraction (Fig. 5).

When diagnosing involuntary contractions, it is important that the clinician be certain that the contraction is indeed involuntary. Sometimes a patient may become confused during the study and actually void as soon as they feel the desire. Also urgency and involuntary contractions can sometimes be an "artifact of testing," and it is often worthwhile to repeat the CMG (perhaps at a slower-filling rate) if the patient experiences uncharacteristic symptoms. In the nonneurological patient, it is extremely important to determine whether or not a patient's symptoms are reproduced during the involuntary contraction. If not, then the CMG should be considered to be nondiagnostic. This is not necessarily true in some neurological conditions when the patient may not have symptoms, and detrusor hyperreflexia is potentially dangerous. On the contrary, it is important to realize that if an involuntary contraction is not demonstrated on CMG, it does not rule out its existence, especially

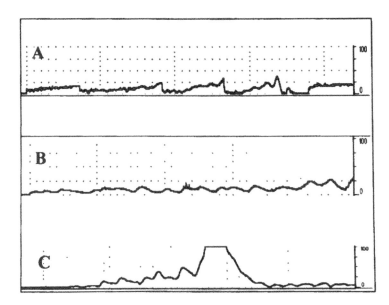

Figure 5 One cannot differentiate between detrusor hyperreflexia and detrusor instability based on the cystometric findings themselves. It is only the history of the neurological lesion that classifies a patient as having hyperreflexia: (A) CMG (detrusor pressure curve) of a teenage male with a tumor involving his sacral spinal cord. Involuntary detrusor contractions are considered hyperreflexia because of the known neurological lesion. (B) CMG (detrusor pressure curve) from an elderly woman with severe frequency, urgency, and urge incontinence. The multiple involuntary contractions throughout filling are classified as detrusor instability because of the lack of a known neurological lesion. (C) CMG (detrusor pressure curve) of a 70-year-old man with frequency, urgency, urge incontinence, and a decreased force of stream. There are multiple involuntary contractions, one of which is of extremely high amplitude. This patient also has bladder outlet obstruction, secondary to benign prostatic hyperplasia, thus the involuntary contractions are classified as detrusor instability, as there is no neurological lesion. (From Ref. 3.)

if the patient's symptoms are not reproduced during the testing period. Strict concentration by the patient during the test will often inhibit the instability that is normally present.

The term *compliance* refers to the change in volume/change in pressure and is expressed in mL/cmH$_2$O. Because the bladder is normally able to hold large volumes at low pressures, it is said to be highly compliant (see Fig. 2). The spherical shape of the bladder as well as the vesicoelastic properties of its components contribute to its excellent compliance, allowing storage of progressive volumes of urine at low pressure. When the pressure begins to rise with increasing volumes, compliance is decreasing or impaired (Fig. 6). Impaired compliance commonly occurs when there is prolonged bladder outlet obstruction. The "overworked bladder" becomes scarred as smooth muscle is replaced by collagen. Also impaired compliance can result from radiation, surgery on the bladder, tuberculosis and other chronic infectious diseases, and other conditions that affect the size, shape, and vesicoelastic properties of the normal bladder.

The calculated value of compliance is probably less important than the actual bladder pressure during filling. This is because compliance value can change, depending on the volume over which it is calculated. This is why compliance, despite being a well-known

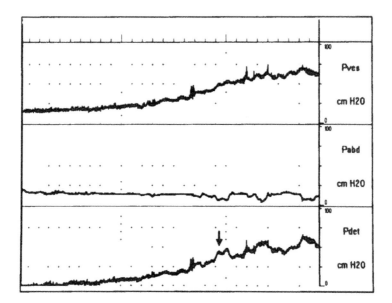

Figure 6   Poorly compliant bladder with prolonged high-pressure storage: At arrow, detrusor pressure exceeds 40 cmH$_2$O and remains above 40 cmH$_2$O for the rest of the filling. P_{ves}, total vesical pressure; P_{abd}, total abdominal pressure; P_{det}, subtracted detrusor pressure.

and accepted parameter, is rarely reported in terms of a discrete or well-defined value in the urological literature. Normal compliance has been difficult to establish. Toppercer and Tetreault evaluated a group of normal asymptomatic women and women with stress incontinence and found mean compliance to be 55.71 ± 27.37 (9). Therefore, if two standard deviations are used, normal would be between 1 and 110 mL/cmH$_2$O. When compliance is calculated as a single point on the pressure–volume curve, it makes it a "static" property. However, this oversimplifies the concept of compliance and may lead to potentially erroneous conclusions (10). McGuire and associates have shown that sustained pressures of 40 cmH$_2$O or higher during storage can lead to upper tract damage (11). Clearly, storage pressures in this range are dangerous, regardless of the volume in the bladder or calculated compliance value. In poorly compliant bladders in children, Churchill and associates have suggested determining compliance between initial filling and the point at which detrusor pressure exceeds 35 cmH$_2$O (10). More recently, these investigators have applied the concept of dynamic compliance and argue that the amount of time spent with bladder compliance less than 10 mL/cmH$_2$O (an empirically derived value) will strongly influence upper tract deterioration (12). We would certainly agree that prolonged high-pressure storage is an ominous urodynamic finding, independent of any discrete value of compliance (see Fig. 6). As with involuntary contractions, impaired bladder compliance may also result from abnormal urethral function (anatomical or functional obstruction). Impaired compliance may also occur in association with involuntary detrusor contractions. In such cases, involuntary contractions can occur with a rising baseline pressure (Fig. 7).

3.   Storage

Urinary incontinence is the end result of failure to store urine. It can occur as a result of sphincter or bladder dysfunction. To store urine properly, the bladder and urethral sphincter must work as a unit to accommodate increasing amounts of urine, even when subjected

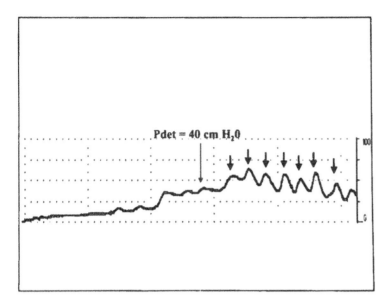

Pdet = 40 cm H$_2$O

Figure 7 Impaired compliance with involuntary contractions: There is impaired compliance with storage detrusor pressures more than 40 cmH$_2$O. There are also superimposed uninhibited contractions (arrows). In this study, only the detrusor pressure curve is shown.

to rises in intra-abdominal pressure. The critical factor for the bladder is the maintenance of low intravesical pressures. Increases in pressure owing to impaired compliance or involuntary contractions may result in incontinence. The urethral sphincter must have enough intrinsic tone and pressure to resist changes in intra-abdominal pressure, yet still be able to "relax" properly during voluntary voiding.

Abnormalities in various components of this bladder–urethral sphincter unit can result in faulty urinary storage. Measurements of intravesical and intra-abdominal pressure during episodic urinary incontinence can reveal the site (bladder vs. urethra) of the functional or anatomical abnormality. These "leak point pressures" measure the resistance of the urinary sphincter to detrusor or abdominal expulsive forces (13). There are two distinct types of leak point pressures. Detrusor or *bladder leak point pressure* (BLPP) reflects the detrusor pressure required to generate leakage. Valsalva or *abdominal leak point pressure* (ALPP) indicates the ability of the urethral sphincter to resist leakage as a result of increases in intra-abdominal pressures.

Bladder leak point pressure is a measure of the bladder's response to abnormally high urethral resistance. This resistance can be anatomical (urethral stricture, prostatic obstruction, posterior urethral valves), or functional (detrusor external sphincter dyssynergia, dysfunctional voiding). As described earlier, changes in detrusor compliance and involuntary contractions can occur as a result of abnormal urethral resistance, leading to lower urinary tract symptoms and upper urinary tract damage. When detrusor pressures generated as a result of impaired detrusor compliance or involuntary detrusor contractions overcome urethral resistance, leakage occurs. When such pressures are high and persistent, this can lead to progressive and upper and lower urinary tract deterioration (11). Therefore, BLPP is a truly a measure of the underlying abnormality in urethral resistance (Fig. 8).

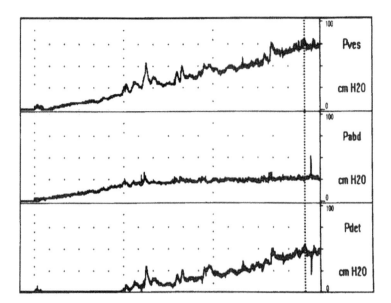

Figure 8 Bladder leak point pressure: Urodynamic study of a patient with spina bifida and urinary incontinence; note the impaired compliance. Leakage occurs at broken line (P_{det} = 52 cmH$_2$O). Note there is no increase in abdominal pressure. P_{ves}, total vesical pressure; P_{abd}, total abdominal pressure; P_{det}, subtracted detrusor pressure.

Abdominal leak point pressure is a measure of the competence of the urethral sphincter in the face of increased intra-abdominal pressures (14). Thus, it is useful for cases of decreased urethral resistance (i.e., stress urinary incontinence). The ALPP is a reflection of urethral sphincter function, and not bladder function or the bladder's response to decreased urethral resistance. This measurement provides information on the magnitude and type of urethral sphincter incompetence, which guides appropriate treatment (Fig. 9). In cases of female stress urinary incontinence, the ALPP has been used as a guide to determine the amount of intrinsic sphincter deficiency. Although there are no absolute measures for the diagnosis of ISD using ALPP, most experts would agree that ALPP less than 60 cmH$_2$O is a definite indication of ISD, and ALPP less than 90 cmH$_2$O indicates at least a component of ISD.

4. Pelvic Floor Electromyography During Filling and Storage

The response of the external urethral sphincter and pelvic floor during the micturition cycle can be monitored by electromyography (EMG). This can be done by applying surface electrodes to each side of the perianal area or by placing needle electrodes into the anal or urethral sphincter. Most urodynamics laboratories will use surface electrodes as a way to determine external sphincter response during filling, storage, and emptying, and needle electrodes when detailed information about those responses is necessary. A more detailed description of EMG techniques and interpretation is provided elsewhere (15).

During normal bladder filling there is a constant low level of EMG activity present in the striated sphincter. This activity will increase slightly as the volume in the bladder increases. Also with coughing or other increases in intra-abdominal pressure, EMG activity will also increase (Fig. 10). During involuntary detrusor contractions in the neurologically normal patient, EMG activity usually increases as the patient attempts to inhibit the un-

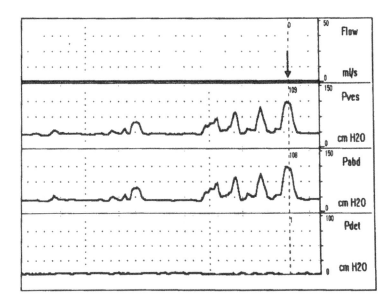

Figure 9 Abdominal leak point pressure: Urodynamic study of a woman with stress urinary incontinence. Leakage occurs with increase in abdominal (and total vesical pressure) without a rise in detrusor pressure (arrow). Abdominal leak point pressure is 109 cmH$_2$O as determined by the P_{ves} tracing. P_{ves}, total vesical pressure; P_{abd}, total abdominal pressure; P_{det}, subtracted detrusor pressure.

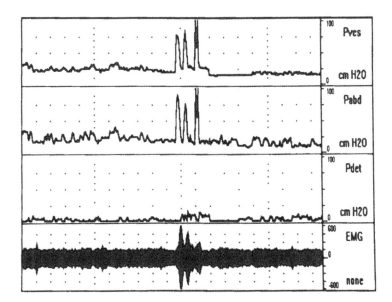

Figure 10 Urodynamic tracing showing increased EMG activity with coughing (i.e., a rise in total abdominal and total vesical pressure): P_{ves}, total vesical pressure; P_{abd}, total abdominal pressure; P_{det}, subtracted detrusor pressure.

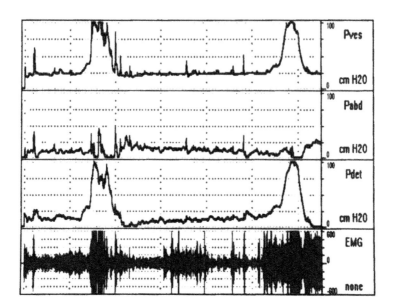

Figure 11   Urodynamic tracing of a young girl with urinary incontinence and tethered cord: There are two episodes of detrusor hyperreflexia accompanied by increased EMG activity. This is true detrusor hyperreflexia with detrusor–external sphincter–dyssynergia: P_{ves}, total vesical pressure; P_{abd}, total abdominal pressure; P_{det}, subtracted detrusor pressure.

wanted contraction (see Fig. 10). The involuntary increase in EMG activity during a hyperreflexic contraction (neurologically mediated involuntary contraction) is termed detrusor–external sphincter–dyssynergia (Fig. 11). The difference between the increased EMG activity with instability and hyperreflexia is that in the former it is voluntary, whereas in the latter it is involuntary.

B.   Parameters of Emptying

1.   Detrusor Contractility and the Pressure Flow Relation

Urodynamic measurements during voiding allow two critical parameters to be determined: detrusor contractility and bladder outlet resistance. In addition coordination between the bladder and urethral sphincters can be assessed. Together these will determine the efficiency of bladder emptying. Impaired detrusor contractility as well as bladder outlet obstruction can cause similar symptoms of decreased force of stream, hesitancy, incomplete emptying, and urinary retention. However, it is not possible to differentiate between bladder outlet obstruction, impaired contractility, and cystometric abnormalities of filling based on symptoms alone (16–18). Noninvasive testing such as uroflowmetry and postvoid residual determination may indicate that there are abnormalities in the voiding phase, but cannot distinguish between obstruction and impaired contractility (19–23). It is only by a complete evaluation of the voiding phase, with simultaneous measurement of voiding pressure and urinary flow rate (and pelvic floor EMG in select cases), that a precise diagnosis of the voiding phase can be obtained.

Normal voiding occurs when cortical inhibitory input is voluntarily "turned off." This results in relaxation of the striated urethral sphincter and a rise in detrusor pressure. Once the detrusor pressure exceeds outlet resistance, urine flow is initiated. This is first seen as a decrease or silencing of EMG activity, which precedes the actual detrusor contraction by as much as a few seconds. The detrusor contraction should be of an adequate magnitude and of sufficient duration to effectively empty the bladder. EMG activity should return to normal after voiding is completed. Figure 12 demonstrates a normal voiding study.

Measuring detrusor pressure and simultaneous uroflow during voiding is the most common way to determine contractility and outlet resistance. When detrusor function is normal, the recorded detrusor pressure is dependent on urethral resistance to flow. The higher the resistance is, the greater the detrusor pressure is (to overcome the resistance) and the lower the flow is. The speed of muscle shortening and, therefore, the generated detrusor pressure is determined by this resistance to flow. Speed of muscle shortening decreases as resistance increases, and increases as the resistance decreases. Detrusor muscle responds to increased resistance to flow by a decrease in speed of contraction, rather than an increase in detrusor strength (24). Thus, for any given bladder, there is a unique bladder output relation that reflects outlet resistance, and the higher the detrusor pressure is, the lower the flow is (25,26). Therefore, detrusor pressure is a function of urethral resistance to flow. Increased resistance (obstruction) encountered during voiding is directly responsible for the elevation of detrusor pressure as the bladder attempts to overcome such resistance. The traditional misconception that high voiding pressure equals a strong bladder must be replaced

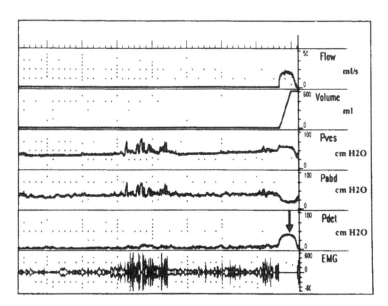

Figure 12 Normal filling and voiding urodynamic study: note the rise in both abdominal and vesical pressures early in the study indicating movement and coughing. With voiding (arrow), there is relaxation of the external sphincter EMG and normal voiding pressure (P_{det} at Q_{max} = 42 cmH$_2$O) and flow (Q_{max} = 22mL/sec): flow, urinary flow rate; volume, volume voided; P_{ves}, total vesical pressure; P_{abd}, total abdominal pressure; P_{det}, subtracted detrusor pressure.

by concepts centered on the balance of voiding, (i.e., the bladder and outlet both contribute to voiding function) (27).

The pressure–flow relation has been studied extensively in males and to a much less degree in females (see later). It has been determined that a detrusor pressure of approximately 20–35 cmH$_2$O of pressure is required to drive urine across the normal male urethra (28). Therefore, voiding detrusor pressures more than 30 cmH$_2$O, which are associated with decreased urinary flow, may indicate the presence of some degree of obstruction in males, and even lower voiding detrusor pressures may indicate obstruction in females. Blaivas has empirically defined *obstruction* as a detrusor contraction of greater than 40 cmH$_2$O associated with a uroflow of less than 12 mL/sec; *impaired contractility* is a detrusor contraction of less than 30 cmH$_2$O associated with an associated uroflow of less than 12 mL/sec; and detrusor pressure between 30 and 40 cmH$_2$O with an associated uroflow of less than 12 mL/sec are considered *indeterminate* (29,30). Although these simple criteria cannot be used in all cases, simple inspection of the pressure flow curve is sometimes all that is necessary to diagnosis obstruction (or impaired contractility) in obvious cases (Figs. 13 and 14).

Simultaneous plots of detrusor voiding pressure and the corresponding flow rates, with pressures on one axis and flow rates on the perpendicular axis, have become a standard way to analyze pressure–flow results. The first of these, the Abrams–Griffiths nomogram, was developed by plotting maximal flow rate and the corresponding detrusor pres-

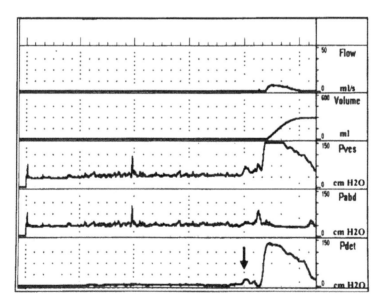

Figure 13 A case of unequivocal bladder outlet obstruction: multichannel urodynamic study of a 72-year-old man with severe lower urinary tract symptoms. Note the extremely high voiding pressure of 140 cmH$_2$O associated with a maximum flow rate of 9 mL/sec. There is also an episode of detrusor instability (arrow), just before voiding. This is obviously bladder outlet obstruction, and no further analysis is required: flow, urinary flow rate; volume, volume voided; P_{ves}, total vesical pressure; P_{abd}, total abdominal pressure; P_{det}, subtracted detrusor pressure.

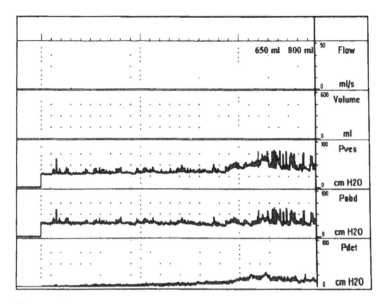

Figure 14 A case of impaired detrusor contractility: multichannel urodynamic study of an 82-year-old man with urinary retention. The study shows low pressure storage up to 650 mL. Between 650 and 800 mL, the patient had an urge to void, and attempted to void mostly by abdominal straining. There is only a slight rise in detrusor pressure: flow, urinary flow rate; volume, volume voided; P_{ves}, total vesical pressure; P_{abd}, total abdominal pressure; P_{det}, subtracted detrusor pressure.

sure at maximal flow rate on separate axes using pressure–flow data from 117 men with possible prostatic obstruction (31). By comparing pressure–flow data among these patients and plotting the maximum flow rate (Q_{max}) on the *x*-axis and the detrusor pressure at maximum flow (P_{det} at Q_{max}) rate on the *y*-axis, they created three zones representing obstructed, unobstructed, and equivocal micturition (Fig. 15). The boundaries of these zones were created by a combination of empiric observations and theoretical considerations, allowing categorization of pressure–flow data for any patient. The upper boundary of the equivocal zone has a slope of 2 cmH$_2$O/mL sec^{-1}. For a patient in the equivocal zone, if the mean slope of the pressure–flow curve is less than 2 cmH$_2$O/mL sec^{-1} and the minimum voiding detrusor pressure is less than 40 cmH$_2$O, the patient is considered unobstructed. However, if either the slope is greater than 2 cmH$_2$O/mL sec^{-1} or the minimum voiding detrusor pressure is greater than 40 cmH$_2$O, the patient is considered obstructed. The Abrams–Griffiths nomogram can be used plotting a single point, Q_{max} and P_{det} at Q_{max} or by plotting the entire voiding cycle (Fig. 16). The latter requires a computer-generated analysis. Two drawbacks of this nomogram are that there is a broad equivocal zone and, conceptually, it does not permit a diagnosis of impaired detrusor contractility, with or without coexisting bladder outlet obstruction. However, this nomogram is quite simple to use and applicable for many clinical situations.

Another popular way to analyze pressure–flow data is the linear passive urethral resistance relation (LinPURR) developed by Schafer. This is a modification of the passive

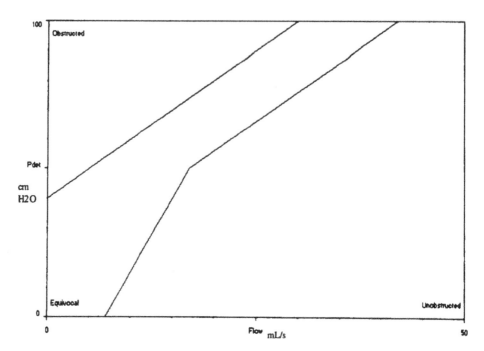

Figure 15 The Abrams–Griffiths nomogram: This was originally described for a single point (Q_{max} and P_{det} at Q_{max}).

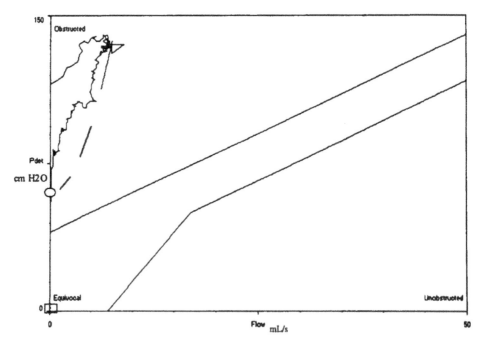

Figure 16 Computer-generated pressure–flow plot from the obstructed patient in Figure 13 plotted on the Abrams–Griffiths nomogram: Note that the entire act of voiding is in the obstructed zone.

urethral resistance (PURR) curve which describes the relation between pressure and flow during the period of lowest urethral resistance (i.e., during complete relaxation) and, therefore, defines the lowest urethral resistance during a single voiding event (32). According to the underlying model, the PURR exactly defines the influence of the passive bladder outlet during voiding when the outlet is maximally open. Typically, the PURR has a minimum opening pressure, which is the intercept of the curve on the pressure axis, and under normal circumstances, has a low value of less than 25 cmH$_2$O. In addition, the PURR has a steep rise in flow rate for a small increase in detrusor pressure, representing a large urethral cross-sectional area (Fig. 17). Therefore, outlet function is characterized by two simple parameters, the minimum-opening pressure, reflecting collapsibility of the tube, and the cross-sectional area of the flow–rate-controlling zone, reflecting extensibility (27). Thus, the PURR curve is a method of assessing the presence or absence of bladder outlet obstruction independent of inherent detrusor strength. The PURR was the first attempt to quantify relevant features of the voiding cycle describing the interplay of detrusor capability and bladder outlet resistance. From the shape of the PURR curve, Schafer defined two types of obstruction, compressive and constrictive. In compressive obstruction, the energy demand for voiding is higher for the initiation and termination of flow as well as during midvoiding. That is, a higher P_{det} minimum void and a normal-shaped PURR curve that is shifted to the right. Conceptually, this means that the urethra is not narrow, but simply requires a higher detrusor pressure for voiding. Thus, there is a proportionately higher minimum detrusor power required to maintain flow. However, once the higher minimum opening pressure is reached, the effective cross-sectional area to which the urethral lumen can extend is unchanged; therefore, the steepness of the curve is usually unchanged (see Fig. 17). The compressive curve is the predominate PURR type seen in prostatic obstruction. Constrictive obstruction can occur as a separate pathophysiological change in outlet resistance, distinct from compressive obstruction. In constrictive obstruction there is a decrease in the urethral cross-sectional area, resulting in a decreased slope of the PURR. There is

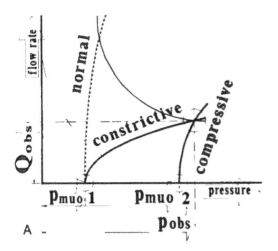

Figure 17 Passive urethral resistance relation (PURR) curve: see text for description. (From Ref. 33.)

usually a plateau-like, low-flow rate curve, especially in the midportion of voiding, despite a high detrusor pressure. Because there is no increased energy requirement at the beginning and termination of flow, P_{det} minimum void is unchanged, and there is less consumption of detrusor muscle strength compared with compressive obstruction (see Fig. 17). Examples of constrictive obstruction are urethral strictures, meatal stenosis, bladder neck sclerosis, and even a small atrophic prostate. Schafer subsequently modified the PURR by using a straight-line instead of a parabolic curve (33). This is done by connecting the maximum flow point (plot of maximum flow rate and detrusor pressure at maximum flow rate) to the detrusor pressure intercept (lowest pressure at which voiding occurs) on the flow versus detrusor pressure graph. Schafer divided this linear PURR curve into seven zones labeled 0–to VI, corresponding to increasing grades of obstruction: grade 0 and 1, no obstruction; grade 2, equivocal or mild obstruction; grades 3–6, increasing severity of obstruction (Fig. 18). The boundary between grades 2 and 3 corresponds to the boundary between equivocal and obstructed in the Abrams–Griffiths nomogram.

The LinPURR method is a coarse stepwise grading of obstruction. The grade of obstruction is not very sensitive to changes in detrusor contractility. For a change in voiding pressure or flow rate to be considered significant, this change has to result in a change in grade or zone of obstruction. Therefore, if what appears to be a large change in voiding pressure or flow rate does not place the maximum flow point in a new zone, the change is not considered significant. Conversely, if a small change results in the maximum flow point shifting to a new zone of obstruction, the change is considered significant. The linear PURR also permits the assessment of detrusor contractility independent of obstruction. Detrusor contractility is classified as strong, normal, weak, and very weak (Fig. 19).

Recently, the International Continence Society has proposed a standard nomogram for the evaluation of pressure–flow studies for clinical and research use (34). It is based on

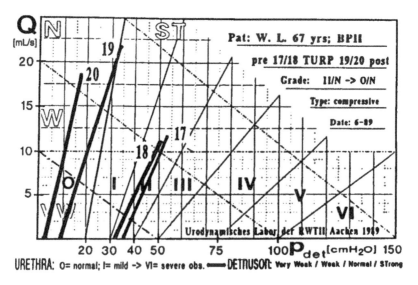

Figure 18   Linear PURR nomogram. (From Ref. 33.)

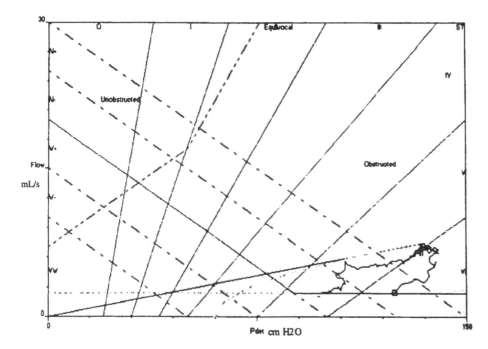

Figure 19 Computer-generated linear PURR nomogram from obstructed patient in Figure 13. Patient is in zone VI (severe obstruction) with normal[+] contractility.

the principles described in the foregoing and designed so that results from different centers can be compared (Fig. 20). A provisional diagnostic may be derived from the single point of Q_{max} and P_{det} at Q_{max} as follows:

If (P_{det} at $Q_{max} - 2*Q_{max}$) is more than 40, the pressure–flow study is obstructed.
If (P_{det} at $Q_{max} - 2*Q_{max}$) is less than 20, the pressure–flow study is unobstructed.
If (P_{det} at $Q_{max} - 2*Q_{max}$) is between 20 and 40, the study is equivocal.

It is important to realize that the foregoing nomograms were derived for men and do not necessarily apply to women. Because of different voiding characteristics of women, for example, the ability to generate normal flow rates by relaxing the pelvic floor with a measurable detrusor contraction, and the lower baseline outlet resistance, pressure–flow analysis that is applicable to men is not so to women. There are no universally accepted pressure–flow criteria for women. Nitti et al. recently proposed videourodynamic criteria for outlet obstruction in women, which include a sustained detrusor contraction of any magnitude with radiographic evidence of obstruction between the bladder neck and urethral meatus (35). With these criteria there is a large overlap between detrusor pressures and maximum flow rates between obstructed and unobstructed women. We concluded that pressure–flow studies alone may not be sufficient to diagnose outflow obstruction in women and may be greatly facilitated by simultaneous voiding cystourethrography (see Sec. III).

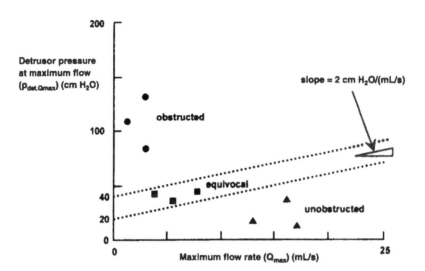

Figure 20 Provisional ICS method for definition of obstruction: the points represent schematically the values of maximum flow rate and detrusor pressure at maximum flow rate for nine different voids, three in each class. (From Ref. 34.)

Standard voiding pressure–flow studies cannot determine the actual site of outflow obstruction, which may be anatomical, or functional (e.g., detrusor—external sphincter—dyssynergia [DESD]). Detrusor hyperreflexia with DESD occurs when there is dyscoordination between the contracting detrusor and the external sphincter owing to a neurological lesion and occurs in association detrusor hyperreflexia. The pontine micturition center allows coordination between detrusor and urethral sphincters, resulting in sphincter relaxation during detrusor contraction. In a suprasacral spinal cord injury, for example, this coordination is lost, and the urethral sphincter may not relax or may even contract during detrusor contraction, resulting in a functional obstruction (36) (see Fig. 11). DESD is a potential dangerous condition, as it can result in excessively high storage pressures and retention of urine, leading to upper tract deterioration. A similar phenomenon, known as pseudodyssynergia or dysfunctional voiding, can also occur in the absence of a neurological lesion, but such cases are caused by a learned behavior; thus, they are not considered true dyssynergia.

III. VIDEOURODYNAMICS

Videourodynamics (VUDS) refers to the simultaneous measurement and display of urodynamic parameters with radiographic visualization of the lower urinary tract. When performing VUDS, radiographic contrast is used as the infusant for cystometry. Urodynamics tests are performed as described in the forgoing (37–41). Because all variables are visualized simultaneously one can better appreciate their interrelations and identify artifacts with ease, making VUDS the most precise diagnostic tool for voiding dysfunction.

Simultaneous fluoroscopic imaging of the bladder and bladder outlet during voiding can aid in the diagnosis and localization of obstruction (Fig. 21). Also external sphincter ac-

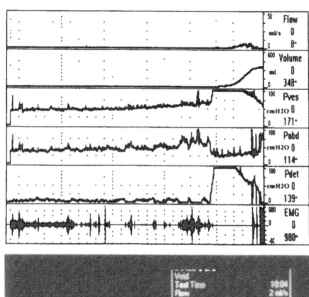

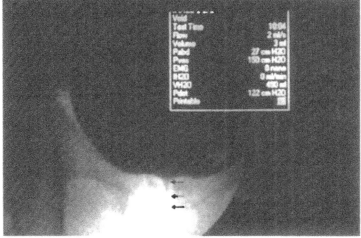

Figure 21 Videourodynamic study of a 40-year-old man with severe lower urinary tract symptoms refractory to medication: (A) Multichannel urodynamic study showing a stable, compliant bladder with high-pressure, low-flow voiding. There is a delay in flow from the onset of the detrusor contraction despite a decrease in EMG activity. Clearly, this is consistent with obstruction. (B) Fluoroscopic image of the bladder outlet with urodynamic parameters (inset) taken during voiding localizes the obstruction to the bladder neck and proximal urethra (arrows). In this case, it was critical to localize the obstruction in this young man as he had failed medical therapy. Successful surgery (a bladder neck incision) was later performed with confidence knowing exactly where the obstruction was located. There is only a slight rise in detrusor pressure: flow, urinary flow rate; volume, volume voided; P_{ves}, total vesical pressure; P_{abd}, total abdominal pressure; P_{det}, subtracted detrusor pressure.

tivity can be monitored fluoroscopically during voiding, which is helpful when EMG is equivocal. Videourodynamics is also useful when vesicoureteral reflux is present, as reflux volumes and pressures can be determined.

Although some clinicians prefer to use VUDS routinely, there are specific circumstances for which this type of testing should always be employed. For example, in patients

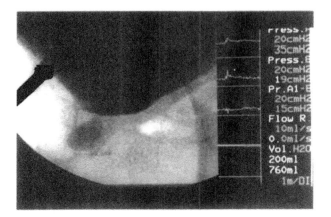

Figure 22 Female bladder outlet obstruction: videourodynamic study of an 85-year-old woman 3 years after excision of a urethral caruncle which resulted in total urinary retention. She was maintained on intermittent self-catheterization. The study shows a sustained, but low-pressure detrusor contraction of 15 cm/H$_2$O. There is an obvious distal urethral obstruction with a very dilated urethra proximal to it. Without the video image, one might be tempted to make a diagnosis of impaired detrusor contractility. At surgery the patient's true urethra was found to be closed off and she was catheterizing through a false passage above the true urethra. After urethral reconstruction, the patient voided spontaneously without residual. Top line on tracing, total vesical pressure; second from top, total abdominal pressure; third from top, subtracted detrusor pressure. (From Ref. 42.)

for whom routine multichannel urodynamics are equivocal or give an incomplete diagnosis, simultaneous fluoroscopic imaging can provide missing information. VUDS is also helpful in cases for whom it is important to visualize anatomy, such as a large cystocele. VUDS also permits an accurate assessment of incontinence and leak point pressures when such measurements are difficult to obtain otherwise. Visualization of the female bladder outlet in cases of suspected obstruction is invaluable when attempting to make such a diagnosis (Fig. 22) (42). Finally, in cases of anatomical abnormalities (e.g., large bladder diverticulum), VUDS can help assess the effect of abnormality on voiding function.

REFERENCES

1. Wein AJ. Classification of neurogenic voiding dysfunction. J Urol 1981; 125:605–609.
2. Nitti VW, Combs AJ. Urodynamics: when, why and how. In: Nitti VW, ed. Practical Urodynamics. Philadelphia: WB Saunders, 1998:15–26.
3. Nitti VW. Cystometry and abdominal pressure monitoring. In: Nitti VW, ed. Practical Urodynamics. Philadelphia: WB Saunders, 1998:38–51.
4. Wein AJ, English WS, Whitmore KE. Office urodynamics. Urol Clin North Am 1988; 15:609–623.
5. Blaivas JG. Multichannel urodynamic studies. Urology 1984; 23:421–438.
6. Abrams P, Blaivas JG, Stanton SL, Andersen JT. The standardization of terminology of lower urinary tract function. Scand J Urol Nephrol Suppl 1988; 114:5–19.
7. Blaivas JG. The neurophysiology of normal micturition: a clinical study of 550 patients. J Urol 1982; 127:958–963.

8. Elbadawi A, Yalla SV, Resnick NM. Structural basis of geriatric voiding, dysfunction. III. Detrusor overactivity. J Urol 1993; 150:1668–1680.

9. Toppercer A, Tetreault JP. Compliance of the bladder: an attempt to establish normal values. Urology 1979; 14:204–205.

10. Gilmour RF, Churchill BM, Steckler RE, Houe AM, Khoury AE, McLorie GA. A new technique for dynamic analysis of bladder compliance. J Urol 1993; 150:1200–1203.

11. McGuire EJ, Woodside JR, Borden TA, Weiss RM. Prognostic value of urodynamic testinc, in myelodysplasic patients. J Urol 1981; 126:205–209.

12. Churchill BM, Gilmour RF, Williot P. Urodynamics. Pediatr Clin North Am 1987; 34:1133–1157.

13. Cespedes RD, McGuire EJ. Leak point pressures. In: Nitti VW, ed. Practical Urodynamics. Philadelphia: WB Saunders, 1998:94–107.

14. McGuire EJ, Fitzpatrick CC, Wan J, Bloom D, Sanvordenker J, Ritchey M, Gormley EA. Clinical assessment of urethral sphincter function. J Urol 1993; 150:1452–1454.

15. O'Donnell PA. Electromyography. In: Nitti VW, ed, Practical Urodynamics. Philadelphia: WB Saunders, 1998:65–77.

16. Nitti VW, Kim Y, Combs AJ. Correlation of the AUA symptom score index with urodynamics in patients with suspected benign prostatic hyperplasia. Neurourol Urodynam 1994; 13:521–529.

17. Yalla SV, Sullivan NT, Lecamwasam HS, Dubeau CE, Vickers MA, Cravalho EG. Correlation of American Urological Association svmptom index with obstructive and nonobstructive prostatism. J Urol 1995; 153:674–680.

18. Sirls LT, Kirkemo AK, Jay J. Lack of correlation of the American Urological Association Symptom 7 Index with urodynamic bladder outlet obstruction. Neurourol Urodynam 1996; 15:447–457.

19. Chancellor MB, Blaivas JG, Kaplan SA, Axelrod S. Bladder outlet obstruction versus impaired detrusor contractility: the role of uroflow. J Urol 1991; 145:810–812.

20. Gerstenberg TC, Andersen JT, Klarskov P, Ramirez D, Hald T. High flow infravesical obstruction in men: symptomatology, urodynamics and the results of surgery. J Urol 1982; 127:943–945.

21. George NJ, Slade N. Hesitancy and poor stream in younger men without outflow tract obstruction—the anxious bladder. Br J Urol 1979; 51:506–509.

22. Griffiths DJ. Pressure-flow studies of micturition. Urol Clin North Am 1996; 23:279–297.

23. Abrams PH, Griffiths DJ. The assessment of prostatic obstruction from urodynamic measurements and from residual urine. Br J Urol 1979; 51:129–134.

24. Coolsaet BLRA, van Venrooij GEPM, Blok C. Prostatism. Rationalization of urodynamic testing. World J Urol 1984; 2:216–221.

25. Griffiths DJ. The mechanics of the urethra and of micturition. Br J Urol 1973; 45:497–507.

26. Griffiths DJ. Urodynamic assessment of bladder function. Br J Urol 1977; 49:29–36.

27. Schafer W. Urodynamics of micturition. Curr Opin Urol 1996; 2:252–256.

28. McGuire EJ. Urodynamic studies in prostatic obstruction. In: Fitzpatrick J, Krane R, eds. The Prostate. New York: Churchill Livingstone, 1989:103–109.

29. Blaivas JG. Multichannel urodynamic studies in men with benign prostatic hyperplasia: indications and interpretation. Urol Clin North Am 1990; 17:543–552.

30. Blaivas JG. Bladder outlet obstruction in men. In: Nitti VW, ed. Practical Urodynamics. Philadelphia: WB Saunders, 1998:156–171.

31. Abrams PH, Griffiths DJ. The assessment of prostatic obstruction from urodynamic measurements and from residual urine. Br J Urol 1979; 51:129–134.

32. Schafer W. Detrusor as the energy source of micturition. In: Hinman F Jr, Boyarsky S, eds. Benign Prostatic Hypertrophy. New York: Springer Verlag, 1983:450–469.

33. Schafer W. Principles and clinical application of advanced urodynamic analysis of voiding function. Urol Clin North Am 1990; 17:553–566.

34. Griffiths D, Hofner K, van Mastrigt R, Rollema HJ, Spangberg A, Gleason D. Standardization of terminology of lower urinary tract function: pressure–flow studies of voiding, urethral resistance, and urethral obstruction. Neurourol Urodynam 1997; 16:1–18.

35. Nitti VW, Tu LM, Gitlin J. Diagnosing bladder outlet obstruction in women. J Urol 1999; 161: 1535–1540.

36. Blaivas JG, Sinha HP, Zayed AA, Labib KB. Detrusor–external sphincter dyssynergia. J Urol 1981; 125:542–544.

37. Bates CP, Corney CE. Synchronous cine/pressure/flow cystography; a method of routine urodynamic investigation. Br J Radiol 1971; 44:44–50.

38. McGuire EJ. Combined radiographic and manometric assessment of urethral sphincter function. J Urol 1977; 118:632–635.

39. Webster GD, Older RA. Videourodynamics. Urology 1980; 16:106–114.

40. Blaivas JG, Fischer DM. Combined radiographic and urodynamic monitoring: advances in techniques. J Urol 1981; 125:693–694.

41. Blaivas JG. Videourodynamic studies. In: Nitti VW, ed. Practical Urodynamics. Philadelphia: WB Saunders, 1998:78–93.

42. Nitti VW, Raz S. Urinary retention. In: Raz S, ed. Female Urology. 2nd ed. Philadelphia, WB Saunders, 1996:197–213.

24

Ambulatory Urodynamic Monitoring

STEPHEN C. RADLEY, DEREK J. ROSARIO, and
CHRISTOPHER R. CHAPPLE

Central Sheffield University Hospitals, Sheffield, England

I. INTRODUCTION

The primary aim of clinical urodynamics is to provide an objective explanation of symptoms with a view to guiding treatment. To this end, tests must be reproducible, reliable, and specific to the condition under investigation. It is over a century since Dubois (1) and Mosso and Pellacani (2) described the measurement of intravesical pressure during filling and voiding, respectively. In the 1950s and 1960s "hydrodynamics" or "urodynamics" gained recognition in clinical practice (3,4). During the 1970s, understanding of outflow obstruction improved with Griffiths' work defining the relation between pressure and flow through distensible tubes (5). Cystometric findings were shown by several workers to be predictive of outcome following outflow surgery in men and continence surgery in women. The techniques and terminology used, in what have now come to be referred to as "conventional" or "static" urodynamic investigation, were standardized by the International Continence Society during the 1980s (6). *Ambulatory urodynamic monitoring* may broadly be defined as any cystometric investigation performed outside the laboratory utilizing "natural" bladder filling. The principal aim of ambulatory urodynamics is to reproduce a patient's symptoms and measure associated detrusor and sphincter function during natural filling in a normal environment. In the adult human, the detrusor is unique as the only involuntary muscle under direct cortical control. Therefore, in addition to the effects of nonphysiological filling, detrusor function may be further influenced by environmental conditions prevalent during conventional testing. Whereas static urodynamic investigation was introduced largely unchallenged as a peerless investigation of lower urinary tract function, ambulatory monitoring must be shown to have clear evidence of clinical benefit before its introduction into mainstream practice. This process has been hindered by a lack of validated protocols for its conduct and interpretation and by concerns over data quality and reliability. The following chapter highlights the advantages and drawbacks of ambulatory monitoring in a range of clinical and research settings, with particular reference to our extensive experience of this modality in our unit.

II. HISTORY

In 1957, Comarr described cystometry using natural filling in patients with neurological injury (7). He reported increased bladder capacity and decreased filling pressure in studies employing diuresis-induced natural filling, compared with artificial filling methods. In 1960 Tsuji reported increased phasic activity in some spinal injury patients studied by natural-filling methods (8). These findings resulted in practical changes in the urodynamic investigation of neuropathic patients, but were not extrapolated to urodynamics in the neurologically intact. In 1978 James described monitoring of detrusor function during physical exercise, using long-term natural fill, and introduced the term *ambulatory monitoring* (9). The technique was limited by the physical constraints of the system. The recording equipment was separated from the patient by a partition in the room, which although affording more privacy, substantially restricted mobility. Nevertheless, the ability to demonstrate abnormal detrusor contractions while reproducing the conditions under which the patient experienced symptoms was clearly demonstrated. The next development was that of a magnetic tape recorder allowing portability (10). This device lacked memory, which limited, among other things, the sampling rate. The conflict between portability and memory capacity has been resolved by the increased power and miniaturization of computer systems. Styles et al. investigated a variety of patient groups using long-term natural-fill ambulatory monitoring, initially using a rather cumbersome system, which limited testing to the bedside (11). Subsequently, a digital system was employed that could truly be regarded to as portable or ambulatory (12). Modern-day recorder units, such as the MMS UPS-2020 are purpose-built, microprocessor units that are lightweight, of a convenient size, and capable of recording continuously on several channels for several hours. Currently, there are at least three different systems available worldwide for ambulatory monitoring.

Various types of pressure transducer have been described for use in ambulatory monitoring. In early systems, pressure was transmitted by water- or saline-filled catheters to externally mounted transducers. These are easily calibrated and zeroed to atmospheric pressure. Once zeroed, the pressure relative to an external reference point (conventionally, the superior border of the pubic symphysis) is measured. With this system, artifact increases considerably with increased patient movement. James approached this problem by employing an air-filled catheter, the principle being that the volume of air in a small-caliber, short, rigid-walled tube is relatively insignificant compared with the volume of the reservoir at the tip (9). Therefore, pressure transmission is not significantly affected by compression, and the accuracy of pressure readings is maintained. This assumption necessitates a catheter of short length, thereby restricting patient mobility. The availability of Luer-lock, mounted micropressure transducers can overcome some of these limitations and have been employed by some units. Microtip transducers mounted on silicone-coated catheters are currently the most popular. Their main advantages are quality of signal and reliability. However, there are disadvantages. Unlike fluid-filled measurement systems, where an external pressure reference point is defined, the zero reference point is the tip of the catheter itself; hence, once the catheter is introduced, zero cannot be reset without removing the catheter. Also as the bladder fills, the position of the transducer may vary, altering the pressure registered without a "true" change in intravesical pressure.

III. THE CONDUCT OF AMBULATORY URODYNAMIC STUDIES

In our unit, ambulatory urodynamic monitoring is performed using an MMS UPS-2020 recording device with pressure sampling at 8 Hz (Fig. 1). We use Gaeltec microtip transducers, end-mounted on a silicone coated 7F catheter. All catheters are presoaked for at least 15 min before their calibration in a 50-cm column of water. The rectal transducer is covered with a prewetted vented finger-cot and both transducers zeroed to atmospheric pressure. The patient initially voids in private, following which urethral and rectal catheters are inserted and recording commenced. Postmicturition residual urine volumes are measured by ultrasound. Patients are administered an oral fluid load of 750 mL (fruit juice or water) at the start of each test. Measured losses during the test are replaced with further oral

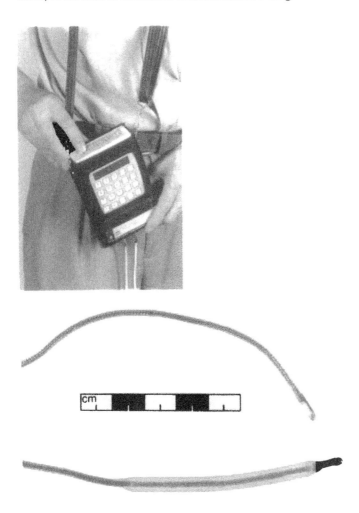

Figure 1   Ambulatory monitoring device (MMS UPS-2020) with solid-state transducers, end mounted on silicone-coated microtip vesical and rectal catheters (Gaeltec).

fluids. Additional food and fluid intake is permitted if requested, avoiding caffeine or alcohol. Instruction is given in the use of a contemporaneous symptom diary, recording symptoms or events during the study, in particular the timing and severity of urinary urgency or leakage. Patients are asked to grade urgency as mild (+), moderate (++), or severe (+++). Event buttons on the top of the ambulatory box are also used to confirm the timing of symptoms, provocative tests, and voids.

Each study is divided into three periods of approximately 1 hr. During the first hour, patients are asked to sit quietly, having consumed the initial fluid load. During the second hour of the test, patients perform normal activities, including climbing one flight of stairs and walking. The third hour of the test includes two periods of provocative testing (Fig. 2), separated by 10–20 min, performed at least 30 min after the previous void.

Provocative exercises include the following:

Standing from the sitting position ten times.
Coughing vigorously ten times.
Bending down and picking up an object from the floor five times.
Handwashing in cold, running water in the women's washroom for 1 min.

During provocative testing, the patient is asked to continue grading, reporting, and recording her symptoms. A weighed, absorbent perineal pad is changed and reweighed after each hour of the test to quantify urinary leakage. Subjects are strongly encouraged to withhold voiding for as long as they feel comfortable, returning when necessary to void in private on a commode equipped with a flow meter connected to the recording device. Checks of correct catheter placement and function are performed using cough tests with on-line observation of vesical and rectal pressure at intervals of approximately 20 min.

An event button is pressed and a cough test performed before and following each void, the time and volume of which are recorded. The study is usually concluded during the

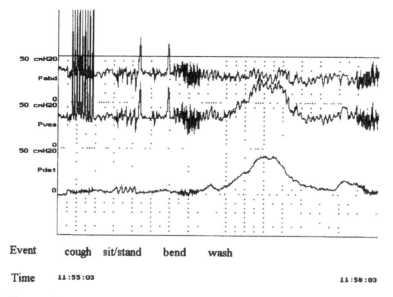

Figure 2   Section of ambulatory urodynamic study during provocative testing including repeated coughs followed by handwashing-provoked detrusor instability.

third hour, provided that the patient has voided during that hour and ideally completed two sets of provocative exercises. Residual urine is again estimated by ultrasound scanning and, when necessary, catheter drainage.

IV. THE INTERPRETATION AND REPORTING OF AMBULATORY URODYNAMIC STUDIES

A. Data Quality

Unlike static urodynamics, ambulatory monitoring relies on reproducing, as far as possible, the natural conditions of filling and voiding. However, ensuring adequate data quality during ambulatory recording requires painstaking attention to detail. During static urodynamics, pressure measurement may be observed continuously by the test supervisor and problems identified and dealt with promptly. Ambulatory monitoring does allow intermittent on-line assessment of transducer function. Nevertheless, a number of investigations will, in retrospect, prove to be uninterpretable for technical reasons alone. Furthermore, the freedom and flexibility afforded by ambulatory monitoring is one of its main attractions and must not be unduly compromised by effectively conducting a prolonged "laboratory" study, reintroducing some of the inherent drawbacks that ambulatory monitoring seeks to avoid.

The test supervisor will himself or herself have an important influence on a patient during the study. The quality of information or instruction given, the prompting of symptoms, and even the degree of embarrassment will potentially affect results and may vary between different investigators. Furthermore, the interpretation of so-called objective cystometric findings is a highly subjective process, as evidenced by high intra- and interobserver variation in reporting of these studies. Ambulatory urodynamics may overcome some of these difficulties, but has its own particular problems of interpretation.

There is no substitute for experience when conducting, interpreting, and reporting urodynamic studies. The use of ambulatory urodynamic protocols should assist in achieving reliable and reproducible measurements, without interfering substantially with the aims of assessing lower urinary tract function in as normal an environment as possible. A rigid protocol will not suit all circumstances and individuals. However, measurements made in a nonstandardized way will be less objective and, therefore, of less clinical value. If a pragmatic approach is applied and guidelines are simple, the overall result should be an improvement in quality. Data quality is dependent not only on the accuracy of pressure measurements themselves, but also the records kept by the subject and the observer, particularly for the recording of symptoms. Studies are rarely if ever perfect. However, poor-quality studies can often yield useful information. Although the detection of detrusor activity and classification of urinary incontinence may be of primary importance, the measurement and reporting of other parameters, such as symptoms, voiding function, cystometric capacity, or residual urine volume must not be overlooked.

B. Data Handling

Recorded data is downloaded to a PC and analyzed with MMS software. Interpretation is undertaken in conjunction with the symptom diary, event markers, and additional documentation made by the test supervisor. The mean fill rate for each filling phase is derived from the initial and final residual urine volumes, the voided volume, and the duration of each cycle. These parameters are then employed to estimate the bladder volume when symptoms and events occurred. The volume at which mild, moderate, or severe urgency were reported is calculated for each filling phase.

C. The Reporting of Symptoms

The accuracy and reliability of symptom diaries and event markers during ambulatory urodynamics is inevitably variable and depends on a patient's ability to understand and comply with instructions, the quality of information and instruction given, and the degree of subsequent supervision. Differences in the subjective interpretation, recording, and grading of symptoms will inevitably be encountered between patients of differing cultural background, mental state, and intellectual ability and may be influenced by past medical history and urodynamic experience, their expectations, and preconceptions.

In some instances, symptom recording may be incomplete, inaccurate, and nonrepresentative. For example, a patient who is experiencing mild urgency, is more likely to accurately record this symptom and its timing than when experiencing urge incontinence, when data collection may be of lesser importance than personal hygiene. Compliance with symptom recording may improve during the course of a particular study, giving the erroneous impression of an increase in symptoms or replacing asymptomatic with symptomatic detrusor overactivity. Conversely, the discomfort associated with urethral catheterization is often reported as "continuous mild urgency," a symptom that usually settles during the early part of the test. Urgency is itself a nonspecific symptom, commonly reported in association with rectal contractions and even genuine stress incontinence. Furthermore, in studies showing involuntary detrusor activity, most urgency symptoms are not associated with detectable detrusor activity.

D. The Detection of Leakage

Urine loss is quantified using preweighed pads, which are replaced hourly. Losses of greater than 1 g/hr are reported as positive (ICS pad test). "Genuine stress incontinence" (GSI) is diagnosed when urine loss is reported and detected in the absence of detrusor instability. In women with coexistent detrusor instability, stress incontinence is diagnosed only when leakage is reported in the absence of detrusor activity and a positive pad test. The addition of an electronic leakage detection device may improve the specificity of the investigation by recording the timing of leakage, particularly if the patient diary is incomplete or unreliable (Fig. 3). These pads add to the cost of the study, may suffer from artifact, and do not accurately quantify the volume of leakage.

E. Detrusor Overactivity

The amplitude and duration of the first and maximum spontaneous detrusor contractions and associated symptoms is reported. Detrusor contractions provoked by handwashing are assessed separately. No arbitrary minimum amplitude is set for the detection of detrusor activity, which, therefore, is determined by the quality and resolution of the subtracted detrusor pressure trace itself. Detrusor instability is diagnosed only if bladder overactivity is associated with symptoms such as urgency or incontinence.

V. ARTIFACTS

The use of catheter-mounted, solid-state microtip transducers during ambulatory monitoring may improve some aspects of data quality, although it is not of itself without some

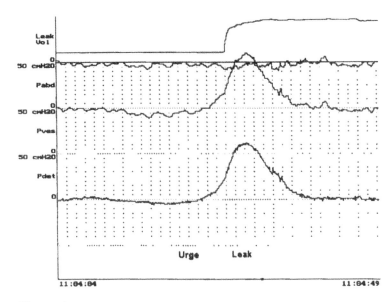

Figure 3 Ambulatory urodynamic study during episode of urge incontinence: electronic leakage detection (upper trace) and detrusor contraction (lower trace).

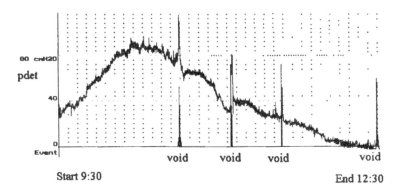

Figure 4 Ambulatory urodynamic study showing subtracted detrusor pressure with large artifactual pressure rise and fall over a 3-hr period of study (transducer malfunction).

drawbacks. These catheters and their transducers ultimately fail, often during a study when the fault may not be fully appreciated until the study has been completed (Fig. 4). Even when a problem has been identified during a study, intervention is limited to adjustments in catheter position. A decision must be made whether to persist with a substandard study or to start afresh with exchange and calibration of new catheters. In the clinical setting, problems detected during the first hour, not remediable by repositioning, warrant radical action, which usually implies removing and changing all catheters. In such circumstances the patient is asked to continue to withhold voiding and the investigator accepts that the first hour of the study, in terms of pressure measurement, is invalid. It should be remembered that assessment of bladder capacity and symptoms during the filling phase are still ongoing. Readings during the first part of any study may be subject to higher degrees of artifact and compliance, with the recording of symptoms being generally poorer. In terms of cystometric data, detrusor overactivity is most commonly seen during the latter stages of the investigation, usually in the third hour and during provocative maneuvers. Continuing with a study with the suspicion of suboptimal transducer function risks an invalid test, which may ultimately need repeating.

Consistent and measurable artifactual changes in baseline pressure may be subtracted to estimate the true amplitude of pressure waves. Such adjustments, nevertheless, demand evidence of otherwise satisfactory transducer function with good subtraction, facilitated by carrying out regular cough tests (at intervals of 10–20 min and before and after voids). If such adjustments to detrusor pressure are made, standardization of method must be established to maintain objectivity.

When attributing apparent pressure changes to either detrusor activity or artifact the morphology of pressure traces gives helpful clues: A sudden straight line rise or fall in pressure may be observed in either vesical or abdominal pressure and is characteristic of artifact owing to change in catheter position in relation to the wall of the viscus (Fig. 5a) or solid material within it. A smoother sinusoidal rectal pressure rise caused by rectal contractions (see Fig. 5b), may lead to the erroneous impression of detrusor activity, especially to the untrained observer. Examples are seen in both ambulatory and conventional cystometry; however, such activity rarely lasts more than a few minutes. This may be critical during medium fill cystometry, but is unlikely to invalidate an entire ambulatory study, a major advantage of ambulatory urodynamics.

Artifactual changes in baseline detrusor pressure are, therefore, observed in a large proportion of studies and can usually be distinguished from actual detrusor activity. However, if uncertainty exists as to the origin and authenticity of apparent detrusor pressure changes, this portion of the study is reported as "inadequate for diagnostic purposes."

VI. STUDIES INVOLVING AMBULATORY URODYNAMIC MONITORING

Although several studies utilizing ambulatory techniques have been reported, to date there has been no standardization of methodology, making comparison of results difficult. Additionally, the issue of data quality has not been adequately addressed, and guidelines are lacking for the conduct and interpretation of these studies. We include here only those studies for which methodology has been adequately described and some attempt made to exclude artifact during analysis.

A. Asymptomatic Volunteers

The largest study to date involving normal female subjects has been carried out by van Waalwijk van Doorn, investigating 50 healthy female volunteers using ambulatory urodynamics, urethral pressure profilometry, and conventional static cystometry (13). Only 36 volunteers were analyzed, 12 being excluded because of symptoms detected on a pretesting questionnaire and 2 because of equipment failure. In these 36, asymptomatic volunteers, the mean duration of ambulatory urodynamics was 4 hr 56 mins. Only 11 (31%) had a completely uneventful trace of vesical pressure (i.e., no detectable detrusor activity). The remainder had between one and four contractions (36%) and five or more contractions (33%). It is important to note, however, that the mean rise in detrusor pressure was only 9.8 cmH_2O and the mean duration only 10.1 secs. It is also noteworthy that the minimum amplitude of contractions recorded was 3 cmH_2O. Most investigators would consider a change of pressure of this magnitude to be within the margins set for movement artifact. Robertson (12) studied 17 volunteers (11 men, 6 women) of whom 16 underwent ambulatory urody-

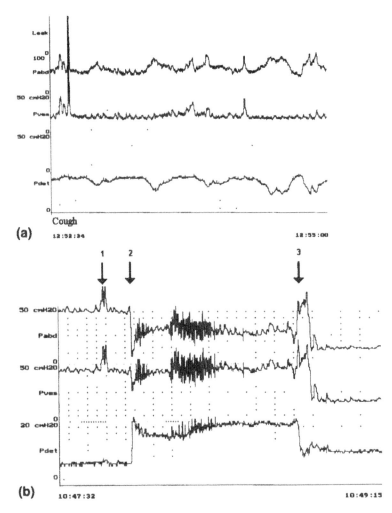

Figure 5 (a) Ambulatory urodynamic study showing artifactual change in subtracted detrusor pressure (lower trace) caused by rectal contractions (upper trace). (b) Ambulatory urodynamic study showing artifactual rise in subtracted detrusor pressure (lower trace) attributed to change in catheter position: 1) cough; 2) artifactual pressure rise; 3) resolution.

namics. Six of these (38%) had detectable detrusor activity during filling of which two (both women) had peak amplitudes of 20 and 25 cmH$_2$O. In an attempt to differentiate between detrusor activity seen in asymptomatic volunteers and in symptomatic patients, van Doorn introduced the concept of a "detrusor activity index." Although this approach has yet to be universally accepted, such activity as detected on ambulatory urodynamics in asymptomatic individuals seems, in most cases, to be qualitatively different from that seen in symptomatic patients (see later discussion).

B. Male Voiding

In the evaluation of normal male voiding function during ambulatory urodynamics, few studies have reported synchronous pressure–flow data. In a group of 18 asymptomatic male

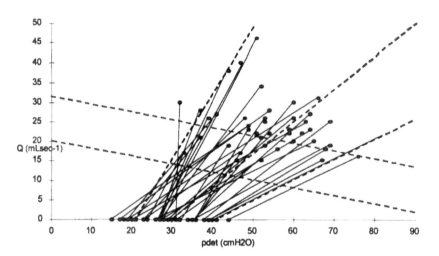

Figure 6 LinPURR plots in young asymptomatic males showing variability in voiding characteristics: Note that several of the voids plot into the minimally obstructed category of Schäfer (grade II) with one even plotting as unequivocally obstructed (grade III).

volunteers between 18 and 40 years of age, we found the mean $P_{det}Q_{max}$ to be 53 cmH$_2$O (range 32–83 cmH$_2$O) with a mean Q_{max} of 24 mL sec^{-1} (range 15–46 mL sec^{-1}) (14). Figure 6 illustrates the variability of the voids for $P_{det}Q_{max}$ against Q_{max} on the Schäfer pressure–flow diagram. Figure 7 illustrates three successive voids in an asymptomatic individual on the ICS nomogram. One of these is unequivocally obstructed and the other two are equivocal for obstruction. There would appear to be considerable variability in voiding pressure both between and within individuals. These findings have implications for the uro-

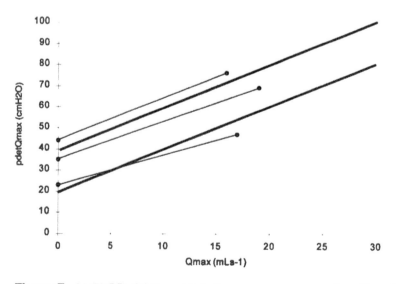

Figure 7 LinPURR of three voids in the same young asymptomatic male demonstrating variability: The voids are plotted on the proposed ICS nomogram for defining male bladder outflow obstruction associated with BPH. (From Ref. 14.)

dynamic definition of abnormal voiding and the clinical application of both static and ambulatory urodynamics in this context.

Robertson studied numerous men undergoing prostatic resection to see whether ambulatory monitoring could assist in the definition of outflow obstruction (15). He found little difference between the two in terms of voiding pressure and concluded that ambulatory monitoring had little to offer in the routine assessment of men with symptoms of bladder outflow obstruction. We used ambulatory urodynamics in low-pressure voiders to examine differences between natural and artificial fill cystometry. In common with previous findings we found no significant difference in detrusor pressure at peak flow. However, the peak flow rate during ambulatory studies was significantly higher than during static cystometry. There was also considerable variability in pressures during voiding, with successive voids tending to be less obstructed than the first void. Several of those with equivocal or even borderline obstruction during static cystometry were reclassified as unobstructed using ambulatory urodynamics (Fig. 8). It would appear from this data that conditions prevalent during urodynamic testing can affect outcome, with some men failing to adequately relax their outlet, resulting in an artifactual degree of obstruction. The poor results of transurethral resection in borderline obstructed men suggest that the addition of ambulatory urodynamics in this selected group may help distinguish truly obstructed from nonobstructed individuals.

C. Female Voiding

In a prospective randomized study comparing static with ambulatory urodynamics in 107 women with urinary urgency, bladder capacity and voiding pressures were not significantly different between the two modalities. However, we found significantly higher flow rates during ambulatory than during conventional cystometry. Residual urine volumes were also less, and the incidence of complete inability to void with catheters in situ was zero during ambulatory, compared with 9% during conventional urodynamics (Table 1).

These findings support the use of ambulatory monitoring in the assessment of female voiding function, with more efficient bladder emptying, reflecting more physiological detrusor and sphincter function. Ambulatory monitoring, therefore, is more likely to yield meaningful voiding data than static cystometry.

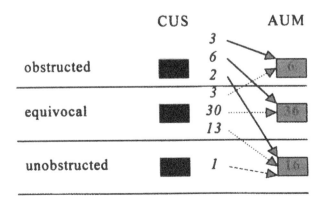

Figure 8 Differences in classification on the Abrams–Griffiths nomogram in 58 borderline obstructed males between conventional static cystometry (CUS) and ambulatory monitoring (AUM). (From Ref. 21.)

Table 1 Voiding Parameters During Ambulatory and Conventional Urodynamics in a Group of 107 Women Referred for Investigation of Urinary Urgency. Paired Prospective Data, Randomized for Study Order.

	Ambulatory monitoring mean (SD)	Static monitoring mean (SD)	p value
Maximum voided volume (mL)	450.0 (149.1)	425.8 (120.6)	0.267[a]
Maximum cystometric capacity (mL)	482.4 (170.4)	442.3 (112.2)	0.047[a]
Q_{max} (mL/sec)	22.73 (10.04)	17.22 (7.05)	<0.001[a]
$P_{det}Q_{max}$ (cmH$_2$O)	33.27 (18.03)	36.13 (19.0)	0.265[a]
P_{detmax}	44.42 (25.42)	45.7 (21.2)	0.689
Incomplete or unable to void	21%	34%	Relative risk = 0.6
Unable to void with catheter in situ	0	9%	

[a]Student t test.

D. Bashful Bladder Syndrome

The bashful bladder is defined as the inability of a male to void when in the presence of others. In a group of 40 consecutive men, unable to void during static cystometry, pressure–flow data were available for 37, with a mean number of 2.72 ± 0.1 storage-void cycles recorded per patient (16). The videocystometrogram of one such man is shown in Figure 9. The trace shows poor activation of the detrusor, abdominal straining, and failure to relax the

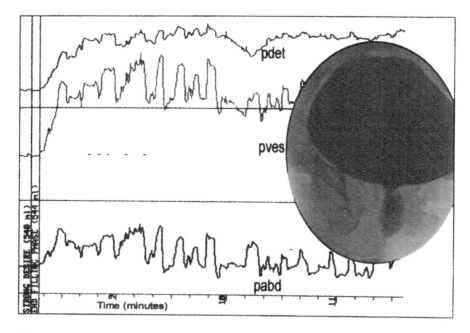

Figure 9 Voiding phase of static video cystometrogram: Note abdominal straining pattern, poor detrusor contractility, and failure to relax the pelvic floor. EMG in such cases typically shows increased activity during voiding.

pelvic floor. In this group, 6 men (15%) were obstructed, all of whom were older than 40 years of age, 6 (15%) had equivocal outflow obstruction, and the remaining 25 were unobstructed. Two of the 6 obstructed men have undergone TURP and one urethrotomy, with good subjective and objective results.

E. Chronic Urinary Retention

The relation between bladder pressure, residual volume, and upper tract changes is a matter of considerable interest. Using natural filling, the high end-filling pressure seen during conventional cystometry can be shown to be artifactual, being replaced with phasic detrusor activity during ambulatory monitoring (11). In those men with upper tract dilation, phasic rises in detrusor pressure are more common and the resting pressure is higher, suggesting that this, rather than an elevated voiding pressure, contributes to upper tract damage.

F. Neuropathic Bladder Dysfunction

It is accepted that in neuropathic patients, artificial filling leads to significant artifact. As previously stated, Comarr reported an increased bladder capacity and lower filling pressures in such patients studied during diuresis-induced natural fill compared with artificial fill cycles (7). In 1960 Tsuji reported increased phasic activity in some patients with spinal injured during natural fill cystometry (8). This work has been further elaborated by Thomas (17), who has developed protocols for the investigation of reservoir and voiding function in subjects with spinal injury, using conventional videourodynamic investigations. Webb et al. carried out both conventional- and natural-fill urodynamic investigation on such patients and found that in a group with low compliance during artificial filling there was a high incidence of phasic activity detected during natural filling, and furthermore this activity correlated well with upper tract changes (18).

G. Drug Evaluation

A high correlation between symptoms and findings on ambulatory monitoring has been reported in several studies, supporting the hypothesis that this technique more accurately reflects lower urinary tract behavior and, therefore, symptomatology, than conventional urodynamics (16,19,20,21). Several studies have employed static cystometry in an attempt to demonstrate quantitative changes in detrusor overactivity. There is no generally accepted cystometric criterion that is reliably related to the severity of detrusor instability. Surrogate endpoints that have been used include volume at first desire to void, maximal detrusor pressure during filling, and maximum cystometric capacity (22–24). The very nature of conventional urodynamics renders such markers not only operator-dependent and, therefore, open to considerable individual bias, but also likely to be influenced by extraneous patient factors, such as embarrassment and anxiety. It is generally accepted by experienced urodynamicists that such time points are highly variable within any one individual and correlate poorly with symptoms. There are considerable difficulties, therefore, in the quantitative interpretation of measurements taken during static urodynamics.

In a small phase III study involving six patients we found that symptom data for individual patients correlated well with urodynamic markers of detrusor activity during ambulatory urodynamic tests. In those reporting symptomatic improvement there was a reduction in almost every parameter measured, whereas in those with no improvement in

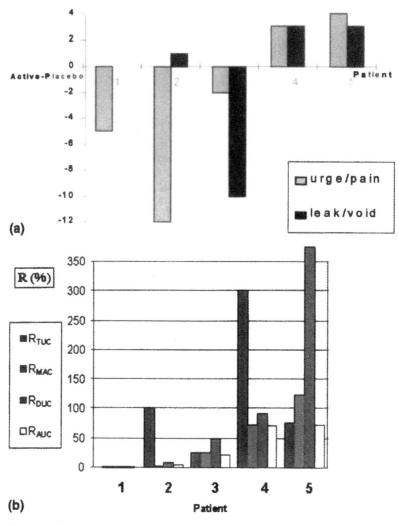

Figure 10   (a) Change in symptoms in five patients on darifenacin or placebo in a randomized controlled trial; (b) Change in detrusor activity in five patients treated with darifenacin:

$$R, Ratio = \frac{activity\ while\ on\ drug}{activity\ while\ on\ placebo} \times 100$$

TUC, total number of unstable contractions; MAC, maximal amplitude; DUC, duration of unstable contraction; AUC, area under the curve. (From Ref. 14.)

symptoms, there was little or no change (Fig. 10). Because this is a small sample, these observations must be viewed with some caution; nevertheless, they support the suggestion that ambulatory urodynamic indices better reflect symptoms than arbitrary markers used during static cystometry (25). These findings are in agreement with those of van Doorn who used ambulatory urodynamics to assess the efficacy of oxybutynin in a similar patient group (26).

H. The Urge Syndrome

The definition of bladder overactivity in terms of urodynamic, rather than clinical terms, has led to confusion in the classification of urinary urgency and urge incontinence. Although characterized by irritative symptoms, these symptoms themselves are not exclusive to, nor diagnostic of bladder overactivity. In the past this observation has provided a compelling argument for the use of urodynamic studies in the investigation of lower urinary tract symptoms. However, several studies have shown that a significant proportion of women suffering from urgency, in whom conventional urodynamics fails to diagnose detrusor instability, will have symptomatic bladder overactivity during ambulatory urodynamics. The definition of detrusor instability per se is based on conventional, not ambulatory, urodynamic parameters. There is, therefore, continuing controversy over the significance and classification of bladder overactivity detected during ambulatory urodynamics. Early comparative studies commonly included heterogeneous groups of patients, selected on the basis of symptoms unexplained by static urodynamics. These observational studies do not allow unbiased comparison of the two tests and cannot determine the true value of ambulatory urodynamics in the clinical setting.

We conducted a randomized prospective study, comparing the results of ambulatory urodynamics with conventional static cystometry. Validated questionnaires (Bristol female lower urinary tract symptoms questionnaire) and standardized protocols (as described in the foregoing) were used for both ambulatory and static urodynamic evaluations in a consecutive series of women referred for investigation of their lower urinary tract symptoms, all of whom had urgency or urge incontinence. Using current ICS standards for urodynamic diagnosis of bladder disorders, our findings are presented here, in particular the detection of detrusor instability and genuine stress incontinence, and the relation of these findings to lower urinary tract symptoms.

The mean patient age was 52 years (range 26–80). Subjects were randomly assigned to undergo either static urodynamics followed 1 month later by ambulatory urodynamics, or vice versa. When cyclical urinary symptoms were described, urodynamic investigations were scheduled to coincide with the phase of the cycle when symptoms were most troublesome. Having completed both studies, all women were asked to complete a follow-up postal questionnaire seeking their views and preferences for the two tests.

The mean fill rate of all ambulatory fill–void cycles studied was 5.23 mL/min (range 1.61–14.81). The fill rates of "stable" and "unstable" cycles were not significantly different. There was no significant difference in maximum voided volume recorded on the frequency volume chart or during ambulatory or static urodynamics (Table 2).

Table 2 Maximum Voided Volume Recorded During 3-Day Frequency Volume Chart Compared with Ambulatory Urodynamics and Static Urodynamics ($n = 97$)

Measured by	Maximum voided volume mean (SD) (95% CI)	p value[a]
Frequency volume chart	426 mL (151) (392 to 460)	—
Ambulatory urodynamics	450 mL (149) (416 to 484)	0.21
Static urodynamics	426 mL (121) (398 to 453)	0.99

[a]Paired samples t test.

Table 3 Ambulatory and Static Urodynamic Findings in 97 Women with Urinary Urgency in a Randomized Prospective Study of Women with Urinary Urgency

Urodynamic diagnosis	Ambulatory	(%)	Static	(%)	p value[a]
Detrusor instability (all)	69	(71.1)	30	(30.9)	<.001
DI only	48	(49.5)	22	(22.7)	—
Mixed DI + GSI	21	(21.6)	8	(8.2)	—
Genuine stress incontinence (all)	34	(35.1)	37	(38.1)	.629
GSI only	13	(13.4)	29	(29.9)	—
Normal study	15	(15.5)	38	(39.2)	<.001
Total	97	(100)	97	(100)	—

[a]McNemar's test for paired nominal data.

The diagnostic findings of the two urodynamic modalities are summarized in Table 3. Detrusor instability was detected in 31% of conventional and 71% of ambulatory urodynamic studies. GSI was detected in 38% conventional and 35% ambulatory studies. A measure of the clinical importance of bladder overactivity detected during ambulatory urodynamics was made by comparing the incidence of associated urge incontinence between groups. This occurred in over 70% of all studies and its incidence was not significantly different in women who had stable or unstable conventional studies (Table 4). Of the 67 women with stable conventional static cystometry, detrusor instability was detected during ambulatory urodynamics in 44, (65.7%), of whom 31 (70.5%) experienced coincident urinary incontinence.

I. Symptoms and Urodynamic Findings

Severe nocturia (three or more episodes per night on average) was not predictive of the subsequent urodynamic detection of detrusor instability or genuine stress incontinence using either ambulatory or static urodynamics.

Increasing severity of urgency and urge incontinence were strongly correlated with the subsequent finding of detrusor instability on ambulatory monitoring, but significantly less so with conventional cystometry (Fig. 11). All ten women who reported that urge incontinence occurring "all of the time" were subsequently found to have detrusor instability during ambulatory urodynamics, whereas only three of this group had detrusor instability detected during conventional studies.

After completed both investigations, 80.5% of women felt that their normal bladder symptoms were reproduced during ambulatory, compared with 66.7% during static urodynamics (p = 0.013 using McNemar's test for paired nominal data).

Table 4 The Detection of Detrusor Instability and Associated Leakage During Ambulatory Urodynamics in Women with Stable or Unstable Static Urodynamics

Parameters	Stable static study	Unstable static study
Total	67	30
Number with DI during AUM	44	25
Number with DI with leakage during AUM (%)	31 (70.5%)	20 (80.0%)

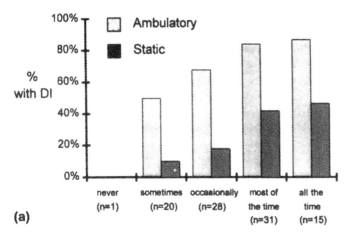

(a)

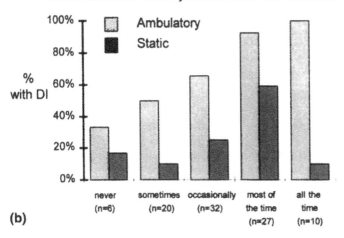

(b)

Figure 11   (a) Symptom of urinary urgency and subsequent ambulatory and static cysto-metric detection of detrusor instability in a randomized prospective study. (b) Symptom of urge incontinence and subsequent ambulatory and static cystometric detection of detrusor instability in a randomized prospective study.

J.   Incontinence

Involuntary detrusor activity is seen in apparently asymptomatic volunteers during both static and ambulatory monitoring; its finding in up to 70% of ambulatory studies has impeded the introduction of this modality into clinical practice. Whether asymptomatic detrusor overactivity is a genuine phenomenon or an artifact is impossible to estimate from these series and is largely esoteric. Most importantly, if bladder overactivity is indeed asymptomatic it may be considered an interesting phenomenon, but clinically irrelevant. In the randomized prospective study described here, the finding of bladder overactivity was interpreted in the context of coincident symptoms. All women recruited to this study complained of urinary urgency; however, the finding of involuntary detrusor contractions alone was not of itself accepted as evidence of clinically important bladder overactivity (detrusor instability). Only when coincident symptoms were noted was detrusor instability diagnosed. Perhaps most importantly, in over 70% of all women with symptomatic bladder overactivity, an episode of such overactivity was associated with urinary leakage; a symptom that cannot be readily dismissed as a variation of normal. In addition, there was no significant difference in the incidence of such urge incontinence between those women with normal detrusor function during static cystometry and those who had detrusor instability during both ambulatory and static cystometry. Quantitative assessment of lower urinary tract dysfunction, particularly in relation to bladder overactivity, is not possible using static cystometric parameters. However, ambulatory urodynamics offers a unique opportunity to correlate symptoms with lower urinary tract function and allows a degree of quantification of these disorders not achievable in the laboratory setting. This objective requires data quality of the highest order, demanding painstaking attention to detail, a time-consuming and, ultimately, expensive investment. Furthermore, much of the valuable information gained during ambulatory monitoring is accrued not only from protracted measurement of bladder pressure, but also the extended time period spent with the patient assessing their symptoms.

K. Patient Preference

Following completion of both ambulatory urodynamics and conventional static cystometry (in random order), of the 76 respondents to a follow-up postal questionnaire, 47.3% stated that if given a choice they would choose static urodynamics, 25% preferred ambulatory urodynamics, and 27.6% expressed no preference. The "bother" attributed to the duration of ambulatory was significantly higher than for static urodynamics ($p < 0.001$). However, other bother factors including embarrassment, catheterization, discomfort, and voiding were not significantly different for the two tests.

VII. CONCLUSIONS

In women presenting with urinary urgency or urge incontinence, ambulatory urodynamics allows greater detection of clinically important bladder overactivity compared with static cystometry. Further support for an environmental influence on detrusor function is gained from the observation during ambulatory urodynamic studies of more efficient and complete voiding and also the potent effect of handwashing. During ambulatory monitoring, handwashing was undertaken using cold running water in a washroom, an environment strongly associated with voiding. In over 70% of subjects this maneuver provoked detrusor contractions, over half of which resulted in urge incontinence. Conversely listening to running water and handwashing in a bowl of cold water during static urodynamics evaluation was relatively ineffective in provoking detrusor instability. The study environment clearly has important influences on detrusor function during cystometry and thereby the provocation and detection of clinically important bladder overactivity.

Although phasic detrusor activity suggestive of detrusor instability occurs more commonly during natural fill than medium fill cystometry, both in symptomatic and asymptomatic individuals, the significance of this finding is unclear (3,12,13). Episodic asymptomatic involuntary detrusor activity may be of little or no importance; however, the detection of bladder overactivity resulting in incontinence during ambulatory monitoring (over 70% in our series), whether spontaneous or provoked, cannot be considered a variation of normal. The current ICS definition of detrusor instability is based on static conventional urodynamic criteria. Our findings refocus attention on the clinical history and symptoms. It is no longer acceptable to declare "the bladder is an unreliable witness" when the current gold standard investigation fails to detect approximately half of all clinically important bladder overactivity.

A. Mixed Urinary Incontinence

Noninvasive forms of assessment can reveal much valuable information: Bladder neck mobility can be assessed by clinical examination; functional bladder capacity by frequency volume chart; residual urine volume by ultrasound or catheter drainage; and a weighed pad test can be used to quantify urinary leakage. Women in whom stress leakage of urine is objectively demonstrable, have a degree of sphincteric insufficiency that may not require cystometric evaluation before treatment. However, such uncomplicated presentations are estimated to represent only a small proportion of all the total caseload (27). It has been suggested that women with more complex urinary symptoms, especially those with recurrent stress incontinence, warrant cystometric assessment. If the rationale for this is to detect detrusor instability that was previously undetected, then conventional static cystometry is not a logical investigation. When detrusor overactivity is suspected as the cause of recurrent incontinence, there is little value in repeating a test that failed to detect the condition in the first place and detects only half of all clinically important detrusor instability in symptomatic patients.

Surgical treatment of stress incontinence in a patient with coexistent detrusor instability carries at best an uncertain outcome and may result in a deterioration in irritative symptoms. When sphincter insufficiency and bladder overactivity coexist, a quantitative assessment of their relative contributions must be made to prescribe the most appropriate treatment. As discussed previously, this is often difficult, if not impossible, using conventional urodynamic parameters. However, the longer period of observation afforded by ambulatory urodynamics allows a degree of quantification of bladder storage disorders and gives greater insight into the pathophysiology of lower urinary tract symptoms, often with surprising results. Van Waalwijk van Doorn combined the frequency, amplitude, duration and area under the curve of uninhibited detrusor contractions during ambulatory monitoring to derive a "detrusor activity index" and suggested that this index was clinically useful in quantifying detrusor overactivity (28). Such an approach may be of particular value in more complex cases and mixed incontinence.

B. Summary and Future Directions

Conventional static cystometry has become established as central in the investigation and management of a wide range of lower urinary tract symptoms and in the classification of storage and voiding disorders. However, evidence from several studies suggests that ambulatory urodynamics better reproduces symptomatology and physiological detrusor and sphincter function than conventional static cystometry. To finally establish the clinical relevance of these observations, longitudinal data are required, assessing the influence of ambulatory urodynamics on subsequent management and outcome. With this caveat in mind, there can be little argument that ambulatory urodynamics can be usefully employed either to supplement conventional static cystometry or as a primary investigation. Compared with the current gold standard investigation, ambulatory urodynamics offers an alternative diagnostic modality, allowing more physiological assessment of lower urinary tract function and symptom reproduction. Furthermore, noninvasive forms of assessment, such as careful and meticulous history taking and examination, pad tests, and frequency volume charts, should not be neglected in favor of invasive and expensive investigations, often without good evidence of their clinical benefit.

REFERENCES

1. Dubois P. Ueber den Druck in der Harnblase. Dtsh Arch Klin Med 1876; 17:148–163.
2. Mosso A, Pellacani P. Sur les functions de la vessie. Arch Ital Biol 1882; 1:97–128, 291–324.
3. Hodgkinson CP, Ayers MA, Drukker BH. Dyssynergic detrusor dysfunction in the apparently normal female. Am J Obstet Gynecol 1963; 87:717–730.
4. Bates, CP, Whiteside CG, Tumer–Warwick RT. Synchronous cine/pressure/flow/cystourethrography with special reference to stress and urge incontinence. Br J Urol 1970; 42:714–723.
5. Griffiths DJ. Urodynamics—The Mechanics and Hydrodynamics of the Lower Urinary Tract. Bristol: Adam Hilger, 1980:107–108.
6. Abrams P, Blaivas JG, Stanton SL, Anderson JT. The standardisation of terminology of lower urinary tract function. Scand J Urol Nephrol Suppl 1988; 114:5–19.
7. Comarr AE. Excretory cystometry: a more physiological method. J Urol 1957; 77:622–633.
8. Tsuji I, Kuroda K, Nakajima F. Excretory cystometry in paraplegic patients. J Urol 1960; 83:839–844.
9. James ED. The behaviour of the bladder during physical activity. Br J Urol 1978; 50:387–394.
10. Bhatia NN, Bradley WE, Haldeman S. Urodynamics: continuous monitoring. J Urol 1982; 128:963–968.
11. Styles RA, Neal DE, Griffiths CJ, Ramsden PD. Long term-monitoring of bladder pressure in chronic retention of urine: the relationship between detrusor activity and upper tract dilatation. J Urol 1988; 140:330–334.
12. Robertson AS, Griffiths CJ, Ramsden PD, Neal DE. Bladder function in healthy volunteers: ambulatory monitoring and conventional urodynamic studies. Br J Urol 1994; 73:242–249.
13. Van Waalwik van Doom ESC, Remmers A, Janknegt RA. Conventional and extramural ambulatory testing of the lower urinary tract in female volunteers. J Urol 1992; 47:1319–1326.
14. Rosario DJ, Potts KL, Woo HH, Chapple, CR. Ambulatory pressure–flow studies in young asymptomatic males. Neurourol Urodynam 1996; 15:278–279.
15. Robertson AS, Griffiths C, Neal DE. Conventional urodynamics and ambulatory monitoring in the definition and management of bladder outflow obstruction. J Urol 1996; 155:506–511.
16. Rosario DJ, Chapple CR, Tophill PR, Woo HH. Urodynamic assessment of the bashful bladder. J Urol 2000; 163:215–220.
17. Thomas DG, O'Flynn KJ. Spinal cord injury. In: Mundy AR, Stephenson TP, Wein AJ eds. Urodynamics. Principles, Practice and Application. 2nd ed. Edinburgh: Churchill Livingstone. 1994:345–358.
18. Webb RJ, Griffiths CJ, Ramsden PD, Neal DE. Ambulatory monitoring in low compliance neuropathic bladder dysfunction. J Urol 1992; 148:1477–1481.
19. Webb RJ, Griffiths CJ, Ramsden PD, Neal DE. Ambulatory monitoring and electronic measurement of urinary leakage in the diagnosis of detrusor instability and incontinence. Br J Urol 1991; 68:148–152.
20. Porru D, Usai E. Standard and extramural ambulatory urodynamic investigation for the diagnosis of detrusor instability-correlated incontinence and micturition disorders. Neurourol Urodynam 1994; 13:237–242.
21. Rosario DJ, MacDiarmid SA, Radley SC, Chapple CR. A comparison of ambulatory and conventional urodynamic studies in men with borderline outlet obstruction. Br J Urol 1999; 83:400–409.
22. Moore KH, Hay DM, Imrie AE, Watson A, Goldstein M. Oxybutynin hydrochloride (3 mg) in the treatment of women with idiopathic detrusor instability. Br J Urol 1990; 66:479–485.
23. Tapp AJ, Cardozo LD, Versi E. The treatment of detrusor instability in post-menopausal women with oxybutynin hydrochloride: a double blind placebo controlled study. Br J Obstet Gynaecol 1990; 97:521–526.

24. Riva D, Casolati E. Oxybutynin chloride in the treatment of female idiopathic detrusor instability. Results from double blind treatment. Clin Exp Obstet Gynecol 1984; 11:37–42.
25. Rosario DJ, Smith DJ, Radley SC, Chapple CR. Pharmacodynamics of anticholinergic agents measured by ambulatory urodynamic monitoring—a study of methodology. Neurourol Urodynam 1999; 18:223–233.
26. Van Waalwijk van Doom ESC, Zwiers W. Ambulant monitoring to assess the efficacy of oxybutynin chloride in patients with mixed incontinence. Eur Urol 1990; 18:49–51.
27. Versi E, Cardozo LD, Anand DD, Cooper D. Symptom analysis for the diagnosis of genuine stress incontinence. Br J Obstet Gynaecol 1991; 98:815–819.
28. Van Waalwijk van Doom ESC, Malone–Lee JG, Janknegt RA. The differentiation of normal and abnormal detrusor contractions on ambulatory urodynamics. Neurourol Urodynam 1995; 14: 531–533.

25

Ultrasound Imaging of the Female Urinary Sphincter*

BERNARD JACQUETIN

Auvergne University, Clermont I, and Auvergne University Hospital, Clermont-Ferrand, France

I. INTRODUCTION

Fleming Mattox (1), in an editorial published in 1994 in *Ultrasound in Obstetrics and Gynecology,* noted that almost all gynecologists and obstetricians use ultrasonography in their everyday practice, but only a few academic centers apply this imaging modality to study stress urinary incontinence (SUI) and pathology of the pelvic floor. He estimated that this was probably because ultrasound could give little additional information, except for postvoid residual determination (which can also easily be done by catheterization) and the position and mobility of the bladder neck (which can be documented with a much better cost/benefit ratio by the Q-tip test).

The aim of this chapter is to evaluate the place of ultrasonography in female SUI, especially for visualizing the urethrovesical junction, its position, and its mobility.

To accomplish this goal, we have so far used the following:

1. Physical examination
2. The Q-tip test of Crystle (2) which, however, has low specificity
3. Voiding cystourethrography (VCUG), which has been well standardized (3–5)
4. Video voiding cystourethrography (VVCUG) and videourodynamics evaluations (6).

---

*Adapted from the French by Erik Schick, MD.

II. HISTORICAL BACKGROUND

It is difficult to identify the first investigator who applied ultrasound in urogynecology. Credit should probably be given to Schaaps and Lambotte (7) from Belgium who, in 1977, described modifications of the pelvic floor in SUI. A few years later, in 1980, Ostergard (8) compared measurable angles in continent and incontinent patients. Other pioneers in the field are mentioned by Dermici (9–21).

In 1985, endocavitary ultrasonography became available, and numerous investigators used this new approach: Beco (10) in Belgium; Porena et al. (11) in Italy; Brown (12), Leonor de Gonzales (13), Richmond (14,15), Gordon (16), and Quinn et al. (17,18) in England; Koelbl (19) in Germany; Shapeero (20), Kohorn (21), and, later on, Bergman (22–24) in the United States. From our institution, Lemery (25) described the morphological and functional anatomy of the normal female urinary tract as it appeared on ultrasonographic exploration.

Bhatia (25a) in 1987, Benson and Summers (26,27) in 1990 and 1991, as well as Ghoniem (28) in 1992 summarized these early experiences. Since then, the development of urogynecological ultrasonography has been rapid, perhaps too rapid, because no standardization of the methodology has been proposed and widely accepted. One of the main difficulties is the problem of artifacts encountered during these explorations. Beco (29) reviewed and summarized these artifacts.

The German Urogynecologic Society organized a Consensus Conference in Zurich in 1995. The conclusions and recommendations of this meeting, dealing only with the perineal and introital approaches, met the approval of the German-speaking scientific community (19,31,32), and they have been published by Schaer (30). These conclusions, however, have been challenged by others (33,34).

More recently, several review articles have been published on this subject (35–42). Textbooks dealing with lower urinary tract (LUT) physiology and physiopathology now contain chapters devoted to ultrasonographic explorations (43,44).

The aim of this chapter is 1) to compare ultrasonography with radiographic imaging; 2) to discuss problems related to different approaches (perineal, introital, or other), artifacts, and methodological variations; 3) to describe physiopathological conditions and clinical applications; and, finally, 4) to review the most recent technical developments in the field of ultrasonography as applied to the LUT.

III. COMPARISON OF IMAGING QUALITY

Conventional radiologic studies include intravenous pyelography (IVP), VCUG, and VVCUG.

A. IVP

Intravenous pyelography (IVP) has limited value in LUT imaging. It can demonstrate bladder diverticulum, bladder wall trabeculations or fistulas, and bladder neck position at rest, but contributes minimally to the exploration of stress incontinence.

B. VCUG

Table 1 compares the advantages and inconveniences of radiologic and ultrasonographic methods. Radiology precisely delineates bony structures, facilitating measurements. How-

Table 1 Advantages and Disadvantages of Vesicourethral Imaging by Radiologic Means and by Ultrasonography

	Radiology	Ultrasonography
Bony structures	Complete view	Partial view
Pubis	Well delimited	Partial view sometimes Precise localization difficult
Erect position	Frequently	Rarely
Bladder	Complete view	Partial view
Urethrovesical junction	Difficult to localize	Strict criteria for localization
Bladder neck incompetence	Well seen	Difficult to see
Urethra	Not visible	Well seen (except distal 1/3 sometimes)
Urethral sphincter	Not visible	Visible
Periurethral soft tissue	Not visible	Visible
Contrast material	Absolutely necessary	Useless (except for bladder neck incompetence)
Irradiation	Yes	No
Opacification of the urethra	Very frequent	Useless almost all the time (sometimes catheter)
Bladder neck mobility	Need video	Real-time images
Control of stress	Difficult	Biofeedback easy (strain, contraction of pelvic floor)
Pelvic organs	Not seen	Important "supplementary" images
Artifacts	Because of superimposition of different plans	Single section, but anatomical consequences of catheter
Operator dependence	Weak	Strong
Simultaneous urodynamics	Possible	Possible
Morbidity	Weak (allergy)	Negligible
Realization of the study	Complex	Slightly invasive
Cost	High	Relatively low
Acceptance	Less than optimal	Good
Repeatability	Difficult (x-rays)	Easy
Reproducibility	Not analyzed	Good

ever, it does not show soft-tissue structures, and the images are in a single plane instead of a tomographic view. Opacification of the urethra remains a problem. It can only be seen on an x-ray film if the bladder neck is open [which does not necessarily mean that the patient is incontinent (45)] or if the patient is effectively incontinent during the examination. The same difficulties are encountered with ultrasonography, except when ultrasonographic contrast material is used (46). However, the urethrovesical junction (UVJ) can be adequately visualized by ultrasound (29). Because of these difficulties, Hodgkinson (4) introduced the "chain cystogram," in which a small chain is placed in the urethral lumen. Later, Green's classification (5) of stress incontinence was based on this technique (5). However, the diagnostic and prognostic significance of the different angles measured remains controversial, whether they are assessed radiographically or by ultrasound.

C. Ultrasonography

Brown (12) was one of the first investigators to propose the replacement of x-rays films by ultrasound. Comparative measurements by x-ray films or ultrasound of the posterior ure-throvesical angle (16,19,20) or mobility of the urethrovesical junction (22,47–49) gave similar results. Ultrasonography was better in visualizing urethral diverticuli (50,51) or urethral obstruction (52).

More recently, Mouritzen and Strandberg (53) compared transvaginal ultrasonography with colpocystourethrography in 44 incontinent females. The degree of agreement between the two methods was only 58%, which is the same as the interobserver variation established previously in radiology. Measurement of bladder neck–pubic bone distance, as well as mobility of the urethrovesical junction, or the angles measured by both methods, gave similar results, with greater variance by radiology. Better "standardization" can be achieved by ultrasonography, probably because an observed dynamic image allows the observer, at the same time, to "guide" the patient during examination. These authors also demonstrated that mobility of the urethrovesical junction is the criterion that correlates best with SUI.

Schaer et al. (54) studied 60 incontinent patients in the upright position. They analyzed the position of the urethrovesical junction, its mobility with the Valsalva maneuver, the posterior urethrovesical angle, and the competence of the bladder neck. X-ray examination demonstrated this latter parameter better. The posterior urethrovesical angle was not very reproducible; there was a difference between the two methods of measurement, probably because intra-abdominal pressure was not standardized with Valsalva, and the "chainette" in the urethra could provoke reflex contraction of the pelvic floor. They concluded that x-ray films are not adequate to appreciate bladder neck mobility under stress conditions.

Comparing introital and perineal ultrasonography, Badzakov (55) obtained a better correlation between the perineal approach and urethrocystography.

D. VVCUG

For many authors, VVCUG remains the gold standard, not only in neurogenic bladder disease, but also in SUI. Coupled with urodynamic studies (6), it is particularly useful when detrusor–external sphincter dyssynergia (DESD) or obstructive uropathy is suspected. However, in the experience of Beness et al. (56), treatment plans were modified in only 6.6% of 150 women when urodynamic studies were added to the more conventional VCUG.

Ultrasonography is more operator-dependent than is radiology. The former, however, allows complete evaluation of the pelvic organs, their position, the anal sphincter, and even the kidneys and ureter.

IV. METHODOLOGICAL CONSIDERATIONS

Ultrasound probes can be applied as external or endocavitary devices. With external probes, the transabdominal route has been abandoned by the majority of investigators (7,13,57), except for certain specific indications (58,59). The choice remains between the perineal route, which gives a complete view of the pubis, and the introital route where the pubis is usually only partially seen. Both of them, however, provide a panoramic view of the entire pelvic cavity.

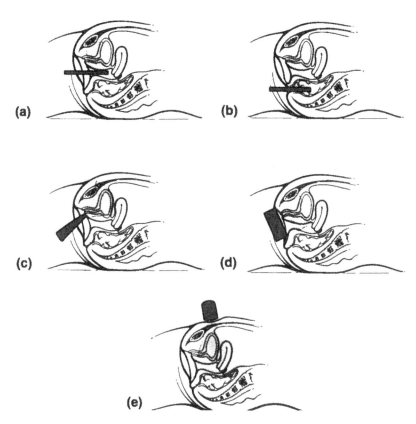

Figure 1 Different ultrasonic routes used during exploration of the urethrovesical region: endocavitary probes: (a) transvaginal (linear); (b) transrectal (linear); external probes, (c) introital (sectorial); (d) transperineal (linear or sectorial); (e) transabdominal (sectorial). (From Ref. 57. Courtesy of J. Beco.)

Endocavitary probes can be placed in the vagina or the rectum and give a view in sagittal section of the pelvis. These techniques, even if they are somewhat more precise and more invasive, probably generate fewer artifacts. Figure 1 illustrates these different approaches according to Beco (57).

A. Perineal Route

The main advantages of this approach are that it is less invasive than endocavitary probes, and provides a panoramic view of the pelvis. It allows the mobility of the urethrovesical junction to be appreciated and, if coupled with urodynamic studies, differentiates between intrinsic sphincter deficiency (ISD) and unstable bladder. This route is probably the one that is best documented in the literature. We found 49 articles dealing with the subject (19,21, 25,30,46,49,50,54,55,60–99).

Table 2 summarizes the advantages of the perineal route. Even if the quality of imaging is less satisfactory, compared with the endocavitary route, it gives a panoramic view of the pelvis, it does not move during stress, it does not interfere with mobility of the urethrovesical junction, does not require, according to the most recent publications, an intraurethral catheter, and is easily applicable, even with significant prolapse.

Table 2 Comparison of Ultrasonographic Methods According to Different Routes

	Abdominal	Perineal	Introital	Transvagina
Type of probe	Linear	Linear (or convex)	Sectorial	Linear
Frequency (MHz)	2.5; 3.5; 5	3.5; 5	5; 7; 7.5	5; 7; 7.5
Patient comfort	++++	+++	+++	++
Operator's comfort	++	++	+	+++
Image quality	+	++	+++	+++
Per-op use	–	–	–	–
Simultaneous urodynamics	+	–	+	+++
Multidisciplinary use of the probe	+++	+++	++	+
Reproducibility	?	+++	?	+++
Modification of bladder neck mobility by probe	No	No	Possibly	Very likely
Displacement of the probe under stress	No	No	Probably	Certainly
Modification of urodynamic parameters by the probe	No	No	No	Probably

Excellent, ++++; very good, +++; good, ++; acceptable, +; inadequate, –.
Source: Ref. 29.

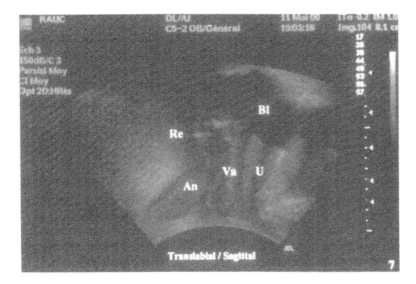

Figure 2 Ultrasonographic colpocystogram: "Translabial" ultrasonography allows a large panoramic view of the pelvic organs as well as the urethral and anal sphincters. Bl, bladder; Re, Retzius space; Va, vagina; U, urethra; An, anus. (Courtesy of D. Lemery.)

B. Introital Route

The probe is positioned just under the urethral meatus or against the distal third of the urethra. Martensson (35) called this the "translabial" route (Fig. 2). Koelbl and Bernascheck (31,32) described and validated the technique. Comparing these observations with urodynamic data and conventional VVCUG, they found introital ultrasonography to be more reliable. It was by this technique that Hanzal (100) demonstrated that intraurethral catheters significantly increased the diameter of the urethra.

One of the advantages of the technique is that it does not need a urethral catheter. However, the probe must be kept immobile during examination and, at the same time, pressure exerted on tissues must be minimal, which is difficult to accomplish (Fig. 3). It becomes almost impossible when simultaneous urodynamic studies are also required. Wise et al. (101) investigated the effect of such probes in the introital position on the parameters of urethral pressure profile (UPP). They demonstrated significant elevations in closure pressure, functional length, and area under the profile curve. Pressure transmission ratios for the first three-fourths of the urethra were also increased. On the other hand, posterior urethrovesical angles decreased by 19% with the probe in place. Results of this magnitude were, however, not reproduced by other investigators. It can be concluded that the method is probably highly operator-dependent. We prefer to use this route, even if it seems less popular in the literature. We found only 18 references dealing with the approach (31,32,35,55, 59,97,100,103–113).

The most important disadvantage of this method is that the whole pubic bone is in the viewing field, which prevents use of the pubic axis as a reference for the horizontal line. However, micturition, contraction of the detrusor, the possibility of blocking voluntarily urine flow, and urine penetration in the urethra can be evaluated adequately (31). Also, bladder neck behavior during uninhibited contraction as well as DESD can be visualized.

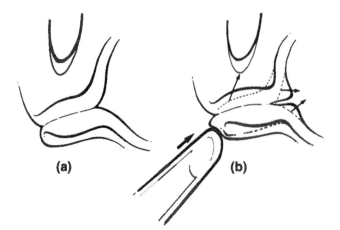

(a)   (b)

Figure 3 Introital route: (a) anatomy without a probe; (b) urethra is "telescoped" inside the bladder and compressed against the arcuate pubic ligament when pressure is exerted on these structures. (From Ref. 57. Courtesy of J. Beco.)

C. Transvaginal Route

As validated by Quinn (17,18), Beco (29,57) considered the transvaginal route to be the method of choice in exploring the LUT. It provides high-quality images (because of the high-frequency used), it is not uncomfortable for the patient, positioning by the operator is easy, it has been validated by inter- and intraobserver repeatability as well as the systematic analysis of artifacts, and finally, it can be coupled relatively easily with urodynamic exploration. This route cannot be used when the vagina is too narrow, too short, or is full of scar tissue, or in case of prolapse (29).

We found 28 references dealing with this approach in the literature (10,17,18,29,34, 35,50,51,53,57,101,114–118,127,131,153–155,178,180). It has also been compared with conventional radiology (53), and artifacts have been studied in detail (115,116) (Fig. 4). Other references focused on clinical applications (114,117). It should be mentioned that Hol (118) compared the transvaginal with the transrectal route.

D. Transrectal Route

In the 1980s, Nishizawa (15) applied this technique in females, and Shapeero (20) in males. In 1985, Brown and Sutherst (12) demonstrated that, in the stress incontinent female, the urethrovesical junction is in a lower position at rest and is more mobile during stress. Bergman (22,23) defined the normal physiological limit of bladder neck mobility to be 1 cm. This value was, however, the median value of his control subjects.

The route has the facility to be combined with urodynamic studies, and DESD can be well visualized (119). Artifacts are less pronounced by the endorectal than by the endovaginal approach (see Fig. 4); the difference, however, does not seem to be significant (118). Also, the endovaginal approach is better accepted by the patient than the endorectal route. Furthermore, the probe in the vagina provokes less reflex contraction of the pelvic floor than if it is in the rectum.

It appears in the literature (11,12,14,15,20–24,40,47,48,52,119–130) that Kuo is the only one who uses this approach routinely (120–122).

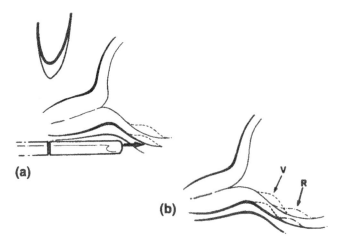

Figure 4 Intravaginal route: distortion of anatomical reference points by the ultrasonic probe: (a) endovaginal probe placed beyond the vesical neck opens the posterior vesicourethral angle and causes distortion of the bladder base (---); (b) distortion of the bladder base by an endorectal probe appears more cranial (R) than the one caused by the vaginal probe (V). (From Ref. 57. Courtesy of J. Beco.)

Given the experience of Beco (57) and Mouritsen (115) with the transvaginal approach, that of Hol (118) with the transvaginal and transrectal route, and of Schaer (90) with the perineal route, a summary of their advantages and inconveniences is presented in Tables 2 and 3.

V. THE ULTRASONOGRAPHIC PROBE EFFECT

The placement of the ultrasonographic probe can induce artifacts, termed the "ultrasonographic probe effect." This has been the subject of considerable debate in the literature.

The transrectal route was advocated by Bergman (22,23). He demonstrated that the Q-tip test was similar, with or without intrarectal probes, even during stress. Richmond and

Table 3 Comparison of Ultrasonographic Methods According to Their Respective Diagnostic Possibilities

	Abdominal	Perineal	Introital	Transvaginal	Transrectal
Study of the sphincter	−	+	++	+++	++
Position of the bladder neck	−	++	++	+++	+++
Posterior urethrovesical angle	+	++	+	−	−
Mobility of the urethro- vesical junction	−	+++	++	+	+
Micturition	−	+	−	++	+++
Postvoid residual	+++	+	+	+	+
Ultrasonic guidance	−	−	−	+++	++

Very good, +++; good, ++; acceptable, +; inadequate, −.
Source: Ref. 29.

Sutherst (123,124) found that cystometry, UPP, and the fluid bridge test were all identical with or without a probe in the rectum. Furthermore, the probe did not provoke detrusor instability or hypertonicity.

We have already mentioned the highly controversial observations of Wise et al. (101), who obtained significantly different urodynamic data with or without the probe in the introital position. The manual pressure exerted by the probe in this study was probably excessive, and only the "probe effect" was evaluated without simultaneous imaging control. Schaer (90) estimated that these authors confounded the introital and vaginal probe positions, while Beco (34) pointed out that it is a "technical bravery" to maintain the probe in the correct introital position, even during stress, and at the same time exert only minimal pressure (so-called "switching off") on tissues.

Three authors studied the influence of intravaginal probes in detail. However, Mouritsen (115) introduced the probe only 1–2 cm deep, Beco (57) 1 cm beyond UVJ, and Hol (118) pushed it "gently" in the vagina, without specifying the exact distance.

Mouritsen (115) noted that while the method used by Wise et al. (101) is subject to criticism, Christensen and Djurhuus (131) confirmed that an increase in maximal urethral pressure provoked by the probe had no effect on urethrovesical mobility, as demonstrated by magnetic resonance imaging (MRI). Mouritsen's probe was small (1.2 cm in diameter), and its viewing angle was specifically oriented at 45 degrees. He compared his results with those obtained by radiology and concluded that, with this special probe, applied almost at the introitus, distortion was minimal, independently of the degree of incontinence. Only the rotational angle of the urethra by Valsalva maneuver was decreased by 20 degrees in case of prolapse. Nevertheless, he estimated that transrectal ultrasound is probably a better alternative when simultaneous urodynamic exploration is planned.

Beco (57) was criticized because his endovaginal probe could logically have a significant "probe effect." To document this effect better, he studied 34 patients, comparing the modifications provoked by the probe on urodynamic parameters and the Q-tip test. In 10 of these patients, in addition to the transvaginal route, he performed transabdominal ultrasonography in the supine position, at rest and during coughing. His conclusions can be summarized as follows:

1. UPP is modified only if the vagina is narrow, (i.e., the distance between the pubic ligament and the probe is less than 12 mm, which happens in 4% of cases); closure pressure will increase by about 5 cmH$_2$O.
2. The Q-tip test is significantly decreased, which suggests that the position and mobility of the urethrovesical junction is modified.
3. Changes at the level of the bladder base (studied by the transabdominal route) are also significant. More specifically, the posterior urethrovesical angle is increased (see Fig. 4) to a point where it can no longer be measured by the transvaginal route. Schaer (90) considered this a major inconvenience of the technique.

Hol et al. (118) studied 160 patients (50 with SUI, 50 controls, and 60 with different LUT symptoms [LUTS], excluding prolapse) in a very strict protocol. The transrectal route was used additionally in 15 patients. Interobserver reproducibility was tested in 20 patients. The examination was carried out with a urethral catheter in place in 20 subjects. They concluded that (1) there is no significant difference between the transvaginal and transrectal routes; (2) interobserver reproducibility is good; (3) no difference is found with the Q-tip test, with or without a urethral catheter. Their study defined the role of patient position during examination, the role of bladder filling, and standardization of the Valsalva maneuver.

Unfortunately, they did not compare their technique with other modalities, such as radiology or external ultrasonography.

Schaer (90) conducted a similar study to test the "probe effect" with the perineal approach. In 31 patients, he focused attention on the difference observed when the probe exerted a strong or only slight pressure on the perineal tissues. He concluded that with strong pressure, the probe displaces the urethrovesical junction in the cranial direction and compresses the urethra at the same time.

From all these studies, it can be concluded that endocavitary probes interfere more with the urethrovesical anatomy than external probes. Endocavitary probes should be the thinnest possible, placed in a vagina that is not too narrow, and without prolapse (57,118). Otherwise, the probe should be withdrawn (115) almost until the introitus where the situation for the examiner becomes particularly "unstable." Under these circumstances, the probe used by Schaer and his German colleagues (30), without excessive pressure on the perineum became the best approach. This is also confirmed by Pajoncini et al. (132).

VI. INFLUENCE OF METHODOLOGY

The type of ultrasound probe and its localization can definitely influence the final result. As emphasized by several authors (9,29,30), other factors should also be considered.

A. Effect of the Patient's Position

The supine position, together with the gynecological position, is probably the most frequently used. The sitting position (66,133) can make micturition easier. The erect position is theoretically the most ideal to detect urine loss (120,121), but it is more difficult to apply the probe, which should then be an external probe (90). The ideal solution is to perform the examination both in the supine and erect (83,89,90,118), or supine and sitting (53,114) positions.

Handa et al. (133), without using ultrasonography, compared the Q-tip test in the supine and erect positions in 46 patients. The test was positive ($\geq 30°$) in the supine position in 34/46 patients, and only 24/46 in the erect position (p < 0.01). None of the negative tests in the supine position became positive in the erect position. The difference between the two positions remained significant when the maximum angle was considered, instead of variations in the angle.

Dietz and Clarke (107), using translabial ultrasound, confirmed the increased mobility of the urethrovesical junction in the supine position in a prospective study of 132 females. Incompetence of the bladder neck, however, could be detected more easily in the erect position, which could be explained by different factors. The urethrovesical junction is already in a lower position when erect, compared with the supine position, which decreases its displacement under stress. Furthermore, the supine position, together with the gynecological position, is more conductive to pelvic floor relaxation.

These observations explain why urethrovesical junction mobility is more pronounced in ultrasonography, when the patient is more often in the supine or sitting position, compared with radiology, where the patient is always erect. However, several authors (103,105, 118) estimate that bladder neck mobility is not significantly affected by position. Hol (118) found a difference of only 0.5 cm between the supine and sitting positions, which disappears with Valsalva and hold maneuvers, the overlap between the values obtained being too great to allow discrimination.

Meyer et al. (83), using Schaer's method, demonstrated a significant difference in bladder neck mobility at rest between the supine and erect positions, especially in women with pure stress incontinence. During the Valsalva maneuver, the bladder neck was situated lower in multiparous women, mainly in those who had forceps applied during delivery, than in nulliparous subjects.

In Schaer's study (90) the major difference between positions was the observation of bladder neck incompetence in the erect position with the Valsalva maneuver.

Mouritsen and Bach (116) compared bladder neck position in the supine and sitting positions by the transvaginal route. They reported that in continent females, the urethrovesical junction is lower in the sitting than in the supine position. This observation was confirmed by Vierhout and Jansen (128). It is also true for incontinent patients, in whom the distance between the bladder neck and the pubis is decreased by 3 mm, whereas the rotational angle is increased by 16 degrees. Furthermore, bladder neck mobility is not affected by position. For some authors, however, this mobility is increased in the supine position.

According to Schaer (90), it can be concluded that the examination should be carried out in the supine position, which is more comfortable for the patient and examiner, and is easily coupled with urodynamic studies. To demonstrate bladder neck incompetence, the erect position is preferred, and to study micturition, the sitting position seems to be the best (94).

B.   Effect of Coughing and Bearing-Down

We found only four studies (57,90,117,121) that explored the effect of coughing. This is mainly because examination under these circumstances is more difficult, as the pelvis and the ultrasonic probe (particularly if endocavitary or introital) move during coughing. It would be a methodological error (29,33,57) to immobilize the probe to maintain the pubic bone as a reference point, since this could interfere with the natural mobility of the bladder neck. The probe must be free and perfectly horizontal if it is in an endovaginal position (Fig. 5).

Furthermore, one must be able to "catch" the moment when the bladder neck is at maximal excursion. This can be realized by video registration and reviewed in slow motion, but has proved to be too fastidious. Beco (29) developed a system for which he coupled a rapid videocamera (≥20 images per second) with urodynamic studies. The data, including the image, are "frozen" automatically at a predetermined pressure level. This allows not only reproducible measurements, but also perfectly standardized efforts (29). Under these circumstances, rapid and repetitive measures can be realized with increasing cough amplitudes. However, Weil (117) found it difficult to interpret these data because of endovaginal probe movements and the difficulty in freezing the image at maximum coughing intensity.

Schaer (90) explored 33 patients and compared coughing with the Valsalva maneuver. He noted that during coughing the bladder neck is displaced less in the posterior direction and more vertically (Fig. 6). Rotational descent is also less pronounced. This tends to confirm the hypothesis that urethrovesical junction mobility is accentuated, with a larger posterior urethrovesical angle, during Valsalva (when the pelvic floor is relaxed) than during coughing (when the pelvic floor is contracted). Furthermore, there is an "effect of inertion" which prevents maximal bladder neck displacement with very brief efforts. In addition, if we consider the difficulty in maintaining urethral image with a perineal or introital

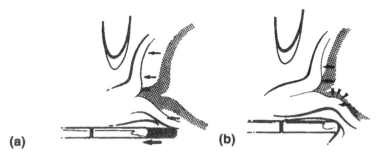

(a)   (b)

Figure 5   Cough effect with intravaginal probe in place: bladder neck mobility is less reduced with (a) freely moving probe than with (b) a fixed probe. (From Ref. 57. Courtesy of J. Beco.)

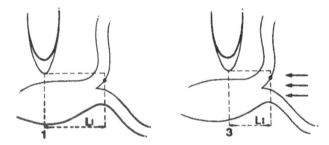

Figure 6   Cough effect: the distance vesical neck–arcuate pubic ligament (L-1) is reduced during cough (L-2). (From Ref. 57. Courtesy of J. Beco.)

probe and avoiding the "pessaire effect" with the intravaginal probe, it becomes clear why clinicians use repetitive coughing less frequently during ultrasonic exploration.

The Valsalva maneuver (Fig. 7a,b) is employed by many investigators (100,118), few of whom have attempted to standardize the method. Hol (118) found significant differences in the parameters evaluated between 30 and 50 cmH_2O pressure generated by Valsalva. He suggested standardization of the effort at 30 cmH_2O, arguing that every women is able to generate such a pressure. This, however, seems to be a very low threshold. The pressure generated can be measured by an intrarectal (100) or intravesical (118) catheter; the best way remains to couple it with urodynamic studies (31). Schaer (33) suggest that, instead of standardizing the pressure, it should rather be monitored; 30 cmH_2O has quite a different meaning from patient to patient, depending on age, weight, physical activity, and such. We feel that the maximum pressure the patient is able to generate should be her reference value and should be used in subsequent evaluations.

C.   Effect of the "Squeezing" Effort

The consequences of "withholding" or "squeezing" (Fig. 7a,c) have rarely been evaluated (53,114–116). This is somewhat surprising, because it is often used during cystourethrography, and it is always integrated in the procedure for colpocystograms. Hol (118) estimates

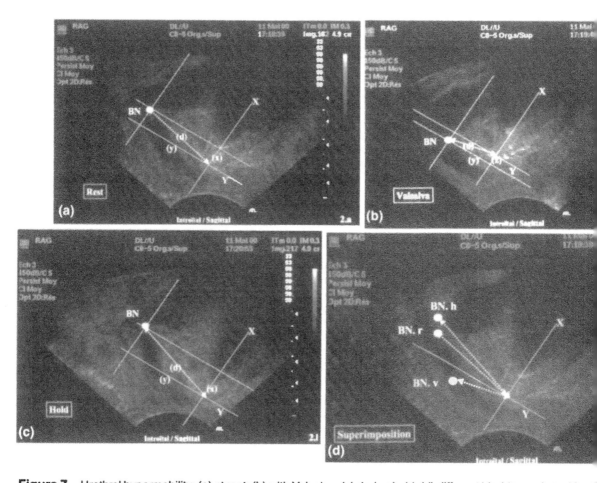

Figure 7 Urethral hypermobility: (a) at rest; (b) with Valsalva; (c) during hold; (d) different bladder neck positions on a single image. Bladder neck position is defined according to X and Y axes, as well as its distance from the ar X, x, Y, y, axes; BN, bladder neck; d, distance between bladder neck and arcuate ligament; BN.h, bladder neck du bladder neck at rest; BN.v, bladder neck with Valsalva. (Courtesy of D. Lemery.)

that this maneuver is valid only during the first two attempts, but nevertheless, adopts it to differentiate continent from incontinent females. Mouritsen (114) also employs it routinely; the bladder neck–pubis distance and rotational angle during Valsalva and "withholding" are significantly different in continent and incontinent patients. Also, the angle decreases as the bladder is filled, and it increases with prolapse (53). Perschers (86) developed this maneuver in a very standardized way to study the consequences of delivery. She measured bladder neck mobility during squeezing to evaluate the contractile capacity of the levator ani muscles. She concluded that contractility is impaired by obstetrical trauma.

D. Effect of Bladder Filling

The consequences of bladder filling (between 50 and 500 mL) have been investigated by several authors (90,116,118). Hol (118) did not find any difference during Valsalva or "squeezing" in ten patients with 250- and 500-mL filling. Mouritsen and Bach (116) tested six patients with 50, 100, and 200 mL of liquid in the bladder. Withholding capacity improved (with a 7% decrease in rotational angle) between 50 and 200 mL. The sensation of full bladder provoked contraction of the levator ani muscles, which was perceptible by the position of the bladder neck at rest. For Schaer (90), the "ideal" bladder volume for exploration would be 300 mL. Further bladder filling might be useful only to detect bladder neck incompetence.

In summary, bladder filling has little influence on the position and mobility of the bladder neck. Mobility seems to be even more pronounced if the bladder is empty (80).

E. Localization of the Urethrovesical Junction

Recent publications suggest that improvement in the resolution of ultrasonographic images makes it unnecessary to localize the bladder neck by special techniques (Fig. 8). Nevertheless, a review of the literature indicates that thin catheters (57,88,89,100,116,121), Foley catheters (66,118), or Q-tips (74) are frequently used (Fig. 9). Very much as in radiology, this tends to prove the difficulty in adequately localizing the bladder neck. Three authors (100,116,121) studied the question in detail. Beco (57) considers localization essential. It does not introduce artifacts if the catheter is small and flexible (Fig. 10). Viewed in full

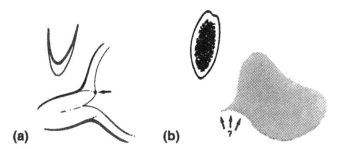

(a) (b)

Figure 8 Ultrasonography locates vesical neck more accurately than x-ray films: (a) anatomical location of the bladder neck; (b) difficulty in locating the bladder neck by cystography, especially in bladder neck incompetence. (From Ref. 57. Courtesy of J. Beco.)

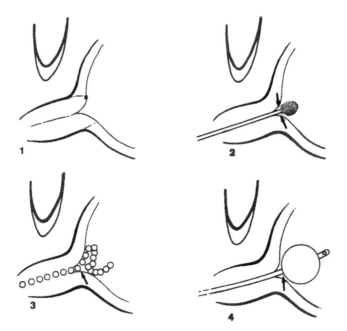

Figure 9   Localization of the bladder neck: (1) based on anatomical elements, junction between the sphincteric zone and the anterior vesical wall; (2) located by the cotton tip of a Q-tip; (3) located by a small chain; (4) balloon of the Foley catheter locates the bladder neck. (From Ref. 57. Courtesy of J. Beco.)

length, it allows confirmation that the plane is perfectly sagittal. This author even makes measurements in relation to the catheter.

It is certainly true that the Q-tip makes the urethra more rigid (74). The Foley catheter is not flexible enough, but its balloon can serve to visualize the horizontal plane (66). Hanzal (100) did not find any difference in mobility of the bladder neck and the posterior vesicourethral angle at rest or "standardized" Valsalva, with or without a 4F urodynamic catheter in the urethra (see Fig. 5a–d). Kuo (121) does not mention artifacts with a catheter when studying frequency–urgency syndrome. A 14F Foley catheter reduces the distance of the urethra to the pubis with larger standard deviations according to Mouritsen and Bach (116).

The ideal situation would be to bypass the bladder neck localization procedure. Beco (29) estimated that visualization of the urethral sphincter allows more precise localization of the urethrovesical junction, between the bulky tissue of the sphincter and the anterior bladder wall, than does radiology. This permits, theoretically at least, differentiation of the vesicourethral junction from the bladder neck, the latter being defined as the more inclined point of the contrast medium, making measurement of bladder neck funneling quite precise. To avoid possible misinterpretation with the bladder base, Vierhout (33) suggested localizing the bladder neck with a catheter and realizing the measurements once it has been withdrawn.

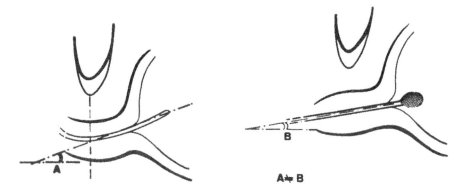

Figure 10 The thin, flexible urethral catheter follows the natural course of the urethra and (A) allows measurement of the real urethrovesical angle; (B) Q-tips render the urethra artificially rigid and straight, modifying the urethrohorizontal angle, which no longer corresponds to the initial angle A. (From Ref. 57. Courtesy of J. Beco.)

F. Geometric Framing of the Ultrasonic Image

Framing includes the determination of 1) reference points (bony or cartilaginous), 2) horizontal lines, 3) the plane of the ultrasonographic section, and 4) distances and angles, to localize the position of the urethrovesical junction.

Almost every author takes the lower edge of the pubic symphysis as a fixed reference point (Fig. 11), without describing in detail how to proceed. However, Beco (57) suggested the largest part of the pubic ligament in the sagittal plane as the reference point. One should read the article and study the illustrations by Beco (29) to be precisely in the median plane at the level of the pubic symphysis and so avoid false measurements. A few millimeters difference in distance can sometimes be significant.

Almost every author considers the pubic axis as the horizontal reference point, but precise descriptions of how to do this are rare (83,86,88–90). Those who use the endovaginal probe take the horizontal position of the probe as the reference (90,117). To do this correctly, the probe should be provided with a level (29) or, instead of the probe, the water level in the Foley balloon (118) can replace the horizontal position of the probe (Fig. 12).

In all other circumstances, the horizontal line must be traced very carefully, and it must be equidistant from the upper and lower limits of the symphysis (90) (Fig. 13). This has the advantage of being rigorously identical in the same patient, because it is not modified by movements of the pelvis or the probe. It implies, however, that the symphysis is seen in its full height, which is rarely possible by the introital route, and in our experience not always possible by the perineal route either. The vertical line is perpendicular to the inferior edge of the arcuate ligament and the UVJ is localized by abscissa and ordinate values (66,69,83,86,88–90,117,118).

Because of these difficulties, several authors prefer to define the mobility of the bladder neck by distance (Fig. 14) and angle (Fig. 15) (53,57,114–116,120,121). Unfortunately, the angle differs from author to author, making valid comparisons between different centers almost impossible. Despite these difficulties, interobserver variation of the measurements remains acceptable (69,89). For those who measure the angles "off-line" on the printed image, the variation in angles measured by the ultrasonographist and the "off-line" reader stays minimal (53,100,114).

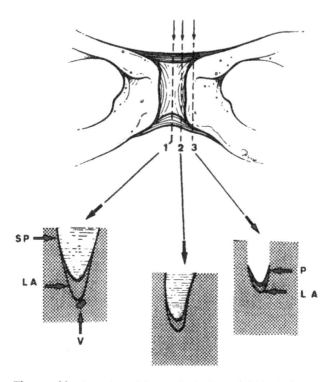

Figure 11   Location of the sagittal plane: (1) ideal plane passes across the thickest part of the arcuate ligament (LA), accompanied by a small vein (V). (2) Parasagittal plane with arcuate ligament less thick, but no hyperechogenic line is visible. The plane still remains in the "symphysial window." (3) Clear hyperechogenic line corresponds to the posterior edge of the pubis and indicates that the plane is transpubic. (From Ref. 57. Courtesy of J. Beco.)

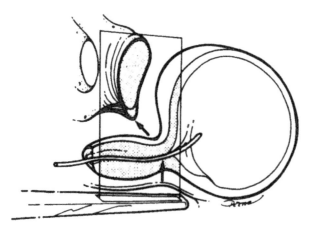

Figure 12   Linear vaginal ultrasonography: To define a section plane, at least one point and one plane must be defined. The point is the posterior edge of the pubic arcuate ligament at its thickest part (arrow). The line is the urethral catheter in its portion above the pubis (arrow). The probe should be perfectly horizontal. (From Ref. 57. Courtesy of J. Beco.)

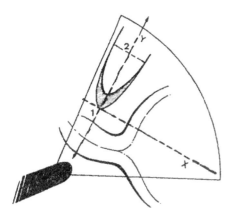

Figure 13 Reference points obtained with sectorial probe applied by perineal route: *y*-axis is defined by the longitudinal axis of the symphysis pubis; *x*-axis is perpendicular to the y-axis at the level of the arcuate ligament. These two axes (*x* and *y*) have the advantage of being independent from patient position, their inconvenience is that they are not directly visible on the screen. (From Ref. 90.)

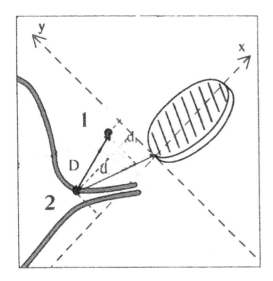

Figure 14 Localization of the urethrovesical junction (UVJ); principal distances: (1) position of the UVJ at rest; (2) position of the UVJ during withhold ($\Delta d = d_2 - d_1$), D = distance between 1 and 2.

Christensen (131) was the first to recognize the necessity of standardizing the practice of urogynecological ultrasound. As mentioned earlier, Beco gave the most complete and detailed description of artifacts (29,34,57).

Hol (118), Schaer (90), Pajoncini (132), and our group (41) applied strictly-defined protocols. German authors (30,105) made recommendations, which met the consensus of their colleagues relative to perineal ultrasonography (Fig. 16).

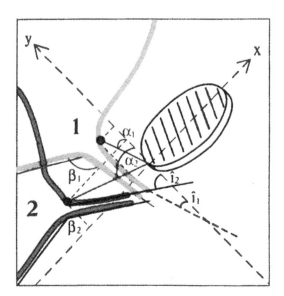

Figure 15   Morphology of the urethrovesical junction (UVJ); principal angles: 1, position of the UVJ at rest; 2, position of the UVJ during withhold; β_1, posterior urethrovesical angle at rest; β_2, posterior urethrovesical angle during stress; α_1, anterior urethrovesical angle at rest; α_2, anterior urethrovesical angle during stress; $\hat{\imath}_1$, angle of inclination at rest; $\hat{\imath}_2$, angle of inclination during stress; $\Delta\hat{\imath} = \hat{\imath}_2 - \hat{\imath}_1$ = rotational angle.

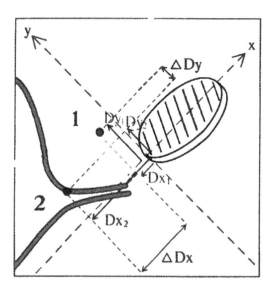

Figure 16   Localization of urethrovesical junction (UVJ) by x–y axes, according to German authors: 1, position of UVJ at rest; 2, position of UVJ during withhold; $\Delta D_y = D_{y1} - D_{y2}$; $\Delta D_x = D_{x1} = D_{x2}$.

In our institution, bladder neck position is categorized as 0 (which is normal), −1 (which is overcorrected), +1, +2, and +3 to characterize the different stages of prolapse. These observations are noted at rest, during coughing, Valsalva, and withholding. Also noted are bladder neck incompetence, a "fixed" urethra, sliding (instead of rotational) descent, urethral distortion, distance and displacement in relation to the symphysis, posterior urethrovesical angle, and variations of all these parameters during different maneuvers.

However, in disagreement with Petri (42), it is our opinion that clinical judgment should be the main factor in establishing indications for surgery. The detection of bladder neck incompetence and the suburethral sling effect appear to be the two major contributions of ultrasonography in SUI. With strictly standardized ultrasonographic methodology, objective pre- and posttreatment evaluations are possible in a given patient. At this time, ultrasonography can not replace urodynamic studies, but may constitute a valuable complement, especially when they are performed simultaneously.

VII. CLINICAL APPLICATIONS

A. Diagnosis and Treatment of SUI

Young et al. (113) studied changes in angle, urethral length, and thickness of the sphincter in 154 continent females. None of these parameters changed with age or the number of deliveries. Only sphincter thickness decreased in nontreated postmenopausal women (p = 0.02). The urethrovesical junction had a lower position during pregnancy and in those with prolapse, but only this latter group had a real hypermobile urethra (Figs. 17 and 18).

1. Comparison Between Continent and Incontinent Females (66,83,103,114,117)

Bader (103) demonstrated that in the continent female, the position of the urethrovesical junction and the posterior urethrovesical angle are related to parity, but are independent of age. Among incontinent patients, cystourethrocele and an increase in posterior vesicourethral angle are significant factors to consider; however, urethral length does not seem to correlate with the severity of incontinence.

Bladder neck position in continent females (grade 0) and incontinent patients up to grade 3 was 20.6, 14.0, 11.0, and 9.4 mm, respectively, at rest. The corresponding figures during Valsalva were 14.0, 1.1, −2.7, and −7.0 mm (p < 0.001). Similarly, the posterior vesicourethral angle changed in continent females up to grade 3 from 96.8 to 112.2 degrees at rest and from 108.1 to 147.7 degrees during Valsalva in incontinent females (p < 0.001). Bladder neck incompetence, never observed by these authors in continent females, was present in the three SUI grades in 8/56, 5/24, and 3/6 of patients, respectively.

Mouritsen (114) measured bladder neck–pubic symphysis distance and the pubourethral angle in 33 continent females, 28 SUI patients, and 39 surgical patients. The continent group had a 90-degree angle at rest, a 2.4-cm distance, and a very slightly mobile bladder neck, whereas the incontinent patients had a 100-degree angle, a distance that decreased to 2.1 cm, and a mobile bladder neck. If the following two out of three criteria are present simultaneously—95-degree angle or more at rest, distance of 2.3 cm or less, and mobility of 20 degrees or more, the diagnosis of incontinence can be made with a sensitivity of 84% and a specificity of 82%.

Weil et al. (117) compared 22 patients with SUI (proved by urodynamic tests) with 33 control subjects, using a vaginal probe. They showed that the position of the bladder

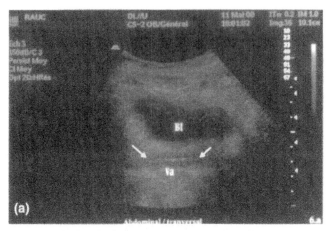

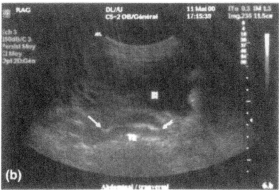

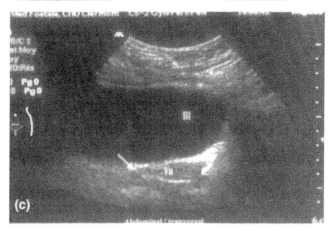

Figure 17 Vaginal "hammock"; indirect visualization of the cervicourethral fascia by the appearance of the lateral fixation of the vagina: (a) normal support of the vagina; (b) paravaginal defect; (c) following surgical correction. B1, bladder, Va, vagina. (Courtesy of D. Lemery.)

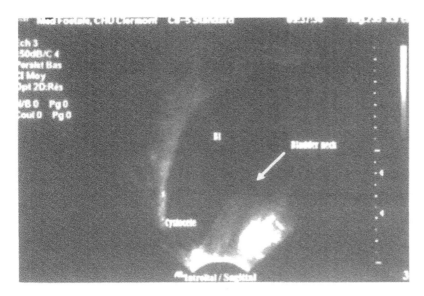

Figure 18   "Pessaire-like" effect of a large cystocele: urethra is pushed upward and kinked. B1, bladder. (Courtesy of D. Lemery.)

neck was different in the two groups (at rest and during stress), but mobility was significantly different only in the craniocaudal direction. Posterior urethrovesical angle had no discriminative power. The authors concluded that SUI can be the consequence of a too low bladder neck or its increased mobility under stress. They also admitted that the numerical values in the two groups overlapped.

Kiilholma (74) correlated the bladder neck mobility (less than 1 cm and more than 1 cm) with the severity of SUI in a small group of patients. This correlation might have existed in the primary SUI group, but not in those who underwent unsuccessful surgery.

Meyer (83) compared 74 continent nulliparous women with 32 genuine SUI patients. If the upper limit of the standard deviation of bladder neck mobility in the continent group (supine position) was exceeded (≥ 14 mm on the x-axis and ≥ 12 mm on the y-axis), the diagnosis of SUI could be made with a sensitivity of 78% for the x-axis and 75% for the y-axis, and with a specificity of 89% for the x-axis and 85% for the y-axis. He thought that bladder neck mobility along the vertical axis alone could be considered without losing important information.

Kuo (121) compared 191 SUI patients with 78 urgency–frequency patients and 27 normal controls. These women were investigated in the upright position. The two main parameters studied were bladder neck–pubis distance and rotational angle in relation to the symphysis (called the pubovesical angle). The rotational angle made discrimination possible between SUI and urgency–frequency patients (angle >20 degrees; angle variation >20 degrees), even if significant overlapping was observed between the two groups. The angle also correlated well with the SUI classes, except for class V. [Kuo's classification (120, 121): class I, bladder neck hypermobility; class II, same as class I but with bladder neck incompetence; class III, same as class II, but with sphincter deficiency; class IV, same as class III, but with cystocele; class V, bladder neck fixed, incompetent, sphincter deficiency]. In urgency–frequency syndrome as well as in normal controls, this angle was less than 10 degrees. Also, bladder neck competence did not discriminate between the latter two groups:

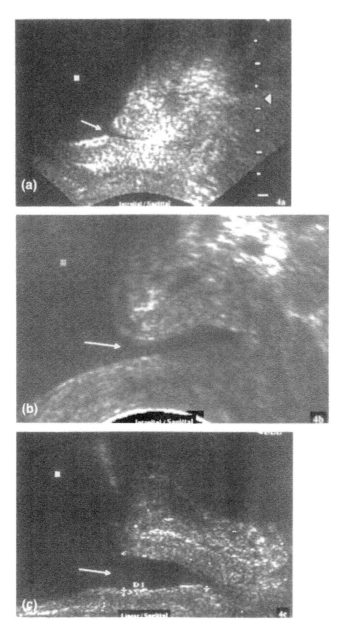

Figure 19 Different stages of bladder neck incompetence: (a) slight "notch" at the bladder base; (b) partial funneling of the bladder neck; (c) large funneling of the proximal urethra. B1, bladder. (a and b: Courtesy of D. Lemery; c: courtesy of C. Jouffroy.)

incompetence was present in 55% of urgency–frequency patients and in 29.6% of asymptomatic nulliparous women. Sphincter weakness was found in 12.8% of the urgency–frequency group, but not in the asymptomatic group (Figs. 19 and 20).

The same author (120) demonstrated in a previous article that bladder neck–pubic bone distance is a function of the suspending structures, and rotational angle depends on the supporting structures, with coaptation of the urethral mucosa remaining the third, inde-

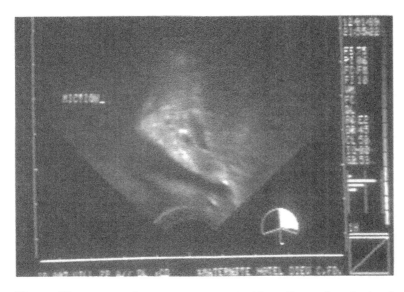

Figure 20   Voiding ultrasonography: urethral funneling and urethral wall are clearly seen. (Courtesy by D. Lemery.)

pendent, factor. Variation in angle is the most important factor. One to three months after surgery, the distance did not change, but the angle decreased significantly. One to three years postsurgery, the angle remained narrow (19 degrees) in those who remained cured, whereas in the recurrent SUI group, the angle became wide-open again (55 degrees). This author suggested different treatments for different classes of SUI. (class I, laparoscopic cure; class II, Marshall–Marchetti–Krantz retropubic urethropexy; class III, Burch colposuspension; class IV, Raz "4-corner suspension"; class V, periurethral bulking injection or suburethral sling).

2.   Effect of Surgery

Together with Kuo (120), two other authors were interested in the effect of SUI surgery (66,114).

 We have mentioned earlier the ultrasonographic criteria of SUI by Mouritsen and Rasmussen (114). Among their 39 surgical patients, those who failed had a shortened bladder neck–pubis distance, increased urethral mobility, and a widened maximum rotational angle (Valsalva angle minus withhold angle). Figure 21 illustrates some of the postoperative observations at the urethrovesical region.

 Because of overlapping values between surgical success and failure groups, the bladder neck–pubis distance has no discriminative power. As far as rotational angle is concerned, it seems that this is more indicative of the type of surgery performed (colposuspension, vaginal colporraphy), than the success or failure of the procedure itself.

 Creighton et al. (66) attempted to define ultrasonographic criteria that could be used in the operating room to define the necessary tension to be applied on the sutures to achieve the desirable position of the bladder neck postoperatively. Using logistic regression analysis, they demonstrated that no single measured factor is significant. The only correlation demonstrated was between the preoperative position of the bladder neck on the x-axis and the patient's age. From this observation, they elaborated a mathematical equation for use in

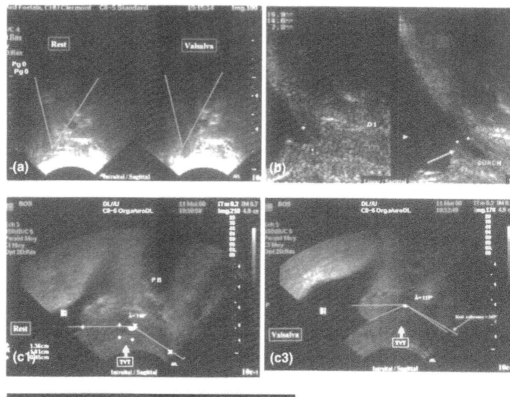

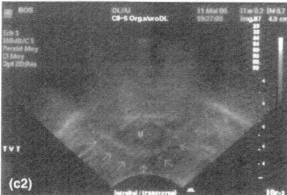

Figure 21 Postoperative appearance of the urethrovesical region: (a) almost no urethral mobility during cough; (b) "spur" beneath the bladder neck following Burch colposuspension; (c1–c3) urethra after TVT-type sling. c1, sagittal section: width of the sling = 0.45 cm, distance from the vesical neck = 1.36 cm, distance from the urethral meatus = 1.61 cm; c2, transverse section at the level of the sling: almost its entire length is seen; c3, sagittal section: urethra is angulated and pushed upward by the Valsalva maneuver. PB, pubic bone; B1, bladder; A, angle; TVT, tension-free vaginal tape; U, urethra. (a and c1–3, Courtesy of D. Lemery; b, courtesy of C. Jouffroy.)

the operating room to define the ideal position of the bladder neck. One of the major criticisms of this method is that perioperative bladder neck position in the anesthetized patient is likely to be quite different from that in routinely performed ultrasonographic examinations. A prospective clinical trial is needed to clarify this point.

B. Consequences of Pregnancy and Delivery

In contrast to other imaging modalities, ultrasonography has the great advantage that it can be done and repeated several times during the course of pregnancy and postpartum, because no radiation is involved. Four authors studied this question in more detail (83,86,104,113).

1. The Role of Pregnancy

Young (113) explored 154 continent women, 46 of them pregnant (16 in the first trimester, 15 in the second trimester, and 15 in the third trimester). When compared with the non-pregnant women, during pregnancy, the urethra became shorter, and the bladder neck was in a lower position at rest and under Valsalva. Its mobility, however, was not increased. These changes were present during the first trimester, and were not influenced by the volume of the uterus, gestational age, or size of the fetus. All of them changes disappeared after delivery. The only modification specific to the first trimester was a decreased posterior urethrovesical angle.

Perschers et al. (86) demonstrated changes in urethral support at the end of pregnancy, but in contrast to the findings of Young et al., they became less pronounced, and did not disappear completely after delivery. The urethrovesical junction was in a lower position than in nulliparous women and women who underwent cesarian section. In this latter group, the bladder neck was 6 mm lower, however, than in the nulliparous group.

In conclusion, it appears that pregnancy, in itself, has a specific influence on urethrovesical anatomy that is independent of the trauma caused by delivery. Whether this is secondary to an increase in intra-abdominal pressure, weight of the fetus, some hormonal effects, or modifications in connective tissue is unknown. However, contraction of the pelvic floor musculature does not seem to be modified.

2. The Role of Delivery

Until ultrasonography became available, evaluation of the consequences of obstetrical trauma was possible only by epidemiological study, rare comparative urodynamic investigations, and invasive electromyographic (EMG) exploration. Because of its nature, radiologic evaluations were always conducted postpartum. Ultrasonography opened the way to quantify this trauma more precisely.

In the study by Perschers et al. (86), ultrasonography was performed at 36–42 weeks of gestation and 6–10 weeks postpartum. The population studied included 25 primigravida, 20 primi- or multiparous (one to three deliveries), 10 cesarian sections, and 25 age-matched nulliparous women serving as control subjects.

The bladder neck was in a lower position at rest after vaginal delivery than in nulliparous subjects or after cesarian section (Fig. 22). Urethrovesical junction mobility was not modified significantly after cesarian section (less than 3-mm difference compared with nulliparous). The difference was significant, however, when compared with primiparous (p = 0.015) or to multiparous (p = 0.001) subjects. There was no difference between the primiparous and multiparous groups (p = 0.70) (Fig. 23). When compared with the predelivery state, reduction of bladder neck elevation greater than 4 mm with the withhold maneuver

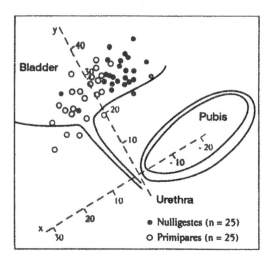

Figure 22 Position of bladder neck at rest in 25 primiparous women, 6–10 weeks follow-ing delivery, compared with 25 age-matched nulligravida. Two primiparous women are at each point defined by 4/25, 6/20, and 8/25. (From Ref. 86.)

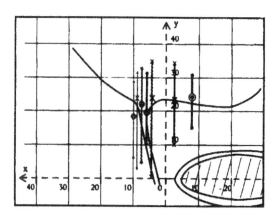

Figure 23 Position of bladder neck at rest before and after delivery, as well as during stress and withhold before and after delivery. Patients in supine position. (From Ref. 86.)

was never observed after cesarian section, and was seen only in 6/25 primiparous and 2/20 multiparous patients. Pelvic floor contractility was completely absent in 2/5 patients in whom forceps were used.

It is suggested that the bladder neck during Valsalva is in a lower position at the end of pregnancy, and this is even enhanced by vaginal delivery. Its displacement during with-hold, which depends on neuromuscular integrity of the pelvic floor, is modified more ran-domly.

Meyer et al. (83), using the same methodology, could not reproduce the results of Peschers et al. (86). Their study population included 74 continent nulliparous controls (group 1), 29 continent primiparous patients (group 2), 64 continent multiparous women (group 3), 16 patients with forceps delivery, and 32 genuine stress incontinent patients who had 2.4 deliveries (mean value) and 9% who had forceps delivery. They concluded that in vaginal delivery (groups 2 and 3), there is no correlation between ultrasonographic parameters, newborn's weight, or mother's weight, nor is there a difference in bladder neck position and number of deliveries, in the supine or erect position. Forceps delivery does not modify bladder neck position at rest or during Valsalva (except in the upright position when it is situated lower than normal). Bladder neck mobility is much more pronounced in patients with genuine stress incontinence than in those with forceps delivery. However, the bladder neck is in a lower position during Valsalva in the erect position, compared with nulliparous subjects.

Bladder neck incompetence and posterior urethrovesical angle were measured by Bader et al. (104) by the introital route in 131 patients during the immediate postpartum period (mean 4.2 days) and compared with 41 asymptomatic nulliparous women. Posterior vesicourethral angle increased more after spontaneous than after forceps delivery, compared with the nulliparous group. After cesarian section, only the angle during Valsalva differed from the controls. The posterior urethrovesical angle increased with the first and second deliveries, but remained stable afterward. In this paper (104), the data differed from those published by the same group during the same year (103).

Similarly, the position of the bladder neck also changes in relation to the mode and number of deliveries. It seems to be in the lowest position during Valsalva after forceps delivery. Also, it tends to be lower at rest, with a rising number of deliveries. According to their observations:

1. Clinically significant SUI increases with the number of deliveries (nulliparous, 2.4%, primiparous, 17.6%; two deliveries, 46.7%; three deliveries or more; 61.1%).
2. The frequency of cystocele increases with the number of deliveries (nulliparous, 0%; cesarian section, 5%; forceps delivery, 11.1%; vaginal delivery, 25.5%) (see Fig. 18). The protective role of forceps in relation to the incidence of cystocele formation is in contrast with what is generally admitted, and might be explained by the small number of cases (nine patients).
3. Bladder neck incompetence is absent in nulliparous subjects and after cesarian section. It has been observed in 11% after forceps, and in 19% after vaginal delivery.

Despite some conflicting observations, it can be concluded from these preliminary studies that

1. There is a "pregnancy effect" on the LUT that is responsible for displacement of the bladder neck. This ptosis is less evident during the first trimester because of the intrapelvic uterus (113), but becomes more manifest in the third trimester when the uterus exerts pressure on the pelvic floor (86).
2. This effect seems to be permanent (86).
3. Compared with cesarian section and with spontaneous delivery, forceps delivery compromises more the supporting structures of the urethra (83).
4. Bladder neck mobility is mainly a function of the position of the urethrovesical junction at rest (86,113) and is less the consequence of damage to supporting structures (as seen during Valsalva) or neuromuscular structures (during withhold).
5. Trauma of the first delivery seems to be of paramount importance (83,86,113). The progression of cystocele or the accentuation of SUI with increasing parity

(104) might be the consequence of aging, or simply a problem of methodology in the investigation of these patients.

6.   The majority of modifications secondary to delivery are virtually identical with those observed in patients with SUI, suggesting a causal relation between delivery and SUI.

C. Progress in Technology

Recent developments in ultrasonographic technology include 1) miniaturized probes for endourethral application, 2) digital imaging for three-dimensional (3-D) reconstruction, 3) ultrasonographic contrast material, and 4) Doppler ultrasonography to study the periurethral circulation.

1.   Endourethral Ultrasonography

Recent technological progress has made possible the construction of ultrasonic probes 1–3 mm in diameter. These high-frequency probes (9–30 MHz) give information not available with computed tomography scan or even MRI. Liu and Goldberg (134) recently summarized the experience gained with the 2-D and 3-D reconstruction of ultrasonographic images obtained by these probes, which provide a 360-degree cross-sectional image of the urethra. There is no need for urethral dilation, because the probes within their sheaths are only 6F–9F. The distance explored from the surface of the urethra is inversely proportional to the frequency of ultrasound (Fig. 24).

We will not comment on the diagnostic possibilities of this probe in cases of urethral diverticulum (135,136), but rather focus our attention on exploring urethra and urinary incontinence. This subject has been reviewed in detail by Heit (137).

Kirschner–Hermanns (139,183) studied the surface and the circumference of the striated urethral sphincter in 32 incontinent and 12 continent control women, using a 9F probe of 20 MHz (15 images per second), which had a depth penetration of 25 mm. The surface (1.03 cm^2 ± 0.3) and circumference (3.61 cm ± 0.5) of the sphincter in continent patients differed significantly from those of the incontinent group (0.73 cm^2 ± 0.5 and 2.97 cm ± 0.7, respectively). They even established a negative correlation between the surface, and circumference and the degree of incontinence. None of the continent patients had a circumference less than 2.8 cm. Unfortunately, these observations were not coupled with urodynamic studies.

Schaer et al. (140) established a parallel between ultrasonographic image and histology in 11 fresh female cadavers. Fischer (141) proved, by needle electromyography (EMG), that the hyperechogenic zone seen by ultrasonography corresponds to the striated urethral sphincter. Also, needle EMG is necessary to differentiate scar tissue from the striated muscle sphincter within the hyperechogenic ring.

Heit et al. (142) measured the circumference of the longitudinal smooth muscle (hypoechogenic) in 10 asymptomatic, 24 incontinent, and 5 ISD women. When Valsalva leak-point pressure passed from more than 60 cmH$_2$O to less than 60 cmH$_2$O, the circumference dropped from 4.17 to 3.78 cm (p = 0.08). Similarly, with maximum urethral closure pressure of more than 20 cmH$_2$O, the circumference was 4.18 cm, and with less than 20 cmH$_2$O, it fell to 3.68 cm (p = 0.04). Finally, with or without bladder neck incompetence, the values were 3.43 and 4.16 cm, respectively (p = 0.03). These values were independent of age, and the authors estimated that the diagnosis of ISD could be made solely by endourethral ultrasonography. A diameter of more than 11.0 mm of the longitudinal smooth muscle elim-

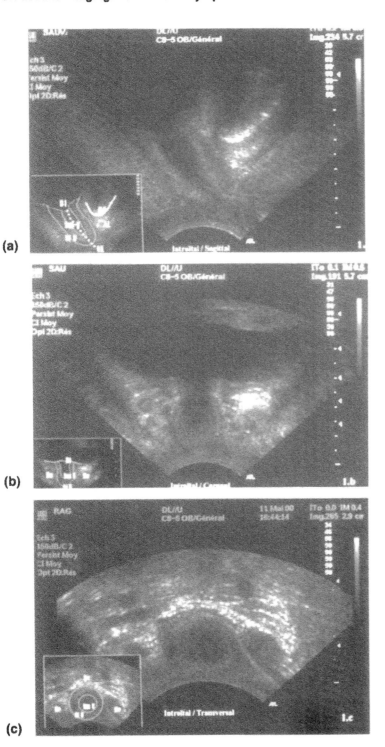

Figure 24 Ultrasonographic appearance of the normal urethral sphincter: (a) sagittal section; (b) coronal section; (c) transverse section. B1, bladder; Smu, smooth-muscle layer of the urethra; Stu, striated muscle layer of the urethra; Re, rectum; AL, arcuate ligament. (Courtesy of D. Lemery.)

inated the possibility of ISD with a negative predictive value of 95%. However, they recognized the wide variability of these hypoechogenic and hyperechogenic layers in the incontinent female.

Frauscher et al. (143) measured the striated sphincter in 34 incontinent and 11 continent patients, with and without voluntary contractions. They found a good correlation with the urodynamic data. Sphincteric function was never decreased with urge incontinence or in the absence of SUI. Furthermore, the correlation was also good with the degree of SUI severity.

Rivas et al. (144), in an animal model, demonstrated that submucosal injection of collagen has the lowest reabsorption rate and is more often colonized by native collagen. Hence, ultrasonography can be a valuable tool to visualize the depth of injection and the amount of collagen to be injected. It remains to be proved whether this approach is better in humans than the classic transparietal or transvaginal route described by Leonhard et al. (145) to control collagen deposition.

In summary, endourethral ultrasonography is an innovative and promising approach to study urethral anatomy and function. At present, preliminary investigations must focus on the reproducibility of measurements on a larger scale, comparing them with urodynamic and electrophysiological data.

2. Urethral Sphincter Measurements by Bi- and Tridimensional Ultrasonography

Classically, urogynecological ultrasonography focused mainly on the position and morphology of the bladder neck and on urethral hypermobility. Endourethral and 3-D ultrasonography allowed more detailed study of the dimensions (length, thickness, circumference, transverse section surface) of the urethral sphincter, making distinctions between smooth and striated muscle elements possible.

Yang (113) revived interest in these studies by using the introital route. He demonstrated a thinner sphincter in postmenopausal than in premenopausal women.

Tunn et al. (112) measured the transverse diameter of the proximal urethra (mean 15.3 mm) in 204 incontinent women. There was no correlation between this diameter and patient age, parity, the use of substitution hormonotherapy, the severity of incontinence, or urethral closure pressure.

When using the perineal and introital routes, Martan et al. (78,80,81) described the striated sphincter as an ovoid structure lying at a distance from the vesical neck. The surface of the sphincter (measured in the sagittal and horizontal plane) was greater in continent, asymptomatic women, whereas its thickness (measured in the sagittal plane) was decreased in incontinent patients. Urethral length had no discriminative value. Intravaginal hormonal treatment had no influence on sphincter thickness, but increased urethral mucosa (79). Bladder volume did not modify surface and thickness measurements (80). Finally, comparing incontinent women with those who underwent Burch colposuspension or vaginal repair for incontinence and prolapse, no significant differences in these parameters could be demonstrated 3–24 months after surgery (81).

Leonor de Gonzales (113) described the female striated sphincter as a "pseudoprostate." Mean values in 97 women were longitudinal length 130 mm, anteroposterior length 46 mm, and transverse length 133 mm.

In 105 SUI patients, Diez and Clarke (67) found a positive correlation between anteroposterior diameter of the midurethra and urethral closure pressure ($p = 0.046$).

The most detailed study on striated and smooth-muscle components of the urethral sphincter was done by Kuo (122) who tested a total of 111 patients, including 14 control subjects. The most significant results are summarized in Table 4.

4 Midurethral Cross-Sectional Area with Its Smooth and Striated Muscle Components in Controls and in Different
ɔgical Situations

s	N	Cross-sectional area (mm² ± 1 SD)		Smooth-muscle component (mm² ± 1 SD)	Striated muscle compe (mm² ± 1 SD)	
s	14	96.4 ± 38.4		42.5 ± 18.3	53.9 ± 35.3	
ɪcy–urgency syndrome	37	107.4 ± 34.6	⎤ p = 0.002	47.4 ± 23.9	59.9 ± 25.9	⎤ p = 0.;002
JIᵃ	42	85.2 ± 27.9	⎦	41.3 ± 16.1	49.3 ± 20.9	⎦
SUI	18	90.3 ± 34.9		49.9 ± 23.9	40.4 ± 20.6	
ɛleᵇ	(9)	75.7 ± 23.1		37.9 ± 12.2	37.8 ± 22.8	
	111	94.8 ± 33.7		44.9 ± 20.6	49.9 ± 25.1	

ɛss urinary incontinence.
ɪce data on patients with cystocele. Differences are not statistically significant, unless otherwise indicated.
Ref. 122.

The normal urethra shows smooth muscle along its entire length, which is in continuity with the detrusor muscle at the bladder neck. There is no striated muscle at the bladder neck, its maximum concentration is at the level of the midurethra. Its distribution around the urethra is variable. Especially in SUI, it is present only laterally on both sides of the urethra, but it is lacking at the anterior and posterior aspects. This kind of distribution was observed in 42% of SUI, and only 15% of normal subjects. Bladder neck incompetence was associated with mild SUI in 63% and severe SUI in 83% of cases. The length of the pubourethral ligament was not modified in the two groups, but the urethropelvic ligaments were thinner in the severe SUI group. The transverse section of the urethra was smaller than normal in SUI; the difference was not significant in the smooth-muscle surface, but it was in the striated muscle surface (42.8 vs. 58.3 mm^2).

In accordance with the observations of Noble et al. (52) and Fischer (141) in patients with urgency–frequency syndrome, the transverse section of the urethra was slightly increased, compared with that of controls, mainly because of marked striated sphincter development.

Since its first application in gynecology in 1994, 3-D ultrasonography has retained the attention of several researchers (147–149). Khullar et al. (150) succeeded in reconstructing a 3-D image of the urethra, using an endorectal 5-MHz probe.

Noble et al. (52) studied patients with obstructive symptoms and abnormal sphincter EMG. They found that sphincter volume was increased by threefold (3.05 cm^3) in this particular group of patients compared with the controls (1.30 cm^3).

Cardozo's group at King's College Hospital, London, recently published an update of their experience with 3-D imaging of the urethral sphincter (43), comparing continent with incontinent patients (150–152), during pre- and postpartum (153–155) and, more specifically, the urethral sphincter in incontinent women (146) (Table 5). The main advantage of 3-D reconstruction of the female urethra is that it allows transverse sections of the urethra to be obtained despite its retropubic position (Fig. 25).

The urethra appears as a target. The inner part (urothelium and smooth muscle) is hyperechogenic, whereas the external part (striated muscle) is hypoechogenic. With aging, however, more echogenic zones are detected, probably because of collagen deposition within the muscle fibers. Echogenecity is probably a function of collagen content and orientation of the muscle fibers in relation to the ultrasonic beam. This might explain why

Table 5 Measurements of the Urethra and Striated Sphincter in a Group of Continent and Incontinent Patients

	Continent ($n = 48$) mean $\pm$ 1 SD	Incontinent ($n = 46$) mean $\pm$ 1 SD	p
Striated sphincter			
Length (mm)	19.2 $\pm$ 3.6	16.9 $\pm$ 1.9	0.001
Thickness (mm)	2.5 $\pm$ 0.4	2.1 $\pm$ 0.5	<0.001
Volume (mL)	1.2 $\pm$ 0.2	0.8 $\pm$ 0.2	<0.001
Urethra			
Maximum transverse section area	1.49 $\pm$ 0.3	1.37 $\pm$ 0.3	NS[a]

[a]NS, Difference not statistically significant.
Source: Ref. 43.

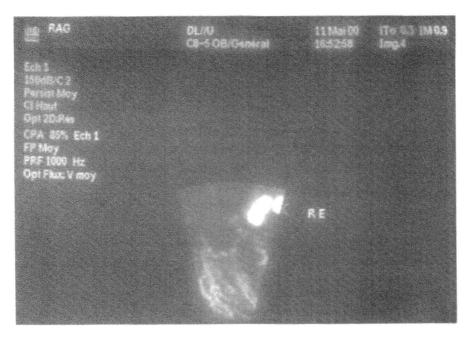

Figure 25 Three-dimensional reconstruction of the urethral vascular network: RE, space of Retzius. (Courtesy of D. Lemery.)

echogenicity varies with the perineal and vaginal routes. The morphology of the sphincter, as depicted by ultrasonography, has been confirmed by MRI which, in turn, has been compared with histology (156) and with dissection of cadavers of different ages (157).

At the bladder neck, the urothelium (hyperechogenic) is surrounded by smooth-muscle fibers (hyperechogenic, irregular ring). At the midurethra, the striated sphincter surrounds the urothelium and the smooth muscle, the latter being responsible for urethral bulkiness at this level. At its distal part, the urethra becomes thinner because of the reduction in smooth (and not striated) muscle. The retropubic space, rich in fascia and vessels, appears hyperechogenic and nonhomogeneous.

The results comparing 46 incontinent patients with 48 continent women are summarized in Table 5. The striated sphincter is shorter, thinner and of smaller volume in incontinent patients than in their continent counterparts. There is no overlapping in volume values between the two groups, and a good correlation is seen between urethral volume and the severity of incontinence, as documented by VVCUG ($r = -0.65$; $p < 0.001$).

Three-dimensional imaging has been proposed to study obstetrical injuries of the anal sphincter (158), congenital anomalies of the pelvic floor, and the anal sphincter in children (126).

To investigate the urethra, the intrarectal route is preferable to the vaginal approach because of less distortion of the urethra. Fecal residue in the rectal ampulla, however, makes the vaginal route more appropriate (127).

In conclusion, 3-D technology can be used with endourethral probes (134), is precise and reliable (159), more so than 2-D evaluations (160). It measures the volume of irregular structures, such as the striated sphincter [validated by in vitro studies (161)], without moving the probe, preventing anatomical distortions. It also has the advantage of demonstrating paraurethral structures as well with a much better cost/benefit ratio than does MRI (39). It has still to confirm its role in surgical prognosis and prove correlations of 3-D "reconstructions" with tissues properties (162).

3.   Opacification of the Bladder Neck

The significance of the open bladder neck has been debated for years. Chapple (45) found an open bladder neck in 29% of 29 nulliparous women, all of them asymptomatic. Four patients with occasional incontinence all had a closed bladder neck. Kim (163) studied 356 females with SUI. With a full bladder, 53.9% had an open bladder neck. There was no correlation with the type of incontinence (110 had ISD), radiologic appearance, hormone status, number of deliveries, or age. An open bladder neck cannot be considered as being diagnostic of ISD. It can have some prognostic value when Valsalva leak-point pressure is in the gray zone (60–90 cmH$_2$O). Nevertheless, an open bladder neck is frequently considered in ultrasonographic evaluations (31,32,49,67,70,103–108,110,112,120–122,132,142) (see Fig. 19).

The screening of bladder neck incompetence by VVCUG is superior to ultrasonography (54,89); the latter is enhanced with patients in the erect position, and with full bladder (90), but diagnosis is only possible in less than 50% of patients (70).

Schaer was the first to use ultrasonographic contrast material (Echovist-300; Schering) to better visualize the bladder neck (91). It is a suspension of galactose, which produces microbubbles under ultrasound. The suspension is prepared on site, must be injected in the bladder (avoiding its dispersion) within 5 min, and ultrasonography performed in the next 5 min. He obtained good results (46): at rest, incompetence was demonstrated in 2 subjects, compared with none without this material, 38 during Valsalva with Echovist, and only 19 without it (Fig. 26). Because of the high cost of this substance, Dietz (164) experimented

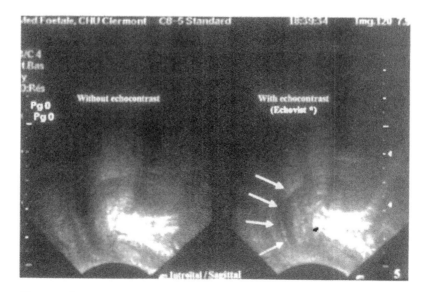

Figure 26   Visualization of the urethra by the ultrasonographic contrast material Echovist. (Courtesy of D. Lemery.)

with oil emulsions in different media (water, normal saline, 5% dextrose in water), but these have not yet been tested in humans.

Masata (82) measured bladder neck diameter with and without contrast material by the perineal route, and then compared these results with Echovist-300, using the perineal and introital routes. He concluded that the diagnostic accuracy obtained by the introital route is almost equivalent to that obtained with contrast material.

Monitoring intra-abdominal and intraurethral pressures by Echovist-300, Schaer et al. (95) demonstrated that increased intra-abdominal pressure during Valsalva or coughing did not influence the importance of bladder neck opening. This study also confirmed the presence of bladder neck incompetence in continent females, except in nulliparas.

These observations suggest that continence can be maintained solely by the distal urethra in continent patients, even with a 19-mm–wide open bladder neck. Also, delivery seems to be the principle responsible for bladder neck incompetence under stress.

In conclusion, measurement of bladder neck incompetence has no diagnostic importance, but might be interesting from the physiopathological point of view, because some surgical procedures, especially slings, correct this incompetence, whereas others (such as tension-free vaginal tape) done under the mid- or distal urethra leave bladder neck incompetence uncorrected.

4. Color Doppler Ultrasonography

Mattox (165) and Khullar (166) made substantial contributions to the understanding of bladder and periurethral vascularization. They demonstrated that (1) bladder vascularization starts to decrease during bladder filling, with a volume as low as 30 mL; (2) vascularization of the bladder base, which is normal in young females and in bladder instability, is decreased in SUI, although intramural blood flow is not significantly modified in these situations; (3) periurethral vascularization decreases with age and in SUI.

Most authors studied the consequences of hormone replacement on periurethral blood flow (79,167–170) and on blood flow within the bladder wall (79). Technical difficulties included localization of the artery in the anterior wall of the urethra, at the midurethral level (170), or at 1 cm distal from the bladder neck (167) (Figs. 27 and 28); as well as determination of the best angle between the vessel and the ultrasonic beam to obtain optimal flow values, particularly at the end of diastole (167); and to calculate the pulsatility index (or Pourcelot's index). These difficulties might explain why different authors obtained different results (79,167–169).

Color Doppler ultrasound has also been proposed to study urine loss, for which it might be an alternative to VVCUG or to distal urethral electric conductance (17), which has a 76% sensitivity for screening SUI. Dietz and Clarke compared color Doppler ultrasound with VCUG in 99 patients. Urine loss was detected in 58 patients by x-ray evaluation and in 56 women with Doppler. The study of urethral blood flow after cardiopulmonary bypass (172,173) has been proposed to explain urethral stenosis secondary to local ischemia. Periurethral vessels have been investigated in pregnant women (174). Following an experimental protocol (175), Doppler was used to determine urine flow velocity and to localize bladder outlet obstruction in males (176,177).

Beco et al. (178) analyzed the submucosal vascular plexus in detail by color Doppler. The plexus started at a mean of 8.8 mm from the bladder neck, and flow was distal, in the direction of the external meatus. In cases where the plexus started at the bladder neck, blood flow was retrograde, in the direction of the bladder, at the first 5 mm of the urethra. These observations are in accordance with the anatomical description of Huisman (176). Beco

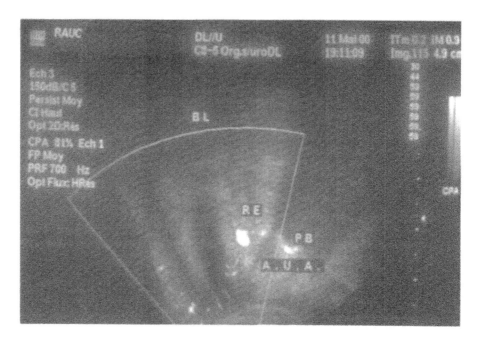

Figure 27   Anterior urethral artery emerging from the retropubic space of Retzius: BL, bladder; RE, space of Retzius; PB, pubic bone; A.U.A., anterior urethral artery. (Courtesy of D. Lemery.)

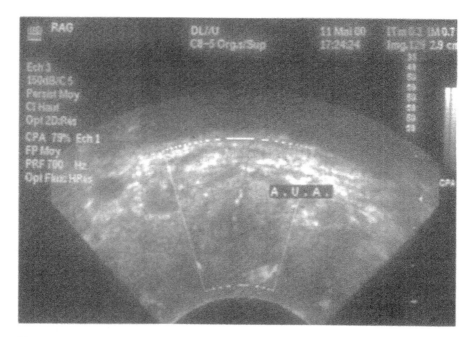

Figure 28   Transverse section of the periurethral vasculature at the level of the anterior urethral artery. A.U.A., anterior urethral artery. (Courtesy of D. Lemery.)

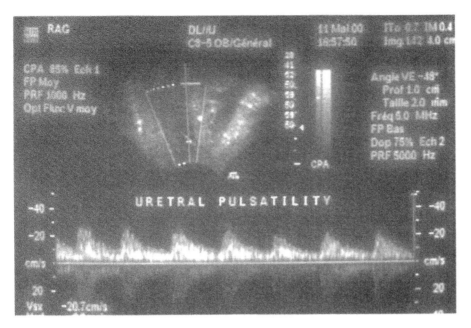

Figure 29 Quantification of urethral pulsations. (Courtesy of D. Lemery.)

(180) also demonstrated that the amplitude of the so-called ultrasonographic urethral pulse (Fig. 29), registered at the thickest part of the sphincter and corresponds to the "urodynamic urethral pulse," correlates well with urethral closure pressure.

Considering patient age, four ultrasonographic parameters and three Doppler parameters, continence was diagnosed in nine of nine patients, and incontinence in 15 of 16 women (p = 0.008). With a simplified approach in which only three parameters were considered [maximum thickness of the vascular plexus, its distance from the bladder neck (Fig. 30), and the distance between the probe and the pubic ligament], the diagnosis of SUI could be made in 22 out of 25 patients (p = 0.003). None of these parameters evaluated bladder neck mobility during stress.

If we accept that the submucosal vascular network is essential for urethral coaptation and represents up to 30% of urethral closure pressure (181), these observations are highly significant. They need, however, to be confirmed by other investigators.

In conclusion, color Doppler might become an interesting tool in functional evaluation of the urethral sphincter. This technology can also be applied to explore the effect of estrogens, α-adrenergic agonists, or vasodilators on the urethra as well as the influence of hormonal variations during the menstrual cycle, during pregnancy, and postpartum. It offers the possibility of evaluating the consequences of periurethral surgery, pelvic vascular surgery, irradiation, and such.

VIII. CONCLUSION

At the end of this updated review on the application of ultrasonography to urinary incontinence, we can conclude on the absolute necessity of standardizing the methodology to be able to compare results from the literature. We should not limit our observations to numeric data alone, which give "static" images of a dynamic process. We should go beyond simple

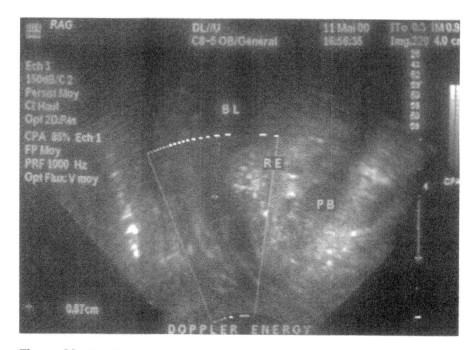

Figure 30 Sagittal section of the periurethral vasculature: the vascular band begins at 0.87 cm from the bladder neck. BL, bladder neck; RE, space of Retzius; PB, pubic bone. (Courtesy of D. Lemery.)

imaging, which is insufficient to explain the mechanism of incontinence and the results of surgery. We should take advantage of the great flexibility of the method to realize pre- and posttreatment comparative studies, longitudinal studies during pregnancy and post partum, and closely follow technological progress in this domain. Improvement in image definition, evaluation of the vascular component, and 3-D image reconstruction will, in the near future, permit conventional radiology to be replaced by ultrasonography and be a real competitor to MRI.

REFERENCES

1. Mattox TF. Ultrasound in urogynecology. Ultrasound Obstet Gynecol 1994; 4:182.
2. Crystle CD, Charme LS, Copeland WE. Q-tip test in stress urinary incontinence. Obstet Gynecol 1971; 38:313–315.
3. Jeffcoate TN, Roberts H. Observation on stress urinary incontinence. Am J Obstet Gynecol 1952; 64:721–738.
4. Hodgkinson CP, Daub HP, Keely W. Urethrocystogram: metallic bead chain technique. Clin Obstet Gynecol 1958; 1:668–677.
5. Green TH. Development of a plan for diagnosis and treatment of urinary stress incontinence. Am J Obstet Gynecol 1962; 83:632–648.
6. Enhoerning G, Miller ER, Hinman F Jr. Urethral closure studies with cineroentgenography and simultaneous bladder and urethral pressure recording. Surg Gynecol Obstet 1964; 118:507–516.

7. Schaaps JP, Lambotte R. Exploration échographique de l'incontinence urinaire de la femme. [Echographic exploration of the female stress urinary incontinence. abstr.] Symposium International d'Échographie Obstetricale; April 22 1977, Paris. Glaxo-Evans Diététique.

8. White RD, McQuown D, McCarthy TA, Ostergard DR. Real-time ultrasonography in the evaluation of urinary stress incontinence. Am J Obstet Gynecol 1980; 138:235–237.

9. Demirci F, Fine PM. Ultrasonography in stress urinary incontinence. Int Urogynecol J Pelvic Floor Dysfunct 1996; 7:125–132.

10. Beco J, Sulu M, Schaaps JP, Lambotte R. Une nouvelle approche des troubles de continence chez la femme: l'échographie urodynamique par voie vaginale. [A new approach to urinary continence disorders in women: urodynamic ultrasonic examination by the vaginal route]. J Gynecol Obstet Biol Reprod (Paris) 1987; 16:987–998.

11. Porena M, Vespasiani G, Virgili G, Lombi R, Mearini E, Rosi P, Micali F. Real-time transrectal monographic voiding cystourethrography. Urology 1987, 30:171–175.

12. Brown MC, Sutherst JR, Murray A, Richmond DH. Potential use of ultrasound in place of x-ray fluoroscopy in urodynamics. Br J Urol 1985; 57:88–90.

13. Leonor de Gonzalez E, Cosgrove DO, Joseph AE, Murch C, Naik K. The appearances on ultrasound of the female urethral sphincter. Br J Radiol 1988; 61:687–690.

14. Richmond DH, Sutherst JR, Brown MC. Screening of the bladder base and urethra using linear array transrectal ultrasound scanning. J Clin Ultrasound 1986; 14:647–651.

15. Nishizawa O, Takada H, Sakamoto F, Matsuo S, Noto H, Kizu N, Harada T, Tsuchida S. Combined urodynamic and ultrasonic techniques: a new diagnostic method for the lower urinary tract. Tohoku J Exp Med 1982; 136:231–232.

16. Gordon D, Pearce M, Norton P, Stanton SL. Comparison of ultrasound and lateral chain urethrocystography in the determination of bladder neck descent. Am J Obstet Gynecol 1989; 160: 182–185.

17. Quinn MJ, Beynon J, Mortensen NN, Smith PJ. Vaginal endosonography in the postoperative assessment of colposuspension. Br J Urol 1989; 63:295–300.

18. Quinn MJ, Beynon J, Mortensen NJ, Smith PJ. Transvaginal endosonography: a new method to study the anatomy of the lower urinary tract in urinary stress incontinence. Br J Urol 1988; 62:414–418.

19. Koelbl H, Bernaschek G, Wolf G. A comparative study of perineal ultrasound scanning and urethrocystography in patients with genuine stress incontinence. Arch Gynecol Obstet 1988; 244:39–45.

20. Shapeero LG, Friedland GW, Perkash I. Transrectal sonographic voiding cystourethrography: studies in neuromuscular bladder dysfunction. Am J Roentgenol 1983; 141:83–90.

21. Kohom EL, Scioscia AL, Jeanty P, Hobbins JC. Ultrasound cystourethrography by perineal scanning for the assessment of female stress urinary incontinence. Obstet Gynecol 1986; 68: 269–272.

22. Bergman A, McKenzie CJ, Richmond J, Ballard CA, Platt LD. Transrectal ultrasound versus cystography in the evaluation of anatomical stress urinary incontinence. Br J Urol 1988; 62: 228–234.

23. Bergman A, Ballard CA, Plan LD. Ultrasonic evaluation of urethrovesical junction in women with stress urinary incontinence. JCU J Clin Ultrasound 1988; 16:295–300.

24. Bergman A, Koonings P, Ballard CA, Platt LD. Ultrasonic prediction of stress urinary incontinence development in surgery for severe pelvic relaxation. Gynecol Obstet Invest 1988; 26: 66–72.

25. Lémery D. Echoanatomie morphologique et fonctionnelle du bas appareil urinaire feminin normal. [Morphological and functional anatomy of the female low urinary tract by echography]. Mémoire pour le diplome d'études et de recherche en biologie humaine; Université René-Descartes, Paris V. 1989:1–55.

25a. Bhatia NN, Ostergard DR, McQuown D. Ultrasonography in urinary incontinence. Urology 1987; 29:90–94.

26. Benson JT, Summers JE. Ultrasound evaluation of female urinary incontinence. Int Urogynecol J 1990; 1:7–11.

27. Benson JT, Summers JE, Pittman JS. Definition of normal female pelvic floor anatomy using ultrasonographic techniques. J Clin Ultrasound 1991; 19:275–282.

28. Ghoniem GM, Shoukry MS, Yang A, Mostwin J. Imaging for urogynecology, including new modalities. Int Urogynecol J 1992; 3:221.

29. Beco J. Reducing uncertainty for vesico-urethral sonography in women. Acta Urol Belg 1995; 63:13–29.

30. Schaer GN, Koelbl H, Voigt R, Merz E, Anthuber C, Niemeyer R, Ralph G, Bader W, Fink D, Grischke E, Hanzal E, Koehler K, Munz E, Perucchini D, Peschers U, Sam C, Schwenke A. Recommendations of the German association of urogynecology on functionnal sonography of the lower female urinary tract. Int Urogynecol J 1996; 7:105–108.

31. Koelbl H, Bernaschek G. A new method for sonographic urethrocystography and simultaneous pressure–flow measurements. Obstet Gynecol 1989; 74:417–422.

32. Koelbl H, Bernaschek G, Deutinger J. Assessment of female urinary incontinence by introital sonography. J Clin Ultrasound 1990; 18:370–374.

33. Vierhout ME. [Letter to the Editor]. Int Urogynecology J 1996; 7:234–235.

34. Beco J. Functional sonography of the lower urinary tract [letter; comment]. Int Urogynecol J Pelvic Floor Dysfunct 1996; 7:270–273.

35. Martensson O, Duchek M. Translabial sonography in evaluating the lower female urogenital tract—pictorial essay. AJR Am J Roentgenol 1996; 166:1327–1331.

36. Demirci F, Fine PM. Ultrasonography in stress urinary incontinence. Int Urogynecol J Pelvic Floor Dysfunct 1996; 7:125–132.

37. Peck RJ. Has ultrasound a role in the functionnal assessment of the bladder and urethra. Curr Opin Obstet Gynecol 1994; 4:189–191.

38. Sanders RC, Genadry R, Yang A. Imaging of the female urethra. Ultrasound Obstet Gynecol 1994; 12:167–170.

39. Koelbl H, Hanzal E. Imaging of the lower urinary tract. Curr Opin Obstet Gynecol 1995; 7: 382–385.

40. Khullar V, Cardozo L. Imaging in urogynaecology. Br J Obstet Gynaecol 1996; 103:1061–1067.

41. Jacquetin B. Intérêt de l'échographie dans l'incontinence urinaire d'effort de la femme. [Is ultrasonography interesting in evaluation of female stress urinary incontinence?]. Constat 1998; 8:11–18.

42. Petri E, Koelbl H, Schaer G. What is the place of ultrasound in urogynecology? A written panel. Int Urogynecol J Pelvic Floor Dysfunct 1999; 10:262–273.

43. Khullar V, Cardozo L. Ultrasonography. In: Appell RA, Bourcier AP, LaTorre F, eds. Pelvic Floor Dysfunction: Investigations and Conservative Treatment. Rome: CESI, 1999:107–114.

44. Lapray JF. Echographie. In: Lapray JF, ed. Imagerie de la Vessie et de la Dynamique Pelvienne de la Femme. Paris: Masson, 1999:194–205.

45. Chapple CR, Helm CW, Blease S, Milroy EJ, Rickards D, Osborne JL. Asymptomatic bladder neck incompetence in nuiliparous females. Br J Urol 1989; 64:357–359.

46. Schaer GN, Koechli OR, Schuessler B, Haller U. Improvement of perineal sonographic bladder neck imaging with ultrasound contrast medium. Obstet Gynecol 1995; 86:950–954.

47. Bandi G, Larizza U, Rodolico R, Giuberchio C, Bagliani F. [Transrectal echography and cystography in the assessment of female stress urinary incontinence]. Radiol Med (Torino) 1990; 79:228–232.

48. Braccini G, Pannocchia P, Alderigi L, Gigoni R, Calderazzi A. [Comparison of colpocystourethrorectography and transrectal ultrasonography in the assessment of female urinary incontinence]. Radiol Med (Torino) 1991; 82:101–106.

49. Dietz HP, Wilson PD. Anatomical assessment of the bladder outlet and proximal urethra using ultrasound and videocystourethrography. Int Urogynecol J Pelvic Floor Dysfunct 1998; 9: 365–369.

50. Siegel CL, Middleton WD, Teefey SA, Wainstein MA, Mcdougall EM, Klutke CG. Sonography of the female urethra. AJR Am J Roentgenol 1998; 170:1269–1274.

51. Fontana D, Porpiglia F, Moffa I, Destefanis P. Transvaginal ultrasonography in the assessment of organic diseases of female urethra. J Ultrasound Med 1999; 18:237–241.

52. Noble JG, Dixon PJ, Rickards D, Fowler CJ. Urethral sphincter volumes in women with obstructed voiding and abnormal sphincter electromyographic activity. Br J Urol 1995; 76:741–746.

53. Mouritsen L, Strandberg C. Vaginal ultrasonography versus colpo-cysto-urethrography in the evaluation of female urinary incontinence. Acta Obstet Gynecol Scand 1994; 73:338–342.

54. Schaer GN, Kochli OR, Hutzli C, Fink D, Haller U. Comparison of lateral urethrocystography and perineal ultrasound—are there differences—a prospective study. Geburtsh Frauenheilk 1994; 54:75–79.

55. Badzakoft N, Lazarevski MB, Chakmakov D, Iliev V. A comparison study of introital and perineal ultrasonography versus colpocystography in patients with genuine stress incontinence. Int Urogynecol J 1998; 9:339–339.

56. Benness CJ, Bamick CGW, Cardozo LD. Is there a place for routine videocystourethrography in the assessment of lower urinary tract dysfunction? Neurourol Urodynam 1989; 8:301–302.

57. Beco J, Leonard D, Lambotte R. Study of the artefacts induced by linear array transvaginal ultrasound scanning in urodynamics. World J Urol 1994; 12:329–332.

58. Ostrzenski A, Osborne NG. Ultrasonography as a screening tool for paravaginal defects in women with stress incontinence: a pilot study. Int Urogynecol J Pelvic Floor Dysfunct 1998; 9:195–199.

59. Jolic V, Gilja I. Vaginal vs. transabdominal ultrasonography in the evaluation of female urinary tract anatomy, stress urinary incontinence and pelvic organs static disturbances. Zentralbl Gynakol 1997; 119:483–491.

60. Bernstein I, Juul N, Gronvall S, Bonde B, Klarskov P. Pelvic floor muscle thickness measured by perineal ultrasonography. Scand J Urol Nephrol Suppl 1991; 137:131–133.

61. Bernstein IT. The pelvic floor muscles: muscle thickness in healthy and urinary-incontinent women measured by perineal ultrasonography with reference to the effect of pelvic floor training. Estrogen receptor studies. Neurourol Urodynam 1997; 16:237–275.

62. Caputo RM, Benson JT. The Q-tip test and urethrovesical junction mobility. Obstet Gynecol 1993; 82:892–896.

63. Chen GD, Su TH, Lin LY. Applicability of perineal sonography in anatomical evaluation of bladder neck in women with and without genuine stress incontinence. J Clin Ultrasound 1997; 25:189–194.

64. Chen GD, Wu GS, Lin LY, Lee HS, Chung SL, Lee YY. The determined factors of the bladder neck mobility. Int Urogynecol J 1997; 8:S32.

65. Creighton SM, Pearce JM, Stanton SL. Perineal video-ultrasonography in the assessment of vaginal prolapse: early observations. Br J Obstet Gynaecol 1992; 99:310–313.

66. Creighton SM, Clark A, Pearce JM, Stanton SL. Perineal bladder neck ultrasound—appearances before and after continence surgery. Ultrasound Obstet Gynecol 1994; 4:428–433.

67. Dietz BP, Clarke B. The urethral pressure profile and ultrasound parameters of bladder neck mobility. Neurourol Urodynam 1998; 17:374–375.

68. Dietz HP, Haylen BT, Broome J. The quantification of uterovaginal prolapse by ultrasound: a comparison with the ICS prolapse assessment system. Neurourol Urodynam 1999; 18:306–307.

69. Fink D, Schaer G, Kochli OR, Perucchini D, Haller U. Perineal ultrasound examination: are the results reproducible? Geburtsh Frauenheilk 1995; 55:699–702.

70. Fink D, Schaer G, Perucchini D, Haller U. Gynecological and perineal monographic examinations of women with stress incontinence: a comparison aim. Ultraschall Med 1996; 17:285–288.

71. Halaska M, Martan A, Voigt R, Masata J, Otcenasek M. Ultrasound: GSI surgery outcome monitoring. Int Urogynecol J Pelvic Floor Dysfunct 1998; 9:322.

72. Hextall A, Bidmead J, Cardozo L, Boos K, Mantle J. Assessment of pelvic floor function in women with genuine stress incontinence: a comparison between ultrasound, digital examination and perineometry. Neurourol Urodynam 1999; 18:325–326.

73. Khullar V, Toozs–Hobson P, Boos K, Hextall A, Cardozo L. Re: the pelvic floor muscles: muscle thickness in healthy and urinary-incontinent women measured by perineal ultrasonography with reference to the effect of pelvic floor training. Estrogen receptor studies. Neurourol Urodynam 1999; 18:69–70.

74. Kiiiholma PJ, Makinen JI, Pitkanen YA, Varpula MJ. Perineal ultrasound—an alternative for radiography for evaluating stress urinary incontinence in females. Ann Chir Gynaecol Suppl 1994; 208:43–45.

75. Lukanovic A, Kralj B, Barbic M. Transperineal ultrasound evaluation of urethrovesical junction mobility in female stress urinary incontinence. Int Urogynecol J Pelvic Floor Dysfunct 1998; 9:352–352.

76. Martan A, Halaska M, Drbohlav P, Voigt R. [Ultrasound of the urinary bladder neck: changes before and after pelvic floor muscle exercise]. Ceska Gynekol 1994; 59:121–124.

77. Martan A, Drbohlav P, Masata M, Halaska M, Voigt R. [Changes in the position of the urethra and bladder neck during pregnancy and after delivery]. Ceska Gynekol 1996; 61:35–39.

78. Martan A, Masata D, Halaska M, Voigt R. Ultrasound of the urethral sphincter. Neurourol Urodynam 1997; 16:389–390.

79. Martan A, Masata J, Halaska M, Voigt R. Ultrasound of the lower urinary tract in women with stress or mixed incontinence before and after intra vaginal Ovestin administration. Urogynecol J Pelvic Floor Dysfunct 1998; 9:322–322.

80. Martan A, Masata J, Halaska M, Voigt R. The effect of bladder volume in patients with GSI on the changes of ultrasound parameters of the lower urinary tract. Int Urogynecol J 1999; 10(supp 1):S106.

81. Martan A, Masata J, Halaska M, Voigt R. Is the position of UV junction after operation important for the effect of this operation? Int Urogynecol J Pelvic Floor Dysfunct 1999; 10 (supp 1):S116.

82. Masata J, Martan A, Halaska M, Voigt R. Ultrasound imaging of urethral tunnelling. Neurourol Urodynam 1999; 18:317–318.

83. Meyer S, De Grandi P, Schreyer A, Caccia G. The assessment of bladder neck position and mobility in continent nullipara, multipara, forceps delivered and incontinent women using perineal ultrasound: a future office procedure? Int Urogynecol J Pelvic Floor Dysfunct 1996; 7:138–146.

84. Meyer S, Bachelard O, De Grandi P. Do bladder neck mobility and urethral sphincter fimction differ during pregnancy compared with during the non-pregnant state? Int Urogynecol J Pelvic Floor Dysfunct 1998; 9:397–404.

85. Meyer S, Schreyer A, Degrandi P, Hohlfeld P. The effects of birth on urinary continence mechanisms and other pelvic-floor characteristics. Obstet Gynecol 1998; 92:613–618.

86. Peschers U, Schaer GN, Anthuber C, Delancey JOL, Schuessler B. Changes in vesical neck mobility following vaginal delivery. Obstet Gynecol 1996; 88:1001–1006.

87. Schaer GN, Kochli OR, Schussler B, Haller U. The nature of urethral pressure variations: simultaneous evaluation by perineal videosonography and urethrocystometry. Neurourol Urodynam 1994; 13:359–360.

88. Schaer GN, Koechli OR, Schuessler B, Haller U. Simultaneous perineal ultrasound and urodynamic assessment of female urinary incontinence: initial observations. Int Urogynecol J 1995; 6:168–174.

89. Schaer GN, Koechli OR, Schuessler B, Haller U. Perineal ultrasound for evaluating the bladder neck in urinary stress incontinence. Obstet Gynecol 1995; 85:220–224.

90. Schaer GN, Koechli OR, Schuessler B, Haller U. Perineal ultrasound: determination of reliable examination procedures. Ultrasound Obstet Gynecol 1996; 7:347–352.

91. Schaer GN, Koechli OR, Schuessler B, Haller U. Usefulness of ultrasound contrast medium in perineal sonography for visualization of bladder neck funneling—first observations. Urology 1996; 47:452–453.

92. Schaer GN, Koechli OR, Schuessler B, Haller U. Can simultaneous perineal sonography and urethrocystometry help explain urethral pressure variations? Neurourol Urodynam 1997; 16: 31–38.

93. Schaer GN. Ultrasonography of the lower urinary tract. Curr Opin Obstet Gynecol 1997; 9: 313–316.

94. Schaer GN, Siegwart R, Perucchini D, Delancey JOL. Examination of voiding in seated women using a remote-controlled ultrasound probe. Obstet Gynecol 1998; 91:297–301.

95. Schaer GN, Perucchini D, Munz E, Peschers U, Koechli OR, Delancey JOL. Sonographic evaluation of the bladder neck in continent and stress- incontinent women. Obstet Gynecol 1999; 93:412–416.

96. Sener T, Ozalp S, Hassa H, Yalcin OT, Zeytinoglu S. Preoperative and postoperative transperineal ultrasonographic assessment of the posterior urethrovesical angle in stress incontinent women. J Gynecol Surg 1997; 13:109–115.

97. Voigt R, Halaska M, Michels W, Martan A, Voigt P, Wilke I. [Perineal sonography and introitus sonography in diagnosis of urinary incontinence in women]. Gynakol Geburtshilfliche Rundsch 1993; 33(suppl 1):68–69.

98. Wijma J, Tinga DJ, Visser GH. Perineal ultrasonography in women with stress incontinence and controls: the role of the pelvic floor muscles. Gynecol Obstet Invest 1991; 32:176–179.

99. Yamashita T, Ogawa A. Transperineal ultrasonic voiding cystourethrography using a newly devised chair. J Urol 1991; 146:819–823.

100. Hanzal E, Joura EM, Haeusler G, Koelbl H. Influence of catheterization on the results of sonographic urethrocystography in patients with genuine stress incontinence. Arch Gynecol Obstet 1994; 255:189–193.

101. Wise BG, Burton G, Cutner A, Cardozo LD. Effect of vaginal ultrasound probe on lower urinary tract function. Br J Urol 1992; 70:12–16.

102. Cougard P, L'Helgouarc'h JL, Benoit L, Goudet P. Intraperitoneal polyglactine 910 absorbable mesh. Is it a risk-free attitude? Ann Chir 1999; 53:529–530.

103. Bader W, Degenhardt F, Kauffels W, Nehls K, Schneider J. Ultrasonographic parameters for the assessment of female urinary stress incontinence. Ultraschall Med 1995; 16:180–185.

104. Bader W, Kauffels W, Degenhardt F, Schneider J. Post-partum introital sonography of the lower urinary tract. Geburtshilfe Frauenheilkd 1995; 55:716–720.

105. Bader W, Schwenke A, Leven A, Schussier M, Hatzmann W. Proposal for the standardisation of introital sonography. Geburtshilfe Frauenheilkd 1997; 57:193–197.

106. Dietz BP, Clarke B. A new imaging method in urogynaecology: translabial colour doppler. Neurourol Urodynam 1999; 18:309–310.

107. Dietz BP, Clarke B. The influence of posture on the position and mobility of the bladder neck. Int Urogynecol J Pelvic Floor Dysfunct 1999; 10(suppl 1):S107.

108. Elia G, Bergman A. Periurethral collagen implant: ultrasound assessment and prediction of outcome. Int Urogynecol J Pelvic Floor Dysfunct 1996; 7:335–338.

109. Niemeyer R, Pracht S, Kirsch M, Petri E. Introital sonography in sphincter incompetence and after surgery. Int Urogynecol J 1998; 9:330.

110. Pessarrodona A, Cassado J, Lafont M, Huguet E, Jorda I, Fresnadillo A. Suburethral ultrasound in diagnosis and post surgical evaluation of woman stress urinary incontinence. Int Urogynecol J 1999; 9:335.

111. Tsia–Shu LO, Wang AC. Assessment of bladder neck mobility in stress urinary incontinent women during pregnancy using introital sonography. Int Urogynecol J Pelvic Floor Dysfunct 1998; 9:334.

112. Tunn R, Bettin S, Fischer W. Urethral assessment by extented introitus ultrasound before and after surgery for urinary incontinence and uterine prolapse. Int Urogynecol J Pelvic Floor Dysfunct 1997; 8:S64.

113. Yang JM. Factors affecting urethrocystographic parameters in urinary continent women. J Clin Ultrasound 1996; 24:249–255.

114. Mouritsen L, Rasmussen A. Bladder neck mobility evaluated by vaginal ultrasonography. Br J Urol 1993; 71:166–171.

115. Mouritsen L, Strandberg C, Frimodt–Moller C. Bladder neck anatomy and mobility: effect of vaginal ultrasound probe. Br J Urol 1994; 74:749–752.

116. Mouritsen L, Bach P. Ultrasonic evaluation of bladder neck position and mobility: the influence of urethral catheter, bladder volume, and body position. Neurourol Urodynam 1994; 13: 637–646.

117. Weil EH, Vandoom ES, Heesakkers JP, Meguid T, Janknegt RA. Transvaginal ultrasonography: a study with healthy volunteers and women with genuine stress incontinence. Eur Urol 1993; 24:226–230.

118. Hol M, van Bolhuis C, Vierhout ME. Vaginal ultrasound studies of bladder neck mobility. Br J Obstet Gynaecol 1995; 102:47–53.

119. Shabsigh R, Fishman IJ, Krebs M. Combined transrectal ultrasonography and urodynamics in the evaluation of detrusor–sphincter dyssynergia. Br J Urol 1988; 62:326–330.

120. Kuo HC, Chang SC, Hsu T. Application of transrectal sonography in the diagnosis and treatment of female stress urinary incontinence. Eur Urol 1994; 26:77–84.

121. Kuo HC. Transrectal sonography of the female urethra in incontinence and frequency urgency syndrome. J Ultrasound Med 1996; 15:363–370.

122. Kuo HC. Transrectal monographic investigation of urethral and paraurethral structures in women with stress urinary incontinence. J Ultrasound Med 1998; 17:311–320.

123. Richmond DH, Sutherst J. Transrectal ultrasound scanning in urinary incontinence: the effect of the probe on urodynamic parameters. Br J Urol 1989; 64:582–585.

124. Richmond DH, Sutherst JR. Burch colposuspension or sling for stress incontinence? A prospective study using transrectal ultrasound. Br J Urol 1989; 64:600–603.

125. Richmond DH, Sutherst JR. Clinical application of transrectal ultrasound for the investigation of the incontinent patient. Br J Urol 1989; 63:605–609.

126. Stuhldreier G, Kirschner HJ, Astfalk W, Schweizer P, Huppert PE, Grunert T. Three-dimensional endosonography of the pelvic floor: an additional diagnostic tool in surgery for continence problems in children. Eur J Pediatr Surg 1997; 7:97–102.

127. Umek W, Kratochwil A, Obemair A, Stutterecker D, Hanzal E. 3 Dimensional ultrasound of the female urethra comparing trans vaginal and trans rectal scanning. Int Urogynecol J 1999; 10(supp 1):S109.

128. Vierhout ME, Jansen H. Supine and sitting rectal ultrasound of the bladder neck during relaxation, straining and sqeezing. Int Urogynecol J 1992; 2:141–143.

129. Vierhout ME, Van de Plas de Koning YW. Diagnosing enterocele by rectal ultrasound; a confirmation study. Int Urogynecol J Pelvic Floor Dysfunct 1998; 9:334.

130. Yamada T, Mizuo T, Kawakami S, Watanabe T, Negishi T, Oshima H. Application of transrectal ultrasonography in modified Stamey procedure for stress urinary incontinence. J Urol 1991; 146:1555–1558.

131. Christensen LL, Djurhuus JC. Vaginal endosonography of the lower urinary tract in women: are anatomy and urodynamics affected by the procedure? Proceedings 21st Annual Meeting of the International Continence Society (ICS), Hannover, 1991:45.

132. Pajoncini C, Rosi P, Morcellini R, Costantini E, Guercini F, Porena M. SUI and pelvic floor disease: the best ultrasound scanning approach. Neurourol Urodynam 1998; 17:371–373.

133. Handa VL, Jensen JK, Ostergard DR. The effect of patient position on proximal urethral mobility. Obstet Gynecol 1995; 86:273–276.

134. Liu JB, Goldberg BB. 2-D and 3-D endoluminal ultrasound: vascular and nonvascular applications. Ultrasound Med Biol 1999; 25:159–173.

135. Chancellor MB, Liu JB, Rivas DA, Karasick S, Bagley DH, Goldberg BB. Intraoperative endo-luminal ultrasound evaluation of urethral diverticula. J Urol 1995; 153:72–75.

136. Phillips JL. Fogarty catheter extraction of unusual urethral foreign bodies. J Urol 1996; 155:1374–1375.

137. Heit M. Endoluminal ultrasonography of the urethra; a new technology awaiting further in-vestigation. J Pelvic Surg 1999; 5:22–31.

138. Klein HM, Kirschner–Hermanns R, Lagunilla J, Gunther RW. Assessment of incontinence with intraurethral US: preliminary results. Radiology 1993; 187:141–143.

139. Kirschner–Hermanns R, Klein HM, Müller U, Schäfer W, Jakse G. Intra-urethral ultrasound in women with stress incontinence. Br J Urol 1994; 74:315–318.

140. Schaer GN, Schmid T, Peschers U, Delancey JO. Intraurethral ultrasound correlated with ure-thral histology. Obstet Gynecol 1998; 91:60–64.

141. Fischer JR, Heit NM, Benson JT. Correlation of intraurethral ultrasound with needle EMG of the urethra. Int Urogynecol J Pelvic Floor Dysfunct 1999; 10:87.

142. Heit M, Goldsmith LJ, Newton M. Intraurethral ultrasound: correlation of urethral sphincter morphology with functional urodynamic parameters in stress incontinent women. Int Urogy-necol J Pelvic Floor Dysfunct 1997; 8:252.

143. Frauscher F, Helweg G, Strasser H, Enna B, Klauser A, Knapp R Colleselli K, Bartsch G, Zur Nedden D. Intraurethral ultrasound: diagnostic evaluation of the striated urethral sphincter in incontinent females. Eur Radiol 1998; 8:50–53.

144. Rivas DA, Chancellor MB, Liu JB, Hanau C, Bagley DH, Goldberg B. Endoluminal ultra-sonographic and histologic evaluation of periurethral collagen injection. J Endourol 1996; 10:61–66.

145. Leonhardt C, Krysi J, Arenson AM, Herschorn S. Periurethral injection of collagen in the treat-ment of urinary stress incontinence: ultrasonographic appearance. Can Assoc Radiol J 1995; 46:189–193.

146. Athanasiou S, Khullar V, Boos K, Salvatore S, Cardozo L. Imaging the urethral sphincter with three-dimensional ultrasound. Obstet Gynecol 1999; 94:295–301.

147. Jurkovic D, Jauniaux E, Campbell S. Three-dimensional ultrasound in obstetrics and gynecol-ogy. In: Kurjak A, Chervenak FA, eds. The Fetus as a Patient. Carnforth U.K.: Parthenon, 1994:135–140.

148. Steiner H, Staudach A, Spitzer D, Schaffer H. Three-dimensional ultrasound in obstetrics and gynaecology: technique, possibilities and limitations. Hum Reprod 1994; 9:1773–1778.

149. Platt LD, Santulli T Jr, Carlson DE, Greene N, Walla CA. Three-dimensional ultrasonography in obstetrics and gynecology. Preliminary experience [discussion]. Am J Obstet Gynecol 1998; 178:1199–1206.

150. Khullar V, Salvatore S, Cardozo L, Hill S, Kelleher CJ. Three dimensional ultrasound of the urethra and urethral sphincter: a new diagnostic technique. Neurourol Urodynam 1994; 13: 352–354.

151. Athanasiou S, Boos K, Khullar V, Anders K, Cardozo L. Pathogenesis of genuine stress in-continence and urogenital prolapse. Neurourol Urodynam 1996; 15:339–340.

152. Khullar V, Athanasiou S, Cardozo L, Salvatore S, Kelleher CJ. Urinary sphincter volume and urodynamic diagnosis. Neurourol Urodynam 1996; 15:334–336.

153. Toozs–Hobson P, Athanasiou S, Khullar V, Anders K, Cardozo L. Why do women develop in-continence after childbirth? Neurourol Urodynam 1997; 16:384–386.

154. Toozs–Hobson P, Boos K, Cardozo L, Anders K, Khullar V. Changes in the urethral sphincter in relation to childbirth and the development of stress incontinence. Br J Obstet Gynaecol 1998; 105:1220.

155. Toozs–Hobson P, Khullar V, Cardozo L, Boos K. Predicting incontinence six months after childbirth: does urethral sphincter volume help? Neurourol Urodynam 1998; 17:369–370.

156. Strohbehn K, Quint LE, Prince NM, Wojno KJ, Delancey JOL. Magnetic resonance imaging anatomy of the female urethra: a direct histologic comparison. Obstet Gynecol 1996; 88:750–756.

157. Perucchini D, Delancey JOL, Ashton–Miller JA. Regional striated muscle loss in the female urethra: where is the striated muscle vulnerable? Neurourol Urodynam 1997; 16:407–408.

158. Wisser J, Schar G, Kurmanavicius J, Huch R, Huch A. Use of 3D ultrasound as a new approach to assess obstetrical trauma to the pelvic floor. Ultraschall Med 1999; 20:15–18.

159. Marks LS, Dorey FJ, Macairan NE, Park C, deKernion JB. Three-dimensional ultrasound device for rapid determination of bladder volume. Urology 1997; 50:341–348.

160. Riccabona M, Nelson TR, Pretorius DH, Davidson TE. In vivo three-dimensional sonographic measurement of organ volume: validation in the urinary bladder. J Ultrasound Med 1996; 15: 627–632.

161. Hosli IM, Tercanli S, Herman A, Kretschmann M, Holzgreve W. In vitro volume measurement by three-dimensional ultrasound: comparison of two different systems. Ultrasound Obstet Gynecol 1998; 11:17–22.

162. Duan NX–H, Ashton Miller JA, Delancey JOL. Effect of tissue property changes on female mid-urethral MUCP: a 3-D biomechanical analysis. Neurourol Urodynam 1998; 17:367–369.

163. Kim SJ, Choi JH, Kim DK, Lee KS. The significance of an open bladder neck in the evaluation of the female stress urinary incontinence. Neurourol Urodynam 1999; 18:314–315.

164. Dietz HP, Ellin KE, Rades T, Wilson PD. The development of an ultrasound contrast medium for incontinence diagnosis. Neurourol Urodynam 1997; 16:390–392.

165. Mattox TF, Sinow R, Renslo R, Bhatia NN. The physiology of periurethral vasculature using colorflow doppler. Proceedings 22nd Annual Meeting of the ICS, Halifax, Nova Scotia, 1992: 161.

166. Khullar V, Cardozo LD, Kelleher CJ, Abbott D, Boume TH. Blood flow in the lower urinary tract in women with genuine stress urinary incontinence and detrusor instability. Ultrasound Obstet Gynecol 1993; 3(suppl 2):105–106.

167. Jackson S, McDonnell C, James M, Shepherd A, Abrams P. Is postmenopausal urethral blood flow affected by hormone replacement therapy? A placebo controlled study. Neurourol Urodynam 1997; 16:352–353.

168. Girao MJBC, Jarmy–Di Bella ZIK, Sartori MGF, et al. Power color Doppler velocimetry of peri-urethral vessels before and during estrogen therapy in post-menopause incontinent patients. Int Urogynecol J Pelvic Floor Dysfunct 1998; 9:329.

169. Castillo E, Saibene H, Regueira M, Souza M. Doppler velocimetry of periurethral vessels is efficient in the evaluation of local estrogen therapy in the genuine stress incontinence. Int Urogynecol J Pelvic Floor Dysfunct 1998; 9:336.

170. Kobata SA, Girao MJBC, Sartori MGF, Kawakami FT, Baracat EC, Rodrigues De Lima G. Doppler velocimetry of periurethral vessels in post menopausal women using topical estrogen therapy; preliminary results. Int Urogynecol J Pelvic Floor Dysfunct 1998; 9:338.

171. Adekami OA, Reed H, Freeman RM. The distal urethral electric conductance test revisited: does it improve the detection of female stress and urge incontinence? Int Urogynecol J Pelvic Floor Dysfunct 1999; 10(supp 1):S17.

172. Bamshad BR, Poon MW, Stewart SC. Effect of cardiopulmonary bypass on urethral blood flow as measured by laser Doppler flowmetry. J Urol 1998; 160:2030–2032.

173. Mani P. Effect of cardiopulmonary bypass on urethral blood flow as measured by laser Doppler flowmetry. J Urol 1999; 162:168.

174. Kawakami FT, Girao MJBC, Sartori MGF, et al. Color Doppler evaluation of periurethral vessels in pregnant women. Int Urogynecol J Pelvic Floor Dysfunct 1998; 9:339.

175. Ozawa H, Kumon H, Yokoyama T, Watanabe T, Chancellor MB. Development of noninvasive velocity flow video urodynamics using Doppler sonography—part 1: experimental urethra. J Urol 1998; 160:1787–1791.

176. Ozawa H, Kumon H, Yokoyama T, Watanabe T, Chancellor MB. Development of noninvasive velocity flow video urodynamics using Doppler sonography. Part H: clinical application in bladder outlet obstruction. J Urol 1998; 160:1792–1796.

177. Marconi F, Decastro R. Re: secondary reconstruction of abdominal wall defects associated with exstrophy of the bladder. Ann Plastic Surg 1994; 32:652–653.

178. Beco J, Leonard D, Leonard F. Study of the female urethra's submucous vascular plexus by color Doppler. World J Urol 1998; 16:224–228.

179. Huisman AB. Aspects on the anatomy of the female urethra with special relation to urinary continence. Contrib Gynecol Obstet 1983; 10:1–31.

180. Beco J. Une exploration nouvelle est arrivie: "l'échographie urodynamique".[A new exploration: "urodynainic echography"]. Contracept Fertil Sexual 1992; 20:479–484.

181. Rud T, Andesson KE, Asmussen M, Hunting A, Ulmsten U. Factors maintaining the intra urethral pressure in women. Invest Urol 1980; 17:343–347.

26

Voiding Cystourethrography and Magnetic Resonance Imaging of the Lower Urinary Tract

GARY E. LEMACK and PHILIPPE E. ZIMMERN

The University of Texas Southwestern Medical Center at Dallas, Dallas, Texas

I. INTRODUCTION

Radiologic assessment of bladder and urethral function encompasses several technologies varying in invasiveness, availability, expense, and sensitivity. Although sonography is the least invasive of these modalities, perhaps the most extensive clinical experience is with voiding cystourethrography (VCUG), which remains a reliable extension of physical examination several decades after its introduction. Easily performed, and relatively easily interpreted, there is little argument that VCUG is an important part of any clinician's assessment of lower urinary tract pathology. More recently, advances in magnetic resonance imaging (MRI) technology have broadened the use of this technique to include evaluation of the bladder and urethra, although a clear consensus for indications of its use remains evasive. This chapter describes the current roles of VCUG and MRI in the evaluation of patients with voiding dysfunction.

II. CYSTOURETHROGRAPHY

A. Introduction

Bladder and urethral imaging by cystourethrography has been performed since the turn of the century, and techniques have varied considerably over the years. Previously, for example, the bead chain cystogram was employed routinely to evaluate stress urinary incontinence (SUI) (1,2). Today, cystourethrographic evaluation of urinary incontinence has been helped by the use of Foley catheters to delineate urethral anatomy, together with improved techniques for imaging patients in the standing position and during straining maneuvers.

B. Technique

The patient is instructed to empty her bladder so that a scout film (KUB) image can be obtained. The entire pelvis, extending to at least 5 cm below the lower edge of the ischial tuberosities, should be included in this image. A Foley catheter is inserted into the urethra and the bladder is filled slowly (by gravity) with a high-contrast material. After the bladder is comfortably full, anteroposterior (AP) films are taken with the patient standing, and then lateral spot films are imaged with the catheter in place, with and without straining. The catheter is then removed, and lateral, resting, and straining views are repeated. The patient is asked to void, and fluoroscopy-guided lateral voiding views are obtained, in the standing position. A final AP postvoid film is then taken. Antibiotic prophylaxis may be administered during the 72-hr periprocedural period.

A small suprapubic (SP) catheter is preferable to a urethral catheter in some patients, such as in men with significant bladder outlet obstruction (BOO). Likewise, in some women with urethral pain, or when there is clinical suspicion of urethral stricture, passage of a Foley catheter may be ill-advised. In these situations, we normally leave the SP tube in place for use during urodynamic studies as well.

C. Risks

There is a small, but definite risk, of anaphylactic or vagal reactions following the administration of intravesical contrast agents. One study of 783 patients undergoing VCUG or retrograde pyelography revealed a contrast reaction incidence of 26% (3). High-pressure or large-volume infusions are thought to predispose to contrast reactions in susceptible patients. Therefore, careful attention should be paid to proper infusion techniques, and possible prophylaxis (corticosteroids or histamine blockers) may need to be considered in individuals at risk.

D. Indications

In patients presenting to the clinician with voiding dysfunction, VCUG may not be initially indicated. In fact, recent guidelines from the Agency for Health Care Policy and Research (4) suggest that the primary evaluation of these patients should consist of a history, physical examination, urinalysis, and noninvasive measurement of flow rate. Further evaluation, either urodynamic studies or radiologic imaging, is not indicated at initial presentation. For example, a multigravid patient with SUI, with no previous surgery and without a complex medical history, may require no further workup before discussing treatment options. When the diagnosis is in doubt, if the patient has had previous procedures, or a large prolapse is present, VCUG may be quite helpful. VCUG is also useful to determine if unsuspected reflux or urethral diverticuli are responsible for recurrent urinary tract infections. Finally, if a fistula is suspected on the basis of history and physical examination, then VCUG may be quite helpful in defining its location and guiding surgical planning.

E. Normal Findings

The normal bladder should accommodate 300–500 mL in women. At capacity, the bladder should have a smooth contour, free from trabeculations and diverticuli. The bladder neck should also be smooth and located above the inferior portion of the pubic ramus; this is often best seen on lateral views. The urethral axis can be evaluated from the angle formed by extending a perpendicular line from the urethral catheter to the horizontal axis, at the inferior ramus of the symphysis pubis. In asymptomatic women, this angle is normally 0–30 degrees, and does not vary much with straining or voiding (Fig. 1). However, many women demonstrate hypermobility of this angle with no complaint of urinary leakage. Similarly, although most continent women have a closed bladder neck when straining, some demonstrate funneling (Fig. 2). Taken together, these findings indicate that bladder neck support, urethral position, and intrinsic sphincteric mechanisms contribute, at least partly, to continence in women.

F. Abnormal Bladder Findings

1. Elevated Intravesical Pressures

Findings suggestive of high intravesical pressures include bladder wall trabeculations, diverticula, and vesicoureteral reflux. Whether these symptoms reflect true anatomical obstruction from a urethral stricture, iatrogenic obstruction (such as that found after previous anti-incontinence surgery), or neurogenic obstruction (detrusor–sphincter dyssynergia) can be clarified by case history and further urodynamic evaluation.

2. Cystocele

Bladder descent (cystocele) is well demonstrated by standing VCUG. Correlation of the standing cystogram image with supine physical examination allows grading of the cystocele much more accurately than does an examination alone. In general, any bladder descent below the inferior pubic ramus is indicative of cystocele, although clearly, not all patients

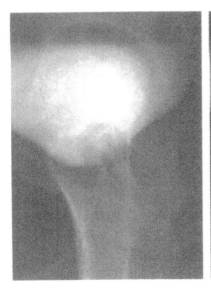 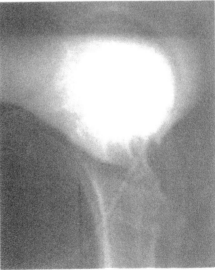

Figure 1 Lateral view voiding cystourethrogram with urethral catheter in place: the image on the left is performed at rest, and on the right, with straining. There is little change in the angle created by the vertical line drawn from the inferior-most aspect of the pubis (outlined) and the catheter (urethral angle).

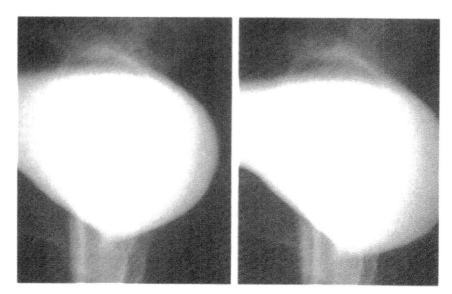

Figure 2   Lateral view voiding cystourethrogram: (left) the bladder neck is open at rest, although no leakage is seen; (right) leakage into the urethra is apparent with straining.

with minor cystoceles (grade 1) are symptomatic, nor are they necessarily at risk for rapid progression. Grade 2 cystoceles, which extend 2–5 cm below the inferior ramus and arrive at the introitus are normally associated with urethral hypermobility, unless previous suspension procedures have addressed this condition. Grade 3 cystoceles extend beyond the introitus and can have either a moderately narrow neck (Fig. 3) or a very broad-based herniation (Fig. 4). Often, the ureterovesical junction and the bladder base are exteriorized owing to the extent of the prolapse. Consequently, we recommend an upper tract study (ultrasound or intravenous pyelogram) to assess for hydroureteronephrosis before embarking on major pelvic surgery to correct the herniation responsible for prolapse. The well-described compressive effect of a large cystocele on the urethra can also be demonstrated on VCUG (Fig. 5); the surgical plan can be tailored to provide bladder neck and proximal urethral support at the time of cystocele repair. Finally, VCUG may be used as a postsurgical outcome measure following correction of urethral hypermobility, particularly in patients who report ongoing leakage postoperatively.

3.   Previous Repairs

Iatrogenic effects of previous anti-incontinence procedures on the bladder neck and urethra can easily be demonstrated on VCUG. For example, significant bladder neck elevation may be apparent on lateral views following multiple previous surgical attempts to correct SUI (Fig. 6). In other cases, more subtle indentations at the bladder neck or proximal urethra may be evident after suspension procedures. Occasionally, the urethrovesical angle will appear overcorrected after surgical repair (Fig. 7).

4.   Fistulas

Fistulas most commonly develop after bladder injury during laparoscopic, vaginal, or open surgical procedures. Vesicovaginal and vesicourethral fistulas are best seen on lateral films by VCUG. Although these entities may be suspected on a purely clinical basis, precise anatomical localization often relies on more than just a carefully obtained history and a

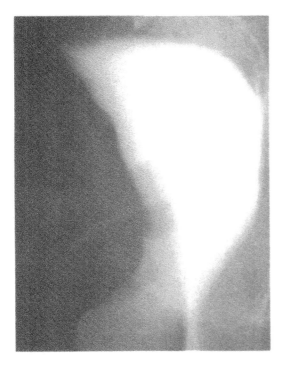

Figure 3   Lateral view cystourethrogram: grade 4 cystocele. The neck of herniation is of moderate size, consistent with a central defect.

thorough physical examination. Both cystourethroscopy and vaginoscopy may reveal the site and extent of the fistula, but both for the purposes of documentation and surgical planning (i.e., vaginal versus abdominal approach), VCUG is a useful adjunct to endoscopy when a fistula is suspected clinically (Fig. 8). Postoperatively, successful fistula closure is important for assessment by VCUG, and is often necessary for medicolegal documentation.

G. Abnormal Urethral Findings

1. Urethral Position

Abnormalities of urethral position are well delineated during standing VCUG. As described in the foregoing, poor urethral support is illustrated by an exaggerated urethrovesical angle on lateral film, both at rest and with straining (Fig. 9). Restoration of urethral support will eliminate this hypermobility and incontinence, provided that the intrinsic sphincteric mechanism is intact. With straining or coughing, urine leak is often seen in women complaining of incontinence. One cannot, however, conclude that SUI is present, unless detrusor pressure monitoring simultaneously rules out active bladder contraction. Alone, therefore, VCUG can not make the diagnosis of SUI or intrinsic sphincteric deficiency (ISD). Nonetheless, a persistently open, fixed, well-supported urethra seen on several views is highly suggestive of ISD, and treatment should be tailored accordingly.

2. Scarring

Urethral fibrosis from previous pelvic surgery for lower urinary tract symptoms or incontinence can also result in urethral narrowing, which can be demonstrated by voiding studies. Frequently, constriction secondary to prior suspension procedures is demonstrated along

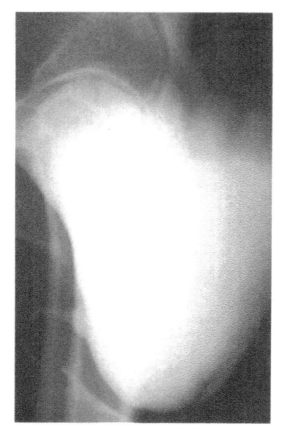

Figure 4 Lateral view cystourethrogram: the neck of herniation is large, suggestive of lateral and central defects.

much of the urethral length (Fig. 10). Often, these patients describe a very abnormal, interrupted flow pattern while straining or bending over to void. Mid- or distal narrowing with proximal urethral ballooning may be seen when a distal stricture is present (Fig. 11); this is also apparent, albeit rarely, in patients with known neurological disorders showing urodynamic evidence of ISD. Although idiopathic distal stricture is rare in women, we have found that those whose only previous intervention was repeated urethral dilations during physical examinations sometimes develop radiological features resembling periurethral fibrosis.

3. Diverticuli

Urethral diverticuli most commonly arise in the middle third of the urethra and are well visualized by VCUG. Although cystoscopy may aid in identifying the neck of the diverticulum, it provides no details of its extent or precise location. Typically, urethral diverticuli arise in periurethral glands and extend posteriorly toward the vagina. In some cases, however, a complex configuration may be present, and VCUG will reveal several pockets in the diverticulum (Fig. 12) that can extend circumferentially around the urethra. Similarly, VCUG may provide additional information on the presence of a diverticular tumor or stone, and multiple diverticuli. In patients with incontinence or pseudoincontinence, films demonstrating urethral hypermobility would support a decision for concomitant bladder neck suspension at the time of diverticulectomy.

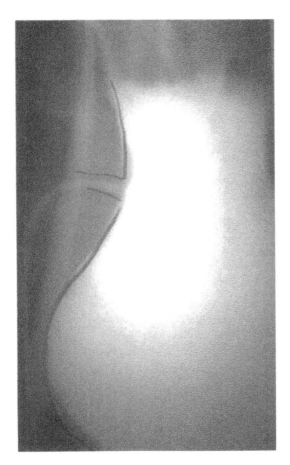

Figure 5 Lateral view cystourethrogram: grade 4 cystocele. Note the severe angulation at the vesicourethral junction created by the cystocele.

H. Conclusion

Standing VCUG represents a logical extension of physical examination. The images give a better assessment of the patient's anatomy than the examiner can achieve while the patient is in a lithotomy position. The effects of gravity are seen by supine VCUG, and thus, it may be possible to establish the nature of the patient's complaints during her normal activities. VCUG is readily available, safe, and easily tolerated. Even though the lack of simultaneous intravesical pressure monitoring render it virtually impossible for this technique to definitively pinpoint the cause of urinary leakage, the clarity of the images and the cost-effectiveness make VCUG extremely useful, particularly when videourodynamic studies are unwarranted or unavailable.

III. MAGNETIC RESONANCE IMAGING

A. Introduction

The use of MRI for imaging of the lower urinary tract in incontinent females remains in its infancy, and its place among all the available imaging modalities has yet to be determined.

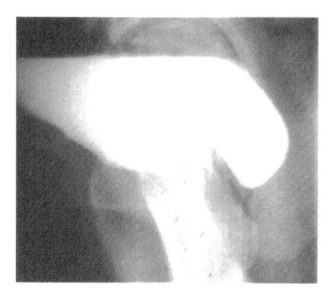

Figure 6 Lateral view cystourethrogram from a woman with multiple sclerosis who presented with severe incontinence 3 months after the fascial sling procedure. The sling has migrated up into the trigone, pulling the bladder neck open and preventing its closure.

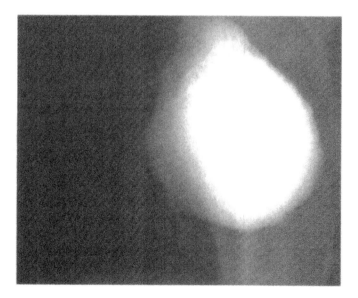

Figure 7 Lateral view cystourethrogram from a woman with severe urgency and frequency who required straining and bending to urinate, several years after the Marshall–Marchetti–Krantz procedure was performed. Note the bladder trabeculations and overcorrection of the urethra.

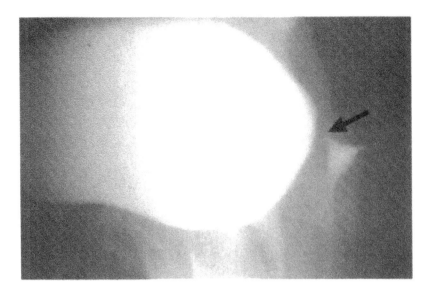

Figure 8   Lateral view cystourethrogram of a vesicovaginal fistula: note the contrast filling in the vagina.

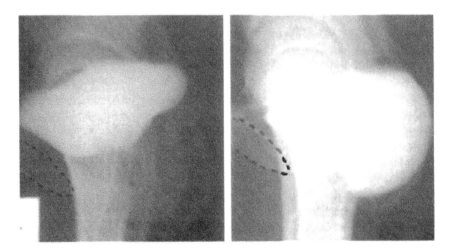

Figure 9   Lateral view cystourethrogram (left) at rest and (right) with straining in a woman with significant urethral hypermobility.

Recent advances in imaging techniques and the use of dynamic MR images have heightened interest in MRI in the field of female urology. Because of the precise anatomical information generated by MRI, its widened availability, and the increased complexity of bladder neck and urethral disorders following failed surgical endeavors, it may become a useful tool in the assessment of pelvic floor disorders in the near future.

B.   Evaluation of the Normal Lower Urinary Tract

Early studies using MRI to evaluate the lower urinary tract in women centered on establishing standards, and began the process of comparing these standards with patients with

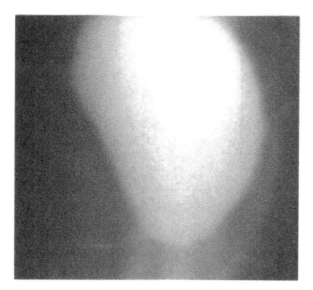

Figure 10 Lateral view of a voiding film from a woman with an obstructive voiding pattern after several surgical procedures for incontinence: note the narrowing along the entire urethral length suggestive of diffuse periurethral fibrosis.

known voiding dysfunction. For instance, Klutke et al. (5) demonstrated the complex fascial and ligamentous support of the bladder neck and proximal urethra in normal women, and compared them with cadaver dissections. These authors described the importance of the urethropelvic ligaments, which represent the medial extension of the levator ani musculature to the bladder neck and proximal urethra. They also reported disruption of this support in women who had undergone unsuccessful anti-incontinence procedures. Similarly, Hricak et al. (6) described normal and abnormal urethral findings, and contributed greatly to the understanding of urethral cross-sectional anatomy. Specifically, they demonstrated the MRI appearance of the three histologically distinct layers in the human urethra: the mucosa, submucosa, and outer muscularis.

Strohbehn et al. (7) further established the role of MRI by subsequently performing trichrome and immunohistochemical staining of harvested cadaver urethral tissue. They correlated the MRI appearance of the striated sphincter with histological evidence of the striated musculature. The sphincter was more prominent ventrally than laterally and appeared as the outermost ring of low-signal intensity on T_2-weighted images.

C. Evaluation of Urethral Abnormalities

MRI appears to be particularly suited to imaging urethral anomalies. Areas of fibrosis, scarring, inflammation, and urinary pooling are well visualized by MRI, whereas conventional techniques often fall short of providing complete information. Staging of urethral carcinoma is well achieved by MRI, although distinction between benign and malignant processes is not always possible (2). The fate of intraurethral collagen injections for stress incontinence has also been documented by endorectal coil MRI techniques (Fig. 13) (8). Although a correlation was noted between the volume of collagen injected and the volume visualized on MRI, neither the position of the collagen nor its volume seen on MRI were predictive of the clinical response. Nurenberg and Zimmern (9) used a transrectal coil to investigate urethral abnormalities in a group of women with voiding dysfunction and were

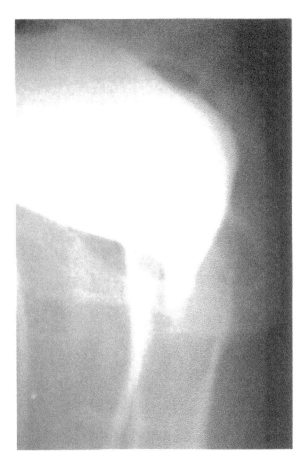

Figure 11   Distal urethral stricture: note the proximal urethral ballooning. The patient had a history of prior urethral dilations and urodynamically proved outlet obstruction.

able to identify the causes of failed periurethral fat and collagen injections. Periurethral fibrosis (Fig. 14) was also easily demonstrated and complex urethral diverticuli, not well-visualized on voiding cystography, were completely characterized with the transrectal coil (Fig. 15). Defining the extent of "saddle bag" diverticuli before embarking on surgical excision was easily accomplished by endorectal MRI (10). Intraurethral wall diverticuli, which may be impossible to see on VCUG, have also been described recently using MRI technology (11). In all the cases described, MRI diagnosis affected the treatment plan. Clearly, when the diagnosis or etiology are in question, MRI has a role in imaging the urethra and periurethral tissues.

D.   Evaluation of the Pathogenesis of Stress Incontinence

Several studies have focused on the role of MRI in evaluating pelvic floor anatomy in an attempt to further understand the pathogenesis of urinary incontinence. A detailed description of the anatomy of the levator ani musculature was published recently (12). In this study, MR images from patients were compared with dissection data from female cadavers. Unfortunately, motion artifacts obscured the MRI data; technical improvements are necessary if MRI is to be clinically useful for incontinence investigation. Kirschner–Hermanns

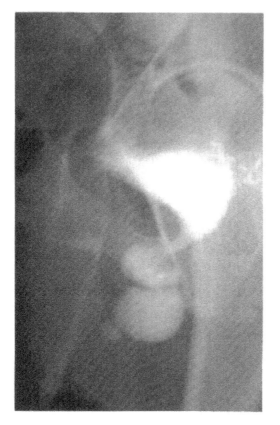

Figure 12   Voiding cystogram demonstrating multiple pockets of complex urethral diverticulum.

et al. (13) used a body coil to examine the pelvic floor anatomy of 24 incontinent women and healthy volunteers. Incontinence was associated with a loss of angulation of the levator sling, perineal tears, and evidence of muscle degeneration in many of the incontinent women, although no details of normal angles or muscle thickness were provided.

Recently, Christensen et al. (14) demonstrated the ability of MRI to distinguish bladder and vaginal ascent during pelvic floor contraction. They found younger women had significantly increased bladder and urethral displacement with pelvic floor contraction than older women.

In summary, the ability of MRI to detect subtle details of pelvic floor anatomy may be useful in the management of complicated cases of incontinence. Still, largely owing to its expense, MRI use in incontinent patients remains mainly experimental.

E.   Dynamic MRI

The development of dynamic MRI over the last several years has opened the door for a unique application of this technology. Yang et al. (15) studied 26 women with clinical evidence of pelvic prolapse by dynamic fast-scan imaging of pelvic floor descent. By using views of the pelvis, both at rest and with straining, these authors noted an increase in the distance from the pubococcygeal line at maximal strain in prolapse patients compared with

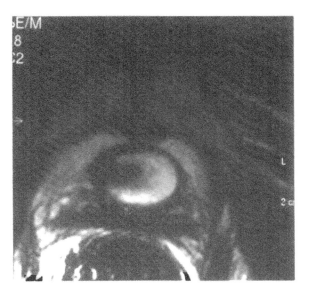

Figure 13   Endorectal coil MR image of the urethra taken 3 months after periurethral collagen injection: collagen is bright on this image, and the urethral lumen is compressed toward the patient's right.

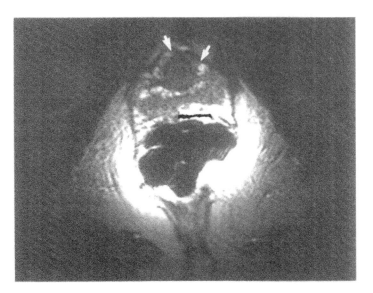

Figure 14   Endorectal coil MRI of the urethra demonstrating periurethral fibrosis (arrows) in a young woman with significant clinical obstructive symptoms and reduced force of stream: note the attenuation of normally bright periurethral fat in this area.

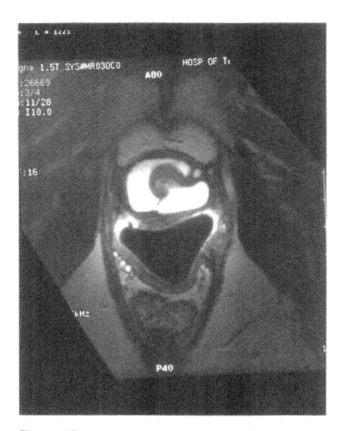

Figure 15   Exact extension and location of complex urethral diverticulum demonstrated by endovaginal coil MRI and confirmed surgically. (Courtesy of Daniel Blander.)

normal controls; in later work, they further characterized the compartmentalization of prolapse (16). In their hands, the use of dynamic images with provocative maneuvers, such as straining, decreased the chance of missing areas of prolapse before surgical repair.

The most recent work involving MRI to evaluate women with voiding dysfunction has centered on advances in techniques that improve the acquisition of detailed anatomical images. Gouse et al. (17) utilized dynamic HASTE (half-Fourier-acquisition single-shot turbospin echo) sequence MRI to evaluate 50 women, and noted unsuspected pelvic pathology in 13 of them. Although conventional-imaging modalities may have uncovered most of these findings, some of the more occult cases of rectocele and enterocele would certainly have been missed by other available modalities. Because the cost was reasonable, and the need for other imaging modalities to exclude associated pelvic pathology (i.e., ultrasound) was negated, the authors advocate using dynamic HASTE MRI over pelvic ultrasonography in the evaluation of female pelvic pathology.

F.   Conclusions

Magnetic resonance images of the pelvis provide the most precise anatomical information currently available, and the possible influence of MRI on clinical decision-making is a fertile ground for research and new developments. However, as costs are a predominant driving force in the delivery of medical care, detailed cost–benefit analysis will be required before more routine use of MRI can be accepted. Certainly, the urethral and periurethral images captured by MRI technology are unparalleled. Moreover, the use of dynamic MRI to evaluate complex cases of pelvic prolapse may be justified before performing major surgical interventions. As technological advances continue, we may expect to learn more about the anatomy of pelvic floor disorders through the use of MRI.

REFERENCES

1. Stevens WE, Smith SP. Roentgenological examination of the female urethra. J Urol 1950; 37: 194–197.
2. Shingleton HM, Barkley KL, Talnbert LM. Management of stress urinary incontinence in the female. Use of the chain cystogram. South Med J 1966; 59:547–552.
3. Weese DL, Greenberg HM, Zimmern PE. Contrast media reactions during voiding cystourethrography or retrograde pyelography. Urology 1993; 41:81–84.
4. Urinary Incontinence Guideline Panel. Urinary Incontinence in Adults: Clinical Practice Guidelines. Rockville, MD: Agency for Health Care Policy and Research, Public Health Service, US Department of Health and Human Services, AHCPR Publication 92-0038, 1992.
5. Klutke C, Golomb J, Barbaric Z, Raz S. The anatomy of stress incontinence: magnetic resonance imaging of the female bladder neck and urethra. J Urol 1990; 143:563–566.
6. Hricak H, Secaf E, Buckley DW, Brown JJ, Tanagho EA, McAninch JW. Female urethra: MR imaging. Radiology 1991; 178:527–535.
7. Strohbehn K, Quint LE, Prince MR, Wojno KJ, DeLancey JO. Magnetic resonance imaging anatomy of the female urethra: a direct histologic comparison. Obstet Gynecol 1996; 88:750–756.
8. Carr LK, Herschorn S, Leonhardt C. Magnetic resonance imaging after intraurethral collagen injected for stress urinary incontinence. J Urol 1996; 155:1253–1255.
9. Nurenberg P, Zimmern PE. Role of MR imaging with transrectal coil in the evaluation of complex urethral abnormalities. AJR Am J Roentgenol 1997; 169:1335–1338.
10. Blander DS, Broderick GA, Rovner ES. Images in clinical urology: magnetic resonance imaging of a "saddle bag" urethral diverticulum. Urology 1999; 53:818–819.
11. Daneshgari F, Zimmern PE, Jacomides L. Magnetic resonance imaging detection of symptomatic noncommunicating intraurethral wall diverticula in women. J Urol 1999; 161:1259–1262.
12. Strohbehn K, Ellis JH, Strohbehn JA, DeLancey JO. Magnetic resonance imaging of the levator ani with anatomic correlation. Obstet Gynecol 1996; 87:277–285.
13. Kirschner–Hermanns R, Wein B, Niehaus S, Schaefer W, Jakse G. The contribution of magnetic resonance imaging of the pelvic floor to the understanding of urinary incontinence. Br J Urol 1993; 72:715–718.
14. Christensen LL, Djurhuus JC, Constantinou CE. MRI imaging of the pelvic floor in the axial sagittal and coronal planes: influence of age on the range of bladder/urethal/levator ani displacement [abstr]. Urodynamics Society 1998.
15. Yang A, Mostwin JL, Rosenshein NB, Zerhouni EA. Pelvic floor descent in women: dynamic evaluation with fast MR imaging and cinematic display. Radiology 1991; 179:25–33.
16. Yang A, Mostwin J, Genadry R, Sanders RZ. Patterns of prolapse demonstrated with dynamic fastscan MRI; reassessment of conventional concepts of pelvic floor weaknesses. Neurourol Urodynam 1993; 12:310–311.
17. Gousse AE, Barbaric ZL, Safir MH, Raz S. Dynamic "haste" MRI sequence in the evaluation of all female pelvic pathology [abstr]. Urodynamics Society 1998.

27

Electrophysiological Evaluation of Genitourinary Nervous Pathways

REINIER-JACQUES OPSOMER

Cliniques Saint-Luc, University of Louvain, Brussels, Belgium

I. INTRODUCTION

Electrophysiological tests have been widely used in clinical neurophysiology for over half a century. They were first applied in the lower genitourinary tract, to study sacral reflexes (1–4). The genitourinary tract has double innervation: somatic and autonomic nerves are distributed to specific areas of the urinary and genital organs. Whereas the investigation of sensory and motor somatic nerves is easy and reproducible (5,6), the testing of autonomic nerves is rather difficult. Investigating sensory–autonomic pathways from the urinary tract is feasible, but rather invasive (6–9), whereas testing motor–autonomic pathways controlling the corpora cavernosa of the penis and the detrusor muscle remains experimental (10–13).

We review here currently available electrophysiological tests that are useful for accurately investigating the level and extent of the neurological damage in various disorders, including spinal cord lesions, multiple sclerosis, and diabetes mellitus. In clinical practice, they provide objective information on the functionality of the nerve trunks and muscles controlling the genitourinary tract. Furthermore, these tests can contribute to our knowledge of spinal and supraspinal control over the lower genitourinary tract. In this chapter, we will review tests evaluating the somatic and autonomic nervous pathways to the genitourinary organs, and consider their clinical contribution and relevance.

II. EVALUATION OF SOMATIC NERVOUS PATHWAYS

A. Electromyography of the Urethral Sphincter

Electromyography (EMG) is the recording of electrical potentials generated by muscle fibers. Unlike striated muscles, the urethral and anal sphincters show spontaneous electrical activity at rest. During micturition, the urethral sphincter has no electrical activity in normal subjects. In contrast, in patients with a suprasacral lesion, it may present dyssynergic behavior. This results in concomitant contraction of the urethral sphincter and the detrusor muscle, elevating pressure in the bladder, and leading, sooner or later, to severe alterations of the urinary tract. The EMG activity of the sphincters, and the pelvic floor musculature in general, is evaluable either from a dynamic and physiological point of view, or from an analytical and electrophysiological point of view. In the former case, an integrated EMG of the sphincters is recorded on urodynamic investigation, whereas the latter involves conventional EMG study.

1.   Dynamic EMG Study of the Urethral Sphincter Combined with Urodynamic Investigation

An EMG study is performed either by inserting a concentric EMG needle electrode into the urethral sphincter or by applying surface electrodes to the perianal or perineal skin. The activity of the urethral sphincter can also be recorded with a ring electrode mounted on a Foley catheter and inserted into the urethra. The EMG signal is integrated and rectified to give a global EMG activity pattern that is recorded throughout the urodynamic investigation: before and during filling of the urinary bladder and during micturition. In normal subjects, during bladder filling, there is a gradual increase in EMG activity of the urethral sphincter (guarding reflex), whereas during micturition the sphincter is electrophysiologically silent. EMG activity resumes after micturition. The urethral sphincter and the detrusor muscle act synergistically in normal subjects: during detrusor contraction, the urethral sphincter relaxes and vice versa. In the event of a suprasacral lesion (located between the sacral micturition center and the brain stem), the pelvic floor and the detrusor muscle may behave in a dyssynergic way, contracting simultaneously. Closure of the sphincter during micturition impedes bladder emptying and thus increases intravesical pressure.

2.   Analytical EMG Study of the Urethral Sphincter

Analytical EMG investigation is performed with a concentric EMG needle electrode (or single-fiber EMG needles) inserted into the urethral sphincter. Few studies have been conducted on normal volunteers. Fowler and Fowler (14) established reference parameters for the urethral sphincter: normal motor units have a characteristic appearance, with a duration of less than 6 msec and an amplitude of between 0.15 and 0.5 mV. Normal units have up to five turns (phase reversals).

B.   Evoked Potentials

1.   Evaluation of Afferent Pathways

Pudendal Somatosensory-Evoked Potentials
        AIM OF THE TEST.   *Somatosensory-evoked potentials* (SEPs) are defined as a transient electroencephalographic alteration following peripheral nerve stimulation. They provide objective information about the afferent volley from the peripheral nerve to the cortex. Pudendal SEPs were first described in the early 1980s (5–7,14–16).
        METHOD.   The technique consists of electrical stimulation of the dorsal nerve of the penis or clitoris (sensory branch of the pudendal nerve) while recording evoked responses over the spine and scalp (Cz – 2 = 2 cm behind the central vertex). First, the sensitivity threshold is measured; this is defined as the lowest perceivable sensation of electrical current at the point of stimulation (17) (Table 1). An electrical current equivalent to two to three

Table 1   Genitourinary Sensitivity Thresholds: Reference Data

	Sensitivity thresholds (mA)	
Stimulation site (Ref.)	Median	Range
Urinary bladder (6,17)	20.0	17.0–26.0
Proximal urethra (6,17)	8.5	7.0–10.1
Penis/clitoris (5,6)	3.0	2.0–5.0

times the sensitivity threshold is then applied. Several thousand stimuli are delivered, and 500 artifact-free responses are registered. The spinal response consists of a positive deflection, whereas the cortical response comprises a series of positive and negative peaks. The latency of the response is measured both at the onset of the response and at the mean peak of the first reproducible deflections (Fig. 1).

    RESULTS.   The mean reference latency for the spinal response is 13.5 msec. In males, the mean latencies of the cortical peaks are 35 msec and 43 msec for onset and top of P1 deflection, respectively (5–7,15) (Table 2).

2.   Evaluation of Efferent Pathways

Pudendal Motor-Evoked Potentials

    AIM OF THE TEST.   Motor-evoked potentials (MEPs) explore the efferent pathways (pyramidal tracts) from the brain to the target muscle (6,15,16).

    METHOD.   The technique consists of stimulating the motor cortex and sacral roots by a magnetoelectric stimulator. For brain stimulation, the posterior edge of the coil is applied

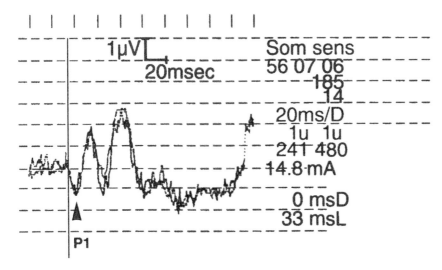

Figure 1   Pudendal SEPs, cortical response: The response starts with a latency of 33 msec (onset marked by the vertical line). The latency of the first positive deflection (P1) is 42 msec. The tracing consists of alternating positive and negative peaks.

Table 2 Pudendal Somatosensory-Evoked Potentials: Reference Latencies of Three Successive Peaks Recorded from the Cortex

Stimulation site	Latencies (msec)		
	Onset	P1	N1
Penis	35.1	43.4	55.0
Clitoris	32.6	39.9	49.9

Source: Ref. 5.

2 cm behind the vertex. For sacral root stimulation, the coil is applied laterally to the spine at the level of the iliac crest. The response is picked up from the sphincters or the bulbo-cavernosus muscles with coaxial electromyographic (EMG) needle electrodes. Brain stimulation is performed, first at rest, and then during a voluntary contraction of the pelvic floor (facilitation procedure). Sacral root stimulation is performed only at rest. The response is measured at the onset of the first reliable deflection.

RESULTS. The mean latencies measured in the bulbocavernosus muscles are 28 msec (brain stimulation, patient at rest), 22 msec (brain stimulation, patient contracting the pelvic floor), and 7 msec (sacral root stimulation). The facilitation procedure induces a shortening of latency and an increase in the amplitude of the response (Table 3).

C. Sacral Reflexes

1. Somatosomatic Sacral Reflex

AIM OF THE TEST. This test examines the sensory and motor branch of the pudendal nerve and the S2-S3-S4 segments (3,4,6,15).

METHOD. The technique consists of stimulating the dorsal nerve of the penis or clitoris and recording the response from the sphincters or the bulbocavernosus muscles. The response usually consists of two deflections (Fig. 2).

RESULTS. The mean latency of the first deflection is 31 msec in the bulbocavernosus muscle (Table 4). A late deflection is often observed at 60 msec (3,4,6,15).

Table 3 Pudendal Motor-Evoked Potentials: Reference Latencies Recorded from the Bulbocavernosus Muscle

		Latency (msec)	
		Mean	SD
Brain stimulation	Patient at rest	28.8	2.6
	Facilitation procedure	22.5	2.7
Sacral root stimulation		7.2	1.0

Source: Ref. 15.

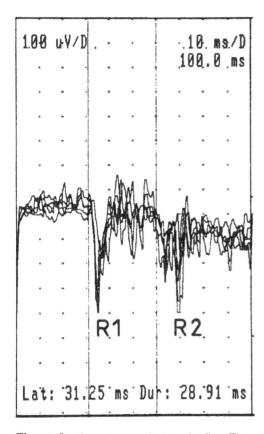

Figure 2 Somatosomatic sacral reflex: The response consists of two deflections (R1 and R2). The latency of the early deflection (R1) is 31.25 msec. The latency of the late deflection (R2) is 60.1 msec.

Table 4 Somatosomatic Sacral Reflex: Reference Latencies Recorded from the Bulbocavernosus Muscle

Stimulation site	Latencies (msec)	
	Mean	Range
Penis	31.4	4.2

Source: Ref. 15.

III. EVALUATION OF AUTONOMIC NERVOUS PATHWAYS

A. Electromyography

1. EMG of the Corpus Cavernosum

AIM OF THE TEST.   The corpus cavernosum consists of a tight network of smooth-muscle fibers and vessels. Wagner et al. (10) were the first to investigate the electrical activity generated by the smooth-muscle fibers of the corpus cavernosum. They demonstrated bursts of electrical activity during flaccidity and detumescence, and a silent period during erection. Stief (11) demonstrated the possibility of recording single electrical potentials from the corpus cavernosum (single potential analysis of cavernosal electrical activity) (11).

METHOD.   EMG activity from the corpus cavernosum is recorded with a mono- or bipolar needle electrode inserted into both corpora cavernosa. Some physicians use surface electrodes. First, resting activity is recorded for about 20–30 min. The patient is then given mild intellectual work; alternatively, provocative tests, such as the Valsalva maneuver, hyperventilation, or needle pricking, are conducted to evaluate the responsiveness of neuromuscular control of the corpora cavernosa.

RESULTS.   Stief (11) described specific patterns in patients with upper and lower motor neuron lesions. A multicentric, international study is in progress to gather reference data (12).

2.   EMG of the Detrusor Muscle

Recording EMG activity from the detrusor muscle is notoriously difficult. Several research groups have spent a great deal of time and energy trying to obtain reproducible tracings and eliminate recording artifacts (18,19). Detrusor EMG is likely to offer a tool for differentiating detrusor myopathies from abnormalities of peripheral innervation (14). A new wave of interest in recording smooth-muscle activity in the urinary and genital tracts is currently apparent among urological researchers (20).

B.   Evoked Potentials

1.   Evaluation of Afferent Pathways from the Urinary Tract

Urinary Somatosensory-Evoked Potentials

AIM OF THE TEST.   The aim is to evaluate afferent volleys from the sensory nerve terminals, located in the urinary tract (bladder wall, proximal urethra), to the brain (6–9).

METHOD.   The technique consists of electrical stimulation of the bladder mucosa or the proximal urethra with a bipolar ring electrode (Dantec 21 L11), placed under the balloon of a Foley catheter. Bladder stimulation is achieved by inserting the Foley catheter completely into the bladder. The balloon of the catheter is not inflated, and slight suction is applied through the catheter to ensure good contact between the bladder mucosa and the stimulating electrode. Proximal urethra stimulation is performed with the catheter balloon inflated and retracted against the bladder neck.

A constant-current stimulator is used. Stimulation consists of rectangular pulses of 0.2 msec in duration, applied at a frequency of 1.5 Hz. The intensity of the current is slowly increased until the subject reports a tingling sensation. The sensitivity threshold is defined as the lowest perceivable intensity (see Table 1). Five successive readings are made and their median is charted (6,7,17). Several thousand electrical stimuli of supramaximal intensity are then delivered. The intensity necessary to obtain a reproducible cortical response is generally equivalent to three times the sensitivity threshold. The responses are recorded 2 cm behind the central vertex with a frontal reference electrode. Five hundred artifact-free responses are averaged. Two tracings are superimposed to check the reproducibility of the response (6–9).

RESULTS.   Reference sensitivity thresholds following bladder and proximal urethra stimulation are presented in Table 1. Sensitivity thresholds from the urinary tract are sig-

Table 5 Urinary Somatosensory-Evoked Potentials: Reference
Latencies of Three Successive Peaks Recorded from the Cortex

	Latencies (msec)		
Stimulation site (Ref.)	Onset	P1	N1
Urinary bladder (7)	57.6	67.3	75.2
Bladder neck (9)	54.3	64.3	91.4
Proximal urethra (7)	59.2	68.0	75.6
Proximal urethra (8)	56.3	72.0	102.1
Proximal urethra (6)	55.4	70.2	82.6

nificantly higher than those from the penile skin, which is innervated by somatic nerve endings (5–7,17).

Urinary SEPs consist of a series of positive and negative peaks. Several authors have
obtained reference data from control subjects. Table 5 summarizes the latency of the early
cortical peaks (6–9). The mean latency of the P1 deflection is approximately 70 msec. The
amplitude of urinary SEPs is lower than that of pudendal SEPs.

2. Evaluation of Efferent Pathways to the Urinary Tract

Detrusor MEPs

AIM OF THE TEST. Bemelmans et al. (13) reported preliminary results with MEPs
recorded from the detrusor muscle following spinal stimulation for which a special electrode was designed.

METHOD. A magnetoelectric stimulator is used. Stimulation is applied over the
L4–L5 intervertebral space with a 90-mm–diameter coil. The response is recorded from the
detrusor muscle by an electrode fixed to an ureteral stent and introduced transurethrally (13).

RESULTS. Bemelmans et al. (13) investigated 12 patients with detrusor hyperreflexia
and recorded latencies of detrusor MEPs ranging from 26 to 50 msec (with a mean latency
of 36 msec). These results await confirmation by other groups before the technique can be
recommended for detrusor hyperreflexia.

3. Evaluation of Efferent Pathways to the Sweat Glands

Sympathetic Skin Responses (SSRs)

AIM OF THE TEST. The test's aim is to record the electrical activity generated from
the sympathetic nerve terminals controlling the sweat glands of the skin following stimulation of any peripheral nerve trunk.

METHOD. The dorsal nerve of the penis is stimulated by means of two ring electrodes wrapped around the penile shaft, the cathode being proximal. Stimulation consists
of single electrical pulses applied at a rate of 0.05 Hz. Sympathetic skin responses are
recorded from the hand, foot, and perineum with disk electrodes affixed to the skin. Two
tracings are superimposed to check the reproducibility of the response (Fig. 3). The right or
left median nerve is then stimulated at the wrist, and SSRs are recorded from the hand, foot,
perineum, and penis (21,22).

RESULTS. The mean latencies of hand, foot, and perineum SSRs following stimulation of the dorsal nerve of the penis are 1.40, 2, and 1.4 sec, respectively (Table 6). After
median nerve stimulation, the latency of penile SSRs is 1.50 sec (21).

ELECTRICAL
STIMULUS

<5 sec Pre-stimulus baseline >

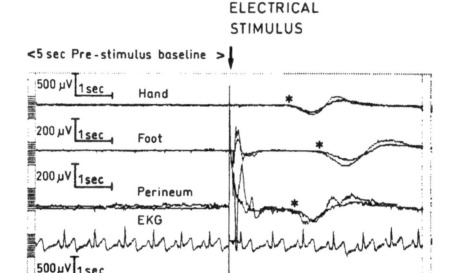

Figure 3 Sympathetic skin responses (SSRs) recorded from hand, foot, and perineum: two tracings are superimposed. The bottom tracing is the ECG recording. The electrical stimulus is applied over the right median nerve (at the wrist) after a 5-sec prestimulus baseline resting period. Note that the foot SSRs are of a longer latency than those recorded from the hand and the perineum.

Table 6 Sympathetic Skin Responses
Following Stimulation of the Dorsal Nerve of the
Penis: Reference Latencies

	Latencies (sec)	
Recording site	Mean	SD
Hand	1.40	0.10
Foot	1.98	0.15
Perineum	1.43	0.20

Source: Ref. 16

C. Sacral Reflexes

1. Viscerosomatic Sacral Reflex

AIM OF THE TEST.   The test is designed to evaluate the peripheral sensory autonomic pathways from the urinary tract (bladder mucosa or proximal urethra), the sacral cord, and the motor branch of the pudendal nerve.

METHOD.   The bladder wall and proximal urethra are stimulated with a ring electrode, as described for urinary sensitivity thresholds and urinary SEPs. The stimulation parameters, too, are identical. The motor threshold (the intensity necessary to obtain the reflex response) is reached by increasing the current up to three times the sensitivity threshold. Supra-maximal stimuli are then applied to obtain responses with a minimal latency and a stable

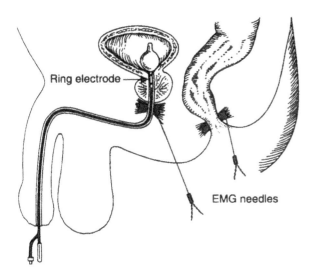

Figure 4 Viscerosomatic sacral reflex; principle of the technique: Electrical stimulation of the urethral mucosa, using a ring electrode mounted on a Foley catheter. The response is recorded from the periurethral striated musculature and the anal sphincter with coaxial EMG needle electrodes.

Table 7 Viscerosomatic Sacral Reflex: Reference Latencies

	Latencies (msec)	
Stimulation site (Ref.)	Mean	Range
Urinary bladder (23)	60	46–75
Proximal urethra (1)	(—)	50–70
Proximal urethra (4)	60	53–64 (males)
	68	60–75 (females)

configuration. Five to 20 stimuli are applied to obtain the reflex and to check the reproducibility of the response. The reflex response is recorded by coaxial needle electrodes inserted into the periurethral sphincter mechanism or the anal sphincter (Fig. 4).

RESULTS. Reference latency values have been established by several others (1–4, 6,7,23), and their results are summarized in Table 7. The latency of the response ranges from 50 to 75 msec.

IV. DISCUSSION

Electrophysiological tests are useful to explore the neurophysiology and pathophysiology of urinary and genital functions. However, the clinical contribution of these tests in neurourological practice is controversial (14,24). We will discuss here their relevance to study the somatic and autonomic genitourinary nervous pathways.

The contribution of the somatic nerves to innervation of the lower genitourinary tract is rather limited compared with that of the autonomic nerves. From a technical point of view, however, the somatic nerves are easily accessible, whereas evaluation of the autonomic genitourinary pathways requires invasive measures. For this reason, most studies rely exclusively on the somatic nerves to reflect the integrity of the genitourinary nervous pathways as a whole. In some cases, this leads to simplistic and erroneous conclusions. For instance, in several neurourological disorders, localized lesions are present in one set of nerves, but not the other. Such is true after abdominoperineal extirpation of the rectum; patients may have bladder areflexia (due to autonomic denervation) while somatic innervation of the penile skin or the pelvic floor musculature remains intact.

A. Evaluation of Somatic Nervous Pathways

The combination of pudendal SEPs, pudendal MEPs and the somatosomatic sacral reflex provides a comprehensive evaluation of somatic fibers controlling genitourinary functions. Testing of the sensory–somatic fibers is easy, but is of limited interest in the evaluation of urinary symptoms; in patients with sexual disorders, however, it may help disclose a neurological deficit. Evaluation of the motor–somatic tracts is more valuable, as the motor branch of the pudendal nerve controls the pelvic floor musculature, including the anal and the urethral sphincters. These muscles are directly involved in the mechanisms of anal and urinary continence. Furthermore, the ischio- and bulbocavernosus muscles are responsible for the prograde expulsion of sperm during sexual activity.

1. Pudendal SEPs

The technique has several limitations: it is difficult to perform unilateral stimulation of the dorsal nerve (especially in women), to position the electrode correctly, and the amplitude of the spinal responses is low. However, by performing dorsal nerve SEPs (of penis or clitoris), afferent volleys from S4 to the somatosensory cortex can be explored. By stimulating the anal margin, the entire spinal cord can be investigated. Our results (25) on electrical brain mapping validate the use of the Cz-2 scalp location to obtain optimal cortical pudendal SEPs.

2. Pudendal MEPs

After transcranial stimulation, the responses recorded from the pelvic floor muscles are of low amplitude, compared with those gathered from the upper or lower limb muscles. The intensity of transcranial stimulation necessary to obtain motor responses from the pelvic floor muscles ranges between 80 and 90% of the stimulator's output. Its intensity is significantly higher than that which elicits MEPs in the upper limb. This may be due to representation of the urogenital structures deep within the motor strip of the interhemispheric fissure (6,15,16).

3. Somatosomatic Sacral Reflex

This technique provides information on the functionality of the pelvic floor muscles, including the urethral sphincter. The test is useful in the investigation of continence problems as well as sexual (ejaculatory) disorders.

B. Evaluation of Autonomic Nervous Pathways

1. Urinary Sensitivity Threshold Measurements

In this semiobjective technique, the patient has to collaborate actively in the test by reporting when he or she starts to feel the stimulation. The test is repeated several times to check the reliability of the measurement and patient alertness (6,7,17). Electrical stimulation of the urinary tract is invasive, requiring urethral catheterization. For this reason, the technique has not been widely used. Electrical stimulation of the bladder mucosa with a ring electrode mounted on a Foley catheter carries some methodological uncertainties, because the investigator does not know exactly which part of the bladder wall is being stimulated. The alternative is to use a needle electrode affixed on a stent inserted under direct vision, but this would be even more invasive.

Stimulation of the proximal urethra is also problematic from a methodological point of view, because the transition between autonomic and somatic innervation in the urethra is variable. Therefore, in some subjects, especially in women, electrical stimulation of the proximal urethra will activate fast-conducting somatic fibers, leading to relatively low sensitivity thresholds and short latencies of the viscerosomatic reflex and urinary SEPs.

Wyndaele (26) investigated a large series of patients with congenital or acquired spinal cord lesions: he confirmed the value of urinary sensitivity threshold measurements in the investigation and follow-up of patients with neurological disorders.

2. Urinary SEPs

The latencies of the different cortical peaks of urinary SEPs are longer than those of pudendal SEPs (6,7,25). However, these differences in latency are rather small (20–30 msec; see Tables 2 and 5). Because autonomic nerves have low conduction velocities, we would expect urinary SEP latencies to be more than 100 msec. Therefore, autonomic as well as somatic fibers may probably contribute to urinary SEPs (and to the viscerosomatic sacral reflex) (25).

It is possible to construct an electrical map of brain activity following urinary stimulation by recording urinary SEPs from 10 to 16 cortical sites. The stimulation technique is the same as that for urinary SEPs, the responses being recorded with an array of 16 electrodes applied over the scalp. Maximal activity is recorded around the central vertex (Cz) and just behind it (Cz-2) (25).

3. Viscerosomatic Sacral Reflex

This test explores the peripheral sensory urinary (autonomic) pathways and the motor branch of the pudendal nerve. The latency of the viscerosomatic sacral reflex is longer than that of the somatosomatic sacral reflex (following stimulation of the dorsal nerve of the penis): indeed, the mean latency of the somatosomatic sacral reflex is 32 msec, whereas that of the viscerosomatic reflex ranges from 50 to 75 msec (see Tables 4 and 7) (2,3,6,23).

4. Detrusor MEPs

The technique is invasive as it requires urethral catheterization and insertion of a needle electrode into the detrusor muscle. Careful validation by neurophysiologists is needed, as previous studies recording detrusor EMG activity were subsequently found to be unsatisfactory. If the technique proves reliable, it may open new vistas in electrophysiology.

5. Sympathetic Skin Responses

Sympathetic skin responses (SSRs) can be obtained from most skin areas following electrical stimulation of any somatic nerve. The pathway of the reflex consists of an afferent somatic limb, an intracerebral loop, and an efferent sympathetic limb. To differentiate a lesion affecting the afferent (somatic) limb from a lesion of the efferent (sympathetic) limb, at least two different nerves should be stimulated while recording the responses from several skin areas. Sympathetic skin responses recorded from the perineum and the penis are useful in evaluating erectile and ejaculatory dysfunctions. Indeed, sympathetic fibers to the eccrine glands of the perineum follow the same pathway (at least in their proximal course) as those innervating the urinary bladder and the corpora cavernosa (21,22,27).

Latencies of foot SSRs are longer than those of the hand or perineal SSRs. Amplitudes of hand SSRs are invariably higher than those of the foot (21,22).

6. Corpus Cavernosum EMG

If confirmed, this technique will improve our understanding of the physiology of erection and detumescence (12). It will also be useful for evaluating patients with possible lesions of the autonomic nerves to the corpora cavernosa (11,12).

V. CONCLUSION

Genitourinary electrophysiological tests are of interest for evaluating pelvic organ innervation. The clinician should be aware, however, of the lack of reproducibility or of the invasiveness of some of the tests; in many cases, it may be undesirable to subject patients to these investigations. In addition to the clinical use of these tests, they are of interest as a research model, for they offer a unique opportunity for neurophysiologists to explore autonomic nerves.

REFERENCES

1. Bradley WE. Urethral electromyelography. J Urol 1972; 10:563–564.
2. Andersen JT, Bradley WE, Timm GW. Electrophysiological techniques for the study of urethral vesical innervation. Scand J Urol Nephrol 1976; 10:189–194.
3. Siroky MB, Sax DS, Krane RJ. Sacral signal tracing: the electrophysiology of the bulbocavernosus reflex. J Urol 1976; 122:661–664.
4. Nordling J, Andersen JT, Walter S, Meyhoff HH, Hald T, Gammelgaard PA. Evoked responses of the bulbocavernosus reflex. Eur Urol 1979; 5:36–38.
5. Opsomer RJ, Guérit JM, Wese FX, Van Cangh PJ. Pudendal cortical somatosensory evoked potentials. J Urol 1986; 135:1216–1218.
6. Opsomer RJ, Amarenco G. Les tests électrophysiologiques en neuro-urologie. In: Monographie de la SIFUD, Paris: FIIS, 1990; 2:161–216.
7. Gerstenberg TC, Klarskow P, Hald T. Pudendal somatosensory urethral and bladder wall evoked potentials in normals. 12th Annual Meeting of the International Continence Society, 1982:150–151.
8. Hansen MV, Ertekin C, Larsson LE. Cerebral evoked potentials after stimulation of the posterior urethra in man. Electroencephalogr Clin Neurophysiol 1990; 77:52–58.
9. Sarica Y, Karacan I. Cerebral responses evoked by stimulation of the vesico-urethral junction in normal subjects. Electroencephalogr Clin Neurophysiol 1986; 65:440–446.
10. Wagner G, Gerstenberg TC, Levin R. Electrical activity of corpus cavernosum during flaccidity and erection of the human penis: a new diagnostic method? J Urol 1989; 142:723–725.
11. Stief CG. Single potential analysis of cavernous electrical activity. In: Jonas U, Thon WF, Stief CG, eds. Erectile Dysfunction. Berlin:Springer-Verlag, 1991:194–203.
12. Jünemann KP, Bührle CP, Stief CG. Current trends in corpus cavernosum EMG. Conclusions of the first International Workshop on Smooth Muscle EMG Recordings/Leiomyogram. Int J Impot Res 1993; 5:105–108.
13. Bemelmans BLH, Van Kerrebroeck PH, Notermans SLH, Wijkstra H, Debruyne FMG. Motor evoked potentials from the bladder on magnetic stimulation of the cauda equina. J Urol 1992; 147:658–661.

14. Fowler C, Fowler CH. Clinical neurophysiology. In: Torrens M, Morrison JFB, eds. The Physiology of the Lower Urinary Tract. London: Springer Verlag, 1987:309–332.
15. Opsomer RJ, Caramia MD, Zarola F, Pesce F, Rossini PM. Neurophysiological evaluation of central-peripheral sensory and motor pudendal fibres. Electroencephalogr Clin Neurophysiol 1989; 74:260–270.
16. Opsomer RJ, Guérit JM, Van Cangh PJ, Zarola F, Romani GL, Rossini PM. Electrophysiological assessment of somatic nerves controlling the genital and urinary functions. In: Rossini PM, Mauguière F, eds. New Trends and Advanced Techniques in Clinical Neurophysiology. Electroencephalogr Clin Neurophysiol Suppl. 1990; 41:298–305.
17. Opsomer RJ, Gerstenberg TC, Klarskov P, Hald T. The electric sensibility threshold in the bladder and the urethra. 2nd Joint Meeting of the International Continence Society and the Urodynamics Society, 1983:196–198.
18. Boyce WH. Bladder electromyography: a new approach to the diagnosis of urinary bladder dysfunction. J Urol 1952; 67:650–668.
19. Stanton SI, Hill DW, Williams JP. Electromyography of the detrusor muscle. Br J Urol 1973; 45:289–298.
20. Jünemann KP, Scheepe J, Persson–Junemann C, Schmidt P, Abel K, Zwick A, Tschada R, Alken P. Basic experimental studies on corpus cavernosum electromyography and smooth-muscle electromyography of the urinary bladder. World J Urol 1994; 12:266–275.
21. Opsomer RJ, Boccasena P, Traversa R, Rossini PM. Sympathetic skin responses from the limbs and the genitalia: normative study and contribution to the evaluation of neurourological disorders. Electroencephalogr Clin Neurophysiol 1996; 101:25–31.
22. Ertekin C, Ertekin N, Mutlu S, Almis S, Akçam A. Skin potentials (SP) recorded from the extremities and genital regions in normal and impotent subjects. Acta Neurol Scand 1987; 76:28–36.
23. Anten H, Van Waalwijk ESC, Debruyne FMJ. Clarification of neurogenic lesions in the urogenital system of EMG and evoked responses. 3rd Joint Meeting of the International Continence Society and the Urodynamics Society, 1986:98–100.
24. Beck R, Fowler CJ. Clinical neurophysiology in the investigation of genitourinary tract dysfunction. In: Rushton DN, ed. Handbook of Neuro-Urology. New York: Marcel Dekker, 1994: 151–180.
25. Opsomer RJ, Guérit JM. Electrical brain mapping following genitourinary and posterior tibial nerve stimulation. Neurourol Urodynam 1991; 10:383–384.
26. Wyndaele JJ. Evaluatie van twee methoden toegepast in de urologische kliniek bij het onderzoek naar gevoel in de lagere urinewegen. Ph.D. dissertation, University of Ghent, Belgium, 1993.
27. Vas CJ. Sexual impotence and some autonomic disturbances in men with multiple sclerosis. Acta Neurol Scand 1969; 45:166–183.

28

Lifestyle Interventions in the Treatment of Urinary Incontinence

INGRID NYGAARD

University of Iowa College of Medicine, Iowa City, Iowa

I. INTRODUCTION

Various lifestyle factors may play a role in either the pathogenesis or, later, the resolution of incontinence. Although published literature about lifestyle factors and incontinence is sparse, alterations in lifestyle are frequently recommended by health care professionals and lay people alike. Interventions often recommended by physicians include weight loss, changing activity, smoking cessation, and decreasing or changing fluid intake. In this chapter, the published evidence for recommending these and other lifestyle interventions will be addressed.

II. WEIGHT LOSS

Growing evidence suggests that obesity is a strong independent risk factor for urinary incontinence in women (1–5). Recently, Brown et al. (6) assessed risk factors for daily urinary incontinence in a large group of 7949 women. In this multivariate analysis, which controlled for age, parity, and other factors, the prevalence of daily incontinence increased by an odds ratio of 1.6:5 BMI (body mass index, kg/m^2) units. Similarly, controlling for other risk factors, Foldspang and Mommsen (7) found that the odds ratio for urinary incontinence increased by 1.07 for each BMI unit.

In a mailed questionnaire, Rasmussen et al. (8) compared the prevalence of incontinence in obese (BMI of at least 30) and normal weight women 6–18 months after delivery. Of the obese women, 29.1% reported at least weekly stress incontinence, compared with 11.7% of normal weight controls.

Although weight loss is probably the intervention most frequently recommended to obese women with incontinence, no prospective randomized trials that evaluate weight loss as an intervention have yet been performed.

Two prospective cohort studies (9,10) evaluated the effect of weight loss in morbidly obese women. Massive weight reduction, accomplished by surgical procedures, resolved incontinence in most of these women. Deitel et al. (10) followed 138 women with a mean weight and age of 124 kg and 35 years, respectively, before bariatric surgery. Mean weight after stabilization was 79 kg. When asked in a questionnaire whether they leaked urine with coughing, laughing hard, or straining, 61.2% answered affirmatively before the surgery. After weight stabilization, only 11.6% noted such leakage. In a later prospective study that evaluated the subjective and objective effects of massive weight loss, Bump et al. (9) found resolution of urinary incontinence in 9 of 12 women 1 year after bariatric surgery. In addition, objective parameters, including measures of vesical pressure, magnitude of bladder pressure increases with coughing, urethral axis mobility, and pressure transmission ratios, all changed. In this group, mean weight changed from 131.5 kg preoperatively to 88.1 kg postoperatively.

Although the data do strongly suggest that weight loss reduces incontinence in morbidly obese women, no studies have evaluated this intervention in the more commonly seen, moderately obese woman. Thus, this recommendation, if made to a patient, should be tempered with a statement summarizing the facts. Given current evidence, maintaining normal weight through adulthood may be an important factor in the prevention of incontinence.

III. PHYSICAL FORCES (EXERCISE, WORK)

The definition of genuine stress incontinence (urine loss associated with increased abdominal pressure in the absence of detrusor contraction) suggests that this condition is associated with physical activity. Certainly, one would expect stress incontinence to be a minimal problem for a hypothetical sedentary woman who refrains from coughing, straining, brisk walking, lifting, or other normal daily activities. Obviously, it is neither realistic nor desirable to recommend to an incontinent woman that she give up all movement as part of her treatment program. However, a question often raised is whether more strenuous activities may be associated with incontinence.

The symptom of stress incontinence is common in young, exercising women (11–13). We surveyed 144 college varsity athletes (14). Overall, 28% reported urine loss while participating in their event. The rate was highest in women participating in activities such as gymnastics (67%) and basketball (66%) that involve jumping and high-impact landings. Similarly, Bø et al. (12) found that 31% of physical education students who exercised at least three times a week reported urinary incontinence, compared with 10% of sedentary nutrition students.

For most of these women, the leakage was of very small volume and generally did not represent a problem. There is little available information on whether strenuous exercise or activity done when young can cause more severe, problematic incontinence later in life. In a questionnaire study of women who were Olympians approximately 25 years ago, those who competed in gymnastics or track and field were not more likely to currently report daily or weekly incontinence than Olympians who competed in swimming (15). However, certain provocations may cause stress incontinence: a recent report described six nulliparous infantry trainees who developed stress incontinence and pelvic floor defects for the first time during airborne training, which included parachute jumping (16).

Another area about which little is known is the relation, if any, between heavy work and urinary incontinence or the related condition of pelvic organ prolapse.

In a case–control study, Jörgensen et al. (17) compared the prevalence of surgery for incontinence and/or pelvic organ prolapse in 28,619 Danish nursing assistants (who were presumably exposed to frequent heavy lifting) with 1,652,533 general population controls. The nursing assistants were 1.6-fold more likely to undergo such surgery than women in the general population. However, as this study was unable to control for parity, the strength of the conclusion is limited. Previously, Spernol et al. (18) found that women with uterine prolapse were more likely to report a heavy work history than controls: 40% of women with prolapse reported a history of heavy work, compared with 17% of women without prolapse. This risk increase remained after controlling for childbirth. In this study, women were asked to subjectively assess whether their past work history had included light, medium, or heavy work; these parameters were not further quantified, nor were the questions validated. The findings were limited by the general, subjective nature of the questions used.

Particularly problematic for clinicians and their patients is the issue of what postoperative recommendations to give women who had successful surgical treatment for incontinence or prolapse. In a rare study that addressed this topic, Maleika–Rabe et al. (19) assessed factors related to surgical failure at least 18 months after surgery for incontinence or prolapse. Forty percent of women required to lift weights of more than 5 kg at work were cured, compared with 57% of those who refrained from lifting.

Given the large proportion of women who are employed in various occupations that require heavy lifting and the paucity of scientific data about the association of such exertions and incontinence, this should be investigated further. Specifically, research must establish whether heavy exertion is an etiological factor in the pathogenesis of incontinence or pelvic organ prolapse, whether changing exertions can alleviate these conditions, and whether heavy exertion reduces the effectiveness of various surgical procedures.

IV. SMOKING

Nicotine produces phasic contraction of isolated bladder muscle probes in vitro (20,21). However, in vivo, there is no strong evidence that associates smoking and incontinence in humans. In a case–control study comparing smoking behavior in 160 continent and incontinent women, Tampakoudis et al. (22) reported that smokers were more likely to report incontinence than nonsmokers. In contrast, a large cross-sectional study that evaluated multiple risk factors for incontinence observed no such relation (6). In another case–control study (23), incontinent smokers had stronger urethral sphincters and lower overall risk profiles than incontinent nonsmokers. Smokers may have a mechanism different from that of nonsmokers that causes their incontinence.

No data have been reported concerning the effects of smoking cessation on incontinence.

V. DIETARY FACTORS

No randomized trials have assessed the efficacy of caffeine restriction, fluid management, or dietary changes in the treatment of incontinence.

Creighton and Stanton (24) compared the effect of caffeine on 30 women with either detrusor instability or no bladder abnormality. After ingesting caffeine tablets, women with detrusor instability had increased detrusor pressure on bladder filling, whereas continent women had no such abnormality. In Brown's multivariate analysis of incontinence risk factors in 7949 women (6), no association was found between either coffee or alcohol drinking and the outcome parameter of daily incontinence.

Decreasing fluid intake is often recommended to avoid urinary leakage or nocturia. In a study of older individuals, Griffiths et al. (25) found a strong relation between evening fluid intake, nocturia, and nocturnal voided volume; this relation was weaker for diurnal intake and voiding. Wyman et al. (26) reported a modest positive relation between fluid intake and the severity of incontinence in older women with stress incontinence; fluid intake accounted for 14% of the explained variability in the number of incontinent episodes. However, no such correlation was observed in women with detrusor instability. Conversely, Dowd et al. (27) suggest that incontinence may be improved by increasing fluid intake. They note that restricting fluid intake concentrates the urine and decreases the functional capacity of the bladder, increasing the likelihood of more incontinent episodes. In a study of 32 women who kept voiding diaries for 5 weeks, 20 women felt that incontinence decreased after increasing fluid intake.

Anecdotal evidence suggests that eliminating dietary factors, such as artificial sweeteners, carbonated beverages, or certain foods, may play a role in continence. There are no published studies that objectively assess this.

The sparse available data suggest that caffeine and fluid intake play a minor, if any, role in the pathogenesis of incontinence. Given that decreasing fluids may lead to urinary tract infections, constipation, or dehydration, this intervention should be reserved for patients with abnormally high fluid intakes. Caffeine consumption is pervasive in many societies. Randomized trials to assess the effect of caffeine and other dietary factors are feasible and important.

VI. CONSTIPATION

There may be an association between straining and pudendal nerve function. Lubowski et al. (28) reported that the mean pudendal nerve terminal motor latency increased after straining, correlated with the amount of descent, and returned to the resting level by 4 min after the effort. However, Jorge et al. (29) found evidence of pudendal neuropathy in only 25% of 213 women with abnormal perineal descent. In this large group of patients with defecating dysfunction, no relation was seen between neuropathy and pelvic descent, leading to the conclusion that pelvic descent and neuropathy may be two independent findings.

In an observational study of 73 women, 30% of subjects with stress incontinence and 61% of those with uterovaginal prolapse reported straining at stool time as young adults, compared with 4% of women without urogynecological symptoms (30). Diokno et al. (31) in a population-based study of 1154 women older than the age of 60 years, found that women with urinary incontinence were slightly more likely to report constipation than those who were continent (31.6 vs. 24.7%). Neither of these studies clarified whether constipation causes urinary incontinence (presumably by deterioration of pudendal nerve function from straining), or whether the two problems share a common etiology.

There are no intervention trials that address the effect of resolving constipation or urinary incontinence. Further research is needed to delineate the role of straining in the pathogenesis of incontinence. If the association holds, public education, particularly of parents and pediatricians, is required to make an impression on the common problem of straining in children.

VII. OTHER FACTORS

Norton and Baker (32) rigorously assessed urine loss during various postural changes and concluded that stress incontinence can be significantly decreased by crossing the legs or by crossing the legs and bending forward. No study has evaluated whether postural changes constitute a satisfactory form of treatment outside of the laboratory setting.

Other incontinence interventions suggested either by health care professionals or the lay press include timed voiding, reducing stress, wearing nonrestrictive clothing, utilizing a bedside commode, decreasing lower extremity edema, treating allergies and coughs, wearing cotton underwear, and increasing sexual activity. None of these has been evaluated in a controlled fashion in the nongeriatric population.

VIII. CONCLUSION

At this time, little research has been directed at the role that lifestyle plays in promoting or treating urinary incontinence. Areas of particular interest, because of their high prevalence in modern society, include obesity, caffeine intake, heavy physical labor, and constipation. Further research will aid clinicians in counseling incontinent women.

REFERENCES

1. Wilson PD, Herbison RM, Herbison GP. Obstetric practice and the prevalence of urinary incontinence three months after delivery. Br J Obstet Gynecol 1996; 103:154–161.
2. Mommsen S, Foldspang A. Body mass index and adult female urinary incontinence. World J Urol 1994; 12:319–322.
3. Dwyer PL, Lee ETC, Hay DM. Obesity and urinary incontinence in women. Br J Obstet Gynecol 1988; 95:91–96.
4. Kölbl H, Riss P. Obesity and stress urinary incontinence: significance of indices of relative weight. Urol Int 1988; 43:7–10.
5. Yarnell JWG, Voyle GJ, Sweetnam PM, Milbank J, Richards CJ, Stephenson TP. Factors associated with urinary incontinence in women. J Epidemiol Community Health 1982; 36:58–63.
6. Brown JS, Seeley DG, Fong J, Black DM, Ensrud KE, Grady D. Urinary incontinence in older women: who is at risk? Obstet Gynecol 1996; 87:715–721.
7. Foldspang A, Mommsen S. Overweight and urinary incontinence in women. Ugeskr Laeger 1995; 157:5848–5851.
8. Rasmussen KL, Krue S, Johansson LE, Knudsen HJ, Agger AO. Obesity as a predictor of postpartum urinary symptoms. Acta Obstet Gynecol Scand 1997; 76:359–362.
9. Bump RC, Sugerman HJ, Fantl JA, McClish DK. Obesity and lower urinary tract function in women: effect of surgically induced weight loss. Am J Obstet Gynecol 1992; 167:392–399.
10. Deitel M, Stone E, Kassam HA, Wilk EJ, Sutherland DJA. Gynecologic–obstetric changes after loss of massive excess weight following bariatric surgery. J Am Coll Nutr 1988; 7:147–153.
11. Nygaard IE, DeLancey JO, Arnsdorf L, Murphy E. Exercise and incontinence. Obstet Gynecol 1990; 75:848–851.
12. Bø K, Mæhlum S, Oseid S, Larsen S. Prevalence of stress urinary incontinence among physically active and sedentary female students. Scand J Sports Sci 1989; 11:113–116.
13. Bø K, Stien R, Kulseng-Hanssen S, Kristofferson M. Clinical and urodynamic assessment of nulliparous young women with and without stress incontinence symptoms: a case–control study. Obstet Gynecol 1994; 84:1028–1032.
14. Nygaard IE, Thompson FL, Svengalis SL, Albright JP. Urinary incontinence in elite nulliparous athletes. Obstet Gynecol 1994; 84:183–187.

15. Nygaard IE. Does prolonged high-impact activity contribute to later urinary incontinence? A retrospective cohort study of female Olympians. Obstet Gynecol 1997; 90:718–722.

16. Davis GD, Goodman M. Stress urinary incontinence in nulliparous female soldiers in airborne infantry training. J Pelvic Surg 1996; 2:68–71.

17. Jörgensen S, Hein HO, Gyntelberg F. Heavy lifting at work and risk of genital prolapse and herniated lumbar disc in assistant nurses. Occup Med 1994; 44:47–49.

18. Spernol R, Bernaschek G, Schaller A. Entstehungsursacher des deszensus. [Etiology of uterine prolapse]. Geburtshilfe Frauenheilkd 1983; 43:33–36.

19. Maleika–Rabe A, Wallwiener D, Grischke EM, Solomayer E, Bastert G. Long-term outcome of incontinence and prolapse surgery with reference to multiple endogenous and exogenous risk factors for the female pelvic floor. Zentralbl Gynakol 1998; 120:176–182.

20. Hisayama T, Shinkai M, Takaynagi I, Toyoda T. Mechanism of action of nicotine in isolated bladder of guinea-pig. Br J Pharmacol 1988; 95:465–472.

21. Koley B, Koley J, Saha JK. The effects of nicotine on spontaneous contractions of cat urinary bladder in situ. Br J Pharmacol 1984; 83:347–355.

22. Tampakoudis P, Tantanassis T, Grimbizis G, Papeletsos M, Mantalenakis S. Cigarette smoking and urinary incontinence in women—a new calculative method of estimating the exposure to smoke. Eur J Obstet Gynecol Reprod Biol 1995; 63:27–30.

23. Bump RC, McClish DM. Cigarette smoking and pure genuine stress incontinence of urine: a comparison of risk factors and determinants between smokers and nonsmokers. Am J Obstet Gynecol 1994; 170:579–582.

24. Creighton SM, Stanton SL. Caffeine: does it affect your bladder? Br J Urol 1990; 66:613–614.

25. Griffiths DJ, McCracken PN, Harrison GM, Gormley EA. Relationship of fluid intake to voluntary micturition and urinary incontinence in geriatric patients. Neurourol Urodynam 1993; 12:1–7.

26. Wyman JF, Elswick RK, Wilson MS, Fantl JA. Relationship of fluid intake to voluntary micturitions and urinary incontinence in women. Neurourol Urodynam 1991; 10:463–473.

27. Dowd TT, Campbell JM, Jones JA. Fluid intake and urinary incontinence in older community-dwelling women. J Community Health Nurs 1996; 13:179–186.

28. Lubowski DZ, Swash M, Nicholls RJ, Henry MM. Increase in pudendal nerve terminal motor latency with defaecation straining. Br J Surg 1988; 75:1095–1097.

29. Jorge JMN, Wexner SD, Ehrenpreis ED, Norgueras JJ, Jagelman DG. Does perineal descent correlate with pudendal neuropathy? Dis Colon Rectum 1993; 36:475–483.

30. Spence–Jones C, Kamm MA, Henry MM, Hudson CN. Bowel dysfunction: a pathogenic factor in uterovaginal prolapse and urinary stress incontinence. Br J Obstet Gynecol 1994; 101:147–152.

31. Diokno AC, Brock BM, Herzog AR, Bromberg J. Medical correlates of urinary incontinence in the elderly. Urology 1990; 36:129–138.

32. Norton PA, Baker JE. Postural changes can reduce leakage in women with stress urinary incontinence. Obstet. Gynecol 1994; 84:770–774.

29

Pelvic Floor Muscle Exercises

KARI BØ

Norwegian University of Sports and Physical Education, Oslo, Norway

I. PHYSICAL THERAPY OR PHYSIOTHERAPY FOR PELVIC FLOOR TRAINING

The World Confederation for Physical Therapy (WCPT) gave the following description of physical therapy/physiotherapy at its 14th General Meeting in May 1999: Physical therapy/physiotherapy is providing services to people and populations to develop, maintain, and restore maximum movements and functional ability throughout their lifespan. Physical therapy includes the provision of services in circumstances when movement is threatened by the process of aging or that of injury or disease. Physical therapy/physiotherapy is concerned with identifying and maximizing movement potential, within the spheres of

- Promotion
- Prevention
- Treatment
- Rehabilitation

Physical therapy is an essential part of health services delivery system. Physical therapists practice independently of other health care providers and also within interdisciplinary rehabilitation–habilitation programs for the restoration of optimal function and quality of life in individuals with loss and disorders of movement. The WCPT states that physical therapy is the service provided *only* by, or under the direction and supervision of, a physical therapist and includes assessment, diagnosis, planning, intervention, and evaluation.

A. Assessment

Assessment includes both the examination of individuals or groups with actual or potential impairments, functional limitations, disabilities, or other conditions of health by history taking, screening, and the use of specific tests and measures, and evaluations of the results of examination through analysis and synthesis within a process of clinical reasoning. In incontinence, the physical therapist will, after thorough history taking, assess the function of the pelvic floor by observation, vaginal palpation, and measurement of muscle activity (vaginal or urethral squeeze pressure, electromyography, ultrasound, magnetic resonance imaging).

B. Diagnosis

In carrying out the diagnostic process, physical therapists may need to obtain additional information from other professionals. Diagnosis in urinary incontinence often cannot be based on physical therapy assessment alone. Collaboration with, and referral from, an urologist or gynecologist with access to clinical, urodynamic, and other laboratory examinations, provide the best basis for physical therapy assessment and decision making.

C. Planning

An intervention plan includes measurable outcome goals negotiated in collaboration with the patient/client, family, or caregiver. Alternatively, it may lead to referral to another agency in cases that are inappropriate for physical therapy.

D. Intervention

In general, physical therapy intervention is implemented and modified to reach agreed on goals and may include manual handling; movement enhancing; physical, electrotherapeutic and mechanical agents; functional training (muscle strength and endurance, coordination, motor control, body awareness, flexibility, relaxation, cardiorespiratory fitness); provision of aids and appliances; patient/client-related instruction and counseling; documentation and coordination; and communication. In treating urinary incontinence, the mainstay of physical therapy is pelvic floor muscle exercises, with or without the use of biofeedback or, in some instances, electrical stimulation. Equally important are awareness and relaxation exercises for the pelvic floor.

Interventions may also be aimed at prevention of impairments, functional limitations, disability, and injury, including the promotion and maintenance of health, quality of life, and fitness in all ages and populations. To treat urinary incontinence, teaching of pelvic floor exercises in pregnancy and after childbirth is essential. The choice of interventions should be based on the highest level of evidence available (optimally, results from several randomized, controlled trials).

E. Evaluation

Reevaluating, using the same outcome measures before and after treatment, is mandatory to assess outcomes. To treat urinary incontinence, the physical therapist evaluates pelvic floor muscle strength and function, the degree of leakage (leakage episodes, pad tests, instruments for patient description of symptoms), and quality of life. Collaboration with urologists and gynecologists is essential to be able to make proper evaluations at the pathophysiological or impairment level. The effect of new treatment modalities and procedures should be tested in randomized clinical trials before widely implemented to clinical practice.

Kegel (1) was the first to report that pelvic floor muscle (PFM) exercises were effective in treating urinary incontinence (UI) in women. In uncontrolled, nonrandomized studies, he claimed an 84% cure rate in a variety of incontinent types. Since then, several randomized controlled trials (RCTs) have demonstrated that PFM exercise is more effective than no treatment (2–7), electrical stimulation (3,5), or cones (5) in treating genuine stress incontinence (GSI).

The PFMs are one of many factors contributing to the urethral closure mechanism (8). Other important factors are contraction of the smooth and striated muscles within the urethral wall, blood flow, and intact ligaments and fasciae keeping the bladder and urethra in an optimal position during increased intra-abdominal pressure. PFM training may be unsuccessful if factors other than the function of the PFM are the cause of incontinence; for example, if the urethral ligaments are totally ruptured during childbirth. However, because the PFM are untrained in most individuals, training them holds great potential for improvement. Most likely, strengthening and improving PFM function can compensate for other nonfunctioning factors (8).

It has been demonstrated that voluntary contraction of the PFM causes synergistic contraction of the urethral sphincter muscles in women (9), and PFM training produces a significant increase in maximum urethral resting pressure (10,11). Voluntary PFM contraction augments urethral pressure (12) twice as effectively as electrical stimulation (13).

The World Health Organization (WHO) has developed the International Classification of Impairment, Disability and Handicap (ICIDH) system for the evaluation of rehabilitation interventions (14). Pathophysiology is kept outside this classification. The causes of nonoptimal PFM functioning, for example, muscle and nerve damage during vaginal birth, can be classified at the pathophysiological level, and a nonfunctioning PFM can be categorized at the impairment level. The actual leakage and trouble it causes the individual are at the disability level, whereas problems participating in society and quality of life issues are at the handicap–participation level. Physical therapy and PFM exercise are aimed at making changes at all these levels, and the theory behind strength training is that by changing PFM dysfunction, leakage will be stopped or strongly reduced so that the patient can function more adequately with an enhanced quality of life. A higher cure rate after PFM exercise can be expected if the treatment is based on a more exact diagnosis at the pathophysiological level.

In healthy subjects, the PFM is contracted simultaneously with, or precedes, the increase in intra-abdominal pressure as an unconscious cocontraction. Voluntary contraction is most likely mass contraction of the three muscle layers that can be described as an inward movement squeezing around the pelvic openings (15). Magnetic resonance imaging (MRI) studies have demonstrated that during contraction the coccyx is moved ventrally toward the pubic symphysis. Thus, the PFM contract concentrically. During straining, the coccyx is pressed dorsally (16). A correct PFM contraction does not involve any visible movement of the pelvis or outer part of the body. A correct contraction can be felt by vaginal palpation and observed as a movement of the perineum in a cranial direction. Submaximum contractions can be performed in isolation. Most likely, however, maximum PFM contraction is not possible without cocontraction of the abdominal muscles, especially the transverse abdominal muscle (17). In lean subjects, this can be observed as a tiny dorsal movement of the abdomen, with no movement of the pelvis.

As the PFM are situated below the pelvis, and are seldom used consciously, many women do not know how to contract them. Several studies have shown that approximately 30% do not contract correctly at their first consultation, even after thorough individual instruction (10,18,19). Bump et al. (12) reported that after verbal instruction only 50% were able to contract the PFM in a way that increased urethral pressure. No such studies have been performed in men. Physical therapists are trained in functional anatomy, assessment of muscle function, muscle physiology, and motor theory to teach muscle control (see Chap. 5).

Most women learn how to contract very quickly. In an earlier study (11), only 4 of 52 patients were unable to learn how to contract correctly during a 6-month period. Although some women have problems learning how to contract the PFM, it is important to emphasize that 70% are able to do so at the first consultation. Therefore, only a few patients need manual techniques and electrical stimulation after the first consultation. The four elements of PFM training are 1) search, 2) find, 3) control, and 4) train. This chapter focuses on PFM training.

II. EXERCISE SCIENCE RELATED TO PFM TRAINING

The focus of this chapter is effective PFM training to reduce urinary leakage. There are many misconceptions about exercise science in this area; therefore, a brief introduction to strength training theory is warranted. Body awareness, coordination, as well as proprio- and exteroception are covered in Chapter 30, on manual techniques.

Muscle strength is defined as the maximum force that a muscle or muscle group can generate (20). Maximum strength is often referred to as the maximum weight an individual can lift once. This is called the one-repetition maximum or 1RM. Power is the explosive aspect of strength and is the product of strength and speed of movement [power = (force × distance)/time]. Power, the key component in the functional application of strength, is important for the development of PFM function. Speed, however, changes little with training; thus, power is changed almost exclusively through gains in strength.

Muscular endurance can be classified as

1. The ability to repeatedly develop near maximal or maximal forces, determined by assessing the maximum number of repetitions that can be performed at a given percentage of 1RM.
2. The ability to sustain near maximal or maximal forces, assessed by the time it takes to sustain fixed or static muscle actions.

A. Specificity, Overload, Progression, and Maintenance: The Main Principles for Effective Exercise

1. Specificity

Strength training is specific to the area of the body being trained, and unused muscles are prone to atrophy. Many women contract other muscles instead of the PFM (e.g., the abdominal muscles, the gluteal and hip adductor muscles). In addition, they use these muscles simultaneously with PFM contraction (17,19). By using the strong outer pelvic muscles together with the relatively weak and untrained PFM, patients may mask the PFM contraction and believe that they are contracting hard when they are not. We, therefore, recommend concentration on isolated PFM contraction except for transverse abdominal muscle (see p. 445). However, if the patient is unable to contract the PFM at all, contraction of other pelvic muscles may be one way of teaching PFM contraction.

Specificity also means that the muscles should be trained in terms of the functions and positions in which they are supposed to contract. Hence, the PFM should be trained during different tasks (e.g., during lifting and coughing) and in different positions (e.g., standing and sitting) (5,11).

2. Overload and Progression

Muscular strength and endurance are developed by progressive overload principles (21,22). To obtain measurable strength gain, the muscles have to be used more and harder than what is required during daily tasks. Muscle strength is best developed by contractions that require maximum or close to maximum tension with few repetitions, and muscular endurance is best developed by using no or less weights with a greater number of repetitions (20,22). To elicit improvements in both muscular strength and endurance, 8–12 repetitions per set have been recommended (22). A lower repetition range with heavier weight or closer to maximum contraction (e.g., 6–8 repetitions) may optimize strength and power. Heavier resistance to maximal or near maximal loads will elicit a significantly greater training effect. The intensity and volume of the training program can be manipulated by varying the weight load, repetitions, rest interval between exercises and sets, and the number of sets completed. For the PFM, a proper outer weight load is difficult to obtain. Strong encouragement for maximal contraction, longer holding periods, and shorter resting intervals between contractions can be used to overload and make progress in PFM training (11). Another suggestion is to try to hold back a cone when pulling it out. So far, this has not been tried out in an exercise protocol.

3. Maintenance

The general recommendation for maintaining muscle strength is a series of 8–12 contractions twice a week (22). So far, no studies have evaluated how many contractions have to be performed to maintain PFM strength after cessation of organized training. We have shown that PFM strength is maintained for up to 5 years after the cessation of organized training with 70% exercising more than once a week (23). One series of 8–12 contractions can easily be taught in aerobic dance classes or recommended as part of women's general strength-training programs.

Improvement in strength is affected by the initial level of strength and genetic potential for improvement. During the first 6–8 weeks of strength training, the strength gain is due to neural adaptations, such as higher frequency of excitation and recruitment of more effective motor units. Thus, tremendous strength gain can be achieved without hypertrophy. Building of muscle mass is a much slower process and usually starts after 6–8 weeks. This building of muscle volume can go on for years. There is a fixed recruitment pattern during contraction. Slow-twitch (ST) fibers are recruited during light contractions. When more resistance is added, more fast-twitch (FT) fibers are recruited. FT fibers possess a low oxidative capacity and fatigue easily. However, they are needed during rapid movements and close to maximum contractions. All muscle fibers will hypertrophy, but FT fibers possess a higher potential for hypertrophy than ST fibers. The distribution of ST and FT fibers is inherited, and changes in humans have been observed only within each subgroup (e.g., from FTa to FTb) (20). As the strongest stimulation for increased strength is the intensity of contraction (as close to maximum as possible), the main focus is to recruit as many motor units as possible, regardless of whether they are ST or FT fibers. To enhance the potential for strength gain, PFM exercise should be conducted over a length of time so that both neural adaptation and hypertrophy can occur. The American College of Sports Medicine has recommended exercise interventions lasting for at least 5 months (21).

Greater than 100% strength gain has been shown after 8–12 weeks of training (22). The average improvement in sedentary young and middle-aged men and women for up to 6 months of training is 25–30%. As the PFM are totally untrained in most persons, there is a great potential for strength improvement. We have demonstrated a 100% strength increase after 1 month of training (11), with maximum strength continuing to improve in the intensive exercise group (Fig. 1). The group that was left alone with no encouragement for maximal contraction did not show any further improvement.

III. EFFECT OF PFM TRAINING TO TREAT GSI

The aim of this training is to increase muscle strength and power to

1. Build structural support (anatomical location of the muscles, proper attachment, tone, hypertrophy) for the bladder and urethra.
2. Prevent descent of the bladder neck and urethra and close the urethra during abrupt increases in intra-abdominal pressure by automatic, quick, and strong PFM contraction.
3. Make subjects able to voluntarily contract with enough strength and power to close the urethra before intra-abdominal pressure is increased.

The latter objective has been part of PFM training in clinical physical therapy practice for many years. Miller et al. (24) have shown women how to contract, and taught them within a week how to contract before sneezing, coughing, and lifting to significantly reduce urinary leakage. This should, therefore, be recommended in all PFM exercise regimens. However, in continent subjects, PFM contraction is an automatic response without con-

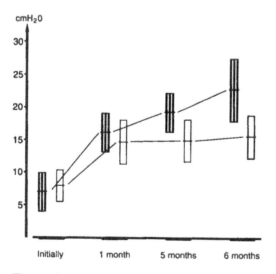

Figure 1 Maximal pelvic floor muscle strength before, after 1 month, after 5 months, and after 6 months of treatment. Columns illustrate 95% confidence intervals of the means. Means are given as horizontal lines. II, intensive exercise group; □, home exercise group. Both groups had increased muscle strength significantly at 1 month (p < 0.01). At 6 months, there was a significant difference in muscle strength between the two groups (p < 0.01). Note that there is no significant difference between the groups after 1 month. (From Ref. 11.)

scious voluntary contraction before activity. In addition, such precontractions are only possible before single bouts of physical exertion. Nobody can run or dance over a long time period of and contract the PFM voluntarily continuously. Therefore, the main goal of PFM training is to build the muscles to reach the automatic response level.

Several RCTs have demonstrated that PFM exercise is better than no treatment (3,5, 25). Because of different outcome measures and instruments to measure PFM function, it is impossible to compare results among studies and to conclude which training regimen is the more effective. However, instructor-followed training is significantly more effective than home exercise (11,26). We combine individual assessment and teaching of correct contraction (Fig. 2) with strength training in groups (5,11) (Fig. 3). Strength training in groups is motivating both for the participants and the therapist. It is cost- and time-effective, and general beneficial health training (strength training of abdominals, back, and thigh muscles, relaxation, lifting techniques, and cardiovascular training) can be incorporated into the program. In our study (11), there was a huge difference in increased strength favoring those who had exercised in groups with a physical therapist, compared with home-training individuals (see Fig. 1). A significant reduction of urinary leakage, measured by the pad test with standardized bladder volume, was demonstrated only in the intensive exercise group (Fig. 4). In addition, the percentages of continent or almost continent subjects were 60% and 17% in the exercise- and home-training groups, respectively. This study demonstrated that a huge difference in outcome can be expected according to the intensity and follow-up of the training program, with little effect after home training.

Typically, the subjective cure rate after PFM exercise varies between 60 and 75% (6). In two studies (5,11) using the same exercise protocol, 60 and 44% of women, respectively,

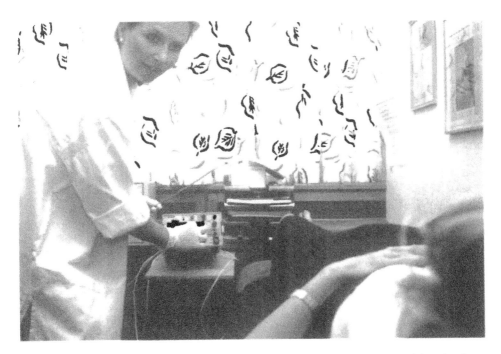

Figure 2 Need for individual teaching, assessment, and feedback of PFM function by a skilled physical therapist.

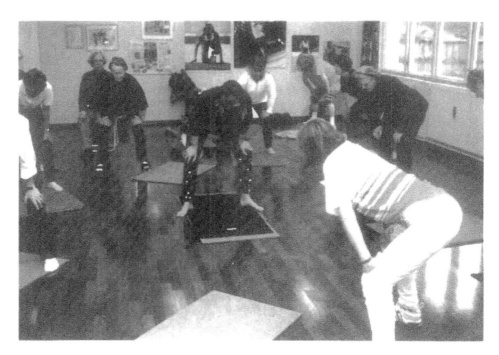

Figure 3 Intensive strength training to contract the PFM correctly can be effectively taught in groups. Exercise classes are motivating for both participants and the physical therapist, who can encourage maximum contractions. Strength training for abdominal, back, and thigh muscles; ergonomic training; relaxation and breathing exercises can be conducted in the interval between series of PFM contractions.

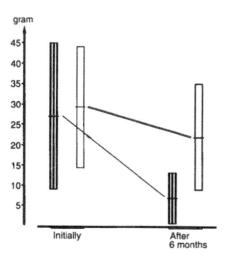

Figure 4 Pad test before and after treatment: columns illustrate 95% confidence intervals of the means. Means are given as horizontal lines. II, intensive exercise group; □, home exercise group. Only the intensive exercise group reduced leakage significantly (p < 0.1). (From Ref. 11.)

no longer had leakage during provocative pad tests after 6 months of intensive training. The lowest cure rate was obtained when the training protocol was administered in a multicenter study (5,11). In these two studies, the patients were tested both subjectively and objectively during physical activity. The effect was, therefore, most likely due to improved automatic muscle function and not only to the ability to contract before increased intra-abdominal pressure.

Several researchers have investigated the factors that influence the outcome of PFM exercise on urinary incontinence (6). No single factor was found to predict outcome, and it was concluded that many factors traditionally supposed to affect outcomes, such as age and the severity of incontinence, may be less crucial than previously thought. The factors that appear to be most associated with positive outcomes are motivation or compliance with the intervention (6). No side effects have been seen after PFM exercise (5,6).

No studies have proved any additional effect of electrical stimulation, cones or bio-feedback synergizing PFM exercise (4–6,27,28). However, these investigations were flawed by small numbers, and future RCTs with better methodological quality should be repeated (4). There are expectations that individually followed training with biofeedback may reinforce strength training without monitoring if general strength training principles are followed. Biofeedback may be important in motivating and enhancing patient effort.

In one RCT, PFM exercise proved to be significantly more effective in improving muscle strength and reducing urinary leakage in GSI women than electrical stimulation, cones, and no treatment (Figs. 5 and 6) (5). In addition, PFM exercise had no side effects and was well-tolerated by all patients.

The use of cones can be questioned from an exercise science perspective (29). Holding the cone for as long as 15–20 min, as recommended (30), may cause decreased blood supply, reduced oxygen consumption, muscle fatigue, and pain, with recruitment of muscles other than the PFM. In addition, many women report that they dislike using cones (5). On the other hand, the cones may add benefit to the training protocol if employed in a different way: the subjects can be asked to contract around the cone and simultaneously try to

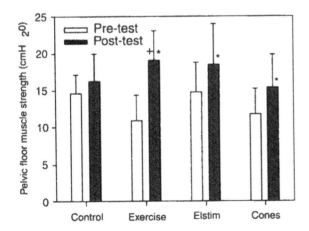

Figure 5 The strength-training group was the only one demonstrating statistically significant improvement in muscle strength when compared with an untreated control group (p < 0.001). (From Ref. 5.)

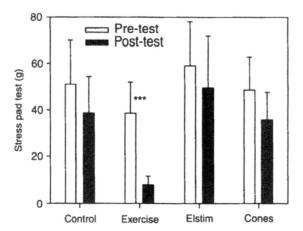

Figure 6   Only the PFM strength training group showed statistically significant improvement in urinary leakage measured by the pad test with standardized bladder volume when compared with untreated controls, electrical stimulation, and vaginal cones (p < 0.01). (From Ref. 5.)

pull it out in a supine or standing position, with 8–12 repetitions in three series per day. In this way, general strength training principles are followed, and progression can be added to the training.

IV.   LONG-TERM EFFECT OF PFM EXERCISE

Several studies have examined the long-term effect of PFM exercise (23,31–33). However, very few of them have undertaken clinical examination of actual urinary leakage (23,31). In a 5-year follow-up, urinary leakage increased significantly after cessation of organized training. However, 56% of subjects still had positive closure pressure during coughing, and 75% had no visible leakage (23). Seventy percent of patients were satisfied with the results and did not want another treatment, and 70% were still exercising the PFM more than once a week. To date, there are no data on how much training is needed to maintain strength. However, in strength training of other skeletal muscles, it generally takes a lot more effort to build than to maintain muscle strength.

V.   URGE INCONTINENCE

As the cause of detrusor instability is often unknown, it is difficult to design an effective exercise protocol. The cause may be disturbances in nerves supplying the bladder wall and the detrusor muscle. However, because detrusor contraction is preceded by an appreciable fall in urethral pressure, some authors have suggested that the cause of bladder overactivity may be the PFM (34,35).

The rationale for using PFM exercise to treat urge incontinence is to teach the patient to contract during urgency, thereby inhibiting the urge to void and detrusor contraction. Such inhibition may give the patient time to reach the toilet, thus preventing urge incontinence. How strong the voluntary contraction has to be to effectively inhibit detrusor contraction is unknown. More basic research is needed to determine how morphological and neurophysiological changes after long-term PFM training may affect bladder instability symptoms.

It is difficult to conclude from the literature whether PFM exercise is effective in treating symptoms of bladder overactivity. Few studies are found in the literature, and most of them are flawed by weak research design, inclusion of several types of incontinence, and use of several treatment modalities (36). In an uncontrolled investigation by Flynn et al. (37), a group of 32 women and 5 men performed 25 repetitions of PFM contraction twice daily for 12 weeks in combination with promotion of bowel regularity, diet, and hydration counseling. Fifty-one percent had urge, and 49% mixed incontinence. The results showed a significant increase in time between voiding with an 80% reduction in the number of overall incontinence episodes. In a RCT, Nygaard et al. (38) reported their results separately for detrusor instability, comparing the effect of exercise with and without an audiotape. Significant improvement was noted in incontinence episodes per day, voids per night, and urge score. However, these results were not compared with untreated controls.

In a well-designed RCT by Burgio et al. (39), 197 women were randomized to either PFM exercise in combination with urge strategies and relaxing exercise, oxybutynin, or placebo. All three groups had the same follow-up and attention during the 8-week–trial period. The results showed a statistically significant reduction in the number of incontinence episodes and subjective improvement in the exercise group.

VI. PFM EXERCISE FOR PRIMARY PREVENTION OF UI

Pregnancy and vaginal delivery have been considered the main risk factors in the development of UI. As early as 1948, Kegel (1) emphasized the value of PFM exercise in restoring function after childbirth. Women in most industrialized countries have been encouraged to engage in postpartum PFM exercise to prevent and treat UI. However, despite the passage of some 50 years, the effect of prevention is sparsely documented.

Sleep and Grant (40) found no significant difference in reported UI after 4 weeks of PFM training postpartum. However, Wilson et al. reported (41) a 10% reduction in the prevalence of UI in women who were training compared with untreated controls. In a matched-pair, controlled, primary prevention study, we (42) demonstrated a 50% decrease in the prevalence of UI in the training group versus the controls. The exercises were performed from 8 to 16 weeks postpartum with 8–12 contractions twice a day and group exercises with a physical therapist once a week. The results were the same at 1-year follow-up (43). This study showed that more intensive follow-up is needed than the written information given postnatally in most hospitals today.

Few investigations have evaluated the effect of PFM exercise during pregnancy. In a RCT, Samselle et al. (44) demonstrated that there were fewer incontinence episodes in a group of primagravidas who had been training the PFM during pregnancy than in a control group. The exercise group was asked to perform 30 close-to-maximum contractions per day, and the final evaluation was 12 months postpartum. However, they had a huge dropout rate for clinical assessment of PFM function, and no conclusion could be drawn on the effect of exercises on PFM strength. More RCTs are needed to evaluate the effect of preventive PFM exercise.

VII. PFM EXERCISE IN MEN

Studies on men are flawed by the inclusion of several diagnoses and the use of many treatment modalities for the same intervention. Subjective improvement rates vary between 60 and 82% in uncontrolled investigations (45–48). Only two RCTs have been conducted on the effect of PFM exercise in men (49,50). Both of them evaluated the effect of PFM exercise on stress UI after radical prostatectomy. The results were contradictory. Moore et al. (49) did not demonstrate any effect after 3 months of PFM exercise or a combination of PFM exercise and electrical stimulation, compared with an untreated control group.

On the other hand, Van Kampen et al. (50) found that the duration of urge and stress incontinence in men was significantly shorter in the exercise group versus the controls. In addition, significant differences were noted in favor of the experimental group in two aspects of quality of life: hobbies and physical well-being. Their program was individually designed and consisted of PFM exercise with the addition of electrical stimulation or bladder training, if needed. Exercises were given as long as the patients needed them and the follow-up period was 12 months. To date, no firm conclusion can be drawn on the effect of PFM exercise in men. There is a need for high-quality RCTs, with sufficient samples, because the use of theory-based exercise protocols in homogeneous diagnostic groups does not provide reliable and valid outcome measures.

VIII. CONCLUSION

PFM exercise with or without biofeedback has been effective in treating female GSI. They have no known side effects, and women should be motivated to perform intensive PFM exercises as the first choice of treatment. However, more than 30% do not contract correctly at their first consultation, and thorough individual instruction is needed. Manual techniques and electrical stimulation can be used to teach women how to contract. Three sets of 8–12 close-to-maximum contractions every day or every second day are recommended. Most people need motivation and encouragement to perform hard strength training. This can be achieved in individual-training sessions or in specifically designed PFM exercise classes. When sufficient function has been achieved, PFM strength has to be maintained by further training, but with lower frequency. More research is needed to find out how much exercise will maintain sufficient PFM function and to evaluate the effect of PFM exercise in men and in urge patients.

REFERENCES

1. Kegel AH. Progressive resistance exercise in the functional restoration of the perineal muscles. Am J Obstet Gynecol 1948; 56:238–249.
2. Fantl JA, Newham DK, Colling J, DeLancey JO, Keeys C, Loughery R, Mcdowell BJ, Norton P, Ouslander J, Schnelle J, Staskin D, Tries J, Urich V, Vitousek SH, Weiss BD, Whitmore K. Urinary Incontinence in Adults: Acute and Chronic Management. Rockville, MD: National Institute of Health, Department of Health and Human Services, Public Health Service, Agency for Health Care Policy and Research, 2.update. 1996.

3. Henalla S, Hutchins C, Robinson P, MacVicar J. Non-operative methods in the treatment of female genuine stress incontinence of urine. J Obstet Gynaecol 1989; 9:222–225.

4. Berghmans LCM, Hendricks HJM, Bø K, Hay–Smith EJ, de Bie RA, van Waalwijk van Doorn ESC. Conservative treatment of stress urinary incontinence in women. A systematic review of randomized clinical trials. Br J Urol 1998; 82:181–91.

5. Bø K, Talseth T, Holme I. Single blind, randomised controlled trial of pelvic floor exercises, electrical stimulation, vaginal cones, and no treatment in management of genuine stress incontinence in women. Br Med J 1999; 318:487–493.

6. Wilson D, Hay–Smith J, Bø K, Wyman J, Nygaard I, Staskin D, Bourchier A. Conservative treatment for women. WHO 1st Consultation for Continence. WHO 1999:579–636.

7. Lagro–Janssen AL, Debruyne FM, Smiths AJ, Van Weel C. The effects of treatment of urinary incontinence in general practice. Fam Pract 1992; 9:284–289.

8. Lose GL. Simultaneous recording of pressure and cross-sectional area in the female urethra: a study of urethral closure function in healthy and stress incontinent women. Neurourol Urodynam 1992; 11:54–89.

9. Bø K, Stien R. Needle EMG registration of striated urethral wall and pelvic floor muscle activity patterns during cough, Valsalva, abdominal, hip adductor, and gluteal muscles contractions in nulliparous healthy females. Neurourol Urodynam 1994; 13:35–41.

10. Benvenuti F, Caputo GM, Bandinelli S, Mayer F, Biagini C, Somavilla A. Reeducative treatment of female genuine stress incontinence. Am J Phys Med 1987; 66:155–168.

11. Bø K, Hagen RH, Kvarstein B, Jørgensen J, Larsen S. Pelvic floor muscle exercise for the treatment of female stress urinary incontinence: 111. Effects of two different degrees of pelvic floor muscle exercise. Neurourol Urodynam 1990; 9:489–502.

12. Bump R, Hurt WG, Fantl JA, Wyman JF. Assessment of Kegel exercise performance after brief verbal instruction. Am J Obstet Gynecol 1991; 165:322–329.

13. Bø K, Talseth T. Change in urethral pressure during voluntary pelvic floor muscle contraction and vaginal electrical stimulation. Int Urogynecol J Pelvic Floor Dysfunct 1997; 8:3–7.

14. International Classification of Impairment, Disability, and Handicap (ICIDH). Zeist, The Netherlands. WHO. 1997; ICIDH-2-beta-1 draft.

15. Kegel AH. Stress incontinence and genital relaxation. Ciba Clin Symp 1952; 2:35–51.

16. Bø K, Lilleas F, Talseth T. Dynamic MRI of pelvic floor and coccygeal movement during pelvic floor muscle contraction and straining [abstr]. Neurourol Urodynam 1997; 16:409–410.

17. Bø K, Kvarstein B, Hagen RR, Larsen S. Pelvic floor muscle exercise for the treatment of female stress urinary incontinence: II. Validity of vaginal pressure measurements of pelvic floor muscle strength and the necessity of supplementary methods for control of correct contraction. Neurourol Urodynam 1990; 9:479–487.

18. Hesse U, Schussler B, Frimberger J, Obernitz N, Senn E. Effectiveness of a three step pelvic floor reeducation in the treatment of stress urinary incontinence: a clinical assessment. Neurourol Urodynam 1990; 9:397–398.

19. Bø K, Larsen S, Oseid S, Kvarstein B, Hagen R, Jørgensen J. Knowledge about and ability to correct pelvic floor muscle exercises in women with urinary stress incontinence. Neurourol Urodynam 1988; 7:261–262.

20. Wilmore J, Costill L, eds. Physiology of Sport and Exercise. Champaign, IL: Human Kinetics, 1994.

21. American College of Sports Medicine Position Stand. The recommended quantity and quality of exercise for developing and maintaining cardiorespiratory and muscular fitness in healthy adults. Med Sci Sports Exerc 1990; 22:265–274.

22. Pollock M, Gaesser G, Butcher J, Despres J, Dishman R, Franklin B, Ewing Garber C. The recommended quantity and quality of exercise for developing and maintaining cardiorespiratory and muscular fitness, and flexibility in healthy adults. Med Sci Sports Exerc 1998; 30:975–991.

23. Bø K, Talseth T. Long term effect of pelvic floor muscle exercise five years after cessation of organized training. Obstet Gynecol 1996; 87:261–265.

24. Miller JM, Ashton–Miller JA, DeLancey JO. A pelvic muscle precontraction can reduce cough-related urine loss in selected women with mild SUI. J Am Geriatr Soc 1998; 46:870–874.

25. Lagro–Janssen TLM, Debruyne FMJ, Smits AJA, Van Weel C. Controlled trial of pelvic exercises in the treatment of urinary stress incontinence in general practice. Br J Gen Pract 1991; 41:445–449.

26. Wilson PD, Samarrai TA, Deakin M, Kolbe E, Brown ADG. An objective assessment of physiotherapy for female genuine stress incontinence. Br J Obstet Gynaecol 1987; 94:575–582.

27. Laycock J, Knight S, Naylor D. Evaluation of neuromuscular electrical stimulation in the treatment of genuine stress incontinence. Physiotherapy 1998; 84:61–71.

28. Berghmans LCM, Frederiks CMA, deBie RA, Weil EHJ, Smeets LWH, van Waalwijk van Doorn ESC, Janknegt RA. Efficacy of biofeedback, when included with pelvic floor muscle exercise treatment, for genuine stress incontinence. Neurourol Urodynam 1996; 15:37–52.

29. Bø K. Vaginal weight cones. Theoretical framework, effect on pelvic floor muscles strength and female stress urinary incontinence. Acta Obstet Gynecol Scand 1995; 74:87–92.

30. Plevnik S. A new method for testing and strengthening of pelvic floor muscles [abstr]. Proc Int Continence Soc 1985; 267–268.

31. Klarskov P, Nielsen KK, Kromann–Andersen B, Maegaard E. Long-term results of pelvic floor training for female genuine stress incontinence. Int Urogynecol J 1991; 2:132–135.

32. Mouritsen L, Frimodt–Møller C, Møller M. Long term effect of pelvic floor exercise on female urinary incontinence. Br J Urol 1991; 68:32–37.

33. Hahn I, Milsom I, Fall M, Eklund P. Long-term results of pelvic floor training in female stress urinary incontinence. Br J Urol 1993; 72:421–427.

34. Mattiasson A. Management of overactive bladder—looking to the future. Urology 1997; 50(suppl 6A):111–113.

35. Artibani W. Diagnosis and significance of idiopathic overactive bladder. Urology 1997; 50(suppl 6A):25–32.

36. BøK, Berghmans L. Overactive bladder and its treatments. Non-pharmacological treatments: pelvic floor exercises. (in press).

37. Flynn L, Cell P, Luisi E. Effectiveness of pelvic muscle exercises in reducing urge incontinence among community residing elders. J Gerontol Nurs 1994; 23–27.

38. Nygaard IE, Kreder KJ, Lepic MM, Fountain KA, Rhomberg AT. Efficacy of pelvic floor muscle exercises in women with stress, urge, and mixed urinary incontinence. Am J Obstet Gynecol 1996; 174:120–125.

39. Burgio KL, Locher JL, Goode PS, Hardin JM, McDowell BJ, Dombrowski M, Candib D. Behavioral vs drug treatement for urge urinary incontinence in older women. A randomized controlled trial. JAMA 1998; 280:1995–2000.

40. Sleep J, Grant A. Pelvic floor exercises in postnatal care. Midwifery 1987; 158–164.

41. Wilson PD, Herbison GP, Glazener CM, Lang G, Gee H, MacArthur C. Postnatal incontinence: a multicentre, randomised, controlled trial of conservative treatment. Neurourol Urodynam 1997; 16:349–350.

42. Mørkved S, Bø K. The effect of postpartum pelvic floor muscle exercise in the prevention and treatment of urinary incontinence. Int Urogynecol J Pelvic Floor Dysfunct 1997; 8:217–222.

43. Mørkved S, Bø K. Effect of postpartum pelvic floor muscle training in prevention and treatment of urinary incontinence—a one year follow up. Br J Obstet Gynaecol 1999; In Press.

44. Sampselle CM, Miller JM, Mims BL, DeLancey JO, Ashton–Miller JA, Antonakos CL. Effect of pelvic muscle exercise on transient incontinence during pregnancy and after birth. Obstet Gynecol 1998; 91:406–412.

45. Burgio KL, Stutzman RE, Engel BT. Behavioral training for post-prostatectomy urinary incontinence. J Urol 1989; 141:303–306.

46. Jackson J, Emerson L, Johnston B, Wilson J, Morales A. Biofeedback: a noninvasive treatment for incontinence after radical prostatectomy. Urol Nurs 1996; 16:50–54.

47. Libert MH, Steckelmacher P, Jennes M, Fontinoy AM. Rééducation de l'Incontinence masculine après chirurgie de la prostate. Résultats chez 35 patients. Acta Urol Belg 1991; 59:83–92.

48. Meaglia JP, Joseph AC, Chang M, Schmidt JD. Post-prostatectomy urinary incontinence: response to behavioral training. J Urol 1990; 144:674–676.
49. Moore KN, Griffiths D, Hughton A. Urinary incontinence after radical prostatectomy: a randomized controlled trial comparing pelvic muscle exercises with or without electrical stimulation. Br J Urol Int 1999; 83:57–65.
50. Van Kampen M, De Weerdt W, Van Poppel H, De Ridder D, Feys H, Baert L. The effect of pelvic floor re-education on the duration and the degree of incontinence after radical prostatectomy: a randomised controlled trial. Lancet 2000; 355:98–102.

30

Pelvic Floor Reeducation: A Practical Approach

CLAUDIA BROWN

Physiothérapie Polyclinique Cabrini, Montreal, Quebec, Canada

I. INTRODUCTION

Pelvic floor rehabilitation is an increasingly popular, noninvasive approach in the treatment of sphincteric dysfunction, its objectives being the education of the patient and the functional reeducation of the pelvic floor unit. It has been established that the position and relationships between the urinary sphincter, the connective tissue, and the striated musculature of the pelvic floor are important, and that pelvic floor muscle contractility and tone will affect sphincteric activity and urethral closure (1–3).

Prior to the setup of an optimal and individualized treatment program, the patient undergoes a detailed physiotherapy evaluation, including a questionnaire and an examination of the pelvic floor and its related structures.

II. HISTORY

The questionnaire provides valuable information about the presumed diagnosis, history, and symptomatology; evacuation habits for urine and stool; and the effect that the patient's problem has on his or her lifestyle. Also, it is during this initial interview that the relationship of confidence is established between the therapist and the patient, essential for optimum success of the training regimen.

III. PHYSICAL EXAMINATION

The physical examination includes a postural assessment, an evaluation of the movement of the spine and bony pelvis, and a detailed evaluation of the pelvic floor structures. Proprioception and sensation, pelvic floor muscle tone and contractility, elasticity of tissue, and relations between the pelvic floor musculature and adjacent pelvic viscera are assessed, as well as the presence of pain or prolapse. Through surface palpation and internal palpation at the vagina and at the anus, the experienced physiotherapist is able to obtain an impression of the tonus of the superficial layer of perineal musculature, and to evaluate muscular activity and tonus of the left and right portions of the pubococcygeus sling, as differentiated from the left and right iliococcygeus and coccygeus muscles in most patients (4). As the coccyx is an important point of attachment for the pelvic floor musculature and its related fascia (5), the coccygeal position and mobility are also assessed. Pelvic floor response during changes in intra-abdominal pressure is evaluated, with an impression of the production and direction intra-abdominal forces. The downward (inferior) movement of the viscera during increases in intra-abdominal pressures should not be excessive, and the upward (superior) movement should be visible during a pelvic floor contraction and during maneuvers that decrease intra-abdominal pressures (4).

IV. AIMS OF TREATMENT

The goals of physiotherapy treatment are established according to the evaluation. For example, typical goals of treatment for a patient with sphincteric deficiency might be the following:

  To improve dietary and micturition routine, to improve bladder function
  To improve proprioception and body awareness of the pelvic floor, to enable the patient to properly exercise his or her musculature
  To strengthen the pelvic floor muscular contraction, improve contraction speed and endurance, to ameliorate the effect of a pelvic floor contraction on sphincteric closure
  To increase muscle tone
  To optimize functional use of the pelvic floor contraction

In some cases, an adequate pelvic floor contraction may not be obtained because of excess tone or guarding owing to pain, or because of scarring or fibrosis of the surrounding tissues, and the treatment must be adapted to address these issues (6,7). Of equal concern is the resultant vector of force exerted onto the pelvic floor from increases in intra-abdominal pressures. The aim is to decrease the magnitude of the force and to direct it posteriorly, to decrease the transmission of pressures over the bladder and the more anterior portion of the pelvic floor (4).

For sphincteric hypertonicity or dyssynergy, the physiotherapist will again aim to improve the patient's proprioception and body awareness at the pelvic floor level, this time with the purpose of teaching the patient to relax the pelvic floor and voluntary sphincter for micturition. It may also be necessary to decrease any associated hypertonicity or pain in the pelvic floor musculature to achieve the goal of voluntary pelvic floor relaxation.

V. THERAPEUTIC MODALITIES

To achieve the functional rehabilitation of the pelvic floor, there are several modalities that can be employed. These modalities include education, exercise, manual techniques, biofeedback, and electrical stimulation, and all are modalities traditionally used by the physiotherapist in the functional retraining of striated musculature.

A. Education

With the use of a pelvic model, diagrams, literature, and the micturition diary, the patient is given a basic understanding of the urinary system and its function. Taken in consideration of the patient's own symptomatology, this will help motivate the patient for his or her functional rehabilitation. Combined with pelvic floor retraining, this knowledge will allow the patient to learn how and when to use his or her musculature for continence and for micturition.

Patients are advised to avoid the use of bladder stimulants in the diet, especially those containing caffeine (8). The importance of an adequate daily intake of water is underlined, to avoid the likelihood of a more concentrated urine and to maintain a healthy functional bladder capacity (9). This will also decrease the tendency toward constipation, which correlates with urinary incontinence (10–12).

Straining during defecation is discouraged, to decrease undue pressure on the bladder, the pelvic floor, the pudendal nerve, and its branches (13). Patients who have difficulty in evacuating without straining are instructed to use an evacuation technique that encourages relaxation at the anal sphincter combined with the use of the respiratory diaphragm as a piston to gently increase the intra-abdominal pressure (14). This technique alone often results in successful evacuation, but if more pressure is necessary, patients are taught to use the transversus abdominus musculature to increase the pressure and to direct the force posteriorly. Use of the transversus abdominus musculature is also encouraged posturally and for stabilization during strenuous activities (15,16).

The micturition diary is used as a tool for evaluation, as seen in a previous chapter, and also as a learning and training guide (8). These are several formats available. Typically, patients are asked to note the hour and quantify for each micturition on a 24-hr basis, over a period of several days. Episodes of leakage and of urgency are noted, with some detail of the circumstances thereof (e.g., coughing, washing hands). In some cases, fluid intake is also noted. In reviewing the diary with the patient, patterns can be recognized and modified. For example, a patient with a diary showing micturition every hour during the morning, but not in the afternoon, may realize the effect her early coffee intake has on her urinary pattern, and subsequently see the changes caused by abstaining from drinking coffee in the morning. Or, a patient with pollakiuria may see that, of the 21 visits she made to the washroom in 1 day, as many as five were for minimal quantities of urine, whereas her bladder was able to hold quite large quantities on other occasions. This will give her confidence in her bladder's ability to retain urine, and subsequently allow her to wait for longer periods of time between each micturition. Patients with stress incontinence may see the effect of therapy on their urinary diary, in that the episodes of leakage are less frequent or that leakage occurs only during the more strenuous of activities (Fig. 1).

Micturition diaries are also used in institutions to recognize the patient's urinary pattern with the intent of finding a means of control. Timed toileting may be one of these means, whereby the patient is periodically taken to the toilet for micturition to prevent episodes of leakage. Bladder retraining can also be done, by slowly and progressively increasing the period of time between visits to the toilet, helping the patient control for progressively larger quantities of urine (17–19).

The pelvic floor contraction is instrumental in the control of urine, owing to its in-

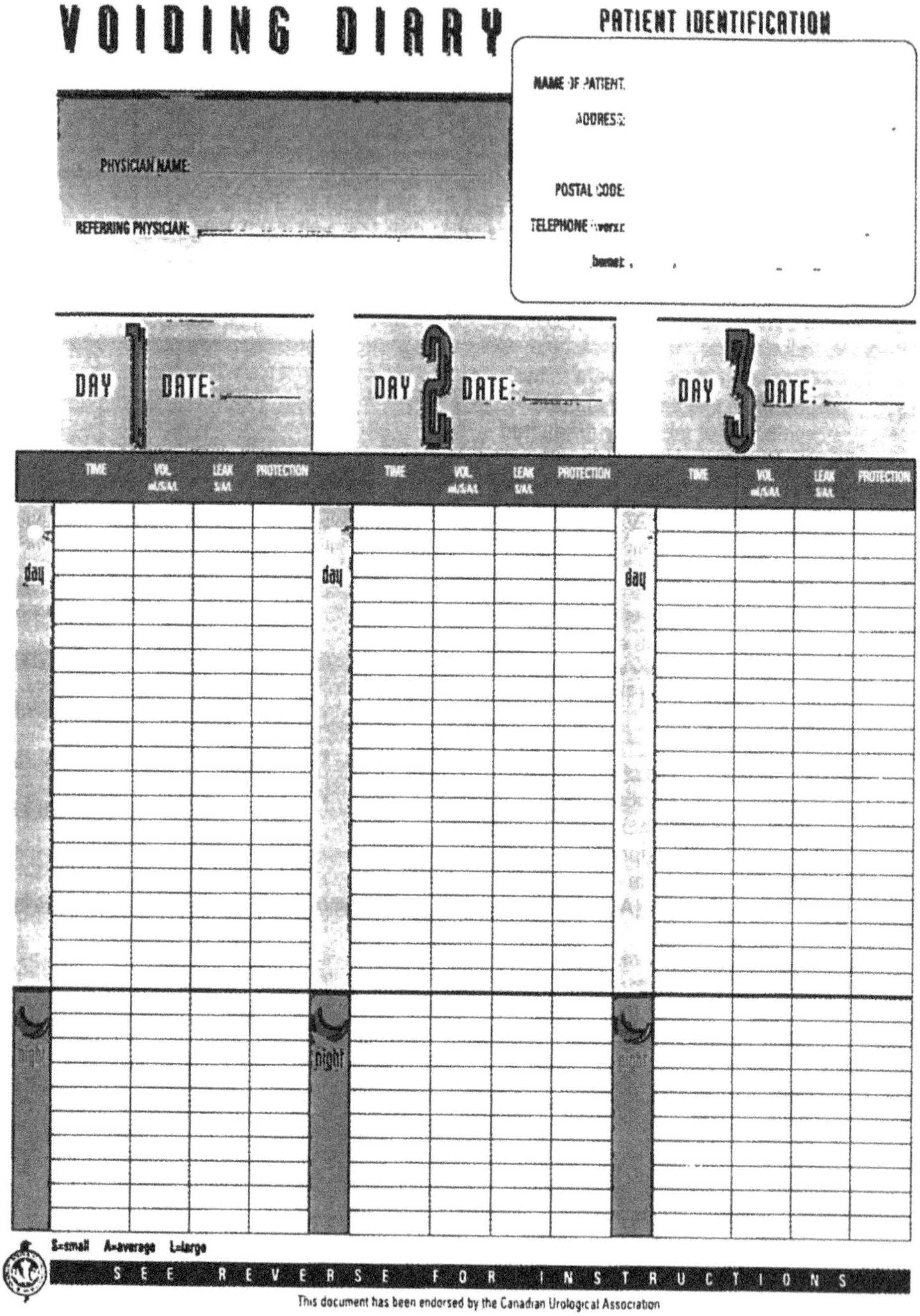

VOIDING DIARY

PHYSICIAN NAME:

REFERRING PHYSICIAN:

DAY 1 DATE:				DAY 2 DATE:				DAY 3 DATE:			
TIME	VOL. mL/S/A/L	LEAK S/A/L	PROTECTION	TIME	VOL. mL/S/A/L	LEAK S/A/L	PROTECTION	TIME	VOL. mL/S/A/L	LEAK S/A/L	PROTECTION
day				day				day			
night				night				night			

S=small A=average L=large

SEE REVERSE FOR INSTRUCTIONS

This document has been endorsed by the Canadian Urological Association

Figure 1 Micturition diary.

hibitory effect on the detrusor muscle and its effect on sphincteric closure (20). Muscle re-training is achieved through a personalized exercise program, which may be augmented by manual techniques, biofeedback, or electrical stimulation.

B. Manual Techniques

The manual physiotherapy techniques used for the pelvic floor musculature are similar to those used for muscle and tissue elsewhere in the body. They can be done on the surface of the perineum, and internally, by vaginal or anal palpation. Techniques such as massage, transverse frictions, proprioceptive stimulation, myofascial release, trigger point pressures, myotatic reflex, muscle energy, mobilizations, passive movements, and manual resistance are used, for a variety of purposes.

Perineal massage, which may be performed internally or externally, helps improve circulation, decrease pain, release adherences, relax the musculature, and improve proprioceptive awareness. It may include transverse frictions, which are done in a direction perpendicular to the muscle fiber to decrease adhesions and pain, and to improve mobility (7). Manual proprioceptive stimulation aims to improve the patient's ability to contract the pelvic floor and may be achieved through directed pressures, stroking or tapping on the skin surface, or internally on the muscle belly. Myofascial release is another manual technique whereby gentle pressure is applied into the direction of fascial restrictions to improve the mobility and function of the myofascial component of the tissue. It is often used in conjunction with trigger-point pressures, which are instrumental in pain relief and the restoration of normal function (6). The bulbocavernosis reflex is used to elicit a myotatic reflex contraction of the pelvic floor by a quick stretch at the introitus, and is used for proprioception and facilitation. With muscle energy techniques, the patient's active contraction is used against a certain resistance to decrease muscular restrictions. Manual resistance is also used for proprioception and for strengthening, and may be applied internally to individual muscle groups as the patient contracts her pelvic floor musculature against pressure exerted by the physical therapist's digits. Mobilizations and passive movements may be performed to decrease pain or improve the mobility and function of the pelvic floor and sacrococcygeal joints (Fig. 2).

These manual techniques are often used in combination to achieve particular goals. Table 1 summarizes some of these goals and the corresponding techniques.

For example, the evaluation of a patient with an incompetent sphincter may demonstrate a very weak pelvic floor contraction, and a lack of proprioception and awareness of the pelvic floor musculature. Useful manual techniques in this case would be those that facilitate a contraction, such as directive pressures, tapping, and the use of the stretch reflex. Another patient, with a hypertonic sphincter, may have hypertonicity in the pubococcygeus portion of the levator ani group. For this patient, techniques such as massage, myofascial release, and trigger point pressures would be employed, to help decrease the tension and promote relaxation of the musculature (6).

C. Biofeedback

Many patients have some difficulty in correctly performing a pelvic floor contraction. This may be due to a lack of understanding of the orientation and function of these muscles, or because of weakness, injury, or dysfunction. Additional factors include social taboos and the relatively hidden location of these muscles. Biofeedback enables patients to visualize

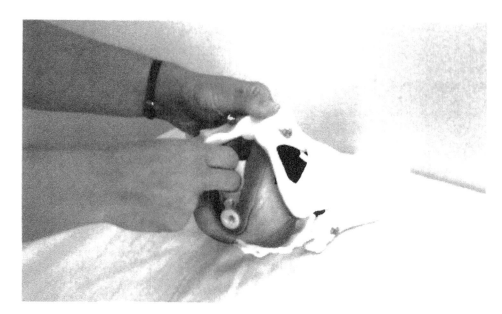

Figure 2   Manual technique demonstrated on pelvic model.

musculature, and see immediately the changes that they are able to effect on their muscular activity. For many, biofeedback makes pelvic floor training more interesting and easier to perform (Fig. 3).

During biofeedback, a physiological response is monitored and displayed. As the patient attempts to change that response, the difference is immediately measured and displayed back to the patient. For pelvic floor retraining, muscular activity can be monitored through its electromyographic (EMG) activity, registered by surface electrodes placed on the perineum or with the use of an intracavity vaginal or anal probe. A mechanical probe can also be used in the vagina or in the anal canal to detect changes in pressure as a result of changes in pelvic floor musculature activity. Various means used to display changes in activity include sound, light bar, digital readout, or through graphics on the screen of a computer monitor (21).

Many patients inadvertently overuse the abdominal muscles in attempting a pelvic floor contraction. For this reason, EMG surface electrodes may be placed on the abdomen, to screen for unwanted contractions of these muscles. Further on, this electrode placement may also be used to help train abdominopelvic synergies, as in ensuring a pelvic floor contraction during increases in intra-abdominal pressures, such as coughing or actively contracting the abdominals (Figs. 3 and 4).

Throughout the training and in planning the exercise regimen, the physiotherapist may want to improve the speed and the endurance, as well as the strength of the contraction to optimize the function of the fast- and slow-twitch muscle fibers. Biofeedback can be particularly useful in these instances. For example, it may be easier for a patient to train for the strong pelvic floor contraction required to prevent leakage during a cough, if she is able to see the increased activity on the biofeedback screen. Or, a patient who requires endurance training will better understand the concept if she sees the activity of her lower-grade and longer-duration contraction displayed in front of her. And, the speed of muscle

Table 1 Manual Physiotherapy Techniques Used in Pelvic
Floor Reeducation

1. Facilitation of the muscular contraction
   Proprioceptive techniques (e.g., directive pressures, tapping)
   Massage
   Manual resistance
   Myotatic reflex
   Passive movements
2. Mobilization
   Osteoarticular: sacrococcygeal
      Passive movements
      Muscle energy
      Joint mobilizations
   Skin, muscle, fascia
      Massage
      Myofascial release
      Stretch
      Muscle energy
3. Strengthening
   Facilitation techniques (for lower muscle testing grades), see above
   Manual resistance
      Pubovaginalis, puborectalis, pubococcygeus bands
      Posterior vaginal wall
      Anorectal angle
      Posterior fibers of pelvic floor (iliococcygeus, coccygeus)
4. Normalization of tone
   Hypotonicity
      Facilitation techniques
      Manual resistance
   Hypertonicity
      Muscle energy techniques
      Massage
      Proprioceptive techniques
      Trigger-point pressures
      Myofascial release
5. Pain modification
   Muscle energy techniques
   Massage
   Proprioceptive techniques
   Trigger-point pressures
   Myofascial release

fiber recruitment can be more easily trained by attempting quick, successive contractions within a time frame clearly defined on the monitor.

With more sophisticated biofeedback units, patients may train by following a pre-programmed activity. The therapist may modify the program to suit the patient's individual requirements, which may change during the course of treatment. This increases the enjoyment of training for many patients, and may be used as a means of evaluating the patient's progress (Figs. 5 and 6).

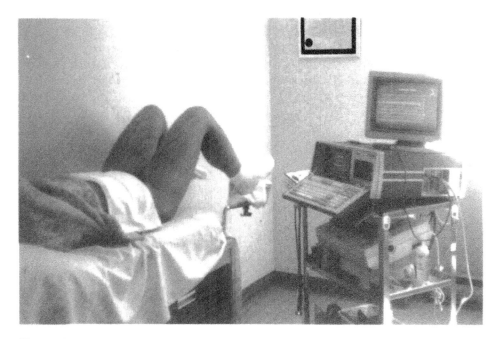

Figure 3   Biofeedback setup.

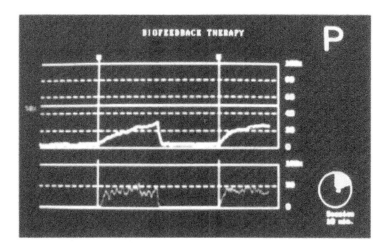

Figure 4   Pelvic activity shown on upper grid; unwanted abdominal activity shown on lower grid.

With surface EMG and intracavity (vaginal or anal EMG), the biofeedback display will vary according to tissue impedance, electrode placement, intracavity electrolyte balance, contact medium, and grounding, among other factors. Accordingly, readouts may also differ from one apparatus to the next. Because of this, absolute values obtained during different treatment protocols cannot readily be used for evaluation or comparison with others, and outcome measures cannot easily be based on these data.

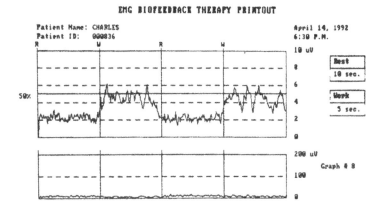

Figure 5 Pelvic activity shown on upper grid; abdominal activity decreased after training.

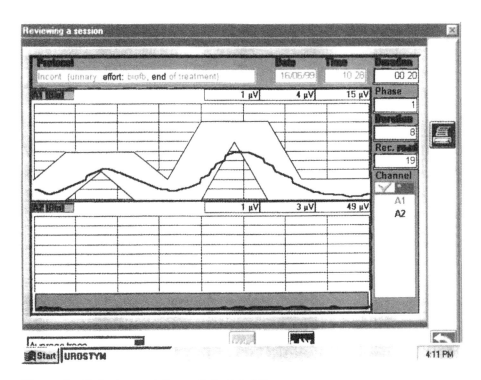

Figure 6 Patients may follow activity template.

D. Electrical Stimulation

Electrical stimulation is used to develop and improve the proprioceptive awareness of the pelvic floor musculature and to facilitate recruitment of muscle fibers. The application of electric current to the pelvic floor musculature produces a reflex muscle contraction by depolarizing the muscle cell membrane (22). In this manner, the patient may experience the sensation of a pelvic floor contraction without having attempted to perform it actively by herself, and may thereby learn to contract it by "imitation." This leads to an improved comprehension of the activity of these muscles and, subsequently, a better active contraction. Also, some muscle fibers that may not respond to an active command, owing to guarding or decreased proprioception, may respond reflexively to electrical stimulation, and recruitment may subsequently be improved through a retraining of neural pathways (23).

With modern muscle stimulation units, the different parameters of the stimulus may be varied. These parameters are waveform, intensity of the current, pulse width, and frequency, ramping of impulses, and on–off timing.

WAVEFORM.   This is the shape of the impulse, depicted on a graph as it relates to a zero line with its positive and negative components. The typical waveform used for muscle stimulation is a rectangular, bipolar, and biphasic waveform. This type of waveform has little or no ionization effect on the tissues and, therefore, will not result in tissue damage.

INTENSITY.   This is the magnitude of current used, depicted on a graph as the height (amplitude) of the curve. It is measured in milliamps (mA), and is often displayed on the apparatus as a percentage of the total available amperage. The typical intensity range for pelvic floor stimulation is from 5 to 35 mA, and will vary with electrode placement and tissue impedance.

PULSE WIDTH (DURATION).   This is the length of time that each individual impulse lasts, measured in milliseconds (msec) or microseconds. It is seen on the graph as the width of the impulse, and for pelvic floor treatment ranges between 0.5 and 5.0 msec.

FREQUENCY.   This is the speed at which the electrical impulses are delivered, and is measured in herz (Hz) or pulses per second (pps). There is much discussion concerning optimal stimulation frequencies for urinary incontinence, as the lower ranges (5–10 Hz) will inhibit the contraction of the detrusor muscle during the stimulation time, and the higher ranges (50–100 Hz) are optimum for urethral closure (24,25). The higher-frequency ranges will often produce a smoother and more comfortable contraction, which may lead to a better learning of the activity.

RAMPING OF IMPULSES.   This is the means by which the height (intensity) of each individual impulse is progressively increased within a train of impulses. This may allow a more comfortable contraction as well as a more natural recruitment pattern.

ON–OFF TIME.   This is the length of time that a train of impulses is delivered, and the rest time between each train. It is suggested that for stimulation at higher frequencies the off time is double that of the on time to allow for adequate recovery between contractions and, thereby, reduce the incidence of fatigue. On–off times are often varied according to each individual patient's tolerance and fatigability.

ELECTRODES.   Delivery of the electric current to the tissues is by an electrode, which

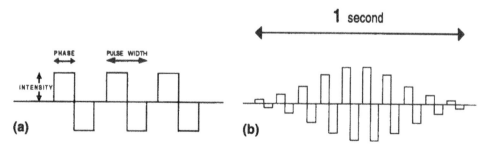

Figure 7   Electrical stimulation parameters: (a) symmetical bypolar biphasic rectangular waveform; (b) 10-Hz frequency, ramped up/down (ampitude modulation).

may be intracavitary (vaginal or anal probe), or on the surface of the skin, usually perianally (Fig. 7).

All the foregoing parameters are preset for the treatment session, except for the intensity. Some apparatus allows an automatic variation of certain parameters within the treatment protocol (e.g., the frequency may be set at a certain level or at a range "sweep" of varying frequencies). The intensity is then increased according to patient tolerance. The patient may feel a tingling sensation, and the sensation of a muscle contraction. This usually coincides with some movement of the probe electrode, caused by the contraction of the stimulated muscle. The aim is to produce a maximal painfree contraction, perceptible by the patient and by the therapist. With the vaginal probe, lower-intensity levels will be required to produce a contraction if the probe is angulated toward the pudendal nerve in Alcock's canal, at an angle of 45-degrees laterally and 45-degrees posteriorly inside the vagina.

It is my opinion that candidates who will most benefit from electrical stimulation are the neurologically intact, who demonstrate little or no active contraction of the pelvic floor, and who have a decreased proprioceptive awareness of the area. Those with a stronger contraction may also benefit from the aforementioned proprioceptive and recruitment advantages. Electrical stimulation is best used in conjunction with an education and exercise program, biofeedback, and manual treatment techniques. The contraindications and precautions to consider in relation to electrical stimulation are summarized in Table 2.

VI. RESULTS

There is no absolute-treatment protocol that is ideal for all patients. Typically, however, patients requiring strengthening may undergo two treatments weekly for 5–6 weeks, in addition to a daily home exercise program. Those requiring pelvic floor relaxation may be seen once or twice weekly for a longer period, again with a home exercise program being of great importance. Patients with comparable evaluation findings may not respond similarly to treatment, and what is successful for one patient may not necessarily be successful for another. Motivation is of utmost importance, as patients are required to undertake much of the training process on their own, and home training must continue once the actual treatment series has finished. The physiotherapist treating pelvic floor disorders should have undergone specialized training for this purpose, and have contact and supportive liaison with other professionals in the field.

Numerous studies attest to the success of exercise and education (26–28), biofeedback (29–31), and electrical stimulation (32–42) in the treatment of urinary incontinence, as well as to the success of different combinations of the aforementioned therapeutic

Table 2 Contraindications and Precautions for Use of Electrical Stimulation

Contraindications to electrical stimulation
   Cardiac pacemaker
   Active vaginal or urinary tract infection
   Active carcinoma in the area
   Pregnancy
Precautions when using electrical stimulation
   Sensory deficit
   Metal implant
   Menstruation (sensation changes, electrode hygiene)
   Fissures

modalities (43–45). However, there is a lack of well-controlled, randomized clinical trials in the literature that give a precise idea of the benefit patients can have using these different treatment modalities (46,47).

The subcommittee on the Conservative Management in Women presented a comprehensive review on the results of conservative management of the incontinent female at the First International Consultation on Incontinence in Monaco in 1988 (48). The following loosely summarizes its findings*:

A. Lifestyle Interventions

It seems reasonable to assume that weight loss of a morbidly obese patient, restriction in physical exercises or heavy lifting activities, treatment of chronic constipation and associated chronic straining, modification of some dietary habits (fluid overload, caffeine consumption, and such) might help reduce urinary incontinence. No scientifically valid article can be found in the literature to substantiate this. Only associations of these factors with incontinence have been reported. Cessation of heavy exercises, caffeine, and massive fluid intake has not been reported to attenuate or prevent urinary incontinence. Surgically induced massive weight loss in the morbidly obese patient may resolve incontinence. Chronic straining associated with constipation may be a risk factor for the development of urinary incontinence.

B. Physical Therapies

The lack of standardization of pelvic floor exercise protocols makes the estimation of the efficacy of exercise difficult. Furthermore, the association of pelvic floor muscle training with other forms of therapies, and the lack of distinction in the reports between cure and improvement make the task even more complicated.

From the published literature, it is estimated that pelvic floor training alone for incontinence (stress, urge, and mixed) is better than no treatment, and that the expected short-term cure improvement rate is in the range of 65–75%. Improvement in symptoms seems more common than cure. No significant difference has been demonstrated in the effectiveness of pelvic floor exercises, with or without biofeedback or intravaginal resistance devices, although possible advantages of these adjuncts may be in terms of teaching, motivation, and compliance.

Probably because of the great variety of devices used and parameters applied in different clinical situations, at this moment there is insufficient evidence to determine whether electrical stimulation is better than no stimulation for women with stress, urge, or mixed incontinence. Results comparing electrical stimulation with sham electrical stimulation are contradictory. Also, it is unclear from the literature whether any particular stimulation protocol is more effective than any other.

The single factor that appears to be most associated with positive outcomes (when using physical therapies) is greater motivation or compliance with the intervention.

---

*The subcommittee on "Conservative Management of Women" presented at the First International Consultation on Incontinence (Monaco, 1998). The subcommittee was chaired by P.D. Wilson (New Zealand), and the members were K. Bø (Norway), A. Bourcier (France), J. Hay–Smith (New Zealand), D. Staskin (USA), I. Nygaard (USA) and J. Wyman (USA). A. Shepherd (U.K.) participated as a consultant. This is the most comprehensive, extensive, and updated review on the results of conservative management of the incontinent female available at the present time. Those who are interested in more details, and wish to consult the relevant bibliography, are kindly requested to consult the original document.

C. Bladder Training

Bladder retraining has been used in the treatment of detrusor instability, genuine stress incontinence, mixed incontinence, and urge incontinence with stable bladder or urodynamic studies. Some evidence in the literature suggests that bladder retraining in these circumstances is an effective treatment, and appears to have benefits similar to drug therapy and may have a greater long-term benefit.

D. Anti-incontinence Devices

More study is required to attest to the success of these devices for conservative management of incontinence.

VII. CONCLUSIONS

In spite of the lack of clear evidence from the published literature, the First International Consultation on Incontinence held in Monaco in 1998 recommended that conservative treatment options should be included in the counseling of incontinent women. And; based on a multidisciplinary panel's analysis of extensive literature reviews, public testimony, and consultant information, the 1996 AHCPR Clinical Practice Guideline for Urinary Incontinence in Adults (26) clearly endorses the use of techniques, such as bladder retraining and pelvic muscle rehabilitation, as "effective, low-risk interventions that can reduce incontinence significantly in varied populations."

There exists an urgent need to elaborate more detailed, randomized, and controlled treatment protocols and to apply these to well-defined, homogeneous patient populations, to conclusively demonstrate the efficacy of the various approaches within the conservative realm of treatment.

REFERENCES

1. Delancey JO. Functional anatomy of the female lower urinary tract and pelvic floor. Ciba Found Symp 1990; 151:57–76.
2. Delancey JO. Structural support of the urethra as it relates to stress urinary incontinence: the hammock hypothesis. Am J Obstet Gynecol 1994; 170:1713–1723.
3. Sampselle CM, Delancey JO. Anatomy of female continence. J Wound Ostomy Continence Nurs 1998; 25:63–70, 72–74.
4. Caufriez M. Thérapies Manuelles et Instrumentales en Urogynecologie, Tome2, Bruxelles: Maite, 1989:9–48, 94–123.
5. Netter FH. Atlas of Human Anatomy. New Jersey: Ciba-Geigy 1989:337–338.
6. Steege, Metzger, Levy. Chronic Pelvic Pain. Philadelphia, Saunders, 1998, pp. 251–254.
7. Travell J. Myofascial Pain and Dysfunction. Baltimore: William & Wilkins; 1983:14–20.
8. Chalker R, Whitmore KE. Overcoming Bladder Disorders. Vol 2. New York: Harper Perennial, 1991.
9. Dowd TT, Campbell JK Jones JA. Fluid intake and incontinence in older community-dwelling women. J Community Health Nurs 1996; 13:179–186.
10. Kerrigan DD, Lucas MG, Sun WM, Donnelly TC, Read NW. Idiopathic constipation associated with impaired urethrovesical and sacral reflex function. Br J Surg 1989; 76:748–751.
11. Meunier P. Syndrome du périnée descendant. Med Digest Nutr 1987; 61:22–26.
12. Bannister JJ, Lawrence WT, Smith A, Thomas DG, Read NW. Urological abnormalities in young women with severe constipation. Gut 1988; 29:17–20.

13. Lubowski DZ, Swash M, Nicholls RJ, Henry MM. Increase in pudendal nerve terminal motor latency with defecation straining. Br J Surg 1988; 475:1095–1097.

14. Valancogne G. Ré-éducation en Colo-proctologie. Paris: Masson, 1993:64–70.

15. Hodges PW. Is there a role for transversus abdominalis in lumbo-pelvic stability? Man Ther 1999; 4:74–86.

16. Hodges PW. Transversus abdominalis and the superficial abdominal muscles are controlled independently in a postural task. Neurosci Lett 1999; 265:91–94.

17. Jarvis GJ, Millar DR. Controlled trial of bladder drill for detrusor instability. Br Med J 1980; 281:1322–1323.

18. Hadley EC. Bladder training and related therapies for urinary incontinence in older people. JAMA 1986; 256:372–379.

19. Burgio KL, Burgio LD. Behavior therapies for urinary incontinence in the elderly. Clin Geriatr Med 1986; 2:809–827.

20. Bradley WE, Rockswold GL, Timm GW, Scott FB. Neurology of micturition. J Urol 1976; 115:481–486.

21. Villet R, Buzelin JM, Lazorthes F. Les Troubles de la Statique Pelvi-perinéale de la Femme. Paris: Vigot, 1995:182–183.

22. Fall M, Lindstrom S. Electrical stimulation: a physiologic approach to the treatment of urinary incontinence. Urol Clin North Am 1991; 18:393–407.

23. Tanagho EA. Electrical stimulation. J Am Geriatr Soc 1990; 38:352–355.

24. Ohlsson B, Lindstrom S, Erlandson BE, Fall M. Effects of some different pulse parameters on bladder inhibition and urethral closure during intravaginal electrical stimulation: an experimental study in the cat. Med Biol Eng Comput 1986; 24:27–33.

25. Erlandson BE, Fall M, Carlsson CA. The effects of intravaginal electrical stimulation on the feline urethra and urinary bladder: electrical parameters. Scand J Urol Nephrol Suppl 1977; 44: 5–18.

26. Fantl JA, Newman DK, Colling J, et al. Urinary incontinence in adults: acute and chronic management. Clinical Practice Guideline, No. 2, 1996 Update. Rockville, MD: U.S. Department of Health and Human Services. Public Health Service, Agency for Health Care Policy and Research. AHCPR Publication. 96-0682. March 1996.

27. Lagro–Janssen TL, Debruyne FM, Smits AJ, van Weel C. Controlled trial of pelvic floor exercises in the treatment of urinary stress incontinence in general practice. Br J Gen Pract 1991; 41:445–449.

28. Bø K, Hagen RH, Kvarstein B, Jørgensen J, Larsen S. Pelvic floor muscle exercise for the treatment of female stress urinary incontinence. III: Effects of two different degrees of pelvic floor muscle exercise. Neurourol Urodynam 1990; 9:489–502.

29. Burgio KL, Robinson JC, Engel BT. The role of biofeedback in Kegel exercise training for stress urinary incontinence. Am J Obstet Gynecol 1986; 154:58–64.

30. Stein M, Discippio W, Davia M, Taub H. Biofeedback for the treatment of stress and urge incontinence. J Urol 1995; 153:641–643.

31. Burns PA, Pranikoff K, Nochajski T, Desotelle P, Harwood MK. Treatment of stress incontinence with pelvic floor exercises and biofeedback. J Am Geriatr Soc 1990; 38:341–344.

32. Bent A, Sand D, et al. Transvaginal electrical stimulation in the treatment of genuine stress incontinence and detrusor instability. Int Urogynecol J 1993; 4:9–13.

33. Caputo RM, Benson JT, McClellan E. Intravaginal maximal electrical simulation in the treatment of urinary incontinence. J Reprod Med 1993; 38:667–671.

34. Eriksen BC, Eik–Nes SH. Long-term electrostimulation of the pelvic floor: primary therapy in female stress incontinence? Urol Int 1989; 44:90–95.

35. Eriksen BC, Mjolnerod OK. Changes in urodynamic measurements after successful anal electrostimulation in female urinary incontinence. Br J Urol 1987; 59:45–49.

36. Fall M. Does electrostimulation cure urinary incontinence? J Urol 1984; 131:664–667.

37. Fall M, Erlandson BE, Nilson AE, Sundin T. Long term intravaginal electrical stimulation in urge and stress incontinence. Scand J Urol Nephrol Suppl 1978; 44:55–63.

38. Kralj B. Conservative treatment of female stress urinary incontinence with functional electrical stimulation. Eur J Obstet Gynecol Reprod Biol 1999; 85:53–56.

39. McGuire EJ, Zhang SC, Horwinski ER, Lytton B. Treatment of motor and sensory detrusor instability by electrical stimulation. J Urol 1983; 129:78–79.

40. Sand PK, Richardson DA, Staskin DR, Swift SE, Appel RA, Whitmore KE, Ostergard DR. Pelvic floor electrical stimulation in the treatment of genuine stress incontinence: a multicenter, placebo-controlled trial. Am J Obstet Gynecol 1995; 173:72–79.

41. Yamanishi T, Yasuda K. Electrical stimulation for stress incontinence. Int Urogynecol J Pelvic Floor Dysfunct 1998; 9:281–290.

42. Yamanishi T, Yasuda K, Sakakibara R, Hattori T, Ito H, Murakami S. Pelvic floor electrical stimulation in the treatment of stress incontinence: an investigational study and a placebo controlled double-blind trial. J Urol 1997; 158:2127–2131.

43. Blowman C, Pickles C, Emery S, Created V, Towell L, Blackburn N, Doyle N, Walkden O. Prospective double blind controlled trial of intensive physiotherapy with and without stimulation of the pelvic floor in treatment of genuine stress incontinence. Physiotherapy 1991; 77:661–664.

44. Cammu H, Van Nylen M, Derde NT, De Bruyne R, Amy JJ. Pelvic physiotherapy in genuine stress incontinence. Urology 1991; 38:332–337.

45. Valiquette L, Paquin JM, Perreault JP, Guertin B, Simard J, Trudel C. La rééducation périnéale dans l'incontinence urinaire d!effort. Ann Chir (Paris) 1991; 45:816–821.

46. Berghmans LC, Hendriks HJ, Bø K, Hay–Smith EJ, de Bie RA, van Waalwijk van Doorn ES. Conservative treatment of stress urinary incontinence in women: a systematic review, of randomized clinical trials. Br J Urol 1998; 82:181–191.

47. Bø K. Effect of electrical stimulation on stress and urge urinary incontinence: clinical outcome and practical recommendations based on randomized controlled trials. Acta Obstet Gynecol Scand 1998; 77(suppl 168):3–11.

48. Wilson DP, Bø K, Bourcier A, Hay–Smith J, Staskin D, Nygaard I, Wyman J. Conservative management in women. In: Abrams P, Khoury S, Wein A, eds. Incontinence. WHO First International Conference on Incontinence, Monaco, 1998. Plymouth: Health Publication 1999:579–636.

31

Intermittent Catheterization

ANANIAS C. DIOKNO

William Beaumont Hospital, Royal Oak, Michigan

BRUCE E. LUNDAK

Bergen Mercy Hospital, Omaha, Nebraska

I. INTRODUCTION

The introduction of intermittent catheterization as a management option for a multitude of urinary bladder or sphincter dysfunctions has changed the practice of urology to a remarkable degree over the past 29 years. The technique involves emptying the bladder (or other urine storage reservoir) on a regular basis with a catheter inserted by the patient or caregiver. The catheter is removed when the bladder is empty. When performed at regular intervals, this technique prevents overdistension of the bladder with urine, while allowing the patient to remain free of a chronically indwelling catheter or other drainage device. Intermittent catheterization is appropriate for children as well as adults, and is applicable to the management of urine storage dysfunction as well as urine emptying dysfunction (1–3). Intermittent catheterization has proved to be a safe, effective, and widely used management option for a variety of urological conditions.

Before the introduction of clean intermittent catheterization (CIC) by Lapides et al. (4) in 1972, sterile intermittent catheterization had been practiced in specialized clinical settings for patients with spinal cord injury and resultant voiding dysfunction, with good results (5,6). However, the fear of repeated introduction of bacteria into the bladder, with subsequent recurrent or chronic urinary tract infection, prevented the application of intermittent catheterization to a wider population. Lapides et al. (4), however, theorized that a well-vascularized urinary tract should have sufficient resistance to bacteria to prevent clinical infection. Bladder overdistension and elevated intravesical pressure decrease blood flow to the bladder mucosa, thereby increasing the risk of infection. They felt that regular bladder emptying by intermittent catheterization would avoid overdistension and high pressures, allowing the bladder to tolerate any bacteria introduced by catheterization (4). They tested this theory on patients of both sexes and with a variety of voiding dysfunctions, and in 1972 released excellent results.

Although seemingly simple in concept, CIC has had a widespread and dramatic influence on urology. Patients with urinary retention caused by neurogenic causes or obstruction can be safely managed with CIC, avoiding chronic indwelling catheters or surgery. Patients with bladder–sphincter dyssynergia can be managed with CIC and anticholinergic therapy, thereby remaining continent and avoiding elevated intravesical pressures. The concept of CIC has been applied to urinary diversions as well, and has allowed the development of continent catheterizable urine reservoirs for both adults and children. In short, CIC has now become a mainstay of urological management.

II. CANDIDATES FOR CIC

Anyone with a bladder or sphincter dysfunction that prevents normal bladder emptying may be a candidate for CIC. The dysfunction may be chronic, as in spinal cord injury, or temporary, as a result of surgery or illness.

Patients who may temporarily require CIC include women with urinary retention after bladder suspension surgery, or men with baseline bladder outlet obstructive symptoms who undergo some type of surgery that results in postoperative urinary retention (e.g., hemorrhoidectomy, herniorrhaphy.) These patients can be expected to have urinary retention of limited duration, and CIC allows them to remain free of an indwelling catheter. These patients may perform their own voiding trials and postvoid residual checks, and in this sense are much more involved in their own recovery than are patients with indwelling catheters (7).

Patients who have a diagnosis of surgically treatable bladder outlet obstruction as a cause of urinary retention may use CIC until the surgery can be performed, or in place of surgery, if they are otherwise poor surgical candidates. A woman awaiting repair of a prolapsing cystocele, or a man planning to undergo transurethral resection of the prostate, for example, could thus be managed. This management may actually reduce the incidence of postoperative infection in comparison with indwelling catheterization.

Chronic bladder emptying dysfunction, often of a neurological etiology, constitutes a common indication for CIC. Patients with neurological conditions, such as myelodysplasia or spinal cord injury, may have a life-long need for CIC. Myelodysplastic children (or their parents) can start CIC at an early age and thereby prevent upper tract damage (8). The advent of CIC has spared many of these patients from invasive surgery, external drainage appliances, and chronic indwelling catheters. Not only has this increased their life expectancy, but CIC allows them to maintain a heightened self-image and sense of control (2,3).

Conditions of a more insidious onset may eventually lead to a neurogenic bladder and the need for CIC. Multiple sclerosis and diabetic peripheral neuropathy are two such diseases. Occasionally, patients who have had a cerebrovascular accident develop an areflexic bladder and, therefore may require CIC.

Chronic, nonneurological conditions may ultimately result in urinary retention and the need for CIC. Patients with chronic bladder outlet obstruction or poor bladder-emptying habits may develop a decompensated, atonic bladder that cannot empty adequately by spontaneous voiding, even after bladder outlet obstruction has been relieved or ruled out.

Some types of incontinence may also be treated with CIC. Obviously, overflow incontinence can be controlled by regular bladder emptying by CIC, if necessary. Patients with detrusor instability or hyperreflexia and resultant incontinence are often managed with anticholinergic therapy, and perhaps an α-adrenergic agonist to improve urinary sphincter tone. If this causes urinary retention, CIC is indicated. Most such patients accept CIC as a preferable alternative to incontinence.

Patients who require urinary diversion for a variety of reasons now have many more options available to them because of CIC. A continent, catheterizable urinary reservoir avoids the need for both a stomal appliance and an indwelling catheter. These principles have been applied to myelodysplastic children and to adults who require cystectomy. The reservoir may be catheterizable through a continent stoma, as in an Indiana or Koch pouch, or through the urethra, as in an orthotopic neobladder. The advent of CIC virtually opened the door to a new phase of reconstructive urological surgery.

In summary, a tremendous spectrum of bladder or sphincter dysfunction can be managed with CIC. The patient must be physically and mentally capable of catheterization on a regular basis, unless a caregiver is willing and able to perform CIC for the patient. While spontaneous, noninstrumented bladder emptying is preferred, CIC provides a safe and effective alternative.

III. NONCANDIDATES FOR CIC

Obviously, a patient must be physically capable of self-catheterization to perform CIC. Quadriplegic patients or those with other conditions that impair manual dexterity may not be able to catheterize themselves. Obesity or other alterations of body habits may also lead to an inability to catheterize. Patients who do not have the mental capacity to understand the rationale and technique of CIC are not good candidates.

CIC may be an option for patients who cannot catheterize themselves, provided they have reliable, around-the-clock caregivers. In such situations, the patient is completely dependent on the caregiver. The provision and reliability of this care should be carefully assessed before prescribing a CIC regimen.

Urethral stricture disease, bladder outlet obstruction, or false passages that prevent safe passage of a urethral catheter are contraindications to CIC. In many such cases, the underlying pathology can be managed such that a catheter can eventually be passed atraumatically. Any continent reservoir that needs catheterization to be emptied, but can no longer be catheterized, requires prompt, continuous drainage by other means until the problem is corrected.

The presence of genitourinary prostheses is not a contraindication to CIC. When properly instructed, patients with a penile prosthesis or an artificial urinary sphincter can catheterize safely (9).

IV. EVALUATION OF POTENTIAL CANDIDATES

The goals of CIC are continent, low-pressure storage of urine for reasonable intervals, with preservation of the upper tracts and ease of catheterization. Evaluation of patients for a CIC regimen should aim at ascertaining that these goals can be met.

Renal function, as measured by serum creatinine levels, should be assessed before and during CIC to monitor for any upper tract involvement.

Cystoscopy and urethroscopy are important to rule out any obstacles to catheterization, including urethral strictures, bladder neck contractures, or false passages. Assessment of the bladder should include the general appearance of the mucosa and detrusor, and the presence of any trabeculation. Bladder calculi or large diverticuli, which may predispose to urinary tract infection, should be managed before beginning CIC. The general appearance of the bladder and urethra should be well documented so that subsequent follow-up cysto-scopic findings can be compared with baseline.

Upper tract imaging should initially include renal ultrasound to rule out any hy-dronephrosis or hydroureter. Ultrasound also permits the assessment of renal parenchyma. If present, the cause of upper tract dilation must be delineated. Hydronephrosis could be due to obstructive uropathy or high-pressure urine storage, but ureteral obstruction or reflux could be another cause. Intravenous pyelography and/or retrograde cystography should, therefore, be performed if the renal ultrasound reveals hydronephrosis. Again, baseline renal ultrasound can be compared with future follow-up ultrasound studies to assess the patient's progress on the CIC regimen.

Urodynamic testing is an important part of the evaluation, and the patient's history and indications for CIC should help determine the extent to which urodynamic studies should be pursued. Bladder capacity is an important factor to document in any patient. For example, a small, contracted bladder of low capacity cannot be expected to store urine at low pressure for reasonable intervals. Such patients may require augmentation cystoplasty in addition to CIC. On the other hand, an atonic bladder can reasonably be expected to store moderate amounts of urine at low pressure.

Intravesical pressures during filling, storage, and voiding, and the presence of unin-hibited bladder contractions are important factors in patients with neurogenic bladder dys-function. Pharmacological therapy with anticholinergic agents may be necessary in these pa-tients to achieve continent, low-pressure urine storage. Repeated urodynamic testing while receiving medical therapy may be undertaken to prove the effectiveness of the therapy.

Sphincter competence and leak-point pressures can also be assessed during urody-namic testing. An insufficient sphincter may not allow continent urine storage between catheterizations. This situation can be managed with α-adrenergic agonists, or surgical therapy if necessary.

The patient's ability to understand and perform CIC is as important as his or her anatomical and physiological parameters on a CIC regimen. The patient should demon-strate not only the skills necessary for catheterization, but knowledge of the importance of catheterization at regular, predictable intervals, and a motivation to rigorously adhere to the regimen. If the catheterization is to be done by a parent or a caregiver, the reliability of these parties should be similarly assessed. A CIC regimen, although well-tailored for a particular patient, can easily fail because of noncompliance. This is best avoided through proper pa-tient selection and instruction.

V. CIC TECHNIQUE AND INSTRUCTION

Physicians and other properly trained health care professionals can instruct patients on the technique of CIC as well as the regimen appropriate for the individual patient. The instruc-tor is an invaluable part of the program, and should provide support and encouragement to the patient as well as technical instruction. The patient should be made to feel that he or she is integral to his or her own care, and that the CIC regimen is important, acceptable, and de-sirable. With training, virtually all properly selected patients should be able to learn CIC.

CIC instruction should include the selection of size, shape, and composition of the catheter that will be the most appropriate and comfortable for the patient. Although a straight 14 or 16F catheter is used most commonly, modifications may be made for children or wheelchair-bound patients. The instructor should be familiar with the various catheters available, and able to help the patient select one that most comfortably meets his or her needs. Use of a water-soluble lubricating agent can also decrease the patient's discomfort.

Patients should be instructed to wash the catheter and their hands with soap and water before and after catheterization. After cleaning, the catheter should be placed in a clean place, such as a plastic bag or carrying pouch, until the next use. It is frequent bladder emptying, rather than catheter sterility, that prevents urinary infection. Therefore, a new, sterile catheter need not be used each time; catheters can be exchanged at 2- to 4-week intervals in most cases.

The catheterization regimen should be tailored to the particular patient. In general, a program should be chosen that ensures storage volumes of less than 400 mL, with catheterization intervals of 3–6 hr. The patient should be educated on the effect that changes in fluid intake or diuretic medications can have on urine output, and the potential need to modify the regimen to accommodate these factors. Anticholinergic medications can be used, as necessary, in appropriate patients to help maintain continence between catheterizations. Finally, patients should be placed on a daily prophylactic dose of antibiotics for the first month of the regimen; this can generally be discontinued thereafter.

VI. FOLLOW-UP

Once on a CIC regimen, periodic assessment of the patient is essential to ascertain that the goals of the regimen are being met. The patient's history can serve to assess continence, catheterization intervals as well as volumes, and ease of catheterization. It is helpful for follow-up if the patient keeps a diary to record this information. The patient should be queried about any symptoms suggestive of urinary tract infection.

Physical examination is essential to rule out signs of significant infection or local complications. It may be helpful to have the patient catheterize in the physician's presence to assess ease of catheterization and the patient's technique. Urinalysis should be performed to examine for abnormally high pyuria or hematuria. A urine culture should be obtained when a clinically significant urinary tract infection is suspected.

Cystourethroscopy is an important element of follow-up, as it allows assessment of the urethra for significant trauma, and of the bladder for stones, foreign bodies, or tumors. Changes indicative of high-pressure storage, such as diverticuli or marked trabeculation, should also be assessed.

Preservation of upper urinary tract function, another goal of CIC, must also be carefully monitored. Serum creatinine level and renal ultrasonography are simple initial measures of this function. More detailed upper tract imaging, such as an intravenous pyelogram, may be necessary if the renal ultrasound suggests significant changes (e.g., hydronephrosis). Nuclear renal scanning may be used to more sensitively evaluate possible renal deterioration (10). Finally, creatinine clearance can accurately assess renal function if the serum creatinine level is abnormal.

The patient's particular history and circumstances should help dictate the required frequency of these follow-up modalities. Initially, patients on a CIC regimen should be seen approximately every 6 months to assure that the regimen is appropriate, and that the patient is comfortable and compliant. After that, annual assessment is usually adequate. Patients with recurrent significant infections, or with a history of high-pressure storage or vesicoureteral reflux, may require more frequent assessment of the upper urinary tract in comparison with patients with low-pressure urinary retention.

VII. COMPLICATIONS

A carefully selected CIC regimen in an appropriately selected patient with proper follow-up should provide safe and effective management of the patient's voiding dysfunction

(11–17). As with nearly any therapy, there can be complications with CIC. Follow-up visits should be aimed at identifying any such complication and addressing it promptly.

A. Urinary Tract Infection

Asymptomatic bactiuria is common in patients on CIC and can generally be ignored. Clinically significant urinary tract infections (UTI) are those that cause signs or symptoms of infection. The true incidence of UTI is difficult to determine when comparing studies on this subject, because of a broad range in the definition of symptoms, and variable patient populations. For example, a patient with intact sensation may have the normally expected signs and symptoms of UTI, whereas a patient with spinal cord injury may exhibit increased spasticity, autonomic dysreflexia, cloudy urine, hematuria, or pyuria. One study on this subject reported an incidence of 44% for clinically significant UTI, 26% for serious UTI (i.e., pyelonephritis, prostatitis), and 3% for urosepsis (18). Other studies have shown a lower incidence of significant UTI in patients on CIC (19,20). One clear risk factor for febrile UTI in patients on CIC is vesicoureteral reflux (21).

Methods of avoiding significant UTI include frequent catheterization, complete bladder emptying, rinsing of catheters with an aseptic solution, or using sterile, disposable catheters (18). Prophylactic antibiotics and antibiotic therapy for asymptomatic bactiuria are generally not warranted (22). Significant infections should be treated with short courses (3 days) of antibiotic therapy, whereas more serious infections such as pyelonephritis require longer courses (10–14 days) of antibiotics. Patients with recurrent, clinically significant UTI, or with vesicoureteral reflux, may benefit from prophylactic antibiotics.

B. Renal Deterioration

An appropriate CIC regimen should rarely contribute to upper urinary tract deterioration. Patients with detrusor hyperreflexia and detrusor–sphincter dyssynergia are obviously more at risk for upper tract damage than are patients with low-pressure urinary retention. Many studies have proved the efficacy of CIC in preserving or improving renal function in these at-risk groups (8,12–14). Such patients may require adjuvant therapy, such as anticholinergics or bladder augmentation, to promote low-pressure urine storage. The periodic assessment of renal function and architecture, by serum creatinine measurement and renal ultrasonography, as discussed previously, is essential to monitor for upper urinary tract changes.

C. Urethral Trauma

Urethral trauma is uncommon in CIC, and occurs mainly in males (11,23). Trauma can cause false passages, stricture disease, urethritis, hematuria, or bladder perforation. In most instances, the trauma is minor and can be managed with an indwelling catheter for a short period.

D. Calculi

Bladder calculi are occasionally seen in patients on CIC. This is frequently due to inadvertent retrograde introduction of a pubic hair into the bladder during catheterization (24). The hair then serves as a nidus for stone formation. Patients should be instructed to carefully avoid such hair introduction during catheterization. Persistent pyuria, hematuria, or recurrent UTI may be signs of a bladder calculus. Such stones can be treated either endoscopically or with open cystolithotomy.

E. Epididymitis

Epididymitis can occur in male patients on CIC, although it is uncommon (20,22). It should easily be treated with oral antibiotics. Patients, especially those with diminished sensation owing to illness or injury, should be instructed to monitor for scrotal changes consistent with epididymitis, and seek treatment promptly.

VIII. SUMMARY

CIC is a safe, effective management option for a spectrum of urological conditions. It may be temporary or chronic, and is useful in children as well as adults. A properly selected CIC regimen in an appropriate patient should permit continent urine storage with upper urinary tract preservation. CIC may be combined with other management modalities, including surgery or medications. The technique is relatively simple to learn and to teach, and with careful follow-up, complications should be few.

REFERENCES

1. Lyon RP, Scott MP, Marshall S. Intermittent catheterization rather than urinary diversion in children with meningomyelocele. J Urol 1975; 113:409–417.
2. Hendren WH. Urinary tract refunctionalization after prior diversion in children. Ann Surg 1974; 180:494–510.
3. Mitchell ME. Urinary tract diversion and undiversion in the pediatric age group. Surg Clin North Am 1981; 61:1147–1164.
4. Lapides J, Diokno AC, Silber SJ, Lowe BS. Clean, intermittent self-catheterization in the treatment of urinary tract disease. J Urol 1972; 107:458–461.
5. Bors E. Intermittent catheterization in paraplegic patients. Urol Int 1967; 22:236–249.
6. Guttmann L, Frankel H. The value of intermittent catheterization in the early management of traumatic paraplegia and tetraplegia. Paraplegia 1966; 4:63–84.
7. Furuhata A, Ogawa K, Saito K, Yamagushi T. Preoperative intermittent catheterization in patients with prostatic hypertrophy. Clin Ther 1988; 10(special ed.):47–51.
8. Kasabian NG, Bauer SB, Dyro FM, Colodny AH, Mandell J, Retik AB. The prophylactic value of clean intermittent catheterization and anticholinergic medication in newborns and infants with myelodysplasia at risk of developing urinary tract deterioration. Am J Dis Child 1992; 146: 840–843.
9. Diokno AC, Sonda LP. Compatibility of genitourinary prostheses and intermittent self-catheterization. J Urol 1981; 125:659–660.
10. Lloyd LK, Kuhlmeier KV, Fine PR, McEachran AB, Stover SL. Prediction of pyelocaliectasis in follow-up of patients with spinal cord injury. Br J Urol 1987; 59:122–126.
11. Lapides J, Diokno AC, Lowe BS, Kalish MD. Follow-up on unsterile, intermittent self-catheterization. J Urol 1974; 111:184–187.
12. Diokno AC, Sonda LP, Hollander JB, Lapides J. Fate of patients started on clean intermittent self-catheterization therapy ten years ago. J Urol 1983; 129:1120–1122.
13. McGuire EJ, Savastano JA. Long-term follow-up of spinal cord injury patients managed by intermittent catheterization. J Urol 1983; 129:775–776.
14. Lin–Dyken DC, Wolraich ML, Hawtrey CE, Doja MS. Follow-up of clean intermittent catheterization for children with neurogenic bladders. Urology 1992; 40:525–529.
15. Whitelaw S, Hammonds JC, Tregellas R. Clean intermittent self-catheterization in the elderly. Br J Urol 1987; 60:125–127.
16. Hill VB, Davies WE. A swing to intermittent clean self-catheterization as a preferred mode of

management of the neuropathic bladder for the dextrous spinal cord patient. Paraplegia 1988; 26:405–412.

17. Robinson RO, Cockram M, Strode M. Severe handicap in spina bifida: no bar to intermittent self-catheterization. Arch Dis Child 1985; 60:760–762.

18. Berkov S, Das S. Urinary tract infection and intermittent catheterization. Infect Urol 1998; 11: 165–168.

19. Bakke A, Digrames A. Bacteriuria in patients treated with clean intermittent catheterization. Scand J Infect Dis 1991; 23:577–582.

20. Bakke A, Vollset SE, Hoisaeter PA, Irgens LM. Physical complications in patients treated with clean intermittent catheterization. Scand J Urol Nephrol 1993; 27:55–61.

21. Kass EJ, Koff SA, Diokno AC, Lapides J. The significance of bacilluria in children on long-term intermittent catheterization. J Urol 1981; 126:223–225.

22. Mohler JL, Cowen DL, Flanigan RC. Suppression and treatment of urinary tract infection in patients with intermittently catheterized neurogenic bladder. J Urol 1987; 138:336–340.

23. Maynard F, Diokno AC. Clean intermittent catheterization for spinal cord injury patients. J Urol 1982; 128:477–480.

24. Solomon MH, Koff SA, Diokno AC. Bladder calculi complicating intermittent catheterization. J Urol 1980; 124:140–141.

32

Treatment of the Sphincter: Medical Therapy

SCOTT E. LITWILLER

Oklahoma University and St. Francis Memorial Hospital, Tulsa, Oklahoma

I. INTRODUCTION

Medical treatment for sphincteric pathology is often pursued as a first-line approach for the patient with either incontinence or obstructive voiding. The decision to pursue medical therapy may be patient-driven and based on the desire to avoid more aggressive invasive procedures. Alternatively, the decision may be physician-driven and possibly prompted by these same desires. The basis for the medical approach stems from the qualities that the sphincter possesses, both as an autonomically innervated organ (internal sphincter) and a skeletal muscle (external sphincter). The distinction should be made when approaching therapy between whether the target of treatment is the smooth internal sphincter (bladder neck) or the striated external sphincter. The medical approach to the treatment of the dysfunctional sphincter may be divided practically into medications to either enhance sphincteric function (as in stress incontinence) or weaken sphincteric function (as in dyssynergia or voiding dysfunction) and promote bladder emptying. The knowledge of these types of therapies, their benefits and risks, therefore, is essential for the clinician who cares for any patient with incontinence, voiding dysfunction, or neurogenic bladder.

II. MEDICAL THERAPY FOR THE HYPERACTIVE SPHINCTER

The general approach to the overactive sphincter must take into account the potential pathophysiology and level of obstruction. Obstruction to flow at the level of the sphincter may result from neurogenic as well as functional causes (1,2). As obstruction may occur at the level of the internal sphincter (bladder neck) or the external sphincter (striated sphincter) (3), proper diagnosis of the level of obstruction as well as the etiology of obstruction is essential for effective treatment. Traditionally, intermittent catheterization has been the standard for treatment of the hyperactive or dyssynergic sphincter. However, many patients cannot personally perform intermittent catheterization and may not have an appropriate caregiver who can perform it for them. The Crede maneuver has been advocated, but it is an inefficient method of bladder emptying even when accompanied by voiding (4). Conversely, many patients with hyperactive sphincter activity may be bothered by symptoms, but do not feel their case significant enough to warrant intermittent catheterization. These patients obviously will benefit most from a conservative medical regimen to assist their voiding dysfunction. See Appendix at the end of this chapter.

A. At the Smooth (Internal) Sphincter Level

1. Physiologic Considerations

In 1973, Krane and Olsson presented the concept of an internal physiological sphincter located in the bladder neck and proximal urethra (5,6). This sphincter was felt to be under tonic control of the sympathetic nervous system. Since that time, the use of α-adrenergic antagonists has extended into treatment of benign prostatic hyperplasia (BPH) as well as experimental use for smooth and striated sphincteric dyssynergia (7).

The rationale for the use of α-adrenergic antagonists in treating sphincteric dysfunction is based on a number of principles. In patients with neurogenic dysfunction, parasympathetic decentralization can account for an increased adrenergic innervation of the bladder and proximal urethra (8,9). α-Receptor supersensitivity was noted in the bladder neck and proximal urethra of patients with neurogenic bladders. Experimental evidence has also supported the activity of central noradrenergic neurons in mediating the tonic facilitation of sympathetic and somatic activity to the pelvic floor (10,11). The importance of central α-receptor function on sphincteric activity is further supported by the action of clonidine on the pelvic visceral sympathetic tone and urethral pressure profile (12). However, probably the most widely recognized effect of α-blockers (α_1) on the internal sphincter is their direct effect on smooth-muscle relaxation at the level of the bladder neck and proximal urethra (5,6,13–15). Thus, in patients with obstruction at the level of the bladder neck (internal sphincter), α-blocker therapy may represent a viable treatment option. There does exist, however a subset of younger male patients with vesical neck obstruction for whom α-blocker therapy fails and for whom endoscopic incision provides good results (3).

2. α-Adrenergic Blockers

Phenoxybenzamine was the first α-receptor blocker used for the treatment of voiding dysfunction. It possesses both α_1 and α_2 properties and is usually given in doses from 10 to 20 mg/day. Its use has been significantly curtailed, because a experimentally it causes peritoneal sarcomas, lung tumors, and gastrointestinal tumors in rats (16). Prazosin was the first widely used α_1-specific receptor blocker. It selectively inhibits α-adrenergic receptors in the proximal urethra and prostate and is dosed three times per day (17). Side effects are primarily due to its α_1 blockade and include asthenia, dizziness, dry mouth, syncope, and palpitations. Some patients experience a first-dose phenomenon caused by acute postural hypotension. This problem may be lessened, however, by administering the first dose at bedtime and by starting at an initial dose of 1 mg. Although the maximal dose is 20 mg/day, doses commonly range between 9 and 12 mg/day. Newer long-acting ($t_{1/2}$ = 12 hr) postsynaptic α_1-antagonists, such as terazosin and doxazosin, have been developed and are given once per day (bedtime) (18). Doses usually range from 5 to 10 mg/day for terazosin and 4 to 10 mg/day for doxazosin. These agents have been widely successful and their convenient dosage has greatly facilitated patient compliance. Side effects are similar to prazosin and, although these two drugs are fairly similar, terazosin is said to have a fourfold greater affinity for α_1-receptors than doxazosin (19). Alfuzosin and tamsulosin are new superselective α-antagonists that reportedly have a greater affinity for α_1-receptors in the prostatic capsule and urethra. They are reported to have a better side effect profile than traditional α-blockers, but may sacrifice efficacy in some patients owing to their diminished central α-effects. Doses range from 7.5 to 10 mg/day in three divided doses for alfuzosin and 0.4 mg/day for tamsulosin.

B. At the Level of the Striated Sphincter

At present, there is no class of drugs that selectively inhibit the external sphincter or the pelvic floor. Most attempts to accomplish this function make use of generalized antispasticity drugs or muscle relaxants: benzodiazepines, dantrolene, and baclofen (20). Although effective for generalized spasticity, the side effect profile of these drugs often limits their use relative to the control of external sphincter spasm. The use of α-adrenergic blockers, although relatively innocuous, has met with mixed results. Consequently, new drug delivery systems (baclofen pumps), injectable agents (botulinum toxin, phenol block) and intraurethral agents (capsaicin) are being pursued in an attempt to better treat external sphincter spasm in a conservative fashion (21–25).

1. α-Adrenergic Blockers

The extent to which α-adrenergic agent's peripheral effect is attributable to an action on the striated sphincter or merely the bladder neck is debated. Initially described in the cat, El-badawi reported adrenergic innervation to the striated sphincter (26). However, subsequent studies by Wein (27), failed to support this finding. In work by Crowe, (28), using the glyoxylic acid method to visualize catecholamines, adrenergic nerve fibers were found around and along the edge of striated muscle bundles. Additionally, blood vessels in the region of both sphincters were innervated by adrenergic nerves (28). In work by Thind et al. (29), prazosin (α_1-selective) decreased urethral closure pressure in the area of the high-pressure zone, but not the entire course of the skeletal muscle bundles, suggesting an effect at the level of the urethral sphincter.

    The importance of central nervous system (CNS) α-receptor activity on external sphincter function has been supported by both Gajewski (30) and Pederson (31) in separate studies using both prazosin and thymoxamine. In these studies, the effect of α-blockade on the external urethral sphincter was felt to be mediated by central α-adrenergic effects, with only modest peripheral effects. These effects may be mediated by inhibition of central sympathetic and somatic outflow on the lower urinary tract. Additionally, beneficial effects may arise from the central action of nonselective α_1-blockers, with or without a decrease in perineal striated muscle activity (10). The importance of central α-receptor effects is further supported by the fact that clonidine, a centrally presynaptic α-agonist, decreases electromyographic (EMG) activity in both urethral and anal sphincters, an effect that is reversible by norepinephrine and yohimbine (32).

    In a study by Herman et al. (33), clonidine not only decreased detrusor sphincter dyssynergia, but also decreased detrusor pressure and systemic blood pressure.

    Phentolamine (which crosses the blood–brain barrier) but not phenoxybenzamine (which does not) decreases external sphincter activity. This further supports the central role of α-receptor activity in affecting sphincteric function (12). Nanninga et al. (34), however, demonstrated that EMG activity of the external sphincter decreased after phentolamine administration in three paraplegic patients, and they attributed this action to a direct sympathetic effect on external sphincter. This data is in contrast with that of Rossier and co-workers (35), who used pudendal nerve blocks and phentolamine to study the activity of the external sphincter in external sphincter dyssynergia. They concluded that there was no sympathetic innervation of the striated sphincter in humans and that sphincter dyssynergia was mediated through pudendal nerves through spinal reflex arcs. They also concluded that the effects of α-receptor blockers were mediated through their effects on pelvic sympathetic ganglions and secondarily by their depressant effects on the bladder smooth muscle (35).

The degree to which these investigational findings translate into practical clinical scenarios, however, is debated. Reported results vary greatly and range from 17 to 80% in various series (7,36,37). Studies by Chancellor (38) found that the α_1-selective blocker terazosin had no effect on the striated sphincter function in spinal cord-injured patients. In this study, 15 patients with a videourodynamic diagnosis of external sphincter dyssynergia, but internal sphincter synergy were treated with terazosin (5 mg/day) and voiding pressures were assessed before and after terazosin therapy. Voiding pressures averaged 92 ± 17 cmH$_2$O before therapy and 88 ± 27 cmH$_2$O after therapy (p = 0.48) (38). The underlying etiology behind an individual patient's voiding dysfunction may, however, play a crucial role in the outcomes obtained with α-blocker therapy because O'Riordan found α-blockers to have some limited use in male patients with obstruction from multiple sclerosis (37). Although the use of α-blockers for external sphincter dysfunction, is limited, they may represent a reasonable initial treatment for patients who are not candidates for other methods of therapy.

2. Benzodiazepines

Traditionally used as antianxiolytics and antispasmodics, benzodiazepines potentiate the action of γ-aminobutyric acid (GABA) at both presynaptic and postsynaptic sites in the brain and spinal cord (39). Benzodiazepines potentiate the affinity of GABA receptor sites on CNS membranes as well as augmenting presynaptic inhibition of neurotransmitter release. Glycine and GABA are recognized as the primary inhibitory transmitters in the spinal cord, and their potentiation by benzodiazepines has had a beneficial effect on skeletal muscle spasticity (39,40). Some, however, feel that the muscle relaxant effects, seen with benzodiazepines are primarily due to their CNS depressant effects, as these same medications are commonly used to treat anxiety disorders, insomnia, and serve as preoperative sedatives (41).

Few studies have critically evaluated the use of benzodiazepines for the treatment of external sphincter dyssynergia. Anecdotal reports have encouraged the use of diazepam in small doses (2 mg) every 2–3 hr (42). However, there are no clinical trials to support this rationale for treatment. In a small study, diazepam was helpful in promoting postoperative voiding in females undergoing bladder neck suspension; however, the mechanism for this effect was not determined (43).

Perhaps the best use for oral benzodiazepines is in the case of functional voiding disorders in neurologically intact patients (44). This clinical entity, also known as pseudodyssynergia, nonneurogenic neurogenic bladder, Hinman–Allen syndrome, or pelvic floor dysfunction, is defined as voluntary striated sphincter and perineal pelvic floor contraction during micturition or attempts to initiate micturition. It may be differentiated from true dyssynergia by the absence of neurological deficit and may be considered a functional or learned behavior (1,2,45,46). Again, clinical trials to support efficacy in these patients are lacking, and the basis for this use may be largely intuitive. Whether improvement in these instances is due to the antianxiety effect of these drugs or to an actual effect on the striated skeletal muscle of the sphincter remains debated. Side effects of benzodiazepines include fatigue, weakness, tachyphylaxis, somnolence, and addiction. Consequently, their use for the treatment of voiding dysfunction should be carefully monitored.

3. β-Adrenergic Agents

The basis for the use of β-adrenergic agents on the sphincter lies in their ability to produce relaxation in slow-twitch skeletal muscles (47). As the outermost portion of the sphincter consists of slow-twitch fibers, β-agonists may have a theoretical effect on sphincteric function (48). β-Adrenergic stimulation has experimentally decreased urethral resistance and urethral closure pressure (terbutaline) (49,50). Other authors have found conflicting data; namely, that β-agonists potentiate the contractility of fatigued urethral muscle (51). Clinically, β-adrenergic agents have little use in the treatment of sphincteric dysfunction, and their use is not widely accepted.

4. Dantrolene Sodium

Dantrolene sodium is a skeletal muscle relaxant that dissociates excitation contraction coupling by inhibiting calcium release at a site distal to the motor end plate in the sarcoplasmic reticulum (52). It preferentially affects fast-twitch skeletal muscle fibers and reduces reflex more than voluntary contractions. In contrast, dantrolene has no effect on detrusor muscle function (53).

Dantrolene has been used to treat external sphincter dyssynergia for over 20 years. Murdock (54) first reported its use in six patients with clinical dyssynergia. Of these patients, five responded clinically with decreased postvoid residuals and improved voiding, as seen on cystourethrography. Voiding pressures were not, however, assessed. In subsequent studies by Hackler (55), 8/15 patients with external sphincter spasm responded to dantrolene with improvement in their postvoid residuals and urethral pressure profiles. Dosages in this study started at 25 mg/day and titrated up to 400 mg/day. Dosages were further increased to 600 mg/day if there was no evidence of clinical efficacy. In this study, 12/15 patients reported significant weakness, malaise, fatigue, and dizziness (55).

Side effects of dantrolene are not limited solely to somatic complaints. Fatal hepatitis has been noted in 0.1–0.2% of patients treated for more than 2 months. Nonfatal hepatitis has been reported in 0.5% and liver function abnormalities in 1%. These risks are approximately doubled in females (56).

Consequently, the most common current use of dantrolene is in the treatment of malignant hyperthermia, a rare hereditary condition characterized by excess release of calcium from the sarcoplasmic reticulum. Patients with this condition develop shaking skeletal muscle contractions accompanied by life-threatening hyperthermia (56).

5. Botulinum Toxin

Botulinum toxin is a naturally occurring inhibitor of acetylcholine release at the striated neuromuscular junction. Its use for the treatment of skeletal muscle spasm has varied widely, and it has been used for the treatment of external sphincter dyssynergia for over 10 years (57). During treatment, botulinum toxin is injected directly into the external sphincter by a transurethral or transperineal route (23,58). Although both routes seem equally efficacious, a study by Schurch (58) revealed an advantage in favor of the transurethral route.

Detailed gadopentetate-enhanced magnetic resonance imaging (MRI) reveals that EMG-directed injection of botulinum toxin is localized to the area of the external sphincter and does not diffuse into the surrounding tissues (59).

A variety of treatment regimens have been used, and dosages range from 25 to 250 international units (IU) (58). The dosing interval has also varied greatly, however, in a randomized comparison study by Schurch, three successive injections of 250 IU at 1 month was most efficacious (58). Urodynamic studies in patients with detrusor–sphincter dyssynergia (DSD) have shown favorable responses in 88–100% of patients (57,58). Primary endpoints include up to a 50% decrease in voiding pressure and amplitude of unstable contractions. Although the efficacy of botulinum toxin A has met with good success, results are temporary and require repeat periodic injections. Neurologically normal patients or those with complex repetitive discharges of the urethra have responded poorly to botulinum toxin A (60). With repetitive use, patients may form antibodies to this toxin. However, there has been no correlation noted between the amount of antibodies present and length of treatment.

6. Phenol Block

The concept of percutaneous nerve blockade is not, however, limited to botulinum toxin A. Success with botulinum toxin A has led some to investigate a more permanent pharmacological blockade of external sphincter activity (61). In a small study of seven patients, 7% phenol was injected directly into the pudendal nerve with EMG localization. Results with this treatment are limited, and further follow-up is clearly needed.

7. Baclofen

Originally thought to function as a classic GABA(A) agonist (20,39), baclofen is currently felt to act as a GABA(B) agonist in the brain and spinal cord. Baclofen inhibits mono- and polysynaptic reflexes by producing presynaptic hyperpolarization of dorsal root terminals, thereby increasing the threshold for excitation of primary afferent nerve terminals in the spinal cord (62). These specific effects are thought to be mediated by modulation of potassium conductance and calcium influx. Additionally, baclofen may antagonize substance P-induced depolarization of spinal cord motor neurons (63). Its direct effect on spasticity is related to its normalizing interneuron activity and decreasing motor neuron activity in the spinal cord (64).

Traditionally, baclofen has been used to treat neurogenically mediated skeletal muscle spasticity (20). Its use in DSD and voiding dysfunction draws its basis from experimental data showing that activation of GABA receptors in the pons and sacral spinal cord may inhibit external sphincter activity (65,66). These effects are accomplished at the rhabdosphincter by depressing pudendal–pudendal and pelvic–pudendal nerve reflexes (67).

Although used for over 20 years, oral baclofen's role in the treatment of sphincteric dysfunction is rather limited because its difficulty in passing through the blood–brain barrier necessitates higher doses that are often accompanied by significant systemic side effects, such as weakness, dizziness and drowsiness, rash and pruritis, and hallucinations (68). In a study by Leyson et al. (69), baclofen was beneficial in reducing the postvoid residuals of 73% of patients, but at a dose of over 120 mg/day (20 mg every 4 hr). Hachen found daily doses of 75 mg ineffective in treating voiding dysfunction in the spinal cord injury population but 20 mg IV was very effective (70).

Consequently, the use of intrathecal baclofen delivery systems has received a great deal of attention for the treatment of spasticity (71). Baclofen has distinct effects on both bladder and external sphincter function (24,34,72). In these studies, the number of patients with external sphincter dyssynergia ranged from one to four, making statistical analysis difficult. There was, however, a consistent trend toward improvement in sphincter function. In a study of ten patients by Steers (72), three patients demonstrated DSD, and all noted improvement in sphincter activity. In a number of patients, this improvement in sphincter function was accompanied by a decrease in bladder contractility and an increase in postvoid residual (72). Consequently, the use of intrathecal baclofen solely for the purpose of reducing sphincteric function is not well supported.

III. MEDICAL THERAPY FOR THE INCOMPETENT SPHINCTER

Incontinence and social distress from an incompetent sphincter is a significant clinical problem for a large percentage of the adult population. In a study supported by the National Institute on Aging, Diokno and colleagues (73) conducted a longitudinal and cross-sectional study on 1955 elderly respondents, age 60 and older. In this study, the prevalence of incontinence was 37.6% overall and the prevalence of female stress incontinence was 26.7% (73). Many of these patients have mild degrees of incontinence, do not desire aggressive treatment measures, or are elderly and are poor operative candidates. The economic significance of incontinence is further supported by the more than 1 billion dollars that are spent on adult diapers and absorbent products per year (74). Many patients with these symptoms seek conservative measures to treat their incontinence. The physician who is called on to treat these symptoms, therefore, must be familiar with the current medical and conservative therapy available for the treatment of sphincteric weakness or stress incontinence. See Appendix at the end of this chapter.

A. α-Adrenergic Agonists

The smooth and striated sphincters posses α-adrenergic receptors which, when stimulated, produce an increase in urethral pressure and resistance (29). Clinically, treatment with α-adrenergic agonists produces an increase in maximal urethral pressure (MUP) and maximal urethral closure pressure (MUCP) (75). These qualities have been effectively utilized to treat stress incontinence for over 50 years (ephedrine) (76). A variety of α-agonists exist. Most are available as over-the-counter preparations of decongestants or appetite suppressants. Although efficacy varies with the drug and dosage used, all share a similar side effect profile. Side effects include hypertension, anxiety, tremor, anorexia, palpitations, respiratory difficulties, and cardiac arrhythmia. Accordingly, they should be used with caution in patients with cardiovascular disease and hypertension.

    Ephedrine is a noncatecholamine sympathomimetic that enhances the peripheral release of norepinephrine and directly stimulates both α- and β-adrenoceptors. Although tachyphylaxis has been reported as a result of continued use (from depletion of norepinephrine stores), a study reported maximal results only after 2 weeks of use (77). In a placebo-controlled, randomized study by Diokno, 27 of 38 patients reported a good to excellent response when treated with ephedrine sulfate. Patients in this study with more severe degrees of incontinence, however, fared worse than those with mild to moderate degrees of incontinence (78). Obrink, however, noted no significant change in urethral pressure in patients taking 100 mg/day of norephedrine and did not consider it an alternative to therapy (79). Pseudoephedrine is a stereoisomer of ephedrine and is a commonly used substitute for it. Its efficacy and side effects are similar to ephedrine. The adult dosage of both ephedrine and pseudoephedrine is 30–60 mg three to four times per day, and it is available without a prescription.

    Phenylpropanolamine hydrochloride (PPA) is also an α-agonist with effects similar to those of ephedrine and pseudoephedrine. Its primary advantage is that is causes less central stimulation and may have a more advantageous side effect profile. It also is available without prescription and has been used in the treatment of stress incontinence for over 20 years (80). Numerous studies have reported the effects of PPA on urodynamic parameters (MUCP, MUP) and on mild stress incontinence (81,82). The AHCPR guideline panel (Urinary Incontinence Guideline Panel, 1992) reports eight randomized studies with PPA for stress incontinence in female patients. The results obtained (minus placebo response) were reported: cure(0–14%), improvement (19–60%), side effects (5–33%), and dropouts (0–4.3%) Preparations of PPA are often formulated as decongestants (Ornade) and sometimes contain an antihistamine (chlorpheniramine), but the dose of PPA is usually 50–75 mg twice per day. The reported side effects with PPA vary, and although some cite a concern over blood pressure elevation (83), larger studies have found little or no significant cardiovascular or autonomic side effects with the use of PPA (84,85). When side effects were present, however, they were more commonly seen with the sustained-release preparation (75 mg) over the regular 25-mg dose.

B. Imipramine

In addition to its well-recognized effect on detrusor activity, imipramine is noted to have specific α-adrenergic effects on the sphincter as well (86). In the presynaptic cleft, imipramine blocks reuptake of released amine neurotransmitters (norepinephrine and serotonin) There is direct in vitro evidence that the effect of imipramine on norepinephrine reuptake occurs in the lower urinary tract as well as sphincter, thus accounting for its α-agonistic properties (87). Clinically, the use of imipramine has largely been limited to the conservative treatment of stress incontinence and nocturnal enuresis (88). In a study by Castledon (89), 60% (6/10) of elderly patients became continent when taking imipramine. In posttreatment studies, maximal urethral pressure (MUP) increased by a mean of 30 cmH$_2$O. In this study, a nighttime dosage of 25 mg was increased by 25 mg every 3 days until continence was achieved or side effects precluded further escalation (89). Although imipramine may be used for its α-adrenergic activity, side effects may limit its full use. These are most commonly seen in the elderly and consist of weakness, fatigue, somnolence, and postural hypotension. Imipramine also may produce cardiac arrhythmias; consequently, its use in patients with cardiac disease is cautioned. Abrupt cessation of this drug in patients receiving high doses may result in abdominal pain, nausea, vomiting, headache, and lethargy. Thus, patients should be weaned slowly if a decision is made to discontinue its use (90).

C. Estrogen Therapy

The use of estrogen therapy to augment sphincteric function is based on a variety of experimental studies documenting the presence of estrogen receptor activity in both the smooth and striated sphincters (91,92). α-Receptors in the rabbit urethra were found by Hodson to demonstrate estrogen sensitivity and could be decreased by castration. This effect, however, was, reversed by readministration of estrogen (93). In a similar study, Larsson reported that estrogen treatment of the isolated rabbit urethra caused an increased number and sensitivity of α-receptors to norepinephrine (94). Additional in vitro effects of estrogens include the hyperpolarization of urethral smooth muscle and the blockade of extraneuronal reuptake of catecholamines, thereby potentiating α-agonist effects (95,96).

The additive effect of estrogens on α-agonists for the treatment of stress incontinence was supported in a study by Beisland (97). Patients were randomized to phenylpropanol-amine (PPA), 50 mg twice daily, or estriol suppositories 1 mg/day. Patients then crossed-over and received both PPA and estriol suppositories. Although improvement was noted with both individual therapies, combination therapy was the most beneficial.

Conflicting studies exist and, in some cases, fail to show any significant effect of es-trogen therapy. Bump reported (98) that estrogen administered to castrate female baboons enhanced the urethral sphincter mechanism as a whole, but the effects were not due to stri-ated muscle effects. He concluded that changes may be related to smooth-muscle changes, mucosal changes, or a combination of both. In a urodynamic study by Rud (99), 4 and 8 mg of estriol were administered to 27 patients. No significant changes in urethral closure pres-sure were noted, there was no correlation between objective improvement and urodynamic criteria and only 8 patients noted subjective improvement. A metaanalysis of clinical stud-ies evaluating estrogen therapy was performed by Fantl and the members of the Hormones and Urogenital Therapy Committee co-workers in 1994 (100). Of 166 published series only 23 met the strict criteria for analysis. This analysis found a significant subjective effect at-tributable to estrogen therapy ($p < 0.01$), but showed no improvement in the amount of fluid lost or in maximal urethral closure pressure (MUCP). Delivery of estrogen therapy may take a variety of forms. Oral therapy is perhaps the most popular. Doses vary from 2 to 4 mg/day of conjugated estrogens. Doses of up to 8 mg/day have been studied without any additional benefit (99). Vaginal estrogens can be an effective method of delivery, for the vaginal epithelium facilitates the conversion of estrone to estriol to a greater degree than oc-curs in the gastrointestinal tract. Thus, the hormonal effect of vaginal administration may indeed be superior to oral equivalents (101). The advantages of vaginal administration of estrogen are improved local effects on vaginal and urethral tissues; avoidance of the en-terohepatic circulation; and lack of effect on coagulation factors, HDL, cholesterol, and triglycerides (102). In some cases, however, systemic absorption may occur, suppressing the secretion of gonadotropins by up to 30% (103). One risk of vaginally administered es-trogens is thus erratic absorption and endometrial stimulation that may predispose patients to the development of endometrial carcinoma. The dosage for vaginally administered es-trogens varies, but an initial dose of 1–2 mg/day may be used initially, followed by a simi-lar maintenance dose two to three times per week. Recently, vaginal estrogen rings have been developed that release a constant level of estrogens, locally into the vagina for a pe-riod of 3 months. These rings appear to be well tolerated, and they avoid the potential for endometrial stimulation that exists with vaginally administered estrogens (104,105).

Although estrogen therapy has been used for the treatment of incontinence for over 60 years, debate still exists on its merits and mechanism of action (106,107). Clearly, oral and topical estrogen has an effect on the mucosa of the female urethra, but the extent to which estrogen exerts a defined clinical effect on smooth or striated sphincter tissue re-mains debated (107).

IV. CONCLUSION

The use of drug therapy for the treatment of sphincteric dysfunction represents an increas-ingly important means for treating both patients with storage and emptying difficulties. For the smooth sphincter, α-adrenergic agonists and antagonists represent an effective way to modulate sphincteric function. Although many different drugs have tried to target striated sphincteric dysfunction, few have been selective enough to warrant widespread clinical use. Too commonly, adverse systemic side effects limit their clinical effectiveness. For a select group of patients, however, these drugs allow them to overcome striated sphincteric dysfunction without resorting to surgery or ablative procedures. Future research efforts will undoubtedly look toward drugs that exert selective effects on the sphincter while subjecting the patient to minimal systemic side effects.

REFERENCES

1. Siroky MB, Krane R. Psychogenic Voiding Dysfunction. New York: Macmillan, 1986.
2. Siroky MB. Clinical characteristics of pseudodyssynergia. Neurourol Urodynam 1986; 5:317–319.
3. Kaplan SA, Te AE, Jacobs BZ. Urodynamic evidence of vesical neck obstruction in men with misdiagnosed chronic nonbacterial prostatitis and the therapeutic role of endoscopic incision if the bladder neck. J Urol 1994; 152:2063–2065.
4. Barbalias GA, Klauber GT, Blaivas JG. Critical evaluation of the Crede maneuver: a urodynamic study of 207 patients. J Urol 1983; 130:720–723.
5. Krane RJ, Olsson CA. Phenoxybenzamine in neurogenic bladder dysfunction: II. Clinical considerations. J Urol 1973; 110:653–656.
6. Krane RJ, Olsson CA. Phenoxybenzamine in neurogenic bladder dysfunction: I. A theory of micturition. J Urol 1973; 110:650–652.
7. Buczynski A. Urodynamic studies in evaluating detrusor sphincter dyssynergia and their effects on treatment. Paraplegia 1984; 22:168–173.
8. Koyanagi T. Further observation on the denervation supersensitivity of the urethra in patients with chronic neurogenic bladders. J Urol 1979; 122:348–351.
9. DeGroat WC, Kawatani M, Hisamitsu T, Cheng CL, Ma CP, Thor K, Steers W, Roppolo JR. Mechanisms underlying recovery of urinary bladder function following spinal cord injury. J Auton Nerv Syst 1990; 30(suppl):S71–S77.
10. Danuser H, Thor KB. Inhibition of central sympathetic and somatic outflow to the lower urinary tract of the cat by the alpha-1 adrenergic receptor antagonist prazosin. J Urol 1995; 153:1308–1312.
11. Ishizuka O, Persson K, Mattiasson A, Naylor A, Wyllie M, Andersson K. Micturition in conscious rats with and without bladder outlet obstruction: the role of spinal alpha-1 adrenoreceptors. Br J Pharmacol 1996; 117:962–966.
12. Nordling J, Meyhoff HH, Hald T. Sympatholytic effect on the striated urethral sphincter. A peripheral or central nervous system effect? Scand J Urol Nephrol 1981; 15:173–180.
13. Schurch B, Yasuda K, Rossier AB. Detrusor bladder neck dyssynergia revisited. J Urol 1994; 152:2066–2070.
14. Kunisawa Y, Kawabe, Niijima T, Honda K, Takenaka T. A pharmacological study of alpha adrenergic receptor subtypes in smooth muscle of human urinary bladder base and prostatic urethra. J Urol 1985; 134:396–398.
15. Caine M. The present role of alpha adrenergic blockers in the treatment of benign prostatic hypertrophy. J Urol 1986; 136:1–4.
16. Hoffman B, Lefkowitz R. Adrenergic Receptor Antagonists. New York: Pergamon, 1990.
17. MacGregor RJ, Diokno AC. The alpha adrenergic blocking action of prazosin hydrochloride on the canine urethra. Invest Urol 1981; 18:426–429.
18. Taylor SH. Clinical pharmacotherapeutics of doxazosin. Am J Med 1989; 87:2S–11S.
19. Wilde MI, Fitton A, Sorkin EM. Terazosin: a review of its pharmacodynamic and pharmacokinetic properties and therapeutic potential in benign prostatic hyperplasia. Drugs Aging 1993; 3:258–277.
20. Cedarbaum J, Schleifer L. Drugs for Parkinson's disease, spasticity and acute muscle spasms. In: Goodman and Gillmans, eds. Pharmacologic Basis of Therapeutics, 8th ed. New York: Pergamon, 1990; pp. 463–484.

21. Parlani M, Conte B, Goso C, Szallasi A, Manzini S. Capsaicin induced relaxation in the rat isolated external urethral sphincter: characterization of the vanilloid receptor and mediation by CGRP. Br J Pharmacol 1993; 110:989–994.

22. Nanninga JB, Frost F, Penn R. Effect of intrathecal baclofen on bladder and sphincter function. J Urol 1989; 142:101–105.

23. Dykstra DD, Sidi AA. Treatment of detrusor sphincter dyssynergia with botulinum-A toxin: a double blind study. Arch Phys Med Rehabil 1990; 71:24–26.

24. Bushman W, Steers WD, Meythaler JM. Voiding dysfunction in patients with spastic paraplegia: urodynamic evaluation and response to continuous intrathecal baclofen. Neurourol Urodyn 1993; 12:163–170.

25. Elbadawi A, Schenk EA. A new theory of the innervation of the bladder musculature. 2. Innervation of the vesicourethral junction and external urethral sphincter. J Urol 1974; 111: 613.

26. Gallien P, Robineau S, Verin M, Lebot MP, Nicolas B, Brissot R. Treatment of detrusor sphincter dyssynergia by transperineal injection of botulinum toxin. Arch Phys Med Rehabil 1998; 79:715–717.

27. Wein AJ, Benson GS, Jacobowitz D. Lack of evidence for adrenergic innervation of the external urethral sphincter. J Urol 1979; 121:324–326.

28. Crowe R, Burnstock G, Light JK. Adrenergic innervation of the striated muscle of the intrinsic external urethral sphincter from patients with lower motor spinal cord lesion. J Urol 1989; 141:47–49.

29. Thind P, Lose G, Colstrup H, Andersson KE. The effect of alpha adrenoreceptor stimulation and blockade on the static urethral sphincter function in healthy females. Scand J Urol Nephrol 1992; 26:219–225.

30. Gajewski J, Downie JW, Awad SA. Experimental evidence for a central nervous system site of action in the effect of alpha-adrenergic blockers on the external urinary sphincter. J Urol 1984; 133:403–409.

31. Pederson E, Torring J, Klemar B. The effect of the alpha adrenergic blocking agent thymoxamine on the neurogenic bladder and urethra. Acta Neurol Scand 1980; 61:107–114.

32. Downie JW, Bialik GJ. Evidence for a spinal site of action of clonidine on somatic and viscerosomatic reflex activity evoked on the pudendal nerve in cats. J Pharmacol Exp Ther 1988; 246:352–358.

33. Herman RM, Wainberg MC. Clonidine inhibits vesico-sphincter reflexes in patients with chronic spinal lesions. Arch Phys Med Rehabil 1991; 72:539–545.

34. Nanninga JB, Kaplan P, Lal S. Effect of phentolamine on perineal muscle EMG activity in paraplegia. Br J Urol 1977; 49:537–539.

35. Rossier A, Fam BA, Lee IY, Sarkarati M, Evans DA. Role of striated and smooth muscle components in the urethral pressure profile in the traumatic neurogenic bladder: a neuropharmacological and urodynamic study. Preliminary report. J Urol 1982; 128:529.

36. Hachen HJ. Clinical and urodynamic assessment of alpha adrenolytic therapy in patients with neurogenic bladder dysfunction. Paraplegia 1980; 18:229–240.

37. O'Riordan J, Doherty C, Javed M, Brophy D, Hutchinson M, Quinlan D. Do alpha blockers have a role in lower urinary tract dysfunction in multiple sclerosis. J Urol 1995; 153:1114–1116.

38. Chancellor MB, Erhard MJ, Rivas DA. Clinical effect of alpha-1 antagonism by terazosin on external and internal urinary sphincter function. J Am Paraplegia Soc 1993; 16:207–214.

39. Davidoff RA. Antispasticity drugs: mechanisms of action. Ann Neurol 1985; 17:107–116.

40. Bloom F. Neurohumoral Transmission and the Central Nervous System. New York: Pergamon, 1990.

41. Lader M. Clinical pharmacology of benzodiazepines. Annu Rev Med 1987; 38:19–28.

42. Madersbacher H. Management of striated sphincter dyssynergia. Neurourol Urodynam 1986; 5:307–315.

43. Stanton SL, Cardozo LD, Kerr–Wilson R. Treatment of delayed onset of spontaneous voiding after surgery for incontinence. Urology 1979; 13:494–496.

44. Raz S, Smith RB. External sphincter spasticity syndrome in female patients. J Urol 1976; 115: 443–446.

45. Siroky MB, Goldstein I, Krane RJ. Functional voiding disorders in men. J Urol 1981; 126:200–204.

46. Hinman F Jr. Non-neurogenic neurogenic bladder (the Hinman syndrome)—15 years later. J Urol 1986; 136:769–777.

47. Olsson A, Swanberg E, et al. Effects of adrenoreceptor agonists on airway smooth muscle and on slow contracting skeletal muscle: in vitro and in vivo results compared. Acta Pharmacol Toxicol 1976; 44:272–276.

48. Gosling J, Dixon JS, Critchley HO, Thompson SA. A comparative study of the human external sphincter and periurethral levator ani muscles. Br J Urol 1981; 153:35–41.

49. Thind P, Lose G, Colstrup H, Andersson KE. The influence of beta adrenoceptor and muscarinic receptor agonists and antagonists on the static urethral closure function in healthy females. Scand J Urol Nephrol 1993; 27:31–38.

50. Vaidyanithan S, Rao S, Bapna BC, Chary KS, Palaniswamy R. beta Adrenergic activity in the human proximal urethra: a study with terbutaline. J Urol 1980; 124:869–871.

51. Yamanashi T, Yasuda K, Hattori T, Sakakibara R, Shimazaki J. Effects of beta-2 stimulants on contractility and fatigue of canine urethral sphincter. J Urol 1994; 151:1066–1069.

52. Bianchine J. Drugs for Parkinson's disease: centrally acting muscle relaxants. In: Goodman and Gillmans, eds. The Pharmacologic Basis for Therapeutics. New York: Macmillan, 1980; 8: 475–493.

53. Harris JD, Benson GS. Effect of dantrolene sodium on canine bladder contractility. Urology 1980; 16:229–231.

54. Murdock MM, Sax D, Krane RJ. Use of dantrolene sodium in external sphincter spasm. Urology 1976; 8:133–137.

55. Hackler R, Broecker BH, Klein FA, Brady SM. A clinical experience with dantrolene sodium for external sphincter hypertonicity in spinal injured patients. J Urol 1980; 124:78–81.

56. Ward A, Chaffman MO, Sorkin EM. Dantrolene: a review of its pharmacodynamic and pharmacokinetic properties and therapeutic use in malignant hyperthermia, the neuroleptic malignant syndrome and an update of its use in muscle spasticity. Drugs 1986; 32:120–124.

57. Dykstra DD, Sidi AA, Scott AB, Pagel JM, Goldish GD. Effects of botulinum-A toxin on detrusor–sphincter dyssynergia in spinal cord injury patients. J Urol 1988; 139:919–922.

58. Schurch B, Hauri D, Rodic B, Curt A, Meyer M, Rossier AB. Botulinum-A toxin as a treatment of detrusor sphincter dyssynergia: a prospective study in 24 spinal cord injury patients. J Urol 1996; 155:1023–1029.

59. Schurch B, Hodler J, Rodic B. Botulinum A toxin as a treatment of detrusor sphincter dyssynergia in patients with spinal cord injury: MRI controlled transperineal injections. J Neurol Neurosurg Psychiatry 1997; 63:474–476.

60. Fowler CJ, Betts CD, Christmas TJ, Swash M, Fowler CG. Botulinum toxin in the treatment of chronic urinary retention in women. Br J Urol 1992; 70:387–389.

61. Ko HY, Kim KT. Treatment of external urethral sphincter hypertonicity by pudendal nerve block using phenol solution in patients with spinal cord injury. Spinal Cord 1997; 35:690–693.

62. Duncan GW, Shahani BT, Young RR. An evaluation of baclofen treatment for certain symptoms in patients with spinal cord lesions: a double blind crossover study. Neurology 1976; 26:441–446.

63. Saito K, Konishi S, Otsuka M. Antagonism between Lioresal (baclofen) and substance P in rat spinal cord. Brain Res 1975; 97:177–180.

64. Milanov IG. Mechanisms of baclofen action on spasticity. Acta Neurol Scand 1992; 85:305–310.

65. Maggi CA, Furio M, Santicioli P, Conte B, Meli A. Spinal and supra spinal components of GABAergic inhibition of the micturition reflex in rats. J Pharm Exp Ther 1987; 240:998–1005.

66. Kontani H, Kawabata Y, Koshiura R. In vivo effects of gamma-amino butyric acid on the urinary bladder contraction accompanying micturition. Jpn J Pharmacol 1987; 45:45–53.

67. Teague CT, Merrill DC. The effect of baclofen and dantrolene on bladder in stimulator induced detrusor sphincter dyssynergia in dogs. Urology 1978; 11:531–535.

68. Roy CW, Wakefield IR. Baclofen pseudo psychosis: case report. Paraplegia 1986; 24:318–321.

69. Leyson JF, Martin BF, Sporer A. Baclofen in the treatment of detrusor dyssynergia in spinal cord injury patients. J Urol 1980; 124:82–84.

70. Hachen HJ, Krucker V. Clinical and laboratory assessment of the efficacy of baclofen Lioresal on urethral sphincter spasticity in patients with traumatic paraplegia. Eur Urol 1977; 3:237–240.

71. Loubser PG, Narayan RK, Sandin KJ, Donovan WH, Russell D. Continuous infusion of intrathecal baclofen: long term effects on spasticity in spinal cord injury. Paraplegia 1991; 29:48–64.

72. Steers W, Meythaler JM, Haworth C, Herrell D, Park TS. Effects of acute bolus and chronic continuous intrathecal baclofen on genitourinary dysfunction due to spinal cord pathology. J Urol 1992; 148:1849–1855.

73. Diokno AC, Brock BM, Brown MB, Herzog AR. Prevalence of urinary incontinence and other urological symptoms in the noninstitutionalized elderly. J Urol 1986; 136:1022–1025.

74. Rohner T, Rohner J. Urinary Incontinence in America: The Social Significance. St Louis, MO: Mosby-Yearbook, 1997.

75. Ek A, Andersson KE, Gullberg B, Ulmsten U. The effects of long-term treatment with norephedrine on stress incontinence and urethral closure pressure profile. Scand J Urol Nephrol 1978; 12:105–110.

76. Rashbaum M, Mendelbaum C. Non-operative treatment of urinary incontinence in women. Am J Obstet Gynecol 1948; 56:777.

77. Lose G, Lindholm P. Clinical and urodynamic effects of norepinephrine in women with stress incontinence. Urol Int 1984; 39:298–302.

78. Diokno AC, Taub M. Ephedrine in the treatment of urinary incontinence. Urology 1975; 5:624–625.

79. Obrink A, Bunne G. The effect of alpha adrenergic stimulation on stress incontinence. Scand J Urol Nephrol 1978; 12:205–208.

80. Awad SA, Downie JW, Kiriluta HG. alpha-Adrenergic agents in urinary disorders of the proximal urethra. Part 1. Sphincteric Incontinence. Br J Urol 1978; 50:332–335.

81. Stewart BH, Banowsky LH, Montague DK. Stress incontinence: conservative therapy with sympathomimetic drugs. J Urol 1976; 115:558–559.

82. Collste I, Lindskog M. Phenylpropanolamine in treatment of female stress incontinence. Double-blind placebo controlled study in 24 patients. Urology 1987; 30:398–403.

83. Biaggioni I, Onrot J, Stewart CK, Robertson D. The potent pressor effect of phenylpropanolamine in patients with autonomic impairment. JAMA 1987; 258:236–239.

84. Blackburn GL, Morgan JP, Lavin PT, Noble R, Funderburk FR, Istfan N. Determinants of the pressor effect of phenylpropanolamine in healthy subjects. JAMA 1989; 261:3267–3272.

85. Liebson I, Bigelo WG, Griffiths RR, Funderburk FR. Phenylpropanolamine: effects on subjective and cardiovascular variables at recommended over-the-counter dose levels. J Clin Pharmacol 1987; 27:685–693.

86. Richelson E. Pharmacology of antidepressants: characteristics of the ideal drug. Mayo Clin Proc 1994; 69:1069–1081.

87. Foreman MM, Mc Nulty AM. Alterations in K(+)-evoked release of ^{3}H-norepinephrine and contractile responses in urethral and bladder tissues induced by norepinephrine reuptake inhibition. Life Sci 1993; 53:193–200.

88. Mahony DT, Laferte RO, Mahoney JE. Observations on sphincter augmenting effect of imipramine in children with urinary incontinence. Urology 1973; 2:317–323.

89. Castleden CM, George CF, Renwick AG, Asher MJ. Imipramine: a possible alternative to current therapy for urinary incontinence in the elderly. J Urol 1981; 125:318–320.

90. Baldessarini R. Drugs at the treatment of psychiatric disorders. In: Goodman and Gillmans, eds. Pharmacologic Basis of Therapeutics, 8th ed. New York: Pergamon, 1990; pp. 383–399.

91. Dube JY, Lesage R, Tremblay RR. Androgen and estrogen binding in rat skeletal and perineal muscles. Can J Biochem 1976; 50:54–55.

92. Dionne FT, Lesage RL, Dube JY, Tremblay RR. Estrogen binding proteins in rat skeletal and perineal muscles: in vitro and in vivo studies. J Steriod Biochem 1988; 11:1073–1080.

93. Hodgson BJ, Dumas S, Bolling DR, Heesch CM. Effect of estrogen on sensitivity of rabbit bladder and urethra to phenylephrine. Invest Urol 1978; 16:67–69.

94. Larsson B, Andersson KE, Batra S, Mattiasson A, Sjogren C. Effects of estradiol on norepinephrine induced contraction, alpha adrenoceptor number and norepinephrine content in the female rabbit urethra. J Pharmacol Exp Ther 1984; 229:557–563.

95. Callahan S, Creed KE. The effects of estrogens on spontaneous activity and responses to phenylephrine of the mammalian urethra. J Physiol 1985; 358:35–46.

96. Iverson L. Role of transmitter uptake mechanisms in synaptic transmission. Br J Pharmacol 1971; 41:571.

97. Beisland HO, Fossberg E, Moer A, Sander S. Urethral sphincteric insufficiency in post-menopausal females: treatment with phenylpropanolamine and estriol separately and in combination. A urodynamic and clinical evaluation. Urol Int 1984; 39:211–216.

98. Bump RC, Freidman CI. Intraluminal urethral pressure measurements in the female baboon: effects of hormonal manipulation. J Urol 1986; 136:508–511.

99. Rud T. The effects of estrogens and gestagens on the urethral pressure profile in urinary continent and stress incontinent women. Acta Obstet Gynecol Scand 1980; 59:265–270.

100. Fantl JA, Cardozo L, McClish DK. Estrogen therapy in the management of urinary incontinence in post menopausal women: a meta-analysis. First report of the Hormones and Urogenital Therapy Committee. Obstet Gynecol 1994; 83:12–18.

101. Whitehead M, Minardi J, et al. Systemic Absorption of Estrogen from Vaginal Cream. Lancaster, UK: MTP Press, 1978.

102. Campagnoli C, Tousijn LP, Belforte P, Ferruzzi L, Dolfin AM, Morra G. Effects of conjugated equine estrogen and oestriol on blood clotting, plasma lipids, and endometrial proliferation in postmenopausal women. Maturitas 1981; 3:135–144.

103. Rigg LA, Hermann H, Yen SS. Absorption of estrogen from vaginal creams. N Engl J Med 1978; 298:195–197.

104. Lippert TH, Seeger H, Mueck AO. Estradiol metabolism during oral and transdermal estradiol replacement in post menopausal women. Horm Metab Res 1998; 30:598–600.

105. Nash HA, Brache V, Alvarez–Sanchez F, Jackanicz TM, Harmon TM. Estradiol delivery by vaginal rings: potential for hormone replacement therapy. Maturitas 1997; 26:27–33.

106. Salmon U, Walter R, et al. The use of estrogen in the treatment of dysuria and incontinence in post-menopausal women. Am J Obstet Gynecol 1941; 42:845.

107. Cardozo L. Role of estrogens in the treatment of female urinary incontinence. J Am Geriatr Soc 1990; 38:326–328.

APPENDIX

Table 1 Drug Therapy for the Hyperactive Sphincter

	Site of action	Mode of action	Route	Side effec
Alpha antagonists	Smooth sphincter	Relaxes smooth muscle of urethra/bladder neck	Oral	Asthenia, weaknes tic
	? Striated sphincter	Inhibits central sympathetic outflow		Hypotension, dizzi
Benzodiazepines	Striated sphincter	Potentiates GABA, augments presynaptic inhibition of neurotransmitters	Oral	Drowsiness, fatigu dence, tachyphy
Beta agonists	Striated sphincter	Decreases urethral resistance and closure pressure	Oral	Tachycardia, anxie tions
Dantrolene	Striated sphincter	Inhibits Ca^{++} release from sarcoplasmic reticulum	Oral	Hepatitis, weaknes dizziness
Botulinum toxin A	Striated sphincter	Inhibits acetylcholine release at neuromuscular junction	IM	Antibody formatio rary effect
Phenol block	Striated sphincter	Permanent nerve ablation	IM	Infection, necrosis
Baclofen	Striated sphincter	GABA(b) agonist, causes presynaptic hyperpolarization of dorsal nerve root terminals	PO	Weakness, rash, di drowsiness, prui cinations
			Intrathecal pump	Infection, meningi ness, rash, dizzi drowsiness, prui cinations

Table 2 Drug Therapy for Sphincteric Deficiency

	Site of action	Mode of action	Route	Side e
Alpha agonists	Smooth sphincter ? Striated sphincter	Contract smooth muscle of urethra/bladder neck, augment central sympathetic outflow	Oral	Urinary retention tachycardia, pa
Tricyclic anti-depressants	(Same as alpha agonists)		Oral	Weakness, fatigu postural hypot arrhythmia, wi toms upon cess
Estrogen	Smooth sphincter Striated sphincter	Questionable effects: hyperpolarization of urethral smooth muscle, blockade of extraneuronal reuptake of catecholamines	Oral Vaginal	Increased risk for cancer, alterati tropic axis, vag dysmenorrhea

33

Urethral Injection Treatment for Stress Urinary Incontinence

ELMER B. PINEDA, JR., and H. ROGER HADLEY

Loma Linda University Medical Center, Loma Linda, California

I. INTRODUCTION

Urethral injectable agents have been used to treat urinary incontinence resulting from intrinsic sphincteric deficiency (ISD). In the past, operative procedures that are known to be effective in treating this disorder are the placement of an artificial urinary sphincter and the insertion of an urethral sling. Unlike these operations, however, the injection of bulking agents into the urethra is a minimally invasive procedure that can be done in the physicians office. In this chapter, we will discuss the proposed mechanism of action of urethral injectable agents, the selection of the appropriate patient, various types of bulking agents, nuances of injection technique, and the outcomes in different patient groups.

Injecting agents into the urethra to improve stress urinary incontinence (SUI) is not a novel concept. The first reported injectable agent into the urethra was performed by Murless in 1938. He induced an inflammatory response that compressed the urethra by injecting sodium murrhate, a sclerosing agent, into the anterior vaginal wall (1). This procedure was abandoned because of unacceptable complications, including postoperative pulmonary embolism (2). Since the 1960s, other investigators have tried different sclerosing and bulking agents (2,3). Polytetrafluoroethylene (Teflon) as a bulking agent was introduced by Lopez et al. in 1964 and popularized by Berg and Politano in the 1970s (5,6). The use of Teflon paste, however, has fallen out of favor because of the theoretical risks of granuloma formation, as well as systemic migration to the spleen, liver, and lung (7). In the United States, it is not approved for the treatment of urinary incontinence by the U.S. Food and Drug Administration (FDA).

Currently, the two most commonly used urethral injectable agents are glutaraldehyde cross-linked collagen and autologous fat. These two substances, therefore, will be the primary focus of discussions in this chapter.

II. MECHANISM OF ACTION

Factors that allow continence to occur are active and passive contraction of the muscles in the urethral sphincter, a well-supported bladder neck, and a functional urethral seal mechanism. The urethral seal component of continence is the factor addressed when treating incontinent patients with urethral bulking agents. The urethral seal mechanism promotes continence by its inherent ability to increase resistance by increasing the opening urethral pressure. Increases in intravesical pressure (coughing and straining), therefore, are less likely to cause leakage because of the increase in urethral resistance. Urodynamically, this means the abdominal pressure necessary to open the urethra (abdominal leak-point pressure) is increased even though there is no appreciable change that occurs in the closure pressure of the urethra. Compromise of the mucosal seal mechanism, therefore, may lead to stress incontinence. Indeed, many experts believe that damage to the seal mechanism is the most important factor in the cause of stress incontinence. Because the seal mechanism is dependent on the suppleness of the urethral tissues, common reasons for failure of the urethral seal mechanism are scarring from previous operative procedures, birth trauma, lack of adequate estrogens, or pelvic radiotherapy.

The goal of urethral bulking agents is to prevent urinary leakage without causing urinary obstruction, thereby providing for socially acceptable continence. Urethral bulking agents accomplish this by improving coaptation at the proximal urethra to help restore the mucosal seal mechanism of the bladder neck. McGuire and Appell note that urethral bulking agents, such as glutaraldehyde cross-linked collagen, improve the ability of the urethra to resist abdominal pressure as an expulsive force without changing the voiding pressure or detrusor pressure at the time of leakage (8). Several other investigators studying glutaraldehyde cross-linked collagen have also shown that the Valsalva leak-point pressure (LPP) increases owing to an increase in the functional urethral length, resulting from the coaptation of the bladder neck and proximal urethra (9–13). According to Benshushan et al. (14), periurethral injections result in the cephalad elongation of the urethra, with a concomitant increase in pressure transmission ratio in the first quarter of the urethral length. To accomplish this goal of increasing the functional urethral length, bulking agents should ideally be placed just distal to the urethral–vesicle junction at the bladder neck or proximal urethra. Deposition in the distal urethra will unlikely increase the functional urethral length or prevent bladder neck opening during episodes of stress (14).

III. PATIENT SELECTION

Candidates for urethral bulking agents must undergo a customary history and physical examination to evaluate for stress urinary incontinence. Most authors employ a urodynamic evaluation or radiographic studies to document bladder function, anatomical support of the bladder neck, and functioning of the proximal urethral sphincter both at rest and with "stress testing."

The ideal female candidate for urethral bulking agents is the patient with demonstrable stress urinary incontinence, intrinsic urethral sphincteric deficiency, a well-supported bladder neck, and a stable bladder. Numerous clinical conditions can result in intrinsic sphincteric deficiency and include prior anti-incontinence procedures, peripheral or autonomic neuropathy, pelvic trauma, chronic catheter drainage, and myelodysplasia (13,15). In females, a pelvic examination that shows minimal urethral hypermobility with straining or coughing, in conjunction with a positive "stress test," during which leakage is seen to occur when the subject coughs or strains with a moderately full bladder, constitutes presumptive evidence of intrinsic sphincteric deficiency (8).

Identification of the appropriate male patient for bulking agents requires that the diagnosis of ISD be made. Leakage demonstrable (direct vision or radiographically) with coughing, straining, or exercise in the presence of a stable bladder is sufficient evidence to judge that intrinsic deficiency is present (8). Men can present with intrinsic sphincteric deficiency after prostate operations, such as a radical prostatectomy or transurethral resection of the prostate (TURP), as well as from neuropathic causes.

Children with ISD secondary to a neuropathic sphincter from myelomeningocele or the exstrophy-epispadias complex may benefit from periurethral bulking agents. However, stress incontinence in these children is often complicated by detrusor dysfunction (16).

Contraindications to urethral injection include untreated urinary tract infection, unmanaged detrusor instability, or known hypersensitivity to bovine collagen (17). The presence of detrusor instability itself, however, does not preclude the use of urethral bulking agents.

IV. TECHNIQUE FOR URETHRAL INJECTION

Periurethral collagen injection is an outpatient procedure performed either in a day surgery center or in the physician's office. Although some urologists prefer to give the patient a preoperative sedative, the procedure is commonly accomplished with only a local (periurethral) or no anesthetic (transcystoscopic). Because of its minimal invasive nature, collagen injection in the doctor's office does not need the preoperative assessments, laboratory studies, or routine radiographic evaluations that are customarily required for procedures performed in an operating room facility. However, an intradermal skin test is performed a few weeks before the urethral injection of collagen to check for collagen hypersensitivity.

On arrival at the doctor's office, the patient is escorted to the patient room where cystoscopies are routinely done. After the patient removes his or her clothes from the waist down, he or she is placed in the lithotomy position. Preparation includes a 1-min antiseptic cleansing of the external genitalia and meatus. A clean drape is placed over the patient with access to the urethra. Depending on the urologist's preference, either a transcystoscopic or periurethral technique may be used in women. In men, urethral collagen injection is performed transcystoscopically.

The transcytoscopic technique does not require a local anesthetic other than intraurethral lidocaine lubricant. It is important that the urologist has the appropriate cystoscope that enhances the ease of the procedure. One may utilize a specialized scope with a specific working element for control of an attached needle device. As an alternative to these potentially expensive cystoscopes, the urologist may use a standard scope with a narrow sheath that is just large enough to allow the long injection needle to pass. By minimizing the free side-to-side movement of the injection needle, the small sheath facilitates the urologist's ability to control the needle while placing it in the suburethral tissue (Fig. 1).

In women, the cystoscope is passed into the bladder and the needle advanced just beyond the sheath where it can be visualized. The cystoscope is withdrawn back to the distal urethra and the needle is inserted into the layer just under the urothelium in either the 3- or

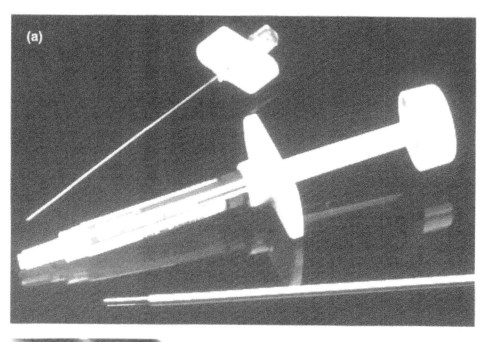

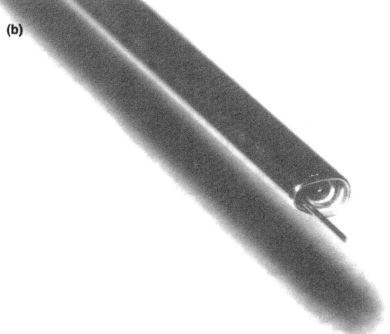

Figure 1   (a) Glutaraldehyde cross-linked collagen delivery system; (b) collagen injection needle through a cystoscope.

9-o'clock position. The needle is advanced up to the bladder neck and a test injection given. There should be immediate inward movement of tissue toward improved coaptation. The lack of an immediate response should prompt the physician to replace the needle in a more superficial position. Once determined that the needle is in a suitable position, the agent is best injected slowly to avoid rupturing the expanding urothelium. The injection is continued until no further inward movement is detected or the urothelium is rapidly thinning and revealing the distinctive white collagen agent. The procedure is repeated on the opposite side. Women rarely use more than 2.5 mL per procedure (Fig. 2).

Before the transcystoscopic approach in men, 2% lidocaine jelly is applied transurethrally and left in place a few minutes. The proximal urethra is visualized using a standard cystoscope with a narrow sheath and a 0- or 30-degree lens. The collagen injection needle is placed through the working element, and into the urethra just proximal to the external sphincter. The injection needle should not be placed directly through the external sphincter to avoid pudendal nerve spasm (17). Under direct visualization, collagen is delivered into the layer just under the urothelium to raise a urethral bleb. This is performed circumferentially in four quadrants until coaptation of the the urethral lumen occurs. The injection pressure needed to raise a urethral bleb and the total volume of collagen used to coapt the urethra tend to be greater in men than in women. This is attributed mostly to iatrogenic scarring of the proximal urethra from prior operations or procedures (i.e., radical prostatectomy, TURP, radiation therapy).

The injection technique for autologous fat generally involves two stages: (1) harvesting of abdominal fat and (2) transcystoscopic/periurethral injection of the fat. Different variations in the harvesting of fat exist ranging from aspiration with a large-bore needle to liposuction (15,18,19). The transcystoscopic or periurethral injection of the harvested fat is similar to that described in the foregoing.

V. INJECTABLE AGENTS

A. Autologous Fat

Fat tissue transplants were first used for filling scars and subsequently had several uses in plastic or reconstructive surgery (20). Fat provides the advantages of being readily avail-

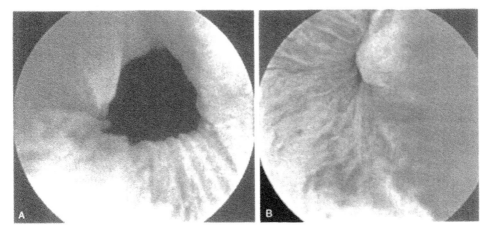

Figure 2 Cystoscopic appearance of bladder neck (a) before and after (b) urethral collagen injection. (From Ref. 32.)

able, biocompatible, and inexpensive (18). The main disadvantage of using fat as a urethral bulking agent, however, is the variability of reabsorption and the degree of eventual connective tissue replacement. Long-term resorption rates of fat grafts of 30–60% have been reported (21). Although there is no scientific evidence to explain how fat resorption occurs, persistence of saline, blood, or anesthetic solution with the injected fat may increase resorption (22,23). Also, despite the fat being injected through a large-bore needle some adipose cells are damaged, thus increasing local resorption. One study revealed that 40% of aspirated fat cells had a defective cell membrane on microscopic examination despite the use of atraumatic harvesting techniques (20). Several techniques aimed at improving graft survival have been attempted, including mixing the harvested fat with Ringer's solution or insulin before injection, cutting harvested fat into "pearls," or minimizing trauma to aspirated fat. No method has been shown to improve graft survival consistently or to minimize resorption, nor has there been any explanation for the wide variations seen in graft survival (23,24).

The fate of autologous fat has been studied histologically by Chajchir and Benzaquen (25). They reported on a 4-year follow-up of pathology specimens from patients who underwent fat injection for soft-tissue augmentations. Specimens obtained 3 months postoperatively revealed zones of cystosteatonecrosis, lipophagic granulomas, lymphocytes, adipocytes, giant cells, and new vessel formation. Biopsies 1 year later revealed large amounts of connective tissue and a fibrotic reaction as the final result. The tissue that followed the cystosteatonecrotic process demonstrated a cicatricial reaction that maintained the desired volume of the area for a considerable period (25).

B. Glutaraldehyde Cross-Linked Collagen

Glutaraldehyde cross-linked collagen is a highly purified suspension of bovine collagen in normal saline containing at least 95% type I collagen and 1–5% type III collagen. It is prepared by selective hydrolysis of the telopeptides of the collagen molecules. Because these telopeptides are the antigenic markers of collagen, their removal decreases its antigenicity (26). Cross-linking collagen to glutaraldehyde makes the collagen more stable and durable by increasing its resistance to the fibroblast-secreted collagenase. The glutaraldehyde cross-linking also decreases the collagen's antigenicity, thereby reducing its hypersensitivity (26,27). Because localized hypersensitivity reactions associated with transient elevation in serum antibodies specific for commercial collagen implants have been reported, an intradermal skin test with collagen is performed a few weeks before injection (28–30). The serum antibody titers typically become undetectable within 1 year, and the antibodies are IgG type which do not cross-react with host collagen (31). This allergic reaction to glutaraldehyde cross-linked collagen occurs in 1–3% of patients (32).

Glutaraldehyde cross-linked collagen stimulates fibroblast infiltration and neovascularization, resulting in host collagen deposition at the implantation site. The collagen material begins to degrade 12 weeks after implantation, and is usually cleared in 9–19 months (33,34). The injected collagen may persist for longer periods, however, as evidenced by magnetic resonance imaging (MRI) studies of injected areas of urethra up to 22 months after treatment (35). Evaluation of ureteric and vesical injection sites after failed endoscopic antireflux procedures revealed no significant foreign body giant cell reaction in response to the implanted collagen after 12 and 19 months. A minimal inflammatory response, however, may result from this noncytotoxic material (36).

Similar to autologous fat, collagen has been used in plastic surgery to correct facial and bodily contour defects with minimal local or systemic reactions. Glutaraldehyde cross-linked collagen was approved for use in the treatment of intrinsic sphincteric deficiency by the U.S. Food and Drug Administration in October 1993 after studies revealed early efficacy and safety. The advantages of collagen include its ease of use, availability, and safety profile. It is a nontoxic substance that appears to have minimal systemic and local side effects. Currently, there is no evidence of distal migration of glutaraldehyde cross-linked collagen. The disadvantages of collagen include concerns over its long-term durability, need for multiple injections, and cost.

VI. TREATMENT GROUPS

A. Women

1. Glutaraldehyde Cross-Linked Collagen

Women with genuine stress urinary incontinence from intrinsic sphincteric deficiency constitute the group most commonly treated with urethral bulking agents. Investigators report success rates ranging from 55 to 86%, with follow-up between 3 and 46 months (Table 1). Caution should be exercised in interpreting these results, or the results of any anti-incontinence procedure, because there is no standardization for the definition of success among these studies.

Several authors have tried to determine if any prognostic factors exist preoperatively in patients undergoing urethral injection therapy. With urodynamic studies, some authors report that there are no preoperative parameters that can determine the success or failure of collagen injections (37,38). Some authors have found that patients who underwent prior anti-incontinence surgery tended to do better that those without previous operations. They hypothesized that this success may be related to the support of the periurethral tissues and a less mobile bladder neck from scarring (39,40). Others have shown that the accurate placement of the injection needle to obtain adequate submucosal bulking without extravasation was associated with a favorable outcome (37). In a study by Smith and Appell, patients achieving continence with collagen received one to three injections and wore three pads per day (ppd) before the study, whereas those who failed received four or more injections of collagen and wore six ppd. Other investigators, however, did not find any relation between the severity of urinary incontinence preoperatively and success rate (41,42).

In other series, detrusor instability before treatment has decreased the effectiveness of collagen injections (10,11,41,43). A study by Herschorn et al. (41) has shown a statistically significant increase in the number of failed collagen injections in patients with preoperative detrusor instability. Smith and Appell (43) have found that the group who failed collagen injection in their series had a higher percentage of patients with preoperative detrusor instability. Although preoperative detrusor instability may decrease the success rate of collagen injection, it is not a contraindication to treatment, especially if adequate bladder stability can be achieved with medications (e.g., anticholinergics). In a few studies, patients with some degree of urethral hypermobility had results comparable with those patients with a well-supported or fixed bladder neck (37,38,41,42).

The most common complications of urethral collagen injection include temporary urinary retention, urinary tract infection, and transient hematuria (Table 2). These are usually few, minor, and self-limited. In one study, however, Stothers et al. (44) studied 337 women who received periurethral collagen injection for the treatment of stress urinary incontinence and noted an overall 20% incidence of complications in any given individual. De novo urinary urgency with incontinence was the most frequent and serious complication, occurring in 12.6% of patients, which may not resolve in all patients (44). There has

1 Results of Glutaraldehyde Cross-Linked Collagen in Women

	Number of patients[a]	Follow-up (mo)	Results	Avg. number injections	Me
...d et al., 1991	25 (SUI—type not specified)	3	Dry 64%, improved 16% (overall success 80%)	—	
...tter et al., 1992	16 (SUI—type not specified)	15 (10–22)	3 mo: cured 44%; improved 39% (overall success 83%); failed 17% 9 mo: cured 39%; improved 44% (overall 83%); failed 17%	—	
...r et al. 1993 (40)	50 (ISD)	11 (1–21)	Cured 42%; improved 40% (overall success 82%); failed 14% Awaiting further injections 4%	1.9	
...d—multicenter ..., 1993 (67)	88 (ISD)	24	Overall success (cured/improved); 78%; not improved/worse 21.6%	3	
...re/Appell, 1994	154 (17 mobile urethra) (137 ISD)	>12	Mobile: dry 47%; improved 17% (overall success 64%); failed 35% ISD: dry 46%; improved 34% (overall success 80%); failed 19%	—	
...nell et al., 1995	44 (ISD)	(longest = 7 mo)	Dry 45%; improved 18% (overall success 63%)	1.5	
...son et al., 1995	42 (ISD)	46 (10–66)	Cured 40%; greatly improved 12%; improved 31% (overall success 83%); unchanged 7%; worse 10%	2.4 (Cured/gr. impr.) 4.1 (impr./no change/wrs.)	17.5 (C... 39... ch...
... et al., 1995 (37)	59 (SUI—type not specified)	3	Subjective improved/cured 86%; objective cured 61%		
	54	12	Subjective improved/cured 77%; objective cured 54%	3	
	29	24	Subjective improved/cured 68%; objective cured 48%		

t al., 1996	181 (124 mobile urethra) (64 ISD) (6 neurogenic incont.)	22 (4–69) (patients cured/impr.)	Cured 23%; improved 52% (overall success 75%); failed 25%	2.5 (success) 2 (failure)	9.65 (su 7.8 (fa
l, 1997 (43)	94 (ISD)	14	Dry 38%; socially continent 29% (overall success 67%); failed 33%	2.1 (success) 3.2 (failure)	11.9 (su 16.1 (fa
., 1997 (42)	59 (not specified)	3	61% success	—	—
		12	54% success		
., 1997 (38)	107 (SUI—not specified)	38 (24–70)	Cured 25%; improved 40% (overall success 65%)	1.7	(12
l., 1997 (69)	28 (SUI—not specified)	12	Subjective cured/improved 79% (objective cured 50%)	1.5	17
	26	24	Subjective cured/improved 69% (objective cured 54%)		
., 1997, abstr	30 (27 type I; 14 type II; 9 type III SUI)	(Follow-up period over 45 mo)	Cured 27%; improved 36% (overall success 61%); failed 27%	(In first 3 mo of tx) Cured: 2.3 (1–4); improved: 1.8 (1–3); failed: 2.4 (1–4)	(In first of tx) Cu (1.5–15); i 9.6 (2.5–2 8.8 (4
1997, abstr	22 (ISD)	(Minimum 12 mo)	Cured 45%; improved 10% (overall success 55%); no change 45%	1.8	6.
1997 (15)	22 (ISD)	>7	Overall success (dry/improved) 86%; subjective improvement 64%	1.9	(13.

rinary incontinence; ISD, intrinsic sphincteric deficiency; tx, treatment.

Table 2 Adverse Events Reported During a Multicenter Study of 382 Patients Treated with GAX-Collagen

Adverse events	Treatment-related		Nontreatment-related	
	Events n (%)	Patients n (%)	Events n (%)	Patients n (%)
Urinary retention	36(15)	31(8)	2(1)	1(<1)
Urinary tract infection	14(6)	14(4)	92(38)	63(16)
Hematuria	8(3)	8(2)	0	0
Injection site injury	5(2)	5(1)	0	0
Urinary outlet obstruction	2(1)	2(<1)	5(2)	4(1)
Accidental injury, urinary	3(1)	3(1)	0	0
Pain at injection site	3(1)	3(1)	0	0
Balanitis	1(<1)	1(<1)	4(2)	3(1)
Urinary urgency	1(<1)	1(<1)	1(<1)	1(<1)
Urethritis	1(<1)	1(<1)	0	0
Epididymitis	1(<1)	1(<1)	0	0
Bladder spasm	1(<1)	1(<1)	0	0
Abscess injection site	1(<1)	1(<1)	0	0
Vaginitis	0	0	1(<1)	1(<1)
Vesicovaginal fistula	0	0	1(<1)	1(<1)

been an occasional case report of other more serious complications associated with urethral collagen injections, such as urethral prolapse (45) and osteitis pubis (46). In general, however, collagen injection is a well-tolerated procedure with minimal morbidity, and the side effects are usually temporary.

2. Autologous Fat

Autologous fat has also been used to treat women with stress urinary incontinence since its introduction by Garibay et al. in 1989 (47). It has the advantages of being readily available, biocompatible, and inexpensive. The main disadvantages is its variability of resorption. Success rates vary from 43 to 86% (Table 3). These studies, however, have relatively shorter-term follow-up (range 7–18 months) than those with collagen injections. Overall, the success rates of autologous fat appear to be inferior to those of collagen. Haab et al. (15) prospectively compared the efficacy of autologous fat and collagen to treat incontinence related to intrinsic sphincteric deficiency. Forty-five women received fat injections and 22 women received collagen injections. At a mean follow-up of 7 months, the dry or improved rate for collagen was 86% and that of autologous fat was 43.2%. In addition, there was a significant difference in the subjective improvement of the collagen group compared with the autologous fat group (64 vs. 22%, respectively). They concluded that collagen is more effective than fat in treating women with intrinsic sphincteric deficiency. Although the autologous fat is less effective, it is felt to be a reasonable option in patients allergic to collagen (15).

The complications of autologous fat injections are similar to those of collagen injections: temporary urinary retention, transient hematuria, and urinary tract infection. As with collagen, these are usually few and self-limited. There have also been case reports of more unusual complications, such as a urethral pseudolipoma after injection of autologous fat (48). Unlike collagen, however, complications relating to the fat-harvesting procedure from

Table 3 Results of Autologous Fat in Women

Author	Number of patients[a]	Follow-up (mo)	Results	Avg. number injections	Mea v
Cervigni/Panei, 1993, abstr (64)	14 (ISD)	10 (3–19)	Cured 57%; improved 29% (overall success 86%); failed 14%	—	
Blaivas/Dmochowski, 1994, abstr (56)	51 (6 mobile urethra, 42 ISD, 3 combined)	12 (1–40)	Overall success (cured/improved) 70%	2.7	
Santarosa/Blaivas, 1994 (19)	15 (12 ISD, 1 mobile urethra, 2 combined)	18 (12–30) (7 patients)	Overall success 57% (84% if exclude patients who chose not to continue collagen secondary to personal reasons)	2.4	
Palma et al., 1997 (48)	30 (ISD) (13—single injection at space of Retzius) (17—repeated injections within urethral muscular envelope)	12	Single injection: 31% dry; 38% improved (overall success 69%) Multiple injections: 64% dry; 12% improved (overall success 76%)	1 2	
Haab et al., 1997 (15)	45 (ISD)	>7	Overall success (dry/improved) 43%; subjective improved 22%	1.7	
Su et al., 1998 (65)	26 (ISD)	12	Dry 50%; improved 15% (overall success 65%)	1	

[a] ISD, intrinsic sphincteric deficiency.

the abdominal wall exist (i.e., abdominal wall hematoma). This complication has been reported to occur in 1–2% of patients (15,18). Thus, possible contraindications to autologous
fat injection include bleeding diathesis and chronic anticoagulation. It is important to in-
form the patient of donor-site pain, bruising, and rarely, a hematoma or infection before of-
fering autologous fat injection. Furthermore, situations in which patients have suboptimal
fat for harvest (e.g., short-gut syndrome) may also be a contraindication (22).

B. Men

Stress urinary incontinence in men is usually iatrogenic (i.e., radical prostatectomy, TURP).
Glutaraldehyde cross-linked collagen has been used to treat this population, although it is
not as effective as it is in women. Overall success rates vary between 36 and 85%, with a
mean follow-up between 6 and 26 months in several series (Table 4). Several authors at-
tribute poorer results to the fixed, nonpliable and scarred proximal urethra that makes it difficult to raise a urethral bleb, thus decreasing the ability of the urethral mucosa to coapt
(9,11,49,50). Those who have severe bladder neck scarring or who have undergone a
transurethral resection or incision of a bladder neck contracture generally have poorer outcomes (9,49,51). In addition, radiation therapy has been shown by some authors to be a
poor prognostic factor as it adds to scarring at the bladder neck (52,53).

The type of surgical treatment an incontinent patient received before injection therapy appears to have a bearing on success rates. Although the numbers in their study were
too few to make any firm conclusions, Smith and Appell found that their patients who have
undergone TURPs had a higher overall success rate compared with those who had radical
prostatectomies (63 vs. 35%, respectively) (51). Similarly, Griebling et al. have shown that
most of the radical prostatectomy patients failed (13/18), whereas all of the patients who
underwent a TURP had minimal or significant improvement (4/4) (54). As in female patients, detrusor instability appeared to be a negative prognostic factor in several series
(10,11,53). In a study by Martins et al. (53), preoperative detrusor hyperactivity was a statistically significant factor in the outcome of collagen injection therapy in postradical
retropubic prostatectomy patients. In their study of 46 postradical retropubic prostatectomy
patients, the percentage of those with detrusor instability who were dry, significantly improved, or failed was 0, 14, and 79%, (53). If detrusor instability is present, it should be
treated with anticholinergics. Appropriately treated, it should not be a contraindication to
injection therapy.

Unlike the studies in women, most authors have shown that the preoperative severity
of male incontinence had a negative effect on the success rates of collagen injection
(43,49,52,53). Smith and Appell have found that patients who used more than three ppd or
wore an external device (e.g., condom catheter or penile clamp) preoperatively for urinary
incontinence had an overall success rate of 28% (vs. 50% in those patients using only one
ppd) (43). The experience by Appell et al. has also shown that men with a history of urine
leakage from a recline position and those with an open bladder neck greater than 1 cm on
fluoroscopic imaging are seldom treated successfully (55). As in women, urethral injection
therapy in men carries similar few, self-limited complications: transient urinary retention,
urinary tract infection, or worsened detrusor instability (11,49,53,54). One patient in a
study by Herschorn et al. suffered acute bacterial prostatitis (11).

In general, the results of Contigen injections in male patients appear somewhat disappointing compared with that in women. Patients can achieve some degree of improvement, but the chance of cure appears to much less, especially in those with significant scarring at the bladder neck or severe preoperative urinary incontinence.

of Glutaraldehyde Cross-Linked Collagen in Men

	Number of patients[a]	Follow-up (mo)	Results[a]	Avg. number injections	Mea vo
9	16 (6 TURP, 10 RP)	(Range 9–23)	Cured 19%; improved 31% (overall success 50%) No change 38%; worse 6% Expired 6% (not related to treatment)	—	
02	10 (4 TURP, 2 RP, 4 NP)	6 (3–11)	Cured 20%; improved 40% (overall success 60%)	6	
94	151 (17 XRT, 134 ISD)	>12	XRT: dry 12%; improved 47% (overall success 59%); no improvement 41% ISD: dry 17%; improved 52% (overall success 69%); no improvement 31%	—	
(9)	33 (22 RP, 11 NP)	65 days	RP: cured 5%; improved 46% (overall success 51%); no change 41%; worse 9% NP: cured 9%; improved 91% (overall success 100%)	—	
ter	60 (ISD)	>24	Cured 25%; improved 47% (overall success 72%); no change 25%; worse 3%	—	
96	15 (RP)	10 (3–15)	Dry 21%; improved 37% (overall success 58%); failed 42%	1.8 (success) 2.4 (failure)	13.8 17.4
(52)	88 (85 RP, 2 NP, 1 trauma)	10 (6–12)	Cured 47%; improved 38% (overall success 85%); no improvement 15%	3.4	
7	25 (18 RP, 4 TURP, 2 salvage RP, cysto-prostatectomy 1)	13	Significantly improved 8%; minimally improved 32%; (overall success 40%) No improvement 60%	2.6	
(53)	46 (RP)	26 (8–44)	Dry 24%; improved 46% (overall 70%); failed 30%	2.3 (dry) 2.5 (improved) 3 (failure)	3 32 (i 48
,	31 (RP)	15 (3–31)	Dry 7%; improved 29% (overall success 36%)	2.6	

omy; XRT, radiation therapy; ISD, intrinsic sphincteric deficiency; TURP, transurethral resection of prostate; NP, neuropathic.

There are very few studies evaluating the use of autologous fat for stress urinary incontinence in men, and the results thus far have been disappointing (19,56). However, urethral injection treatments are minimally invasive and will not interfere with subsequent surgical procedures (i.e., placement of artificial urinary sphincters) (54).

C. Children

In treating incontinence in children, we must consider their longer life expectancy, smaller size, and growth potential. Any intervention should pose minimal risk, be simple to perform, and not affect possible future operative procedures (12). Furthermore, many of these patients (i.e., children with myelodysplasia) have neurogenic bladders, and the ideal treatment should preserve bladder function in a way that is most conducive in protecting the upper urinary tract from damage. The mechanism of action of urethral injectable agents is to prevent urine leakage relative to increases in abdominal pressure by increasing Valsalva LPP. Because there is an unlikely increase in detrusor LPP, urethral injection of agents (i.e., glutaraldehyde cross-linked collagen) is less likely to cause bladder or upper tract deterioration as reported in the more aggressive treatments, such as artificial urinary sphincters or urethral slings (16). These latter modalities increase the detrusor LPP and bladder-emptying pressure. Studies have confirmed that children with improvement in urinary continence after collagen injection usually have increased Valsalva LPP, not resting LPP (12,57,58). In a series by Bomalaski et al. (59), no patient who underwent treatment with urethral collagen injections had urodynamic, radiographic, or clinical evidence of bladder or upper urinary tract deterioration.

The success rate of collagen injection in children ranges from 30 to 88%, with a mean follow-up of 10–24 months (Table 5). In one study, eight patients who were followed for a mean of 4.5 years had durable responses to Contigen with a cure or improvement rate of 86% (59). The population that appears to be best suited for urethral injection of collagen are those with intrinsic sphincteric deficiency from neuropathic causes (i.e., myelodysplasia) or congenital sphincteric deficiency (i.e., exstrophy–epispadias complex) (16,59). In a study by Sundaram et al. (60), their success rates in children (30% overall success rate) were poorer than other studies. They proposed that most of the children in other series had undergone previous anti-incontinence operations (i.e., Young–Dees–Leadbetter procedure), whereas only 10% of the children in their study underwent previous surgery (60). Other favorable patient factors for collagen injection include an adequate bladder capacity with good compliance and stability, and a narrow bladder neck (16,58,61). However, children with detrusor instability who are adequately treated with anticholinergics can subsequently be treated with urethral collagen injections (16). In a study by Chernoff et al. (58), a Valsalva LPP less than 45 cmH$_2$O is associated with a successful outcome. They noted that the coaptation of the urethra is at a maximum in patients with a higher Valsalva LPP and urethral collagen injections would most likely not improve incontinence in these patients (58).

As in adults, the complications of urethral collagen injections in children are mild and self-limited: meatitis, transient worsening of incontinence, temporary urinary retention, and febrile urinary tract infection (12,61). It is usually is not effective as a primary treatment modality for urinary incontinence. It can, however, be used in conjunction with bladder neck reconstruction or when improvement, and not a cure, is the objective (60). Moreover, the children undergoing clean intermittent catheterizations before treatment must continue it afterward (16).

ble 5 Results of Glutaraldehyde Cross-Linked Collagen in Children

athor	Number of patients	Follow-up (mo)	Results	Avg. number injections	Mean vo
an et al., 1992 (12)	8 (6 neuropathic, 1 bilateral ectopic ureter, 1 epispa-dias)	10 (6–33)	Cured 63%; improved 25% (overall success 88%)	2.1	(5-
pozza et al., 1995 (57)	25 (9 neuropathic) (16 exstrophy)	(9–36)	Dry 20%; improved 56% (overall success 76%); failed 24%	—	
n-Chaim et al., 1995 (62)	19 (16 exstrophy, 3 epispadias)	26 (9–84)	Improved 53%; no change 42%; mild improvement (with concomitant fascial sling) 5%	—	
malaski et al., 1996 (59)	40 (25 spina bifida, 12 exstrophy/epispadias, 2 continent reservoirs, 1 bi-lateral ureteral ectopia)	25 (3–75)	Cured 22%; improved 54% (overall success 76%); no change 24%	1.75	(1
onard et al., 1996 (16)	14 (6 neuropathic, 6 extrophy, 1 ectopic urete-rocele excision, 1 trauma)	15 (5–21)	Dry 36%; improved 28% (overall success 64%); failed 36%	—	7 (
rez et al., 1996 (61)	32 (25 neuropathic, 7 exstrophy/epispadias	10 (3–19)	Neuropathic: dry 20%; improved 28% (overall success 48%) Exstrophy/epispadias: dry 43%; im-proved 14% (overall success 57%)	—	Neur 10 Exstro 7.5
ndaram et al., 1997 (60)	20 (15 neuropathic, 4 exstrophy, 1 posterior urethral valve)	15.2 (9–23)	Dry 5%; improved 25% (overall 30%); transient improved (50%); no change 20%	—	
ernoff et al., 1997 (58)	11 (8 neuropathic, 2 exstrophy/epispadias, 1 urogenital sinus defect)	14.4 (4–20)	Dry 36%; improved 19% (overall success 55%); failed 45%	2.5	

VII. SUMMARY

The urethral injection of glutaraldehyde cross-linked collagen or autologous fat has a role in the treatment of urinary incontinence in properly selected patients. It appears to be best suited for patients who have intrinsic sphincteric deficiency associated with minimal urethral hypermobility, an adequate bladder capacity, and a stable detrusor muscle. The treatment responses of urethral injectable agents are best in females, but appear to be less successful than the surgical procedures designed to correct intrinsic sphincteric deficiency. The results are somewhat disappointing in men, which may be related to scarring of the treatment area. In children, the few initial results appear encouraging in select populations (i.e., myelodysplasia, children with exstrophy–epispadias), but the long-term results have yet to be determined.

Importantly, many patients require multiple urethral injections to achieve or maintain improvement of continence. This may be related to several factors including resorption of the injectable agent, inability to determine in advance the volume of substance needed in an individual patient, the unmasking of detrusor abnormalities with improvement of urethral closure, and the increased activities a patient attempts once he or she has become more continent (17). Cost of urethral injection therapy (especially with glutaraldehyde cross-linked collagen) may be a limitation for some patients. Although collagen and autologous fat have been of benefit in treating different patient populations with urinary incontinence, the search for the "ideal" urethral injectable agent continues. This substance must have the following properties: 1) easy to instill, 2) durable, 3) biocompatible, 4) biodegradable, and 5) cost-effective.

Urethral injectables have several distinct advantages. The injection of collagen or autologous fat into the urethra does not create substantial scarring to the area. Furthermore, the procedure is well tolerated by patients and is associated with minimal morbidity, which is usually transient. Thus, this minimally invasive procedure can offer hope for those patients who are elderly or are poor surgical candidates, and will not preclude a surgical procedure for those who desire a more aggressive treatment for their urinary incontinence in the future.

REFERENCES

1. Murless BC. The injection treatment of stress incontinence. J Obstet Gynaecol 1938; 45:67–73.
2. Sasche H. Die Behandlung der Haminkontinenz mit der Sklerotherapie. Urol Int 1963; 15:225.
3. Quackels R. Deux incontinences après adénonectomie guéries par injection de paraffine dans le périnée. Acta Urol Belg 1955; 23:259–262.
4. Lopez AE, Padron OF, Patsias G, Politano VA. Transurethral polytetrafluoroethylene injection in female patients with urinary incontinence. J Urol 1993; 150:856–858.
5. Berg S. Polytef augmentation urethroplasty. Correction of surgically incurable urinary incontinence by injection technique. Arch Surg 1973; 107:379–381.
6. Politano VA. Periurethral polytetrafluoroethylene injection for urinary incontinence. J Urol 1982; 127:439–442.
7. Malizia AA, Reiman HM, Myers RP, Sande JR, Barham SS, Benson RC, Dewanjee MK, Utz WJ. Migration and granulomatous reaction after periurethral injection of polytef (Teflon). JAMA 1984; 251:3277–3281.
8. McGuire EJ, Appell RA. Transurethral collagen injection for urinary incontinence. Urology 1994; 43:413–415.
9. Nataluk EA, Assimos DG, Kroovand RL. Collagen injections for treatment of urinary incontinence secondary to intrinsic sphincter deficiency. J Endourol 1995; 9:403–406.

10. Shortliffe LM, Freiha FS, Kessler R, Stamey TA, Constantinou CE. Treatment of urinary incontinence by the periurethral implantation of glutaraldehyde cross-linked collagen. J Urol 1989; 141:538–541.

11. Herschorn S, Radomski SB, Steele DJ. Early experience with intraurethral collagen injections for urinary incontinence. J Urol 1992; 148:1797–1800.

12. Wan J, McGuire EJ, Bloom DA, Ritchey ML. The treatment of urinary incontinence in children using glutaraldehyde cross-linked collagen. J Urol 1992; 148:127–130.

13. Richardson TD, Kennelly MJ, Faerber GJ. Endoscopic injection of glutaraldehyde cross-linked collagen for the treatment of intrinsic sphincter deficiency in women. Urology 1995; 46:378–381.

14. Benshushan A, Brzezinski A, Shoshani O, Rojansky N. Periurethral injection for the treatment of urinary incontinence. Obstet Gynecol Surv 1998; 53:383–388.

15. Haab F, Zimmern PE, Leach GE. Urinary stress incontinence due to intrinsic sphincteric deficiency: experience with fat and collagen periurethral injections. J Urol 1997; 157:1283–1286.

16. Leonard MP, Decter A, Mix LW, Johnson HW, Coleman GU. Treatment of urinary incontinence in children by endoscopically directed bladder neck injection of collagen. J Urol 1996; 156:637–641.

17. Appell RA. Collagen injection therapy for urinary incontinence. Urol Clin North Am 1994; 21:177–182.

18. Palma PC, Riccetto CLZ, Herrmann V, Netto NR. Repeated lipoinjection for stress urinary incontinence. J Endourol 1997; 11:67–70.

19. Santarosa RP, Blaivas JG. Periurethral injection of autologous fat for the treatment of sphincteric incontinence. J Urol 1994; 151:607–611.

20. Horl HW, Feller AM, Biemer E. Technique for liposuction fat reimplantation and long-term volume evaluation by magnetic resonance imaging. Ann Plast Surg 1991; 26:248–258.

21. Pinski KS, Roenigk HH. Autologous fat transplantation: long-term follow-up. Dermatol Surg Oncol 1992; 18:179–184.

22. Trockman BA, Leach GE. Surgical treatment of intrinsic urethral dysfunction: injectable fat. Urol Clin North Am 1995; 22:665–671.

23. Ersek RA. Transplantation of purified autologous fat: a 3-year follow-up is disappointing. Plast Reconstr Surg 1991; 87:219–227.

24. Gasperoni C, Salgarello M, Emiliozzi P, Gargani G. Subdermal liposuction. Aesthetic Plast Surg 1990; 14:137–142.

25. Chajchir A, Benzaquen I. Fat-grafting injection for soft-tissue augmentation. Plast Reconstr Surg 1989; 84:921–934.

26. Remacle M, Bertrand B, Eloy P, Marbaix E. The use of injectable collagen to correct velopharyngeal insufficiency. Laryngoscope 1990; 100:269–274.

27. Remacle M, Declaye XJ. GAX-collagen injection to correct an enlarged tracheoesophageal fistula for a vocal prosthesis. Laryngoscope 1988; 98:1350–1352.

28. Cooperman L, Michaeli D. The immunogenicity of injectable collagen. I. A 1-year prospective study. J Am Acad Dermatol 1984; 10:638–646.

29. Cooperman L, Michaeli D. The immunogenicity of injectable collagen. II. A retrospective review of seventy-two tested and treated patients. J Am Acad Dermatol 1984; 10:647–651.

30. Siegle RJ, McCoy JP, Schade W, Swanson NA. Intradermal implantation of bovine collagen. Humoral immune responses associated with clinical reactions. Arch Dermatol 1984; 120:183–187.

31. DeLustro F, Condell RA, Nguyen MA, McPherson JM. A comparative study of the biologic and immunologic response to medical devices derived from dermal collagen. J Biomed Mater Res 1986; 20:109–120.

32. Winters JC, Appell R. Periurethral injection of collagen in the treatment of intrinsic sphincteric deficiency in the female patient. Urol Clin North Am 1995; 22:673–678.

33. McPherson JM, Ledger PW, Sawamura S, Conti A, Wade S, Reinhanian H, Wallace DG. The preparation and physicochemical characterization of an injectable form of reconstituted, glutaraldehyde cross-linked, bovine corium collagen. J Biomed Mater Res 1986; 20:79–92.

34. McPherson JM, Sawamura S, Armstrong R. An examination of the biologic response to injectable, glutaraldehyde cross-linked collagen implants. J Biomed Mater Res 1986; 20:93–107.

35. Carr LK, Herschorn S, Leonhardt C. Magnetic resonance imaging after intraurethral collagen injected for stress urinary incontinence. J Urol 1996; 155:1253–1255.

36. Leonard MP, Canning DA, Epstein JI, Gearhart JP, Jeffs RD. Local tissue reaction to the subureteral injection of glutaraldehyde cross-linked bovine collagen in humans. J Urol 1990; 143: 1209–1212.

37. Monga AK, Robinson D, Stanton SL. Periurethral collagen injections for genuine stress incontinence: a 2-year follow-up. Br J Urol 1995; 76:156–160.

38. Swami S, Batista JE, Abrams P. Collagen for female genuine stress incontinence after a minimum 2-year follow-up. Br J Urol 1997; 80:757–761.

39. Eckford SD, Abrams P. Para-urethral collagen implantation for female stress incontinence. Br J Urol 1991; 68:586–589.

40. Stricker P, Haylen B. Injectable collagen for type 3 female stress incontinence: the first 50 Australian patients. Med J Aust 1993; 158:89–91.

41. Herschorn S, Steele DJ, Radomski SB. Follow-up of intraurethral collagen for female stress urinary incontinence. J Urol 1996; 156:1305–1309.

42. Monga AK, Stanton SL. Urodynamics: prediction, outcome and analysis of mechanism for cure of stress incontinence by periurethral collagen. Br J Obstet Gynaecol 1997; 104:158–162.

43. Smith DN, Appell RA, Winters JC, Rackley RR. Collagen injection therapy for female intrinsic sphincteric deficiency. J Urol 1997; 157:1275–1278.

44. Stothers L, Goldenberg SL, Leone EF. Complications of periurethral collagen injection for stress urinary incontinence. J Urol 1998; 159:806–807.

45. Harris RL, Cundiff GW, Coates KW, Addison WA, Bump RC. Urethral prolapse after collagen injection. Am J Obstet Gynecol 1998; 178:614–615.

46. Matthews K, Govier FE. Osteitis pubis after periurethral collagen injection. Urology 1997; 49: 237–238.

47. Gonzales de Garibay S, Castro Morrondo J, Castillo Jimeno JM, Sanchez Robles I, Sebastian Borruel JL. Endoscopic injection of autologous adipose tissue in the treatment of female incontinence. Arch Esp Urol 1989; 42:143–146.

48. Palma PC, Riccetto CL, Netto NR. Urethral pseudolipoma: a complication of periurethral lipoinjection for stress urinary incontinence in a woman. J Urol 1996; 155:646.

49. Cummings JM, Boullier JA, Parra RO. Transurethral collagen injections in the therapy of postradical prostatectomy stress incontinence. J Urol 1996; 155:1011–1013.

50. Sanchez–Ortiz RF, Broderick GA, Chaikin DC, Malkowicz SB, Van Arsdalen K, Blander DS, Wein AJ. Collagen injection therapy for post-radical retropubic prostatectomy incontinence: role of Valsalva leak point pressure. J Urol 1997; 158:2132–2136.

51. Smith DN, Appell RA, Rackley RR, Winters JC. Collagen injection therapy for postprostatectomy incontinence. J Urol 1998; 160:364–367.

52. Aboseif SR, O'Connell HE, Usui A, McGuire EJ. Collagen injection for intrinsic sphincteric deficiency in men. J Urol 1996; 155:10–13.

53. Martins FE, Bennett CJ, Dunn M, Filho D, Keller T, Lieskovsky G. Adverse prognostic features of collagen injection therapy for urinary incontinence following radical retropubic prostatectomy. J Urol 1997; 158:1745–1749.

54. Griebling TL, Kreder KJ, Williams RD. Trans-urethral collagen injection for treatment of postprostatectomy urinary incontinence in men. Urology 1997; 49:907–912.

55. Appell RA, McGuire EJ, DeRidder PA, Bennett AH, Webster GD, Badlani G, Bennett JK, Green B. Summary of effectiveness and safety in the prospective, open, multicenter investigation of Contigen implant for incontinence due to intrinsic sphincteric deficiency in males. AUA 89th Annual Meeting, San Francisco, CA, May 14–19, 1994.

56. Blaivas JG, Heritz D, Santarosa RP, Dmochowski R, Ganabathi K, Roskamp D, Leach G. Peri-urethral fat injection for post-prostatectomy sphincteric incontinence. AUA 89th annual meeting, San Francisco, CA, May 14–19, 1994.

57. Capozza N, Caione P, De Gennaro M, Nappo S, Patricolo M. Endoscopic treatment of vesico-ureteric reflux and urinary incontinence: technical problems in the paediatric patient. Br J Urol 1995; 75:538–542.

58. Chemoff A, Horowitz M, Combs A, Libretti D, Nitti V, Glassberg KI. Periurethral collagen injection for the treatment of urinary incontinence in children. J Urol 1997; 157:2303–2305.

59. Bomalaski MD, Bloom DA, McGuire EJ, Panzl A. Glutaraldehyde cross-linked collagen in the treatment of urinary incontinence in children. J Urol 1996; 155:699–702.

60. Sundaram CP, Reinberg Y, Aliabadi HA. Failure to obtain durable results with collagen implantation in children with urinary incontinence. J Urol 1997; 157:2306–2307.

61. Perez LM, Smith EA, Parrott TS, Broecker BH, Massad CA, Woodard JR. Submucosal bladder neck injection of bovine dermal collagen for stress urinary incontinence in the pediatric population. J Urol 1996; 156:633–636.

62. Ben-Chaim J, Jeffs RD, Peppas DS, Gearhart JP. Submucosal bladder neck injections of glutaraldehyde cross-linked bovine collagen for the treatment of urinary incontinence in patients with the exstrophy/epispadias complex. J Urol 1995; 154:862–864.

63. Bard CR Inc. PMAA submission to United States Food and Drug Administration for IDE G850010, 1990.

64. Cervigni M, Panei M. Periurethral autologous fat injection for type III stress urinary incontinence. AUA 88th Annual Meeting, San Antonio, TX, May 15–20, 1993.

65. Su TH, Wang KG, Hsu CY, Wei HJ, Yen HJ, Shien FC. Periurethral fat injection in the treatment of recurrent genuine stress urinary incontinence. J Urol 1998; 159:411–414.

66. Kieswetter H, Fischer M, Wober L, Flamm J. Endoscopic implantation of collagen (GAX) for the treatment of urinary incontinence. Br J Urol 1992; 69:22–25.

67. Contigen Bard Collagen Implant Product Monograph. Covington, GA: Bard Urological Division, CR Bard, Inc, 1993.

68. O'Connell HE, McGuire EJ, Aboseif S, Usui A. Transurethral collagen therapy in women. J Urol 1995; 154:1463–1465.

69. Stanton SL, Monga AK, Incontinence in elderly women is periurethral collagen an advance? Br J Obstet Gynaecol 1997; 104:154–157.

70. Corcos J, Fournier C. 4 year follow-up of collagen injection for urinary stress incontinence. AUA 92nd Annual Meeting, New Orleans, LA, April 12–17, 1997.

71. Weil D, Hadley HR, Dickinson M. Collagen injection for female incontinence: results after a minimum of one year follow-up. AUA 92nd Annual Meeting, New Orleans, LA, April 12–17, 1997.

34

The Artificial Urinary Sphincter

STEVEN E. MUTCHNIK and TIMOTHY B. BOONE

Baylor College of Medicine, Houston, Texas

I. HISTORY

The concept of an artificial device for treating urinary incontinence dates back to 1947 when Foley described and patented an inflatable cuff that wrapped around the bulbous urethra and was inflated by an externalized pump (1,2). Other authors described devices in the 1970s that never gained wide popularity either because of high mechanical failure rates, no human data, or lack of controlled compression of the urethra (3,4).

In 1976, Rosen described a prosthesis containing two fluid-filled components: an inflatable perineal occluder, which was placed anterior to the bulbar urethra and compressed the urethra against two contramember strut arms placed posteriorly, and a scrotal reservoir/pump with a deflation valve. The patient inflated the perineal occluder to a pressure sufficient for continence and deflated the occluder to allow bladder emptying (5). Initial reports with this device were positive, with 11 of 16 patients continent and no cases of pressure necrosis of the urethra (6). However, with the patient allowed to regulate the degree of urethral closure pressure, the devices were often overinflated, eventually resulting in high rates of urethral erosion. The Rosen device was never extensively implanted and is now only of historical value (7).

Experience with these early devices led investigators to realize that the pressure exerted by the compressive cuff was the key element to a successful device. Aggressive urethral or bladder neck compression, while providing excellent continence, inevitably leads to pressure necrosis and erosion; inadequate closure pressures are safe, but do not provide sufficient compression for satisfactory urinary control. The evolution of the American Medical Systems (AMS) series of artificial sphincter devices is the result of attempts to achieve continence with acceptable rates of pressure necrosis.

Scott described the first-generation artificial sphincter, the AMS 721, in 1973 (8). The device consisted of an occlusive inflatable cuff, an abdominal fluid reservoir, and separate

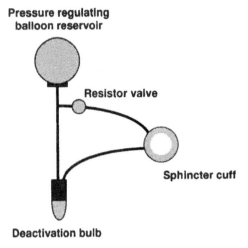

Pressure regulating
balloon reservoir

Resistor valve

Sphincter cuff

Deactivation bulb

AMS 742A

Figure 1   American Medical Systems artificial urinary sphincter model 742A, used from 1974 to 1979: a scrotal/labial pump forced fluid from the cuff to the balloon reservoir. Refilling was controlled by a resistor valve in the tubing from the reservoir to the cuff.

inflation and deflation bulbs. Pressure was regulated by the inflation–deflation bulbs and thus erosion rates were unacceptably high owing to poor regulation of the pressure in the system. Subsequently, the AMS 742 and 761 models were developed (Fig. 1). These models took advantage of a design concept critical to the long-term success seen with the artificial sphincter. An elastic pressure-balloon reservoir was used to provide constant, predetermined pressure within the system. Balloon reservoirs of various pressures (51–60 cmH$_2$O, 61–70 cmH$_2$O, and 71–80 cmH$_2$O) can be selected based on the clinical situation and location of the cuff. A resistor valve was also developed to regulate flow back from the cuff to the reservoir on refilling, giving the patient 3–5 min to void. Further modifications were made to all components of the AMS artificial urinary sphincter (AUS) that greatly increased the reliability, success, and ease of implantation of the device. The AMS 791 and 792 models contained a control assembly in the balloon reservoir tubing that controlled directional fluid flow and refilling (Fig. 2).

The concept that delayed activation of the AUS after implantation can decrease rates of pressure necrosis and cuff erosion, particularly in previously radiated or operated on fields, was introduced as early as 1981 by Furlow (9). Many patients are unable to use the AUS immediately in the postoperative period because of scrotal edema or tenderness. As the AMS 791/792 had no mechanism for extended deactivation, a two-stage implantation procedure was required. The cuff, balloon, and pump were implanted in one setting, followed a few months later by insertion of the control assembly and activation. The ability to deactivate the AUS without an operation is beneficial in patients who are to undergo urethral catheterization or instrumentation. This can limit pressure-induced ischemia, cuff erosion, and urethral trauma.

The AMS 800, introduced in 1983, contains all control mechanisms in the scrotal pump component (Figs. 3 and 4). This pump includes a deactivation button permitting simple device deactivation by the physician. AUS implantation can therefore be accomplished in a single procedure in all patients, and the cuff can be left in a deflated state for any rea-

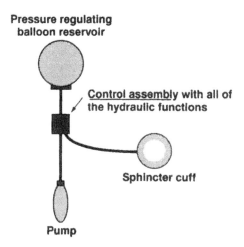

Figure 2 American Medical Systems artificial urinary sphincter model 791/792, used from 1979 to 1983: a single control assembly contained all filling and refilling functions.

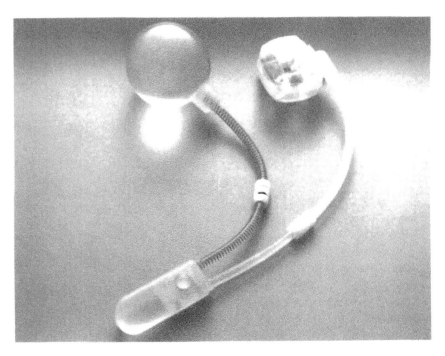

Figure 3 American Medical Systems artificial urinary sphincter model 800, used from 1983 to present: all hydraulic functions, including the deactivation button, are now contained in the scrotal or labial pump.

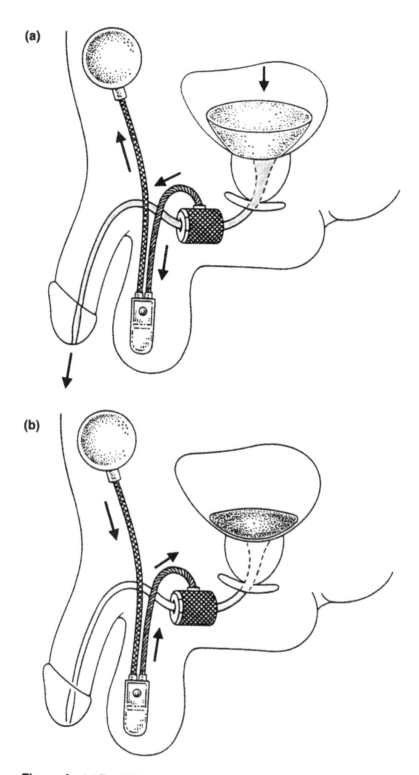

Figure 4 (a) To void the patient squeezes the pump to move fluid from the cuff to the pressure-regulating balloon. (b) After voiding the fluid automatically returns from the pressure-regulating balloon to the cuff. (Courtesy of American Medical Systems.)

son postoperatively. The AMS 800 cuff includes a lubricant coating to prevent leaks at folds in the deflated cuff, and narrow backing to prevent urethral erosion at the edges of the cuff.

II. PATIENT SELECTION

Any patient with urinary incontinence secondary to urethral sphincteric deficiency can be considered a candidate for AUS implantation. No specific limits on severity of leakage are required. It is our belief that a patient's bother and lifestyle issues should be the determinant of whether incontinence is severe enough to warrant AUS placement, and no absolute quantitated minimum amount of leakage is necessary. Before recommending an AUS to an incontinent patient, however, an appropriate evaluation is required to determine if this therapy is warranted.

A. History and Physical Examination

Critical data to be obtained include the etiology of the incontinence (prostatectomy, myelodysplasia, previous bladder or urethral surgery, spinal cord injury, trauma, radiotherapy, or other), severity of the leakage, effect on the quality of life of the patient, and character of the incontinence (continual, stress, urge, mixed, or other). The patient's motivation to undergo surgical therapy for incontinence and the cognitive capacity to operate the device must be determined. Women must be counseled on the limited data relative to pregnancy and childbirth in female AUS patients.

The physical examination should concentrate on the lower abdomen and genitalia. Patients must be able to undergo a lower abdominal incision for balloon reservoir placement. The scrotum or labia must be able to accommodate the pump control assembly. The male perineum should be free of induration and the skin must be free of cutaneous infection if a bulbar urethral cuff is planned, particularly in previously irradiated patients. Urethral meatal stenosis should be noted because it must be repaired before AUS placement. In women, a vaginal examination is mandatory to determine the quality of tissues adjacent to the urethra and bladder neck and to assess concurrent prolapse that may require simultaneous repair.

B. Cystourethroscopy

All candidates for an AUS should undergo endoscopic examination of the lower urinary tract. Intravesical pathology, such as tumors, calculi, foreign body, and inflammatory lesions, should be managed with appropriate follow-up before implantation. The urethra should be examined for stricture disease. Anastomotic strictures are not uncommon in men with postprostatectomy incontinence. It is our view that these strictures should be opened and rechecked at least 2–3 months later before AUS placement. In patients with recurrent stricture disease after repeated endoscopic treatment, we have staged reconstruction by successfully placing a urethral stent(s) (UroLume, American Medical Systems) followed by AUS placement several months later when the stent has epithelialized. Managing proximal urethral strictures after AUS implantation can be extremely difficult, with a high risk of infection, erosion, and perforation of the cuff.

C. Videourodynamics

Data obtained from the urodynamic evaluation are of critical importance in the evaluation of an incontinent patient for possible AUS implantation. Valsalva leak-point pressures should be obtained to ensure intrinsic sphincteric deficiency as the primary etiology of the incontinence. Severe detrusor instability or hyperreflexia is a relative contraindication to AUS placement and may, in fact, worsen postoperatively. Milder degrees of detrusor overactivity should be treated with pharmacological therapy; such patients with a good response may be successfully treated with an AUS.

Impaired detrusor compliance may coexist with sphincteric insufficiency and rarely responds to medical therapy. As compliance may worsen after AUS implantation relative to increased bladder outlet resistance, augmentation cystoplasty may be required either before or simultaneous with AUS placement. Failure to address a noncompliant bladder can lead to recurrent incontinence or upper urinary tract damage.

Patients should be able to demonstrate adequate bladder emptying. Elevated residual volumes place the patient at increased risk of urinary tract infections, calculi, and overflow incontinence. Such patients must be able and willing to perform clean, intermittent self-catheterization after AUS placement. Similarly, any degree of bladder outlet obstruction noted urodynamically by elevated voiding pressures should be investigated and managed before surgery.

Simultaneous radiographic imaging of the lower urinary tract is helpful in the evaluation of AUS candidates. Abnormalities requiring attention before sphincter placement, which can be seen fluoroscopically, include bladder diverticuli, vesicoureteral reflux, detrusor–sphincter dyssynergia, bladder outlet obstruction, and urethral anomalies. The decision to perform ureteral reimplantation before AUS implantation in patients with vesicoureteral reflux should be individualized and based on patient age, history of urinary tract infections, grade of reflux, and associated anatomical anomalies.

Patients with impaired bladder compliance, congenital anomalies of the urinary tract, renal insufficiency, or complicated urological history should undergo upper urinary tract imaging as part the evaluation. This can be accomplished with intravenous–retrograde ureteropyelography or renal sonography. Upper tract imaging is probably not necessary in men with uncomplicated postprostatectomy incontinence.

III. OPERATIVE TECHNIQUE

Patients must have sterile urine before surgery. Urinary tract infections must be treated with culture-specific antimicrobials and eradication of the organism confirmed by a negative culture or bacteriuria screen within a few days of the scheduled procedure. Cutaneous dermatitis and candidiasis are also common in incontinent patients. These skin conditions should be resolved before surgery. Foley catheterization for 1–2 weeks can often be helpful in keeping the perineum dry and allowing skin infection to clear.

Patients are admitted to the hospital on the morning of surgery. They are given broad-spectrum intravenous antibiotics preoperatively covering gram-positive and enteric gram-negative organisms. The operative field is shaved immediately before the skin preparation. The patient is positioned in the lithotomy position if a bulbar urethral cuff is to be placed and in a low lithotomy or frog-leg position if a bladder neck cuff is to placed. Skin preparation is performed with iodophor-based solution for a full 10 min and females receive a vaginal preparation as well.

A. Bulbar Urethral Cuff Technique

We place a 12F coude catheter to ensure bladder emptying throughout the procedure and to assist with urethral dissection (Fig. 5). A midline perineal incision is made with the mid-

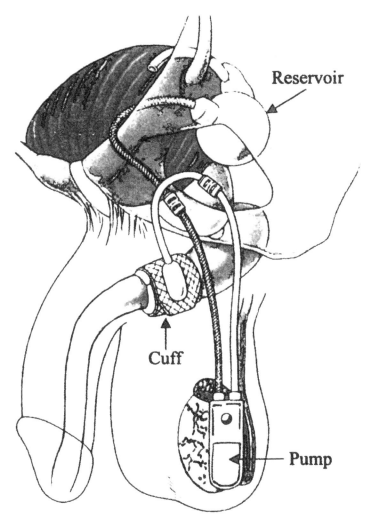

Figure 5 The artificial urinary sphincter with the cuff around the urethra, pump in the scrotum, and reservoir implanted behind the rectus muscle. (Courtesy of American Medical Systems.)

point of the incision placed at the level of the turn of the bulbar urethra as it enters the urogenital diaphragm. A second incision is made in the suprapubic area, usually through the patient's previous surgical scar, if present. A Scott ring retractor (Lone Star Medical Products, Houston, TX) is useful for perineal exposure. Sharp dissection is used to expose the bulbocavernosus muscle approximately 1–2 cm distal to the turn of the urethra. This muscle is incised longitudinally in the midline with care to preserve the muscle bellies bilaterally for subsequent closure over the cuff. The bulbar urethra is identified and circumferentially mobilized. A Babcock clamp gently placed around the anterior wall of the urethral and the catheter can assist in exposure to the posterior wall. Because no defined plane exists between the posterior wall of the urethra and the tunica albuginea of the corpora cavernosa, care must be taken not to perforate the urethra at this level. It is our contention that any urethral injury noted intraoperatively necessitates termination of the procedure because of the greatly increased risk of infection or erosion if an AUS is placed, even if the perforation is repaired primarily. Smaller urethral perforations can be detected by the forceful injection of antibiotic irrigation into the meatus alongside the catheter. A right-angle clamp is passed behind the urethra and the circumference of the urethra is measured with measuring tape. Most patients will be properly fit with a 4.5-cm cuff, although smaller or larger urethras will occasionally be encountered and required a 4.0- or 5.0-cm cuff, respectively. The cuff is passed around the urethra by grasping the noninflating tab with the right-angle clamp. Care must be taken not to grasp the silicone component of the cuff, not to kink the cuff through an inadequate space posterior to the urethra, and to be sure the tab is completely fastened around the cuff button. A knitting needle instrument is used to pass the cuff tubing through the bulbocavernosus muscle and anteriorly into the superficial tissues of the suprapubic incision. The tubing should be directed laterally so as not to leave tubing directly abutting the base of the penis, which can be uncomfortable in the postoperative period.

Through a separate suprapubic incision the rectus fascia is divided sharply for a few centimeters and the retropubic space is entered sharply deep to the rectus abdominis muscle. Blunt dissection should be avoided, for the bladder is often adherent anteriorly to the rectus muscle. The pressure-regulating balloon reservoir is placed in the retropubic pocket, and the tubing is brought through a separate stab wound in the anterior rectus sheath. Typically, a 61- to 70-cmH$_2$O balloon is used, although patients at high risk for urethral erosion are better mananged with a 51- to 60-cmH$_2$O balloon. The rectus fascia is reapproximated with a running, absorbable suture.

A long, curved hemostat is passed from the inferior margin of the suprapubic incision into the anterior hemiscrotum of choice based on the handedness of the patient. Again, this subcutaneous tunnel should course at least 1 cm lateral to the base of the penis and stay anteriorly in the scrotum. Once this clamp has created a scrotal pocket in the most dependent portion of the scrotum, it is replaced with a long nasal speculum. The pump control assembly can be passed between the spread jaws of the speculum and into the scrotal pocket. A babcock clamp is used to gently hold the pump in place while the procedure is completed.

The retropubic balloon reservoir is filled with 22 mL of an appropriate solution. Normal saline is most frequently used, although various iso-osmotic mixtures of contrast material can also be created that will allow radiography of the AUS postoperatively. Table 1 lists the various contrast materials and their appropriate dilution ratios. After ensuring no air, serum, or debris is present in any of the components, the tubing from the pump-control assembly is connected to the cuff and reservoir in the suprapubic area. Either straight or right-angle connectors can be used and secured with the quick-connect system. AMS advises the connections be hand-tied with 2-0 or 3-0 prolene suture on revision cases. The device should be cycled under direct vision to be sure the cuff inflates and deflates properly. All components and surgical fields should be copiously irrigated with antibiotic irrigation solution and both incisions closed in layers with absorbable suture. The AUS is deactivated using the pump control assembly button with the cuff deflated. Patients with a bulbar urethral cuff can usually have the urethral catheter removed and be discharged from the hospital within 24 hr.

B. Bladder Neck Cuff Technique, Suprapubic Approach

A Foley catheter is placed under sterile conditions to assist in bladder drainage and bladder neck dissection. A low midline or Pfannenstiel incision is made and exposure of the ex-

Table 1   Contrast Media and Their Dilution Ratios as Recommended by American Medical Systems, Inc.

Solution	Amount (mL)		Sterile H_2O (mL)
Cysto Conray II	60	+	15
Hypaque 25%	50	+	60
Urovist Cysto	50	+	50
Cystografin Dilute	60	+	13
Isopaque Cysto	60	+	27
Hypaque–Meglumine 30%	60	+	56
Conray FL	58	+	42
Telebrix 12	53	+	47
Urografin 30%	49	+	51
Dip Conray 30%	47	+	50
Omnipaque 180	60	+	15
Omnipaque 240	60	+	35
Omnipaque 300	57	+	60
Omnipaque 350	48	+	60
Iopamiro 300	53	+	60
Iopamiro 200	60	+	23
Iopamiro 370	38	+	60
Solutrast 300	53	+	47
Solutrast 200	60	+	22
Cystografin 14%	62	+	59

traperitoneal retropubic space is obtained by sharp and blunt dissection. The inferior bladder segment is mobilized and the endopelvic fascia exposed. The endopelvic fascia is then sharply incised bilaterally and the bladder neck and posterior urethra are mobilized. Sharp dissection is employed to develop the plane posterior to the bladder neck and anterior to the vagina in the female or rectum in male patients. A pack in the relevant structure is helpful in this dissection, which can be difficult in the previously operated on field. A high cystotomy can also be created to assist in finding the plane posterior to the bladder neck, with no increased risk of infection or erosion.

A 2-cm–wide window posterior to the bladder neck is adequate for cuff placement, and a right-angle clamp is used to pass the measuring tape around the bladder neck. The bladder is then filled with antibiotic solution through the Foley catheter. Any small perforations can be closed with absorbable suture. Similarly, vaginal perforations, if small, can be closed primarily. Rectal injuries, however, require aborting the procedure. The appropriate-sized cuff can then be passed and secured around the bladder neck. Bladder neck cuff sizes range from 6 to 11 cm, depending on patient age, gender, size, and quality of tissues. The cuff tubing is brought out through the rectus muscle and fascia through a separate stab wound at least 5 cm superior to the pubis.

The pressure-regulating balloon reservoir is placed in the retropubic space, with its tubing also penetrating the rectus muscle and fascia near the cuff tubing. A 71- to 80-cmH_2O balloon is typically used, although a 61- to 70-cmH_2O balloon can be used in selected, high-risk patients. The anterior rectus sheath is closed with heavy absorbable suture. The balloon reservoir is filled with 22 mL of normal saline. The pump control assembly component is placed in a dependent subcutaneous position in the scrotum or labium, as described in the foregoing, for the bulbar urethral cuff AUS. Connections are made in the suprapubic area and after the wound is copiously irrigated with antibiotic solution the incision is closed in layers. The AUS is deactivated with the cuff deflated at the termination of the procedure. The Foley catheter is removed 24 hr postoperatively.

C.   Bladder Neck Cuff Technique, Transvaginal Approach

With the patient in the dorsal lithotomy position, a weighted vaginal speculum is placed in the vagina. A 16F Foley catheter is then placed in the bladder. An inverted U incision is made in the anterior vaginal wall with the apex centered in the midurethra. This vaginal wall flap is dissected free of the underlying urethra and bladder neck. The endopelvic fascia is then perforated with scissors bilaterally and the bladder neck and proximal urethra are dissected free of surrounding adhesions. The anterior plane between the bladder and the underside of the pubic bone is developed bluntly, and the measuring tape is passed to select a cuff of the appropriate circumference. The cuff is placed and rotated so that the cuff tubing exits laterally. The bladder is filled with antibiotic solution to check for small, unrecognized perforations, and cystoscopy is performed to ensure that cuff placement is distal to the ureteral orifices.

A suprapubic incision is made and the balloon reservoir and labial pump assembly are prepared and placed as described earlier. The cuff tubing is passed through the retropubic space and through a separate stab wound in the rectus muscle and fascia. After the balloon is filled, tubing connections are made, and the device is cycled under direct vision. The cuff is then deflated, the device deactivated, and the wounds irrigated. The vaginal and suprapubic incisions are closed in layers with absorbable suture and an antibiotic-soaked vaginal pack is placed.

IV.   POSTOPERATIVE CARE

Patients are given routine postoperative instructions on discharge from the hospital. Oral, broad-spectrum antibiotics are continued for 1 week, and patients are advised that their incontinence should not vary considerably from the preoperative state. Most patients find that most swelling and tenderness occur at the scrotal or labial control pump site. For this reason, and to allow for full healing of incisions, activation is typically delayed for 4–6 weeks. It is advised to have the patient periodically pull down on the pump to keep it in a dependent scrotal or labial position. At this time, if tenderness surrounding the pump is resolved, the device is activated by forceful compression of the pump. This will pop the deactivation button back into the activated position and the occlusive cuff will inflate. We always observe whether patients successfully operate the artificial sphincter before allowing them to go home with the activated device.

The AUS 800 device requires between one and three pumps to fully decompress the cuff, depending on the size of the cuff used. Patients have 2–3 min within which to empty the bladder until the cuff automatically reinflates. They are instructed to simply depress the control pump again if complete bladder emptying did not occur before refilling.

Some implanters instruct all AUS patients on how to deactivate the device by depressing the deactivation button on the control-pump assembly and advise patients who are continent at night to deactivate the device while asleep. All patients should be instructed that the AUS 800 can and should be deactivated by medical personnel familiar with the device before any urethral catheterization or manipulation. Patients are also instructed to notify their physician immediately with symptoms of urinary tract infection, hematuria, or increasing pain or swelling around any of the components.

V. RESULTS

As the AMS 800 AUS has now been commercially available for over 15 years, several large series have examined the long-term success rates as well as reoperation rates using this device. Elliott and Barrett reviewed the Mayo Clinic experience of 323 patients implanted with the AMS 800 (10). Mean follow-up was 68.8 months. These investigators found that the narrow-back cuff modification of the AMS 800 has resulted in dramatically reduced mechanical failure, nonmechanical failure, and reoperation rates. Only 17% of patients with the narrow-back cuff design required reoperation and the mechanical failure rate has been reduced to 7.6%. Among all 323 patients, 72% required no surgical intervention after implantation.

Fulford et al. reviewed their results of 68 patients implanted with the AMS 800 with more than 10-years follow-up on all patients (11). Overall, 75% of these patients reported satisfactory continence, but at the expense of a high complication and reoperation rate; only 13% were continent with their original device. These data emphasize that the modifications in cuff design of the AMS 800 have led directly to decreased mechanical complication and reoperation rates.

The most common indication for placement of an AUS is male postprostatectomy incontinence. Several series describe their results with the device for this indication with more than 1-year follow-up. Marks and Light from Baylor were the first to report such a series in 1989. These investigators describe satisfactory "social continence" of 94.5% (12). Litwiller et al. similarly found a higher than 90% satisfaction rate with the AUS in a group of men with severe postprostatectomy incontinence at mean 23.4-months follow-up (13). They noted, however, that up to 50% of the men did have some leakage of a few drops daily, and that the complete continence rate was only 20%. With a minimum of 3.5-years follow-up Haab et al. described social continence in 54 of 68 men, with a revision rate in later AMS 800 devices of only 12.5% (14). Klijn et al. reported a similar 81% satisfaction rate at a mean of 35 months, but predicted, based on Kaplan–Meier curves, a 50% success rate with the original device at 5 years (15). Overall, the literature suggests that, although many patients continue to have some urine leakage and can expect a surgical revision rate of 10–30% at 5 years, an extremely high patient satisfaction rate can be achieved with the AUS for postprostatectomy incontinence.

Published data examining the results of the AUS in women with the latest device modifications are less replete, most likely secondary to other successful alternative treatments for female incontinence (sling procedures and injectables). A recent review on this topic was published by Elliott and Barrett of the Mayo Clinic (16). They report that only 3% of 400 patients in their AUS series were women. In these patients with incontinence secondary either to resection of gynecological or gastrointestinal malignancy or myelodysplasia, a 72% product survival rate and a 67% pad-free rate were achieved. They state that although the indications for AUS placement in incontinent women are extremely rare, long-term success can be achieved in carefully selected patients. It has been demonstrated that women with an AUS have no increased complications during pregnancy with either spontaneous vaginal or cesarean section delivery (17).

Review of the literature reveals a vast experience with the AUS for incontinent children. The majority of children have meningomyelocele and a neurogenic bladder. A large series from Simeoni et al. described the results of AUS placement in 107 children with a mean 5-years follow-up. Eighty-one percent of patients kept their devices, and 83% of these were completely continent (18). However, over 50% of these children required surgical revision, emphasizing the need for continued close follow-up. Levesque et al. confirmed an 82% continence rate in the 61% patients who kept their implants longer than 6 years post-AUS placement owing to persistent incontinence (19). These investigators reported a high rate of augmentation cystoplasty being required after AUS implantation because of decreased bladder compliance with recurrent incontinence or upper tract changes. DeBadiola et al. emphasized the importance of preoperative urodynamic testing before AUS implantation in children with neurogenic incontinence (20). Patients with both normal and small bladder capacities had a satisfactory outcome. In contrast, patients with bladder compliance less than 2 mL/cmH$_2$O almost uniformly required augmentation enterocystoplasty. In general, patients with previous bladder neck reconstructive procedures in general had poor continence and a high complication rate after AUS implantation.

Whereas it is generally agreed that bowel augmentation of the bladder and AUS placement are compatible in terms of both infection and erosion rates and continence, simultaneous augmentation cystoplasty with AUS placement is more controversial. Miller et al. reported infection requiring AUS removal in only 2 of 29 patients with good continence rates (21). However, Light et al. had a 50% prosthetic infection rate from simultaneous procedures and 9.5% from staged procedures; the authors thus recommended that a staged procedure be performed (22). The discrepancy between these two articles is unclear, and more experience will be required before a definite conclusion can be reached. What has been well-substaniated with clinical experience is that clean intermittent catheterization is a safe and effective means of bladder emptying across an AUS cuff and should not be a contraindication to AUS implantation.

VI. COMPLICATIONS

As stated in detail previously in this chapter, the complication rates of the AUS decreased dramatically with the advent of the AMS 800 series. The most common complications, their detection, and management are now discussed.

A. Pressure Atrophy

This is now the most common complication seen with AUS placement with long-term follow-up (23). The pressure-regulating balloon maintains a steady pressure of 61- to 70 or 71- to 80-cmH$_2$O pressure for the bulbar urethral or bladder neck cuff, respectively. These pressures have acceptable continence and cuff erosion rates. However, some degree of urethral atrophy is inevitable after AUS placement. As the urethra atrophies, more fluid is required in the cuff to maintain the desired pressure. This extra fluid in the cuff occurs at the expense of the pressure-regulating balloon volume. At some point the pressure in the balloon becomes too small to maintain urethral coaptation owing to tissue loss, and recurrent incontinence results.

As more of the device fluid is used to fill the cuff in severe pressure atrophy, the number of pumps required to deflate the cuff becomes greater. Each pump transmits approximately 0.75 mL of fluid from the cuff to the balloon reservoir. A properly positioned cuff will hold about 0.75 mL at the bulbar urethra and 2.0 mL at the bladder neck. Therefore, if a patient who previously reported requiring one to three pumps to empty his cuff now complains of needing four to six pumps, either pressure atrophy or a device leak probably has occurred. Cystoscopy demonstrating a lack of urethral or bladder neck compression on cuff filling also suggests pressure atrophy.

Management of pressure atrophy is surgical. Replacing the pressure-regulating balloon reservoir with a balloon of higher pressure will not always increase cuff pressure, may increase the risk of cuff erosion, and is generally not recommended. Replacing the oversized cuff with a smaller, more properly fitting cuff is an appropriate first step in management, although overall success rates are unclear. Other options include repositioning of the cuff, either proximally or distally, or placing a second bulbar urethral cuffs in tandem to the original cuff. One series reported an 83% satisfactory continence rate with no urethral erosion at mean follow-up of 1 year with proximal repositioning of the bulbar urethral cuff (24).

In 1993, Brito et al. described the use of tandem bulbar urethral cuffs for the treatment of persistent incontinence after AUS placement (25). The second cuff is placed 1–2 cm distal to the original cuff and a Y-connector is used either in the perineum or in the suprapubic area to connect the tubing from both cuffs to the pump tubing (Fig. 6). This modification raised the continence rate in this series from 85% to greater than 95%. The cuff erosion rate was 10.5% (26). These results have been confirmed in other series (27).

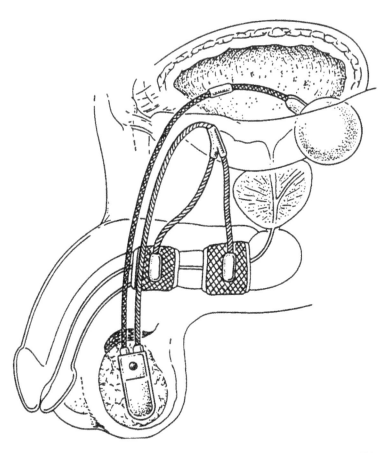

Figure 6   American Medical Systems model 800 with "tandem cuff."

B. Device Leak

Before the introduction of the silicone coating and the narrow-backed cuff with the AMS 800 model in 1983, cuff leaks were a common complication of the AUS. Light reported on 75 devices implanted after 1983 with no leaks and mean 3-year follow-up. Any component of the device may leak, however, and this leak may be gradual or dramatic. Most commonly, patients note a decreased number of pumps required to empty the cuff or of a flat pump. The diagnosis of a device leak can be confirmed by a plain abdominal radiograph in patients with a system filled with radiopaque fluid. Other causes of decreased device fluid volume are inadequate instillation of fluid during implantation and use of a hypotonic fluid mixture with osmotic fluid loss across the reservoir wall.

C. Occlusion

Fluid passage through the three-piece device must be unimpeded for proper AUS function. Large air bubbles, serum, blood, and debris, all can cause obstruction to fluid flow and, therefore, inadequate cuff filling. Usually, these substances are introduced at the time of implantation, but small device leaks can allow introduction of foreign materials into the device. Tube kinking or inappropriately placed connections are also a potential cause of device occlusion. Device occlusion can manifest itself as consistent or intermittent incontinence or slow refilling of the cuff after voiding. The introduction of kink-resistant tubing markedly reduced the incidence of tubing occlusion.

D. Restrictive Balloon Reservoir Pseudocapsule

It is not uncommon for a fibrous pseudocapsule to form around the balloon postoperatively. If this capsule becomes restrictive, complete transfer of fluid from the cuff to the balloon will not occur. This will manifest itself clinically by difficulty squeezing the pump, difficulty voiding past an incompletely deflated cuff, or both. Patients should be encouraged to fully deflate the cuff on each void after initial device activation.

E. Altered Detrusor Characteristics

Changes in detrusor behavior after AUS implantation have been well described in the literature (28,29). These changes are especially noted in neurogenic bladder patients. First, pre-existing detrusor hyperreflexia can worsen after implantation and can lead to incontinence if detrusor pressures exceed cuff pressure. Light et al. noted (29) that the exaggerated hyperreflexia can improve over time and will respond well to antispasmodic medication. More ominous are patients with detrusor areflexia and diminished compliance, often leading to accelerated compliance loss after AUS implantation. Loss of bladder compliance can lead to recurrent incontinence or hydroureteronephrosis. Scott et al. found (28) that only 3.3% of neurogenic bladder patients had progressive upper tract dilation. However, these authors do emphasize the requirement of eliminating any outlet obstruction and the need for close, long-term follow-up. The physiological mechanism for these changes in detrusor behavior after AUS implantation are not well elucidated, but are thought to be due to altered afferent signals from increased bladder distension.

F. Infection and Erosion

Infection of an AUS may present dramatically or gradually, but in almost all cases it is a serious condition and necessitates removal of the device. The most common clinical manifestations of AUS infection are pain, swelling, and erythema around the scrotal pump. Occasionally, similar findings are seen in the perineum surrounding a bulbar urethral cuff. Of note, AUS infections often lack the common clinical findings of fever, leukocytosis, and malaise; thus, a high index of suspicion must be held by the clinician caring for an AUS patient with vague complaints of pain, tenderness, discoloration, or swelling. Infection of any device component, in general, requires removal of the entire device. However, successful reimplantation of an AUS after total removal for infection or erosion has been reported (30).

The most common isolate from AUS infections is *Staphylococcus epidermidis*. The significance of this organism is clinical device infections is unclear, however. Licht et al. (31) prospectively performed quantitative cultures of 22 AUS devices at the time of reoperation for reasons other than infection; *S. epidermidis* was isolated from 36% of these sphincters, but only 9% of these developed clinical infection at a later date. Furthermore, Martins and Boyd reviewed the culture results from a group of patients with AUS infection and found enteric gram-negative, gram-positive, and anaerobic organisms (32). Thus, the microbiology of AUS infection is complex and is most likely due to the route of introduction of organisms.

Cuff erosion is the endpoint of cuff atrophy as well as traumatic injury to the urinary tract and is a common cause of AUS infection. Sterile erosions (erosion with no clinical evidence of infection and a negative urine culture) can occur and do not absolutely require removal of the entire device. Motely and Barrett managed 38 patients by cuff removal and plugging the cuff tubing followed several weeks later by reimplantation of the cuff at another site (33). These authors reported an 84% success rate with this protocol.

Preimplantation risk factors for AUS erosion and infection include radiotherapy and urethral reconstructive surgery; postimplantation risk factors include urethral catheterization or instrumentation and immediate AUS activation. All of these elements have the common result of decreasing blood supply to the urethra and bladder neck. Therefore, it is imperative that patients are instructed to immediately notify all health care providers of the presence of an AUS and to limit any urological instrumentation to personnel familiar with the proper use of the device. Delayed activation of an AUS implant is now broadly recommended, particularly in high-risk patients. Motley and Barrett reported (33) a decrease in the cuff erosion rate from 18 to 1.3% using a delayed activation protocol.

G. Intraoperative Injuries

Injuries to the bulbar urethra in the placement of the AUS in men generally mandates termination of the procedure owing the increased risk of erosion or infection of the cuff even if such an injury is recognized and repaired. On the contrary, injuries during retropubic dissection, particularly in women, can often be repaired and the procedure continued. Salisz and Diokno reported (34) on 6 of 57 women with injuries to the vagina (4), urethra (1), or bladder (1) during difficult AUS placement. With careful primary closure of injuries, antibiotics, and delayed AUS activation 5 patients were continent at mean follow-up of 32 months and no infectious complications occurred.

H. Silicone Shedding

Reinberg et al. (35) examined bladder neck pericapsular tissues and lymph nodes in pediatric patients undergoing AUS revision. They found evidence of silicone particles, with a resultant inflammatory reaction in the pericuff tissues in 50% of the children. There were no changes noted in regional lymph nodes. No clinical syndromes or sequelae of silicone shedding have yet been reported; hence, the clinical importance of this finding is unclear.

VII. CONCLUSION

The artificial urinary sphincter is an effective long-term therapy for incontinence secondary to sphincteric deficiency, with acceptable morbidity and complication rates. Men with postprostatectomy incontinence are the most common patients receiving implants, but carefully selected children and women can have good results as well.

REFERENCES

1. Hajivassiliou CA. The development and evolution of artificial urethral sphincters. J Med Eng Technol 1998; 22:154–159.
2. Foley EBF. An artificial sphincter: a new device and operation for control of enuresis and urinary incontinence. J Urol 1947; 58:250–295.
3. Kosters S, Das SP, Raz S, Kaufman JJ. Prosthetic management of urinary incontinence following prostatectomy with special reference to Kaufman's prosthesis. Z Urol Nephrol 1977; 70: 561–567.
4. Swenson O. An experimental implantable urinary sphincter. Invest Urol 1976; 14:100–103.
5. Rosen M. A simple artificial implantable sphincter. Br J Urol 1976; 48:675–680.
6. Small MP. The Rosen incontinence procedure: a new artificial urinary sphincter for the management of urinary incontinence. J Urol 1980; 123:507–511.
7. Scott FB, Bradley WE, Timm GW. Treatment of urinary incontinence by an implantable prosthetic sphincter. Urology 1973; 1:252–259.
8. Goldwasser B, Ramon J. Prosthetics for urinary incontinence. In: Webster G, Kirby R, King L, Goldwasser B, eds. Recontructive Urology. Boston: Blackwell Scientific, 1983:805–816.
9. Furlow WL. Implantation of a new semiautomatic artificial genitourinary sphincter: experience with primary activation and deactivation in 47 patients. J Urol 1981; 126:741–744.
10. Elliott DS, Barrett DM. Mayo Clinic long-term analysis of the functional durability of the AMS 800 artificial urinary sphincter: a review of 323 cases. J Urol 1998; 159:1206–1208.
11. Fulford SC, Sutton C, Bales G, Hickling M, Stephenson TP. The fate of the "modern" artificial urinary sphincter with a follow-up of more than 10 years. Br J Urol 1997; 79:713–716.
12. Marks JL, Light JK. Management of urinary incontinence after prostatectomy with the artificial urinary sphincter. J Urol 1989; 142:302–304.
13. Litwiller SE, Kim KB, Fone PD, White RW, Stone AR. Post-prostatectomy incontinence and the artificial urinary sphincter: a long-term study of patient satisfaction and criteria for success. J Urol 1996; 156:1975–1980.
14. Haab F, Trockman BA, Zimmern PE, Leach GE. Quality of life and continence assessment of the artificial urinary sphincter in men with minimum 3.5 years of follow-up. J Urol 1997; 158:435–439.
15. Klijn AJ, Hop WC, Mickisch G, Schroder FH, Bosch JL. The artificial urinary sphincter in men incontinent after radical prostatectomy: 5 year actuarial adequate function rates. Br J Urol 1998; 82:530–533.
16. Elliott DS, Barrett DM. The artificial urinary sphincter in the female: indications for use, surgical approach and results. Int Urogynecol J Pelvic Floor Dysfunct 1998; 9:409–415.
17. Fishman IJ, Scott FB. Pregnancy in patients with the artificial urinary sphincter. J Urol 1993; 150:340–341.
18. Simeoni J, Guys JM, Mollard P, Buzelin JM, Moscovici J, Bondonny JM, Melin Y, Lortat–Jacob S, Aubert D, Costa F, Galifer B, Debeugny P. Artificial urinary sphincter implantation for neurogenic bladder: a multi-institutional study in 107 children. Br J Urol 1996; 78:287–293.

19. Levesque PE, Bauer SB, Atala A, Zurakowski D, Colodny A, Peters C, Retik AB. Ten-year experience with the artificial urinary sphincter in children. J Urol 1996; 156:625–628.
20. de Badiola FI, Castro–Diaz D, Hart–Austin C, Gonzales R. Influence of preoperative bladder capacity and compliance on the outcome of artificial sphincter implantation in patients with neurogenic sphincter incompetence. J Urol 1992; 148:1493–1495.
21. Miller EA, Mayo M, Kwan D, Mitchell M. Simultaneous augmentation cystoplasty and artificial urinary sphincter placement: infection rates and voiding mechanisms. J Urol 1998; 160: 750–753.
22. Light JK, Lapin S, Vohra S. Combined use of bowel and the artificial urinary sphincter in reconstruction of the lower urinary tract: infectious complications. J Urol 1995; 153:331–333.
23. Light JK. Complications of surgery for male urinary incontinence. In: Smith RB, Ehrlich RM, eds. Complications of Urologic Surgery: Prevention and Management. Philadelphia: WB Saunders, 1990:518–525.
24. Couillard DR, Vapnek JM, Stone AR. Proximal artificial sphincter cuff repositioning for urethral atrophy incontinence. Urology 1995; 45:653–656.
25. Brito CG, Mulcahy JJ, Mitchell ME, Adams MC. Use of a double cuff AMS 800 urinary sphincter for severe stress incontinence. J Urol 1993; 149:283–285.
26. Kowalczyk JJ, Spicer DL, Mulcahy JJ. Erosion rate of the double cuff AMS 800 artificial urinary sphincter: long-term follow-up. J Urol 1996; 156:1300–1301.
27. Kabalin JN. Addition of a second urethral cuff to enhance performance of the artificial urinary sphincter. J Urol 1996; 156:1302–1304.
28. Scott FB, Fishman IJ, Shabsigh R. The impact of the artificial urinary sphincter in the neurogenic bladder on the upper urinary tracts. J Urol 1986; 136:636–642.
29. Light JK, Peitro T. Alteration in detrusor behavior and the effect on renal function following insertion of the artificial urinary sphincter. J Urol 1986; 136:632–635.
30. Kowalczyk JJ, Nelson R, Mulcahy JJ. Successful reinsertion of the artificial urinary sphincter after removal for erosion or infection. Urology 1996; 48:906–908.
31. Licht MR, Montague DK, Angermeier KW, Lakin MM. Cultures from genitourinary prostheses at reoperation: questioning the role of *Staphylococcus epidermidis* in periprosthetic infection. J Urol 1995; 154:387–390.
32. Martins FE, Boyd SD. Post-operative risk factors associated with artificial urinary sphincter infection–erosion. Br J Urol 1995; 75:354–358.
33. Motley RC, Barrett DM. Artificial urinary sphincter cuff erosion. Experience with reimplantation in 38 patients. Urology 1990; 35:215–218.
34. Silisz JA, Diokno AC. The management of injuries to the urethra bladder or vagina encountered during difficult placement of the artificial urinary sphincter in the female patient. J Urol 1992; 148:1528–1530.
35. Reinberg Y, Manivel JC, Gonzalez R. Silicone shedding from artificial urinary sphincter in children. J Urol 1993; 150:694–696.

35

Intravaginal and Intraurethral Devices for Stress Incontinence

DAVID R. STASKIN

Harvard Medical School and Beth Israel Deaconess Medical Center Continence Center, Boston, Massachusetts

ROXANE GARDNER

Brigham and Women's Hospital, Boston, Massachusetts

MATTHEW L. LEMER

College of Physicians and Surgeons of Columbia University, New York, New York

I. INTRODUCTION

Recent technological advances, and the adaptation of products that have traditionally been employed for other purposes, have provided interesting options for the nonsurgical management of urinary loss in female patients. These devices include those that are placed: 1) externally to the urethral meatus, and accomplish urinary collection; 2) intravaginally beneath the bladder neck, and give anatomical support; or 3) outside or within the urethra, and occlude egress of urine either at the external meatus or within the urethra.

A 1970–1999 Medline search identified devices that have been described or studied in the peer-reviewed literature. Many devices currently in use have not been investigated objectively, especially those employed traditionally for other purposes. Many of the published reports describe devices that were never marketed or are not marketed currently.

Genuine stress incontinence (GSI) results from underactivity of the bladder outlet. The pathophysiology of GSI in the female patient may be secondary to either intrinsic sphincter deficiency (GSI–ISD) or abnormal anatomical support of the bladder neck (GSI–A). The bladder outlet or intrinsic sphincteric mechanism in the female is composed of the bladder neck, proximal urethra, and region of the external sphincter. These sphincteric structures are anatomically supported by the vaginal wall, vaginal attachments, and the levator ani complex.

The GSI type (e.g., GSI–A vs. GSI–ISD) may affect the efficacy of a device supporting the bladder neck, rather than an occlusive device compensating for low urethral resistance. GSI in combination with detrusor overactivity (urge incontinence) or underactivity (urinary retention) is clinically important when utilizing devices that function by increasing urinary outlet resistance.

II. EXTERNAL COLLECTION DEVICES

External collection devices are usually placed over the urethral meatus or within or around the introitus and secured with adhesives, special straps, or by suction. The most common collection methods are diapers, pads, and incontinence pants. The devices reviewed are those that collect urine in an external drainage bag. In female patients, forming an efficient seal around the urethral meatus has been the greatest challenge. Variations in anatomical shape of the perimeatal area make it difficult to standardize or individualize collecting devices.

Adhesives that are strong enough to secure the device are prone to causing epithelial irritation. The degree of suction used is proportional to the reported amount of periurethral edema and tissue damage. The combination of an extrameatal plate with an intravaginal component to secure the device has not proved to be efficient or comfortable. Abdominal or gluteal straps are cumbersome and ineffective in securing the meatal portion of the device. No tested method has been successful in ambulatory patients, and few devices have been clinically applicable, even in bedridden nursing home patients. Most published articles on external collection devices have been the result of small descriptive studies of patients in rehabilitation centers or nursing homes (1–5).

III. OCCLUSIVE DEVICES

Occlusive devices block urinary leakage at the external urethral meatus. Several of them are currently marketed, but their success and presence in the peer-reviewed literature are limited.

Only one peer-reviewed study was published in 1996 (6). Eckford et al. investigated 19 women with symptoms of stress incontinence who used an external urethral occlusive pad (6). The soft occlusive foam-like pad was secured by an adhesive hydrogel over the urethral meatus and was removed for voiding and replaced. The median age of the 19 women was 45 years, range 36–72 years. Continence data were collected using pad tests, urinary diaries, and symptom review. Seventeen women reported a cure or improvement measured by the number of incontinence episodes per week. There was a significant decrease in both the number of episodes ($p < 0.001$) and pad test leakage ($p < 0.002$) when using the device. The ability to place and remove the device was a major difficulty.

The same device was studied by Brubaker et al. (7), who analyzed its efficacy and safety in 356 women (there were 12 withdrawals for device problems and 24 for protocol issues) with a minimum of three leakage episodes per week. The investigation was designed for minimal patient training in anticipation of "over-the-counter" patient acquisition of the product. The number of leakage episodes was analyzed by use of a voiding diary, subjective severity of urinary leakage, incontinence impact scores, and pad testing. Safety was evaluated by symptom assessment, urinalysis and culture, postvoid residual, vulvar cytology, vaginal culture, and cystometric testing. Objectively, the barrier was effective in reducing urine loss episodes from a baseline mean of 14.2 ± 12.3 (median 10.0) to 4.9 ± 6.9

(median 3.0) at week 17, and urinary loss "severity" from a baseline mean of 10.1 ± 5.1 (median 9.0) episodes to 3.5 ± 4.3 (median 2.0) at week 17. The device was concluded to be a safe, nonsurgical alternative in patients with mild or moderate stress incontinence.

This device was marketed as a prescription device (Impress) by Uromed in the United States without commercial success, but may be released again by Johnson & Johnson as an over-the-counter product after regulatory approval.

Several other commercial products occlude urinary loss at the meatus by either a simple barrier effect, or by compression of the distal urethra. Peer-reviewed literature is not available. Most are "cap" products made of silicone or plastic that adhere primarily by mild suction.

IV. INTRAVAGINAL DEVICES TO SUPPORT THE BLADDER NECK

Support of the bladder neck to improve stress urinary incontinence has been achieved, with varying degrees of success, with tampons, pessaries, contraceptive diaphragms, and intravaginal devices not specifically designed for such support. The quality of the data varies, depending on the individual device studied. Many abstracts have been presented at national and international meetings, but the data are limited by short-term or laboratory use only. Nygaard (8) performed a prospective, randomized, laboratory-based study of 18 patients using a Hodge pessary with support, a super tampon, or no device. All patients performed three standardized 40-min aerobics sessions. Both devices decreased the amount of urine loss, but half of the tampon users were either continent or had only mild leakage of less than 4 g.

Pessaries to correct prolapse have been tested to identify women with coexisting, but unsuspected, stress incontinence. In studies conducted by Bhatia et al. (9,10), the Smith–Hodge pessary was used for brief testing, as opposed to long-term treatment, in 12 women who underwent urodynamic investigation (uroflowmetry, postvoid residual, functional urethral length, urethral closure pressure, urethral closure pressure profile, and cough pressure profile), as well as Q-tip testing. Ten of the 12 patients became continent in the laboratory. Long-term clinical data were not obtained. Later, 30 women were evaluated with a pessary in the hope of identifying a more clinically useful test than the Bonney test. The pessary equalized pressure transmission in 26 of the 30 women, 21 of whom were continent in the standing position. Long-term treatment data were not reported.

Realini and Walters (11) analyzed the benefit of a coil-type diaphragm ring, softer than a pessary, in ten women with incontinence. The women used the diaphragm for 1 week and recorded events in a urinary diary. A 2-hr pad test was performed. Six patients reported subjective improvement, four experienced no change in symptoms, and none became worse. Objectively, 40% of them responded with a 50% reduction on the pad test and a 50% decrease in leakage episodes per week.

Suarez (12) studied the efficacy of a 60- to 70-mm contraceptive diaphragm in 12 patients. Urodynamic tests were performed with and without the device in place. Flow decreased (29 to 24 mL/sec) and resting maximal urethral pressures increased (37.5 to 81.0 cm H_2O), consistent with the investigator's desire to place a device large enough to cause compression of the urethra against the posterior aspect of the symphysis pubis. One woman was not continent, 2 women discontinued the device because of discomfort, 9 were continent and without complaints of either obstruction or urinary tract infection.

V. DEVICES DESIGNED SPECIFICALLY FOR BLADDER NECK SUPPORT

The use of a pubovaginal spring device was described and studied by Edwards (13) in 1971. The device, which was not available commercially, was inserted into the vagina to apply pressure on the urethra through the vaginal wall and was removed for voiding. It was some-what cumbersome to use and 1 of 43 women developed vaginal ulceration.

Bonnar (14) and Cardozo (15) tested the same inflatable device with two horns of flexible silicone which projected laterally. When inserted into the vagina, it was positioned in the lateral fornices, and an inflatable balloon was placed anteriorly at the midline to support the upper urethra and bladder neck. Deflating the device permitted voiding. Bonnar reported a 40% success rate in 60 women. Cardozo investigated 33 patients for 1 month, 20 of whom completed the study. Two of these 20 women chose to continue with the device after the study was terminated. Four patients, who were cured of incontinence, felt the device was too cumbersome to use because of size, discomfort, and difficulties with insertion and inflation. The 14 women who were not cured felt that the problems with the device outweighed its usefulness.

Davila and Osterman (16,17) and Bernier and Harris (18) reported on the same patient group in three separate publications. Thirty-two physically active women were enrolled, 30 of whom completed the protocol. The majority of these women were dry with the device in place during stress testing. Urodynamic testing with and without the device demonstrated significant changes in functional urethral length, pressure transmission ratio, and Q-tip angle, with no evidence of urethral obstruction. There was a documented decrease in the number of weekly incontinence episodes from 10 to 3 ($p < 0.05$) over a 4-week period of observation. The device was acceptable, convenient, and comfortable for most of these women. Davila et al. (19) studied a separate group of 53 women (29 with pure stress and 24 with mixed incontinence) with 7-day bladder diaries and standardized pad tests. A statistically significant improvement was seen on pad testing with the device (16.6-g–average loss) versus no device (46.6-g–average loss) in the stress incontinence group, and with the device (6.8-g–average loss) versus no device (31.9-g–average loss) in the mixed incontinence group.

Thyssen (20) reported on the use of a disposable polyurethane vaginal device in 22 of 26 patients between the ages of 27 and 69 years who completed a 3-day diary, 24-hr home pad test, and urodynamic testing (uroflowmetry and postvoid residual). Urine and vaginal cultures were obtained over a 1-month–study period. The diaries showed that 41% of patients were subjectively cured 45% improved, and 14% were unchanged. All patients manifested objective improvement with a decrease in urinary leakage, but only 1 of 19 patients was dry. Three of four patients with greater than 100 mL urine loss without the device showed a 50% reduction in leakage. There were no urinary tract infections and no problems with bladder emptying.

VI. INTRAURETHRAL DEVICES

Intraurethral devices to block urinary leakage are inserted into the urethra. Their efficacy and safety require the prevention of intravesical migration, which is usually accomplished with a meatal plate. The devices must physically block urinary leakage, usually with an inflatable balloon, sphere, or flange. They achieve bladder emptying, either by their removal, voiding through them, or by a pumping mechanism. Some devices are indwelling, with insertion by a physician for 28 days or longer, whereas others are single-use, disposable devices that are inserted and removed by the patient before voiding.

Single-use devices with spheres were studied by Neilsen et al. (21–23) between 1990 and 1995. These urethral plug devices had an oval meatal plate, a soft stalk with a removable semirigid guide pin (removed after insertion), and either one or two spheres along the stalk with fixed distances between the meatal plate and the spheres. One-sphere (original) and two-sphere (improved) devices were tested. Eighteen of 40 patients completed the study. Most of them (17/18 = 94.4%) were subjectively and objectively continent or improved; most preferred the two-sphere device. Urinary tract infections in 6 of 18 and migration of the device into the bladder in 2 of 18, necessitating cystoscopic removal, were major complications experienced with it.

Peschers et al. (24) screened 53 patients with GSI, and 21 of them agreed to participate in their study of a two-sphere urethral plug device. Fourteen of these 21 patients completed the 4-month–long investigation. Seven of the 14 subjects experienced no improvement in their symptoms. Urinary tract infection and device migration were major complications with this device.

We reported on a group of 135 out of 215 patients who were observed during a 4-month multicenter study (25). The intraurethral device consisted of a disposable balloon-tipped urethral insert made of a thermoplastic elastomer. The balloon was inflated with an applicator after insertion and deflated by pulling a string at the meatal plate for removal and to permit voiding. Urodynamic testing excluded patients with urge incontinence and classified the study population into anatomical hypermobility and intrinsic sphincter deficiency. Complete dryness was reported by 72%, with 17% improvement, on diary entry, and 80% with complete dryness and 15% improvement (80% decrease in measured urine loss) on pad weight testing. There was a decrease from 43.2 mL without the device to 2.3 mL with the device. Treatment for positive urine cultures was undertaken in 20% of symptomatic and 11% of asymptomatic patients. Thirty-nine percent of subjects had positive cultures, but were not treated, and 30% had negative cultures at all monthly intervals during the 4-month study. The main reason for dropout was discomfort with the device.

Miller and Bavendum (26) reported on 63 of 135 patients from the aforementioned cohort who used the balloon-tipped intraurethral device for 1 year. Of these 63 patients, 79% reported complete dryness and 16% significant improvement on objective pad weight testing. These findings were consistent with improvement in subjective diaries ($p < 0.0001$). The patients reported increased comfort and ease of use over time, with sensation of device presence decreasing from 35% at week 1 to 7% at 12 months. The most common morbidities were one or more episodes of gross hematuria (24%), cystoscopic findings of mucosal irritation at 4 or 12 months (9%), and symptomatic bacteriuria on monthly cultures (30%) over the 1-year study period. This device is no longer commercially available.

Intraurethral inserts have demonstrated their efficacy in the control of urinary incontinence. The morbidity associated with their use varies with design. There have been no long-term studies on devices that are not removed at each voiding. The morbidity associated with usage should be considered when patients are interested in the effectiveness of such devices.

VII. SUMMARY

Technological advances will continue to supply workable alternatives in the nonsurgical treatment of the underactive bladder outlet. More long-term outcome research is needed to identify which device or devices provide optimal convenience, efficacy, and the lowest morbidity in the nonsurgical correction of GSI.

REFERENCES

1. Crowley IP, Cardozo LJ, Lawrence LC. Female incontinence: a new approach. Br J Urol 1971; 43:492–498.
2. Johnson DE, Muncie HL, O'Reilly JL, Warren JW. An external urine collection device for incontinent women. Evaluation of long-term use. J Am Geriatr Soc 1990; 38:1016–1022.

3. Johnson DE, O'Reilly JL, Warren JW. Clinical evaluation of an external urine collection device for nonambulatory incontinent women. J Urol 1989; 14:535–537.

4. Pieper B, Cleland V, Johnson DE, O'Reilly JL. Inventing urine incontinence devices for women. Image Nurs Sch 1989; 21:205–209.

5. Pieper B, Cleland V. An external urine-collection device for women: a clinical trial. J ET Nurs 1993; 20:51–55.

6. Eckford SD, Jackson SR, Lewis PA, Abrams P. The continence control pad—a new external urethral occlusion device in the management of stress incontinence. Br J Urol 1996; 77:538–540.

7. Brubaker L, Harris T, Gleason D, Newman D, North B. The external urethral barrier for stress incontinence: a multicenter trial of safety and efficacy. Miniguard Investigators Group. Obstet Gynecol 1999; 93:932–937.

8. Nygaard I. Prevention of exercise incontinence with mechanical devices. J Reprod Med 1995; 40:89–94.

9. Bhatia NN, Bergman A, Gunning JE. Urodynamic effects of a vaginal pessary in women with stress urinary incontinence. Am J Obstet Gynecol 1983; 147:876–884.

10. Bhatia NN, Bergman A. Pessary test in women with urinary incontinence. Obstet Gynecol 1985; 65:220–226.

11. Realini JP, Walters MD. Vaginal diaphragm rings in the treatment of stress incontinence. J Am Board Fam Pract 1990; 3:99–103.

12. Suarez GM, Baum NH, Jacobs J. Use of a standard contraceptive diaphragm in management of stress urinary incontinence. Urology 1991; 37:119–122.

13. Edwards L. The control of incontinence of urine in women with a pubovaginal spring device: objective and subjective results. Br J Urol 1971; 43:211–225.

14. Bonnar J. Silicone vaginal appliance for control of stress incontinence. Lancet 1977; 2:1161.

15. Cardozo LD, Stanton SL. Evaluation of female urinary incontinence device. Urology 1979; 13:398–401.

16. Davila GW, Ostermann KV. The bladder neck support prosthesis: a nonsurgical approach to stress incontinence in adult women. Am J Obstet Gynecol 1994; 171:206–211.

17. Davila GW. Introl bladder neck support prosthesis: a nonsurgical urethropexy. J Endourol 1996; 10:293–296.

18. Bernier F, Harris L. Treating stress incontinence with the bladder neck support prosthesis. Urol Nurs 1995; 15:5–9.

19. Davila GW, Neal D, Horbach N, Peacher J, Doughtie JD, Karram M. A bladder-neck support prosthesis for women with stress and mixed incontinence. Obstet Gynecol 1999; 93:938–942.

20. Thyssen H, Lose G. New disposable vaginal device (continence guard) in the treatment of female stress incontinence. Design, efficacy and short term safety. Acta Obstet Gynecol Scand 1996; 75:170–173.

21. Neilsen KK, Kromann–Andersen B, Jacobsen H, Nielsen EM, Nordling J, Holm HH, Larsen JF. The urethral plug: a new treatment modality for genuine urinary stress incontinence in women. J Urol 1990; 144:1199–1202.

22. Neilsen KK, Walter S, Maegaard E, Kromann–Andersen B. The urethral plug II: an alternative treatment in women with genuine urinary stress incontinence. Br J Urol 1993; 72:428–432.

23. Neilsen KK, Walter S, Maegaard E, Kromann–Andersen B. The urethral plug—an alternative treatment of women with urinary stress incontinence. Ugeske Laeger 1995; 157:3194–3197.

24. Peschers U, Zen Ruffinen F, Schaer GN, Schussler B. The VIVA urethral plug: a sensible expansion of the spectrum for conservative therapy of urinary stress incontinence? Geburtshilfe Frauenheilkd 1996; 118–123.

25. Staskin DR, Bavendam T, Miller J, Davila GW, Diokno A, Knapp P, Rappaport S, Sand P, Sant G, Tutrone R. Effectiveness of a urinary control insert in the management of stress urinary incontinence: early results of a multicenter study. Urology 1996; 47:629–636.

26. Miller JL, Bavendum T. Treatment with the Reliance urinary control insert: one-year experience. J Endourol 1996; 10:287–292.

36

Sacral Nerve Neuromodulation and Its Effects on Urinary Sphincter Function

J. L. H. RUUD BOSCH

Erasmus University Rotterdam and Academic Hospital Rotterdam, Rotterdam, The Netherlands

I. INTRODUCTION

Since the early 1980s, sacral nerve neuromodulation has been explored as a treatment for various voiding dysfunctions, such as urge incontinence, urge–frequency syndromes, urinary retention, and pelvic pain (1). In this context, the word *neuromodulation* means that patients who are refractory to conservative treatments are treated with continuous electrical stimulation of the sacral nerves. These patients first undergo percutaneous nerve evaluation to test the integrity of their sacral nerves (2).

In typical situations, electrical stimulation of the S3 sacral nerve is marked by contraction of the levator ani, flexion of the great toe, and a pulling sensation in the rectum. Stimulation of the S2 nerve leads to contraction of the sphincter ani and the calf muscles, and gives a pulsating sensation in the vagina or scrotum. Stimulation of S4 usually leads to more posteriorly based contraction of the levator ani only (3). These efferent effects, which are a result of stimulation of myelinated α-motor nerve fibers, serve as a biological marker for the correct placement of test electrodes.

The therapeutic effects of neuromodulation are thought to be due to the concomitant activation of sensory afferent nerve fibers. As will be discussed in this chapter, the stimulation of sensory afferent nerve fibers can lead to inhibition of the bladder. Because of the stimulation parameters used in neuromodulation (i.e., low amplitudes and pulse frequencies less than 20 Hz), unmyelinated nerve fibers are not stimulated. It is also less likely that lightly myelinated nerve fibers are stimulated. Therefore, these stimulation parameters will not stimulate parasympathetic motor fibers to the bladder or pain fibers.

The choice of stimulation parameters and the absolute value of the different parameters create a therapeutic window for this type of neuromodulation. A test electrode is inserted percutaneously in one of the sacral foramina (usually S3) once the integrity of the nerve has been ascertained. Over a period of 4–7 days, the S3 nerve is stimulated continuously with an external nerve stimulator. A permanent implant is considered if the patient responds with more than 50% improvement of the voiding dysfunction during this subchronic test phase. The response is confirmed by the comparison of voiding–incontinence diaries that the patients keep at baseline and during the test period.

A permanent implant (Fig. 1) consists of a foramen electrode that is connected to a pulse generator by an extension cable (Medtronic Interstim) (4). The precise mechanism of

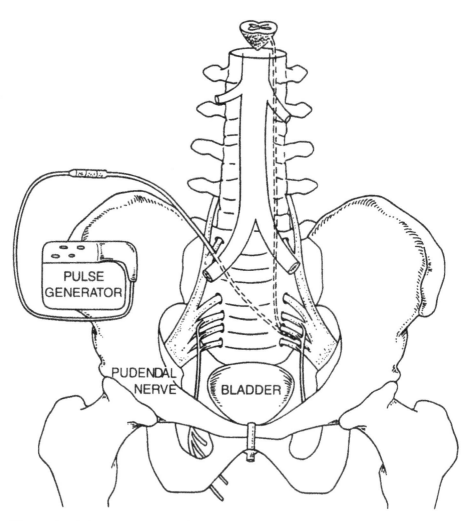

Figure 1 Schematic representation of a permanent foramen S3 neuroprosthetic implant consisting of a foramen S3 electrode, which is connected to the pulse generator by an extension cable. The extension cable is tunneled subcutaneously to a subcutaneous pocket for the pulse generator. This subcutaneous pocket is situated in the left or right lower abdominal quadrant.

action of neuromodulation remains to be determined. This chapter will outline our present understanding of its mechanism, with an emphasis on the role of the urethral sphincter. This understanding is based on neurophysiological studies in animals, brief electrophysiological studies in normal humans and patients with neurological disease, as well as urodynamic or electrophysiological studies in patients with permanent electrode implants.

II. RELEVANT ANATOMY OF THE URINARY SPHINCTER AND THE PELVIC FLOOR IN RELATION TO NEUROMODULATION

Some anatomical and functional aspects of the urethral sphincter are relevant to understanding the possible effects of sacral nerve neuromodulation on the closure mechanism of the lower urinary tract. Over the years, the neuromuscular anatomy of the external urethral sphincters has been the subject of hot debate. Even now, a generally accepted concept has not emerged.

Functionally, the striated muscular closure mechanism of the lower urinary tract is composed of several components. Together, these components are called the external urethral sphincter (5). However, only the intrinsic striated rhabdosphincter around the membranous urethra is a true sphincter. The extrinsic components, which together form the pelvic floor, are actually not a true sphincter. Even the intrinsic rhabdosphincter is characterized by an uneven distribution of its muscular mass. Most of the mass of this Ω-shaped muscle is located anteriorly, whereas no striated muscle fibers are found on the midposterior aspect of the urethra (6).

The neuromuscular anatomy has been revisited in recent years. Detailed anatomical dissections have yielded interesting results. Juenemann et al. (7) observed that the intrinsic external urethral rhabdosphincter, which is found in the membranous urethra, and the extrinsic urethral "sphincter," which is mainly composed of the levator ani and the transversus perinei profundus muscles, are innervated by somatic nerve fibers derived from sacral roots S2 and S3. Somatic fibers of sacral roots S2–S4 form the pudendal nerve. En route to the peripheral muscles, however, some somatic fibers branch away from the ventral roots before the pudendal nerve is formed. These branches innervate the levator ani muscle and the intrinsic striated rhabdosphincter around the membranous urethra.

With use of electrical stimulation of the S2 and S3 sacral ventral roots, Juenemann et al. (7) performed studies in quadriplegic and paraplegic patients who had undergone various types of neurotomies peripheral to the point of stimulation. These studies suggested that about 70% of the pressure of the external urethral sphincter was derived from impulses from the S3 ventral root (the somatic fibers of which innervate mainly the intrinsic rhabdosphincter and the levator ani muscle). Neuronal impulses from the S2 ventral root, which is the main contributor of pudendal nerve fibers, supplied the remaining 30%. In addition, the authors contended that fibers from S2 and S3 crossed over and partially innervated the other component of the external sphincter. These studies indicate that, of the sacral nerves, S3 is the best target for neuromodulation of sphincter function.

In a more recent anatomical study from the same institution, Zvara et al. (8) confirmed that the intrinsic external sphincter has dual innervation. Apart from the extrapudendal nerves that run above the levator ani muscle, there are terminal branches of the pudendal nerve that enter the sphincter from the perineal side (8). Strasser et al. (6) also identified fibers coursing to the rhabdosphincter after the pudendal nerve had left Alcock's canal. These fibers appear to be different from those that were identified by Zvara et al. (8). Interestingly, Zvara et al. (8) also identified branches entering the striated sphincter from the purely sensory, dorsal penile nerve. They believe that these branches represent part of the sensory afferent pathway of the micturition reflex. There is evidence from animal models that pudendal nerve afferents play an important role in regulation of the micturition reflex. In anesthetized, neurologically intact dogs, electrical stimulation of S2 (which is equivalent to S3 in humans) leads to simultaneous contraction of the bladder and the sphincter mechanism. We (9) found that when total bilateral pudendal neurotomy was performed in the ischiorectal fossa, the urethral responses to S2 ventral root stimulation were decreased by almost 80%. Interestingly, the bladder response also decreased in most of the dogs that were subjected to this type of pudendal neurotomy. Nishizawa et al. (10) made a similar observation: they found overflow incontinence in 7 of 16 dogs after pudendal neurotomy. High-frequency urethral contractions often occur in dogs during stimulated micturition. These contractions, which may have a role in territory-marking behavior, seem to be an essential component of a positive-feedback mechanism that keeps the bladder contracting.

Functional studies performed in patients with spinal cord injuries can define the result of stimulation of several nerve roots and branches because they deal mainly with efferent effects. In neurologically intact humans, the consequences of stimulation of the same nerves may be quite different, because the stimulation of afferent pathways can dramatically modulate functional effect.

III. IMPROVEMENT OF STORAGE FUNCTION OF THE LOWER URINARY TRACT BY NEUROMODULATION

Tanagho and Schmidt (11) contended that activation of the external urethral sphincter could provoke reflex inhibition of detrusor overactivity. They based this assertion on the fact that, during the initiation of voiding, relaxation of the urethral sphincter precedes bladder contraction (12). There are indications, however, that the urethral sphincter or pelvic floor musculatures are not activated at the level of stimulation used to achieve a therapeutic response in sacral neuromodulation (13). Furthermore, the results of detailed neurophysiological investigation of peripheral nerve responses suggest that modulation of afferent pathways is the primary mechanism of sacral neuromodulation (14). These findings are concordant with observations in the cat model for which stimulation of pelvic floor muscle afferents did not inhibit the bladder (15).

The bladder can be inhibited by stimulation of muscle afferents from the limbs that inhibit parasympathetic motor neurons through interneurons (16). Vodusek et al. (17) have shown that electrical stimulation of nonmuscular sacral somatic nerve afferents in the pudendal nerve can induce bladder inhibition in patients whose detrusor hyperreflexia is due to traumatic spinal cord injury, multiple sclerosis, or cerebrovascular accident (18). Most of these pudendal nerve fibers reach the spinal cord through the dorsal roots of the sacral nerves. Of the sacral spinal nerves, S3 is the most practical one for use in permanent electrical stimulation (3). In the cat, stimulation of afferent anorectal branches of the pelvic nerve and afferent dorsal penile or dorsal clitoral branches of the pudendal nerve results in strong inhibition of the detrusor muscle (15). These afferents can centrally activate the sympathetic nervous system; β-adrenergic receptor activation can suppress bladder activity (Edvardsen's reflex) (19), but it is unclear if this reflex plays an important role in humans.

In summary, in patients with urge incontinence caused by bladder instability, sacral neuromodulation seems to act primarily by activation of nonmuscular afferent sacral somatic nerve fibers that inhibit parasympathetic motor neurons through interneurons. However, in vivo electrophysiological studies directly exploring these mechanisms at the spinal cord level are lacking. Therefore, other mechanisms remain possible.

IV. IMPROVEMENT OF EMPTYING FUNCTION OF THE LOWER URINARY TRACT BY NEUROMODULATION

Neuromodulation has also been beneficial in patients with urinary retention. Several theories have attempted to explain its efficacy in these patients.

A. Excitation of Mechanoreceptors

Ebner et al. (20) have shown that intravesical electrical stimulation in cats activates A-delta mechanoreceptor afferents, which leads to central reflex activation of the detrusor. This mechanism is often quoted as an explanation for the effect of neuromodulation in retention patients. It is somewhat difficult to understand, however, why the same type of stimulation protocol inhibits the micturition reflex in one category of patients and stimulates the bladder in others. Furthermore, it is unlikely that the lightly myelinated A-delta fibers are stimulated by parameter settings that are common in neuromodulation.

B. "Rebound" Phenomenon

Schultz–Lampel et al. (21) studied a cat model and concluded that a rebound phenomenon occurring after the cessation of stimulation was responsible for the initiation of detrusor contraction. Although this effect may well play some role in humans, there is evidence that other factors are more important (13,14,22). Furthermore, the effects of neuromodulation would be easier to understand if a common mechanism existed for patients with bladder instability and those with retention. The urethral sphincter, for example, might be a candidate for mediating such a common mechanism.

C. Increased Awareness of the Pelvic Floor Musculature

In women with chronic retention, the restoration of voiding following neuroprosthetic implantation has been attributed to increased awareness of the pelvic floor musculature, caused by the sensation of stimulation (22). According to this theory, the muscles to be relaxed are "pointed out" by the electrical stimulation. These authors (22) believe that the acontractile state of the bladder is due to the inhibitory effect of sphincteric contraction. Neuromodulation would then restore voluntary relaxation of the pelvic floor muscles, releasing bladder inhibition.

D. Afferent–Mediated Sphincter Relaxation

Goodwin et al. (14) studied the effect of S3 sacral neuromodulation on urinary retention in women suffering from the Fowler syndrome. This is a syndrome that occurs in young women, who present urinary retention and typical electromyographic (EMG) abnormalities of the striated urethral sphincter (23). Some of these women also have polycystic ovaries (24). Their EMG activity resembles myotonia: a state of sustained striated muscle activity following a contraction. Although the authors of this study were not able to identify the precise mechanism of action of neuromodulation in the women, the latencies of anal sphincter contraction following S3 stimulation were so prolonged that they implicated an afferent-mediated reflex. These results are at variance with the theory that a rebound phenomenon is responsible for the restoration of voiding in these patients. The initially good clinical results reported by some authors in retention patients without the Fowler syndrome are not explained by these neurophysiological responses. Furthermore, De Ridder et al. (25) found that, in a group of female patients with retention, who were treated with a permanent S3 electrode implant, excellent sustained results were obtained in a much higher percentage of those with the Fowler syndrome than the non-Fowler syndrome. They concluded that the non-Fowler syndrome retention patients should be excluded from this expensive therapy.

V. URODYNAMIC EVIDENCE OF THE EFFECTS OF NEUROMODULATION ON SPHINCTER FUNCTION DURING THE FILLING PHASE

Hyperactivity of the urethral sphincter during the filling phase of the bladder has been implicated as a possible cause of the so-called urethral syndrome (26). Symptoms that correlate with the abnormal activity of the urethral sphincter, such as urgency, frequency, and pain or discomfort, can respond favorably to electrical stimulation of the S3 nerves.

Schmidt (26) stated that the ability of neuromodulation to fatigue the sphincter musculature is the basis of its usefulness in treating the urethral syndrome. He contended that this effect is selective in the sense that hyperreflexive sphincter behavior is fatigued, but not the tone of the intrinsic sphincter. This explanation could be valid only if the tone of the urethral sphincter were regulated by smooth-muscle activity. However, firm evidence that this is indeed true has yet to be presented. Others have stated that striated muscle fatigue during stimulation occurs only with excessively high pulse frequencies (27). Because neuromodulation typically uses frequencies in the 10- to 20-Hz range, it seems unlikely that muscle fatigue would explain the beneficial effects of neuromodulation in urethral syndrome patients. Clear urodynamic evidence of the disappearance of urethral hyperactivity during the filling phase under the influence of electrical stimulation of the S3 nerve has not yet appeared in the peer-reviewed literature.

VI. URODYNAMIC EVIDENCE OF THE EFFECTS OF NEUROMODULATION ON SPHINCTER FUNCTION DURING THE VOIDING PHASE

Electrical stimulation of S3 will lead to contraction of the levator ani muscle if the amplitude is high enough. Given the results of Juenemann et al. (7), it is likely that the intrinsic urethral rhabdosphincter is also activated. Patients with a permanent implant can attempt to void with the stimulator on or off. The effects of unilateral S3 stimulation on urethral pressure profile parameters, urethral resistance, and bladder contraction strength can thus be examined in patients with a permanent S3 electrode implant. Such studies can help us better understand the role of the pelvic floor muscles in this treatment modality.

We (13) investigated 17 women, with a mean age of 46 years, who had a permanent implant because of detrusor instability-induced refractory urge incontinence. In all patients, unilateral contraction of the levator ani muscle was visible during low-frequency (2-Hz) electrical stimulation. The stimulation parameters had been adjusted during the first months after implant to achieve an optimal symptomatic result at 6 months follow-up.

Urodynamic studies, including pressure flow and urethral pressure profile, have been performed before the implant was put in and at 6 months follow-up, with the pulse generator in the on as well as in the off mode. The urethral resistance parameter (URA) and the bladder contraction strength parameter were calculated from the pressure–flow data (28). Maximum urethral closure pressure (MUCP) and functional urethral length (FUL) were determined from the urethral pressure profile. Compared with preimplant measurements, bladder contraction strength at 6 months follow-up was significantly higher, regardless of whether the IPG was in the on or off mode. Apparently, the micturition reflex was either inhibited to a lesser degree or facilitated, compared with preimplant measurements. If a rebound phenomenon did exist in this situation, it would have been likely that bladder contraction strength was higher during voiding with the stimulator in the off mode. Urethral resistance, measured at 6 months follow-up with stimulation off, was no different from preimplant values. When the subjects voided with stimulation on, however, urethral resistance was significantly lower than both preimplant values and values measured at 6 months with stimulation off. This counterintuitive finding can be explained by improved relaxation of the pelvic floor musculature, perhaps owing to the ability to better identify these muscles as a result of the electrical stimulation that is perceived in the pelvic floor (22). Alternatively, it could be explained by an afferent-mediated mechanism, as suggested by Goodwin et al. (14). The urethral pressure profile parameters (MUCP and FUL) did not show a significant increase with stimulation switched on (Fig. 2).

Given the aforementioned stimulation parameters, this suggests that the putative afferents responsible are not secondarily activated muscle afferents from the pelvic floor. Figure 3 presents an example of the effect of neuromodulation on urodynamic voiding studies in a man with incontinence caused by detrusor instability, with coexisting, incomplete emptying of the bladder owing to sphincter hyperactivity in the voiding phase. After the permanent implant was put in place, the spasticity of the pelvic floor musculature during voiding disappeared and the incontinence improved more than 50%. Accordingly, his flow pattern improved significantly, as can be seen in Figure 4.

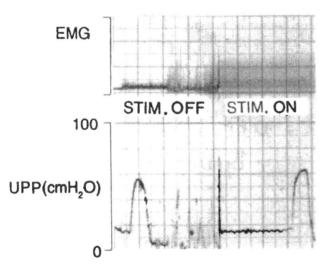

Figure 2 Urethral pressure profiles in a 54-year-old woman with multiple sclerosis and a permanent S3 foramen electrode implant. The left profile is drawn with the pulse generator in the off mode, and the right profile with the pulse generator in the on mode. There is no stimulation effect on the profile parameters.

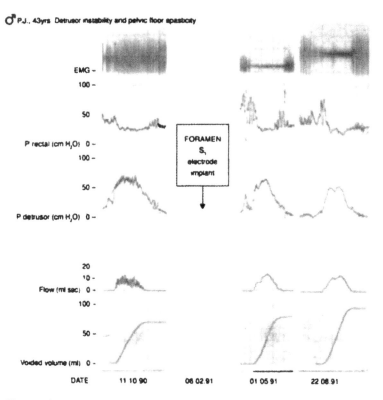

♂ P.J., 43yrs Detrusor instability and pelvic floor spasticity

Figure 3 Urodynamic pressure–flow studies in a 43-year-old man with bladder instability and pelvic floor spasticity. The left panel shows the situation before the S3 implant. Note the high pelvic floor EMG activity during voiding. This goes hand-in-hand with a sawtooth pattern of the flow curve. The right panel shows the situation after implant. Pressure–flow studies with stimulation in the off mode were performed 3 months and 6 months after the implant was put in and showed improved pelvic floor relaxation, increased flow rate, and decreased detrusor pressure at maximum flow.

VII.   ASSOCIATION BETWEEN PELVIC FLOOR OVERACTIVITY AND OVERACTIVE BLADDER

Many investigators accept that outflow tract obstruction may lead to detrusor instability in a certain proportion of male benign prostatic hyperplasia patients. In some series, 50–80% of the men with signs of benign prostatic hyperplasia showed urodynamic evidence of detrusor instability (29). In the rat, a link between outlet obstruction and central neural plasticity has been established, with long-standing outflow obstruction leading to structural deformation of the bladder smooth musculature which, in turn, elicited increased production of nerve growth factor (30). Nerve growth factor induces neuronal enlargement and enhancement of the spinal micturition reflex. Evidence that increased urethral resistance during voiding can also be associated with detrusor instability in female patients has recently been presented (31). In this study, urethral resistance in women with idiopathic detrusor instability was clearly higher than in groups with stress incontinence, mixed incontinence, or no incontinence.

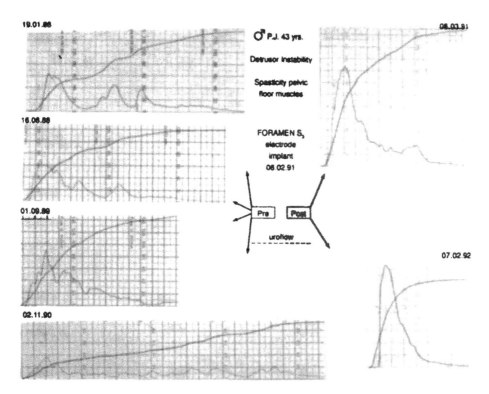

Figure 4 Multiple flow rate recordings of the same patient as in Figure 3 show deterio-rating flow rate patterns over a period of almost 3 years. The flow rate pattern normalizes after implant. The last recording presented was produced 1 year after the implant was put in place.

It can be speculated that the increased urethral resistance is due to a training effect in women who activate their pelvic floor muscles frequently in an attempt to inhibit unstable contractions. Alternatively, increased urethral resistance may result from overactivity of the sphincteric mechanism and may be the cause of detrusor instability. To firmly prove these hypotheses, it would be necessary to conduct a prospective study on the effects of neuro-modulation in women with increased urethral resistance and detrusor instability to show that disappearance of detrusor instability strongly correlates with a decrease in urethral re-sistance. A common mechanism for urge incontinence and urinary retention in patients re-sponding to neuromodulation could then be confirmed. If this were shown, it would sug-gest that the efficacy of neuromodulation in both incontinence and retention involves a pivotal role of the urethral sphincter.

From the considerations outlined in this chapter, it is difficult to define the exact role of the urethral sphincter in neuromodulation as well as the therapeutic effects of neuro-modulation on the urethral sphincter, or more widely, on the closure mechanism of the lower urinary tract. This is because nerve stimulation makes it impossible to study the di-rect action on EMG of the urethral sphincter or the pelvic floor. Only EMG changes that might remain after stopping the stimulation for a while would be detectable. Effects on the sphincter during stimulation can be studied only indirectly by urodynamic techniques.

REFERENCES

1. Schmidt RA. Applications of neurostimulation in urology. Neurourol Urodynam 1988; 7:585–592.
2. Markland C, Bradley W, Chou S, Merrill D, Westgate H. Sacral nerve stimulation: a diagnostic test of bladder innervation. Br J Urol 1971; 43:453–459.
3. Schmidt RA, Senn E, Tanagho EA. Functional evaluation of sacral nerve root integrity. Report of a technique. Urology 1990; 35:388–392.
4. Siegel SW. Management of voiding dysfunction with an implantable neuroprosthesis. Urol Clin North Am 1992; 19:163–170.
5. Dixon J, Gosling J. Structure and innervation in the human. In: Torrens M, Morrison JFB, eds. The Physiology of the Lower Urinary Tract. London: Springer-Verlag, 1987:3–22.
6. Strasser H, Klima G, Poisel S, Horninger W, Bartsch G. Anatomy and innervation of the rhabdosphincter of the male urethra. Prostate 1996; 28:24–31.
7. Juenemann K–P, Lue TF, Schmidt RA, Tanagho EA. Clinical significance of sacral and pudendal nerve anatomy. J Urol 1988; 139:74–80.
8. Zvara P, Carrier S, Kour N–W, Tanagho EA. The detailed neuroanatomy of the human striated urethral sphincter. Br J Urol 1994; 74:182–187.
9. Bosch RJ, Benard F, Aboseif SR, Schmidt RA, Tanagho EA. Perineal pudendal neurotomy versus selective neurotomy of the S2 somatic contribution to the pudendal nerve: effects on sacral–root-stimulated bladder and urethral responses in the dog. Urol Int 1992; 48:48–52.
10. Nishizawa O, Satoh S, Harada T, Nakamura H, Fukuda T, Tsukada T, Tsuchida S. Role of the pudendal nerves on the dynamics of the micturition of the dog evaluated by pressure flow EMG and pressure flowplot studies. J Urol 1984; 132:1036–1039.
11. Tanagho EA, Schmidt RA. Electrical stimulation in the clinical management of the neurogenic bladder. J Urol 1988; 140:1331–1339.
12. Tanagho EA, Miller ER. Initiation of voiding. Br J Urol 1970; 42:175–183.
13. Bosch R, Groen J. Effects of sacral segmental nerve stimulation on urethral resistance and bladder contractility: how does neuromodulation work in urge incontinence patients? Neurourol Urodynam 1995; 14:502–504 (abstr 62).
14. Goodwin RJ, Swinn MJ, Fowler CJ. The neurophysiology of urinary retention in young women and its treatment by neuromodulation. World J Urol 1998; 16:305–307.
15. Lindström S, Sudsuang R. Functionally specific bladder reflexes from pelvic and pudendal nerve branches: an experimental study in the cat. Neurourol Urodynam 1989; 8:392–393.
16. Mc Guire EJ, Zhang SC, Horwinski ER, Lytton B. Treatment of motor and sensory detrusor instability by electrical stimulation. J Urol 1983; 129:78–79.
17. Vodusek DB, Light JK, Libby JM. Detrusor inhibition induced by stimulation of pudendal nerve afferents. Neurourol Urodynam 1986; 5:381–389.
18. Vodusek DB, Plevnik S, Vrtacnik, P, Janez J. Detrusor inhibition on selective pudendal nerve stimulation in the perineum. Neurourol Urodynam 1988; 6:389–393.
19. Edvardsen P. Nervous control of the urinary bladder in cats 1: the collecting phase. Acta Physiol Scand 1968; 72:157–171.
20. Ebner A, Jiang C, Lindström S. Intravesical electrical stimulation—an experimental analysis of the mechanisms of action. J Urol 1992; 148:920–924.
21. Schultz–Lampel D, Jiang C, Lindström S, Thüroff JW. Experimental results on mechanisms of action of electrical neuromodulation in chronic urinary retention. World J Urol 1998; 16:301–304.
22. Vapnek JM, Schmidt RA. Restoration of voiding in chronic urinary retention using the neuroprosthesis. World J Urol 1991; 9:142–144.
23. Fowler CJ, Kirby RS, Harrison MJG. Decelerating burst and complex repetitive discharges in the striated muscle of the urethral sphincter associated with urinary retention in women. J Neurol Neurosurg Psychiatry 1985; 48:1004–1009.
24. Fowler CJ, Christmas TJ, Chapple CR, Parkhouse HF, Kirby RS, Jacobs HS. Abnormal elec-

tromyographic activity of the urethral sphincter, voiding dysfunction and polycystic ovaries: a new syndrome? Br Med J 1988; 297:1436–1438.

25. De Ridder D, Van Cleynenbreugel B, Baert L. Sacral nerve stimulation for the female urinary retention: a two year follow-up. Eur Urol 1999; 35(suppl 2):17 (abstr 67).

26. Schmidt RA. The urethral syndrome. Urol Clin North Am 1985; 12:349–354.

27. Gleason CA. Electrophysiological fundamentals of neurostimulation. World J Urol 1991; 9:110–113.

28. Bosch RJ, Griffiths DJ, Blom JH, Schroeder FH. Treatment of benign prostatic hyperplasia by androgen deprivation: effects on prostate size and urodynamic parameters. J Urol 1989; 141: 68–72.

29. Andersen JT. Prostatism: clinical, radiologic and urodynamic aspects. Neurourol Urodynam 1982; 1:241–293.

30. Steers WD, de Groat WC. Effect of bladder outlet obstruction on micturition reflex pathways in the rat. J Urol 1988; 140:864–871.

31. Bosch R, Groen J. Urethral resistance is related to type of incontinence: changing etiologic concepts in female incontinence. Neurourol Urodynam 1998; 17:386–388.

37

Neurostimulation

PHILIP E. V. VAN KERREBROECK

University Hospital Maastricht, Maastricht, The Netherlands

I. INTRODUCTION

Dysfunction of the urinary sphincter is a common finding in various neurogenic diseases. Any injury or disease that is associated with paralysis of the lower limbs can affect the behavior of the urinary sphincter.

In patients with spinal cord injury, the inability to control the body's autonomic functions, especially the storage and evacuation function of the lower urinary tract, is a major aspect of their handicap.

Besides these problems with a proved neurological basis, a vast number of patients suffer from lower urinary tract dysfunction, including sphincter dysfunction without an evident neurological cause. These are patients with different forms of so-called idiopathic dysfunctional voiding syndromes and incontinence problems. Because the cause of these abnormalities is unknown, specific therapy is difficult. For these persons and their doctors, therapy becomes frustrating and often leads to mutilating derivation surgery.

In patients with evident neurogenic bladder dysfunction, incontinence and poor evacuation of urine with residual urine and recurrent urinary tract infections can cause significant morbidity. The relation between lower urinary tract dysfunction and upper urinary tract problems is evident and is influenced by the quality of bladder and sphincter control (1). Therefore, adequate treatment of bladder and urethral sphincter dysfunction is one of the most important prognostic tools for approaching upper urinary tract problems (2).

Two major types of urethral dysfunction can be distinguished: urinary sphincter overactivity and hypoactivity. In general, urinary sphincter overactivity is present in combination with lack of relaxation during voiding owing to dyssynergia and will cause incomplete emptying or urinary retention. Urinary sphincter hypoactivity will produce a variable degree of incontinence, depending on the remaining resting activity and recruitment during bladder filling.

Classic therapeutic modalities are limited. Moreover, long-term treatment and careful follow-up are often necessary (3). For patients with poor voiding or retention, the introduction of regular clean intermittent catheterization (CIC) has reduced the rate of urological complications, including urinary tract infections (4). However, many patients are not able to catheterize themselves or are unwilling to be dependent on catheterization (5). Even with a good technique, recurrent urinary tract infections can occur and remain a major problem (6). Chronic catheterization can induce severe infectious complications and urethral strictures (7,8).

Pharmacological treatment is not particularly effective in the correction of abnormal urinary sphincter behavior. Moreover, lifelong continuation of therapy is a major issue, mainly because of side effects (9). In most patients, especially in females, incontinence remains a problem, even with maximal pharmacological treatment. Medication that can produce a significant amelioration of urine evacuation by decreasing outlet resistance is limited (10).

The failure of pharmacological manipulation has led to the development of surgical approaches for abnormal urinary sphincter function. Different forms of neural ablation to reduce detrusor and urinary sphincter activity have been tried, with variable results (11). Sphincteric incisions can be made to control urine evacuation in case of severe sphincter spasticity, but with lifelong incontinence as a consequence (12). An artificial sphincter can be used to restore insufficient closure function. However, because bladder activity is also abnormal in many patients with abnormal sphincter function, increased outlet resistance is a delicate compromise between relief of incontinence and protection of the upper urinary tract (13).

A considerable percentage of patients with lower urinary tract dysfunction continue to have significant urological problems, even with maximal classic therapy. Therefore, newer approaches have been tried. The use of electronic means to control storage and evacuation of urine has become an important tool in urological treatment.

II. BACKGROUND OF ELECTRICAL STIMULATION IN LOWER URINARY TRACT CONTROL

The ultimate goal of treatment to manage neurogenic lower urinary tract dysfunction must be to restore the storage and evacuation capacity of the lower urinary tract as closely as possible to the physiological state. Different pathological entities with consequences for the filling or voiding phase of the bladder, or for the whole micturition cycle, can be present in cases of neurogenic bladder dysfunction. Depending on these pathological entities, the clinical goals of electrical stimulation in dysfunction of the lower urinary tract can be divided into four categories:

1. To treat incontinence caused by lack of activity of the striated muscles of the urethral closure mechanism by improving contraction of the sphincter mechanism
2. To overcome incontinence caused by detrusor hyperactivity or urethral instability by reducing detrusor instability or controlling urethral activity
3. To permit urine evacuation in patients with a paraplegic bladder by provoking detrusor contractions
4. To manage micturition in the hyperreflex bladder by combining dampening of spontaneous reflex excitability of the bladder with controlled activation of the detrusor

These aims can be fulfilled by three different forms of electrical stimulation:

1. Direct stimulation of the efferent nerves to the lower urinary tract with a direct cause and effect
2. Activation of reflex activity by the stimulation of afferent nerves
3. An indirect or modulatory effect on the behavior of some elements of the lower urinary tract by the electrical stimulation of other structures.

In patients with complete spinal cord injury and bladder hyperreflexia, the complete micturition cycle must be controlled. This means that supplementary to electrostimulation for evacuation, an increase in bladder capacity and compliance must be realized by other methods. Only under these conditions will both evacuation and storage of urine be controlled in a way such that the physiological mechanisms are imitated.

The importance of different urological problems in neurogenic lower urinary tract dysfunction has been the basis of extensive research in the field of electrical stimulation during the last four decades. General interest in neurostimulation for the treatment of various functional problems has helped in the development of different systems of electrical stimulation as a therapeutic tool. Most systems that are meant to produce electrical stimulation of the lower urinary tract will have an effect on the bladder as well as on the urinary sphincter.

In general, distinction can be made between devices that are not surgically implanted and implantable neuroprostheses. Many forms of electrical stimulation with urological applications have been studied, and an impressive number of different systems have been presented. Few methods, however, have survived and proved their benefits with reasonable follow-up.

Surface electrodes are used as nonimplantable devices (transcutaneous electrical nerve stimulation; TENS) for the treatment of pain caused by striated muscle spasticity in the pelvic region (14). Insertable plugs in the anal canal or the vagina are applied to treat incontinence (15–17). Intravesical electrostimulation has been tested in children with spina bifida (18). Implantable prostheses are available to induce bladder contraction to evacuate urine in paraplegic bladders or to control detrusor contraction in hyperreflex bladders (19–21). Another application of electrical stimulation is the modulation of symptomatic voiding dysfunctions such as urgency, frequency, urge incontinence, and functional obstructive problems (22,23).

III.   HISTORY OF ELECTRICAL STIMULATION

The first mention of the use of bioelectrical activity with the intention of curing disease is found in an Egyptian papyrus of 2750 BC (24). For centuries, various forms of natural electrical current have been applied as an empirical treatment for a broad group of human diseases.

Better knowledge of the neurophysiological backgrounds of electrical stimulation started with the frog experiments of Galvani, showing that a muscle contracts after electrical stimulation of the nerve. The invention of the dry battery by Volta made artificial electricity available as a therapeutic tool in human medicine.

In the beginning of the 19th century, great interest was drawn to the effects of electricity on the human body. At the same time, better knowledge of basic neurophysiology has been gained, permitting us to understand the specific innervation of different organs and to explain the activity of electricity on biological processes. The work of Bell (25) and Magendie (26), in particular, demonstrated that the roles of the posterior spinal roots as sensory afferent pathways and of the anterior spinal roots as motoric pathways were very important for this.

In 1864, Budge (27) showed that a detrusor contraction could be evoked by direct stimulation of the ventral portion of the sacral spinal cord. Therefore, the bladder was the first organ ever to be submitted to direct electrical stimulation.

The first experiments to develop a system that could permit continuous direct electrical stimulation of the lower urinary tract originated in 1940 (28). The advent of the transistor made continuous electrical stimulation possible, and the cardiac pacemaker became available. At the same time, experiments were started to develop a bladder pacemaker.

The first direct bladder stimulator was implanted in humans in 1954 (29). Electrodes were placed directly on the bladder wall and stimulated with transcutaneous wires. Further technical development permitted the construction of a stimulator consisting of electrodes that were implanted on the bladder wall and controlled by a subcutaneous receiver. Different models of this type of stimulator have been developed (30–33). Maximal bladder pressures of 55 cmH$_2$O were reached, but owing to the lack of bladder neck relaxation, evacuation of urine without a reduction of outflow resistance was not possible. The spread of current to other pelvic structures, the stimuli thresholds of which were lower than that of the bladder, often resulted in abdominal, pelvic, and perineal pain (35,36). Furthermore, the simultaneous desire to defecate, contraction of the pelvic and leg muscles, and erection and ejaculation in men prevented the long-term use of these stimulators (37). Many technical problems, especially detachment of the electrode from the bladder wall or erosion through the bladder, were encountered with these systems, and this method of bladder stimulation was abandoned completely.

Burghele et al. (38) tried to stimulate the bladder in patients with spinal cord injury by planting electrodes on the pelvic splanchnic nerves. Very limited clinical results were published on this technique (39). The fact that the pelvic splanchnic nerves are usually plexiform in humans makes it difficult to apply electrodes. Stimulation of the splanchnic nerves can produce good bladder emptying only if no sympathetic fibers are stimulated simultaneously, to prevent contraction of the bladder neck at the moment of detrusor contraction. Possibilities with this type of electrical stimulation seem limited, and no system for clinical use is yet available.

Electrical stimulation was applied directly to the spinal cord by Nashold et al. (40), taking advantage of the remaining intact motor pathways to initiate micturition. Although good results were published with a short follow-up (41), many of the side effects seen with direct bladder stimulation were encountered (42). Side effects with this form of stimulation included high outflow resistance, needing sphincterotomies, sweating, and piloerection, penile erection in males, and movements of the lower limbs. Enthusiasm for this technique has waned considerably, but a conus implant for bladder stimulation is still available, and long-term results in a limited number of patients seem to be interesting (43).

Tanagho's team (44) from San Francisco started their research also with direct spinal cord stimulation, but found a very high rise in outlet resistance during stimulation. Although some emptying occurred, high intravesical pressure against high outflow resistance was registered with voiding only at the end of stimulation, when outlet resistance decreased. They concluded that, at the spinal cord level, it was not possible to separate a bladder center from a striated sphincter center. Therefore, an extensive series of experiments was started to achieve maximal specific detrusor stimulation with minimal sphincter activation (45,46). This research showed that separation of the dorsal component from the ventral component of the sacral roots involved was necessary, together with eventual sectioning of the somatic fibers of the sacral ventral roots to be stimulated (47). These experiments finally resulted in an extradural sacral anterior root stimulator for patients with spinal cord injury that is available for clinical research (48). In this treatment, bladder stimulation is combined with partial sacral rhizotomies to control reflex bladder activity.

Brindley (49,50), from London, started with animal experiments to develop a system for intradural sacral anterior root stimulation in 1969 and achieved implant-driven voiding in normal and paraplegic baboons in 1972. The first successful sacral anterior root stimulator for a patient with traumatic paraplegia was implanted in 1978 (51). Since then, more than 700 patients have been implanted worldwide (52). Clinical results have been largely improved since the introduction by Sauerwein (53), in 1986, of complete intradural sacral posterior root rhizotomies to control the reservoir function of the bladder in combination with implantation of the sacral posterior root stimulator.

Stimulators of sacral segmental nerves at the level of the sacral foramen were introduced by Habib (54) in 1967. Although this type of stimulator was likely to produce the same effects as anterior sacral root stimulators, the results were poor, probably because of inhibition by simultaneous stimulation of the afferent fibers. This work, however, was the basis of further research by Schmidt (55) and produced the sacral foramen stimulator for the treatment of functional lower urinary tract disorders.

Simultaneously with the development of systems for direct bladder stimulation, implantable stimulators were introduced to treat incontinence. Caldwell (56) was the first to introduce a direct sphincter stimulator. This type of stimulator and later related ones were used continuously throughout the day and sometimes at night, except during voiding. Their aim was to improve the tonic activity of the striated muscles of the urethra. The stimulation electrodes were placed near the distal sphincter, and stimulation probably occurred either by stimulation of the motor fibers to the sphincter, by the initiation of reflex activity, or by a mixture of both, depending on the strength of the currents used. Permanent stimulation effective in increasing intraurethral pressure seems to have been problematic because all surgeons who formerly used this type of stimulator have ceased to do so.

Nonsurgically implanted anal or vaginal electrodes have been tried for many years in different forms of lower urinary tract problems with variable success. The anal plug originally designed for the treatment of fecal incontinence was also applied for the treatment of urinary incontinence. It probably stimulates some motor fibers of the pudendal nerves, and the therapeutic effect results from reflex consequences of the stimulation of these afferent fibers. Vaginal devices resembling the anal plug have been developed for the treatment of stress incontinence (57,58). Work from Scandinavian authors has extended the treatment of detrusor instability with these devices (59,60). For all these probes, therapeutic activity is presumably related to the reflex consequences of stimulation of afferent nerve fibers. The use of these types of stimulators is limited. In patients with neurogenic problems, and well-controlled trials are difficult to organize. Some patients probably can benefit to a certain degree, but the cost–benefit analysis is weak.

In the treatment of neurogenic lower urinary tract dysfunction after spinal cord injury, only stimulation of the sacral anterior roots is now of clinical use. For the various forms of functional disorders, including those related to neurological diseases, sacral foramen stimulation seems to be an interesting option for the future.

IV. ELECTRICAL STIMULATION IN SPINAL CORD INJURY

The development of systems for electrical stimulation of the lower urinary tract in spinal cord injury coincided with better knowledge of the pathophysiology of neurogenic lower urinary tract dysfunction. The risks of untreated high-pressure detrusor contractions led to the application of aggressive anatomical approaches. These realized an important decrease in mortality from 90% after World War II to 2% in the 1970s (61). However, treatments such as urinary diversion and sphincterotomy are important compromises in terms of quality of life. Therefore, treatment with electrical stimulation of the bladder in spinal cord injury must achieve low-pressure detrusor storage and convenient evacuation of urine. Only then are the survival risks minimized and a good quality of life guaranteed at the same time.

Two approaches to stimulation of the bladder in patients with spinal cord injury are actually available, one of which is intradural, and the other, extradural.

Actual systems for electrical stimulation in spinal cord injury consist of a radiotransmitter applied to the skin over a buried receiver that is connected to the electrodes. This principle was already described in 1934 to stimulate a monkey's brain (62). The same principle was first used in 1962 by Bradley et al. to stimulate the bladder (30).

The problems, however, with direct bladder stimulation and stimulation of the conus medullaris have oriented attempts to gain electronic control over the bladder and the urethra through the sacral roots. Habib (54) first used the sacral roots for stimulation in animals and in humans. Sacral root stimulators were originally designed and developed as devices that would activate either the bladder or the striated sphincter and the pelvic floor according to the stimulus parameters employed. It was originally expected that many patients would use both the bladder-emptying mode to lower residual urine and the sphincter-activating mode to assist continence. In practice, the bladder-emptying mode has been of great value, but the sphincter-activating mode is seldom used because of the need for continuous stimulation and the poor results owing to striated muscle fatigue. Appropriate stimulation of the sacral roots will also activate the smooth muscle of the colon and the rectum and can have an influence on the defecation process. Furthermore, continuous stimulation of the sacral roots can induce penile erection in males.

Habib's experiments with sacral segmental stimulation proved that stimulation of the bladder was possible at this level (54). However, to permit complete evacuation, it became evident that afferent stimulation must be limited. Therefore, Brindley (49) started animal experiments to develop a system for implant-driven micturition that could be applied to the intradural part of the sacral roots. Because of the anatomical features of the sacral roots, separation of the anterior (motoric) part and the posterior (sensory) part of the sacral roots is possible in their intradural part. The first animal experiments were performed in baboons, and in 1971, the first micturition by sacral root stimulation in bursts was realized (49). Stimulation in bursts was necessary because stimulation of the sacral anterior roots resulted in simultaneous activation of the striated muscles of the pelvic floor, the urinary sphincter, and the detrusor. Stimulation in bursts, however, permitted the different characteristics of the smooth and striated muscles to be used. The striated muscle of the outlet contracts rapidly and the smooth muscle of the detrusor slowly. In the gap between bursts, the outlet relaxes rapidly, whereas the slower-reacting detrusor is still in contraction, resulting in poststimulus voiding (63).

As these prostheses remained usable for up to 4.5 years, a model for implantation in humans was built and implanted successfully in 1978 (51). Good initial clinical results were achieved, and the first urodynamic results were published (64). In 1986, the results on the first 50 patients were reported (20). The results of these series were very much influenced by the number of rhizotomies performed. Initially, no rhizotomies were done. After the first incidental rhizotomies in 1979, a significant increase in bladder capacity was noted, and in later operations in patients with a complete spinal cord lesion, bilateral posterior rhizotomies at the S3 level were undertaken. These roots are considered to contain the main afferent fibers from the bladder and, therefore, should be cut to increase bladder capacity (65). Further experience, however, showed that parasympathetic innervation of the bladder is not consistent in every patient and that S2, S4, and eventually, S5 roots can contain afferent parasympathetic fibers. These are not necessarily active at the moment of surgery, but can become so afterward, which explains the high recurrence rate of detrusor hyperreflexia following partial sacral posterior rhizotomies (66). This possibility of reinnervation of the bladder by higher or lower sacral segments after partial rhizotomies was already demonstrated in 1975 (67). Parasympathetic reinnervation, however, has never been encountered at a level above S2 (68). Therefore, complete parasympathetic deafferentation of the bladder, necessary for a high-capacity, high-compliance bladder reservoir, should include complete posterior rhizotomies from S2 to S4–S5. The urodynamic results in patients submitted to complete deafferentation before implantation of an anterior root stimulator proved this with a permanent change in bladder behavior (69).

Therefore, the actual technique of intradural sacral anterior root stimulation in the treatment of neurogenic bladder dysfunction after spinal cord injury consists of combining complete posterior rhizotomies with implantation of Finetech–Brindley electrodes on the remaining anterior roots (70). With this technique, more than 1000 patients have been operated on worldwide. In a personal overview of 184 patients from different centers, more than 80% were able to achieve sufficient intravesical pressure and efficient voiding. Different reasons can prevent use of the implant, among them pain in patients with a partial lesion and without rhizotomies, nerve root damage, or electronic component failure. In nearly all patients with a functioning implant, the incidence of infections is decreased. In patients who have had posterior rhizotomies, the occurrence of reflex uninhibited detrusor contractions is abolished as the reflex arc is no longer intact (71). As a result, patients have an increased functional capacity without involuntary detrusor contractions. Therefore, continence can be achieved in most patients without previous surgery, reducing urethral closure function (72). Most patients will become appliance-free, which enhances dignity and self-image.

Another type of sacral root stimulation for the evacuation of urine in spinal cord injury was developed by a San Francisco group of researchers (55). As a result of their research, they placed the electrodes extradurally and combined the implantation of electrodes on sacral roots S3 or S4, or both, with selective posterior rhizotomies. The extradural approach has the advantage of easier surgical technique, with less risk of cerebrospinal fluid leakage. However, exact separation of the anterior and posterior parts of the sacral roots is more difficult in the extradural segment of S3, and it is nearly impossible at the S4 level. Moreover, the crossing of anterior and posterior nerve fibers can occur at this level (73).

To overcome any residual concomitant striated muscle contraction of the urethra, selective division of the urethral nerve fibers traveling with the pudendal nerve was undertaken by Schmidt in 1988 (55). In a total group of 22 patients, he realized complete success in 8 (42%), meaning normal reservoir function, continence, and evacuation of urine with electrical stimulation (74). Voiding with this type of stimulation is claimed to be synchronous and to occur with low voiding pressure. The extradural stimulation system has not been commercialized, and the results of further experimental and clinical work are not available.

V. INDICATIONS FOR ELECTRICAL STIMULATION IN SPINAL CORD INJURY

Three different types of patients with spinal cord injury can be distinguished in terms of electrical stimulation:

1. Patients with a lesion that has destroyed the efferent innervation of the detrusor: These patients have bladder areflexia, and sacral anterior root stimulators are useless because the fibers that they are designed to stimulate have been destroyed. It is unlikely that any other kind of electrical implant will be successful.
2. Patients with a complete spinal cord lesion that leaves the sacral segments of the cord intact: After the phase of spinal shock, these patients will have detrusor hyperreflexia. Even if this reflex activity of the bladder is inefficient for complete evacuation of urine, owing to the insufficient duration of reflex activity or to detrusor–sphincter dyssynergia, those patients can be candidates for treatment with sacral anterior root stimulation.
3. Patients with an incomplete lesion: Patients with a stationary incomplete lesion could be candidates for sacral anterior root stimulation if no pelvic sensitivity is preserved. If pelvic sensitivity is preserved, stimulation for urine evacuation can be so painful that it cannot be used. Furthermore, sacral rhizotomies before implantation of the stimulator will abolish perineal sensitivity, which can be very important in these wheelchair-bound patients.

Patients with slowly progressive lesions could be suitable candidates for electrical stimulation alone without rhizotomies. Some patients with multiple sclerosis have been treated with sacral root stimulation, but their number is too limited to draw conclusions. With the actual techniques, only patients with a stable complete spinal cord injury are ideal candidates for sacral anterior root stimulation and posterior root rhizotomies. In patients with preserved sensitivity, the stimulation parameters used in Finetech–Brindley bladder control can induce pain sensation that prevents normal use of the stimulator.

VI. FUTURE POSSIBILITIES

The experience with electrically stimulated graciloplasty for fecal incontinence has proved that training of the striated muscle is possible, transforming it to produce long-lasting tonic activity. Initial experiments with gracilis muscle plasty to create a neosphincter have been performed with variable results.

Future developments will see the improvement of electronic means to control voiding and continence, with more computerization and perhaps less invasiveness. More patients with various forms of neurogenic lower urinary tract dysfunction could probably benefit from these techniques and regain more normal control of the lower urinary tract with less morbidity.

REFERENCES

1. McGuire EJ, Woodside JR, Borden TA, Weiss RM. Prognostic value of urodynamic testing in myelodysplastic patients. J Urol 1981; 126:205–209.
2. McGuire EJ, Woodside JR, Borden TA. Upper urinary tract deterioration in patients with myelodysplasia and detrusor hypertonia: a follow-up study. J Urol 1983; 129:823–826.

3. Burke MR, Hicks AF, Robins M, Kessler H. Survival of patients with injuries of the spinal cord. JAMA 1960; 172:121–124.
4. Guttmann L. The value of intermittent catheterisation in the early management of traumatic paraplegia and tetraplegia. Paraplegia 1966; 4:63.
5. Lapides J, Diokno AC, Silber SJ. Clean, intermittent self catheterisation in the treatment of urinary tract disease. J Urol 1972; 107:458–461.
6. Maynard FM, Diokno AC. Urinary infection and complications during clean intermittent catheterisation following spinal cord injury. J Urol 1984; 132:943–946.
7. Blacklock NJ. Catheters and urethral strictures. Br J Urol 1986; 58:475–478.
8. Hardy HG. Complications of the indwelling urethral catheter. Int J Paraplegia 1968; 6:5.
9. Thompson IM, Lauvetz R. Oxybutinine in bladder spasm, neurogenic bladder and enuresis. Urology 1976; 8:452–454.
10. Krane RJ, Olsson CA. Phenoxybenzamine in neurogenic bladder dysfunction: clinical considerations. J Urol 1973; 110:653–656.
11. Torrens M, Hald T. Bladder denervation procedures. Urol Clin North Am 1979; 6:283–293.
12. Ross JC, Gibbon NO, Sunder GS. Division of the external urethral sphincter in the neuropathic bladder—a twenty years review. Br J Urol 1976; 48:649–656.
13. Light JK, Scott FB. Total reconstruction of the lower urinary tract using bowel and the artificial sphincter. J Urol 1984; 131:953–956.
14. Bradley WE, Timm GW, Chou SN. A decade of experience with electronic stimulation of the micturition reflex. Urol Int 1971; 26:283.
15. Godec C, Cass AS, Ayala GF. Electrical stimulation for incontinence: technique, selection and results. Urology 1976; 7:388–397.
16. Merrill DC. The treatment of detrusor incontinence by electrical stimulation. J Urol 1979; 122:515–517.
17. Fall M. Does electrical stimulation control incontinence? J Urol 1984; 131:664.
18. Katona F. Stages of vegetative afferentiation in reorganization of bladder control during intra_vesical electrotherapy. Urol Int 1975; 30:192–203.
19. Caldwell KP. Urinary incontinence following spinal injury treated by electronic implant. Lancet 1985; 1:846.
20. Brindley GS, Polkey CE, Rushton DN, Cardozo L. Sacral anterior root stimulators for bladder control in paraplegia. The first 50 cases. J Neurol Neurosurg Psychiatry 1986; 49:1104–1114.
21. Tanagho EA, Schmidt RA, Orvis BR. Neural stimulation for control of voiding dysfunction: a preliminary report in 22 patients with serious neuropathic voiding disorders. J Urol 1989; 142:340–345.
22. Markland C, Merrill D, Chou S, Bradley W. Sacral nerve root stimulation: a clinical test of detrusor innervation. J Urol 1972; 107:772–776.
23. Schmidt RA. Advances in genitourinary neurostimulation. Neurosurgery 1986; 19:1041–1044.
24. Kellaway P. The part played by electric fish in the early history of bioelectricity and electrotherapy. Bull Hist Med 1946; 20:112.
25. Bell C. Idea of a New Anatomy of the Brain. London: Stratham & Preston, 1811.
26. Magendie F. Expérience sur les fonctions des racines des nerfs rachidiens. J Physiol 1822; 2:276.
27. Budge J. Uber den Einfluss des Nervensystems auf die Bewegung der Blase. Z Rationelle Med 1864; 21:1.
28. Dees JE. Contraction of the urinary bladder produced by electrical stimulation: preliminary report. Invest Urol 1965; 15:539–547.
29. Boyce WH, Lathem JE, Hunt LD. Research related to the development of artificial electrical stimulator for the paralysed human bladder. J Urol 1964; 91:41–51.
30. Bradley WE, Wittmers LE, Chou SN, French LA. Use of radio transmitter receiver unit for the treatment of neurogenic bladder: a preliminary report, J Neurosurg 1962; 19:782–786.
31. Hald T, Meier W, Khalili A, Agrawal G, Benton J, Kantrowitz A. Clinical experience with a radio-linked bladder stimulator. J Urol 1967; 97:73–78.

32. Stenberg CC, Burnette HW, Bunts RC. Electrical stimulation of human neurogenic bladders: experience with 4 patients. J Urol 1967; 97:79–84.

33. Susset JG, Boctor ZN. Implantable vesical stimulator: clinical experience. J Urol 1967; 98:673–678.

34. Halverstadt DB, Leadbetter WF. Electrical stimulation of the human bladder: experience in three patients with hypotonic neurogenic bladder dysfunction. Br J Urol 1968; 40:175–182.

35. Merrill DC, Conway CJ. Clinical experience with the Mentor bladder stimulator. I. Patients with upper motor neuron lesions. J Urol 1974; 112:52–56.

36. Merrill DC. Clinical experience with the Mentor bladder stimulator in patients with vesical hypotonia. J Urol 1975; 113:335–337.

37. Halverstadt DB, Parry WL. Electronic stimulation of the human bladder: nine years later. J Urol 1975; 113:341–344.

38. Burghele T, Ichim V, Demetresco M. Etude expérimentale sur la physiologie de la miction et l'évacuation électrique de la vessie chez les traumatisés médullaires. Exp Surg 1967; 1:156.

39. Kaeckenbeeck B. Electrostimulation de la vessie des paraplégiques. Technique de Burghele–Ichim–Demetrescu. Acta Urol Belg 1979; 47:139–140.

40. Nashold BS, Friedman H, Glenn JF, Grimes JH, Barry WF Avery R. Electromicturition in paraplegia. Implantation of a spinal neuroprothesis. Arch Surg 1972; 104:195–202.

41. Nashold BS, Friedman H, Grimes J. Electrical stimulation of the conus medullaris to control the bladder in paraplegia: a ten year review. Appl Neurophysiol 1982; 45:40–43.

42. Sarramon JP, Lazorthes Y, Sedan R, Leandri P, Lhez JM. Neurostimulation médullaire dans les vessies neurogènes centrales. Acta Urol Belg 1979; 47:129–138.

43. Dobelle WH. Avery Laboratories Conus Implants for bladder stimulation in spinal cord injuries. Personal communication, 1992.

44. Jonas U, Jones LW, Tanagho EA. Controlled electrical bladder evacuation via stimulation of the sacral micturition centre or direct detrusor stimulation. Urol Int 1976; 31:108–110.

45. Thüroff JW, Bazeed MA, Schmidt RA, Wiggin DM, Tanagho EA. Functional pattern of sacral root stimulation in dogs: I. Micturition. J Urol 1982; 127:1031–1033.

46. Thüroff JW, Bazeed MA, Schmidt RA, Wiggin DM, Tanagho EA. Functional pattern of sacral root stimulation in dogs: II. Urethral closure. J Urol 1982; 127:1034–1038.

47. Schmidt RA, Bruschini H, Tanagho EA. Feasibility of inducing micturition through chronic stimulation of sacral roots. Urology 1978; 12:471–477.

48. Tanagho EA, Schmidt RA. Electrical stimulation in the clinical management of the neurogenic bladder. J Urol 1988; 140:1331–1339.

49. Brindley GS. Experiments directed towards a prosthesis which controls the bladder and the external sphincter from a single site of stimulation, Proceedings Biological Engineering Society 46th Meeting, Liverpool, 1972.

50. Brindley GS. Emptying the bladder by stimulating sacral ventral roots. J Physiol 1973; 237:15–16.

51. Brindley GS, Polkey CE, Rushton DN. Sacral anterior root stimulators for bladder control in paraplegia. Paraplegia 1982; 20:365–381.

52. Van Kerrebroeck PE, Debruyne FM. World-wide experience with the Finetech–Brindley sacral anterior root bladder stimulator. Neurourol Urodynam 1993; 12:497–503.

53. Sauerwein D. Die operative Behandlung der spastischen Blasenlahmung bei Querschnittlahmung. Urologe 1990; A29:196–203.

54. Habib HN. Experience and recent contributions in sacral nerve stimulation for voiding in both human and animal. Br J Urol 1967; 39:73–83.

55. Schmidt RA. Applications of neurostimulation in urology. Neurourol Urodynam 1988; 7:585–592.

56. Caldwell KP. The electrical control of sphincter incontinence. Lancet 1963; 2:174–175.

57. Hopkinsons BR, Lightwood R. Electrical treatment of incontinence. Br J Surg 1967; 54:802–805.

58. de Soldenhoff R, McDonnell H. New device for control of female urinary incontinence. Br Med J 1969; 4:230.

59. Alexander S, Rowan D. Electrical control of urinary incontinence by radio implant: a report of 14 patients, Br J Urol 1968; 55:358–364.

60. Fall M, Erlandson BE, Nilson AE, Sundin T. Long term intravaginal electrical stimulation in urge and stress incontinence. Scan J Urol Nephrol 1978; 44:55–63.

61. Fall M, Erlandson BE, Sundin T, Waagstein F. Intravaginal electrical stimulation. Clinical experiments on bladder inhibition. Scand J Urol Nephrol 1978; 44:41–47.

62. Swain A, Grundy D, Russel J. A.B.C. of spinal cord injury at the accident. Br Med J 1985; 291: 1558–1560.

63. Chaffey EL, Light RU. Radiofrequency link to stimulate the monkey brain, Yale Biol Med 1934; 7:83.

64. Brindley GS. An implant to empty the bladder or close the urethra. J Neurol Neurosurg Psychiatry 1977; 40:358–369.

65. Cardozo L, Krishnan KR, Polkey CE, Rushton DN, Brindley GS. Urodynamic observations on patients with sacral anterior root stimulators. Paraplegia 1984; 22:201–209.

66. Meirowsky AM, Scheibert CD, Hinchey TR. Studies on the sacral reflex arc in paraplegia. II. Differential sacral neurotomy. An operative method. J Neurosurg 1950; 7:39.

67. Rockswold GL, Chou SN, Bradley WE. Re-evaluation of differential sacral rhizotomy for neurological bladder disease. J Neurosurg 1978; 48:773–778.

68. Toczek SK, McCullough DC, Gargour GW, Kachman R, Baker R, Luessenhop AJ. Selective sacral rootlet rhizotomy for hypertonic neurogenic bladder. J Neurosurg 1975; 42:567–574.

69. De Groat WC, Nadelhaft I, Milne RJ, Booth AM, Morgan C, Thor K. Organisation of the sacral parasympathetic reflex pathways to the urinary bladder and large intestine. J Auton Nerv Syst 1981; 3:135–160.

70. Van Kerrebroeck PE, Koldewijn EL, Wijkstra H, Debruyne FM. Urodynamic evaluation before and after intradural posterior sacral rhizotomies and implantation of the Finetech–Brindley anterior sacral root stimulator. Urodinamica 1992; 2:7.

71. Van Kerrebroeck PE, Koldewijn E, Wijkstra H, Debruyne FM. Intradural sacral rhizotomies and implantation of an anterior sacral root stimulator in the treatment of neurogenic bladder dysfunction after spinal cord injury. World J Urol 1991; 9:126–132.

72. O'Flynn KJ, Grant J, MacDonagh R, Thomas DG. The effect of sacral rhizotomy on lower urinary tract function in spinal injury patients. Eur Urol 1990; 18:8.

73. MacDonagh RP, Forster DM, Thomas DG. Urinary continence in spinal injury patients following complete sacral posterior rhizotomy. Br J Urol 1990; 66:618–622.

74. d'Avella D, Mingrino S. Microsurgical anatomy of lumbosacral spinal roots, J Neurosurg 1979; 51:819–823.

38

Sphincterotomy and Sphincter Stent Prosthesis Placement

DAVID A. RIVAS

Jefferson Medical College, Thomas Jefferson University, Philadelphia, Pennsylvania

MICHAEL B. CHANCELLOR

University of Pittsburgh, Pittsburgh, Pennsylvania

I. INTRODUCTION

Approximately 10,000 new spinal cord injuries (SCI) occur each year. Eighty-five percent of the patients are men and 58% result in quadriplegia (1,2). Many of these patients develop neurogenic lower urinary tract dysfunction (detrusor hyperreflexia; DH) associated with detrusor–external sphincter dyssynergia (DESD) (3–5). DH in conjunction with DESD, resulting in elevated intravesical pressure, can result in a 50% or greater long-term urological complication rate. The associated morbidity includes sepsis, hydronephrosis, vesicoureteral reflux, nephrolithiasis, renal insufficiency, and even renal failure (5–8).

External sphincterotomy has been the treatment of choice for over 30 years for those afflicted with SCI or other neurological impairment associated with DH and DESD who are unable to perform clean, intermittent catheterization (CIC). Sphincterotomy permits low-pressure urinary drainage, which often significantly reduces postvoid residual urine volumes (9). Urinary collection is accomplished using an external condom catheter after sphincterotomy, although total dribbling incontinence is unusual unless the bladder neck and prostatic urethra have also been previously surgically compromised.

Sphincterotomy has been proved by several investigators to be an efficacious treatment for men with SCI afflicted with DH and DESD. In one study, 22 spinal cord-injured men with videourodynamically verified DESD underwent external urinary sphincter ablation using the contact Nd:YAG laser. Three patients afflicted with bladder neck obstruction required concurrent contact–laser incision of the bladder neck.

The mean duration of surgery was 45 ± 21 min. Bladder voiding pressure decreased from 87 ± 23 preoperatively to 47 ± 11 cmH$_2$O at 12 months (p < 0.01). Residual urine volume decreased significantly from 122 ± 77 to 33 ± 19 mL at 12 months (p < 0.01) whereas bladder capacity remained unchanged at 174 ± 84 and 230 ± 92 mL (p = 0.57). Three patients had recurrent sphincter obstruction 1 year after laser sphincterotomy. Two patients experienced complications associated with condom catheter urinary drainage and returned to the use of an indwelling catheter. One patient experienced diminished reflex erectile function postoperatively. No patient required blood transfusion. No deleterious effects on renal function or symptoms of autonomic dysreflexia were noted (10).

The complications, hospitalization requirement, and cost of irreversible surgical external sphincterotomy have prompted investigations into other treatments. These have included balloon dilation (11,12), or the placement of intraurethral wire mesh stent prosthesis at the level of the membranous urethra, as alternatives to defeating the function of the external sphincter (13). A major potential advantage of sphincter stent placement is that the treatment is reversible; sphincter function returns when the stent is removed.

In this chapter, we will briefly present the results of the multicenter North American clinical experience with UroLume (American Medical Systems, Minnetonka, MN) sphincter stent prosthesis placement, discuss the complications encountered and their treatment, and the reversibility of sphincter stent therapy for DESD. In addition, the results of a randomized, prospective multicenter trial, which compared conventional sphinterotomy with sphincter stent prosthesis placement, will be used to illustrate the efficacy and safety of these two procedures in the treatment of DESD.

II. EXTERNAL SPHINCTEROTOMY

Sphincterotomy has traditionally been performed endoscopically using electrosurgical applications, although more recently this technique has been supplanted with a contact neodymium: yittrium aluminum garnet (Nd:YAG) laser to accomplish sphincter incision (14). The sphincterotomy procedure requires that the patient be placed in the dorsal lithotomy position after the induction of spinal or general anesthesia. Rigid cystoscopy is performed to examine the bladder and urethra. The sphincter is visualized, the extent of laser treatment determined, and the contact Nd:YAG laser (Surgical Laser Technologies, Oaks, PA) with a cutting chisel tip is placed through the working channel of the cystoscope (15).

The external sphincter is vaporized in a deep groove under direct vision, with the laser set at 40–50 W of power, using a combined retraction and forward pressure maneuver. An incision of at least 4 cm from the proximal bulbous to the midprostatic urethra is created. In younger men without prostatic or bladder neck obstruction, an incision at the endoscopic 12 o'clock position is ideal. This location avoids damage to the penile arteries and nerves, which run more laterally. In patients with concomitant bladder neck obstruction, an additional incision at the 6 o'clock position of the bladder neck is performed using the contact laser tip, similar to that performed for a conventional transurethral incision of the prostate. After the sphincter has been incised, a 22F continuous-irrigation catheter is inserted transurethrally.

Continuous irrigation of the urethral catheter is performed for up to 24 hr when hematuria is evident. The patient is maintained as an inpatient until hematuria has cleared, usually 24–48 hr postoperatively, then discharged with the catheter in place. Replacement with condom catheter urinary collection is undertaken 7–10 days postoperatively in an outpatient setting (10).

The complications associated with conventional external sphincterotomy include a reoperation rate, ranging from 12 to 26% (16), hemorrhage requiring blood transfusion in 5–23% of cases (17), and erectile dysfunction (either complete or partial loss of erection) in 2.8–64% of patients (18–22).

III. SPHINCTER STENT PROSTHESIS PLACEMENT

The UroLume prosthesis is inserted in lengths of 2, 2.5, and 3 cm by a standard technique, with a purposely designed endoscopic insertion tool (Fig. 1). The UroLume stent, made from a nonmagnetic superalloy woven into a tubular mesh, is a biocompatible and inert structure. Its unique properties permit it to expand the membranous urethra and, at the same time, permit the urethral epithelial cells to infiltrate its interstices so that the stent becomes completely epithelialized.

The sphincter stent prosthesis is packaged preloaded within its 21F insertion tool. This device accommodates a 0 degree cystoscopic telescope, with the delivery system functioning much as a conventional rigid cystoscope. Thus, the prosthesis is placed under direct vision, such that its proximal margin covers the distal one-half of the veru montanum. The

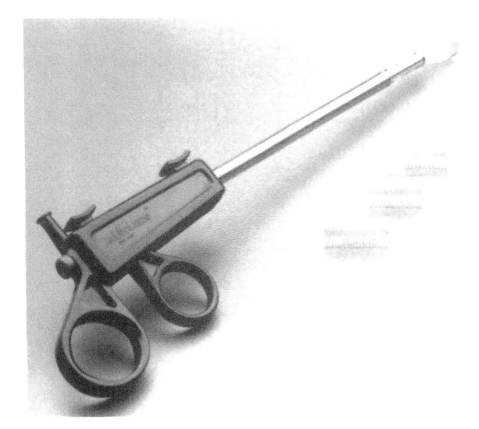

Figure 1   (a) Preloaded insertion device; (b) partial deployment of the prosthesis: The 0-degree cystoscopic lens can move in and out of the insertion tool to inspect the proximal and distal margins to ensure precise placement before the prosthesis is released.

distal end of the prosthesis should extend at least 5 mm into the bulbous urethra, well beyond the distal aspect of the external sphincter (Fig. 2; see color insert). In cases of a relatively long membranous urethra, an additional overlapping stent may be placed to ensure that the external sphincter is completely expanded by the device (Fig. 3). A condom catheter is used immediately for urinary collection postoperatively. A temporary suprapubic tube cystostomy may be deployed in the initial perioperative period to assure urinary drainage, as urethral catheter insertion may displace a newly positioned urethral stent (23). The stent position is then confirmed radiographically (24).

IV. THE MULTICENTER NORTH AMERICAN TRIAL

One hundred and sixty men with SCI, who had stable neurological injury and urodynamically confirmed DH and DESD, were entered into this experimental study at 15 North American centers to determine the usefulness of sphincter stent prosthesis placement as a treatment of DESD (25).

A. Sphincter Stent Trial: Methods

Each patient underwent preoperative evaluation, which included a medical history, physical examination, urinalysis and culture, serum chemistry evaluation, complete blood

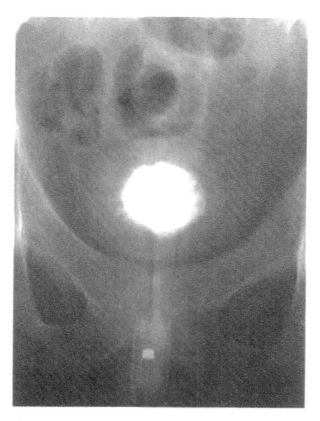

Figure 3 Voiding cystourethrogram (VCUG) 12 months after sphincter prosthesis placement: During a reflex involuntary detrusor contraction, the external sphincter is open.

count, urodynamic study, and upper tract imaging, with either a renal ultrasound, intravenous urogram, or radioisotope renal scan.

The presence or absence of subjective symptoms of autonomic dysreflexia (AD) was recorded before stent insertion and at each postoperative period. The patients were generally aware of their history of AD as manifested by headache, diaphoresis, and previously documented paradoxical hypertension and bradycardia, especially during urological manipulation.

Urodynamic evaluation included measurement of voiding pressure, urethral pressure, maximal cystometric capacity, residual urine volume, and sphincter electromyography (EMG). Patients who demonstrated EMG and manometric evidence of DESD during involuntary detrusor contraction were considered candidates for sphincter stent placement. Concomitant documented bladder neck dysfunction or prostatic enlargement resulting in bladder outflow obstruction served as exclusion criteria.

B. Therapeutic Results

1. Patient Demographics

The patients ranged in age from 16 to 74 (mean, 36.3 ± 12.1) years. Neurogenic lower urinary tract dysfunction was attributed to SCI in 150 patients (93.8%), multiple sclerosis (MS) in 8 patients (5%), spinal vascular accident in 1 patient (0.6%), and spinal cord tumor in 1 (0.6%). The mean duration of SCI or neurological disease was 9.0 ± 9.4 years. Forty-six of the 160 patients (28.8%) had undergone at least one previous external sphincterotomy, with a mean number of 1.7 ± 1.0 sphincterotomies. In addition, 11 patients (6.9%) had been treated with a previous transurethral prostatectomy, 11 patients (5.9%) underwent bladder neck resection, and 4 patients (2.5%), a bladder neck incision.

2. Urodynamic Results

A statistically significant decrease in voiding pressure occurred in patients with matched data from preinsertion to postinsertion values at each follow-up period (Table 1). The data have been reanalyzed relative to the two subgroups, specifically those patients with or without a prior sphincterotomy. No statistically significant differences were evident between the two groups relative to their preoperative urodynamic parameters, except that patients without previous sphincterotomy demonstrated a higher voiding pressure ($80.6 \pm 26.7 \, cmH_2O$) than those with prior sphincterotomy ($62.6 \pm 27.8 \, cmH_2O$), $p = 0.001$. During the follow-up period, all urodynamic parameters were similar between the two groups, except for two isolated data points, voiding pressure at 3 months and residual urine volume at 1 and 2 years. By 3 years of follow-up, no differences were documented between patients with and without prior external sphincterotomy when all three urodynamic parameters were compared.

3. Hydronephrosis

Postoperatively, all but 1 patient demonstrated improvement or stabilization of hydronephrosis, that was present before stent placement. Hydronephrosis actually resolved in 22 of 28 patients (78.6%) after stent placement. In the remaining patients, stable renal function was observed.

Table 1 Sphincter Stent Trial: Comparative Urodynamic Parameters Outcome with Matched Data Sets

Time period	Voiding pressure (cmH$_2$O)		Residual urine volume (mL)		Cystometric capacity (mL)
3-mo	Pre: 74.3 ± 28.0	n = 112	Pre: 197 ± 147	n = 111	Pre: 271 ± 157
	Post: 41.8 ± 24.6	p < 0.001*	Post: 105 ± 116	p < 0.001*	Post: 237 ± 145
6-mo	Pre: 74.0 ± 26.7	n = 109	Pre: 205 ± 148	n = 106	Pre: 272 ± 159
	Post: 39.6 ± 23.3	p < 0.001*	Post: 118 ± 154	p < 0.001*	Post: 241 ± 145
1-yr	Pre: 77.1 ± 26.0	n = 99	Pre: 198 ± 140	n = 100	Pre: 260 ± 155
	Post: 38.3 ± 24.0	p < 0.001*	Post: 113 ± 125	p < 0.001*	Post: 248 ± 153
2-yr	Pre: 75.6 ± 22.0	n = 79	Pre: 204 ± 136	n = 76	Pre: 268 ± 156
	Post: 38.2 ± 20.5	p < 0.001*	Post: 105 ± 101	p < 0.001*	Post: 270 ± 158
3-yr	Pre: 76.0 ± 22.6	n = 62	Pre: 198 ± 111	n = 59	Pre: 278 ± 164
	Post: 41.6 ± 27.8	p < 0.001*	Post: 135 ± 112	p < 0.001*	Post: 259 ± 129
4-yr	Pre: 78.7 ± 22.4	n = 42	Pre: 202 ± 98	n = 38	Pre: 258 ± 152
	Post: 44.5 ± 26.1	p < 0.001*	Post: 135 ± 113	p < 0.001*	Post: 260 ± 135
5-yr	Pre: 78.5 ± 22.4	n = 27	Pre: 209 ± 151	n = 31	Pre: 250 ± 141
	Post: 44.6 ± 28.7	p < 0.001*	Post: 124 ± 105	p < 0.001*	Post: 285 ± 157

4. Autonomic Dysreflexia

One hundred and fifteen patients (71.9%) reported symptoms of AD on entering this clinical study. One year after stent insertion and condom catheter urinary drainage were established, 70% of patients reported the resolution of AD symptoms (p = 0.0001). Only 3 of 36 patients (8.3%) without AD symptoms before stent insertion reported AD 2 years later. The improvement in AD was maintained at 2-year (p = 0.0000), 3-year (p = 0.0002), 4-year (p = 0.0004), and 5-year (p = 0.05) follow-up evaluations.

5. Stents Required

Of 160 patients, 115 (71.9%) required a single insertion procedure to adequately assure patency of the entire external sphincter. Thirty-five patients (21.9%) needed two, and 10 patients (6.2%) required three or more insertion procedures. Eighty-three patients (52%) needed a single 3-cm stent to adequately cover the external sphincter. Forty-eight patients (30.0%) required two prostheses, and 11 patients needed three stents (6.9%).

6. Epithelialization, Hyperplasia, and Encrustation

Cystoscopically, epithelialization of the device appears to be initiated shortly after sphincter stent placement. At 3 months, 47.1% of patients demonstrated 90–100% stent epithelialization, whereas at 1 year, 82.7% of patients had established 90–100% epithelialization, which persisted throughout follow-up.

Epithelial hyperplasia within the stent lumen may occur after urethral stent insertion. During the follow-up period, 34–44.4% of patients were observed to have this tissue response during cystoscopic evaluation. The tissue response was seen to be only mild in 71.4–93.3% of these patients. Stenosis within the sphincter stent occurred in only five cases (3.1%) in this multicenter trial. Encrustation within the stent was rarely observed in the series. Only one patient after 1 year (0.8%), three patients at 2 years (3.0%), three patients at 3 years (4.0%), two patients at 4 years (3.4%), and three patients at 5 years (6.0%) demonstrated encrustation. Actual stone formation within the stent did not occur in this series.

7. Urinary Tract Colonization

A history of urinary tract infections (UTI) was reported in 153 patients (96%) at the time of preinsertion evaluation, with a mean number of 4.6 ± 3.0 UTIs per year (minimum = 1, maximum = 17 infections per year). Routine urine cultures obtained at each follow-up period revealed a similar percentage of patients with a positive urine culture before and after stent insertion (Table 2). To correlate positive urine culture with symptomatic UTI, patients were asked if they had symptoms of UTI at the time urine cultures were obtained. The investigation of this parameter was initiated after the study had already begun; therefore, some values were missing from before and shortly after stent insertion.

8. Complications Associated with Stent Insertion

Perioperative or postoperative hemorrhage requiring transfusion, soft-tissue erosion, or stone formation did not occur in any patient as a result of sphincter stent prosthesis placement. Although two patients were noted to have encrustation of the stent at 3 months and one patient at 12 months, none required treatment, and none were obstructed by urodynamic criteria. Subjective erectile function was not adversely altered in any patient.

Twenty-four patients (15%) underwent device explantation during the follow-up period, but 4 of the 24 (16.7%) were reimplanted with another stent prosthesis. Seven explan-

Table 2 Routine Urine Culture Result[a] at Each Follow-Up Period and Correlation with Patient Symptoms

	Urine culture		UTI symptoms		
Time period	Positive urine culture n (%)	Valid value (V) missing value (M)	Symptoms n (%)	Asymptomatic n (%)	Valid value (V) missing value (M)
Preinsertion	79 (52.3)	V = 151, M = 9			
1-mo	72 (61.0)	V = 118, M = 42			
3-mo	67 (51.1)	V = 131, M = 29			
6-mo	69 (53.5)	V = 129, M = 31	2 (7.7)	24 (92.3)	V = 26, M = 134
1-yr	72 (60.5)	V = 119, M = 41	3 (6.3)	45 (93.8)	V = 48, M = 112
2-yr	53 (60.2)	V = 88, M = 72	2 (4.0)	48 (96.0)	V = 50, M = 110
3-yr	42 (58.3)	V = 72, M = 88	4 (10.5)	34 (89.5)	V = 38, M = 122
4-yr	28 (65.1)	V = 43, M = 117	1 (3.7)	26 (96.3)	V = 27, M = 133
5-yr	16 (50.0)	V = 32, M = 128	0 (0.0)	15 (100)	V = 15, M = 145

[a]McNemar exact two-tailed test.

tations were required because of stent migration, 3 of which occurred at the time of the initial insertion procedure. One explantation was performed because of pain and urethral edema. Another stent was removed because of incomplete epithelialization, secondary bladder neck contracture, and worsening hydronephrosis after 1 year. The remaining explantation was undertaken 1 year after insertion because the patient experienced persistent difficulty maintaining condom catheter coverage.

Hematuria occurred in 53 patients (33.0%) during the study. Temporary catheterization was reported necessary for 10 patients with hematuria. Edema of the penis occurred in 1 patient. Another patient noted a superficial penile ulcer from excessive force used in condom catheter application. Three patients developed a urethrocutaneous fistula caused by excessive condom catheter pressure at the base of the penis. The small fistulae healed spontaneously in 2 patients and the third required urethroplastic closure of the fistula.

Two patients experienced epididymo-orchitis, which resolved with oral antibiotics. Three patients with preexisting vesicoureteral reflux demonstrated persistent reflux and clinical pyelonephritis postoperatively. This occurred despite proper prosthesis location and a documented decrease in voiding pressure. Two patients with persistent reflux underwent ureteral reimplantation, and the third patient was managed with indwelling urethral catheterization. Two patients were rehospitalized 1 week after stent insertion for a febrile pseudomonas UTI.

There have been 42 reported cases (26.3%) of bladder neck obstruction after stent placement. The bladder neck obstructions were managed in 20 of 47 cases (42.6%) with bladder neck incision, in 10 cases (21.3%) with drug therapy (α_1-blockade), in 8 cases (17.0%) with intermittent catheterization, and no treatment was reported in 9 cases (19.1%).

9. Stent Removal and Sphincter Function

Four patients (three quadriplegic and one paraplegic) underwent permanent sphincter stent explantation 6 months or longer after insertion without either stent replacement or surgical sphincteric ablation. Three patients required stent removal because of device migration, and one patient required explantation because of difficulty maintaining condom catheter urinary collection.

Each patient was evaluated with cystoscopy and renal ultrasound before sphincter stent insertion, immediately before sphincter stent removal, and 1 year after stent removal. Mean voiding pressure of 62.5 ± 39.4 cmH$_2$O before stent implantation decreased to 20.7 ± 6.5 cmH$_2$O after stent insertion. One year after stent explantation, mean voiding pressure increased to 58.5 ± 21.5 cmH$_2$O.

All stents were completely removed cystoscopically, using a combination technique of neoepithelial resection and forceps extraction, without perioperative complications. Neither stress urinary incontinence nor urethral stricture has developed in any patient, with over 1 year of follow-up since stent removal. Urethral catheterization and cystourethroscopy can be performed in each patient without difficulty. Furthermore, no changes in symptoms of AD, renal function, or erectile function have developed in these patients.

One patient subsequently underwent a cutaneous ileocystostomy 6 months later. Urodynamic and cystourethroscopy demonstrated no permanent injury to the membranous urethra. The urethral mucosa appeared normal without stricture, and voiding pressure was quantified at 65 cmH$_2$O 6 months after explantation versus 75 cmH$_2$O before initial stent insertion. The patient did not leak urine per urethra after his urinary ileostomy procedure.

10. Subjective Outcome

Overall, more than 80% of patients reported that they were somewhat much better after UroLume stent placement, and the investigators reported that they felt the treatment was successful in over 84% of patients in the follow-up period.

V. SPHINCTEROTOMY VERSUS SPHINCTER STENT PROSTHESIS PLACEMENT

Multicenter trials have demonstrated the efficacy of stenting the dyssynergic external sphincter in cases of DESD, yet the question remains whether the stent procedure should eclipse sphincterotomy as the treatment of choice for those afflicted with this lower urinary tract dysfunction. A randomized, prospective multicenter trial was undertaken to determine whether the efficacy and safety of potentially reversible sphincter stent prosthesis placement actually superceded that of irreversible conventional sphincter ablation procedures.

A. Sphincterotomy Versus Sphincter Stent Trial: Methods

A total of 57 SCI patients with urodynamically verified sphincter dysfunction were entered into this study comparing sphincter stent placement and external sphincterotomy at three Model SCI Centers, with follow-up scheduled at 3, 6, 12, and 24 months postoperatively (26). Each initial patient evaluation included a medical history, physical examination, urinanalysis and culture, serum chemistry analysis, complete blood count, urodynamic study, and upper urinary tract imaging with renal ultrasonography, intravenous urography, or a radioisotope renal scan. The presence or absence of subjective autonomic dysreflexia was recorded before the operative intervention and at each postoperative period.

Each patient was evaluated urodynamically with fluoroscopy, and maximum detrusor pressure, maximal cystometric capacity, residual urine volume, and sphincter EMG were recorded according to the standards of the International Continence Society. Patients who demonstrated electromyographic and manometric evidence of DESD during involuntary detrusor contractions were considered candidates for this study. Concomitant documented bladder neck obstruction or prostatic obstruction served as exclusion criteria. Patients were then randomized to receive either conventional sphincterotomy or sphincter stent prosthesis placement as treatment for dyssynergic sphincter function.

An initial postoperative evaluation was performed 1 month after the sphincter-defeating procedure. This included physical examination, urinanalysis and culture, and a repeat pelvic radiograph in stent patients only. Follow-up cystoscopy, pelvic radiography (stent only), urine culture, and urodynamics were performed at 3, 6, 12, and 24 months. Renal ultrasonography, intravenous urography, or nuclear medicine renal scanning provided upper tract imaging at 6, 12, and 24 months postoperatively. The primary outcome parameter was urodynamic maximum detrusor pressure. Secondary urodynamic parameters of bladder capacity and residual urine volume were compared between sphincterotomy and stent patients pre- and postoperatively at 3, 6, 12, and 24 months. In addition, patients completed questionnaires concerning voiding sensation and quality of life issues at each follow-up visit.

B.   Sphincterotomy Versus Sphincter Stent Trial: Therapeutic Results

1.   Patient Demographics

The mean age of the sphincterotomy group ($N = 26$) was 34.5 ± 9.9 years and that of the sphincter stent group ($N = 31$) was 39.1 ± 11.8 years (p = 0.124). The mean duration of SCI was 8.7 ± 6.6 years for sphincterotomy and 8.0 ± 5.3 years for stent patients (p = 0.641). Cervical level SCI accounted for 70% of injuries whereas the remaining 30% suffered from thoracic level injuries. Prior urological intervention included 1 patient in each group previously undergoing transurethral prostatectomy. Three sphincterotomy patients and 1 stent patient had previously undergone bladder neck incision. Five sphincterotomy patients and 1 stent patient had undergone prior external sphincterotmy (p = 0.083).

2.   Stents Required

Of 31 sphincter stent patients, 31 (77.4%) required one insertion procedure. Six (19.4%) and 1 (3.2%) required two and three insertion procedures, respectively. The total number of stents implanted per patient was one stent in 21 of 31 patients (67.7%) to bridge the external sphincter, whereas two stents were required in 9 patients (29.0%), and 1 patient (3.2%) needed three stents.

3.   Urodynamic Results

The preoperative urodynamic parameters were similar between the sphincterotomy and stent prosthesis groups (Table 3). Each urodynamic parameter was compared between matched data from preprocedure to each of the follow-up periods at 3, 6, 12, and 24 months.

Table 3   Sphincterotomy Versus Sphincter Stent Trial: Preoperative Urodynamic Parameters

Urodynamic parameter	Sphincterotomy ($n = 26$)	Sphincter stent ($n = 31$)	
Maximum detrusor pressure (cmH_2O)	98.3 ± 27.6	95.7 ± 27.7	p = 0.73
Residual urine volume (mL)	212 ± 163	168 ± 114	p = 0.33
Cystometric capacity (mL)	245 ± 158	251 ± 145	p = 0.87

The urodynamic parameters at each time period were also compared between the sphincterotomy and stent placement patient groups, at the 3-, 6-, 12-, and 24-months evaluation. The urodynamic parameters at each time period were also compared between the sphincterotomy and stent placement patient groups. At the 3-, 6-, 12-, and 24-month evaluations, a significant decrease in maximum detrusor pressure occurred in both the sphincterotomy and stent placement patient groups (Table 4). No significant change in bladder capacity was noted in either sphincterotomy or stent placement patients throughout follow-up. Residual urine volume decreased significantly in both sphincterotomy and stent placement patients at some, but not all, of the follow-up evaluations. Changes in urodynamic parameters were equivalent in patients treated with either sphincterotomy or stent placement.

4. Hydronephrosis

Hydronephrosis was evaluated radiographically before and after stent insertion. Each renal unit (right and left) was monitored individually for it. Therefore, a total of 114 renal units were evaluated among the 57 patients. Preoperatively, 5 of 52 renal units (9.6%) demonstrated hydronephrosis in the sphincterotomy group, and 9 of 69 evaluated renal units (15.3%) in stent placement patients were hydronephrotic. At the 12-month follow-up, 4 sphincterotomy and no stent renal units demonstrated hydronephrosis, whereas at 24 months, 3 sphincterotomy renal units and 1 stent renal unit were hydronephrotic.

5. Vesicoureteral Reflux

Vesicoureteral reflux was evaluated before and after stent insertion. Each ureter (right and left) was counted individually for reflux. Preoperatively, 6 of 52 ureters (11.5%) demonstrated reflux in the sphincterotomy group, and 5 of 59 evaluated ureters (8.5%) in stent placement patients demonstrated reflux. After 12 months, vesicoureteral reflux resolved in all ureters of patients treated with sphincterotomy, and reflux resolved in 4 of 5 ureters in stent placement patients. At 24 months, reflux resolution was universal.

6. Autonomic Dysreflexia

A history of AD symptoms was reported in 16 (61.5%) of sphincterotomy (11 mild, 4 moderate, and 1 severe) and 18 (58.1%) stent (7 mild, 8 moderate, and 3 severe) patients before treatment. Of the 16 sphincterotomy patients who had baseline AD 9 (56.3%) improved after treatment. Of the 16 sphincterotomy patients who had baseline AD, 6 did not report any AD at their last follow-up visit. Of the 18 stent patients who had baseline AD, 13 (72.2%) improved after treatment, of the 18 sphincterotomy patients who had baseline AD did not report any AD at their last follow-up visit. The foregoing results are evidence that the incidence of AD is reduced in more than half of the patients with DESD treated with sphincterotomy or a sphincter stent.

7. Stents Required

Thirteen of 26 (50%) sphincterotomy and 22 of 31 (71%) stent patients required indwelling catheterization management before the study. At 3 months postoperatively, 3 sphincterotomy and 1 stent patient could not void without catheterization, whereas at 6 months, 4 sphincterotomy and no stent patients required catheterization. After 12 months, 2 sphincterotomy patients and 1 stent patient required catheters. At 24 months, only 1 sphincterotomy and 2 stent patients need catheters.

Table 4 Sphincterotomy Versus Sphincter Stent Trial: Comparative Urodynamic Parameters Outcome

Time period	Maximum detrusor pressure (cmH$_2$O)		Residual urine volume (mL)		Cystometric cap
3-mo					
Sphincterotomy	Pre 100.2 ± 28.6	p = 0.000[a]	Pre 188 ± 172	p = 0.428	Pre 258 ± 159
n = 19	3-mo 57.4 ± 23.0		3-mo 156 ± 197		3-mo 237 ± 172
Sphincter stent	Pre 93.7 ± 27.2	p = 0.000[a]	Pre 180 ± 118	p = 0.001[a]	Pre 265 ± 156
n = 24	3-mo 53.7 ± 25.0		3-mo 85 ± 71		3-mo 244 ± 160
	sphincterotomy vs. stent p = 0.572		sphincterotomy vs. stent p = 0.299		sphincterotomy vs. s
6-mo					
Sphincterotomy	Pre 98.9 ± 27.1	p = 0.000[a]	Pre 221 ± 187	p = 0.346	Pre 259 ± 171
n = 17	6-mo 58.9 ± 29.8		6-mo 172 ± 185		6-mo 280 ± 168
Sphincter stent	Pre 99.2 ± 30.9	p = 0.000[a]	Pre 178 ± 115	p = 0.07	Pre 262 ± 164
n = 20	6-mo 55.5 ± 26.5		6-mo 115 ± 139		6-mo 298 ± 133
	sphincterotomy vs. stent p = 0.516		sphincterotomy vs. stent p = 0.781		sphincterotomy vs. s
12-mo					
Sphincterotomy	Pre 97.2 ± 26.9	p = 0.000[a]	Pre 200 ± 139	p = 0.029[a]	Pre 228 ± 165
n = 17	12-mo 48.9 ± 16.4		12-mo 98 ± 70		12-mo 225 ± 98
Sphincter stent	Pre 95.2 ± 31.6	p = 0.000[a]	Pre 191 ± 127	p = 0.832	Pre 254 ± 135
n = 20	12-mo 52.6 ± 31.6		12-mo 184 ± 218		12-mo 270 ± 149
	sphincterotomy vs. stent p = 0.287		sphincterotomy vs. stent p = 0.421		sphincterotomy vs. s
24-mo					
Sphincterotomy	Pre 90.6 ± 25.1	p = 0.000[a]	Pre 218 ± 150	p = 0.008[a]	Pre 242 ± 186
n = 14	24-mo 41.6 ± 16.3		24-mo 112 ± 106		24-mo 220 ± 135
Sphincter stent	Pre 101.9 ± 30.0	p = 0.010[a]	Pre 164 ± 132	p = 0.181	Pre 258 ± 138
n = 20	24-mo 71.6 ± 43.8		24-mo 132 ± 159		24-mo 262 ± 134
	sphincterotomy vs stent p = 0.131		sphincterotomy vs. stent p = 0.725		sphincterotomy vs. s

t-test for equality of means two-tail.
[a]Statistical significance.

8. Epithelialization, Hyperplasia, and Encrustation

After 6 months of follow-up, cystoscopic examination revealed that 82.6% of the stents were covered 90% or more by epithelium. By 24 months, 95.0% of the stents were 100% covered, and the remaining 5.0% had 90–99% coverage. The tissue response within the stent lumen was assessed in all stented patients. At 12 months, 36.4% of patients had no response, and 63.6% had a mild to moderate response. At 24 months, 50% had no response, and 50% had a mild to moderate tissue response. No functional obstruction occurred as a result of the tissue response. Neither encrustation of the stent nor stone formation within the stent was observed in any patient.

9. Urinary Tract Colonization

A history of UTI was reported in nearly half of the patients during the initial evaluation in both groups. Routine urine cultures were obtained at each follow-up period. A similar percentage of patients from each treatment group developed positive urine cultures before and after stent insertion or sphincterotomy. To differentiate positive urine cultures from symptomatic UTI, patients were asked if they felt that they had symptoms of UTI at the time urine cultures were obtained. Most cases of bacteriuria were asymptomatic in both sphincterotomy and stent patients.

10. Complications

Six of 31 stent patients (19%) required stent explantation. Stent migration occurred in 3 of 6 patients detected at the 3-month follow-up in each group. All were removed without difficulty or long-term complications. One case of stent explantation was due to stent misplacement at the time of insertion. One patient requested stent removal because he did not like using the condom catheter to collect his urine. The remaining patient developed pain and symptoms of dysreflexia during reflex voiding.

Bladder neck obstruction requiring treatment developed in 12 patients (6 in each group). Nine of the bladder neck obstructions were treated with an oral α-adrenergic antagonist, 2 were treated with transurethral incision of the bladder neck, and 1 was treated with bladder neck dilation. Urethral stricture requiring urethrotomy developed in 5 patients (4 stent, 1 sphincterotomy) during the 2-year follow-up. The strictures were treated with transurethral visual internal urethrotomy. Restenosis of the sphincter was documented in 2 sphincterotomy patients (8%) and they were treated with another sphincterotomy at 6 months postoperatively.

The length of hospitalization was analyzed and categorized to 1 day versus 2 or more days for each treatment group. Of the sphincter stent group, a significantly greater percentage of patients (36.7%) were discharged after 1 day versus the sphincterotomy group (11.5%; p = 0.036). The sphincter stent and sphincterotomy patients experienced similar perioperative bleeding, quantified by comparison of preoperative hemoglobin value with that of the first postoperative day hemoglobin (p = 0.189).

11. Quality of Life Issues

The patients were surveyed concerning their ability to empty their bladder and questions about their quality of life relative to urological condition. Between 80 and 90% of the patients who received either sphincterotomy or sphincter stent placement reported that they were somewhat better to much better in terms of bladder-emptying ability postoperatively.

Preoperatively, 77% of sphincterotomy and 81% of sphincter stent patients stated that they worried somewhat to a lot about their DESD. Two years after surgery, only 35% of sphincterotomy and 35% of sphincter stent patients worried about their health because of DESD. Preoperatively, 62% of sphincterotomy and 77% of sphincter stent patients had somewhat to a lot of bothersome trouble with urination. Postoperatively, only 14% of sphincterotomy and 14% of sphincter stent patients complained of somewhat to a lot of bothersome trouble with urination.

Preoperatively, 58% of sphincterotomy and 61% of sphincter stent patients reported that they were kept from doing usual things because of their sphincter dyssynergia somewhat to a lot of the time. Postoperatively, only 14% of sphincterotomy and 38% of sphincter stent patients complained that they were kept from doing usual things somewhat to a lot of the time.

Preoperatively, 50% of sphincterotomy and 58% of sphincter stent patients reported that their urological condition interfered with their social life somewhat to a lot of the time. Postoperatively, only 14% of sphincterotomy and 21% of sphincter stent patients complained of their condition interfering with their social life somewhat to a lot of the time. No alterations in erectile function or the ability to ejaculate were appreciated in men undergoing either sphincterotomy or sphincter stent placement at any timepoint.

12. Defeating Sphincter Function with Sphincter Stenting Versus Sphincter Incision

The endoluminal wire mesh stent was first employed in the urinary tract as treatment for bulbous urethral strictures in 1988 (27). Additional reports used the stent prosthesis for treatment of benign prostatic hyperplasia and neurogenic vesical dysfunction have been encouraging (22,28–30).

In the report from the North America Multicenter Trial of the UroLume stent for the treatment of DESD, of 160 SCI patients treated at 15 centers, the stent achieved clinical success in approximately 85% of patients after 5 years of follow-up (25). In the latest report on the efficacy and safety of the sphincter stent versus conventional sphinteric incision, the sphincter stent has demonstrated its usefulness as reversible treatment for those afflicted with DESD (26).

Patients with SCI prefer the use of the sphincter stent prosthesis to conventional sphincterotomy because of the sphincter stent's potential reversibility. Milroy and Chapple (30) reported the uncomplicated removal of three stents that were completely epithelialized 1 year after insertion, and Chancellor et al. (12) reported removal of five stents, which had been in situ for over 1 year, from SCI patients. Indeed, long-term follow-up after stent removal has revealed that the urinary sphincter returned to its baseline obstructive condition without the development of associated urethral strictures. In those patients who required stent removal in this series, the procedure was performed without difficulty, despite epithelialization. No patient has suffered adverse sequelae secondary to stent removal.

Most patients with SCI who where studied were able to dispose of indwelling catheter management after either sphincterotomy or sphincter stent insertion. Both sphincterotomy and sphincter stent prosthesis placement significantly decreased maximum detrusor pressure without an adverse effect on cystometric bladder capacity. This decrease in maximum detrusor pressure has been sustained in the patients who have completed 2 years of follow-up. No differences between the two treatment groups were recognized in terms of maximum detrusor pressure at each evaluation period.

Residual urine decreased in some, but not all, patients. This may be accounted for by the difficulty in determining the occurrence of spontaneous voiding in patients with SCI, as they do not sense micturition. Furthermore, bladder contraction duration is variable in SCI patients, yielding different measurements for residual urine volume in the same patient under different conditions. Hydronephrosis improved and vesicoureteral reflux resolved in most patients after either sphincterotomy or sphincter stent insertion.

The presence of intermittently positive urine cultures continued throughout the follow-up periods in this patient population. This was not unexpected because the majority of patients collect their urine using condom catheters, which have been associated with a higher rate of positive urine cultures. This does not bear clinical relevance (31). Over 89% of the patients were aymptomatic for infection at the time of positive urine cultures and required no treatment. It is noteworthy that there have been no reports of abscess development or infected tissue at the site of the prosthesis in the external sphincter associated with positive urine cultures. The epithelialization process appears to provide adequate tissue coverage along the length of the prosthesis and serves as a barrier against its infection.

The complications identified during the comparison study of sphincter stent versus sphincterotomy included device removals, additional insertions procedures, bladder neck obstruction, and the use of catheters to empty the bladder. Device removals were primarily attributed to stent migration that may result from inadvertent stent manipulation during digital bowel evacuation, aftercare management of the patients, or as a result of poor stent seating because of scarring and fixation of the proximal urethra caused by previous transurethral sphincterotomy. Prosthesis migration was easily diagnosed in all cases. Explantation did not induce any adverse sequelae.

Twenty-one percent of patients were treated for bladder neck obstruction after sphincterotomy or sphincter stent placement. This internal sphincter dysfunction has been previously reported to occur in association with external sphincter dyssynergia, and it is often masked by the more dramatic dyssynergia of the external sphincter during initial evaluation (31,32). The relatively low incidence of bladder neck dyssynergia in this series serves to emphasize that, usually, ablation of only external sphincter function is sufficient to normalize maximum detrusor pressure to a nonpathogenic level in patients with SCI and DESD.

The majority of sphincter stent patients required a single-stent insertion at a single-operative setting without complications and a brief hospital stay. Although the prosthesis is manufactured in 2- to 2.5- and 3-cm lengths, the 3-cm–length device is recommended for the treatment of DESD. Neither epithelial hyperplasia causing obstruction, encrustation, nor stone formation occurred in either the mulitcenter trial or the comparative trial of the sphincter stent prosthesis.

Recently, use of the contact YAG laser has been reported for the treatment of DESD. The results are promising and similar to that of conventional sphincterotomy (10,14). However, prospective randomized multicenter assessment of laser sphincterotomy has not been performed.

The prospective multicenter randomized study at three model SCI centers evaluated a new reversible sphincter stent prosthesis as an alternative treatment to conventional irreversible surgical ablation of external urinary sphincter function. It demonstrated that the sphincter stent prosthesis is as safe and effective as external sphincterotomy, which is the current standard of care. The simplicity of placement and minimal associated morbidity establishes the sphincter prosthesis as an attractive alternative to external sphincterotomy for the treatment of DESD.

13. The Sphincter Stent: Maximizing Efficacy

Proper patient selection is most important in achieving a high clinical success rate with sphincter stent implantation. Preoperative urodynamic testing is an absolute necessity. Only patients with DH and DESD should be considered candidates for sphincter stent prosthesis placement. This procedure is contraindicated in patients with detrusor areflexia, significantly diminished compliance, or elevated residual urine volume.

The sphincter stent, even if perfectly placed, will serve as an effective management strategy only if the patient can reliably wear a condom catheter. Patients must be fully counseled and able to demonstrate the effective application and maintenance of an external catheter before considering a sphincter-defeating procedure.

14. The Sphincter Stent: Infertility Concerns

Most men with SCI experience neurogenic ejaculatory failure. The technique of electro-ejaculation is most commonly used to produce a semen specimen, which is then processed to maximize the potential for conception and used for artificial insemination. It is theoretically possible to obstruct the ejaculatory ducts by the proximal edge of the stent. Therefore, great care in proper candidate selection and surgical technique is essential in cases for whom fertility is an important issue. In general, the sphincter stent is not recommended to men who are considering electroejaculation, or in younger men who have not thoroughly considered their fertility potential. However, the recent increasing popularity and success of newer sperm aspiration and intracytoplasmic sperm injection techniques may alleviate some concern over the effect of the sphincter stent on semen parameters.

VI. CONCLUSIONS

The long-term urological needs and costs of SCI care are high. Many patients with SCI are eternally hopeful that a cure for this disorder will be developed, enabling complete restoration of neurological function, including ambulation. With this belief, some patients refuse or defer irreversible treatments, even if the treatment is medically necessary. Patients prefer sphincter stent prosthesis placement to external sphincterotomy in clinical trials because the stent is potentially reversible. Although the sphincter prosthesis is designed as a permanent implant for the treatment of DESD, investigations have demonstrated that it may be removed without sequelae, if deemed necessary.

Sphincter stent prosthesis placement effectively decreases detrusor pressure in patients afflicted with DESD. Given the experience with UroLume stent placement at various levels of the urethra for various reasons, including the bladder neck, prostate, and bulbous urethra, patients undergoing sphincter stent placement have the least complaints postoperatively. These patients are neurologically impaired and most have ejaculatory dysfunction; therefore, few report pain, urinary dribbling, irritation, or hematospermia. Also, the risk of encrustation, stone formation, and incomplete epithelization is minimal in patients with sphincter stent placement when compared with patients with bladder neck or prostate stent placement.

The complications discussed in this chapter are largely associated with the "learning curve" of using a new device. With greater experience, most could be avoided. The device can be completely removed, even after an extended time period and complete epithelization, without causing damage to external sphincter function.

The UroLume stent prosthesis is an effective device for the treatment of DESD. When compared with conventional sphincterotomy, the reversibility of the device dramatically enhances patient acceptability. The decreased cost and complication rate certainly should enhance its utilization by urologists caring for those afflicted with detrusor hyperreflexia associated with detrusor–sphincter dyssynergia.

REFERENCES

1. De Vito MJ, Rutt RD, Black KJ, Go BK, Stover SL. Trends in spinal cord injury demographics and treatment outcome between 1973 and 1986. Arch Phys Med Rehabil 1992; 73:424–430.
2. Stover SL, Fine RR. The epidemiology and economics of spinal cord injury. Paraplegia 1987; 25:225–230.
3. Kaplan SA, Chancellor MB, Blaivas JG. Bladder and sphicter behavior in patients with spinal cord lesions. J Urol 1991; 146:113–117.
4. McGuire EJ, Brady S. Detrusor–sphincter dyssynergia. J Urol 1979; 121:774–777.
5. Yalla SV, Blunt KJ, Fam BA, Constantinople NI, Gittes RF. Detrusor–urethral sphincter dyssynergia. J Urol 1977; 118:1026–1029.
6. Blaivas JG. The neurophysiology of micturition: a clinical study of 550 patients. J Urol 1982; 127:958–963.
7. Bunts RC. Management of urological complications in 1000 paraplegics. J Urol 1958; 79:733–741.
8. Yalla SV, Rossier AB, Fam BA. Dyssynergic vesicourethral responses during bladder rehabilitation in spinal cord injury patients: effects of suprapubic percussion, Crede method, and bethanechol chloride. J Urol 1976; 115:575–579.
9. Perkash I. Modified approach to sphincterotomy in spinal cord injury patients: indications, technique, and results in 32 patients. Paraplegia 1976; 13:247–252.
10. Rivas DA, Chancellor MB, Staas WE, Gomella LG. Contact neodymium:yttrium aluminum–garnet laser ablation of the external sphincter in spinal cord-injured men with detrusor sphincter dyssynergia. Urology 1995; 45:1028–1031.
11. Chancellor MB, Rivas DA, Abdill CK, Karasick S, Ehrlich SM, Staas WE. Prospective comparison of external sphincter balloon dilatation and prosthesis placement with external sphincter in spinal cord injured men. Arch Phys Med Rehabil 1994; 75:297–305.
12. Chancellor MB, Rivas DA, Watanabe T, Bennett JK, Foote JE, Green BG, Killorin EW, Millan R. Reversible clinical outcome after sphincter stent removal. J Urol 1996; 155:1992–1994.
13. Rivas DA, Chancellor MB, Bagley D. Prospective comparison of external sphincter prosthesis placement and external sphincterotomy in men with spinal cord injury. J Endourol 1994; 8:89–93.
14. Perkash I. Laser sphincterotomy and ablation of the prostate using a sapphire chisel contact tip firming neodymium:YAG laser. J Urol 1994; 152:2020–2024.
15. Perkash I, Barret C, Gomella LG, Liberman SN, Chancellor MB. Use of the contact Nd:YAG laser for ablation of the external urethral sphincter. J Urol 1993; 149:358A.
16. Lockhart JL, Vorstman B, Weinstein D, Politano VA. Sphincterotomy failure in neurogenic bladder disease. J Urol 1986; 135:86–89.
17. Kiviat MD. Transurethral sphincterotomy: relationship of site of incision to postoperative potency and delayed hemorrhage. J Urol 1975; 114:399–401.
18. Crane DB, Hackler RH. External sphincterotomy: its effect on erections. J Urol 1976; 116:316–318.
19. Dollfus P, Jurascheck F, Adli G, Chapuis A. Impairment of erection after external sphincter resection. Paraplegia 1976; 13:290–295.
20. Whitmore WF, Fam BA, Yalla SV. Experience with anteromedian (12 o'clock) external urethral sphincterotomy in 100 male subjects with neuropathic bladders. J Urol 1978; 117:489–493.
21. Hacken HJ, Ott R. Late results of bilateral endoscopic sphincterotomy in patients with upper motor neurone lesions. Paraplegia 1976; 13:268–272.
22. Schellhammer PF, Hackler RH, Bunts RC. External sphincterotomy: an evaluation of 150 patients with neurogenic bladder. J Urol 1973; 110:199–202.
23. Sauerwein D, Gross AJ, Kutzenberger J, Ringert RH. Wallstents in patients with detrusor-sphincter dyssynergia. J Urol 1995; 154:495–497.
24. Chancellor MB, Karasick S, Erhard MJ, Abdill CK, Liu J–L, Goldberg BB, Staas WE. Place-

ment of a wire mesh prosthesis in the external sphincter of men with spinal cord injuries. Radiology 1993; 187:551–558.

25. Chancellor MB, Gajewski J, Ackman D, Appell RA, Bennett J, Binard J, Boon TB, Chetner MP, Crewalk JA, Defalco A, Foote J, Green B, Juma S, Jung SY, Linsenmeyer T, McMillan R, Mayo M, Oxawa H, Roehrborn CG, Shenot PJ, Stone A, Vasquez A, Killorin W, Rivas DA. Long-term (5 years) follow-up of the North American Multicenter UroLume trial for the treatment of detrusor–external sphincter dyssynergia. J Urol 1999; 161:1545–1550.

26. Chancellor MB, Bennett C, Simoneau AR, Finocchiaro MV, Kline C, Bennett J, Foote J, Green B, Martin SH, Hudson S, Killorin W, Crewalk JA, Rivas DA. Sphincter stent versus external sphincterotomy in spinal cord injured men: prospective randomized multicenter trial. J Urol 1999; 161:1893–1898.

27. Milroy EJG, Chapple CR, Cooper JE, Eldin H, Wallsten H, Seddon AM, Rowles PM. A new treatment for urethral strictures. Lancet 1988; 1:1424.

28. Shaw PJR, Milroy EJG, Timoney AG, Eldin A, Mitchell N. Permanent external striated sphincter stents in patients with spinal injuries. Br J Urol 1990; 66:297–301.

29. McInerney PD, Vanner TF, Harris SAB, Stephenson TP. Permanent urethral stents for detrusor sphincter dyssynergia. Br J Urol 1991; 67:291–293.

30. Milroy EJG, Chapple CR. Permanent UroLume prostate stent: 3-year experience—indications and problems. J Urol 1992; 147:307A.

31. Gilmore DS, Schick DS, Young MN, Montgomerie JZ. Effect of external urinary collection system on colonization any urinary tract infections with *Pseudomonas and Klebsiella* in men with spinal cord injury. J Am Paraplegia Soc 1992; 15:155–158.

32. Chancellor MB, Rivas DA, Ackman D, Appell RA, Binard J, Boon TB, Roehrborn CG, Chetner MP, Thorndyke WC, Defalco A, Mayo M, Gajewski J, Green B, Bennett J, Foote J, Juma S, Linsenmeyer T, McMillan R, Stone A, Vasquez A. Multicenter trials of UroLume endourethral Wallstent prosthesis for urinary sphincterotomy in spinal cord injured men. J Urol 1994; 152:924–930.

39

Surgery for the Incompetent Urethral Sphincter: Bladder Neck Suspension Procedures

DANIEL S. BLANDER

Southern California Permanente Medical Group, Irvine, California

PHILIPPE E. ZIMMERN

The University of Texas Southwestern Medical Center at Dallas, Dallas, Texas

I. INTRODUCTION

For over 50 years, bladder neck suspension procedures have been performed by urologists and gynecologists for the treatment of urinary incontinence secondary to bladder neck and proximal urethral hypermobility (genuine stress incontinence; GSI). Although the first true retropubic suspension is credited to Marshall and co-workers (1), over the past 50 years, multiple techniques for achieving this same goal have been described. Pereyra (2), Burch (3), Stamey (4), and Raz (5) have been credited with major modifications in the technique of bladder neck suspension (BNS), among others, The purpose of the current chapter is to give an overview of the goal of these procedures, their respective advantages, their long-term results, their potential complications, and their current place in the treatment of stress urinary incontinence (SUI).

A. Indications

Bladder neck suspension procedures are indicated for stress incontinence in several situations. In the simplest case, a patient must have bothersome stress incontinence in conjunction with bladder-neck and proximal urethral hypermobility. The pathophysiology of this condition is discussed elsewhere in this text. The patient's stress incontinence must be demonstrable during physical examination or urodynamic testing. In general, candidates for BNS should have tried nonsurgical therapies, such as medications, Kegel exercises, or biofeedback, with limited success and be desirous of surgical treatment.

In more complex cases involving prolapse, mixed incontinence, or outlet obstruction, the surgical indications for BNS remain controversial. When GSI is associated with a cystocele or vaginal vault prolapse, some authors base their decision to proceed with BNS on the results of urodynamic studies (UDS), performed with or without a vaginal pack or pessary. Others recommend preventatively performing a "light" BNS to support and stabilize the urethra (6). After prior anti-incontinence surgery, GSI may coexist with intrinsic sphincteric deficiency (ISD), and a pubovaginal sling may have to be considered instead of a simple BNS or an anterior vaginal wall sling. If a pubovaginal sling is to be performed, consideration must be given to parameters such as postvoid residual and detrusor contractility, owing to the obstructive nature of this procedure and the risk of long-term urinary retention or de novo detrusor instability. Finally, an individual who has had previous anti-incontinence surgery may have obstructive symptoms (straining or urinary retention) or detrusor instability in conjunction with GSI. Such a patient also requires UDS before repair because urethrolysis may also be indicated at the time of the BNS.

For the purpose of this review, we have divided BNS procedures into four categories: vaginal, retropubic, laparoscopic, and new procedures. The choice of suspension procedure depends on many factors, including previous anti-incontinence surgery, need for concomitant procedures, patient body habitus, and patient preferences (Table 1). Patients who require a lower abdominal incision for ovarian, uterine, or cervical pathology may best be served by the retropubic approach. Individuals with a small vagina or inability to tolerate the lithotomy position because of joint disease may not be candidates for a transvaginal procedure. For the patient who requires a concomitant pelvic prolapse repair from the vaginal approach, a vaginal bladder neck suspension technique might be the procedure of choice. Although individual surgeons may be dogmatic in their beliefs about the superiority of one procedure over another, there is good data to support that there is no single procedure with dramatically greater success or lower complication rate than any other (7).

B. Outcomes

The literature on outcomes of incontinence surgery has recently been addressed by the AUA's Female Stress Urinary Incontinence Clinical Guidelines Panel (7). This group performed a metanalysis of all recent articles (through 1993) that addressed the surgical treatment of female stress urinary incontinence. The panel generated some data that specifically addressed the efficacy of the various procedures for stress incontinence In doing this study, the authors found that only 282 of the 5322 articles in the literature met their criteria for analysis. Although a significant proportion of these articles were rejected for technical reasons (not written in English, using a non–FDA-approved therapy), tremendous inconsistencies in the reporting of outcomes in the stress incontinence literature were observed. One of

Table 1 Conceptual Differences Between Anti-incontinence Procedures

Dissection of retropubic space
Vaginal wall vs. fascia for support
Formation of retropubic scar tissue
Position of suspension sutures in relation to urethra
Adjustment in suture tension

the most significant problems in this arena is that there is no gold standard for assessing surgical outcomes (8).

Therefore, when reviewing the results of stress incontinence surgery, one must keep in mind several factors. Certainly not all surgeons perform a given procedure the way it was described by its original author. Also, diagnostic tests, such as urethral pressure profiles and leak-point pressures, have not been standardized. In addition, the results of an operation for stress incontinence are not necessarily generalizable to individuals with stress incontinence and prolapse. Finally, there is significant variability in the reported follow-up methods. Without standardized outcome instruments and staging, creating a set of guidelines for therapy is a formidable and error-prone task (9).

Several questionnaires for assessing outcomes of stress incontinence surgery have recently been proposed (10,11), but none has yet been widely accepted. According to recent standards proposed by the Urodynamic Society, such a questionnaire should be part of the routine follow-up of patients who have undergone antistress incontinence procedures (12). The necessary elements of adequate pre- and postoperative assessment of patients treated for stress incontinence are summarized in Table 2. Such an assessment needs to evaluate

Table 2 Patient Assessments Before and After Anti-incontinence Surgery

Preoperative patient assessment
   Incontinence severity index
   Cost/year (pads and medications)
   Quality of life and bothersomeness indices
   Patient expectations of surgery
Timing of postoperative assessments
   6 mo
   1 yr
   Longer
Is the patient dry?
   Third-party investigation
   Questionnaires
   Physical examination
   Pad test
   VLPP at full bladder capacity
Is the patient obstructed?
   Obstructive symptoms
   Uroflow
   Postvoid residual
Is the anatomical defect corrected?
   Physical examination
   Q-tip test
   Ultrasound
   VCUG (with lateral views comparing rest and straining)
Have secondary problems been induced?
   Sexual function
   Secondary prolapse
   Repeat operations (persistent incontinence)
   Additional treatment (dilation, repeat BNS, urethrolysis)

symptom severity, influence on the quality of life, and treatment outcome. It is also essential postoperatively to determine whether or not the anatomical defect that the surgery intended to rectify (hypermobility from inadequate urethral support) has been corrected, regardless of any persistent symptomatology.

In general, at least two separate values should be reported in studies of surgery for stress incontinence: one for success, reflecting cure or improvement of stress incontinence; and one for overall patient satisfaction. The latter value usually takes into account such factors as long-term urinary retention, pain, or bothersome urge incontinence, either induced or unmasked by the operation. Cure–dry rates, as reported in the literature, generally do not reflect the presence of urge incontinence, thereby masking that a patient may be cured from SUI, but wet from secondary urge incontinence.

As in the reporting of success rates, there is tremendous variability in the reporting of complications with bladder neck suspension procedures. As good follow-up data for these procedures becomes available, one must keep in mind that although stress incontinence can dramatically alter an individual's quality of life, it is an inherently benign condition; therefore, a high rate of significant complications is unacceptable for any corrective procedure (13).

II. RETROPUBIC SUSPENSIONS

A. MMK Procedure

1. Goal

Although a retropubic sling had been described by Goebel in 1910 (14), the first true retropubic urethropexy was described by Marshall, Marchetti, and Krantz (MMK); (1) in a man who was incontinent after abdominoperineal resection. The goal of the MMK is to fix the proximal urethra and bladder neck in a high retropubic position to prevent descent during stress maneuvers. Despite encouraging initial results, the authors later changed their procedure by placing the supportive sutures away from the urethral wall to avoid secondary obstruction from urethral kinking or distortion (15).

2. Technique

The patient is placed in supine position, with the legs abducted slightly to allow access to the vagina. A Foley catheter is placed in a sterile fashion such that it may be manipulated during the procedure. The space of Retzius is exposed through a transverse or midline incision, and the bladder is dissected away from the pubic bone until the urethrovesical junction is exposed. Dissection anterior to the urethra is unnecessary because the suspension sutures are placed in the periurethral vaginal tissues (16). The bladder neck can easily be identified by palpating the balloon of the Foley catheter. This dissection can be especially tedious in a patient who has previously been operated on. In fact, some authors have recommended opening the bladder at the start of the procedure to facilitate dissection of the plane between the bladder and the pubic symphysis (17).

Once the dissection is completed, absorbable suspension sutures are placed in the periurethral vaginal tissues on each side of the urethra, but carefully excluding the urethral wall. Following placement of all of the sutures in the vaginal wall, each one is passed through its corresponding location in the cartilaginous portion of the pubic symphysis (Fig. 1). In some cases, the most proximal stitch must be passed through the aponeurosis of the rectus muscle, rather than through the symphysis itself. The sutures are tied from distal to

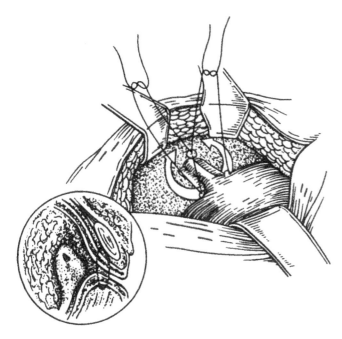

Figure 1 Suture placement for the MMK procedure (inset). The proximal urethra and ure-throvesical junction are elevated under the symphysis pubis. (From Ref. 86.)

proximal, leaving the Foley catheter in place. During the tying of the sutures, the assistant's finger is placed in the vagina, elevating the urethra and taking tension off the stitches. The sutures should be tied in a such manner that they reposition and stabilize the bladder neck and urethra, without being so tight that they obstruct or strangulate the urethra (18). The wound is then closed in a routine fashion, with or without placement of a drain in the space of Retzius.

3. Results

Metanalysis of the MMK operation has revealed an 88% cure rate for SUI in over 2400 pa-tients (19). There is tremendous variation among the outcomes reported by different sur-geons at different institutions. Spencer et al. (20) found a 57% cure rate at 68 months in a group of 54 patients who underwent the MMK operation. In the same cohort, using a ques-tionnaire-based study with a mean follow-up of almost 17 years, Clemens and co-workers (21) found only a 33% cure rate in 36 patients. The Clemens' study represents the longest published follow-up of the MMK procedure.

B. Burch Procedure

1. Goal

The goal of the Burch operation, as described initially, is to suspend the paravaginal fascia to the iliopectineal ligament (Cooper's ligament). This procedure was developed as a mod-ification of the MMK procedure when Burch found that he was unable to secure sutures re-liably in the pubic symphysis. Cooper's ligament is adjacent to the pubic bone and was used instead, Although the initial drawings of this procedure suggested a complete elevation of the anterior vagina to Cooper's ligament, it has now been accepted that adequate support and stabilization of the bladder neck and proximal urethra can be achieved with much less tension.

2. Technique

Dissection and exposure of the retropubic space is identical in the Burch and MMK procedures. The location of the suspension sutures distinguishes these two operations. In the Burch procedure, two or three sets of vaginal sutures are placed, the most proximal sutures at the level of, but significantly lateral to, the urethrovesical junction, and the most distal sutures at the level of the midurethra. The sutures should be taken parallel to the urethra, incorporating the full thickness of the vaginal wall. The depth of the vaginal sutures can be guided by placing a curved clamp in the vagina. Although Burch used absorbable sutures in his original operation, contemporary authors recommend the use of nonabsorbable sutures, such as polypropylene. Because of the relatively lateral position of the suspension sutures in the Burch procedure (compared with the MMK), we advise cystoscopy after intravenous administration of indigo carmine at this point in the procedure to ensure that the ureters have not been compromised, and that no sutures have penetrated the bladder.

Once ureteral integrity has been confirmed, the vaginal sutures are placed through their corresponding locations in Cooper's ligament. The distal sutures are passed medially, and the proximal sutures in a more lateral portion of Cooper's ligament (Fig. 2). When performing this procedure, we loosely pack the vagina while the sutures are being tied. Starting with the most distal sutures, they are tied down gently over the tips of a rubbershod right-angle clamp to prevent oversuspension with subsequent angulation or compression of the urethra.

3. Results

Long-term results of the Burch procedure are summarized in Table 3. In general, with follow-up of over 5 years, the reported cure rates are 60–80%, with de novo urge incontinence rates ranging from 5 to 15%. Five to twenty percent of patients will complain of obstructive symptoms (including hesitancy and straining) at long-term follow-up. Not all of these studies included postoperative urodynamic studies. Most of them reported greater efficacy in patients who were undergoing the Burch operation as their first operative procedure for SUI.

Alcalay and co-workers (25) demonstrated a significant decline of efficacy of the Burch procedure with time in 109 patients, with an average of 13.8 years. These investigators demonstrated cure rates of 94, 90, and 72% at 3, 60, and longer than 120 months, respectively. The patients in this series were assessed objectively with pad tests, urodynamic studies (when indicated), and physical examination to accurately determine continence at follow-up.

C. Paravaginal Fascia Repair

1. Goal

The paravaginal fascia repair was originally described by White (29) as a vaginal procedure, but later a retropubic approach was popularized by Richardson (30). The paravaginal repair is directed at correcting a lateral defect in vaginal wall support. This defect is thought to be the result of attenuation of the pubocervical fascia at or near its attachment to the levator muscles near the lower margin of the superior pubic ramus. The defect is usually unilateral, but can be bilateral. Of four different defects in the pubocervical fascia that can lead to cystocele and SUI, the lateral defect was most commonly found. Therefore, the goal of

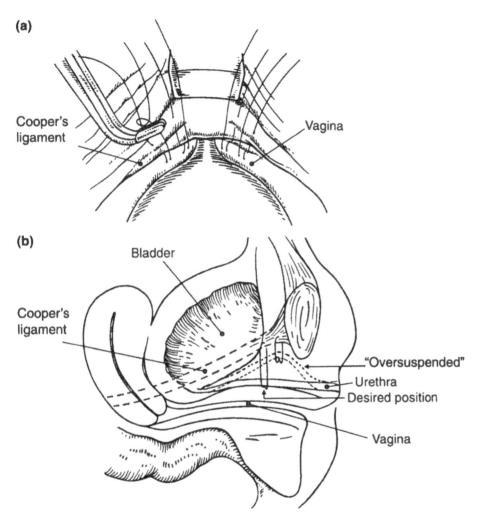

Figure 2   (a) In the Burch procedure, suspension sutures are anchored in Cooper's ligament bilaterally. We grasp the suture with the tips of a rubbershod right-angle clamp and tie
the suture above the clamp, with the bottom of the clamp resting on Cooper's ligament. This
technique prevents oversuspension with subsequent distortion and compression of the urethra. (b) A sagittal view of a patient undergoing a Burch suspension demonstrating the desired amount of urethral support (solid line) as well as an "oversuspended" urethra (dotted
line).

the paravaginal fascia repair is to approximate the endopelvic fascia overlying the superior
lateral sulcus of the vagina to the tendinous arc of the obturator fascia. Significant elasticity of the vaginal wall is essential to perform this procedure, especially for bilateral defects.

2.   Technique

The patient is positioned in low lithotomy, and a lower midline or Pfannenstiel incision is
made. The space of Retzius is developed, exposing the vesical neck and proximal urethra.
From three to six no. 1 absorbable sutures are placed at 1-cm intervals in the paravaginal
fascia and vaginal wall, beginning at the level of the bladder neck. These sutures are then

Table 3 Long-Term Outcome of Burch Suspension Procedure

Author	No. patients	Instrument	Average f/u (yr)	Cure (%)	DI/urgency (%)
Eriksen 1990 (22)	86	ques ± pe/uds	5	87	15
Feyereisl 1994 (23)	87	pe, uds	5–10	82	15
Kjølhede 1994 (24)	232	ques	6	63	nr
Alcalay 1995 (25)	109	pe, pad test	14	73	15
Bergman 1995 (26)	33	pe, uds	5	82	nr
Kinn 1995 (27)	141	ques ± pe/uds	5	78	4
Christensen 1997 (28)	86	ques	7	33	6

DI, detrusor instability; ques, questionnaire; pe, physical examination; uds, urodynamics; nr, not reported.

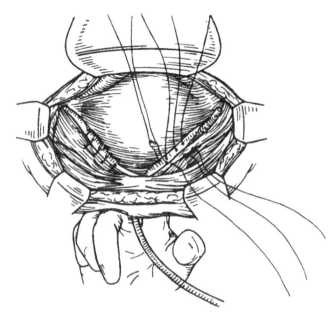

Figure 3   Suture placement for the paravaginal fascial repair approximates the vaginal wall to the tendinous arc on the sidewall of the pelvis. (From Ref. 69.)

passed through the obturator fascia at the arcus tendineus. The sutures are tied, beginning with the ones at the level of the bladder neck, approximating the paravaginal fascia directly to the tendinous arc (Fig. 3).

3.   Results

Considering the length of time that this procedure has been performed, there are few published studies documenting its safety and long-term results in the management of SUI. Richardson initially reported a 92% success rate at an average of 20 months follow-up in 60 patients. In a multicenter study involving 213 patients, Richardson and co-workers later demonstrated an 88% cure rate at 2–8 years follow-up (31). However, in a randomized study comparing the paravaginal defect repair with the Burch procedure in 36 patients, the paravaginal defect repair was significantly less effective, with only a 61% cure rate at 2-year follow-up (32).

D.   Complications of Retropubic Suspensions

A classic complication of retropubic suspensions is bladder outlet obstruction (Fig. 4). Outlet obstruction after bladder neck suspension surgery can manifest as urinary retention, urgency, or urge incontinence. Although the obvious reason for urinary retention is over-tightening the suspension sutures, poor detrusor contractility may also play a role in this condition. Wang (33) has demonstrated urodynamic evidence of obstruction in patients with detrusor instability after bladder neck suspension, and Webster and Kreder (34) showed that urethrolysis of obstructed patients may relieve bladder instability. From the AUA Guidelines Panel, the rates of permanent retention and de novo urgency after retropubic suspension are approximately 5 and 15%, respectively.

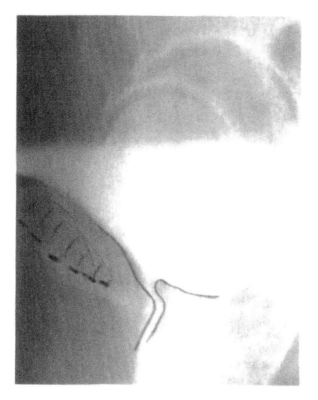

Figure 4 Voiding cystourethrogram of a patient obstructed after a Burch procedure: The urethra has been displaced anteriorly by overtightening the suspension sutures, and now the proximal urethra and bladder neck are severely angulated and distorted.

Bladder and urethral injuries can occur during any of the retropubic suspension procedures, but more commonly during repeat surgery. The key to the management of these injuries is their immediate recognition. Primary repair of such an injury leads to a minimal complication rate (35).

Ureteral injuries are a rare complication of retropubic suspension. Ureteral obstruction results from incorporation of the trigone into the suspension sutures at the level of the bladder neck. Cystoscopic observation of prompt efflux from the ureteral orifices after the administration of intravenous indigo carmine should help the surgeon recognize this complication. Significant hemorrhage is also a rare complication of retropubic suspension techniques. Intraoperative blood loss is poorly quantified in most series. The overall incidence of significant postoperative hematomas is less than 3% (35).

Osteitis pubis, a reactive sclerosis of the pubic bone, occurs postoperatively in up to 10% of MMK procedures. The diagnosis of osteitis pubis can usually be made based on the clinical presentation of pain in the pubic region after this procedure. Use of radionuclide bone scan and plain radiography can aid in the diagnosis of this entity. Most cases resolve with supportive measures and local infiltrations of antibiotics or steroids.

Secondary rectocele or enterocele can occur after retropubic suspension as a result of latent defects in posterior support or excessive elevation of the anterior vaginal wall changing the vaginal axis and exposing the posterior compartment to increases in intra-abdominal pressures. The diagnosis of this condition can be made accurately only by physical examination. Posterior prolapse has been reported, with an incidence as high as 30% after Burch colposuspension (23), but in most series fewer than 10% of patients require a secondary surgical procedure for this condition alone.

E. Needle Suspensions

1. Goal

The goal of needle suspension procedures is to provide the same anatomical support that is created with a retropubic suspension, without creating a lower abdominal incision. These procedures were pioneered by Pereyra (2) and subsequently have undergone many revisions in both technique and equipment. The key instrument in these procedures is the suture passer, which is a cannula approximately 10 in. long that has a sharp end through which one or more sutures can be threaded. Many individuals have developed their own variant of this device.

2. Technique

Pereyra. With the patient in high lithotomy position, a urethral catheter is placed and a weighted speculum exposes the vagina. A small stab wound is made in the midline about 1 in. above the symphysis pubis, The tip of the Pereyra needle is then directed laterally through the subcutaneous tissues, traverses the rectus fascia at the back of the symphysis pubis, and then pierces the vaginal wall in a location just lateral to the bladder neck. The two tips of the trochar exit the vaginal mucosa approximately 1 cm from one another, on the same side of the bladder neck. Pereyra originally described threading a no. 30 stainless steel wire through the ends of the trochar. The trochar is then withdrawn, locking the wire in place, and the device is removed through the suprapubic incision, Another suture is placed on the contralateral side using the same technique.

Once the wires are in place, the surgeon pulls up on them to produce the "desired elevation of the urethra and bladder neck," and the ends are tied together. As described by Pereyra, the suspension result is only temporarily dependent on the splinting effect of the wires. Ultimately, the scar that forms from the wires pulling through the paravaginal tissues produces the support that prevents stress incontinence in the long-term. To aid in the formation of this scar tissue, he recommended cauterizing along the vaginal course of each wire to start the inflammatory process that would lead to the scarring.

Later modifications to the Pereyra procedure utilized a midline vaginal incision to allow the surgeon to pass the sutures from the suprapubic incisions under better control. Pereyra and Lebherz (36) also described using prolene, rather than wire as the suspension suture. In their modified procedure, the vaginal wall is dissected from the underlying tissues at the level of the bladder neck, the endopelvic fascia is detached from the paraurethral tissue, and the surgeon places helical sutures of prolene in the medial edge of the endopelvic fascia

Stamey. Stamey (4) described an endoscopic suspension that brought several modifications to the Pereyra procedure With the patient in the high lithotomy position, two horizontal suprapubic incisions are made, about 2 cm from the midline, two fingerbreadths above the pubic symphysis. The subcutaneous tissues are then dissected down to the rectus fascia. The length of the urethra is measured from the Foley balloon to the urethral meatus, A T-shaped incision is made in the vaginal wall, with the horizontal portion of the T at the level of the midurethra. The anterior vaginal wall is dissected off the underlying fascia. A Stamey needle is then passed from the suprapubic incision into the space of Retzius and then out through the vaginal incision, just lateral to the vesical neck. With the needle in place, cystoscopy is performed to confirm that the needle is in proximity to the bladder neck, and that it was not passed through the bladder wall. A no. 2 monofilament nonabsorbable suture is placed in the needle passer, and then the instrument is withdrawn through the suprapubic incision. In an identical fashion, the Stamey needle is then passed through the space of Retzius, exiting through the vagina 1 cm distal to the first suture, and the other end of the prolene suture is withdrawn through the skin incision.

If the vaginal tissues are of poor quality, a Dacron bolster can be placed inside the loop. The process is repeated on the contralateral side, always using endoscopic guidance to place the sutures close to the vesical neck. The vaginal incision is closed and a suprapubic catheter is inserted. Stamey initially recommended that the suspension sutures be tied with "considerable tension."

Raz.   Another major modification to the Pereyra procedure was described by Raz (5). In this procedure, an inverted U-shaped flap is made in the anterior vaginal wall underneath the urethra and bladder neck. The endopelvic fascia is perforated from the vaginal side using long Metzenbaum scissors, and the retropubic space is entered. Nonabsorbable monofilament sutures are then used to anchor the vaginal wall, without the mucosa, to the deep endopelvic fascia in a helical fashion. A single-pronged needle is then passed, under fingertip control, from a suprapubic incision through to the vaginal incision after draining the bladder, the ligature carrier is then withdrawn, transferring the suspension sutures suprapubically. The sutures are then tied above the rectus fascia.

Gittes.   Gittes and Loughlin (37) described a "no incision" urethropexy, similar to the original Pereyra operation, except that the needle is passed through the lower abdominal wall without making any incision at all. They observed that, over time, exposed sutures cut through the vaginal wall when they were tied under tension and not bolstered. Animal experimentation indicated that a band of scar tissue develops along the path of the suture as it pulls through the vaginal tissues, eventually securing the vaginal tissues to the lower abdominal wall with a "chain" of scar.

3.   Results

Long-term success rates for the various needle suspension techniques are summarized in Table 4. There are significant discrepancies between the original authors' reported success rates and the long-term results reported by other authors. For example, Stamey (38) reported a 91% success rate for his endoscopic needle suspension, yet review of the literature reveals a success rate from 18 to 70%. As proved by multiple authors, the success rates can be dramatically affected by the type of follow-up obtained in these patients (chart review versus questionnaire) (47,48). Contemporary series tend to be more stringent in assessing surgical outcome, than even series from just 5 years ago, so the initial reports are not inaccurate, but simply reflect a different standard of outcome measurement.

In general, studies that assess both patient satisfaction and objective cure demonstrate that patient satisfaction rates obtained by questionnaire are much higher than cure rates for SUI. For example, Kuczyik et al. reported (42) a 62% satisfaction rate, and a 34% cure rate for SUI in 85 women an average of 5 years after a Stamey procedure. Likewise, Mills et al. reported (40) an 83% satisfaction rate at 10 years in 30 patients who had undergone the Stamey procedure, in spite of a 33% cure rate over the same interval.

Table 4 Long-Term Outcome of Vaginal Suspension Procedures

Author	Procedure	No. pts	Instrument	Average f/u	Cure rate (%)
Stamey 1980 (38)		203	nr	16 mo	91
Spencer 1987 (20)	Stamey	41	Chart review	46 mo	61
O'Sullivan 1995 (39)	Stamey	22	Ques	>5 yr	18
Mills 1996 (40)	Stamey	30	Pe/ques	120 mo	33
Conrad 1997 (41)	Stamey	130	Ques	66 mo	50
Kuczyk 1998 (42)	Stamey	85	Ques	61 mo	31
Gofrit 1998 (43)	Stamey	63	Ques	90 mo	70
Kondo 1998 (44)	Stamey	342	Ques	13.8 yr	72
Pereyra 1982 (45)		54	nr	4–6 yr	95
Raz 1992 (46)		206	Chart review	15 mo	83
Sirls 1995 (47)	Modified Pereyra	102	Ques	25 mo	47
		102	Chart review	25 mo	72
Trockman 1995 (48)	Modified Pereyra	125	Ques	9.8 yr	49
Gittes 1987 (37)	Gittes	38	Chart review	2–29 mo	87
Kondo 1998 (44)	Gittes	40	Ques	6.4 yr	37
Elkabir 1998 (49)	Gittes	52	Ques	53 mo	23

Nr, not reported; ques, questionnaire.

Of note, Gofrit and co-workers reported (43) a significantly lower success rate in individuals who had severe urge symptoms preoperatively compared with individuals with mild preoperative urgency (33 vs. 65%). There is significant controversy over this issue in the literature, with multiple nonprospective, nonrandomized trials demonstrating no effect of preoperative urge symptoms on outcome (50). This area might be revisited in future studies using validated questionnaires.

As demonstrated in Table 4, similar trends are seen in long-term follow-up for the modified Pereyra, Gittes, and Raz procedures. Under the scrutiny of objective follow-up instruments, all of these procedures seem to have excellent short-term results, but significant rates of failure more than 2 years postoperatively.

4. Complications

The AUA Guidelines panel reported a 12 and 4% risk of intraoperative bladder injury for the Stamey and modified Pereyra procedures, respectively (7). Performing endoscopy with a 70-degree lens or flexible scope immediately after use of the suture passer can help identify this problem once it has occurred. In the event that this complication is recognized intraoperatively, the suture should be removed and replaced. No retropubic drainage is required in this circumstance (Fig. 5). Significant bleeding requiring transfusion, and ureteral or urethral injuries are rare complications of needle suspension procedures.

Two types of nerve damage can occur with transvaginal suspensions. Because the patient is in the dorsal lithotomy position, neural injuries to the common peroneal, sciatic, femoral, and saphenous nerves have been reported. Avoiding hyperflexion of the thighs over the hips, and the liberal use of padding at pressure points aid in the prevention of this complication. A nerve entrapment can result from compromise of sensory branches of the genitofemoral and ilioinguinal nerves by the sutures as they pass through the rectus fascia. To prevent this complication, the suprapubic incision should be made short and close to the pubic symphysis (one fingerbreadth above) and the ligature carrier should not be passed too

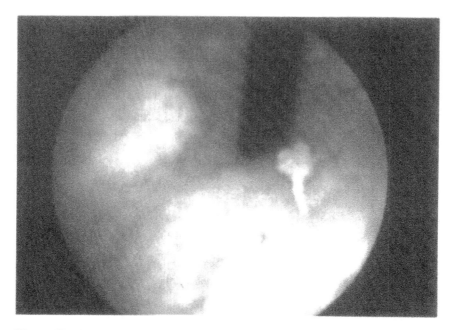

Figure 5   Endoscopic view (using a flexible cystoscope) of a prolene stitch that has penetrated the bladder neck anteriorly during a modified Pereyra bladder neck suspension. Prior rigid cystoscopies with a 30-degree lens had missed this exposed suture.

laterally, Fixation of the suspension sutures directly to the pubic bone has been proposed as a method of prevention (51).

F. Laparoscopic BNS

1. Goal

Laparoscopic techniques have been applied to retropubic suspensions, either transperitoneally as described by Liu and Paek (52) or retroperitoneally (53). The goal of the laparoscopic bladder neck suspension is to suspend the periurethral vaginal tissues to either Cooper's ligament or the pubic periosteum using sutures or even staples with a nonabsorbable mesh, while avoiding a large lower abdominal incision. Balloon dissection of the retropubic space has shortened the operative time of these procedures significantly (54).

2. Technique

Multiple techniques of laparoscopic BNS have been described. Basically, all involve laparoscopic dissection of the space of Retzius, either through the peritoneal cavity, or directly using a balloon dissector. Suspension of the periurethral vaginal tissues to the pubic periosteum or Cooper's ligament is accomplished using either suturing techniques or stapling devices, with or without the incorporation of synthetic mesh. These procedures all closely resemble either the MMK or Burch repairs described earlier.

3. Results

Radomski and Herschorn reported an 95% cure rate in 34 patients with an average of 17 months after a laparoscopic Burch procedure (55). These investigators used nonabsorbable sutures through both extraperitoneal and intraperitoneal approaches. Polascik et al., using a suturing technique through both intraperitoneal and extraperitoneal routes, noted an 83% cure rate at a mean follow-up of 21 months in 12 patients (56). These authors found that the laparoscopic approach led to significantly shorter hospital stays, decreased analgesic requirements, and faster return to normal activity when compared with a Burch bladder neck suspension. In this study, the authors found no difference in the efficacy between the two procedures. Similarly, McDougall and co-workers found no significant difference in success between laparoscopic and transvaginal bladder neck suspension, whereas the laparoscopic procedure allowed patients to return to normal activity and voiding at significantly shorter intervals (57). In that study, 19 patients had the laparoscopic procedure, and of these, 90% were cured at 2 years follow-up.

Blander and co-workers, reporting on a stapling technique using Marlex mesh, found an 80% cure rate and an overall 70% success rate at an average follow-up of 29 months in 20 patients (58). In this study, all patients who reported that they would not elect to have the procedure again had bothersome de novo urge incontinence postoperatively.

4. Complications

The complications of laparoscopic urethropexy are similar to those of any other laparoscopic procedure. Conversion to an open procedure occurs in up to 26% of patients, but this figure is highly dependent on patient selection and the surgeon's experience with the procedure (55). Incidental perforation of the bladder occurs in approximately 5% of cases, and can frequently be managed laparoscopically or with simple prolonged bladder drainage. Conversion to an open procedure owing to a bladder, ureteric, or bowel injury is a relatively rare event (56).

III. NEWER TECHNIQUES

A. Bone Anchors

1. Goal

Benderev described a needle suspension procedure with no vaginal incision. This procedure utilizes bone anchors to suspend the bladder neck and proximal urethra directly to the pubic symphysis (59). The procedure uses a durable, fixed point as the anchor for the suspension with the goal of having a lower long-term failure rate than procedures that use fascia as the point of fixation. Also, by not tying the sutures across the rectus fascia, the surgeon may avoid a nerve entrapment syndrome.

2. Technique

In this procedure, a novel suture-passing device is used to take bites of the pubocervical fascia and of the vaginal wall using a no-incision technique. A simple suture is placed in the vaginal wall with a Z stitch on each side of the bladder neck (Fig. 6). The sutures are tied to bone anchors drilled in the pubic bone bilaterally. The sutures are tied down over a spacer which prevents overtightening and subsequent urethral obstruction.

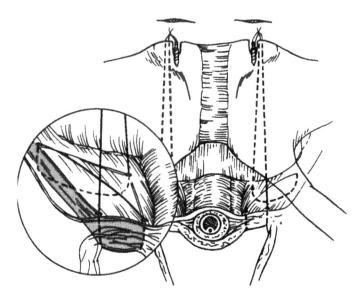

Figure 6 The "Z-stitch" used in bladder neck suspension with bone anchor fixation captures a large amount of pubocervical fascia and vaginal wall. (From Ref. 70.)

3. Results

Appell reported (60) on a series of 71 patients who underwent percutaneous bladder neck stabilization (PBNS) using bone anchors. That study, with a mean follow-up of 3 years, reported an 82% success rate. Successful results were also reported by Nativ et al. (61), who found an 82% short-term (1-year) cure rate in 50 patients using a transvaginal bone anchor system to perform a modified urethropexy. In contrast, Schultheiss et al. reported (62) only a 43% cure rate in 37 patients at 11 months follow-up. Long-term follow-up of this procedure is still lacking.

4. Complications

European series and preliminary United Stated studies have confirmed the short-term safety and ease of the procedure. Although surgeons with significant experience with bone anchor techniques claim minimal complication rates (59,63), reports of significant complications are beginning to accumulate. Although uncommon, complications, such as osteitis pubis, osteomyelitis, and nerve entrapment syndrome, have been described (64,65) (Fig. 7). When any of these complications occur, removal of the bone anchor is indicated. Removal of the bone anchors does not seem to lead to failure of the suspension, but the numbers of these reports are quite small.

B. Intravaginal Slingplasty

1. Goal

Ulmsten and co-workers (66) reported on another minimally invasive procedure called intravaginal slingplasty (IVS). This procedure is the progenitor of the transvaginal tape (TVT) procedure. IVS can be done under local anesthesia in the outpatient setting. Its goal is to correct inadequate urethral support from the pubourethral ligaments. Petros and Um-

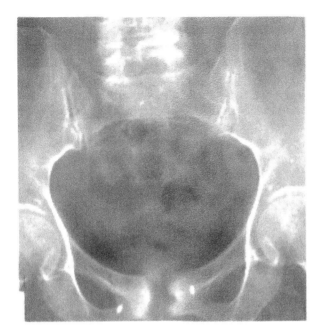

Figure 7 Pelvic plain x-ray film reveals significant changes over the pubic symphysis consistent with osteitis pubis in a patient after BNS with bone anchor fixation.

sten's integral theory of urinary incontinence suggests that these support structures are important in the maintenance of continence during stress maneuvers (67).

2. Technique

The patient is placed in lithotomy position and given intravenous sedation along with local anesthesia to the lower abdominal wall and the anterior vaginal wall. Two 1-cm transverse incisions are made in the lower abdominal wall along the upper margin of the pubic bone, and a 1.5-cm midline vertical incision is made in the vaginal wall starting 0.5 cm from the urethral meatus. One centimeter of blunt dissection is performed on each side of the urethra. With a Foley catheter in place, the bladder neck is moved laterally, and a special needle that is already connected to a tape of prolene mesh is passed up from the vaginal incision to the corresponding abdominal incision. The procedure is repeated on the other side, and then, the plastic covering over the mesh is removed. To ensure that the sling is loosely placed around the urethra, the patient is asked to cough and some leakage should be observed. The abdominal ends are pulled up through the skin incisions, and then the mesh is cut below the skin surface. The sling is held in place only by the friction of the mesh. Cystourethroscopy is performed before removing the plastic cover over the mesh to inspect the integrity of the bladder and urethra. No bladder drainage is required.

3. Results

By using the foregoing technique, Ulmsten and co-workers reported (66) an 84% cure rate in 63 patients at 2 years follow-up, with an 8% failure rate and a 7% rate of urinary tract infections. They reported no rejection or erosion of the sling, and no long-term urinary retention. Although promising and adopted by many European experts, there is currently no long-term follow-up on this simple and rather minimally invasive procedure.

IV. CONCLUSIONS

Bladder neck suspension procedures appear to be safe and effective in the treatment of stress urinary incontinence secondary to urethral hypermobility. Although a wide variety of procedures exist using several different surgical approaches, most authors agree that the best operation to cure a given patient is the first one that is performed. It is prudent for a urologist to have both a retropubic and vaginal BNS procedure in their armamentarium to provide their patients with the best alternatives on an individual basis. Within the different categories of procedures, there are no obviously superior procedures, but in general, long-term follow-up of the retropubic suspension procedures demonstrates a slightly higher cure rate than for the vaginal procedures. The literature on SUI is replete with studies that do not make use of standardized, objective outcome measures, and as mature data becomes available for the newer BNS procedures, surgeons must be very critical of the way in which patients have been evaluated both pre- and postoperatively in such studies.

REFERENCES

1. Marshall FV, Marchetti AA, Krantz KE. The correction of stress incontinence by simple vesicourethral suspension. Surg Gynecol Obstet 1949; 88:509–518.
2. Pereyra AJ. A simplified surgical procedure for the correction of stress incontinence in women. West J Surg Obstet Gynecol 1959; 67:223–226.
3. Burch JC. Urethrovaginal fixation to Cooper's ligament for correction of stress incontinence, cystocele, and prolapse. Am J Obstet Gynecol 1961; 81:281–290.
4. Stamey TA. Endoscopic suspension of the vesical neck for urinary incontinence. Surg Gynecol Obstet 1973; 136:547–554.
5. Raz S. Modified bladder neck suspension for female stress incontinence. Urology 1981; 17:82–85.
6. Zimmern PE, Leach GE, Sirls L. Four-corner bladder neck suspension. Atlas Urol Clin North Am 1994; 2:29–36.
7. Leach GE, Dmochowski RR, Appell RA, Blaivas JG, Hadley HR, Luber KM, Mostwin JL, O'Donnell PD, Roehrborn CG. Female stress urinary incontinence clinical guidelines panel summary report on surgical management of female stress urinary incontinence. J Urol 1997; 158:875–880.
8. Albertsen PC. Outcomes research: a primer for urologists. AUA Update Ser 1998; 17:106–111.
9. Rovner ES, Ginsberg DA. Raz S. Re: female stress urinary incontinence Clinical Guidelines Panel summary report on surgical management of female stress urinary incontinence. J Urol 1998; 159:1646–1647.
10. Uebersax JS, Wyman JF, Shumaker SA, McClish DK, Fantl JA. Continence Program for Women Research Group. Short forms to assess life quality and symptom distress for urinary incontinence in women: the incontinence impact questionnaire and the urogenital distress inventory. Neurourol Urodynam 1995; 14:131–139.
11. Jackson S, Donovan J, Brookes S, Eckford S, Swithinbank L, Abrams P. The Bristol Female Lower Urinary Tract Symptoms Questionnaire: development and psychometric testing. Br J Urol 1996; 77:805–812.
12. Blaivas JG, Appell RA, Fantl JA, Leach G, McGuire EJ, Resnick NM, Raz S, Wein AJ. Standards of efficacy for evaluation of treatment outcomes in urinary incontinence: recommendations of the Urodynamic Society. Neurourol Urodynam 1997; 16:145–147.
13. Fischer–Rasmussen W. Transvaginal needle bladder neck suspension for stress urinary incontinence: practicable methods but not optimal results. Acta Obstet Gynecol Scand Suppl 1998; 168:77:38–43.

14. Goebell R. Zur operativen Beseitigung der Angelborenen Incontinenz Vesicae. Z Gynäkol Urol 1910; 2:187–191.
15. Marchetti AA, Marshall VF, Shultis LD. Simple vesicourethral suspension. Am J Obstet Gynecol 1957; 74:57–63.
16. Tanagho EA. Colpocystourethropexy. In: Raz S, ed. Female Urology. Philadelphia; WB Saunders, 1996:319–324.
17. Lee RA, Symmonds RE. Repeat Marshall–Marchetti procedure for recurrent stress urinary incontinence. Am J Obstet Gynecol 1975; 122:219–225.
18. Penson DF, Raz S. Why anti-incontinence surgery succeeds or fails. In: Raz S, ed. Female Urology. Philadelphia: WB Saunders, 1996:435–442.
19. Jarvis GJ. Stress incontinence. In: Mundy AR, Stephenson TP, Wein AJ eds. Urodynamics: Principles, Practice and Application. New York, Churchill Livingstone, 1994:299–326.
20. Spencer JR, O'Conor VJ, Schaeffer AJ. A comparison of endoscopic suspension of the vesical neck with suprapubic vesicourethropexy for treatment of stress urinary incontinence. J Urol 1987; 137:411–415.
21. Clemens JQ, Stern JA, Bushman WA, Schaeffer AJ. Long-term results of the Stamey bladder neck suspension: direct comparison with the Marshall–Marchetti–Krantz procedure. J Urol 1998; 160:372–376.
22. Eriksen BC, Hagen B, Eik–Nes SH, Molne K, Mjølnerød OK, Romslo I. Long-term effectiveness of the Burch colposuspension in female stress incontinence. Acta Obstet Gynecol Scand 1990; 69:45–50.
23. Feyereisl J, Dreher E, Haenggi W, Zikmund J, Schneider H. Long-term results after Burch colposuspension. Am J Obstet Gynecol 1994; 171:647–652.
24. Kjølhede P, Ryden G. Prognostic factors and long-term results of the Burch colposuspension. Acta Obstet Gynecol Scand 1994; 73:642–647.
25. Alcalay M, Monga A, Stanton SL. Burch colposuspension: a 10–20 year follow up. Br J Obstet Gynecol 1995; 102:740–745.
26. Bergman A, Elia G. Three surgical procedures for genuine stress incontinence: five year follow-up of a prospective randomized study. Am J Obstet Gynecol 1995; 173:66–71.
27. Kinn AC. Burch colposuspension for stress urinary incontinence. 5-year results in 153 women Scand J Urol Nephrol 1995; 29:449–455.
28. Christensen H, Laybourn C, Eickhoff JH, Frimodt–Moller C. Long-term results of the Stamey bladder neck suspension procedure and of the Burch colposuspension. Scand J Urol Nephrol 1997; 31:349–353.
29. White GR. Cystocele: a radical cure by suturing later sulci of vagina to white line of pelvic fascia. JAMA 1909; 53:1707–1710.
30. Richardson AC, Lyon JB, Williams NL. A new look at pelvic relaxation. Am J Obstet Gynecol 1976; 126:568–573.
31. Richardson AC, Edmonds PB, Williams NL. Treatment of stress urinary incontinence due to paravaginal fascial defect. Obstet Gyencol 1981; 57:357–362.
32. Colombo M, Milani R, Vitobello D, Maggioni A. A randomized comparison of Burch colposuspension and abdominal paravaginal defect repair for female stress urinary incontinence. Am J Obstet Gynecol 1996; 175:78–84.
33. Wang AC. Burch colposuspension vs. Stamey bladder neck suspensions comparison of complications with special emphasis on detrusor instability and voiding dysfunction. J Reprod Med 1996; 41:529–533.
34. Webster GD, Kreder KJ. Voiding dysfunction following cystourethropexy: its evaluation and management. J Urol 1990; 144:670–673.
35. Kelly MJ, Zimmern PE, Leach GE. Complications of bladder neck suspension procedures. Urol Clin North Am 1991; 18:339–348.
36. Pereyra AJ, Lebherz TB. The revised Pereyra procedure. In: Buchsbaum H, Schmidt JD, eds. Gynecologic and Obstetric Urology. Philadelphia: WB Saunders, 1978:208–222.

37. Gittes RF, Loughlin KR. No-incision pubovaginal suspension for stress incontinence. J Urol 1987; 138:568–570.

38. Stamey TA. Endoscopic suspension of the vesical neck for incontinence in females. Report of 203 consecutive patients. Ann Surg 1980; 192:465–471.

39. O'Sullivan DC, Chilton CP, Munson KW. Should Stamey colposuspension be our primary surgery for stress incontinence? Br J Urol 1995; 75:457–460.

40. Mills R, Parsad R, Ashken NM. Long-term follow-up results with the Stamey operation for stress incontinence of urine. Br J Urol 1996; 77:86–88.

41. Conrad S, Pleper A, de la Maza SF, Busch R, Huland H. Long-term results of the Stamey bladder neck suspension procedure: a patient questionnaire based outcome analysis. J Urol 1997; 157:1672–1677.

42. Kuczyk MA, Klein S, Grunewaid V, Machtens S, Denil J, Hofner K, Wagner T, Jonas U. A questionnaire-based outcome analysis of the Stamey bladder neck suspension procedure for the treatment of urinary stress Incontinence: the Hannover experience. Br J Urol 1998 82(2):174–180.

43. Gofrit ON, Landau EH, Shapiro A, Pode D. The Stamey procedure for stress incontinence: long-term results. Eur Urol 1998; 34:339–343.

44. Kondo A, Kato K, Gotoh M, Narushima M, Saito M. The Stamey and Gittes procedures: long-term follow-up in relation to incontinence types and patient age. J Urol 1998; 160:756–758.

45. Pereyra AJ, Lebherz LB, Growdon WA, Powers JA. Pubourethral supports in perspective: modified Pereyra procedure for urinary incontinence. Obstet Gynecol 1982; 59:643–648.

46. Raz S, Sussman EM, Erickson DB, Bregg KJ, Nitti VW. The Raz bladder neck suspension: results in 206 patients. J Urol 1992; 148:845–850.

47. Sirls LT, Keoleian CM, Korman HJ, Kirkemo AK. The effect of study methodology on report success rates of the modified Pereyra bladder neck suspension. J Urol 1995; 154:1732–1735.

48. Trockman BA, Leach GE, Hamilton J, Sakamoto M, Santiago L, Zimmern PE. Modified Pereyra bladder neck suspension: 10 year mean follow-up using outcome analysis in 125 patients. J Urol 1995; 154:1841–1847.

49. Elkabir JJ, Mee AD. Long-term evaluation of the Gittes procedure for urinary stress incontinence. J Urol 1998; 159:1203–1205.

50. Trockman BA, Leach GE. Needle suspension procedures: past, present, and future. J Endourol 1996; 10:217–220.

51. Leach GE. Bone fixation technique for transvaginal needle suspension. Urology 1988; 31:388–390.

52. Liu CY, Paek W. Laparoscopic retropubic colposuspension (Burch procedure). J Am Assoc Gynecol Laparosc 1993; 1:31–35.

53. Ou CS, Presthus J, Beadle E. Laparoscopic bladder neck suspension using hernia mesh and surgical staples, J Laparoendosc Surg 1993; 3:563–566.

54. Lose G. Laparoscopic Burch colposuspension. Acta Obstet Gynecol Scand 1998; 168:29–33.

55. Radomski SB, Herschorn S. Laparoscopic Burch bladder neck suspension: early results. J Urol 1996; 155:515–518.

56. Polascik TJ, Moore RG, Rosenberg MT, Kavoussi LR. Comparison of laparoscopic and open retropubic urethropexy for treatment of stress urinary incontinence. Urology 1995; 45:647–652.

57. McDougall EM, Klutke CG, Cornell T. Comparison of transvaginal versus laparoscopic bladder neck suspension for stress urinary incontinence. Urology 1995; 45:641–646.

58. Blander DS, Carpiniello VL, Harryhill JF, Malloy TR, Rovner ES. Extraperitoneal laparoscopic urethropexy with Marlex mesh. Urology 1999; 53:985–989.

59. Benderev TV. A modified percutaneous outpatient bladder neck suspension system. J Urol 1994; 152:2316–2320.

60. Appell RA. The use of bone anchoring in the surgical management of female stress urinary incontinence. World J Urol 1997; 15:300–305.

61. Nativ O, Levine S, Madjar S, Issaq E, Moskovitz B, Beyar M. Incisionless pervaginal bone an-

chor cystourethropexy for the treatment of female stress incontinence: experience with the first 50 patients. J Urol 1997; 158:1742–1744.

62. Schultheiss D, Hoffier K, Oelke M, Grunewald V, Jonas U. Does bone anchor fixation improve the outcome of percutaneous bladder neck suspension in female stress urinary incontinence? Br J Urol 1998; 82:192–195.

63. Leach GE, Appell R. Percutaneous bladder neck suspension. Urol Clin North Am 1996; 23:511–516.

64. Bernier PA, Zimmern PE. Bone anchor removal after bladder neck suspension. Br J Urol 1998; 82:302–303.

65. Matkov TG, Hejna MJ, Coogan CL. Osteomyelitis as a complication of Vesica percutaneous bladder neck suspension. J Urol 1998; 160:1427.

66. Ulmsten U, Henriksson L, Johnson P, Varhos G. An ambulatory surgical procedure under local anesthesia for treatment of female urinary incontinence. Int Urogynecol J Pelvic Floor Dysfunct 1996; 7:81–85.

67. Petros P, Ulmsten U. An integral theory of female urinary incontinence. Acta Scand Obstet Gynecol Suppl. 1990; 53:1–79.

68. Kantz KE. The Marshall–Marchetti–Krantz procedure. In: Stanton SL, Tanagho AE, eds. Surgery of Female Incontinence, 2nd ed. New York: Springer–Verlag, 1986:99.

69. Webster GD, Khoury JM. Retropublic suspension surgery for female sphincteric incontinence. In: Walsh PC, Retik AB, Vaughan ED, Wein AJ, eds. Campbell's Urology. 7th ed. Philadelphia: WB Saunders, 1988:1099.

70. Benderev TV. A modified percutaneous outpatient bladder neck suspension system. J Urol 1994; 152:2317.

40

Surgical Reconstruction of the Bladder Neck

MARC CENDRON

Dartmouth–Hitchcock Medical Center, Lebanon, New Hampshire

I. INTRODUCTION

The principal goal of bladder neck reconstruction is to create bladder outlet resistance to treat urinary incontinence caused by sphincter incompetence. The degree of bladder outlet resistance should compensate for variations in intra-abdominal pressure and permit emptying the bladder during detrusor contraction. Because surgical reconstruction techniques tend to do away with the normal anatomical arrangement of the bladder neck, bladder neck reconstruction is actually a misnomer: the procedure modifies, rather than reconstructs, the bladder neck to create a certain degree of obstruction at the level of the bladder outlet. In Europe, this procedure is called cervicoplasty, which is perhaps more accurate than our own terminology.

Given our current understanding of the anatomy of the bladder neck and our rather gross surgical techniques, reconstruction of the functional unit referred to as the bladder neck is essentially impossible. The surgical procedures described in the literature, therefore, do not reconstruct the bladder neck, but rather, serve to tighten or lengthen the proximal urethra to increase bladder outlet resistance.

The first description of bladder neck reconstruction was published by Young (1) in 1919. The procedure entailed lengthening the most proximal portion of the urethra and tubulizing it, using portions of the detrusor muscle from the funneled part of the bladder base. In Young's procedure, two triangular portions of the posterior bladder neck muscle are excised and the bladder neck is reconstructed by narrowing it with a silver probe of small diameter (Fig. 1). In 1922, Young (2) reviewed a first series of 13 children with epispadias–exstrophy complex. Twelve of these patients were reported continent after a single intervention.

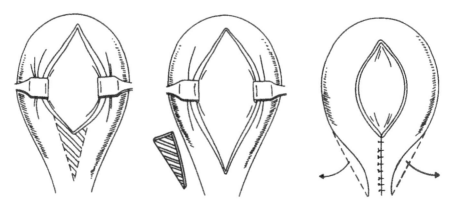

Figure 1   Young's procedure. (From Ref. 29.)

Several modifications of the Young procedure have been described in the literature. In 1949, Dees (3) suggested excising triangular wedges of tissues from the anterior portion of the bladder neck and removing the proximal tissue anteriorly and laterally to the base of the bladder. This was done to tubulize and cinch the proximal urethra and bladder neck, which lengthened the most proximal portion of the urethra (Figs. 2 and 3). The procedure was performed with the insertion of an 8F or 10F catheter. In 1964, Leadbetter (4) modified the Young procedure by reimplanting the ureter to gain length in the most proximal portion of the urethra up into the bladder neck and base (see Fig. 3). In a series of five patients, Leadbetter (4) reported follow-up from 4 months to 2 years, with four patients exhibiting good continence. More than 20 years later, his retrospective review of 34 patients, who were followed-up for up to 2 years, showed that a majority of them (7 adults, 19 children) had a successful outcome, defined as the patient being totally dry and wearing no pad (5).

In 1980, Mollard (6) described a further modification of the procedure. With this technique, muscle flaps of the bladder neck and proximal urethra are cinched around the most proximal portion of the urethra to provide a better continence mechanism (Fig. 4). Lepor and Jeffs (7) added urethral suspension to bladder neck reconstruction. In this procedure, the proximal urethra is tubulized following the Young–Dees–Leadbetter technique

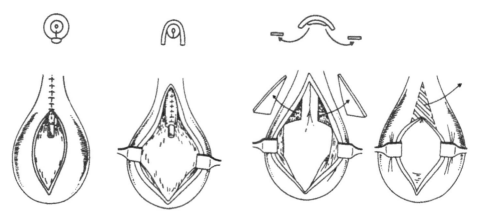

Figure 2   Dee's modifications of Young's procedure.

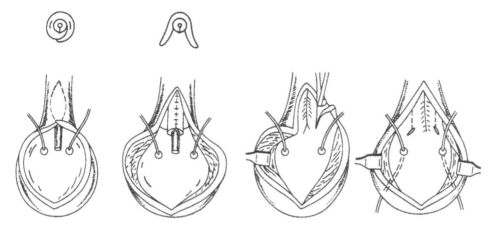

Figure 3 Leadbetter's modification of the Young–Dee procedure using urethral lengthening and reimplantation of the ureters.

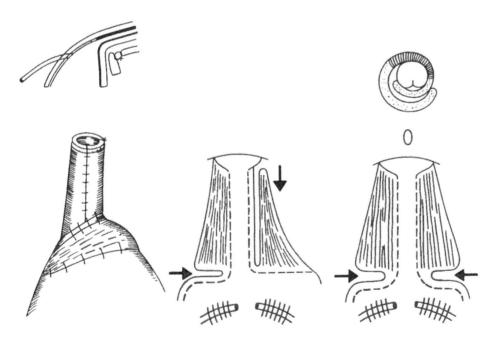

Figure 4 Mollard's modification of the Young–Dee–Leadbetter procedure.

and then suspended from the posterior aspect of the rectus fascia, using the method described by Marshall et al. (8). Careful urethral pressure profilometry is undertaken at the time of the procedure to document and accordingly adjust the amount of urethral resistance (7).

The basic principles of all the procedures based on the Young–Dees–Leadbetter technique are a lengthening of the proximal urethra and narrowing of the bladder neck, to increase bladder outlet resistance. A different way of lengthening the proximal urethra was reported in 1949 by Barnes and Wilson (9), who described the use of an anterior bladder flap to create the most proximal portion of the urethra. Approximately 20 years later, Tanagho et al. (10–12) proposed a technique employing a tubulized segment of the anterior bladder wall to reconstruct the bladder neck. They based their surgical approach on anatomical studies in animals that showed a circular arrangement of muscle fibers at the level of the bladder neck. According to their procedure, the bladder neck and a portion of the proximal urethra are divided, and an anterior bladder wall flap is isolated and tubulized over a 14F–16F catheter, then brought down for reanastomosis with the proximal urethra (Fig. 5). The detrusor tube is also suspended from the anterior abdominal wall or pubic bone. In an heterogeneous group of mostly adult postprostatectomy patients who were followed-up for 10 years, 70% demonstrated good or excellent results (11). In the pediatric age group, in whom the anatomy is such that the posterior bladder wall may be deficient, Williams and Snyder (13) described a modification of the Tanagho procedure, with the distal end of the detrusor flap kept in continuity with the urethra, thus preserving a better blood supply to the detrusor pedicle.

Using the concept of the detrusor flap, Kropp and Angwafo (14) presented a technique that creates a flap-valve mechanism to provide continence at the level of the bladder neck (Fig. 6). In this procedure, a segment of the detrusor, in continuity with the bladder neck, is isolated from either the anterior or posterior aspect of the bladder, and then tubulized with subsequent submucosal reimplantation into the posterior aspect of the bladder. The physiological principle of the flap-valve mechanism relies on compression of the detrusor tube, as intravesical pressure rises with the increasing volume of stored urine. Patients who have undergone this procedure are not able to void spontaneously; therefore, clean intermittent catheterization (CIC) is mandatory. However, CIC is difficult for many of these patients, because the surgical procedure tends to distort the proximal urethral making the passage of the catherter more tortuous. Long-term results have been good for continence. Belman and Kaplan (15) reported that 78% of patients experienced total continence. Modifications of this procedure have since been made (16).

In 1994, Pippi–Salle et al. (17) described the use of an anterior bladder flap to create a flap-valve mechanism at the level of the bladder neck (Fig. 7). With this technique, an anterior bladder flap is isolated carefully, and its blood supply preserved. A posterior bladder wall trough is produced with or without urethral reimplantation, depending on the distance between the bladder neck and the ureteral orifices. The anterior flap is laid into the trough and sewn, to create an intravesical tube from the bladder neck up into the trigone. This intravesical tube is covered by the mucosa of the bladder. CIC is also mandatory for the procedure because it essentially creates a one-way valve mechanism similar to that used with the Kropp technique. Catheterization has been reported to be easier with this than with the Kropp method (18).

Finally, a simplified flap-valve mechanism can be created by constructing a tubulized portion of the trigone and posterior wall in the midline. Koyle (18) reported on three flap-valve procedures that can be used to reconstruct the bladder neck. He concluded that the Kropp technique provided the best means of achieving continence, but was limited by difficulties with catheterization. The Pippi–Salle procedure was less reliable for continence, but easier in terms of catheterization.

Most of these surgical techniques have been developed in children, but are also applicable to the adult population. Evaluation of the patient and careful selection of the appropriate surgical technique will ensure a satisfactory outcome.

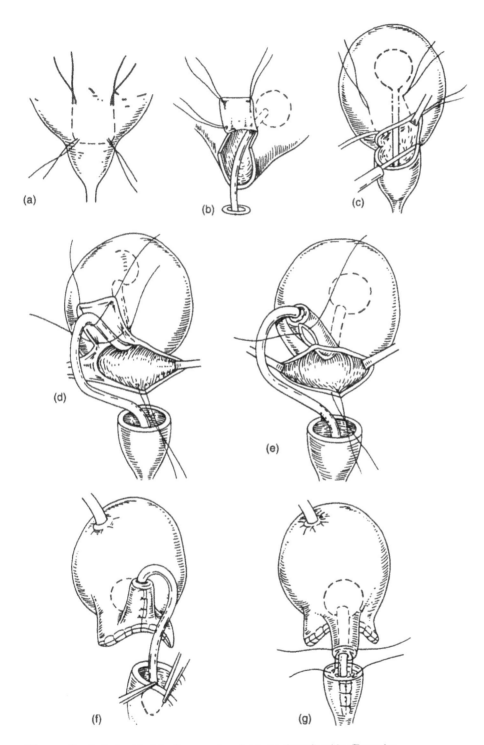

Figure 5   Anterior bladder flap cervicoplasty as described by Tanagho.

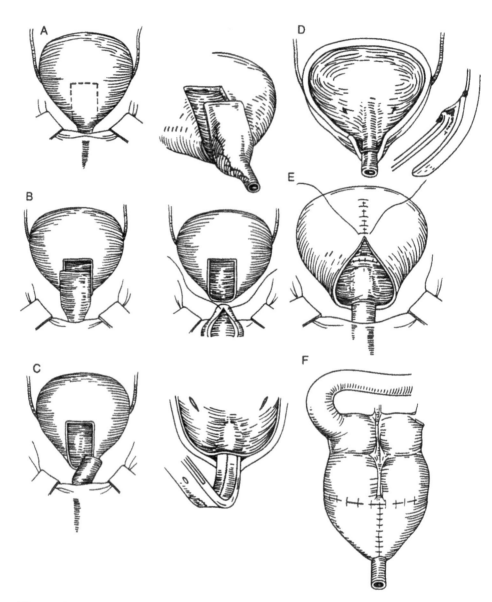

Figure 6 Kropp detrusor flap-valve mechanism for bladder neck reconstruction. (From Ref. 14.)

II. INDICATIONS FOR SURGICAL RECONSTRUCTION OF THE BLADDER NECK

Bladder neck reconstruction should be recommended only for a select group of patients who have a diagnosis of having total urinary incontinence arising from bladder outlet incompetence. Bladder neck incompetence may be due to several factors: congenital disease, such as epispadias–exstrophy complex; neurological diseases, such as myelomeningocele, lipomeningocele, sacral agenesis, or spinal cord injury; or trauma or surgical injuries to the proximal urethra.

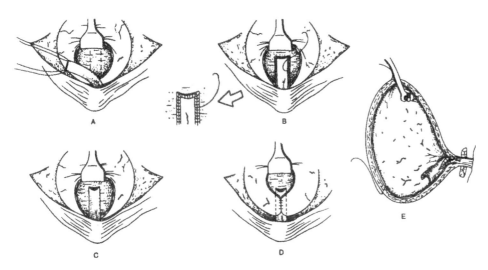

Figure 7   Pippi–Salle procedure with anterior bladder flap. (From Ref. 17.)

Competence of the bladder neck is best identified and diagnosed by videourodynamic studies. Findings consistent with bladder neck incompetence include low leak-point pressure despite preserved bladder compliance and the absence of detrusor instability. On fluoroscopy, a wide-open, patulous bladder neck and proximal urethra can be identified. This will translate into leakage at low volume and very low intravesical pressure.

Surgery should be considered only after failure of medical therapy (usually α-sympathomimetics), cystoscopically injected bulking agents, or bladder suspension procedures (19). Documentation of persistent bladder outlet incompetence after treatment with these forms of therapy must be obtained before surgical reconstruction of the bladder neck.

Each of the aforedescribed procedures applies best to certain clinical situations. In our experience and that of others in pediatric urology, the Young–Dees–Leadbetter procedure is best applied to epispadias–exstrophy patients who may still be able to void spontaneously. The Kropp and Pippi–Salle procedures seem best suited for patients with neurogenic bladder incompetence. In the adult population, reconstruction of the bladder neck should be considered only in cases of spinal cord injury with lower motor neuron lesions, posttraumatic urethral and bladder neck injuries, and failed bladder neck suspension with significant scarring of the proximal urethra. Reconstruction of the bladder neck should also be considered in patients for whom sling procedures have failed, and who have significant distortion of the bladder neck owing to build up of scar tissue and a persistently open bladder outlet. These cases are rare.

Before undertaking bladder neck reconstruction, an important factor to consider is how to achieve appropriate bladder volume and compliance. Tightening of the bladder neck and urethra may cause changes in bladder physiology, which will alter the compliance and capability to accommodate increasing volumes in up to 25% of cases (20). Therefore, it has been our policy to consider bladder augmentation at the time of bladder neck reconstruction. In addition to providing adequate bladder capacity and increased compliance, enterocystoplasty may also produce lower intravesical pressures. Tight reconstruction of the bladder neck, such as in the Kropp procedure, will not allow pop-off mechanisms to vent increased intravesical pressures. Adding a segment of bowel or using a ureter for uretero-cystoplasty may permit better control of intravesical pressures, and thus provide assurance that the upper tracts are not at risk. Some patients may not even require bladder neck procedures if the bladder is made larger and more compliant, as recommended by Hollowel and Ransley (19).

III. OUTCOMES OF BLADDER NECK RECONSTRUCTION

Outcome measures for bladder neck reconstruction are urinary continence and preservation of the upper urinary tract, including renal function. After reviewing the current literature, evaluation of the surgical outcomes of bladder neck reconstruction is difficult.

Articles reviewing the procedures described in this chapter are mainly anecdotal reports, based on relatively small series of patients with relatively short follow-up periods. Most studies involve pediatric patients and few offer follow-up of longer than 10 years.

For achieving continence, however, the literature shows that bladder neck reconstruction has had good overall results (30). Table 1 summarizes studies evaluating continence after the Young–Dees–Leadbetter procedure. Surgical outcomes have also been good following the Kropp–Onlay procedure. Mollard and Mure (21) reported that 86% of patients (6–11 years follow-up) were dry after CIC. These results compare favorably with continence rates reported by Belman and Kaplan (78%) (15) and by Nill et al. (80%) (27). Koyle (18) compared three techniques of bladder neck reconstruction, including Kropp–Onlay, reversed Kropp, and Pippi–Salle. Koyle felt the Kropp–Onlay procedure provided the best continence rate (greater than 95%), followed by the reversed Kropp (82%), and the Pippi–Salle technique: these percentages refer to the success rate after a sin-

Table 1   Summary of Studies Evaluating Urinary Continence After the Young–Dees–Leadbetter Procedure

Author and year	Procedure	Dry interval > 3 hr
Young 1922 (1)	Bladder neck reconstruction	90%
Dees 1949 (2)	Bladder neck reconstruction	85%
Leadbetter 1985 (5)	Bladder neck reconstruction and reimplantation	57% in adults 70% with children
Klauber and Williams 1974 (24)	Bladder neck ± sling procedure	9 of 17 females (52%) 9 of 21 males (43%)
Lepor and Jeffs 1983 (7)	Bladder neck reconstruction and sling	86% success
Mollard 1980 (6)	Bladder neck repair (modified)	65%
Kramer and Kellalis 1982 (25)	Bladder neck repair (epispadias)	83% in males 70% in females
Perlmutter et al. 1991 (26)	Bladder neck repair	41% after single operation
Hollowel and Ransley 1991 (19)	Bladder neck repair plus augmentation cystoplasty	80%
Gearhart et al. 1991 (22)	Bladder neck repair plus augmentation cystoplasty	85%
Donnahoo et al. 1999 (28)	Bladder neck repair plus ± augmentation cystoplasty	70%

gle procedure. One basic goal of bladder neck reconstruction is to provide sufficient outlet resistance, but not so much that high intravesical pressures are created with no pop-off mechanism. Such high intravesical pressures can ultimately jeopardize the upper urinary tract and kidneys. The Kropp technique may not allow for a pop-off mechanism, and patients who undergo this procedure, therefore, are at increased risk. Finally, bladder neck reconstruction can be performed in conjunction with the creation of a catheterizable urinary stoma, as described by Mitrofanoff (23). This will improve the patient's ability to catheterize, thereby increasing compliance. By providing adequate continence and easy catheterization, the overall outcome for these patients is felt to be excellent.

Complications of bladder neck reconstruction can be avoided by appropriate selection of patients, careful surgical technique, and consistent long-term follow-up. Intraoperative complications include bleeding and injuries to adjacent organs. Inadvertent injury to the vagina or bowel will often require further surgical steps and may jeopardize the success of the procedure. Therefore, preoperative bowel preparation and intravenous antibiotics are recommended. Immediate postoperative complications do not differ significantly from those encountered in reconstruction of the lower urinary tract. Long-term complications include persistent incontinence, recurrent urinary tract infections, and upper urinary tract deterioration.

IV. CONCLUSION

Bladder neck reconstruction should be proposed only for patients who have been selected carefully. No surgical procedure has emerged as superior to another, and thus the surgeon must select the one most likely to provide the best outcome and the least upper tract deterioration in a given patient. Surgical reconstruction of the bladder neck represents a solution of last resort for patients who have had no success with prior anti-incontinence procedures. Additional procedures, such as bladder augmentation and ureteral implantation, may also be performed in conjunction with bladder neck reconstruction. This surgery in itself may be challenging if there is extensive scarring from prior surgical procedures. Patients should be aware that CIC may be necessary after surgery. The surgeon should be cognizant of the need for adjunct procedures, such as the creation of a catheterizable urinary stoma, to facilitate CIC.

REFERENCES

1. Young HH. An operation for the cure of incontinence of urine. Surg Gynecol Obstet 1919; 28:84.
2. Young HH. An operation for the cure of incontinence associated with epispadias. J Urol 1922; 7:1.
3. Dees JE. Congenital epispadias with incontinence. J Urol 1949; 62:513.
4. Leadbetter GW. Surgical reconstruction of total urinary incontinence. J Urol 1964; 261:91.
5. Leadbetter GW. Surgical reconstruction for complete urinary incontinence: a 10 to 22 year follow-up. J Urol 1985; 133:205–206.
6. Mollard P. Bladder reconstruction in exstrophy. J Urol 1980; 124:525–529.
7. Lepor H, Jeffs RD. Primary bladder closure and bladder neck reconstruction in classical bladder exstrophy. J Urol 1983; 130:1142–1145.
8. Marshall VJ, Marchetti AA, Krantz KE. The correction of stress urinary incontinence by simple vesicourethral suspension. Surg Gynecol Obstet 1949; 85:590.

9. Bames RW, Wilson WM. Reconstruction of urethra with a tube from the bladder flap. Urol Cutan Rev 1949; 53:604–605.

10. Tanagho EA, Smith DR. The anatomy and function of the bladder neck. Br J Urol 1966; 38:54–71.

11. Tanagho EA, Smith DR, Meyers FH, Fisher R. Mechanism of urinary incontinence: 11 techniques for surgical correction of incontinence. J Urol 1969; 101:305–313.

12. Tanagho EA. Bladder neck reconstruction for total urinary incontinence: ten-year experience. J Urol 1981; 125:321–326.

13. Williams DI, Snyder HM. Anterior detrusor tube repair for urinary incontinence in children. Br J Urol 1976; 48:671–674.

14. Kropp KA, Angwafo FF. Urethral lengthening and reimplantation for neurogenic incontinence in children. J Urol 1986; 135:553–536.

15. Belman AB, Kaplan GW. Experience with the Kropp anti-incontinence procedure. J Urol 1989; 141:1160–1162.

16. Snodgrass W. A simplified Kropp procedure for incontinence. J Urol 1997; 158:1049–1052.

17. Pippi–Salle JL, De Fraga JC, Amarante A, Silveira ML, Lambertz M, Schmidt M, Rosito NC. Urethral lengthening with anterior bladder wall flap for urinary incontinence: a new approach. J Urol 1994; 152:803–806.

18. Koyle MA. Flap valve techniques in bladder neck reconstruction. Dialog Pediatr Urol 1998; 21:6.

19. Hollowel JG, Ransley PG. Surgical management of incontinence in bladder exstrophy. Br J Urol 1991; 68:543–548.

20. Bauer SB, Reda EF, Colodny AH, Retik AB. Detrusor instability: a delayed complication in association with the artificial sphincter. J Urol 1986; 135:1212–1215.

21. Mollard P, Mure PY. Neuropathic bladder: surgery of incontinence. In: Stringer MD, Oldham KT, Mouriquand PDE, et al, eds. Pediatric Surgery and Urology: Long-Term Outcome. London: WB Saunders, 1998; 578–586.

22. Nill TG, Peller PA, Kropp KA. Management of urinary incontinence by bladder tube urethral lengthening and submucosal reimplantation. J Urol 1990; 144:559–563.

23. Mitrofanoff P. Cystotomie transapendiculaire dans le traitements des vessies neurologiques. Chir Pediatr 1980; 21:297–305.

24. Klauber GT, Williams DI. Epispadias with incontinence. J Urol 1974; 111:110–113.

25. Kramer SA, Kelalis PP. Assessment of urinary incontinence in epispadias: review of 94 patients. J Urol 1982; 128:290–293.

26. Perlmutter AD, Weinstein MD, Reitelman C. Vesical neck reconstruction in patients with epispadias–exstrophy complex. J Urol 1991; 146:613–615.

27. Gearhart JP, Canning DA, Jeffs RD. Failed bladder neck reconstruction: options for management. J Urol 1991; 146:1082–1084.

28. Donnahoo KK, Rink RC, Cain MP, Casale AJ. The Young–Dees–Leadbetter bladder neck repair for neurogenic incontinence. J Urol 1999; 161:1946–1949.

29. Gunst MA, Ackerman D, Zingg EG. Eur Urol 1987; 13:62–69.

30. Kryger JV, Gonzales R, Spencer-Barthold J. Surgical management of urinary incontinence in children with neurogenic sphincter incompetence. J Urol 2000; 163:256–263.

41

The Use of Artificial Material in Sling Surgery

MATTHEW L. LEMER

College of Physicians and Surgeons of Columbia University, New York, New York

JONG MYUN CHOE

University of Cincinnati College of Medicine, Cincinnati, Ohio

DAVID R. STASKIN

Harvard Medical School and Beth Israel Deaconess Medical Center Continence Center, Boston, Massachusetts

I. INTRODUCTION

The use of a sling procedure to correct genuine stress urinary incontinence (GSI) in female patients involves placement of autologous or artificial material beneath the bladder neck, the proximal urethra, or both. With the more recent transvaginal tape procedure (TVT), the artificial graft material is placed at the level of the external sphincter.

Sling surgery has been performed classically for severe forms of stress incontinence. The loss of urethral integrity and urethral resistance is now qualified and quantified by the term *intrinsic sphincter deficiency* (ISD), in reference to the lowered urethral closure pressure and lowered urethral resistance. Usually, ISD presents as a well-supported, but open "pipe stem urethra," with or without the loss of bladder neck and urethral support. The etiology of this severe form of urethral dysfunction is associated with denervation or devascularization from conditions such as multiple surgeries, myelodysplasia, or trauma. The concept of urethral dysfunction has evolved and now recognizes the more subtle, complex, and multifactorial etiologies contributing to coaptation, compression, and coordination of the urethral sphincter. More subtle conditions that affect the submucosa, smooth muscle, and skeletal muscle of the sphincter unit are receiving recognition for their contribution to the spectrum of the disorder.

Classically, the sling procedure was thought to work by compressing the urethra. In fact, a "tight" sling was a "good" sling. More recently, it has been recognized that the sling procedure restores continence by a combination of factors, among them (1) suspending the bladder neck and increasing the transmission of intra-abdominal pressure to the proximal urethra, (2) facilitating coaptation of the urethra and increasing intrinsic urethral closure pressure, (3) preventing the "shear force" that is created when the anterior vaginal wall and posterior urethra descend and rotate a greater distance relative to the pubourethral ligaments and anterior urethra, and (4) avoiding "sagging" between the suspension sutures that is occasionally observed with classic repairs and allows persistent bladder neck motion in spite of good paravaginal support.

Patients with deficient periurethral tissue, a condition that predisposes to decreased healing or impaired retropubic scarring, or those who are prone to extreme or chronic increases in intra-abdominal pressure, require a more durable procedure. These patients often have a history of prior vaginal surgery or vaginal atrophy that is secondary to hormonal deprivation. Patients with severe obstructive lung disease or obesity, who challenge classic repairs with frequent, high-pressure "stress" maneuvers, should be considered candidates for sling procedures. Artificial graft material increases the strength of the repair and prevents the erosion of suspension sutures from deficient periurethral or paraurethral tissues.

II. SELECTION OF THE SURGICAL APPROACH

The most logical method of classifying sling procedures with artificial graft material is to consider the sling material and the surgical approach employed. The choice of sling material is covered in a later part of this chapter. Selection of the surgical approach should be made with several considerations: the first is to choose an intervention that minimizes morbidity and ensures optimal success. The surgeon should, therefore, use an anatomically familiar approach. A successful procedure requires accurate placement of the sling beneath the bladder neck and proximal urethra, with a broad base of compression, and the simple and safe passage of the supporting arms of the sling through the retropubic space for attachment. An optimal approach will minimize the risk of damage to the bladder, bladder neck, urethra, and vagina. Surgeons have described abdominal, combined abdominovaginal, and primarily vaginal approaches. A vaginal sling may be a patch sling, with or without perforation, a hemisling, or a complete sling.

The pure abdominal approach involved division of the rectus fascia, entrance into the retropubic space, and placement of the sling beneath the proximal urethra and bladder neck without a vaginal incision. The abdominovaginal approach combines abdominal entrance into the retropubic space with a vaginal incision. Combined vaginal incision aids in accurate placement of the body of the sling beneath the urethra and creates a controlled vaginal opening that is intentionally closed over the graft material. The vaginal approach employs a vaginal incision for placement of the body of the sling, and usually relies on instrument passage of the arms of the sling into the retropubic space to attach to retropubic bone achors, or above the rectus fascia without opening it.

A. The Abdominal Approach

The use of the pure abdominal approach should be limited to those patients for whom the lithotomy position is contraindicated (e.g., decreased mobility of the hip or severe spinal problems), the rare circumstance when a sling is erected intraoperatively (e.g., inability to obtain sufficient periurethral or paraurethral tissue mobilization to perform a classic suspension), or when positioning of the legs in the lithotomy position limits exposure for concomitant abdominal procedures (e.g., bladder augmentation or abdominal hysterectomy). If the lithotomy position is contraindicated, a frog-legged position is preferred, which affords vaginal access for intraoperative palpation of the bladder neck during sling passage.

The tissue superficial to the mid- and distal urethra consists of periurethral fascia and the overlying anterior vaginal wall. There is limited fibroareolar tissue space for dissection in this plane. Anatomically, this space is too distal to be used for sling placement, for postoperative obstruction is the all-too-common result. The proper plane for dissection is at the level of the proximal urethra–vesical neck, in the vesicovaginal plane. If prior incontinence surgery or cystocele repair has been performed, dissection within this plane beneath the bladder neck may be more difficult secondary to scar tissue. During a pure abdominal approach, the bladder should be opened before dissection of the tunnel for the sling. Transvesical exposure of the bladder neck allows palpation during dissection beneath the bladder neck and visualization of the bladder neck area to assure that the sling has not been placed within the bladder or urethra. Early postoperative sling erosion into the urethra is too often a misnomer for a sling that was placed through the urethral wall at the time of surgery. To avoid damage to the urethra or bladder neck, the plane for dissection of the sling tunnel should begin proximal to the level of the bladder neck where the vesical fascia can be separated more easily from the anterior vaginal wall. Distal dissection beneath the urethra is facilitated once this plane has been developed more proximally. In situations during which the plane beneath the bladder neck and proximal urethra is difficult to develop, it may be best to enter the vagina. The vaginal wall will subsequently have to be mobilized to cover the artificial sling as the vagina will not granulate over the foreign material, but this avoids more ominous urethral injury.

B. The Abdominovaginal Approach

The addition of a vaginal counterincision for sling placement is highly recommended when the abdominal approach is used, as it provides improved exposure. The abdominovaginal approach combines an abdominal incision, which is used for dissection within the retropubic space, with an anterior vaginal wall vertical flap incision, which allows direct exposure beneath the bladder neck. This approach permits the formation of paraurethral tunnels by combined abdominal and vaginal routes. A relaxed lithotomy position provides adequate exposure for the abdominal and vaginal portions of the surgery. The ability to pass the sling below the urethra and bladder neck, without fear of unintentionally perforating the anterior vaginal wall, significantly decreases the amount of retropubic space dissection required for exposure of the bladder neck. A vertical or Pfannensteil skin incision can be performed, its size being determined purely by the need for retropubic space exposure. However, the need for an abdominal incision to enter the retropubic space is obviated by the pure vaginal approach.

C. The Vaginal Approach

Similar to the abdominovaginal approach, the vaginal approach uses a vertical or flap incision in the vaginal wall for placement of the sling at the bladder neck under direct vision. With this strategy, the supporting arms of the sling are passed with a clamp, a pilot suture, or a suspension needle through tunnels or canals formed by instrument, or finger dissection within the retropubic space. The tunnels can be formed from above (abdominally to vaginally) or below. The tunneling maneuver eliminates the need for splitting the rectus musculature and opening the retropubic space. A more acute lithotomy position can be employed for improved vaginal exposure. A small abdominal skin incision to the level of the rectus fascia is required for securing the arms of the sling.

The advantage of the vaginal approach is decreased exposure of the retropubic space compared with the previously discussed approaches. The primary disadvantage of the vaginal approach is the increased risk of bladder, bladder neck, or urethral injury during blind passage of the arms of the sling. The vaginal approach will be reviewed in detail later in this chapter.

A vaginal sling may be composed of a simple patch, which is supported by sutures, without perforation of the endopelvic fascia or entrance into the retropubic space. Perforation of the endopelvic fascia and attachment of the graft to these edges is also preferred. With the hemisling technique, the graft material is brought into the retropubic space, but is supported by suture material before attachment. A complete sling is taken completely through the retropubic space and attached above the rectus fascia. Differentiation of a patch, hemisling, and complete sling may not be as important when using artificial graft material as when using fascia, dermis, or another collagen matrix material. The durability and strength of artificial material ensures that a patch sling will not rely on retropubic space scarring for a permanent result. Entrance into the retropubic space is not as critical with artificial graft material. The possibility of infection or degradation of a collagen matrix graft requires scarring within the retropubic space. A hemisling with scarring to the pubic bone or obturators, or an uninterrupted scar bridge with a complete sling, may be the preferred method for collagen-based materials. This principle may also hold true for abdominal or abdominovaginal slings that employ sutures to bridge the gap during collagen-based slings. Erosion of the suture from the sling material, which is not seen with artificial graft material, may result in sling failure if scarring has not already taken place.

III. ADVANTAGES OF ARTIFICIAL SLING MATERIAL

Surgeons now have several options of sling material. The major decision involves the use of organic versus artificial material. Artificial slings have been fashioned as continuous pieces of material that comprise both the body as well as the arms of the sling or, alternatively, as patches or grafts that are placed beneath the urethra with the supporting arms provided by nonabsorbable suture. The choice of artificial sling material simplifies the operative procedure in that the graft is readily available and does not require harvesting from a second operative site. The readiness and ease of preparation decreases operative time, patient discomfort, postoperative complications from a second incision, such as seroma or infection, and difficulty obtaining tissue from an obese patient. Artificial sling material is packaged in several predetermined graft lengths. This ensures adequate sling length intraoperatively and minimizes the possibility that the strip harvested from the rectus fascia or fascia lata will be too short for the intended procedure. Endogenous fascia of a patient undergoing a sling operation and commercially processed allogenic fascia may be weak and suboptimal. The use of man-made material bypasses these potential problems by ensuring uniformity and reliable sling strength.

Acceptable artificial graft materials are chemically and physically inert, durable, and noncarcinogenic. Although the biocompatability of many artificial materials has been demonstrated, their use does increase the risk of infection and possible subsequent erosion into the urethra or vagina. Broad-spectrum intravenous and oral antibiotics, which provide gram-positive, gram-negative, and anerobic coverage thorough preoperative vaginal preparation, can significantly decrease the incidence of infection. Infective risk is also decreased by employing the least amount of foreign material necessary to correct the incontinence and by decreasing intraoperative exposure time of the material. Vaginal erosion may be caused by infection of the artificial material and necessitates removal. Many patients who require excision of the infected or eroded material still remain continent. Presumably, their continence is due to persistent support from scar tissue that has formed.

Contraindications to using artificial graft material include known allergy to inorganic material, a history of previous rejection of artificial material, and lack of patient acceptance. Artificial sling graft material should not be used in the presence of urethral injury from a previous surgery (i.e., fistula or urethral sloughing), or if urethral injury occurs during the course of sling placement. A relative contraindication is the presence of excessively thin hypoestrogenic vaginal mucosa.

IV. ARTIFICAL GRAFT MATERIALS

Choosing which artificial graft material to use is typically based on the surgeon's preference and experience. Most artificial grafts are permanent and nondegradable. Short-term results with polyglactin mesh (Vicryl), an absorbable artificial material, were reported by Fianu and Soderburg (1) and appeared promising, but no further information is available. Absorbable, similar to nonabsorbable, artificial sling material benefits the patient by ease of availability and decreased operative time, but may also provide benefit by reducing the long-term risk of sling infection and erosion from permanent artificial materials. Uniformity and tissue strength have not been clinically proved with available absorbable materials.

The nonabsorbable artificial materials that have been used for suburethral sling procedures include nylon, Perlon, polyethylene terephthalate (Mersilene ribbon or mesh), polypropylene (Marlex mesh), polytetrafluoroethylene (PTFE, Teflon, Gore-tex), and Silastic. These materials differ in composition, weave, porosity, and flexibility. The differences in their chemical and physical properties alter their individual propensities to scarification, injury to surrounding tissues, infection, and rejection.

Mersilene mesh is a polyester mesh composed of multifilament fibers of polyethylene terephthalate. Marlex mesh is a monofilament mesh composed of polypropylene. Gore-tex is expanded Teflon, a multifilament mesh of PTFE, the production of which is a trade secret. The Silastic sheet consists of medical-grade silicone rubber reinforced with woven polyethylene terephthalate.

Theoretically, monofilament mesh withstands infection better than multifilament mesh. The propensity to infection with multifilament fibers is related to the differential entry of small bacteria, compared with larger macrophages and polymorphonuclear leukocytes, into small interstices between filaments. This does not occur with monofilament mesh.

The size, shape, and number of pores, or mesh porosity, influences the development of fibrous scarification to adjacent tissue. Tissue bonding is a double-edge sword, with bonding beneficial to the healing process and in rendering support, the goal of incontinence procedures. On the other hand, intense scarification between the implanted mesh and surrounding tissue can make mesh removal technically difficult. Based on the work of Pourdeyhimi (2), Mersilene is known to have the greatest porosity; therefore, it becomes embedded in fibrous scarification, bonding the mesh firmly to adjacent structures. Likewise, Marlex mesh acts as a scaffold on which connective tissue can grow (3). On the other hand, PTFE mesh bonds poorly to surrounding tissue owing to larger pore size and chemical composition. Mesh flexibility is greatest with Gore-tex and least with Marlex, a fact that may relate to the propensity of Marlex to erode into adjacent tissue (4). Historically, surgeons have looked to alternative, inorganic materials from which to fashion the suburethral sling and give support to the urethrovesical junction. In 1951, Bracht was the first to describe the use of inorganic material, reporting on the use of a nylon cord (5). This was followed by the work of Anselmino, who used Perlon in 1952, and of Zoedler who used nylon in 1961 (5). Williams and Telinde, as well as Ridley, fashioned slings from Mersilene ribbon (6). These early artificial slings caused problems with urethral obstruction, retention, and even urethral transection owing to their cord-like configuration that placed direct pressure on the urethra at a narrow location along its length.

A. Polyethylene Terephthalate (Mersilene)

In 1968, Moir (7) adapted the use of a wider strip of Mersilene mesh to the Aldridge sling procedure that stabilized the suburethral sling graft to the aponeurosis of the abdominal wall. The initial series by Moir reported an 83% cure or substantial improvement in incontinence, but did not specifically mention postoperative complications.

Surgeons have continued to use the Mersilene gauze hammock sling operation over the ensuing 30 years with continued success. Investigators have reported a 73–96% subjective cure rate (8–13). Recently, Young et al. (13) objectively evaluated the Mersilene gauze hammock procedure with pre- and postoperative urodynamic testing, showing a 93% objective cure rate. The study found no significant change in maximum urethral closure pressure postoperatively, except in the subgroup of patients with a preoperative low-pressure urethra. This subset of patients, with a mean preoperative maximum urethral closure pressure of 15 cmH$_2$O showed a mean increase of 8.6 cmH$_2$O (57%) postoperatively. A significant increase in the pressure transmission ratio from a mean of 75% preoperatively to 112% (p < 0.0001) postoperatively was also found.

A lower indication of complications, specifically voiding dysfunction and urinary retention, was noted compared with previously used cord slings. This was attributed to the wider width of the sling graft underlying the bladder neck. However, problems with erosion of the artificial graft into adjacent structures and abscess and sinus formation at vaginal and abdominal sites continued to occur. Patients also experienced urinary retention and voiding dysfunction owing to excessive tension on the graft during placement.

B. Polypropylene (Marlex Mesh)

Following this example of broader bladder neck support, Morgan et al. (14–16) described the use of a wide band of Marlex mesh, placed by a two-team approach through both abdominal and vaginal routes, and attached to the iliopectineal ligament bilaterally. Marlex was chosen as the graft material because of its inert properties and monofilament composition, which were thought to bypass the extensive scarring and infection associated with polyethylene terephthalate.

The Marlex mesh suburethral sling has been used by different centers around the world, with subjective cure rates ranging from 79 to 100% (14–19). One small study performed postoperative urodynamic testing and reported a 70% objective cure at 3 months. Long-term objective cure rates are unknown.

In the initial series of 20 patients, Morgan (14) reported two cases requiring sling removal because of urinary retention in one case and development of a vesicovaginal fistula in the other. Further experience by Morgan and other investigators (14–19) continued to find an increased incidence of infection, sinus formation, urethral obstruction and vaginal or urethral erosion requiring sling revision or removal. Most concerning has been the propensity of Marlex to cause trauma to the urethra (14–19).

C. Polytetrafluoroethylene

The use of Teflon tape to suspend the urethrovesical junction was described in 1981 by Cato (20), but this initial procedure is not considered a sling, as no graft was placed suburethrally. The use of expanded Teflon—Gore-tex—was first reported in 1988 by Horback et al. (21) for a combined vaginal and abdominal approach to placement of a full-circle "standard" strip sling attached to the aponeurosis of the rectus fascia. The investigators employed the suburethral sling specifically for patients with urodynamically diagnosed GSI, with a low-pressure urethra (< 20 cmH$_2$O). Eighty-five percent of patients were subjectively cured at 3 months, with 11 of 13 (84.6%) cured objectively. At 1-year subjective follow-up, 12 of 13 (92%) were continent. Postoperative urodynamic testing revealed an improvement of urodynamic parameters, specifically a significant increase in maximum urethral closure pressure from a mean of 11.4 to 36.1 cmH$_2$O ($p < 0.02$). Patients with a hypermobile urethrovesical junction preoperatively had restoration of normal urethrovesical junction support based on normalization of their Q-tip test.

Summit et al. (22) followed a larger cohort of patient for 10 months and reported an 82% objective cure rate with the suburethral Gore-tex sling. The major postoperative complication experienced was that of delayed return to normal voiding, with a mean time to suprapubic catheter removal of 21.6 days. Two (4.2%) patients required sling revision to relieve outlet obstruction. Delayed complications of vaginal erosion (5, or 10.5%) and sinus tract formation (1, or 2.1%) also resulted in removal of the Gore-tex sling. All patients remained continent following sling removal.

In another study designed to evaluate the long-term clinical and urodynamic outcomes of the Gore-tex suburethral sling, 62 patients were followed for 1 year postoperatively, and urodynamic testing was repeated (23). Seventy-three percent of patients were subjectively cured of stress incontinence and 61% were objectively cured. There was a significant increase in maximum urethral closure pressure postoperatively with a 33% incidence of de novo detrusor instability (DI). The incidence of artificial graft complications requiring partial or complete graft removal was 22%: 10 for sinus tract formation, 4 for persistent vaginal granulation tissue, 3 for anterior vaginal wall erosion, and 1 for persistent groin pain.

In a separate investigation, the same center histologically evaluated slings that were removed because of abdominal or vaginal rejection of the sling material, with nonhealing at that site or the development of a sinus tract (24). Sling rejection or removal occurred in 20 (or 20%) of 115 patients. Histology revealed gram-positive cocci in all Gore-tex patch interstices as well as fibrous tissue, fibroblasts, and collagen. These findings suggest an infective process that begins at or following graft placement that results in nonhealing of the operative site. Interestingly, 75% of patients remained continent following removal of the sling, which was attributed to the characteristic fibrous sheath that forms around Gore-tex after placement and is not removed with the graft.

In trying to minimize the risk of infection and graft rejection, surgeons have tried to decrease the amount of artificial graft material used in the operation. The result has been the evolution of "patch" slings, rather than the more traditional complete sling or hemi-sling. A description of this technique and the results of a series of our patients undergoing a Gore-tex patch sling are detailed later in this chapter.

D. Silastic

Because of difficulties in revising slings once placed, Stanton et al. (25) suggested the use of a medical-grade Silastic sheet for the suburethral sling graft. The tissue reaction to Silastic is minimal, with formation of only a thin fibrous sheath around the graft material. Much like Gore-tex, which exhibits minimal bonding to the surrounding tissue, this characteristic of Silastic allows easy revision or removal of the sling if necessary. In the initial report on the use of Silastic slings, Stanton recorded an 83% objective cure rate at 1 year. Four (13.3%) patients required release or removal of the sling owing to voiding difficulties. The procedure described involves an abdominal approach with creation of a suburethral tunnel for passage of the sling graft. The Silastic graft is attached to the iliopectineal ligament. Other reported complications involve intraoperative entry into the bladder, urethra, and vagina, all of which are related to the surgical abdominal approach.

Chin and Stanton (26) reported long-term results of the Silastic sling procedure in a large cohort of 88 patients. There was no postoperative infection requiring sling removal. However, sling erosion into adjacent structures occurred in 10 patients (11.4%), including the vagina (5%), bladder (4%), and urethra (1%). Four other patients required sling release or removal secondary to voiding difficulties. Other reasons for removal included intractable groin pain (2%) and strangulated hernia (1%). Korda et al. (27,28) reported their experience with the Silastic sling procedure. In spite of a 80.6% subjective cure rate, 24% of patients required sling revision to establish postoperative voiding, 4.5% underwent sling removal for sinus tract formation and for intractable pain, and 3% developed de novo DI.

E. Antibiotic-Treated Synthetic Slings

Two new sling materials consist of synthetic mesh impregnated with collagen and treated with antibiotics. These are Meadox and Protegen, both of which have been used previously as vascular prostheses. These materials have been removed recently from commercial sale by the manufacturer owing to the high rate of vaginal erosion.

F. Bone Anchors

Most reported techniques rely on attachment of the abdominal ends of the sling to the rectus aponeurosis, either in situ as in Aldridge's original description, or, as in more modern descriptions, through small incisions just above the pubic symphysis, and direct suture to the rectus sheath or Cooper's ligament. The abdominal ends of the sling can also be positioned with bone anchors embedded into the symphysis pubis. This is proposed to more accurately reposition the urethra and to provide support at the junction of the proximal urethra.

The concept of a patch sling has been teamed recently with the use of bone anchors in an attempt to provide a fixed site of attachment for the sling. Kovac and Cruikshank (29) reported a 100% subjective cure rate in 25 patients undergoing this procedure with a 4-year follow-up, and no incidence of infection, rejection, or erosion. A 91.4% cure rate at 8 months was found among 35 women undergoing a similar polypropylene mesh patch sling attached to bone anchors embedded in the pubic tubercles (30). Again, no postoperative complications have been experienced that have required revision or removal of the sling. The risk of osteomyelitis from bone anchors has been reported by Maktov et al. (31).

G. Tension-Free Vaginal Tape (TVT) Procedure

This relatively new technique is based on the premise that stress incontinence results from failure of the pubourethral ligaments in the midurethra (32,33), which led to the proposal of "an integrated theory for the maintenance" (34–36) of female stress incontinence. In this model, continence is maintained at the midurethra and not at the bladder neck.

The TVT procedure uses a knitted prolene mesh tape that is covered by a removable plastic sheath and is placed at the midurethra (37) (Fig. 1). The tape is inserted through a small vaginal incision using two 6-mm trocars. Because of the weave of the tape, it is self-retaining. The procedure can be performed under local or regional anesthesia, allowing the position of the tape to be adjusted during a series of coughs, at which time, the plastic sheath is removed and fine adjustments are made. The aim is to have the tape lying free at rest (hence, "tension-free") and to exert only sufficient pressure on the urethra during a cough to prevent leakage of urine.

A multicenter study carried out in six centers in Scandinavia on women with no previous surgery for incontinence shows a 91% cure rate after 1 year (38). In another report, Ulmsten (39) demonstrates an 86% complete cure rate and an 11% significant improvement rate, with no long-term voiding difficulties or de novo detrusor instability at a 3-year follow-up. Other groups using this device have also begun to report their results, with similar outcomes, but a relatively high rate (4–8%) of bladder injury (40–42). Hilton and Ward have recently published results from 50 women, 40% of whom had previously undergone at lease one incontinence operation. Their results show an 88% objective cure rate as a primary procedure and 75% as a secondary procedure. However, 4 women in this study developed long-term voiding difficulties and required CISC (43).

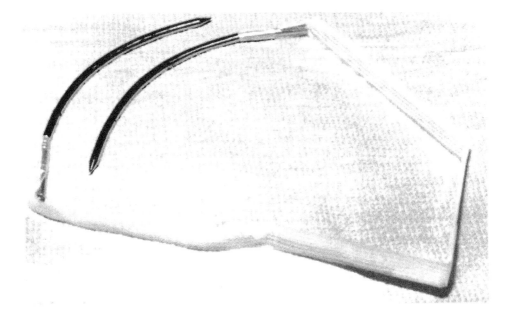

Figure 1 The tension-free vaginal tape (TVT).

The procedure differs from traditional slings in that it is not placed at the bladder neck, but at the midthird of the urethra, replacing the support normally provided by the pub-ourethral ligaments. Although initial reports demonstrate good results, numbers are limited and, even if this technique avoids the need for a suprapubic incision, it also introduces the possibility of complications arising from the use of bone anchoring, in particular os-teomyelitis. It is still unclear whether this technique offers any advantage over fixation of the sling to the abdominal wall.

V. COMPLICATIONS OF SLING SURGERY

A. General Complications

The general surgical complications are no higher with sling surgery than with other vagi-nal or suprapubic operations. Wound hematoma rates of near 3% and postoperative urinary infection of 5% have been reported (44). Pain at the site of sling attachment to the rectus fascia is specific to the sling, although it is rarely reported. Dyspareunia is also very rarely reported.

B. Postoperative Voiding Difficulties

The relatively high incidence of voiding difficulties following sling surgery has been one of the most significant factors preventing more widespread use of this technique (45). Subu-rethral slings are reputed to be more obstructive than other incontinence operations, with an incidence of retention varying from 2.2–16% and 1.5–7.8% requiring long-term self-catheterizations (5).

In a systematic review of surgery for stress incontinence, Jarvis (46) found a mean in-cidence of postoperative voiding disorders of 12.8% (range 2–37%). However, this figure includes one study by Korda et al. (27,28) in which 28% of women required further surgery to reduce sling tension before voiding could take place. When the figures from this study are removed, the result is a mean of 10.8% (range 2–20%).

Postoperative voiding difficulties may occur as a result of either poor detrusor func-tion or as a result of urethral obstruction. Poor detrusor function may be identified preop-eratively using free and pressure–flow studies (47). Women with suboptimal detrusor func-tion need to be warned of the risk of prolonged postoperative voiding difficulties and the potential need for long-term clean intermittent self-catheterization (CISC) (48). Urethral obstruction may occur as a result of excessive sling tension. Hilton (49) found a significant reduction in peak urine flow rate and a small rise in maximum voiding pressure following sling surgery, suggesting that a slight degree of urethral obstruction occurs.

Prolonged catheterization following fascial (10,51) sling placement is 12–60 days, with up to 15% of women performing CISC, whereas, following Mersiline (8) sling place-ment, 11% of women catheterized for longer than 14 days and, after Marlex (17) graft placement, 9% of women catheterized for 3–6 months, and 1% developed permanent re-tention.

Recently, the importance of avoiding excessive sling tension has been recognized, and there is a trend for slings to be placed under less tension or even completely loose (52); this may reduce the incidence of voiding dysfunction. Appell (53) reports only 2% of women required long-term CISC with fascial slings placed under minimal tension.

Prediction of which women are most at risk of developing postoperative voiding dif-ficulties seems difficult. A higher incidence of voiding difficulties has been described following colposuspension in women voiding using a Valsalva maneuver (54). This was not found by McLennan et al. (55) in a study of voiding following fascia lata sling procedures. Age over 65, low urine flow rate (less than 20 mL), and concomitant surgery appeared to increase the risk of delayed spontaneous voiding. The retention rate of 5% was lower in this study than in previous reports. Again, the authors ascribe this to reduced sling tension.

C. Postoperative Detrusor Instability

Detrusor instability arising after bladder neck surgery appears inevitable in some cases. The reported incidence of postoperative symptoms of urge incontinence varies widely, from 3–30%. In a review of published series, the American Urological Association (AUA) found the incidence of de novo DI to be 7% (95% confidence interval [CI] 3–11%) (56). Whether this is due to preexisting DI, undiagnosed by preoperative cystometry, or as has been suggested, owing to denervation following surgical dissection is unclear. Overelevation of the bladder neck, excessive sling tension, and irritation of the bladder neck by synthetic sling materials have also been implicated. It may be significant that one of the studies reporting the highest rate of de novo DI of 33% involved the use of a Gore-tex sling (23). In this study, postoperative urethral pressure measurement showed a significant increase in MUCP. This supports the view that excess tension, combined with the use of an unyielding synthetic material, increases the incidence of de novo DI and voiding difficulties. However, postoperative voiding dysfunction is common to all suburethral sling procedures, and is probably more a reflection of surgical technique than sling material.

Early studies did not investigate the occurrence of urge incontinence symptoms in relation to the sling procedure, so little is known about the incidence with the use of Mersilene and Marlex. In more recent studies assessing the success of Gore-tex, preoperative and postoperative urodynamic testing has been used to indicate clearly the rates of persistent and de novo detrusor instability (21–23,57). These rates are significant, with up to a 77% rate of persistence and a 66% rate of de novo detrusor instability related to the use of standard or patch Gore-tex slings. Subjective rates of persistent and de novo detrusor instability with the use of Silastic slings have similarly been as high as 61.5–100% and 3.7–66.7%, respectively (25–28). Although it may not be possible to eliminate problems from postoperative DI, it seems sensible to attempt to limit this by appropriate preoperative urodynamic investigations, patient selection, and proper sling tension.

D. Postoperative Graft Erosion

Problems related to erosion of the sling material, either through the vagina or urethra, appear to be encountered almost exclusively with artificial sling materials. Although the incidence of such problems is low, graft erosion can pose a formidable management problem. Chronic inflammation around an artificial sling may cause erosion of the adjacent vaginal and urethral epithelial surfaces (58,59), formation of a chronic sinus with persistent vaginal discharge, or a vesicovaginal fistula, and destruction of the urethral sphincter. A chronic inflammatory response occurs either because of the inherent tissue reaction of the material itself, or more probably, owing to chronic infection. Even in an era of easy access to broad-spectrum antibiotic chemoprophylaxis, caution needs to be exercised when insertion of a foreign body into a potentially contaminated wound is contemplated.

An assessment of the true incidence of such problems is difficult; many early reports of new sling techniques do not describe the incidence of sling erosion, even when materials that are now well known to cause problems are used. Gore-tex has been associated with a high rate of local infection and sling removal of up to 23% in some studies (24). It appears that the microporous structure actually inhibits in-growth of fibrous tissue and, possibly, provides areas for bacterial colonization and chronic infection (60) that are inaccessible to antibiotics. Infection rates with Gore-tex may relate to graft size and technique and have been reported in "patch" procedures to be less than 3% (61).

Marlex has a large open weave mesh, which should allow free in-growth of fibrous tissue. Nonetheless, nonhealing of the vaginal wall appears to be a particular problem with this material and is reported as occurring in 6.2 and 7% of cases (17,19). Not all reports, however, demonstrate such high complication rates with Marlex. In a 16-year review of the Marlex sling operation, Morgan et al. (15) report a success rate of 80% with two cases of urethral transection, but no other graft-related complications.

Low rates of erosion and mesh removal of Mersilene mesh have been ascribed to its open weave, flexibility, and thinness. In one study, three women (3.6%) had complications related to mesh erosion after a mean follow-up of 16 months (13). And in another recent study, 7 women (6%) who had undergone Mersilene mesh suburethral sling procedures developed varying degrees of mesh visible in the vagina, 1–3 months after the operation (62). These erosions were treated by conservative surgical management, including trimming of the visible mesh, removal of adjacent granulation tissue, and vaginal wall reapproximation. Six patients (87%) were successfully treated by this conservative management, and only one woman required an additional office-based revision. Urethral transaction with artificial sling materials has also been described. The Mersilene tape was most often associated with this complication, and its use has thus been abandoned (63).

Interestingly, where sling erosion and infection have necessitated resection or division of the sling material, continence is often maintained, reinforcing the view that it is the fibrosis induced by the sling that provides urethral support, rather than the material itself (26).

Complication rates with artificial materials may be underreported because erosion can occur relatively late, at 1–4 years postoperatively (23). Promising early results of surgery are often submitted for publication, and late adverse events are less likely to be reported. As new techniques become more widely used, complications, such as erosion, become more widely encountered. But it is often 10 or more years before the true incidence of such problems becomes apparent. Initial success with a novel artificial graft material, therefore, must be judged cautiously until long-term results are available. Review of the available publications indicates that the incidence of significant problems associated with artificial materials, excluding Gore-tex, appears to be low, in the region of 1–6%. Complications with Gore-tex have been higher, in the region of 3–23%.

VI. GORE-TEX PATCH PLACEMENT USING THE VAGINAL APPROACH

Our preferred sling approach is a vaginal approach, with a Gore-tex patch, which is suspended by two Gore-tex sutures (Figs. 2 and 3) (61,64). We currently perform this procedure without mobilization of the endopelvic fascia ("nonperforated") and with mobilization of the endopelvic fascia. ("perforated"). The nonperforated (see Fig. 2) patch sling is a needle procedure similar to a Stamey. The suspension needles are passed bilaterally, a cystoscopy is performed, and if the needles are not in the bladder, the sutures that were preattached to the sling are transferred through the retropubic space. We use this technique when the patient has stress incontinence caused by urethral hypermobility with classic type II rotation of the bladder neck. The sling stabilizes the periurethral tissue as the urethra rotates posteriorly.

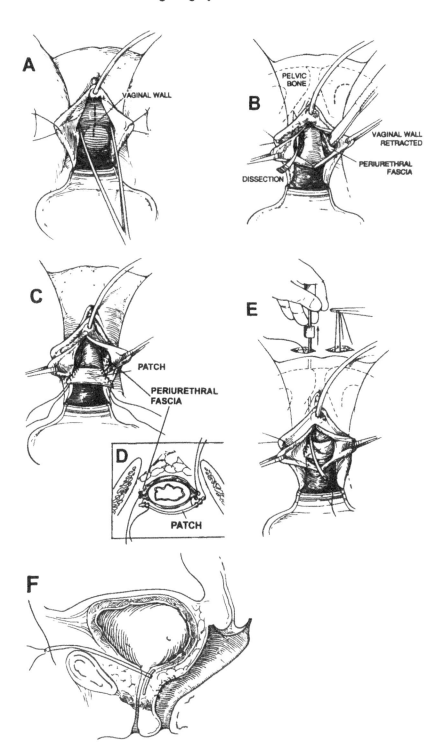

Figure 2 (A–F) Technique of the nonperforated Gore-tex patch sling. Sutures are passed into the retropubic space without breakage of the endopelvic fascia and extensive dissection of the retropubic space. The graft material sits entirely on the vaginal surface of the endopelvic fascia.

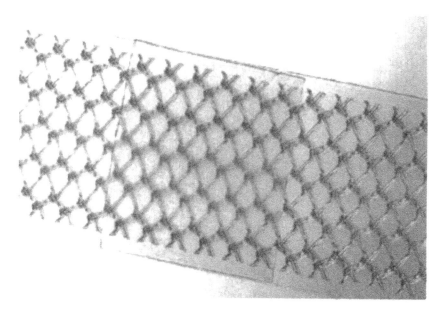

Figure 3   Gore-tex patch material.

The perforated patch sling (not illustrated) is similar to a Raz suspension. The endopelvic fascia is mobilized, the sling is sutured to the edge of the mobilized medial edge of the periurethral tissue, and the suspension needles are then used to transfer the individual sutures through the retropubic space. We employ this technique when there is ISD. Mobilization of the endopelvic fascia provides a "cradling" of the urethra that is not provided without mobilization. This cradling effect has been demonstrated to provide a more efficient "backboard" for urethral pressure transmission in our preliminary urodynamic analysis.

A.   Positioning and Exposure

The patient is positioned in a full lithotomy position. After a weighted vaginal speculum is inserted, a 16F. Foley catheter is placed for drainage. The bladder neck is identified by palpation of the Foley balloon, with care not to place any tension on the catheter. Ten to twenty-five milliliters of sterile saline is injected into the vesicovaginal space, at the level of the bladder neck and laterally, to facilitate dissection. An Allis clamp is placed 2 cm distal to the bladder neck and a 4- to 5-cm longitudinal incision is made. A longitudinal incision is preferred over a U-shaped incision, as it avoids necrosis of the tip of the U caused by devascularization, and avoids having the artificial graft cross the incision twice when the incision is closed. Dissection is undertaken laterally in the vesicovaginal plane, parallel to the periurethral fascia, to the inferior aspect of the pubic rami. [Antibiotic solution is used to irrigate all incisions throughout the surgery. Patients are given gentamicin and ampicillin (or vancomycin) preoperatively.]

B. Formation of the Patch

The width of the patch is determined by placing a large forceps into the paravaginal spaces at the level of the bladder neck. This measurement ensures that the patch width will be adequate for each individual. The patch is standard 1-mm thick Gore-tex, measured to a standard of 2 cm in height. Two 2-0 Gore-tex sutures (THX-26) are used to secure the medial edge of the patch. If a non-perforated patch sling is planned, the needles are removed. If a perforated patch sling is indicated, the needles are left on the suture so that the patch can be secured to the medial edge of the mobilized endopelvic (periurethral) fascia.

C. Nonperforated Sling

At the level of the bladder neck, Metzenbaum scissors are used to perforate the endopelvic fascia with a small hole. Unlike the Raz procedure, the scissors are not opened, and finger dissection is not performed. Through a small suprapubic incision of choice, the suspension needles are passed through the retropubic space onto the finger that is placed at the site of the small perforation.

A cystoscopy is performed and a suprapubic tube is inserted with the suspension needles in place. Sling sutures can be inserted in the suspension needles and brought through the retropubic space if they are not in the bladder. The patch can be centered (it does not need to be secured into place because it cannot migrate through the limited periurethral perforations, and the vaginal wall can be closed immediately.

D. Perforated Sling

After the retropubic space is entered by sharp perforation, the scissors are opened, withdrawn in the opened position, and a limited (enough for the finger to enter) dissection of the periurethral fascia is performed. The retropubic space is not completely mobilized. Blunt perforation is not used, because it creates a defect through the weakest portion of the periurethral tissue, often more medial to the urethra. The pubourethral ligaments may be palpated medial to the dissecting finger, and dissection of these structures or dissection across the midline above these structures is not required. The same maneuver is now performed on the patient's right side. Bleeding encountered during these maneuvers is usually from the edge of the periurethral fascia that has been mobilized from the pubic bone. Attempts to obtain hemostasis by clamping or cauterizing should be reserved until after the sutures have been placed; often, they will incorporate the area responsible for most of the bleeding.

The patch is brought onto the field and the suspension sutures are incorporated into the mobilized edge of the periurethral fascia, as in a Raz procedure. If the periurethral tissue is severely deficient, a "bite" of the posterior surface of the anterior vaginal wall lateral to the incision is taken, to provide a reference point for tension when tying the sutures at the termination of the procedure. The sutures are then passed individually through the retropubic space. The vaginal wall is closed.

E. Suture Tying

The sutures are tied with "no tension." They are pulled up with minimal tension, released, and then tied at that level over the rectus fascia. If the endopelvic fascia has been mobilized, it is possible to overcorrect the bladder neck, even without tension, because the urethra is mobilized. In these patients, a finger is placed in the paravaginal fornix while adjusting sling tension where the aforementioned stitch is located during securing of the patch. When the vaginal finger can feel the fornix begin to elevate, the sling is tied at this level.

VII. RESULTS

Between December 1989 and September 1994, 141 patients with urodynamically documented stress and mixed incontinence underwent a GPS (62). Complete follow-up was available in 90 patients. Forty-three women (30.3%) could not be located. The remaining 8 (5.9%) failed to respond or answer the telephone follow-up. Mean age was 54.2 years (range 32–86). Mean follow-up was 51 months (range 27–84).

Of the 90 patients, 43 (48%) had at least one previous anti-incontinence procedure. Prior endoscopic needle suspensions were reported in 27 patients, retropubic suspensions in 9, and anterior repairs for incontinence in 8. Mean vaginal parity was 2.7 (range 1–11). Thirty-eight (42%) patients had undergone a previous hysterectomy.

Videourodynamic studies revealed that 31 (34%) had pure anatomical urethral hypermobility, 15 (17%) had pure intrinsic sphincter deficiency, and 44 (49%) had combined pathophysiology. Pure stress incontinence was observed in 42 of 90 (46.7%) patients, and mixed incontinence was present in 48 of 90 (53.3%).

Stress incontinence was cured in 80 of the 90 (88.9%) patients. Of the remaining 10 patients, 4 had persistent stress incontinence and 6 manifested mixed (stress and urge) symptomatology. In 4 patients with persistent postoperative stress incontinence, mean daily pad use decreased from 4.4 to 1.8 ($p < 0.05$). On an incontinence scale of 1–5 (5 = severe incontinence), 2 of 4 patients reported a score of 1 of 5, and the group as a whole, had a mean score of 1.5 of 5. The patients recorded an overall improvement score of 68%.

Preoperative urge incontinence resolved in 31 of 48 (65%) patients. De novo urge incontinence developed in 5 of 52 (9.6%). Sixteen patients had pure urge incontinence postoperatively. They reported a decrease in mean pad use from 3.6 to 2.8 ($p < 0.05$). On a scale of 1–5 (5 = severe incontinence), 10 of 16 patients rated their incontinence as 1.5 of 5, and overall mean rating was 2.1 of 5. The patients reported an overall improvement score of 43%.

The suprapubic tube was removed within 1 week of surgery in 81 of 90 (90%) patients. Two patients had urodynamically proved urethral obstruction; both required incision of the sling. Seven patients required temporary clean intermittent catheterization lasting 3 months for urinary retention; incision of the sling was indicated in 2 of 7 patients. All are now voiding spontaneously with residual urine volumes less than 75 mL. The mean time to resumption of normal activity was 3.1 weeks (range 1–12).

Five patients required excision of the sling for persistent nonhealing of the vaginal incision, with the presence of granulation tissue. The mean interval from initial surgery to excision was 8.4 months. Of these five patients, two had recurrent stress incontinence, two had pure urge incontinence, and one remained dry. Transvaginal incision of the sling was indicated in six patients. The mean interval from initial surgery to incision was 2.3 months. Stress incontinence has not occurred in any of the six patients, but one developed pure urge incontinence.

When the patients were surveyed in 1994 (unpublished data), as opposed to 1996 (62), the continence rate for the group was 96 of 121 (88%). The continence rates were similar. In addition, the complication rates were also similar. The results were long-lasting. Of the 11 patients who were reoperated on, 7 were between 1989 and 1992, which may very well reflect the initial learning curve of any sling procedure. The patients who were un-happy acknowledged that the source of their dissatisfaction was postoperative urge incon-tinence, rather than persistent stress incontinence.

VIII. CONCLUSIONS

There is little doubt that sling operations, in expert hands, can produce very good results. The type of sling material chosen probably does not affect outcome in terms of cure rates, provided that the characteristics of the chosen material are considered carefully. The princi-pal difference between organic and artificial material is in the complication rate because of chronic infection or tissue reaction. Some artificial materials appear less likely to cause these problems than others. However, a certain incidence of erosion and related problems is prob-ably inevitable following the insertion of a permanent implant through a potentially con-taminated wound. It appears that the main function of the sling material, whether natural or synthetic, is to provide a framework for fibrosis. Once this has taken place, the sling mate-rial itself is largely redundant. The newer generation of absorbable materials presently being used in sling surgery provide easily available lengths, decrease surgical morbidity, and do not persist beyond the time taken for fibrosis to occur. The use of these materials may be a preferable option in the future. If we are to advance our understanding of new sling tech-niques and materials, thorough evaluation is required of the surgical procedures, objective and subjective outcomes as well as complications with at least a 5-year follow-up.

REFERENCES

1. Fianu S, Soderberg G. Absorbable polyglactin mesh for retropubic sling operations in female urinary stress incontinence. Gynecol Obstet Invest 1983; 16:45–50.
2. Pourdeyhimi B. Porosity of surgical mesh fabrics: new technology. J Biomed Mater Res 1989; 23:145–152.
3. Usher FC. The repair of incisional and inguinal hernias. Surg Gynecol Obstet 1970; 131:525–530.
4. Chu CC, Welch L. Characterization of morphological and mechanical properties of surgical mesh fibers. J Biomed Mater Res 1985; 19:903–916.
5. Ghoniem GM, Shaaban A. Sub-urethral slings for treatment of stress urinary incontinence. Int Urogynecol J 1994; 5:228–239.
6. Iglesia CB, Fenner DE, Brubaker L. The use of mesh in gynecologic surgery. Int Urogynecol J Pelvic Floor Dysfunct 1997; 8:105–115.
7. Moir JC. The gauze–hammock operation. (A modified Aldridge sling procedure). J Obstet Gy-naecol Br Commonw 1968; 75:1–9.
8. Nichols DH. The Mersilene mesh gauze-hammock for severe urinary stress incontinence. Ob-stet Gynecol 1973; 41:88–93.
9. Kersey J. The gauze hammock sling operation in the treatment of stress incontinence. Br J Ob-stet Gynaecol 1983; 90:945–949.
10. Losif CS. Sling operation for urinary incontinence. Acta Obstet Gynecol Scand 1985; 64:187–190.
11. Kersey J, Martin MR, Mishra P. A further assessment of the gauze hammock sling operation in the treatment of stress incontinence. Br J Obstet Gynaecol 1988; 95:382–385.
12. Guner H, Yildiz A, Erdem A, Erdem M, Tiftik Z, Yildirim M. Surgical treatment of urinary stress incontinence by a suburethral sling procedure using a Mersilene mesh graft. Gynecol Obstet In-vest 1994; 37:52–55.

13. Young SB, Rosenblatt PL, Pingeton DM, Howard AE, Baker SP. The Mersilene mesh subu-
    rethral sling: a clinical and urodynamic evaluation. Am J Obstet Gynecol 1995; 173:1719–1726.
14. Morgan JE. A sling operation, using Marlex polypropylene mesh, for treatment of recurrent
    stress incontinence. Am J Obstet Gynecol 1970; 106:369–377.
15. Morgan JE, Farrow GA, Stewart FE. The Marlex sling operation for the treatment of recurrent
    stress urinary incontinence: a 16-year review. Am J Obstet Gynecol 1985; 151:224–226.
16. Morgan JE, Heritz DM, Stewart FE, Connolly JC, Farrow GA. The polypropylene pubovaginal
    sling for the treatment of recurrent stress urinary incontinence. J Urol 1995; 154:1013–1016.
17. Bryans FE. Marlex gauze hammock sling operation with Cooper's ligament attachment in the
    management of recurrent urinary stress incontinence. Am J Obstet Gynecol 1979; 133:292–294.
18. Hilton P, Stanton SL. Clinical and urodynamic evaluation of the polypropylene (Marlex) sling
    for genuine stress incontinence. Neurourol Urodynam 1983; 2:145–153.
19. Drutz HP, Buckspan M, Flax S, Mackie L. Clinical and urodynamic reevaluation of combined
    abdominovaginal Marlex sling operations for recurrent stress urinary incontinence. Int Urogy-
    necol J 1990; 1:70–73.
20. Cato RJ, Murray AG. Teflon tape suspension for the control of stress incontinence. Br J Urol
    1981; 53:364–367.
21. Horbach NS, Blanco JS, Ostergard DR, Bent AE, Cornella JL. A suburethral sling procedure
    with polytetrafluoroethylene for the treatment of genuine stress incontinence in patients with
    low urethra closure pressure. Obstet Gynecol 1988; 71:648–652.
22. Summitt RL, Bent AE, Ostergard DR, Harris TA. Suburethral sling procedure for genuine stress
    incontinence and low urethral pressure: a continued experience. Int Urogynecol J 1992; 3:
    18–21.
23. Weinberger MW, Ostergard DR. Long-term efficacy of the Gore-tex suburethral sling for the
    treatment of genuine stress incontinence. Int Urogynecol J 1993; 4:389.
24. Bent AE, Ostergard DR, Zwick–Zaffuto M. Tissue reaction to expanded polytetrafluoroethyl-
    ene suburethral sling for urinary incontinence: clinical and histological study. Am J Obstet Gy-
    necol 1993; 169:1198–1204.
25. Stanton SL, Brindley GS, Hohnes DM. Silastic sling for urethral sphincter incompetence in
    women. Br J Obstet Gynaecol 1985; 92:747–750.
26. Chin YK, Stanton SL. A follow-up of Silastic sling for genuine stress incontinence. Br J Obstet
    Gynaecol 1995; 102:143–147.
27. Korda A, Peat B, Hunter P. Experience with Silastic slings for female urinary incontinence. Aust
    N Z Obstet Gynaecol 1989; 29:150–154.
28. Korda A, Peat B, Hunter P. Silastic slings for female incontinence. Int Urogynecol J 1990; 1:
    66–69.
29. Kovac SR, Cruikshank SH. Pubic bone stabilization sling for recurrent urinary incontinence.
    Obstet Gynecol 1997; 89:624–627.
30. Hom D, Desautel MG, Lumerman JH, Feraren RE, Badlani GH. Pubovaginal sling using
    polypropylene mesh and Vesica bone anchors. Urology 1998; 51:708–713.
31. Matkov TG, Hejna MJ, Coogan CL. Osteomyelitis as a complication of Vesica percutaneous
    bladder neck suspension. J Urol 1998; 160:1427.
32. Petros P, Ulmsten UL. An integral theory on female urinary incontinence: experimental and
    clinical considerations. Acta Obstet Gynecol Scand Suppl 1990; 153:7–31.
33. Petros P, Ulrnsten UI. An integral theory and its method for the diagnosis and management of
    female urinary incontinence. Scand J Urol Nephrol 1993; 153:1–93.
34. Petros P, Ulmsten U. Urethral pressure increase on effort originates from within the urethra, and
    continence from musculovaginal closure. Neurourol Urodynam 1995; 14:337–350.
35. Petros P, Ulmsten U. Role of the pelvic floor in bladder neck opening and closure: I. muscle
    forces. Int Urogynecol J Pelvic Floor Dysfunct 1997; 8:74–80.
36. Petros P, Ulmsten U. Role of the pelvic floor in bladder neck opening and closure: II. Vagina.
    Int Urogynecol J Pelvic Floor Dysfunct 1997; 8:69–73.

37. Ulmsten U, Petros P. Intravaginal slingplasty: an ambulatory surgical procedure for treatment of female urinary stress incontinence. Scand J Urol Nephrol 1995; 29:75–82.
38. Ulmsten U, Falconer C, Johnson P, Jomaa M, Lanner L, Nilsson CG, Olsson I. A multicentre study of tension-free vaginal tape (TVT) for surgical treatment of stress urinary incontinence. Int Urogynecol J Pelvic Floor Dysfunct 1998; 9:210–213.
39. Ulmsten U, Henriksson L, Johnson P, Varhos G. An ambulatory surgical procedure under local anaesthesia for treatment of female urinary incontinence. Int Urogynecol J Pelvic Floor Dysfunct 1996; 7:81–86.
40. Nilsson CG. The tensionfree vaginal tape procedure (TVT) for the treatment of female stress urinary incontinence. A minimal invasive surgical procedure. Acta Obstet Gynaecol 1998; 168: 34–37.
41. Riva D, Virgano R, Gandini L, Marchiano A, Quellari P, Ferrari A. Tension free vaginal tape for the therapy of stress urinary incontinence: early results and urodynamic analysis. Neurourol Urodynam 1998; 17:351–352.
42. Wang AC, Lo TS. Tension-free vaginal tape. A minimally invasive solution to stress urinary incontinence in women. J Reprod Med 1998; 43:429–434.
43. Ward K, Hilton P. TVT early experience [abstr]. Int Urogynecol J IUGA Meeting, 1998.
44. McGuire EJ. Abdominal procedures for stress incontinence. Urol Clin North Am 1985; 12:285–290.
45. Horback NS. Suburethral sling procedures. In: Ostergard DR, Bent AE, eds. Urogynecology and Urodynamics. 3rd ed. Philadelphia: Williams & Wilkins, 1991:413–421.
46. Jarvis GJ. Surgery for genuine stress incontinence. Br J Obstet Gynaecol 1994; 101:371–374.
47. Webster GD, Kreder KJ. Voiding dysfunction following cystourethropexy: its evaluation and management. J Urol 1990; 144:670–673.
48. Carr LK, Webster GD. Bladder outlet obstruction in women. Urol Clin North Am 1996; 23:385–391.
49. Hilton P. A clinical and urodynamic study comparing the Stamey bladder neck suspension and suburethral sling procedures in the treatment of genuine stress incontinence. Br J Obstet Gynaecol 1989; 96:213–220.
50. McGuire EJ, Bennett CJ, Konnack JA, Sonda LP, Savastano JA. Experience with pubovaginal slings for urinary incontinence in the University of Michigan. J Urol 1987; 138:525–526.
51. Beck RP, McCormick S, Nordstrom L. The fascia lata sling procedure for treating recurrent genuine stress incontinence of urine. Obstet Gynecol 1988; 72:699–703.
52. Blaivas JG, Jacobs B. Pubovaginal fascial sling for the treatment of complicated stress urinary incontinence. J Urol 1991; 145:1214–1218.
53. Appell R. Primary slings for everyone with genuine stress incontinence? The argument for. Int Urogynecol J Pelvic Floor Dysfunct 1998; 9:249–251.
54. Bhatia NN, Bergman A. Urodynamic predictability of voiding following incontinence surgery. Obstet Gynecol 1984; 63:85–91.
55. McLennan MT, Melick CF, Bent AE. Clinical and urodynamic predictors of delayed voiding after fascia lata suburethral sling. Obstet Gynecol 1998; 92:608–612.
56. Leach GE, Dmochowski RR, Appell RA, Blaivas JG, Hadley HR, Luber KM, Mostwin JL, O'Donnell PD, Roehrborn CG. Female Stress Urinary Incontinence Clinical Guidelines Panel summary report on surgical management of female stress urinary incontinence. J Urol 1997; 158:875–880.
57. Sand PK, Utrie J, Summitt RL, Ostergard DR. The effect of a suburethral sling on detrusor instability. Int Urogynecol J 1993; 4:396.
58. Avtan L, Avci C, Bulut T, Fourtanier G. Mesh infections after laparoscopic inguinal hernia repair. Surg Laparosc Endosc 1997; 7:192–195.
59. Miller K, Junger W. Ileocutaneous fistula formation following laparoscopic polypropylene mesh hernia repair. Surg Endosc 1997; 11:772–773.
60. Bent AE, Ostergard DR, Zwick–Zaffuto M. Tissue reaction, to expanded polytetrafluoroethyl-

ene suburethral sling for urinary incontinence: clinical and histologic study. Am J Obstet Gynecol 1993; 169:1198–1204.

61. Choe JM, Staskin DR. Gore-tex patch sling: 7 years later. Urology 1999; 54:641–646.

62. Myers DL, LaSala CA. Conservative surgical management of Mersilene mesh suburethral sling erosion. Am J Obstet Gynecol 1998; 179:1424–1428.

63. Melnick I, Lee R. Delayed transaction of the urethra by Mersilene tape. Urology 1976; 8:580–581.

64. Norris JP, Breslin DS, Staskin DR. Use of synthetic material is sling surgery: a minimally invasive approach. J Endourol 1996; 10:227–230.

42

Fascial Slings

KATHLEEN C. KOBASHI

Virginia Mason Medical Center, Seattle, Washington

GARY E. LEACH

University of Southern California Medical School and Tower Urology Institute for Continence, Cedars-Sinai Medical Center, Los Angeles, California

I. INTRODUCTION

Since the first pubovaginal sling (PVS) was described by Von Giordano in 1907 (Table 1) (1), the PVS has evolved into the gold standard for the surgical treatment of female stress urinary incontinence (SUI) caused by intrinsic sphincter deficiency (ISD), and it is used as a first-line surgical therapy for SUI associated with urethral hypermobility. PVSs are placed beneath the proximal urethra and bladder neck to provide a hammock effect as well as direct urethral compression. The sling serves as a "backstop" to prevent urethral descensus and opening when increased intra-abdominal pressure occurs.

II. INDICATIONS AND PATIENT SELECTION

A. Indications

Slings are the most widely accepted treatment for ISD, and we prefer to use slings for all female patients with any type of SUI should they opt for surgical therapy. However, slings are performed only after confirming the presence of SUI and the absence of detrusor instability or of instability that is controlled by medications. Exceptions include urodynamically demonstrated detrusor instability only at high bladder volumes, or if the instability does not correlate with the patient's symptoms. Pelvic prolapse, if present, must be repaired at the time of sling placement (see later discussion). Conversely, the bladder neck and proximal urethra must be supported at the time of cystocele repair even if preoperative SUI is not demonstrated to prevent the development of SUI postoperatively.

Table 1 Evolving Technique of Sling Surgery

Author	Technique
VonGiordano, 1907 (1)	First sling; gracilis muscle
Stoeckel, 1917 (2)	Plication of "muscular structures"[a] around bladder neck
Price, 1933 (3)	Passage of fascial strip beneath urethra from AP incision and fix to rectus muscle
Aldridge, 1942 (4)	Suture two strips of fascia together beneath urethra
Lytton/McGuire, 1978 (5)	Fix to rectus fascia
Leach, 1988 (6); Appell, 1997 (7)	Bone anchors (suprapubic or transvaginal placement)

[a]Muscles used included gracilis, pyramidalis, levator ani, rectus, and bulbocavernosus.

B. Evaluation and Workup Specific to Slings

A thorough discussion of the preoperative evaluation of incontinent patients is covered elsewhere in this textbook; therefore, this section will cover only the evaluation relevant to the sling.

1. History

A detailed history is essential, and assessment of the impact of the incontinence on the patient's quality of life is important. The SEAPI instrument (see chapter Appendix 1) can be useful for objective evaluation of patient symptoms. Patients should be questioned about the presence or absence of SUI and urgency or urge incontinence. History pertaining to the possibility of neurogenic bladder dysfunction or sacral arc denervation is essential, as this condition puts the patient at higher risk for permanent postoperative urinary retention. Evaluation for neuropathology includes questions concerning the patient's sensation of bladder filling, sensation of complete bladder emptying, and their ability to void spontaneously. Routine questions, such as frequency of urination, degree of leakage, number of pregnancies, and history of infections, are relevant. Past medical history may reveal neurological injury, for example, secondary to cerebrovascular accident or trauma; or to neurological disease, such as multiple sclerosis or Parkinson's disease; or to diabetes mellitus, which can affect bladder function. Past surgical history is also important because previous pelvic or abdominal surgery can affect the difficulty of sling surgery or require urethrolysis if abundant scar tissue is present.

Voiding diaries and pad tests are techniques that may help the clinician objectively quantify a patient's voiding pattern and degree of incontinence.

2. Physical Examination

Pelvic examination is important in the assessment of urethral position, degree of periurethral fibrosis, and urethral mobility, as well as the presence of concomitant prolapse. The current trend is toward placing slings for treatment of all types of SUI, regardless of the Valsalva leak-point pressure or presence of hypermobility. In patient, in whom there is no pelvic prolapse present, cadaveric transvaginal sling (CaTS) is performed with a 2 × 7-cm strip of cadaveric fascia (see section IV). However, collagen injection therapy may also be considered in patients with SUI and a well-supported urethra ("classic" ISD). Conversely, if the urethra is hyperelevated or severely fixed secondary to scarring following previous anti-incontinence procedures, urethrolysis should be performed in conjunction with sling placement to allow adequate urethral compression from the sling.

The degree and location of concomitant pelvic prolapse, if present, must be assessed, for surgical planning. Currently, the authors are utilizing a new technique of simultaneous cystocele repair and pubovaginal sling with a single piece of cadaveric fascia, a procedure entitled *ca*daveric *p*rolapse repair and *s*ling (CaPS).

3. Workup

A urodynamic study is performed to demonstrate SUI and evaluate for bladder "overactivity" (detrusor instability or hyperreflexia). If the patient complains of urgency, but cystometry reveals a stable bladder, the urologist must still take into account the possibility of instability that was not demonstrated in the laboratory-testing situation. Correlation of the urodynamic findings with the patient's history is imperative. Approximately 20–40% of patients will have persistent urgency and 10–12% of patients may develop de novo postoperative urgency.

Preoperative postvoid residual should be determined by a bladder scan or catheterization to evaluate bladder emptying. Patients with incomplete emptying before sling placement are clearly at risk for postoperative urinary retention requiring intermittent catheterization. Nonetheless, the clinician must be aware that postvoid residuals are often falsely elevated in the laboratory. To confirm preoperative incomplete emptying, patients are asked to keep a log of their postvoid catheterized volumes obtained at home before surgery.

Finally, cystourethroscopy is performed to evaluate urethral position and mobility and to exclude bladder pathology such as an intravesical suture, stone, or tumor.

III. TISSUE SOURCES

Numerous materials, including autologous and allogenic tissues as well as synthetic materials, have been used to create slings with varying results (Table 2). Although the short-term results have been comparable between autologous, homologous, and synthetic slings, the literature suggests an overall increased complication rate with synthetic materials. Higher infection and erosion rates have been demonstrated with the synthetic materials, although no statistically significant difference in the erosion rates has been demonstrated (Table 3) (12).

This chapter focuses on fascial slings, such as the rectus fascia and fascia lata. Although harvesting of rectus fascia may cause less pain than that of fascia lata (13), fascia

Table 2 Materials Used to Create Slings

Type	Examples
Autologous	Muscle, rectus fascia, fascia lata, dura mater, tendons, vaginal wall, dermis
Allogenic	Cadaveric fascia lata
Xenografts	Porcine dermis
Synthetic materials	Gore-tex, polyester, nylon, Silastic, polytetrafluoroethylene (PTFE), etc.

Table 3   Comparison of Complications with Synthetic Versus
Autologous Materials (12)

Complications	Autologous materials (*n* = 1715)	Synthetic materials (*n* = 1515)
Vaginal erosion	1 (0.0001)	10 (0.007)
Urethral erosion	5 (0.003)	27 (0.02)
Fistula	6 (0.003)	4 (0.002)

lata is reported to be three to four times stronger than rectus fascia (14). Additionally, harvesting of fascia lata does not require the extensive abdominal dissection that increases the risk of nerve entrapment and postoperative pain associated with rectus fascia harvesting. Moreover, the rectus fascia in patients with a history of multiple abdominal surgeries or radiation therapy may be of poor quality. Cadaveric fascia has recently grown in popularity, as no harvesting of fascia is necessary, thereby shortening operative time, hospital stay, and the recuperation period, as well as significantly decreasing postoperative pain.

Cadaveric tissues are processed by tissue banks licensed by the Food and Drug Administration (FDA). Both freezing and freeze-drying the soft tissue accomplish elimination of antigenicity (15,16), although these processes may compromise the integrity of the fascia. Protection against infection transmission is achieved by careful donor selection, antibody testing, and various sterilization techniques (17). A multistep process is performed to inactivate viral particles (16). The most common sterilizing treatment is gamma radiation (18), which up to 4.0 mrad, has no effect on the tensile strength of the fascia (17,19). There is a wide variability in the processing techniques employed to sterilize the fascia, and there is no standardized method required of all tissue banks. One company has developed a patented procedure for tissue processing. Tissue treated using this sterilization technique has been used in over 500,000 surgical transplant patients, with no reported cases of disease transmission (20).

IV.   SURGICAL TECHNIQUE

A.   Preoperative Preparation

A sterile urine culture is essential before placement of the PVS. Ideally, the patients are taught how to perform self-catheterization before surgery in case of postoperative urinary retention. In patients who are unable to perform self-catheterization preoperatively, a suprapubic tube (SPT) may be placed at the time of surgery. Vaginal preparation with a povidone–Iodine (Betadine) douche is performed by the patient the night before and the morning of surgery. Sterile urine must be confirmed before surgery, and all patients receive perioperative intravenous antibiotics. The authors prefer ampicillin or cefazolin together with gentamicin for approximately 24 hr, with the first dose administered on call to the operating room. If the patient is allergic to penicillin, vancomycin is administered for gram-positive coverage.

Patients are placed on an intravaginal hormonal cream regimen to improve the quality of the vaginal tissue and urethral mucosa before surgery. Timing and dosage of estrogen replacement therapy is controversial. Maximal tissue response to vaginal estrogens takes 3–24 months to achieve (21). The authors recommend starting patients on local estrogen therapy at least 6 weeks before surgery if the tissue is atrophic.

B. Placement of the Fascial Sling

1. Transabdominal Approach

An abdominal incision is made and the proximal urethra is isolated. The fascial strip is passed behind the urethra and secured to the rectus fascia or pubic bone (see later discussion). This technique may be difficult and risks injury to the urethra and bladder, especially in cases of significant pelvic scarring following previous pelvic procedures. For this reason, the authors prefer a transvaginal technique.

2. Combined Abdominal and Transvaginal Approach

The patient is placed in the dorsal lithotomy position and an inverted U-shaped anterior vaginal incision is made, extending from the midurethra to the bladder neck (Fig. 1). Dissection is carried laterally to the ischium, and the endopelvic fascia is perforated. Blunt or sharp dissection is performed to create a tunnel through the retropubic space toward the rectus muscle for the sling (Fig. 2). A short suprapubic incision is made and carried down to the rectus fascia, a 1.5 × 4- to 8-cm strip of the rectus fascia is obtained. The ends of the strip are sutured to prevent separation of the fascia, and the sling is excised. Harvesting of

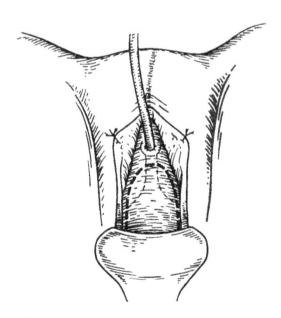

Figure 1   An inverted U-incision is made in the anterior vaginal wall.

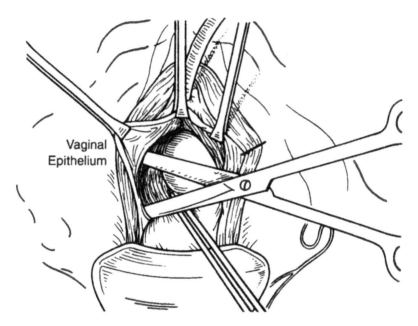

Vaginal
Epithelium

Figure 2   Dissection into the retropubic space is made by a combination of sharp and blunt dissection.

fascia lata involves two or three small incisions in the lateral thigh. A 1.5- to 2-cm–wide fascial segment is harvested. During dissection, extensive distal dissection should be avoided to prevent injury to the common peroneal nerve. Typically, the fascial defect is left open, a drain is placed, and the skin incisions are closed.

A Pereyra needle is used to transfer the prolene sutures, located at the ends of the fascia, from the vagina to the suprapubic incision (Fig. 3). Cystoscopy ensures that no bladder perforation has occurred, and that no suture material has passed through the bladder or urethra. In cases of concomitant pelvic prolapse repair, cystoscopy also allows visualization of urine efflux from the ureteral orifices to confirm ureteral patency following the repair. Sutures are used to fix the sling to the periosteum with a no. 5 Mayo needle (6), or to the rectus fascia. The sling is visualized cystoscopically as the sutures are being secured without excessive tension suprapubically to avoid excessive sling elevation. The free end of the sling is elevated until a minimal indentation of the urethral floor is seen through the 20F female cystoscope with a zero-degree lens. The sling is then secured to the pubic tubercle, with care taken to avoid excessive tension.

3.   Transvaginal (Cadaveric Transvaginal Sling; CaTS)

We prefer the transvaginal approach for the pubovaginal sling because it avoids the pain caused by the passing of the sutures through the abdominal wall. An inverted U-shaped incision is made in the anterior vaginal wall extending from the distal urethra to the bladder neck. The flap is dissected on the white shiny layer on the inside of the vaginal wall. When the correct plane is identified, there is minimal blood loss. The flap is mobilized proximally

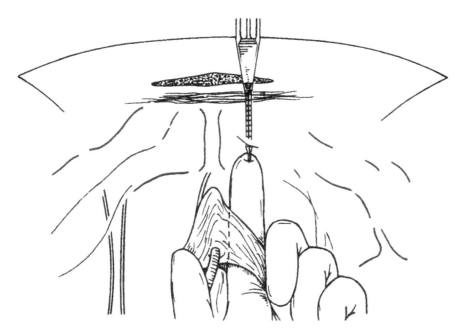

Figure 3   The vaginal sutures are transferred to the suprapubic incision.

to the bladder neck, which is identified by palpation of the Foley catheter balloon (Fig. 4). The pubic bone is exposed lateral to the urethra, and the underside of the bone is cleared of adjacent tissue on the undersurface of the bone. In patients who have undergone previous anti-incontinence surgery, this dissection should be performed sharply to avoid inadvertent perforation of the bladder or urethra. The endopelvic fascia is not routinely perforated unless periurethral scarring is present or in cases in which there is inadequate space for placement of the transvaginal anchor.

Bone anchors are placed transvaginally using a transvaginal anchoring system into the underside of the pubic bone (Fig. 5). The corners of the 2 × 7-cm cadaveric fascia strip are folded over to prevent tearing-through of the sutures (Fig. 6a). The 0-prolene sutures attached to the anchors are passed through the fascia using a straight 18-gauge needle to minimize trauma to the fascia (see Fig. 6b). One side of the sling is tied firmly to the bone. The tension of the sling is determined by placing a small right-angle clamp between the urethra and sling while securing the second side of the fascia in place (Fig. 7). The sling should lie flat and snug against the right angle, such that the right angle can be removed and replaced without a problem. The distal edge of the fascia is tacked to the periurethral tissue using a 2-0 absorbable suture to prevent rolling of the fascial patch toward the bladder neck. Any excess fascia is trimmed, and the vaginal flap is closed with 2-0 Vicryl running stitch. An antibiotic-soaked vaginal packing and a 16F Foley catheter are left in place overnight.

C.   Postoperative Care

The vaginal packing and Foley catheter are removed on the first postoperative day, and the postvoid residual volumes are determined by in-and-out catheterization. If the residuals are more than 100 mL, the technique of CIC is reviewed with the patient before discharge, and she is instructed to continue CIC at home until the PVR is consistently less than 100 mL.

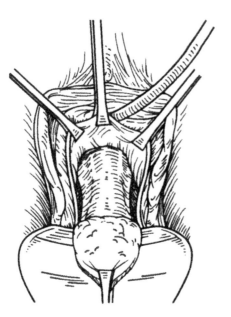

Figure 4   A vaginal flap is created extending from the apex at the distal urethra to the proximal bladder neck.

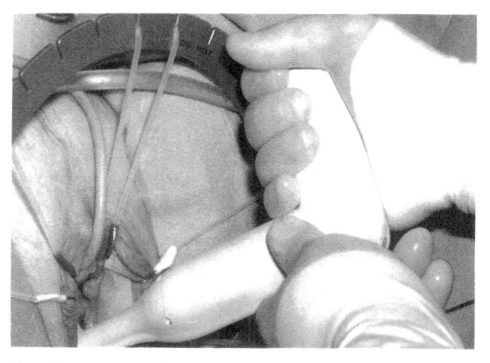

Figure 5   A transvaginal drilling device is used to place bone anchors into the pubic bone.

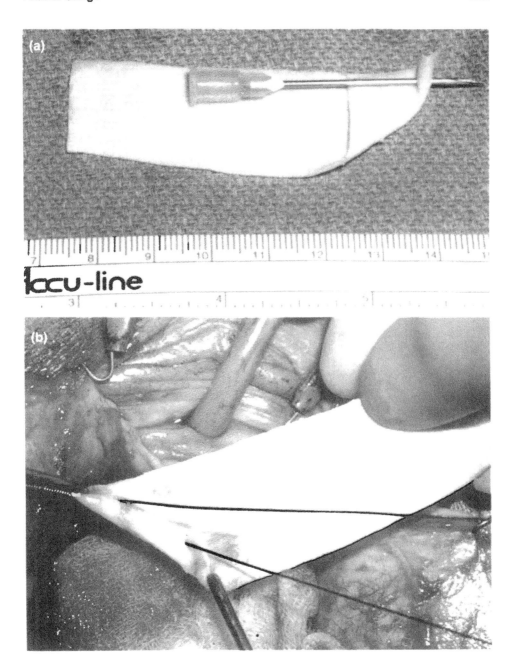

Figure 6 (a) The corners of the fascial strip are folded as illustrated to minimize the risk of the sutures pulling through the fascial fibers. (b) The nonabsorbable suture is passed atraumatically through the fascia using an 18-gauge needle.

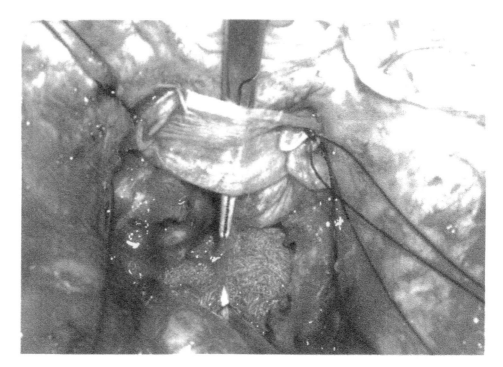

Figure 7 A small right-angle clamp is placed between the urethra and fascia as the second side of the fascia is secured in place. The suture is secured until the sling lies flat and snug on the clamp without excessive tension.

In the rare case in which a patient has an SPT, the PVRs are measured through the SPT and, if necessary, the patient is discharged home with the tube plugged and instructed on how to check the residuals at home.

Routine precautions are taken to prevent infection. Patients receive approximately 24 hr of perioperative intravenous antibiotics, followed by 1 week of oral antibiotics (cephalexin or ciprofloxacin). Most patients need only acetaminophen for adequate analgesia.

V. OUTCOMES AND COMPLICATIONS

Following an extensive literature review covering surgical techniques for treatment of female SUI, the AUA Clinical Guidelines Panel compiled a set of guidelines for the surgical treatment of female SUI (12). Slings and retropubic suspensions had the best long-term results, with an 83–84% cure or dry rate at 48 months, as compared with an only 67% cure or dry rate among patients who had undergone needle suspensions (Fig. 8). The sling appears to be most efficacious over time for all types of recurrent SUI. One must consider that, in the past, slings were used only for the more severe cases of SUI. Yet slings still maintain excellent long-term results, comparable with those of retropubic suspensions that were employed for the less complex cases of SUI.

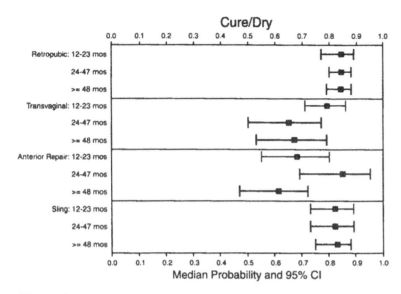

Figure 8   The AUA Clinical Guidelines panel for treatment of female stress urinary incontinence concluded that, based on the literature, slings and retropubic suspensions have the best long-term results.

A.   Based on the Material Used

1.   Autologous Fascia

Use of fascia lata provides several advantages over other autologous fascia and allogenic tissue. Autologous fascia lata reportedly has a higher tensile strength than does rectus fascia (14), and there is no theoretical risk of infection transmission as there may be with cadaveric fascia. The biggest disadvantage of fascia lata is pain at the harvest site. Sixty-seven percent of patients experience pain with walking, although Wheatcroft et al. (22), showed that pain persists for an average of only 1 week postoperatively. In our experience, the pain has persisted for approximately 6 weeks. Cosmetic results are also a consideration. 38% of patients in Wheatcroft's series were unhappy with the appearance of the scar, and Naugle reported the complication of herniation of the muscle belly at the fascial harvest site (23).

Haab et al. (24), studied 40 patients who underwent PVS placement using autologous fascia for treatment of ISD. Questionnaire analysis was used with a mean follow-up of 48.2 months (range 24–60 months). Thirteen patients had a rectus fascia sling, and 27 patients underwent fascia lata PVSs. Patients who had preoperative SUI alone were more likely to be dry than patients with mixed incontinence (67 vs. 36%). Twenty-seven percent ($n = 10$) had recurrent SUI; 62.2% ($n = 23$) had postoperative urgency, including 10% ($n = 4$) patients who experienced the de novo urgency; and 8% ($n = 3$) patients had permanent retention, including 2 with sacral arc denervation who were expected preoperatively to go into retention.

Use of rectus fascia provides the same excellent long-term results as fascia lata. Disadvantages of rectus fascia include development of abdominal hernia and a "pulling" sensation or pain radiating to the groin, presumably caused by the tension of the suspension sutures on the rectus fascia or suprapubic nerve "entrapment" (6).

Carr et al. (25), studied their results with rectus fascia slings in the geriatric patient population by comparing their outcomes in 19 patients older than 70 years of age versus 77 patients younger than 70 years old, all with SUI. Mean follow-up was 22 months (range 3–43 months). The symptoms of SUI resolved in 100% of the geriatric patients and 97% of the patients younger than 70 years of age. Urgency symptoms improved postoperatively in 50% of the geriatric patients and 61% of the control group patients who had preoperative detrusor instability. De novo urgency occurred in 10% of patients in both groups, but was controlled adequately in all patients with anticholinergic medications.

Chaikin et al. (26) studied 251 patients who underwent pubovaginal slings using autologous rectus fascia, with a mean follow-up of 3.1 years (range 1–15 years). Ninety-two percent (231) of the patients were cured or improved after surgery, 3% (7) of the patients had de novo urge incontinence, 23% (58) had persistent urge incontinence, and 2% (4) experienced unexpected permanent urinary retention.

2. Cadaveric Fascia Lata

Early results with the transvaginal approach to placement of cadaveric slings (CaTS) have been excellent. Thus far, the authors have performed 94 CaTS using a transvaginal bone-anchoring system (see Fig. 6a, 6b, and 7), with early follow-up to 10 months. Patients have been evaluated preoperatively and postoperatively using the SEAPI score, with early results revealing a significant decrease in the mean SEAPI scores postoperatively (5.36 vs. 1.27, $p < 0.001$). Less than 50% of patients require temporary intermittent catheterization, but only 1 patient has experienced unexpected permanent postoperative urinary retention (1 patient had expected urinary retention). None of the remaining patients have required intermittent catheterization for longer than 1 week. Of the 92 patients available for follow-up (range 1–10 months), 63 (68.5%) patients are totally dry, 12 (13.0%) have persistent mild SUI, 4 (4.3%) have persistent urge incontinence, 9 (9.8%) have had de novo urge incontinence, and 2 (2.2%) have mixed incontinence. Patients who have undergone CaTS alone (no concomitant procedures) admitted for 23-hr observation to receive intravenous antibiotics. No abdominal or lower extremity incision for graft harvesting or sling fixation is necessary. Therefore, there is little to no postoperative pain and, in our experience, the majority of patients require no more than acetaminophen for analgesia.

There is a minimal risk of infection transmission from the transplanted cadaveric fascia. The risk of acquiring HIV-infected tissue from a properly screened donor is reported to be 1:1,667,600 (27), and the risk of transmission of HIV from banked cadaveric fascia is 1:8 million (28). There is one reported case of HIV transmission from a seronegative donor. Seroconversion occurred only in the recipients of solid organs (4 of 4) and unprocessed fresh-frozen bone (3 of 3). None of the 34 patients who received other tissues, including 3 who received lyophilized soft tissue, became infected with HIV.

Vaginal wound infection or "rejection" has not yet been seen in our experience. Handa reported 2 of 16 (12%) patients developed abdominal wound infections following placement of cadaveric slings (14), comparable with the incidence reported by Beck with autologous fascial slings (28).

Wright et al. (11) evaluated their results in 92 patients with a mean age of 60 years and mean follow-up of 11.5 months. They compared autograft ($n = 33$) versus allograft ($n = 59$) fascial PVSs. Preoperative SEAPI scores, number of previous anti-incontinence procedures, and leak-point pressure were similar between the two groups. The procedures were equally well tolerated, with marked improvement in both groups and without infection or sling erosion. Mean operative time and hospital stay were significantly lower in the allograft patients.

B. How to Avoid and Treat Complications

The etiology of urinary incontinence after PVS placement can be divided into three main categories: (1) persistent stress urinary incontinence, (2) detrusor instability (persistent or de novo), and (3) overflow incontinence. Accurate determination of the cause of incontinence is imperative to restore continence. Evaluation includes postoperative physical examination to assess urethral position, determination of postvoid residuals to evaluate bladder emptying, urodynamic studies, and cystourethroscopy. Multichannel urodynamic studies may demonstrate detrusor instability or persistent SUI. Cystourethroscopy is performed to exclude urethral erosion of the sling or suture material in the bladder.

1. Persistent SUI

Persistent SUI after sling placement is usually due to inadequate tension being placed on the sling or urethral fixation not released by urethrolysis. Physical examination is performed to examine for urethral hypermobility. In patients in whom SUI persists, but urethral hypermobility is absent, collagen injection is a minimally invasive option. Although some sources suggest that injection therapy may be helpful even in cases of SUI involving urethral hypermobility (29), the authors use collagen only in patients with no urethral hypermobility.

2. Persistent or De Novo Detrusor Instability

De novo detrusor instability occurs in 10–12% of patients following placement of a sling (9). Patients with preoperative instability or symptoms of urgency must be counseled on the 20–40% incidence of persistent symptoms (9–11). Postoperative anticholinergic medications may successfully relieve urgency and urge incontinence, although if urgency present preoperatively persists following sling placement, it is often difficult to treat. Combination anticholinergic therapy (two medications) or intravesical anticholinergic instillation should be tried. Biofeedback or neuromodulation may also be helpful. In extreme cases, a patient may eventually require an augmentation cystoplasty.

3. Overflow Incontinence

Postoperative urinary retention following sling placement is most frequently caused by excessive sling tension and outlet obstruction. A 1–2% incidence of permanent urinary retention (9) and up to 60% incidence of temporary retention (10) is reported in the literature. Postoperative overdistension of the bladder must be avoided to prevent myogenic detrusor dysfunction that could contribute to prolonged retention. Additionally, the urologist must be cognizant of the possibility of preoperative poor detrusor function that is evidenced by high preoperative postvoid residual volumes. A preoperative voiding diary and postvoid residual log kept by those patients suspected of having poor emptying is essential to confirm elevated postvoid residual volumes. Finally, in cases of urethral hyperelevation or severe periurethral scarring, urethrolysis with Martius fat pad graft placed around the freed urethra may be required in those patients who have urodynamically demonstrated outlet obstruction (Fig. 9).

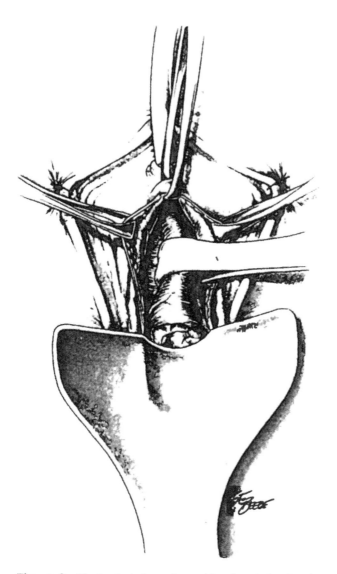

Figure 9 Urethrolysis is performed by sharply freeing the urethra from surrounding scar tissue with two lateral incisions. Care is taken to place the incisions very laterally to avoid injury to the urethra.

VI. CONCLUSIONS

A myriad of techniques for the treatment of female SUI have been described. The current trend in surgical therapy is toward slings for all female patients with SUI. Before sling placement, the surgeon must document the SUI and be aware of potential problems related to detrusor instability or incomplete emptying.

The use of cadaveric fascia avoids complications associated with synthetic slings is safe and avoids the pain and complications from harvesting autologous fascia. Technically, the transvaginal approach is simple and, used together with the cadaveric fascia, decreases postoperative pain, operative time, hospital stay, and recuperation period.

Appendix   SEAPI Incontinence Score

	Subjective	Objective
Stress-related leakage	0 = No urine loss	0 = No leak
	1 = Loss w/strenuous activity	1 = Leak at >80 cmH$_2$O
	2 = Loss w/moderate activity	2 = Leak at 30–80 cmH$_2$O
	3 = Loss with minimal activity	3 = Leak at <30 cmH$_2$O
Emptying ability	0 = No obstructive sxs	0 = 0–60 mL
	1 = Minimal sxs	1 = 61–100 mL
	2 = Significant sxs	2 = 101–200 mL
	3 = Only dribbles or retention	3 = >200 mL or unable to void
Anatomy	0 = No descent w/strain	0 = Above symphysis[a] w/strain
	1 = Descent, not to introitus	1 = <2 cm below symphysis w/strain
	2 = Through introitus w/strain	2 = >2 cm below symphysis w/strain
	3 = Through introitus at rest	3 = >2 cm below symphysis at rest
Protection	0 = Never used	0 = Never used
	1 = Certain occasions	1 = Certain occasions
	2 = Daily, occasional accidents	2 = Daily, occasional accidents
	3 = Continually, frequent accidents or constant leakage	3 = Continually, frequent accidents or constant leakage
Inhibition	0 = No urge incontinence (UI)	0 = No pressure rise
	1 = Rare UI	1 = Rise late filling (>500 mL)
	2 = UI once a week	2 = Medium fill rise (150–500 mL)
	3 = UI at least once a day	3 = Early rise (<150)

Syx, symptoms.
[a]Position of bladder neck (BN).
Source: Ref. 8.

REFERENCES

1. Ridley JH. The Goebel–Stoeckel sling operation. In: Mattingly RF, Thompson JD, eds, TeLinde's Operative Gynecology. Philadelphia: Lippincott, 1985.
2. Stoeckel W. Uber die Verwendung der Musculi pyramidales bei der operativen Behandlung der incontinentia Urinae. Zentralbl Gynakol 1917; 41:11.
3. Price PB. Plastic operations for incontinence of urine and feces. Arch Surg 1933; 26:1043.
4. Aldridge AA. Transplantation of fascia for relief of urinary stress incontinence. Am J Obstet Gynecol 1942; 44:398.
5. Lytton B, McGuire EJ. Pubovaginal sling procedure for stress incontinence. J Urol 1978; 119:82–84.
6. Leach GE. Bone fixation technique for transvaginal needle suspension. Urology 1988; 31:388–390.
7. Appell RA. The use of bone anchoring in the surgical management of female stress urinary incontinence. World J Urol 1997; 15:300–305.
8. Raz S, Stothers L, Chopra A. Anterior vaginal wall sling. In: O'Donnell D, ed. Urinary Incontinence. St Louis; Mosby, 1997:450–451, Appendices F and G.
9. Blaivas JG, Jacobs BZ. Pubovaginal fascial sling for the treatment of complicated stress urinary incontinence. J Urol 1991; 145:1214–1218.

10. Zarazoga MR. Expanded indications for the pubovaginal sling: treatment of type 2 or 3 stress incontinence. J Urol 1996; 156:1620–1622.

11. Wright EJ, Iselin CE, Carr LK, Webster GD. Pubovaginal sling using cadaveric allograft fascia for the treatment of ISD. J Urol 1998; 160:759–762.

12. Leach GE, Dmochowski RR, Appell RA, Blaivas JG, Hadley HR, Luber KM, Mostwin JL, O'Donnell PD, Roehrbom CG. Female SUI clinical guidelines panel summary report on surgical management of female stress urinary incontinence. The American Urological Association. J Urol 1997; 158:875–880.

13. Sirls LT, Leach GE. Use of fascia lata for pubovaginal sling. In: Raz S, ed. Female Urology. Philadelphia: WB Saunders, 1996.

14. Crawford JS. Nature of fascia lata and its fate after implantation. Am J Ophthalmol 1969; 67: 900–907.

15. Cooper JL, Beck CL. History of soft-tissue allografts in orthopedics. Sports Med Arthrosc Rev 1993; 1:2–16.

16. Handa VL, Jensen JK, Germain MM, Ostergard DR. Banked human fascia lata for the suburethral sling procedure: a preliminary report. Obstet Gynecol 1996; 88:1045–1049.

17. Bedrossian EH Jr. HIV and banked fascia lata. Trans Pa Acad Ophthalmol Otolaryngol 1989; 41:831–833.

18. Vangsness CT Jr, Triffon MJ, Joyce MJ, Moore TM. Soft tissue for allograft reconstruction of the human knee: a survey of the American Association of Tissue Banks. Am J Sports Med 1996; 24:230–234.

19. Cutz A, Reid DB, Basu PK. Tensile strength of fascia lata sutures following gamma radiation. Can J Ophthalmol 1977; 12:211–215.

20. Biodynamics International, Inc. Tutoplast Processed Fascia Lata package insert.

21. Semmens JP, Tsai CC, Semmens EC, Loadholt CB. Effects of estrogen therapy on vaginal physiology during menopause. Obstet Gynecol 1985; 66:15–18.

22. Wheatocroft SM, Vardy SJ, Tyers AG. Complications of fascia lata harvesting for ptosis surgery [comments]. Br J Ophthalmol 1998; 82:333–334.

23. Naugle TC Jr, Fry CL, Sabtier RE, Elliott LF. High leg incision fascia lata harvesting. Ophthalmology 1997; 104:1480–1488.

24. Haab F, Trockman BA, Zimmern PE, Leach GE. Results of pubovaginal sling for the treatment of intrinsic sphincteric deficiency determined by questionnaire analysis. J Urol 1997; 158: 1738–1741.

25. Carr LK, Walsh PJ, Abraham VE, Webster GD. Favorable outcome of pubovaginal slings for geriatric women with stress incontinence. J Urol 1997; 157:125–128.

26. Chaikin DC, Rosenthal J, Blaivas JG. Pubovaginal fascial sling for all types of stress urinary incontinence: long-term analysis. J Urol 1998; 160:1312–1316.

27. Simonds RJ, Homberg SD, Hurwitz RL, Coleman TR, Bottenfield S, Conley LJ, Kohlenberg SH, Castro KG, Dahan BA, Schable CA. Transmission of human immunodeficiency virus type 1 from a seronegative organ tissue donor. N Engl J Med 1992; 326:726–732.

28. Beck RP, McCortnick S, Nordstrom L. The fascia lata sling procedure for treating recurrent genuine stress incontinence of urine. Obstet Gynecol 1988; 72:699–703.

29. Herschorn S, Steele DJ, Radomski SB. Followup of intraurethral collagen for female stress urinary incontinence. J Urol 1996; 156:1305–1309.

43

Management of the Incompetent Sphincter: A Synthesis

JACQUES CORCOS

McGill University and Jewish General Hospital, Montreal, Quebec, Canada

ERIK SCHICK

University of Montreal and Maisonneuve–Rosemont Hospital, Montreal, Quebec, Canada

Urethral function is an essential part of the continence mechanism. Its failure leads to what is so-called intrinsic sphincteric deficiency or ISD. The term *intrinsic* suggests that several factors may be responsible for the failed sphincteric function, some of them are structural (e.g., muscular, mucosal, or fascial) others functional (e.g., nerve receptors, neurotransmitters, or hormone sensitive cells) in nature. Detailed pathophysiology of this condition in male and female has been described in Chapter 12.

If the diagnostic tools and approach are similar in men and women, treatment will have to be individualized. Factors such as associated medical conditions (neurological diseases, diabetes, radiation therapy, or other) and past surgical history must be taken into consideration in the choice of therapeutic modalities.

In this chapter we attempted to synthesize the different treatment alternatives from the point of view of the practicing physician. Some of these modalities have been developed in much greater detail in other parts of this book and we will refer to them.

I. CLINICAL ASSESSMENT

A. History

Detailed history focusing on the lower urinary tract must be obtained to analyze the sphincteric component of incontinence, together with other associated factors, such as urgency, increased frequency, abnormal sensations during filling and voiding, that might suggest bladder dysfunction. Different questionnaires can be used to register and analyze clinical symptoms. Several of these instruments have been validated from the methodological point of view and proved to be reliable (1–6).

Past medical and surgical history is of importance (spina bifida, spinal cord lesions, peripheral neuropathy, radical hysterectomy, colorectal surgery, lymph node dissection, previous attempts to cure incontinence, radiation therapy, and so on) because these can explain eventual sphincteric dysfunction and influence therapeutic choice. For instance, artificial sling material will not be used in patients having had pelvic irradiation or in poorly controlled diabetic patients.

B. Quality of Life

The evaluation of the influence of incontinence on the quality of life is an essential part of the history. Different questionnaires can be used to measure this. It is recommended to use a disease-specific questionnaire, such as the Incontinence Impact Questionnaire (IIQ) (7), the King's questionnaire (8), or other, rather than generic questionnaires.

Quality of life (QoL) analysis also allows the physician to evaluate the expectations of the patient. A patient with a poor QoL secondary to a severe incontinence will be satisfied even with an improvement of his or her condition, whereas another incontinent patient with a relatively good QoL will be satisfied only by a complete cure.

Knowing the success rate of each of our treatments, the evaluation of the QoL of our patient provides another dimension to help one choose the best treatment for a given patient.

As for any lower tract urinary complaint, voiding diaries are an essential part of the initial assessment. These diaries have been fully described in Chapter 18.

C. Physical Examination

The aim of this physical examination is obviously to evaluate the urethra, but also the surrounding tissues.

Hormonal content of the vaginal mucosa is an important element to consider. Clinical assessment of tissue softness and mucosal color is usually enough to decide on the need for hormonal replacement therapy. Prolapses (cystocoele, rectocoele, uterine descent, and enterocoele) have to be part of the correction because they interfere with the global pelvic balance. However, these prolapse corrections will have to be carefully planned considering the symptoms they are responsible for and the sexual activity of the patient. A complete correction of the prolapse may lead to a poorly functional vagina, which, in a patient with an active sexual life may have a highly negative effect on the quality of life.

Urethral mobility, its position, or the degree of periurethral fibrosis, all are details to be considered that may modify the treatment plan. For instance, a hypercorrected urethra with severe scarring following a previous anti-incontinence surgery may require urethrolysis at the time of the new correction (9).

Finally, a neurological examination is always mandatory in patients with incompetent sphincter because it may reveal a more widespread neurological involvement that might require a specific management.

Details on the physical examination can be found in Chapters 15 and 17 of this book.

D. Urodynamic Studies

As ISD is poorly understood, its evaluation is difficult. As mentioned previously, ISD is the result of a combination of factors and only global evaluation of the sphincteric capability of the urethra makes sense. If striated muscular deficiency is suspected as the main cause, or at least to be a significant contributory factor in the development of the sphincteric dysfunction, an electromyogram (EMG) may be of great help (10,11). Two tests are mainly used to assess urethral function: urethral pressure profile and the Valsalva leak-point pressure measurements. If the latter is more attractive because it looks more functional, both failed to show a high degree of correlation with clinical symptoms and other measures of the degree of incontinence, such as the pad test (see Chap. 19). A better test, including the muscle function and tissue compliance, to obtain an accurate evaluation of the sphincter is still to be described. Existing urodynamic parameters are studied in more detail in Chapters 21–23.

II. TREATMENT

Treatment of ISD is a challenge to everyone dealing with urinary incontinence. The aim of the treatment must be an improvement of the sphincteric function. However, there is a lack of evidence that muscle exercises, electrical stimulation, or pharmacological manipulation can cure ISD (see Chapters 29, 30, and 32). Surgical treatment usually leads to a cure or to a significant improvement of the condition, but does not really correct ISD.

A. Treatment of IDS in the Male

Most of the ISDs in men are secondary to prostatic surgery. Pathophysiology is not well understood. It seems, however, that although urinary incontinence after simple prostatectomy is more likely due to bladder dysfunction than to pure sphincteric injury (12), after radical prostatectomy it is more likely that sphincteric injury is mainly responsible for incontinence. Appropriate measures to prevent incontinence during prostatic surgery is still debated.

1. Modification in Lifestyle

If the incontinence is mixed with a bladder and a sphincteric component, some changes in lifestyle, such as decreased caffeine consumption, decreased fluid intake, and timed voiding may decrease the leakage. Details on these changes can be found in Chapter 28.

2. Physiotherapy

Physiotherapy directed toward the pelvic floor musculature by means of biofeedback or electrical stimulation, or both are widely used. Several other factors of prognostic value, such as associated bladder instability, patient's age, and severity of incontinence, have to be analyzed. They will help in the selection of patients. Only a few studies on the results of physiotherapy in male incontinence have been published (13–16).

3. Medication

The use of α-adrenergic agonists has been reported, with limited success (17,18). Other medications are reviewed in Chapter 32.

4. Injectables

In general, coaptation of the urethral mucosa is difficult to obtain because of scarring of the proximal urethra. This probably represents the main cause for failure. To improve this coaptation, submucosal injection of glutaraldehyde cross-linked collagen has been widely used, but with poor long-term results, close to the 50% range, including cured and improved patients (19–21). Both retrograde and antegrade approaches were proposes with similar results (22). Other devices or injectables, such as microballoons, fat, Teflon, and silicone, have been used without significantly improving the cure rate. A review of these techniques and their results can be found in Chapter 33.

5. Surgery

Men's ISD usually requires a surgical approach. For more than 20 years an artificial urinary sphincter has been the best option. Very recently slings have been proposed as an alternative to sphincters (23).

Artificial Urinary Sphincter (AUS). Several authors report high long-term success rates and patient satisfaction in the 90% range (24,25), despite persistence of some leakage at the time of significant efforts. Revision rate of AUS is high even in the nonneurological population, varying from 10 to 30%, mainly because of mechanical failure or urethral atrophy (26). An extensive review of AUS is found in Chapter 34.

Fascial Sling. As described by Schaeffer et al. (27), use of the fascial sling has been reported recently by Oefelein (28) who compared it with AUS in a small number of patients; they did not find any significant difference in continence rate between the two techniques at 15-month follow-up. Further studies on a larger number of patients with longer follow-up are obviously necessary.

In conclusion, male sphincteric deficiency leads, most of the time, to an AUS insertion. For patients with a very mild incontinence, biofeedback, associated or not with an α-adrenergic agonist may have some advantages. The role of slings in this indication is promising and has to be more extensively studied. An algorithm for the management of male ISD is proposed in Figure 1.

B. Treatment of ISD in the Female

There is probably more controversy in the treatment of female sphincteric incompetence than in male ISD. This controversy exists because there is a wider variety of available treatments and some of them, because of their low invasiveness may be used even if they do not offer the best results (29).

1. Devices

Except for diapers, pads, and incontinence pants, successful external collection devices have not been well developed for the female because of the anatomical challenge they represent. Adhesive devices and urethral plugs exist, but their use is limited by the local mucosal reaction that occurs and their high rate of associated urinary infection.

Literature is very limited in studies using intravaginal devices despite that in elderly women with high surgical risk they may represent an interesting alternative. An overview of all these devices is available in Chapter 35.

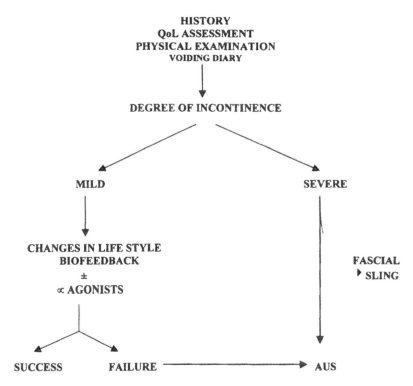

Figure 1 Management of male intrinsic sphincter deficiency.

2. Change in Lifestyle and Physiotherapy

Changes in types of sport activities, diet, management of constipation, and control of fluid intake have some effect on the frequency and the severity of leakage episodes. These techniques are reviewed in Chapter 28.

Physiotherapy, with or without electrical stimulators have to be considered in young or middle-aged patients with mild or moderate incontinence. Large prolapses, scarred periurethral tissues, and a history of radiation therapy are usually poor prognostic factors for the results of physiotherapy. The techniques and results of physiotherapy are reviewed extensively in Chapters 29 and 30.

3. Injectables

Collagen injection received widespread acceptance for treating type 3 stress urinary incontinence in women. Globally, the long-term success rate including cure (20–25%) and improvement (25–40%) varies between 50 and 75%. To obtain these results, several injections are often necessary. However, considering the very low invasiveness of the technique, collagen injection remains an excellent alternative to surgery. Some authors did not find a significant difference in results whether or not ISD was associated with bladder neck hypermobility (29–32).

Fat injection has been more disappointing, mainly because of the relative invasiveness of the fat harvesting, the rapid reabsorption of the injected fat, and the need for repeated injections.

Several other substances are presently being investigated, mainly because it appears that if the technique itself has several advantages, collagen is not the ideal substance to inject. Our present knowledge about injectables is reviewed in Chapter 33.

4. Surgery

Sling.   More than 100 techniques have been described to treat stress urinary incontinence in women. When we speak about sphincteric deficiency there seems to be a consensus that slings probably represent the most efficient technique (33–35).

Most of the authors now recognize that SUI is always associated with a certain degree of ISD, with or without bladder neck mobility. Slings appear then as one of the best surgical approachs to treat SUI. However, the immediate post-operative course following a sling operation is often more complicated than the standard colposuspension procedure.

Different types of slings can be used, depending on their size, length, attachment, and origin. Two chapters address these issues: indications and outcomes of fascial slings are analyzed in Chapter 42, and Chapter 41 reviews use of artificial slings.

Advantages of synthetic slings are essentially their availability and their strength (even if it not sure that this represents a real advantage). Their disadvantages are their cost and their risk of infection, leading to erosion. Cadaveric fasciae are an interesting alternative to artificial slings, eliminating, almost completely, the risk of infection, but sharing with them the problem of their cost. Furthermore, the biological behavior of these cadaveric slings is unknown and some concerns exits for the potential transmission of viral infection.

Finally, despite the problems related to their harvesting, fascial slings and vaginal wall slings appear to be the best choice of material.

Fixation of the slings remains controversial. Some support the initially described technique in which the sling is secured to the Cooper's ligaments, others support the attachment to the anterior abdominal wall, whereas still others prefer the bone anchoring of the graft. According to our knowledge, no randomized studies comparing these techniques exist and the choice is dictated by the surgeon's preference and experience.

Among these sling techniques, one deserves a special mention because it differs from the others in several aspects: it is the tension-free vaginal tape (TVT). A recent, but extremely promising technique if we consider its impressive success rate of 90% at 3 years (36). Until now, no erosion or infection has been reported, despite thousands of operations done worldwide. However, recently a word of caution has been made against too much enthusiasm in relation to a surgical procedure that has no meaningful short- or long-term follow-up (37).

Artifical Sphincter.   If we consider the AUS almost as the gold standard of male ISD, this technique is not widely used to treat female ISD in North America (see Chap. 34).

Salvage Surgery.   In cases of major urethral damage, such as trauma, major complications following surgical failure, radiation therapy, severe congenital abnormality, or other, the urethra may be considered as irremedially lost from the functional point of view. In these circumstances the previously mentioned techniques are not applicable. Urinary diversion remains the only reasonable option. If the bladder has an adequate capacity and compliance, continent diversions using the bladder as a reservoir remains the best approach. A vesicocutaneous continence mechanism may be obtained using the appendix when available (Mitrofanoff technique) (38–40), or a retubularized segment of the small bowel (Monti procedure) (41,42).

Figure 2 summarizes the suggested management for female ISD. It is worthwhile to note, that ISD is not synonymous with stress urinary incontinence. Furthermore, it should be pointed out that following failure of a therapeutic measure, full reevaluation—including urodynamic studies—should be performed before considering another treatment option.

III. CONCLUSION

Intrinsic sphincter deficiency remains a fascinating problem, and our understanding of the exact physiopathological process involved will certainly evolve in the future. There are at least three domains where research should make substantial progress.

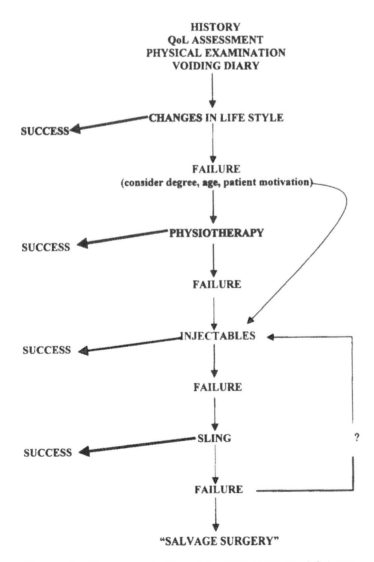

Figure 2 Management of female intrinsic sphincter deficiency.

Pathophsyiology is still poorly understood. This is essential not only for the development of successful treatment strategies but, even more importantly, for adequate measures to be elaborated to prevent the occurrence of ISD.

Research should also address the question of evaluation of this condition. There is no consensus as to what is, or what are, the best tests to investigate these patients. Diagnostic tools should be developed that correlate better with the clinical results of different treatments.

Finally, more research is needed to develop new treatment strategies, giving probably a more significant place to injectables and new sling materials.

REFERENCES

1. Shumaker SA, Wyman JF, Uebersax JS, McClish D, Fantl JA. Health-related quality of life measures for women with urinary incontinence: the Incontinence Impact Questionnaire and the Urogenital Distress Inventory. Qual Life Res 1994; 3:291–306.
2. Jackson S, Donovan J, Brookes S, Eckford S, Swithinbank L, Abrams P. The Bristol Female Lower Urinary Tract Symptoms questionnaire: development and psychometric testing. Br J Urol 1996; 77:805–812.
3. Black N, Griffiths J, Pope C. Development of a symptom severity index and a symptom impact index, for stress incontinence in women. Neurourol Urodynam 1996; 15:630–640.
4. Sandvik H, Hunskaar S, Seim A, Hermstad R, Vanvik A, Bratt H. Validation of a severity index in female urinary incontinence and its implementation in an epidemiological survey. J Epidemiol Community Health 1993; 47:497–499.
5. Bernstein I, Sejr T, Able J, Andersen JT, Fischer–Rasmussen W, Klarskov P, Lose G, Madsen H, Mortensen S, Tetzschner T, Walter S. Assessment of lower urinary tract symptoms in women by a self-administered questionnaire: test–retest reliability. Int Urogynec J 1996; 7:37–47.
6. Gaudenz R. Der Inkontinenz-fragebogen, mit dem neuen Urge-score und Stress-score. Geburtshilfe Frauenheilkd 1979; 39:784–792.
7. Wyman JF, Harkins SW, Choi SC, Taylor JR, Fantl AJ. Psychosocial impact of urinary incontinence in women. Obstet Gynecol 1987; 70:378–381.
8. Kelleher CJ, Cardozo LD, Khullar V, Salvatore S. A new questionnaire to assess the quality of life of urinary incontinent women. Br J Obstet Gynaecol 1997; 104:1374–1379.
9. Cross CA, Cespedes RD, English SF, McGuire EJ. Transvaginal urethrolysis for urethral obstruction after anti-incontinence surgery. J Urol 1998; 159:1199–1201.
10. Dibenedetto M, Yalla SV. Electrodiagnosis of striated urethral sphincter dysfunction. J Urol 1979; 122:361–365.
11. Bump RC. The urodynamic laboratory. Obstet Gynecol Clin North Am 1989; 16:795–816.
12. Seaman EK, Jacobs BZ, Blaivas JG, Kaplan SA. Persistance or recurrence of symptoms after transurethral resection of the prostate: a urodynamic assessment. J Urol 1994; 152:935–937.
13. Burgio KL, Stutzman RE, Engel BT. Behavioral training for post-prostatectomy urinary incontinence. J Urol 1989; 141:303–306.
14. Opsomer RJ, Castille Y, Abi Aad AS, Van Cangh PJ. Urinary incontinence after radical prostatectomy: is professional pelvic floor training necessary? Neurourol Urodynam 1994; 13:382–384.
15. Stewart BH, Banowsky LH, Montague DK. Stress incontinence: conservative therapy with sympathomimetic drugs. J Urol 1976; 15:558–559.
16. Khanna OP. Disorders of micturition: neuropharmacologic basis and results of drug therapy. Urology 1976; 8:316–328.
17. Diokno AC, Taub M. Ephedrine in the treatment of urinary incontinence. Urology 1975; 5:624–625.

18. Awad SA, Downie JW, Kiruluta HG. alpha-Adrenergic agents in urinary disorders of the proximal urethra. Part 1. Sphincter incontinence. Br J Urol 1978; 50:332–335.
19. Deane AM, English P, Hehir M, Williams JP, Worth PH. Teflon injection in stress incontinence. Br J Urol 1985; 57:78–80.
20. Gottfried HW, Maier S, Brandle E, Kleinschmidt K, Hautman R. Transurethral collagen injection for treatment of urinary stress incontinence. Urologe [A] 1997; 36:413–419.
21. Reek C, Noldus J, Huland H. Experience with local collagen injection in male stress incontinence. Urologe [A] 1997; 36:440–443.
22. Loughlin KR, Comiter CV. New technique for antegrade collagen injection for post radical prostatectomy stress urinary incontinence. Urology 1999; 53:410–411.
23. Schreiter F. Surgical therapy of urinary incontinence in the male. Urologe [A] 1991; 30:223–230.
24. Marks JL, Light JK. Management of urinary incontinence after prostatectomy with the artificial urinary spincter. J Urol 1989; 142:302–304.
25. Litwiller SE, Kim KB, Fone PD, White RW, Stone AR. Post-prostatectomy incontinence and the artificial urinary sphincter: a long-term study of patient satisfaction and criteria for success, J Urol 1996; 156:1975–1980.
26. Elliott DS, Barrett DM. The artificial urinary sphincter in the female: indications for use, surgical approach and results. Int Urogynecol J Pelvic Floor Dysfunct 1998; 9:409–415.
27. Schaeffer AJ, Clemens JQ, Ferrari M, Stamey TA. The male bulbo urethral sling procedure for post radical prostatectomy incontinence. J Urol 1998; 159:1510–1515.
28. Oefelein MG. Personnal communication. Dec 1999.
29. Corcos J, Fournier C. Periurethral collagen injection for the treatment of female stress urinary incontinence 4 years follow-up. Urology 1999; 54:815–818.
30. Herschorn S, Steele DJ, Radomski SB. Follow-up of intraurethral collagen for female stress urinary incontinence. J Urol 1996; 156:1305–1309.
31. Monga AK, Stanton SL. Urodynamics: prediction, outcome and analysis of mechanism for cure of stress incontinence by periurethral collage. Br J Obstet Gynaecol 1997; 104:158–162.
32. Smith DN, Appell RA, Winters JC, Rackley RR. Collagen injection therapy for female intrinsic sphincteric deficiency. J Urol 1997; 157:1275–1278.
33. Enzelsberger H, Helmer H, Schatten C. Comparison of Burch and Lyodura sling procedures for repair of unsuccessful incontinence surgery. Obstet Gynecol 1996; 88:251–256.
34. Henriksson L, Ulmsten U. A urodynamic evaluation of the effects of abdominal urethrocystopexy and vaginal sling urethroplasty in women with stress incontinence. Am J Obstet Gynecol 1978; 131:77–82.
35. Richmond DH, Sutherst JR. Burch colposuspension or sling for stress incontinence? A prospective study using transrectal ultrasound. Br J Urol 1989; 64:600–603.
36. Olsson I, Kroon U. A three year post-operative evaluation of tension free vaginal tape. Gynecol Obstet Invest 1999; 48:267–269.
37. Blaivas JG. Physician, heal thyself: caveat emptor [editorial]. Neurourol Urodynam 2000; 19:1–2.
38. Mitrofanoff P. Cystostomie continente transappendiculaire dans le traitement des vessies neurologiques. Chir Pediatr 1980; 21:297–305.
39. Duckett JW, Snyder HM 3d. Use of Mitrofanoff principle in urinary reconstruction. Urol Clin North Am 1986; 13:271–274.
40. Woodhouse CR, Macneily AE. The Mitrofanoff principle: expanding upon a versatile technique. Br J Urol 1994; 74:447–453.
41. Monti PR, deCarvatho JR, Arap S. The Monti procedure: applications and complications. Urology 2000; 55:616–621.
42. Monti PR, Lara RC, Dutra MA, de Carvalho JR. New technique for reconstruction of efferent conduits based on the Mitrrofanoff principle. Urology 1997; 49:112–115.

44

Management of the Dyssynergic Sphincter: A Synthesis

ERIK SCHICK

University of Montreal and Maisonneuve–Rosemont Hospital, Montreal, Quebec, Canada

JACQUES CORCOS

McGill University and Jewish General Hospital, Montreal, Quebec, Canada

Detrusor–sphincter dyssynergia (DSD) implies, by definition, contraction of the detrusor and simultaneous contraction, or at least nonrelaxation, of the urinary sphincter. According to the definition of the International Continence Society (1), when this sphincter contraction occurs at the level of the urethral or periurethral striated muscles, the term *detrusor–external sphincter dyssynergia* or *detrusor–sphincter dyssynergia* should be used. When there is failure of bladder neck opening during a detrusor contraction, the term *detrusor–bladder neck dyssynergia* applies. When overactivity of the urethral sphincter mechanism occurs during voiding in the absence of neurological disease, it is best described as *dysfunctional voiding*.

DSD is harmful, because it represents, in essence, obstructed voiding. When voiding does not take place, the situation might even be worse, with the hyperreflexic detrusor contracting against a closed urethral sphincter. In the short run, first, the detrusor will start to suffer from this situation. It will undergo hypertrophy (increase in mass) (2), with a secondary rise in voiding pressure (3). The contractility of the muscle will be altered. The degree of functional impairment will be directly related to the degree of muscle hypertrophy (4). Figure 1 summarizes, in a schematic way, the factors responsible for deterioration of detrusor function. With progressive loss of bladder contractility and collagen deposition in the bladder wall (5), bladder compliance will decrease progressively and create conditions necessary for the development of a high-pressure system.

The example of a 47-year-old patient with multiple sclerosis illustrates the relatively

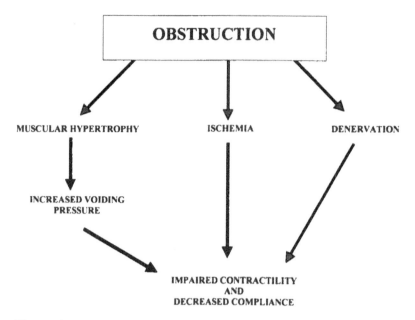

Figure 1 Physiopathological mechanisms by which intravesical obstruction can lead to impaired contractility and decreased compliance.

rapid development of a high-pressure system. The upper urinary tract deteriorated markedly in fewer than 18 months, from September 1985 to February 1987, when the patient underwent an ileocystoplasty (Figs. 2–5). The ureter and ureterovesical junctions were left undisturbed during the surgery. Three months postoperatively, an intravenous pyelogram (IVP) showed significant improvement (Fig. 6). This example also underlines the necessity of following these patients relatively closely.

The exact physiopathological mechanism responsible for the development of a low-compliant bladder is not well known. Sundin et al. (6) observed that parasympathetic injury to the bladder resulted in increased α-adrenergic action, instead of a normal β-adrenergic relaxing effect. Neal et al. (7) demonstrated an augmented number of cholinergic nerve terminals after prolonged parasympathetic denervation. This denervation will also provoke collagen infiltration into the bladder, with thickening and decreased contractility of its wall (8,9). Interruption of the sympathetic nerve supply to the bladder will also reduce its compliance, at least in the cat (10). It is possible that some or all of these factors contribute, in varying degrees, to the decrease in compliance (Fig. 7). Because the ureter is unable to transport urine boluses into the bladder against a pressure gradient greater than 40 cmH₂O for a prolonged period, progressive ureterohydronephrosis will develop, leading ultimately to impairment of renal function (11,12).

Two conditions provoke DSD: a contracting detrusor and a contracting (or nonrelaxing) sphincter. Consequently, therapeutic approaches may be directed toward the detrusor or the urethral sphincter. Eliminating the action of one of these two constituents of the pathological process will make it disappear.

I. ACTIONS DIRECTED TOWARD THE DETRUSOR

The overactive bladder can be controlled by pharmacological or surgical means (Table 1).

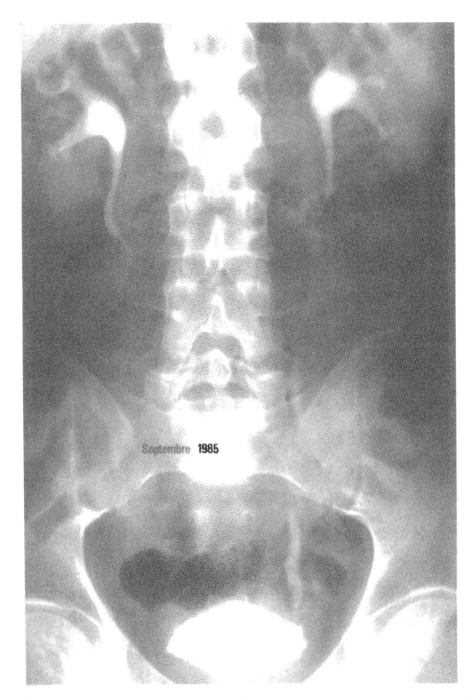

Septembre 1985

Figure 2 Intravenous pyelogram of a 47-year-old wheelchair-bound man with multiple sclerosis. The upper urinary tract is almost normal; slight dilation of the left distal ureter is present.

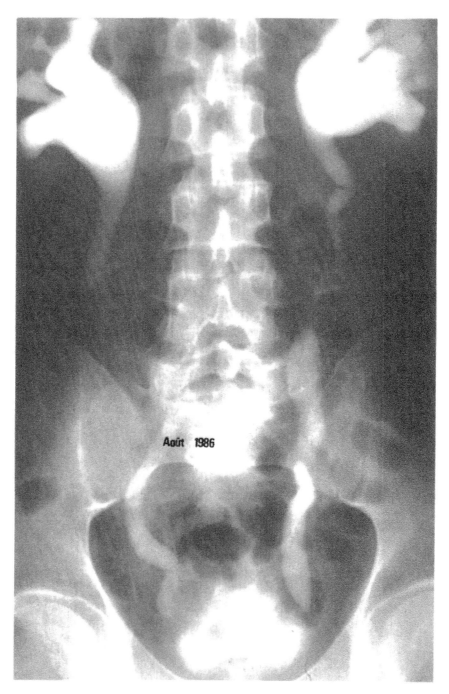

Figure 3 Intravenous pyelogram of the same patient 11 months later: Significant bilateral upper tract dilation is obvious.

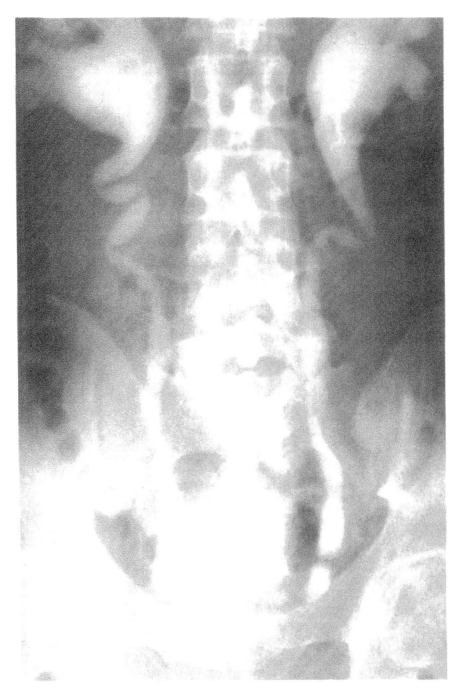

Figure 4   Four months later, bilateral ureterohydronephrosis is even more accentuated.

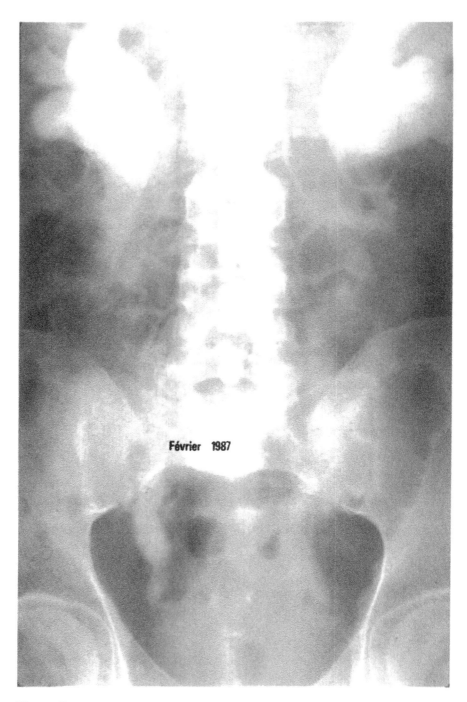

Février   1987

Figure 5   Two months later, the patient is referred to the urologist. The intravenous pyelogram at this time shows an almost completely decompensated upper urinary tract.

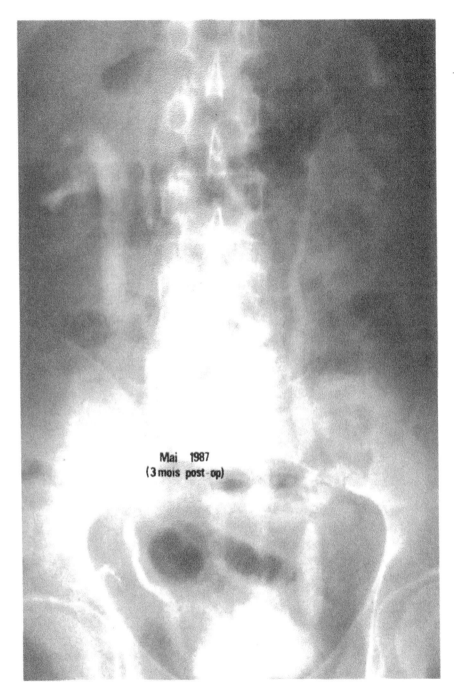

Figure 6   Only 3 months after a clam-ileocystoplasty, ureterohydronephrosis decreased significantly.

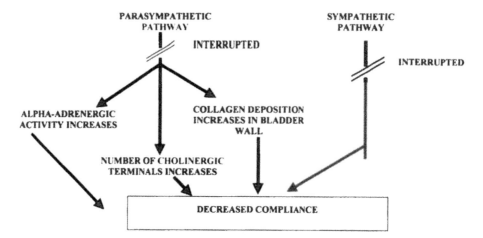

Figure 7 Pathophysiological mechanisms involved in the development of decreased bladder wall compliance when parasympathetic or sympathetic nervous pathways are interrupted.

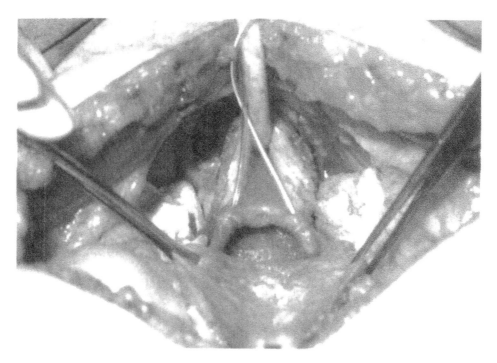

Figure 8 Bladder transection: the bladder is opened, the two ureters are intubated, and the bladder wall is completely transected about 1 cm above the ureteral orifices; the bladder dome (between the Allis clamp) becomes completely detached from the bladder base (the Foley catheter, passed through the urethra, helps to better expose the trigone).

A. Pharmacological Approaches

1. Per Os Medication

Orally administered medication includes mainly anticholinergics (oxybutynin, flavoxate, or tolterodine, or other). Their administration will be successful in about 50% of cases (13).

2. Transcutaneous Route

James and Iacovou (14) used dermal patch nitroglycerin to control unstable bladder contractions. To the best of our knowledge, this has not been tested in neurogenic bladder patients. Some experimental work has been done to explore the possibility of transdermal oxybutynin delivery.

3. Intravesical Route

Successful intravesical administration of oxybutynin to control hyperreflexia has been reported by several authors (15,16). This influences the efferent nerve terminals.

Recently, capsaicin and resiniferatoxin were administered intravesically in preliminary clinical studies to block the fibers of the afferent reflex arc (17,18). McInerney et al. (19) instilled bupivicaine (Marcaine) solution in the bladder and observed the disappearance of ice water in 56% of cases. This reflex is known to be mediated by C fibers (20).

4. Intrathecal Route

Steers et al. (21) administered baclofen, a α-aminobutyric acid (GABA) agonist, intrathecally. Abnormal contractions were abolished in all patients with hyperreflexic detrusor function. A 72% increase in capacity and 16% improvement in compliance were observed when no cervical spinal pathology was present; DSD was abolished in 40% of patients. A similar experience was reported by Kums and Delhaas (22).

Parasympatholytics are certainly a class of pharmacological substances that occupy an important place in treatment of the hyperreflexic or unstable bladder. The main limitation to their use is the relatively high incidence of side effects, which significantly decrease patient compliance. Recently, the pharmaceutical industry developed new anticholinergic substances (e.g., tolterodine) and modified the mode of delivery of some already-existing agents (e.g., oxybutynin SR) that present no, or a much lower incidence of, undesirable side effects. These should improve patient compliance.

There has been no real clinical experience with the transdermal delivery of pharmacological substances in urology. The widespread use of hormone delivery transdermally suggests that there is no theoretical reason to believe that this cannot be accomplished with anticholinergics as well. If the therapeutic effects can be maintained, patient compliance should increase even more.

Intravesical instillation of a pharmacological substances is still in its infancy. Experience gained so far with this approach is promising. There are some limitations, however. At least in our experience, instillation can be reasonably instituted in patients who are on a clean intermittent catheterization regimen, or who have an indwelling catheter. The patient must have manual dexterity as well. Even in these circumstances, instillation is rather cumbersome. It could be greatly facilitated if pharmaceutical companies would market pre-assembled kits for patients.

Intrathecal infusion of baclofen seems to be very efficacious. However, the need for very expensive infusion pumps limits its widespread use.

B.   Surgical Approaches

1.   Bladder Denervation

Spinal blocks, cystolysis, and subtrigonal injection of phenol were all abandoned because of their temporary beneficial effect or the complications encountered.

Bladder transection has been developed to interrupt nervous fibers inside the bladder wall (Figs. 8 and 9). It has been demonstrated in an experimental model that nerve regrowth does not cross the anastomotic line in the detrusor (23). In our experience, 60–65% of patients with unstable bladder will be cured clinically or show significant improvement after this procedure. Similar experience has been reported by others (24). The results seem to be better in the unstable than in the hyperreflexic bladder, but are less favorable with endoscopic transection (25).

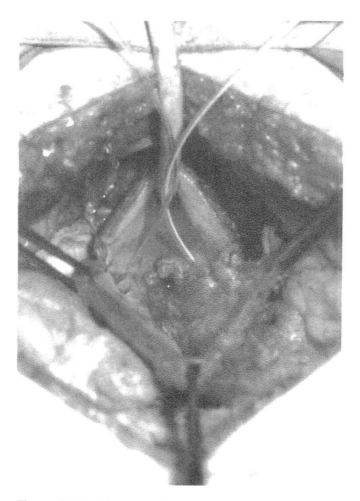

Figure 9   Bladder transection: the posterior wall of the bladder has been reunited; the two ureteral catheters are still in place. They will be withdrawn before the bladder is completely closed. The urethral Foley catheter is left in place for 5–7 days.

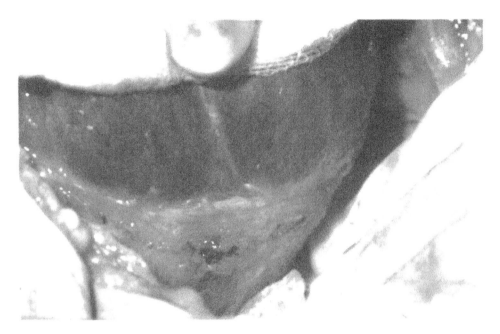

Figure 10   Partial detrusorectomy: limit between the intact bladder wall and the zone where the detrusor has been excised leaves only the intact bladder mucosa behind.

2.   Autoaugmentation

The advantage of bladder autoaugmentation over enterocystoplasty is that obviously no intestinal mucosa will be in contact with urine, no mucus will be excreted in urine, the alimentary tract will remain intact, and the peritoneum is not entered during detrusorectomy, decreasing the morbidity associated with this procedure, in comparison with enterocystoplasty. All our patients who voided spontaneously before surgery did so in the postoperative period.

The rationale behind autoaugmentation (or partial detrusorectomy) is twofold. On the one hand, a substantial part of the abnormally contracting muscle is excised. On the other hand, by leaving the bladder mucosa intact, a diverticulum is created artificially, which acts as a buffer to absorb, or partially decrease, the amplitude of contraction generated by the remaining detrusor (Figs. 10 and 11). Good long-term results were reported recently by Stöhrer et al. (26). In case of failure, enterocystoplasty can still be offered to the patient.

A modification of this technique was reported recently (27) with only a circular vesicomyotomy being performed, leaving the mucosa intact. A psoas-hitch fixed the bladder dome to the psoas muscle. In animal experiments, bladder capacity and bladder compliance increased by 32 and 28%, respectively.

3.   Enterocystoplasty

Incorporation of a detubularized segment of the ileum or colon in the lower urinary tract 1) augments bladder capacity, 2) enhances compliance of the augmented reservoir, 3) transforms a high-pressure system to a low-pressure system, and 4) Significantly decreases the amplitude of uninhibited contractions (Figs. 12 and 13) (28–30).

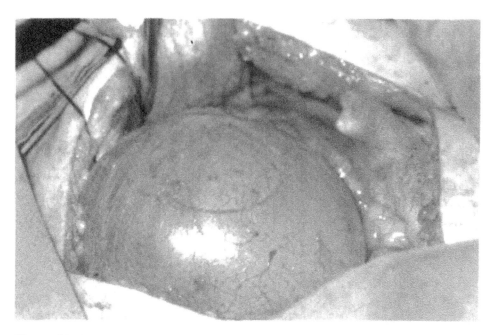

Figure 11 Partial detrusorectomy at the dome of the bladder; an artificial diverticulum has been created, lined only by the thin mucosal layer. The air-bubble at the bladder dome can be seen by transparency.

BLADDER CAPACITY (mL)

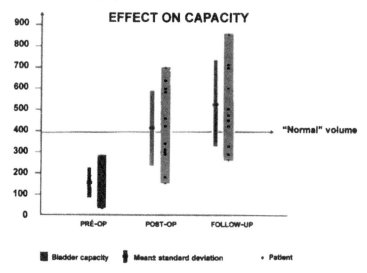

Figure 12 Effect of ileocystoplasty on bladder capacity in a series of 12 patients. Mean capacity before surgery: 160 mL (± 74 mL); mean capacity after surgery (mean: 22.2 months): 508 mL (± 191 mL).

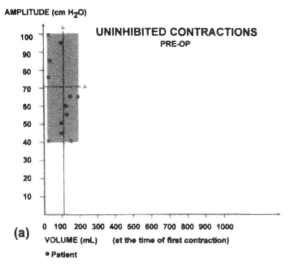

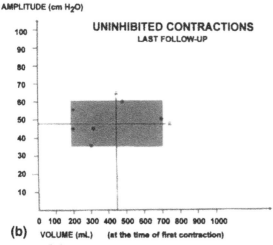

Figure 13   Changes in the amplitude of uninhibited contractions following enterocysto-plasty and the bladder volume at which they occurred: (a) preoperative mean amplitude = 64.5 cmH$_2$O ($\pm$ 21.5 cmH$_2$O); mean volume = 92.1 mL ($\pm$ 58.2 mL); (b) Postoperative mean amplitude = 50.9 cmH$_2$O ($\pm$ 10.9 cmH$_2$O); mean volume = 309.2 mL ($\pm$ 200.5 mL).

Although 15–50% of patients with neurogenic bladder dysfunction will develop vesicoureteral reflux (31), the necessity of performing simultaneous ureteral reimplantation in these patients remains controversial, mainly because the transformation of a high-pressure to a low-pressure system can, by itself, cure reflux (32,33). Others believe, however, that reflux greater than grade I should be reimplanted at the time of enterocystoplasty (34).

It should be pointed out that, in contrast to patients with bladder autoaugmentation, those in whom enterocystoplasty is planned should be able and willing to perform clean intermittent catheterization postoperatively.

Table 1   Pharmacological and Surgical Treatment Alternatives in the Control of the Overactive Bladder

Pharmacology	Per os (anticholinergics)
	Transcutaneous (nitroglycerin)
	Intravesical (capsaicin, resiniferatoxin, oxybutynin, marcain)
	Intrathecal (Baclofen)
Surgery	Denervation (spinal bloc, supraselective sacral rhizotomy, transtrigonal phenol injection, bladder transection)
	Autoaugmentation
	Enterocystoplasty
	Functional electrostimulation of the pelvic floor

4.   Functional Electrical Stimulation of the Pelvic Floor

The rationale and different modalities of this approach have been described elsewhere in the present volume. Here, it should be mentioned only that the technique needs an intact sacral reflex pathway. Stimulation is applied to the afferent nerve terminals of this reflex (vaginal, anal canal, perianal or suprapubic skin, pudendal nerve trunk, or such). These afferent stimuli evoke stimulation of the pelvic floor muscles and striated urethral sphincter. They simultaneously inhibit detrusor contraction. The neurophysiological principles underlying this approach have been summarized by Fall and Lindström (35).

Medication alone frequently does not improve the patient's condition enough. In these circumstances, the surgical approach must be considered. The general rule should be to start with a less invasive procedure, and as the clinical status of the patient warrants, move ahead with more invasive treatments.

Functional electrostimulation of the pelvic floor is a less invasive surgical approach, using a vaginal or anal electrode. However, the stimulating device is rather expensive. Implantation of electrodes around the sacral nerves in almost all centers familiar with the technique is done only in the context of experimental protocols. This limits accessibility of the patient population to this technology.

Among the denervation procedures, bladder transection seems to give the most satisfactory results, even if the final outcome can not be predicted in the individual patient.

This is also true with bladder autoaugmentation. Preoperative urodynamic tests are still not sensitive enough to allow the selection of patients who are more susceptible to a favorable outcome.

The great advantage of these two techniques is that both of them are extraperitoneal procedures, so morbidity is reduced. In our experience, the results are roughly the same: cure and improvement can be expected in about 60–65% of patients. The choice between the two operations is based mainly on preoperative bladder capacity. When it is less than 250–300 mL, we perform bladder autoaugmentation. Above this capacity, bladder transection is offered to the patient.

In a recent study by Leng et al. (36), autoaugmentation and enterocystoplasty had comparable success, or bladder function improved without incurring the significant complication rate of enterocystoplasty. Furthermore, detrusorectomy or bladder transection does not compromise future enterocystoplasty.

II. ACTIONS DIRECTED TOWARD THE URETHRAL SPHINCTER

In DSD, the urethral sphincter, with its uncoordinated function, is responsible for bladder outlet obstruction. Elimination of sphincter contractility will lead to urinary incontinence. Hence, the ideal treatment should be to either bypass the urinary sphincter or influence it in such a way that the urethra will not be obstructed during bladder contraction.

To achieve this goal, pharmacological treatment can be initiated. If unsuccessful, surgery may be necessary (Table 2).

A. Pharmacological Approaches

The α-adrenergic blockers (e.g., prazosin, doxazosin, and tamsulosin, a recently developed α-adrenergic blocker with high uroselectivity) have been disappointing in neurological patients. They are more efficacious in those with dysfunctional voiding.

Table 2 Pharmacological and Surgical Treatment Alternatives for the Uncoordinated Urinary Sphincter

Pharmacology	Per os: alpha-blockers
	In loco: botulinum-A toxin
	Intrathecal: baclofen
Surgery	Clean intermittent catheterization (male and female)
	Balloon dilatation of the striated sphincter (male)
	Overdilatation of the urethra (female)
	Intraurethral stent (male)
	Transurethral incision of the bladder neck (male) and the prostate
	Sphincterotomy (male)

Elsewhere in this volume (see Chap. 45), Zermann and co-workers describe in detail the use of botulinum-A toxin injected transurethrally into the external striated sphincter. The results are encouraging, even if treatment must be repeated from time to time. It is interesting that Fowler et al. (37) injected the toxin in women with nonneurological chronic urinary retention, none of whom improved symptomatically. No significant systemic adverse effects have been reported with the drug.

As mentioned earlier (21), intrathecal infusion of baclofen can eliminate not only undesireable hyperreflexia, but in a significant number of cases (40%), DSD as well.

B. Surgical Approaches

Recognizing that clean but nonsterile, intermittent self-catheterization is not harmful, Diokno et al. (38) made a major contribution to treatment of the neurogenic bladder that revolutionized the day-to-day management of these patients. They have described in detail, elsewhere in this volume (see Chap. 31), the selection and initial evaluation of potential candidates for this form of treatment, the technique itself, eventual complications, and follow-up of these patients.

Successful balloon dilation was reported by Chancellor et al. (39) in 15 out of 17 male patients with DSD. One year after the operation, voiding pressure and postvoid residual decreased significantly. Even autonomic dysreflexia, when present, was improved.

If preoperative evaluation of females demonstrates a closed bladder neck, overdilation of the urethra can be undertaken without fear of subsequent SUI (40). The Crédé maneuver is much more efficacious when the pelvic floor is paralyzed. In these circumstances, the intra-abdominal pressure generated by the maneuver is partially dissipated by the pelvic floor and, consequently, a smaller proportion of this pressure will be transmitted to the proximal urethra, promoting better emptying of the bladder.

Elsewhere in this volume, Rivas and Chancellor (see Chap. 38) have described the experience gained with intraurethral stent placement in a multicenter North American trial.

Transurethral incision of the bladder neck was popularized by Turner–Warwick (41), with excellent results. We had similar experience with this technique.

DSD is one of the principal indications for transurethral sphincterotomy, which improves bladder emptying in 86% of patients with hyperreflexia. It can even be proposed to patients with hypo- or areflexic bladders, improving bladder emptying in 38% of them (42). More details on this technique can be found elsewhere in this volume (see Chap. 38).

Clinical experience suggests that pharmacological manipulation of the urinary sphincter is more successful in dysfunctional voiders than in neurological patients. In the latter, botulinum-A toxin injection is a repeatable and not irreversible procedure. Restrictions for the intrathecal injection of baclofen are the same as those mentioned in the previous section on the hyperreflexic bladder.

From the surgical point of view, whenever possible, clean intermittent catheterization is the treatment of choice In DSD. When this is impossible, and if the male patient accepts wearing a condom catheter permanently, transurethral external sphincterotomy remains an excellent approach. It should be remembered, however, that the placement of an intraurethral stent in some circumstances may replace sphincterotomy. Unfortunately, because no satisfactory external collective device exists at present, these two therapeutic alternatives can hardly be recommended for female patients.

Fortunately, however, because the external striated sphincter in the female is much less powerful than in the male, harmful DSD is much less frequent in women than in men.

REFERENCES

1. Andersen JT, Abrams P, Blaivas JG, Stanton SL. The standardization of terminology of lower urinary tract function. Scand J Urol Nephrol Suppl 1988; 144:5–19.
2. Malkowicz SB, Wein AJ, Elbadawi A, Van Arsdalen K, Ruggieri MR, Levin RM. Acute biochemical and functional alterations in the partially obstructed rabbit urinary bladder. J Urol 1986; 136:1324–1329.
3. Kato K, Wein AJ, Longhurst PA, Haugaard N, Levin RM. Functional effects of long-term outlet obstruction on the rabbit urinary bladder. J Urol 1990; 143:600–606.
4. Levin RM, Wein AJ, Longhurst PA. Neuropharmacology of the lower urinary tract. In: Mundy AR, Stephenson TP, Wein AJ, eds. Urodynamics. Principles, Practice and Application. 2nd ed. Edinburgh: Churchill Livingstone, 1994:29–42.
5. Gilpin S, Gosling J, Barnard J. Morphological and morphometric studies of the human obstructed, trabeculated urinary bladder. Br J Urol 1985; 57:525–529.
6. Sundin T, Dahlström A, Norlin L, Svedmyr N. The sympathetic innervation and adrenoreceptor function of the lower urinary tract in the normal state and after parasympathetic denervation. Invest Urol 1977; 14:322–328.
7. Neal DE, Bogue PR, Williams RE. Histological appearances of the nerves to the bladder in patients with denervation of the bladder after excision of the rectum. Br J Urol 1982; 54:658–666.
8. McGuire EJ, Morrissey SG. The development of neurogenic vesical dysfunction after experimental spinal cord injury or sacral rhizotomy in non-human primates. J Urol 1982; 128:1390–1393.
9. Ghoniem GM, Regnier CH, Biancani P, Johnson L, Susset JG. Effect of bilateral sacral decentralization on detrusor contractility and passive properties in dog. Neurourol Urodynam 1984; 3:23–33.
10. Flood HD, Downie JW, Awad SA. The influence on filling rates and sympathectomy on bladder compliance. Neurourol Urodynam 1987; 6:138–139.
11. McGuire EJ, Woodside JR, Borden TA, Weiss RM. Prognostic value of urodynamic testing in myelodysplastic patients. J Urol 1981; 126:205–209.
12. McGuire EJ, Woodside JR, Borden TA. Upper urinary tract deterioration in patients with myelodysplasia and detrusor hypertonia: a follow-up study. J Urol 1983; 129:823–826.
13. Barrett DM, Wein AJ, Parulkar BG. Surgery for neuropathic bladder. AUA Update Ser 1990; 9(lesson 38):298–303.
14. James MJ, Iacovou JW. The use of GNT patches in detrusor instability: A pilot study. Neurourol Urodynam 1993; 12:399–400.
15. Brandler BCH, Radebaugh LC, Mohler JL. Topical oxybutynin chloride for relaxation of dysfunctional bladders. J Urol 1989; 141:1350–1352.
16. Madersbacher H, Jilg G. Control of detrusor hyperreflexia by the intravesical instillation of oxybutynin chloride. Paraplegia 1991; 29:84–90.
17. Fowler CJ, Beck RO, Gerrard S, Betts CD, Fowler CG. Intravesical capsaicin for treatment of detrusor hyperreflexia. J Neurol Neurosurg Psychiatry 1994; 57:160–173.
18. Chancellor MB, de Groat WC. Intravesical capsaicin and resiniferatoxin therapy: spicing up the way to treat the overactive bladder. J Urol 1999; 162:3–11.
19. McInerney PD, Grant A, Chawla J, Stephenson TP. The effect of intravesical Marcaine instillation on hyperreflexic detrusor contraction. Paraplegia 1992; 30:127–130.
20. Geirsson G, Lindström S, Fall M. The bladder cooling reflex in man: characteristics and sensitivity to temperature. Br J Urol 1993; 71:675–680.
21. Steers WD, Meythaller JM, Haworth C, Herrell D, Park IS. Effects of acute bolus and chronic continuous baclofen on genito-urinary dysfunction due to spinal cord pathology. J Urol 1992; 148:1849–1855.
22. Kums JJM, Delhaas EM. Intrathecal baclofen infusion in patients with spasticity and neurogenic bladder disease. Preliminary results. World J Urol 1991; 9:99–104.

23. Staskin DR, Parson KG, Levin RM, Wein AT. Bladder transection—a functional neurophysiological, neuropharmacological and neuroanatomical study. Br J Urol 1981; 53:552–557.

24. Crooks JE, Khan AB, Meddings RN, Abel BJ. Bladder transection revisited. Br J Urol 1995; 75:590–591.

25. Hassan ST, Robson WA, Ramsden PD, Essenhigh DM, Neal DE. Outcome of endoscopic bladder transection. Br J Urol 1995; 75:592–596.

26. Stöhrer M, Kramer G, Goepel M, Lockner–Ernst D, Kruse D, Rubben H. Bladder auto-augmentation in adult patients with neurogenic voiding dysfunction. Spinal Cord 1997; 35:456–462.

27. Surer I, Elicevik M, Oztork H, Sakarya T, Cetinkursun S. An alternative approach to bladder auto-augmentation. Tech Urol 1999; 5:100–103.

28. Raezer DM, Evans RJ, Shrom SH. Augmentation ileocystoplasty in neuropathic bladder. Urology 1985; 25:26–30.

29. Robertson AS, Davies JB, Webb RJ, Neal DE. Bladder augmentation and replacement: urodynamic and clinical review of 25 patients. Br J Urol 1991; 68:590–597.

30. Luangkhot R, Peng BCH, Blaivas JG. Ileocystoplasty for the management of refractory neurogenic bladder: surgical technique and urodynamic findings. J Urol 1991; 146:1340–1344.

31. Brereton RJ, Narayanan R, Ratnatunga C. Ureteric reimplantation in the neuropathic bladder. Br J Surg 1987; 74:1107–1110.

32. Nasrallah PHF, Aliabadi HA. Bladder augmentation in patients with neurogenic bladder and vesicoureteral reflux. J Urol 1991; 146:563–566.

33. Firlit CF, Sommer JR, Kaplan WE. Pediatric urinary undiversion. J Urol 1980; 123:748–753.

34. Bennett JK, Gray M, Green BG, Foote JE. Continent diversion and bladder augmentation in spinal cord injured patients. Semin Urol 1992; 10:121–132.

35. Fall M, Lindström S. Electrical stimulation. A physiological approach to the treatment of urinary incontinence. Urol Clin North Am 1991; 18:393–407.

36. Leng WW, Blalock HJ, Frederiksson WH, English SF, McGuire EJ. Enterocystoplasty or detrusor myomectomy? Comparison of indications and outcomes for bladder augmentation. J Urol 1999; 161:758–763.

37. Fowler CJ, Betts CD, Christmas TJ, Swash M, Fowler CG. Botulinum toxin in the treatment of chronic urinary retention in women. Br J Urol 1992; 70:387–389.

38. Diokno AC, Sonda P, Hollander JB, Lapides J. Fate of patients started on clean intermittent self-catheterization therapy 10 years ago. J Urol 1983; 129:1120–1122.

39. Chancellor MB, Karasick S, Strup S, Abdill CK, Hirsch IH, Staas WE. Transurethral balloon dilation of the external urinary sphincter: effectiveness in spinal cord injured men with detrusor–external urethral sphincter dyssynergia. Radiology 1993; 187:557–560.

40. Parson KF. Difficulty with voiding or acute urinary retention having previously voided satisfactorily. In: Parson KF, Fritzpatrick JM, eds. Practical Urology in Spinal Cord Injury. London: Springer–Verlag, 1991:27–42.

41. Turner-Warwick R. Bladder outflow obstruction in the male. In: Urodynamics: Principles, Practice and Application. Mundy AR, Stephenson TP, Wein AJ, eds. Edinburgh: Churchill Livingstone, 1984:183–204.

42. Schellhammer FP, Hackler RH, Buntz RC. External sphincterotomy: an evaluation of 150 patients with neurogenic bladder. J Urol 1973; 110:199–202.

45

Management of the Hypertonic Sphincter or Hyperpathic Urethra

DIRK-HENRIK ZERMANN

University Hospital, Friedrich–Schiller-University, Jena, Germany

MANABU ISHIGOOKA

Yamagata University School of Medicine, Yamagata, Japan

RICHARD A. SCHMIDT

University of Colorado Medical School and Rose Hospital, Denver, Colorado

I. INTRODUCTION

The desired goal in the management of an overactive urinary sphincter is to eliminate increased or unstable reflex exciteability that leads to compromised behavior in pelvic organs and is responsible for pain and chronic urinary retention. This can be accomplished by biofeedback therapies, use of drugs such as α-adrenergic blockers—terazosin (Hytrin); prazosin (Minipress); or clonidine (Catapress) (1), or muscle relaxants (diazepam), or a combination of both. In severe pelvic pain, first-line fast relief by a symptomatic approach is mandatory. Other neurophysiological-based treatments include the use of neurotoxin (botulinum toxin A; BTX) and external or sacral neuromodulation (Fig. 1).

II. BIOFEEDBACK

The essential goal of biofeedback is to reestablish the proper dynamic behavior of the pelvic musculature (2,3). Often, patients simply have no concept of how to relax these muscles. They may not even be able to identify these muscles or to exert any voluntary influence on their behavior. The objective of biofeedback is to restore appropriate concepts of

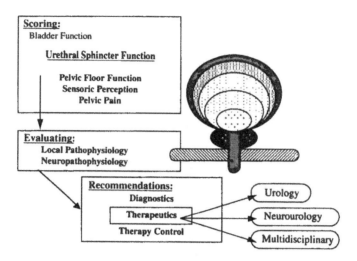

Figure 1 Clinical approach to sphincter and lower urinary tract dysfunction.

pelvic muscle relaxation. This can be as simple as a suggestion to take time with voiding and never to push, strain, or rush the event.

It is important for patients with an overactive urinary sphincter to be made aware of adverse voiding habits or of uncontrolled anxiety states. Patients need to be consciously aware of the goals of biofeedback and to be actively involved on a daily basis with relearning the voiding technique, if long-term success is to be achieved. If awkward voiding methods continue, biofeedback approaches will ultimately fail to affect symptoms. If necessary, the patient should be counseled to deal with stress and with lifestyle patterns that contribute to anxiety, as emotions can affect sphincter tension through the brain stem.

At times, patients will need more specific instruction. Biofeedback equipment and software programs are one option. A simple rectal examination is less expensive and can be very useful in helping patients learn to control their pelvic muscles. Patients are asked to tighten and relax on a rectal balloon or gloved finger so that the physician can assess the efficiency and specificity of these movements. Patients should practice this dynamic, emphasizing relaxation, at regular intervals daily. Progress can be monitored with voiding diaries, repeat rectal examinations, or flow rates. If treatment is successful, there should be a precipitous decline in symptoms (i.e., pain, intermittency, or slowness of the urinary stream). Biofeedback approaches should be combined with medications as well as other treatments for maximum results (Table 1).

Table 1 General Recommendations for Changing Wrong Voiding Behavior

Take time for micturition. Do not rush.
Sit for voiding every time (men also).
No straining.
Timed voiding.

III. ACUPUNCTURE

Acupuncture above the medial malleolus in the inside of the leg, similarly to surface pelvic floor and direct S3 nerve root stimulation, has a suppressive effect on urge-based urinary incontinence and may be promising also in the treatment of a hypertonic sphincter (4–6). The mechanism is probably direct activation of the larger muscle afferents that effectively modulate synaptic transmission in the spinal cord. The technique is simple and complements biofeedback and drug therapy. For reasons that are unclear, it is most effective if the needles are placed through the skin at a point of lowest skin impedance, 4 cm above the medial malleolus and just behind the tibia (posttibial nerve).

IV. α-ADRENERGIC BLOCKERS

It is known that urethral sphincteric overactivity, spasticity, or irritability can result in poor bladder emptying. α-Adrenergic blockers, through their peripheral and central actions, can help lower bladder outlet resistance (Table 2) (1,7). There are no publications on the treatment of hypertonic sphincter in controlled trials.

V. INTERMITTENT SELF-CATHETERIZATION OR LONG-TERM CATHETERS

There are occasions when catheter management is the only option. It is a pure symptomatic treatment option. The method of intermittent self-catheterization is generally preferred over insertion of a long-term catheter. Learning self-catheterization allows the patient to empty the bladder alone, with low risks of side effects. This procedure has to be done on a strong time schedule because bladder sensitivity is missing in most patients who have chronic urinary retention. Patients with a hypertonic urethra have to be aware of possible problems passing the sphincter with the catheter. Skillful catheterization will prevent hematuria, sphincter lesions, and via falsa.

Insertion of a suprapubic or transurethral long-term catheter is an ultima ratio in the management of hypertonic sphincter. Generally, these patients have severe motor disabilities related to central nervous system (CNS) pathology. Long-term catheters are associated with an increased risk of problems, such as recurring infections, sepsis, stones, pain, and cancer. Catheter-related complications are greatly increased by hyperactive, hypertensive, or hypertonic bladders. Patients can do very well if their bladder is kept in a low-pressure, low-activity state, they are well hydrated, and they exercise good perineal hygiene with regular catheter changes. New catheter designs being developed will both facilitate emptying and allow patients more mobility and, hence, a better quality of life.

Table 2   α-Adrenergic Blockers Used in Neurourology

Prazosin (Minipress)
Tamsulosin (Flowmax)
Doxazosin (Cardura)
Terazosin (Hytrin)
Clonidine (Catapres)

VI. TRANSCUTANEOUS NERVE STIMULATION (TENS) THERAPY

The principle of TENS has been established as a valuable tool in the treatment of urinary incontinence and pain over the last 15 years. The technique is simple and virtually risk-free. Electrical stimulation is applied to critical areas within the sacral dermatomes. Sites reported to be associated with beneficial results include the sacral, suprapubic, common perineal, and posterior tibial nerves. Large skin afferents, when stimulated, suppress spontaneous reflex activity within the same dermatome. Vaginal and anal plugs have also been reported to be useful.

Although it is encouraging to know that relatively simple approaches can be effective, there are drawbacks. As a general rule, the effects of neurostimulation do not last, and when it is effective, patients are dependent on frequent, ongoing treatment. In addition, the results of superficial stimulation are rather unpredictable from patient to patient. Vaginal and anal plug devices, or both, have not proved popular with patients in North America and Europe if more than a few sessions of stimulation are necessary. The technique is, however, simple and may be considered in a patient before resorting to destructive surgical procedures.

VII. BOTULINUM TOXIN

Botulinum toxin (BTX) is a potent neurotoxin with a high affinity toward acetylcholine (ACh) receptors. It is produced by the gram-negative, rod-shaped anerobic bacterium *Clostridium botulinum*. The neurotoxin, synthesized in seven different serotypes, acts on peripheral cholinergic nerve endings to inhibit ACh release (8). Although the neurotoxin is most potent at somatic neuromuscular junctions, it does have the ability to inhibit, autonomic cholinergic transmission (9). Therefore, BTX is capable of suppressing transmitter release from pre- and postganglionic cholinergic nerve endings of the autonomic nervous system as well as interfering with smooth-muscle visceral function. Injected BTX attaches quickly to somatic ACh receptors when injected into the target muscle. There is very little risk of it adversely affecting neighboring striated or visceral smooth muscle or even ganglionic transmission. BTX does not penetrate the blood–brain barrier in therapeutic doses. There is, therefore, no significant risk that transmitter function in the CNS will be affected. In doses used clinically, BTX is a highly selective and safe neurotoxin.

The treatment of striated muscle with BTX results in an accelerated loss of junctional ACh receptors (10). Paralysis and near complete decline of miniature end-plate potentials occur within a few hours after its injection (11,12). The muscle becomes functionally denervated, atrophies, and develops extrajunctional ACh receptors (13). The clinical effect is to weaken the injected muscle.

In the early 1980s, BTX was introduced successfully for the treatment of strabismus (14), and its use subsequently expanded to other conditions manifested by involuntary muscle spasm, spasticity, and tremors (15).

Selective urethral sphincter BTX injection can reduce hypertonic and hyperreflexic sphincter activity, with the potential of providing pain relief and improving lower urinary tract symptoms.

Many patients with pelvic pain experience pelvic floor muscle tenderness, myofascial trigger points, and sphincter hypersensitivity, hypertonicity, and hyperactivity (16,17). Clinical examination typically reveals restricted pelvic floor dynamic control (i.e., contraction and relaxation) (see Diagnostics).

Whether pelvic muscular dysfunction is a root cause of pain, or an integral part of CNS failure that underlies pain, addressing the muscular dysfunction directly makes sense. It is a logical step toward reducing the neurogenic cascade of events that can feed inflammation and hypersensitivity in tissue. BTX not only can weaken injected muscle, but it also affects neighboring muscle within the same dermatome (18). This may occur by its local diffusion or by its effect on the spinal reflex regulation of muscle within the dermatome. The latter indirect effect on spinal cord circuits could occur through the intrafusal (19) or extrafusal neuromuscular junction, or both (20,21). An observed change in muscle activity pattern after BTX injection suggests that central reorganization is induced by the therapy. This position is supported by results from a positron emission tomography (PET) study, which showed increased activation within the parietal cortex and the caudal supplementary motor area, after BTX therapy of writer's cramp. The changes that did occur reflected changes in muscle movement strategy and in the associated CNS activation patterns that controlled these muscle activities. These changes could also be explained by cortical reorganization secondary to loss of motoneurons and decreased sensory afferent input (22).

VIII. NEUROMODULATION (SACRAL NERVE STIMULATION)

Stimulation of the sacral nerves evokes striated and smooth-muscle contractions in the pelvis within a pain-free window of applied current. Painful amplitudes of current applied to either the S3 or S4 nerve will produce bladder contraction at thresholds four to five times higher than for the striated pelvic floor muscle. There is, therefore, a tolerable pain-free window for stimulation of the striated pelvic muscle.

S3 nerves supply some branches to the pudendal nerves. However, owing to pre- and postfixation of the spinal nuclei, the significance of this contribution can vary widely among patients. The S3 nerves will predictably supply the more anterior levator muscle systems through pelvic branches that leave the nerve trunk before they contribute to the sciatic and pudendal nerves (i.e., the ischial spine). Direct S3 stimulation will produce visible contraction of the levator muscles (bellows-like movement) and contraction of the large toe or the distal foot (i.e., all toes). Referred sensation to the rectum and scrotum is common. Contraction of the large toe, and less often the forefoot, may be evident along with referred sensation to the scrotum.

S4 nerves do not contribute to pudendal innervation of the pelvis or to the sciatic nerves. Their direct stimulation will produce contraction of the posterior portion of the levator. This is a referred sensation to the rectum or to the tip of the coccyx, or both.

The bladder neck is pulled open by the contracting detrusor body. The longitudinal muscle of the bladder is known to extend down and around the bladder neck, forming the detrusor loops. When the bladder contracts, the loops are pulled back into the body of the bladder, and the neck of the bladder is mechanically opened. This observation does not negate the theory that there is active relaxation of the bladder neck by sympathetics, but it does support a concept wherein the actual funneling of the bladder neck is dependent on cholinergically mediated active smooth-muscle contraction.

Implanted devices have specific advantages and are able to circumvent most of the disadvantages of TENS therapy. Patients who benefit from neurostimulation trials can be helped regardless of the time, place, need, or dependence on neurostimulation. Inefficiencies associated with the delivery of TENS current are minimized with implants because of direct application of current to a specific sacral nerve. Finally, nerve stimulation is the most efficient way to elicit continuous influence over pelvic muscle failure. This, in turn, provides the best hope of regulating striated pelvic floor muscle behavior. It is therapeutically attractive to specifically neutralize hyperreflexic striated sphincter activity, without compromising the reflex contractility of the bladder. Usually, with stimulation of a sacral nerve, a pleasant pulling or tugging in the perineum is felt by the patient.

A period of testing is required to determine if the proper set of nerve fibers can be found for chronic neurostimulation, then if stimulation can be applied on a continuing basis. In this procedure, an insulated needle is positioned in one or more of the sacral foramens. Stimulation is applied, gradually, by increasing (ramping) the current to a comfortable intensity. Usually, the stimulation intensities will be much higher and more comfortable when good muscle contraction is obtained. If it is not, the stimulation will be unpleasant. When it is effective, tenderness will be markedly reduced in tissues during and after stimulation. A temporary electrode is then inserted into the foramen through the test needle and left in place for 3–7 days. If the patient does well during this period of trial stimulation, there is the option of placing the electrode permanently (Fig. 2), or of waiting and repeating the trial. Few patients who benefit from stimulation will remain in remission from their symptoms once stimulation therapy is withdrawn. Trial therapies over several days

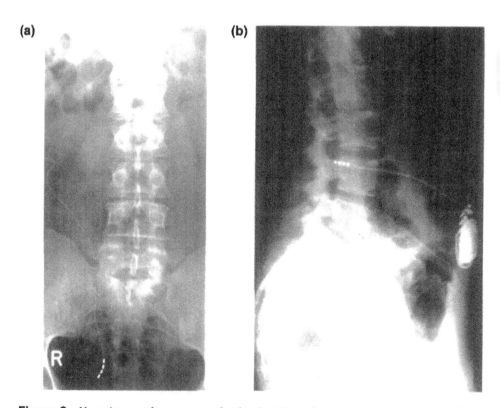

(a)   (b)

Figure 2   X-ray image of os sacrum after implantation of a permanent electrode on S3 for sacral nerve stimulation: (a) sagittal view; (b) lateral view.

have been performed on over 600 nerves for a variety of reasons. Permanent implants were performed specifically for the treatment of pain in 40 patients, none of whom showed evidence of nerve injury (23). Thus, the techniques of evaluation and continuous stimulation, when successful, do not appear to present undue risks. Within this experience, patients who did best were those who had identifiable dysfunction in the pelvic muscles.

REFERENCES

1. Secrest CL, Aldridge JE. Management of the spastic urinary sphincter. Urology 1993; 41:127–129.
2. Oldenburg B, Millard RJ. Predictors of long term outcome following bladder re-training programme. J Psychosom Res 1986; 30:691–698.
3. Hafner RJ. Biofeedback treatment of intermittent urinary retention. Br J Urol 1981; 53:125–128.
4. Dung HC. Acupuncture points of the sacral plexus. Am J Chin Med 1985; 13:145–156.
5. Zhang ZY, Zhang K Wu DZ. [Effect of acupuncture on the pons micturition centre and the related function of the urinary bladder]. Chen Tzu Yen Chiu 1987; 12:116–122.
6. Morrison JF, Sato A, Sato Y, Suzuki A. Long-lasting facilitation and depression of periurethral skeletal muscle following acupuncture-like stimulation in anesthetized rats. Neurosci Res 1995; 23:159–169.
7. Andersson KE, Lepor I–L, Wyllie MG. Prostatic α_1- adrenoceptors and uroselectivity. Prostate 1997; 30:202–215.
8. Simpson LL. The origin, structure, and pharmacological activity of botulinum toxin. Pharmacol Rev 1981; 33:155–188.
9. Girlanda P, Vita G, Nicolosi C, Milone S, Messina C. Botulinum toxin therapy: distant effects on neuromuscular transmission and autonomic nervous system. J Neurol Neurosurg Psychiatry 1992; 55:844–845.
10. Avila OL, Drachman DB, Pestronk A. Neurotransmission regulates stability of acetylcholine receptors at the neuromuscular junction. J Neurosci 1989; 9:2902–2906.
11. Pestronk A, Drachman DB, Griffin JW. Effect of botulinum toxin on trophic regulation of acetylcholine receptors. Nature 1976; 264:787–789.
12. Kao I, Drachman DB, Price DL. Botulinum toxin: mechanism of presynaptic blockade. Science 1976; 193:1256–1258.
13. Borodic GE, Cozzolino D, Ferrante R, Wiegner AW, Young RR. Innervation zone of orbicularis oculi muscle and implications for botulinum A toxin therapy. Ophthalmol Plast Reconstr Surg 1991; 7:54–60.
14. Scott AB. Botulinum toxin injection of eye muscles to correct strabismus. Trans Am Ophthalmol Soc 1981; 79:734–770.
15. Jankovic J, Brin W. Therapeutic uses of botulinum toxin. N Engl J Med 1991; 324:1186–1194.
16. Zermann DH, Ishigooka M, Doggweiler R, Schmidt RA. Postoperative chronic pelvic pain and bladder dysfunction—windup and neuronal plasticity—do we need a more neurourological approach in pelvic surgery? J Urol 1998; 160:102–105.
17. Zermann DH, Ishigooka M, Doggweiler R, Schmidt RA. Neuro-urological insights to the etiology of genitourinary pain in men. J Urol 1999; 161:903–908.
18. Eleopra R, Tugnoli V, Caniatti L, DeGrandis D. Botulinum toxin treatment in the facial muscles of humans: evidence of an action in untreated near muscles by peripheral local diffusion. Neurology 1996; 46:1158–1160.
19. Priori A, Berardelli A, Mercuri B, Manfredi M. Physiological effects produced by botulinum toxin treatment of upper limb dystonia. Changes in reciprocal inhibition between forearm muscles. Brain 1995; 118:801–807.

20. Bertolasi L, Priori A, Tomelleri G, Bongiovanni LG, Fincati E, Simonati A, DeGrandis D, Rizzuto N. Botulinum toxin treatment of muscle cramps: a clinical and neurophysiological study. Ann Neurol 1997; 41:181–186.
21. Gelb DJ, Yoshimura DM, Olney RK, Lowenstein DH, Aminoff MJ. Change in pattern of muscle activity following botulinum toxin injections for torticollis. Ann Neurol 1991; 29:370–376.
22. Ceballos–Baumann AO, Sheean G, Passingham RE, Marsden CD, Brooks DJ. Botulinum toxin does not reverse the cortical dysfunction associated with writer's cramp. A PET study. Brain 1997; 120:571–582.

46

Overview of the ICS Standardization Reports

ERIK SCHICK

University of Montreal and Maisonneuve–Rosemont Hospital, Montreal, Quebec, Canada

One of the prerequisites of communication in general is the use of words, terms, or expressions that are understood by everyone in the same manner, and that have the same meaning for everybody. This is particularly true in the scientific world, and applies to urodynamics as well.

In the early days, when urodynamics left the experimental laboratories and became progressively implanted in clinical practice, new concepts and new phenomena became recognized and started to be explored in different ways, with different words and expressions used by different investigators who often described similar or even identical phenomena.

For instance, to characterize a bladder that escaped from cortical control, investigators used terms such as automatic, spastic, hypertonic, hyperreflexic, unstable, and so on.

At the very beginning of the International Continence Society (ICS), members recognized the need to elaborate some form of uniformity in the vocabulary used. They established, more than 25 years ago in 1973, a committee with a clear mandate to standardize the terminology to be used when studying the function and dysfunction of the lower urinary tract. This committee, known as the "International Continence Society Committee on Standardization of Terminology" published its first report 3 years later, in 1976, and which has been reproduced by four different scientific (urological) journals. All of the reports, except the fifth, dealing with the quantification of urinary loss, which was an internal document of the society, have been approved by the members during the different annual meetings of the ICS.

The first report dealt with urinary incontinence and procedures related to evaluate urine storage (cystometry, urethral closure pressure profile), the second with procedures related to the evaluation of micturition (flow rate, pressure measurements), the third with other aspects of micturition (pressure–flow relations, residual urine), the fourth with the neuro-muscular dysfunction of the lower urinary tract, the fifth, as mentioned, with quantification of urine loss, the sixth more largely with neurophysiological investigations (EMG, nerve conduction studies, reflex latencies, evoked potentials, and sensory testing), and the seventh with lower urinary tract rehabilitation techniques. The subsequent reports do not bear specific numbers.

In 1996, a report was produced about female pelvic organ prolapse and pelvic floor dysfunction. As far as we know, this is the only report that has been elaborated in collaboration of other scientific societies namely the American Urogynecologic Society and the Society of Gynecologic Surgeons.

In the same year another report was published on the assessment of functional characteristics of intestinal urinary reservoirs.

One of the most recent reports, published in 1999 in the Society's journal *Neurourology and Urodynamics,* deals with neurogenic bladder dysfunction. In contrast with previous reports, the subcommittee elaborated some suggestions for diagnostic procedures as well.

The latest report published in March 2000 is the one dealing with the standardization of ambulatory urodynamic monitoring. Part of the report are 11 explanatory examples to facilitate one's ability to interpret these ambulatory urodynamic tracings.

As urodynamics continued to develop, a new subcommittee has been formed, 17 years after the third report was published, to evaluate new procedures related to micturition (pressure–flow studies of voiding, urethral resistance, and urethral obstruction).

In recent years the Standardization Committee decided to look into problems related to outcome measures. They produced a report in 1998 on general principles of outcome studies in patients with lower urinary tract dysfunction. This was followed shortly by three more specific reports on outcome measures for research in adult women, adult males, and frail older persons.

Two "review articles" have been published in which authors merged several reports in one single article.

In December 1976, Hugh J. Jewett, then editor-in-chief of the *Journal of Urology,* asked William E. Bradley to prepare a synopsis of three previous reports on the standardization of terminology of lower urinary tract function as he was member of the subcommittee who prepared the first three ICS reports. This article was published in 1979 in the *Journal of Urology.*

Later on P. Abrams, together with J. G. Blaivas, S. L. Stanton, and J. T. Andersen (who was then the Chairman of the Committee), wrote a synthesis of the six first reports (including also the fifth one on quantification of urine loss), which was published in 1988 simultaneously in a supplement to the *Scandinavian Journal of Urology and Nephrology,* and *Neurourology and Urodynamics.* Among all the standardization reports this article is probably the one that is the more often quoted by different authors.

As English is more and more the most widely used language in medical communication, almost every physician and scientist understands, reads, and is able to write in English. This might explain why there is virtually no translation of these reports in other languages. For example, to the best of our knowledge, no French or German version of these reports exists. We are aware, however, that the review article of P. Abrams et al. and the report on urodynamic equipment has been translated into Hungarian by A. Tanko and was published as an addendum to his book on female urinary incontinence, in 1990.

Finally we should mention two highly technical reports.

The first of these defines some technical aspects of urodynamic equipment. It was published in 1987, and was not produced strictly by the Standardization Committee, but rather, by an ICS Working Party on Urodynamic Equipment. The majority of companies manufacturing urodynamic equipment today tend to conform to these standards.

The second one was published as an appendix to the second report on pressure–flow studies (in 1997), and made some suggestions about ICS standards for digital exchange of pressure–flow study data.

The intention of the International Continence Society instituting the Standardization Committee was not to establish guidelines on how to investigate or how to treat patients with lower tract symptoms, but rather, to allow scientists, clinicians, and researchers to better communicate.

Urodynamics and neurourology are relatively young disciplines within urology. They are constantly evolving and other topics are being considered by the committee (for example, nocturia, quality control of urodynamic studies, etc.). In the light of new research, our understanding of well-known phenomena are changing. This means that previous reports probably need to undergo some degree of revision in the near future.

In the following pages we reproduced the different reports in extenso to give the opportunity to interested readers to find all this information available in a single site.

47

List of the Reports of the ICS Committee on Standardization of Terminology of Lower Urinary Tract Function

The following list has been established with the collaboration of A. Mattiasson, from the University of Lund, Sweden, former chairman of the Standardization Committee.

A. Reports on Standardization

1. Bates P, Bradley WE, Glen E, Melchior H, Rowan D, Sterling A, Hald T.

   First report on the standardization of terminology of lower urinary tract function
   Urinary incontinence
   Procedures related to the evaluation of urine storage:
   Cystometry
   Urethral closure pressure profile
   Units of measurements.
   Brit J Urol 1976; 48:39–42
   Eur Urol 1976; 2:274–276
   Scand J Urol Nephrol 1977; 11:193–196
   Urol Int 1976; 32:81–87

2. Bates P, Glen E, Griffiths D, Melchior H, Rowan D, Sterling A, Hald T.

   Second report on the standardization of terminology of lower urinary tract function
   Procedures related to the evaluation of micturition
   Flow rate
   Pressure measurement
   Symbols
   Acta Urol Jpn 1977; 27:1536–1566
   Br J Urol 1977; 49:207–210
   Eur Urol 1977; 3:168–170
   Scand J Urol Nephrol 1977; 11:197–199

3. Bates P, Bradley WE, Glen E, Griffiths D, Melchior H, Rowan D, Sterling A, Hald T.

    Third report on the standardization of terminology of lower urinary tract function
       Procedures related to the evaluation of micturition:
       Pressure–flow relations
       Residual urine
    Brit J Urol 1980; 52:348–359
    Eur Urol 1980; 6:170–171
    Acta Urol Jpn 1980; 27:1566–1568
    Scand J Urol Nephrol 1980; 12:191–193

4. Bates P, Bradley WE, Glen E, Melchior H, Rowan D, Sterling A, Sundin T, Thomas D, Torrens M, Turner–Warwick R, Zinner NR, Hald T.

    Fourth report on the standardization of terminology of the lower urinary tract function
    Terminology related to neuromuscular dysfunction of lower urinary tract.
    Brit J Urol 1981; 53:333–335
    Urology 1981; 17:618–620
    Scand J Urol Nephrol 1981; 15:169–171
    Acta Urol Jpn 1981; 27:1568–1571

5. Abrams P, Blaivas JG, Stanton SL, Andersen JT, Fowler CJ, Gerstenberg T, Murray K.

    Sixth report on the standardization of terminology of the lower urinary tract function:
       Procedures related to neurophysiological investigations
       Electromyography
       Nerve condustion studies
       Reflex latencies
       Evoked potentials
       Sensory testing
    World J Urol 1986; 4:2–5
    Scand J Urol Nephrol 1986; 20:161–164

6. Andersen JT, Blaivas JG, Cardozo L, Thüroff J.

    Seventh report on the standardization of terminology of lower urinary tract function
       Lower urinary tract rehabilitation techniques.
    Int Urogynecol J 1992; 3:75–80

7. Bump RC, Mattiasson A. Bø K, Brubaker LP, DeLancey JO, Klarskov P, Shull BL, Smith ARB.

    The standardization of terminology of female pelvic organ prolapse and pelvic floor dysfunction
    Am J Obstet Gynecol 1996; 175:10–17

8. Thüroff JW, Mattiasson A, Anders JT, Hedlund H, Hinmann F Jr, Hohenfellner M, Månsson W, Mundy AB, Rowland RG, Steven K.

Standardization of terminology and assessment of functional characteristics of intestinal urinary reservoirs
Neurourol Urodyn 1996; 15:499–511
Brit J Urol 1996; 78:516–523
Scand J Urol Nephrol 1996; 30:349–356

9. Griffiths D, Höfner K, van Mastrigt R, Rollema HJ, Spånberg A, Gleason D.

Standardization of terminology of lower urinary tract function:
Pressure–flow studies of voiding
Urethral resistance
Urethral obstruction
Neurourol Urodynam 1997; 16:1–8

10. Stöhrer M, Goepel M, Kondo A, Kramer G, Madersbacher H, Millard R, Rossier A, Wyndaele JJ.

The standardization of terminology in neurogenic lower urinary tract dysfunction.
(With suggestions for diagnostic procedures.)
Neurourol Urodynam 1999; 18:139–158

11. van Waalwijk van Doorn E, Anders K, Khullar V, Kulseng–Hanssen S, Pesce F, Robertson A, Rosario D, Schäfer W.

Standardisation of ambulatory urodynamic monitoring
Report of the standardization subcommettee of the International Continence Society for ambulatory urodynamics
Neurourol Urodynam 2000; 19:113–125

B. Reports on Outcome Studies

12. Mattiasson A, Djurhuus JC, Fonda D, Lose G, Nordling J, Stöhrer M.

Standardization of outcome studies in patients with lower urinary tract dysfunction
A report on general principles from the standardization committee of the International Continence Society
Neurourol Urodynam 1998; 17:249–253

13. Lose G, Fantl JA, Victor A, Walter S, Wells TL, Wyman J, Mattiasson A.

Outcome measures for research in adult women with symptoms of lower urinary tract dysfunction
Neurourol Urodynam 1998; 17:255–262

14. Nordling J, Abrams P, Ameda K, Andersen JT, Donovan J, Griffiths D, Kobayashi S, Koyanagi T, Schäfer W, Yalla S, Mattiasson A.

Outcome measures for research in treatment of adult males with symptoms of lower urinary tract dysfunction
Neurourol Urodynam 1998; 17:263–271

15. Fonda D, Resnick NM, Colling J, Burgio K, Ouslander JG, Norton C, Ekelund P, Versi E, Mattiasson A.

     Outcome measures for research of lower urinary tract dysfunction in frail older people
     Neurourol Urodyn 1998; 17:273–281.

C. Synthesized Reports

16. Bates P, Bradley WE, Glen E, Griffiths D, Melchior H, Rowan D, Sterling A, Zinner N, Hald T.

     The standardization of terminology of lower urinary tract function.
     J Urol 1979; 121:551–554

17. Abrams P, Blaivas JG, Stanton SL, Andersen JT.

     The standardization of terminology of lower urinary tract function.
     Scand J Urol Nephrol Suppl 1988; 144:5–19
     Neurourol Urodynam 1988; 7:403–417

D. Technical Reports

18. Rowan D, James ED, Kramer AEJL, Sterling A, Suhel PF.

     Urodynamic equipment: technical aspects. (ICS Working Party on Urodynamic Equipment)
     J Med Eng Technol 1987; 11:57–64

19. van Mastrigt R, Griffiths D.

     ICS Standard for digital exchange of pressure–flow study data. (Version 7.1)
     Neurourol Urodynam 1997; 16:9–18

Standardization of Terminology of Lower Urinary Tract Function: Synthesis of First Six Reports

I. INTRODUCTION

The International Continence Society (ICS) established a committee for the standardization of terminology of lower urinary tract function in 1973. Five of the six reports (No. 1–4 and 6) from this committee, approved by the society, have been published. The fifth report, on "Quantification of Urine Loss," was an internal ICS document but appears, in part, in this document.

These reports are revised, extended, and collated in this monograph. The standards are recommended to facilitate comparison of results by investigators who use urodynamic methods. These standards are recommended not only for urodynamic investigations carried out on human patients, but also during animal studies. When urodynamic studies in animals are conducted, the type of any anesthesia used should be stated. It is suggested that acknowledgment of these standards in written publications be indicated by a footnote to Methods and Materials or its equivalent, to read as follows: "Methods, definitions and units conform to the standards recommended by the International Continence Society, except where specifically noted."

Urodynamic studies involve the assessment of the function and dysfunction of the urinary tract by any appropriate method. Aspects of urinary tract morphology, physiology, biochemistry, and hydrodynamics affect urine transport and storage. Other methods of investigation, such as the radiographic visualization of the lower urinary tract are useful as adjuncts to conventional urodynamics.

This monograph concerns the urodynamics of the lower urinary tract.

From Paul Abrams, Jerry G. Blaivas, Stuart L. Stanton, and Jens T. Andersen (Chairman), *International Continence Society Committee on Standardisation of Terminology,* Neurourology and Urodynamics 7:403–427 (1988). Copyright 1988 by Alan R. Liss, Inc.

II. CLINICAL ASSESSMENT

The clinical assessment of patients with lower urinary tract dysfunction should consist of a detailed history, a frequency/volume chart, and a physical examination. In urinary incontinence, leakage should be demonstrated objectively.

A. History

The general history should include questions relevant to neurological and congenital abnormalities, as well as information on previous urinary infections and relevant surgery. Information must be obtained on medication with known or possible effects on the lower urinary tract. The general history should also include assessment of menstrual, sexual, and bowel function, and obstetric history.

The urinary history must consist of symptoms related to both the storage and the evacuation functions of the lower urinary tract.

B. Frequency/Volume Chart

The frequency/volume chart is a specific urodynamic investigation recording fluid intake and urine output per 24-hr period. The chart gives objective information on the number of voidings, the distribution of voidings between daytime and nighttime, and each voided volume. The chart can also be used to record episodes of urgency and leakage and the number of incontinence pads used. The frequency/volume chart is very useful in the assessment of voiding disorders, and in the follow-up of treatment.

C. Physical Examination

Besides a general urological and, when appropriate, gynecological examination, the physical examination should include the assessment of perineal sensation, the perineal reflexes supplied by the sacral segments S2–S4, and anal sphincter tone and control.

III. PROCEDURES RELATED TO THE EVALUATION OF URINE STORAGE

A. Cystometry

Cystometry is the method by which the pressure/volume relation of the bladder is measured. All systems are zeroed at atmospheric pressure. For external transducers, the reference point is the level of the superior edge of the symphysis pubis. For catheter-mounted transducers, the reference point is the transducer itself.

Cystometry is used to assess detrusor activity, sensation, capacity, and compliance.

Before starting to fill the bladder the residual urine may be measured. However, the removal of a large volume of residual urine may alter detrusor function, especially in neuropathic disorders. Certain cystometric parameters may be significantly altered by the speed of bladder filling (see Sec. 6.1.1.4).

During cystometry, it is taken for granted that the patient is awake, unanesthetized, and neither sedated nor taking drugs that affect bladder function. Any variations should be specified.

Specify
    a.   Access (transurethral or percutaneous)
    b.   Fluid medium (liquid or gas)
    c.   Temperature of fluid (state in degrees Celsius)

d. Position of patient (e.g., supine, sitting, or standing)
e. Filling may be by diuresis or catheter. Filling by catheter may be continuous or incremental; the precise filling rate should be stated. When the incremental method is used the volume increment should be stated. For general discussion, the following terms for the range of filling rate may be used:
  i. Up to 10 mL/s is slow-fill cystometry ("physiological" filling).
  ii. 10–100 mL/min is medium-fill cystometry.
  iii. More than 100 mL/min is rapid-fill cystometry.

Technique
a. Fluid-filled catheter—specify number of catheters, single or multiple lumens, type of catheter (manufacturer), size of catheter
b. Catheter tip transducer—list specifications
c. Other catheters—list specifications
d. Measuring equipment

Definitions
Intravesical pressure is the pressure within the bladder.

Abdominal pressure is taken to be the pressure surrounding the bladder. In current practice it is estimated from rectal or, less commonly, extraperitoneal pressure.

Detrusor pressure is that component of intravesical pressure that is created by forces in the bladder wall (passive and active). It is estimated by subtracting abdominal pressure from intravesical pressure. The simultaneous measurement of abdominal pressure is essential for the interpretation of the intravesical pressure tracing. However, artifacts on the detrusor pressure tracing may be produced by intrinsic rectal contractions.

Bladder sensation is difficult to evaluate because of its subjective nature. It is usually assessed by questioning the patient in relation to the fullness of the bladder during cystometry.

Commonly used descriptive terms include the following:

First desire to void

Normal desire to void (this is defined as the feeling that leads the patient to pass urine at the next convenient moment, but voiding can be delayed if necessary).

Strong desire to void (this is defined as a persistent desire to void without the fear of leakage).

Urgency (this is defined as a strong desire to void accompanied by fear of leakage or fear of pain).

Pain (the site and character of which should be specified). Pain during bladder filling or micturition is abnormal.

The use of objective or semiobjective tests for sensory function, such as electrical threshold studies (sensory testing), is discussed in detail in Section 5.5.

The term *capacity* must be qualified:

Maximum cystometric capacity, in patients with normal sensation, is the volume at which the patient feels he or she can no longer delay micturition. In the absence of sensation the maximum cystometric capacity cannot be defined in the same terms and is the volume at which the clinician decides to terminate filling. In the presence of sphincter incompetence, the maximum cystometric capacity may be significantly increased by occlusion of the urethra (e.g., by a Foley catheter).

The *functional bladder capacity*, or voided volume, is more relevant and is assesed from a frequency/volume chart (urinary diary).

The *maximum (anaesthetic) bladder capacity* is the volume measured after filling during a deep general or spinal/epidural anesthetic, specifying fluid temperature, filling pressure, and filling time.

Compliance indicates the change in volume for a change in pressure. Compliance is calculated by dividing the volume change (ΔV) by the change in detrusor pressure (Δ pdet) during that change in bladder volume ($\Delta V/\Delta$ pdet). Compliance is expressed as milliliteres per centimeter H_2O (mL/cmH$_2$O) (see Sec. 6.1.1.4).

B. Urethral Pressure Measurement

The urethral pressure and the urethral closure pressure are idealized concepts that represent the ability of the urethra to prevent leakage (see Sec. 6.1.5). In current urodynamic practice the urethral pressure is measured by a number of different techniques that do not always yield consistent values. Not only do the values differ with the method of measurement, but there is often lack of consistency for a single method; for example, the effect of catheter rotation when urethral pressure is measured by a catheter-mounted transducer.

Intraluminal urethral pressure may be measured

a.   At rest, with the bladder at any given volume
b.   During coughing or straining
c.   During the process of voiding (see Sec. 4.4).

Measurements may be made at one point in the urethra over a time period, or at several points along the urethra consecutively, forming a *urethral pressure profile* (UPP).

STORAGE PHASE.   Two types of UPP may be measured:

a.   Resting urethral pressure profile—with the bladder and subject at rest.
b.   Stress urethral pressure profile—with a defined applied stress (e.g., cough, strain, Valsalva).

In the storage phase the *urethral pressure profile* denotes the intraluminal pressure along the length of the urethra. All systems are zeroed at atmospheric pressure. For external transducers the reference point is the superior edge of the symphysis pubis. For catheter-mounted transducers the reference point is the transducer itself. Intravesical pressure should be measured to exclude a simultaneous detrusor contraction. The subtraction of intravesical pressure from urethral pressure produces the *urethral closure pressure profile*.

The simultaneous recording of both intravesical and intraurethral pressures are essential during stress urethral profilometry.

Specify

a.   Infusion medium (liquid or gas)
b.   Rate of infusion
c.   Stationary, continuous, or intermittent withdrawal
d.   Rate of withdrawal
e.   Bladder volume
f.   Position of patient (supine, sitting, or standing)

Technique

  a. Open catheter—specify type (manufacturer), size, number, position, and orientation of side or end hole.

  b. Catheter-mounted transducers—specify manufacturer, number of transducers, spacing of transducers along the catheter, orientation relative to one another; transducer design (e.g., transducer face depressed or flush with catheter surface); catheter diameter and material. The orientation of the transducer(s) in the urethra should be stated.

  c. Other catheters (e.g., membrane, fiber-optic) specify type (manufacturer), size, and number of channels as for microtransducer catheter.

  d. Measurement technique: for stress profiles the particular stress employed should be stated (e.g., cough or Valsalva).

  e. Recording apparatus: describe type of recording apparatus. The frequency response of the total system should be stated. The frequency response of the catheter in the perfusion method can be assessed by blocking the eyeholes and recording the consequent rate of change of pressure.

Definitions   (Fig. 1: referring to profiles measured in storage phase).

  Maximum urethral pressure is the maximum pressure of the measured profile.

  Maximum urethral closure pressure is the maximum difference between the urethral pressure and the intravesical pressure.

  Functional profile length is the length of the urethra along which the urethral pressure exceeds intravesical pressure.

  Functional profile length (on stress) is the length over which the urethral pressure exceeds the intravesical pressure on stress.

  Pressure "transmission" ratio is the increment in urethral pressure on stress as a percentage of the simultaneously recorded increment in intravesical pressure. For stress profiles obtained during coughing, pressure transmission ratios can be obtained at any point along the urethra. If single values are given, the position in the urethra, should be stated. If several pressure transmission ratios are defined at different points along the urethra, a pressure "transmission" profile is obtained. During "cough profiles" the amplitude of the cough should be stated if possible.

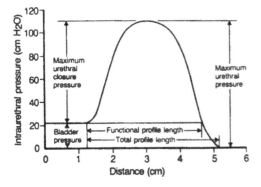

Figure 1   Diagram of a female urethral pressure profile (static) with ICS-recommended nomenclature.

Note: The term *transmission* is in common usage and cannot be changed. However, *transmission* implies a completely passive process. Such an assumption is not yet justified by scientific evidence. A role for muscular activity cannot be excluded. *Total profile length* is not generally considered a useful parameter.

The information gained from urethral pressure measurements in the storage phase is of limited value in the assessment of voiding disorders.

C. Quantification of Urine Loss

Subjective grading of incontinence may not reliably indicate the degree of abnormality. However, it is important to relate the management of the individual patients to their complaints and personal circumstances, as well as to objective measurements.

To assess and compare the results of the treatment of different types of incontinence in different centers, a simple standard test can be used to measure urine loss objectively in any subject. To obtain a representative result, especially in subjects with variable or intermittent urinary incontinence, the test should occupy as long a period as possible, yet it must be practical. The circumstances should approximate those of everyday life, yet be similar for all subjects to allow meaningful comparison. On the basis of pilot studies performed in various centers, an internal report of the ICS (fifth) recommended a test occupying a 1-hr period during which a series of standard activities were carried out. This test can be extended by further 1-hr periods if the results of the first 1-hr test were not considered representative by either the patient or the investigator. Alternatively, the test can be repeated, with the bladder filled to a defined volume.

The total amount of urine lost during the test period is determined by weighing a collecting device, such as a nappy, absorbent pad, or condom appliance. A nappy or pad should be worn inside waterproof underpants or should have a waterproof backing. Care should be taken to use a collecting device of adequate capacity.

Immediately before the test begins the collecting device is weighed to the nearest gram.

Typical test schedule

a. Test is started without the patient voiding.
b. Preweighed collecting device is put on and the first 1-hr test period begins.
c. Subject drinks 500 ml sodium-free liquid within a short period (max. 15 min), then sits or rests.
d. Half-hour period: subject walks, including stair climbing, equivalent to one flight up and down.
e. During the remaining period the subject performs the following activities:
    i. standing up from sitting, ten times
    ii. coughing vigorously, ten times
    iii. running on the spot for 1 min
    iv. bending to pick up small object from floor, five times
    v. wash hands in running water for 1 min
f. At the end of the 1-hr test the collecting device is removed and weighed.
g. If the test is considered representative, the subject voids and the volume is recorded.
h. Otherwise the test is repeated, preferably without voiding.

If the collecting device becomes saturated or filled during the test, it should be removed and weighed, and replaced by a fresh device. The total weight of urine lost during the test period is taken to be equal to the gain in weight of the collecting device(s). In interpreting the results of the test it should be borne in mind that a weight gain of up to 2 g may result from weighing errors, sweating, or vaginal discharge.

The activity program may be modified according to the subject's physical ability. If substantial variations from the usual test schedule occur, this should be recorded so that the same schedule can be used on subsequent occasions.

In principle, the subject should not void during the test period. If the patient experiences urgency, then he or she should be persuaded to postpone voiding and to perform as many of the activities in step e as possible to detect leakage. Before voiding, the collection device is removed for weighing. If inevitable, voiding cannot be postponed, then the test is terminated. The voided volume and the duration of the test should be recorded. For subjects not completing the full test the results may require separate analysis, or the test may be repeated after rehydration.

The test result is given as grams of urine lost in the 1-hr test period in which the greatest urine loss is recorded.

1. Additional Procedures

Additional procedures intended to give information of diagnostic value are permissible, provided they do not interfere with the basic test. For example, additional changes and weighing of the collecting device can give information about the timing of urine loss; the absorbent nappy may be an electronic-recording nappy so that the timing is recorded directly.

2. Presentation of Results

Specify

    a.   Collecting device
    b.   Physical condition of subject (ambulant, chairbound, bedridden)
    c.   Relevant medical condition of subject
    d.   Relevant drug treatments
    e.   Test schedule

In some situations the timing of the test (e.g., in relation to the menstrual cycle) may be relevant.

Findings. Record weight of urine lost during the test (in the case of repeated tests, greatest weight in any stated period). A loss of less than 1 g is within experimental error and the patients should be regarded as essentially dry. Urine loss should be measured and recorded in grams.

Statistics. When performing statistical analysis of urine loss in a group of subjects, nonparametric statistics should be employed, because the values are not normally distributed.

IV. PROCEDURES RELATED TO THE EVALUATION OF MICTURITION

A. Urinary Flow Rate Measurement

Urinary flow may be described in terms of *rate* and *pattern* and may be *continuous* or *intermittent. Flow rate* is defined as the volume of fluid expelled via the urethra per unit time. It is expressed in milliliters per second (mL/s).

Specify
    a.   Voided volume
    b.   Patient environment and position (supine, sitting, or standing)
    c.   Filling
         i.   By diuresis (spontaneous or forced: specify regimen)
         ii. By catheter (transurethral or suprapubic)
    d.   Type of fluid

Technique
    a.   Measuring equipment
    b.   Solitary procedure or combined with other measurements

Definitions
    a.   Continuous flow (Fig. 2)

        Voided volume is the total volume expelled via the urethra.
        Maximum flow rate is the maximum measured value of the flow rate.
        Average flow rate is voided volume divided by flow time. The calculation of average
           flow rate is meaningful only if flow is continuous and without terminal dribbling.
        Flow time is the time over which measurable flow actually occurs.
        Time to maximum flow is the elapsed time from onset of flow to maximum flow. The
           flow pattern must be described when flow time and average flow rate are measured.

    b.   Intermittent flow (Fig. 3)

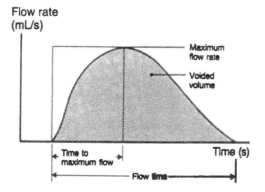

Figure 2   Diagram of a continuous urine flow recording with ICS-recommended nomenclature.

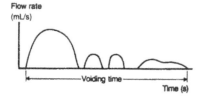

Figure 3   Diagram of an interrupted urine flow recording with ICS-recommended nomenclature.

The same parameters used to characterize continuous flow may be applicable if care is exercised in patients with intermittent flow. In measuring flow time the time intervals between flow episodes are disregarded. *Voiding time* is total duration of micturition (i.e., includes interruptions). When voiding is completed without interruption, voiding time is equal to flow time.

B. Bladder Pressure Measurements During Micturition

The specifications of patient position, access for pressure measurement, catheter type, and measuring equipment are as for cystometry (see Sec. 3.1).

Definitions (Fig. 4).

    Opening time is the elapsed time from initial rise in detrusor pressure to onset of flow. This is the initial isovolumetric contraction period of micturition. Time lags should be taken into account. In most urodynamic systems a time lag occurs equal to the time taken for the urine to pass from the point of pressure measurement to the uroflow transducer. The following parameters are applicable to measurements of each of the pressure curves: intravesical, abdominal, and detrusor pressure.

    Premicturition pressure is the pressure recorded immediately before the initial isovolumetric contraction.

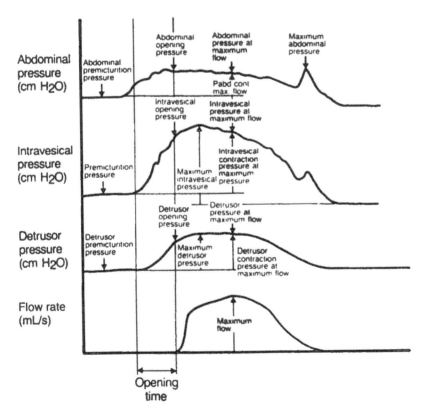

Figure 4 Diagram of a pressure–flow recording of micturition with ICS-recommended nomenclature.

Opening pressure is the pressure recorded at the onset of measured flow.

Maximum pressure is the maximum value of the measured pressure.

Pressure at maximum flow is the pressure recorded at maximum measured flow rate.

Contraction pressure at maximum flow is the difference between pressure at maximum flow and premicturition pressure. Postmicturition events (e.g., after contraction) are not well understood and so cannot yet be defined.

C. Pressure–Flow Relationships

In the early days of urodynamics the flow rate and voiding pressure were related as a "urethral resistance factor." The concept of a resistance factor originates from rigid-tube hydrodynamics. The urethra does not generally behave as a rigid tube as it is an irregular and distensible conduit the walls and surroundings of which have active and passive elements and, hence, influence the flow through it. Therefore, a resistance factor cannot provide a valid comparison between patients.

There are many ways of displaying the relations between flow and pressure during micturition; an example is suggested in the ICS 3rd Report (Fig. 5). Currently available data do not permit a standard presentation of pressure–flow parameters.

When data from a group of patients are presented, pressure–flow relations may be shown on a graph as illustrated in Figure 5. This form of presentation allows lines of demarcation to be drawn on the graph to separate the results according to the problem being studied. The points shown in Figure 5 are purely illustrative and indicate how the data might fall into groups. The group of equivocal results might include either an unrepresentative micturition in an obstructed or an unobstructed patient, or underactive detrusor function, with or without obstruction. This is the group that invalidates the use of "urethral resistance factors."

D. Urethral Pressure Measurements During Voiding (VUPP)

The VUPP is used to determine the pressure and site of urethral obstruction.

Pressure is recorded in the urethra during voiding. The technique is similar to that used in the UPP measured during storage (the resting and stress profiles; see Sec. 3.2).

Specify (as for UPP during storage; see Sec. 3.2). Accurate interpretation of the VUPP depends on the simultaneous measurement of intravesical pressure and the mea-

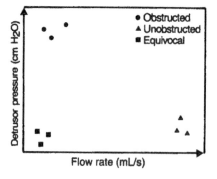

Figure 5   Diagram illustrating the presentation of pressure–flow data on individual patients in three groups of three patients: obstructed, equivocal, and unobstructed.

surement of pressure at a precisely localized point in the urethra. Localization may be achieved by radiopaque marker on the catheter, which allows the pressure measurements to be related to a visualized point in the urethra.

This technique is not fully developed, and several technical as well as clinical problems need to be solved before the VUPP is widely used.

E. Residual Urine Measurement

Residual urine is defined as the volume of fluid remaining in the bladder immediately following the completion of micturition. The measurement of residual urine forms an integral part of the study of micturition. However, voiding in unfamiliar surroundings may lead to unrepresentative results, as may voiding on command with a partially filled or overfilled bladder. Residual urine is commonly estimated by the following methods:

    a. Catheter or cystoscope (transurethral, suprapubic)
    b. Radiography (excretion urography, micturition cystography)
    c. Ultrasonics
    d. Radioisotopes (clearing, gamma camera)

When estimating residual urine, the measurement of voided volume and the time interval between voiding and residual urine estimation should be recorded; this is particularly important if the patient is in a diuretic phase. In the condition of vesicoureteric reflux, urine may reenter the bladder after micturition and may falsely be interpreted as residual urine. The presence of urine in bladder diverticula following micturition presents special problems of interpretation, because a diverticulum may be considered either as part of the bladder cavity or as outside the functioning bladder.

The various methods of measurement each have limitations for their applicability and accuracy in the various conditions associated with residual urine. Therefore, it is necessary to choose a method appropriate to the clinical problems. The absence of residual urine is usually an observation of clinical value, but does not exclude infravesical obstruction or bladder dysfunction. An isolated funding of residual urine requires confirmation before being considered significant.

V. PROCEDURES RELATED TO NEUROPHYSIOLOGICAL EVALUATION OF THE URINARY TRACT DURING FILLING AND VOIDING

A. Electromyography

Electromyography (EMG) is the study of electrical potentials generated by the depolarization of muscle. The following refers to striated muscle EMG. The functional unit in EMG is the motor unit. This is composed of a single motor neuron and the muscle fibers it innervates. A motor unit action potential is the recorded depolarization of muscle fibers that results from activation of a single anterior horn cell. Muscle action potentials may be detected either by needle electrodes or by surface electrodes.

Needle electrodes are placed directly into the muscle mass and permit visualization of the individual motor unit action potentials.

Surface electrodes are applied to an epithelial surface as close to the muscle under study as possible. Surface electrodes detect the action potentials from groups of adjacent motor units underlying the recording surface.

EMG potentials may be displayed on an oscilloscope screen or played through audio amplifiers. A permanent record of EMG potentials can be made only using a chart recorder with a high-frequency response (in the range of 10 kHz).

EMG should be interpreted in the light of the patient's symptoms, physical findings, and urological and urodynamic investigations.

1. General Information

Specify

a. EMG (solitary procedure, part of urodynamic or other electrophysiological investigation)
b. Patient position (supine, standing, sitting, or other)
c. Electrode placement:
   i. Sampling site (intrinsic striated muscle of the urethra, periurethral striated muscle, bulbocavernosus muscle, external anal sphincter, pubococcygeus, or other). State whether sites are single or multiple, unilateral or bilateral. Also state number of samples per site.
   ii. Recording electrode: define the precise anatomical location of the electrode. For needle electrodes, include site of needle entry, angle of entry, and needle depth. For vaginal or urethral surface electrodes, state method of determining position of electrode.
   iii. Reference electrode position. Note: Ensure that there is no electrical interference with any other machines (e.g., x-ray apparatus).

2. Technical Information

Specify

a. Electrodes
   i. Needle electrodes
      • Design (concentric, bipolar, monopolar, single fiber, other)
      • Dimensions (length, diameter, recording area)
      • Electrode material (e.g., platinum)
   ii. Surface electrodes
      • Type (skin, plug, catheter, other)
      • Size and shape
      • Electrode material
      • Mode of fixation to recording surface
      • Conducting medium (e.g., saline, jelly)
b. Amplifier (make and specifications)
c. Signal processing (data: raw, averaged, integrated, or other)
d. Display equipment (make and specifications to include method of calibration, time base, full-scale deflection in microvolts and polarity)
   i. Oscilloscope
   ii. Chart recorder
   iii. Loudspeaker
   iv. Other
e. Storage (make and specifications)
   i. Paper

       ii.   Magnetic tape recorder
      iii. Microprocessor
      iv. Other
   f. Hard-copy production (make and specifications)
       i.   Chart recorder
      ii.   Photographic/video reproduction of oscilloscope screen
      iii. Other

3. EMG Findings

a. *Individual motor unit action potentials.*   Normal motor unit potentials have a characteristic configuration, amplitude, and duration. Abnormalities of the motor unit may include an increase in the amplitude, duration, and complexity of waveform (polyphasicity) of the potentials. A polyphasic potential is defined as one having more than five deflections. The EMG findings of fibrillations, positive sharp waves, and bizarre high-frequency potentials are thought to be abnormal.

b. *Recruitment patterns.*   In normal subjects there is a gradual increase in "pelvic floor" and "sphincter" EMG activity during bladder filling. At the onset of micturition there is complete absence of activity. Any sphincter EMG activity during voiding is abnormal unless the patient is attempting to inhibit micturition. The finding of increased sphincter EMG activity, during voiding, accompanied by characteristic simultaneous detrusor pressure and flow changes is described by the term *detrusor–sphincter dyssynergia.* In this condition a detrusor contraction occurs concurrently with an inappropriate contraction of the urethral and or periurethral striated muscle.

B. Nerve Conduction Studies

Nerve condition studies involve stimulation of a peripheral nerve, and recording the time taken for a response to occur in muscle, innervated by the nerve under study. The time taken from stimulation of the nerve to the response in the muscle is called the "latency." Motor latency is the time taken by the fastest motor fibers in the nerve to conduct impulses to the muscle and depends on conduction distance and the conduction velocity of the fastest fibers.

1. General Information (also Applicable to Reflex Latencies and Evoked Potentials—see following)

Specify

   a. Type of investigation
       i.   Nerve conduction study (e.g., pudendal nerve)
      ii.   Reflex latency determination (e.g., bulbocavernosus)
      iii. Spinal-evoked potential
      iv. Cortical-evoked potential
      v.   Other
   b. Is the study a solitary procedure or part of urodynamic or neurophysiological investigations?
   c. Patient position and environmental temperature, noise level, and illumination.

d. Electrode placement: define electrode placement in precise anatomical terms. The exact interelectrode distance is required for nerve conduction velocity calculations.
    i.   Stimulation site (penis, clitoris, urethra, bladder neck, bladder, or other).
    ii. Recording sites (external anal sphincter, periurethral striated muscle, bulbocavernosus muscle, spinal cord, cerebral cortex, or other). When recording spinal-evoked responses, the sites of the recording electrodes should be specified according to the bony landmarks (e.g., L4). In cortical-evoked responses the sites of the recording electrodes should be specified as in the International 10–20 system (Jasper, 1958). The sampling techniques should be specified (single or multiple, unilateral or bilateral, ipsilateral or contralateral, or other).
    iii. Reference electrode position.
    iv. Grounding electrode site: ideally this should be between the stimulation and recording sites to reduce stimulus artefact.

2. Technical Information (also Applicable to Reflex Latencies and Evoked Potentials—see following)

Specify
    a. Electrodes (make and specifications)—describe separately stimulus and recording electrodes as follows:
        i.   Design (e.g., needle, plate, ring, and configuration of anode and cathode where applicable)
        ii. Dimensions
        iii. Electrode material (e.g., platinum)
        iv. Contact medium
    b. Stimulator (make and specifications):
        i.   Stimulus parameters (pulse width, frequency, pattern, current density, electrode impedance in kΩ. Also define in terms of threshold, e.g., in case of supramaximal stimulation.)
    c. Amplifier (make and specifications):
        i.   Sensitivity (mV–μV)
        ii. Filters—low-pass (Hz) or high-pass (kHz)
        iii. Sampling time (ms)
    d. Averager (make and specifications):
        i.   number of stimuli sampled
    e. Display equipment (make and specifications to include method of calibration, time base, full-scale deflection in microvolts and polarity):
        i.   Oscilloscope
    f. Storage (make and specifications):
        i.   Paper
        ii. Magnetic tape recorder
        iii. Microprocessor
        iv. Other
    g. Hard-copy production (make and specifications):
        i.   Chart recorder
        ii. Photographic/video reproduction or oscilloscope screen

       iii. XY recorder
       iv. Other

3. Description of Nerve Conduction Studies

Recordings are made from muscle and the latency of response of the muscle is measured. The latency is taken as the time to onset, of the earliest response.

    a. To ensure that response time can be precisely measured, the gain should be increased to give a clearly defined takeoff point (gain setting at least 100 μV/div and using a short time base, e.g., 1–2 ms/div).

    b. Additional information may be obtained from nerve conduction studies, if, when using surface electrodes to record a compound muscle action potential, the amplitude is measured. The gain setting must be reduced so that the whole response is displayed and a longer time base is recommended (e.g., 1 mV/div and 5 ms/div). Since the amplitude is proportional to the number of motor unit potentials within the vicinity of the recording electrodes, a reduction in amplitude indicates loss of motor units and, therefore, denervation. (Note: A prolongation of latency is not necessarily indicative of denervation.)

C. Reflex Latencies

These require stimulation of sensory fields and recordings from the muscle that contracts reflexly in response to the stimulation. Such responses are a test of reflex arcs, which are composed of both afferent and efferent limbs and a synaptic region within the central nervous system. The reflex latency expresses the nerve conduction velocity in both limbs of the arc and the integrity of the central nervous system at the level of the synapse(s). Increased reflex latency may occur as a result of slowed afferent or efferent nerve conduction or due to central nervous system conduction delays.

1. General Information and Technical Information

The same technical and general details apply as discussed earlier under nerve conduction studies (see Sec. 5.2).

2. Description of Reflex Latency Measurements

Recordings are made from muscle, and the latency of response of the muscle is measured. The latency is taken as the time to onset, of the earliest response.

    To ensure that reponse time can be precisely measured, the gain should be increased to give a clearly defined takeoff point (gain setting at least 100 μV/div and using a short time base, e.g., 1–2 ms/div).

D. Evoked Potentials

These are potential changes in central nervous system neurons resulting from distal stimulation, usually electrical. They are recorded using averaging techniques. Evoked responses may be used to test the integrity of peripheral, spinal, and central nervous pathways. As with nerve conduction studies, the conduction time (latency) may be measured. In addition, information may be gained from the amplitude and configuration of these responses.

1. General Information and Technical Information

See previous section under Nerve Conduction Studies (Sec. 5.2).

2. Description of Evoked Responses

Describe the presence or absence of stimulus-evoked responses and their configuration.

Specify
   a. Single or multiphasic response.
   b. Onset of response: defined as the start of the first reproducible potential. Because the onset of the response may be difficult to ascertain precisely, the criteria used should be stated.
   c. Latency to onset: defined as the time (ms) from the onset of stimulus to the onset of response. The central conduction time relates to cortical-evoked potentials and is defined as the difference between the latencies of the cortical and the spinal-evoked potentials. This parameter may be used to test the integrity of the corticospinal neuraxis.
   d. Latencies to peaks of positive and negative deflections in multiphasic responses (Fig. 6). P denotes positive deflections, N denotes negative deflections. In multiphasic responses, the peaks are numbered consecutively (e.g., P1, N1, P2, N2 . . .) or according to the latencies to peaks in milliseconds (e.g., P44, N52, P66 . . .).
   e. The amplitude of the responses is measured in µV.

E. Sensory Testing

Limited information, of a subjective nature, may be obtained during cystometry by recording such parameters as the first desire to micturate, urgency, or pain. However, sensory function in the lower urinary tract can be assessed by semiobjective tests by the measurement of urethral or vesical sensory thresholds to a standard applied stimulus such as a known electrical current.

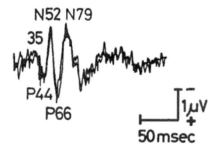

Figure 6 Multiphasic evoked response recorded from the cerebral cortex after stimulation of the dorsal aspect of the penis. The recording shows the conventional labeling of negative (N) and positive (P) deflections with the latency of each deflection from the point of stimulation in milliseconds.

1. General Information

Specify

    a. Patient's position (supine, sitting, standing, other)
    b. Bladder volume at time of testing
    c. Site of applied stimulus (intravesical, intraurethral)
    d. Number of times the stimulus was applied and the response recorded. Define the sensation recorded (e.g., the first sensation or the sensation of pulsing).
    e. Type of applied stimulus
        i. Electrical current: it is usual to use a constant current stimulator in urethral sensory measurement.

- State electrode characteristics and placement as in section on EMG.
- State electrode contact area and distance between electrodes if applicable.
- State impedance characteristics of the system.
- State type of conductive medium used for electrode/epithelial contact.

Note: Topical anesthetic agents should not be used.

- Stimulator make and specifications.
- Stimulation parameters (pulse width, frequency, pattern, duration; current density)

       ii. Other (e.g., mechanical, chemical)

2. Definition of Sensory Thresholds

The *vesical/urethral sensory threshold* is defined as the least current that consistently produces a sensation perceived by the subject during stimulation at the site under investigation. However, the absolute values will vary in relation to the site of the stimulus, the characteristics of the equipment, and the stimulation parameters. Normal values should be established for each system.

VI. A CLASSIFICATION OF URINARY TRACT DYSFUNCTION

The lower urinary tract is composed of the *bladder* and *urethra*. They form a functional unit, and their interaction cannot be ignored. Each has two functions, the bladder to store and void, the urethra to control and convey. When a reference is made to the hydrodynamic function or to the whole anatomical unit as a storage organ—the vesica urinaria—the correct term is the *bladder*. When the smooth-muscle structure known as the m. detrusor urinae is being discussed, then the correct term is *detrusor*. For simplicity, the bladder/detrusor and the urethra will be considered separately so that a classification based on a combination of functional anomalies can be reached. Sensation cannot be precisely evaluated, but must be assessed. This classification depends on the results of various objective urodynamic investigations. A complete urodynamic assessment is not necessary in all patients. However, studies of the filling and voiding phases are essential for each patient. As the bladder and urethra may behave differently during the storage and micturition phases of bladder function it is most useful to examine bladder and urethral activity separately in each phase.

    Terms used should be objective, definable, and ideally, should be applicable to the whole range of abnormality. When authors disagree with the classification presented in the following, or use terms that have not been defined here, their meaning should be made clear.

Assuming the absence of inflammation, infection, and neoplasm, *lower urinary tract dysfunction* may be caused by

   a.   Disturbance of the pertinent nervous or psychological control system
   b.   Disorders of muscle function
   c.   Structural abnormalities.

Urodynamic diagnoses based on this classification should correlate with the patient's symptoms and signs. For example, the presence of an unstable contraction in an asymptomatic, continent patient does not warrant a diagnosis of detrusor overactivity during storage.

A.   The Storage Phase

1.   Bladder Function During Storage

This may be described according to

   1.   Detrusor activity
   2.   Bladder sensation
   3.   Bladder capacity
   4.   Compliance

a.   Detrusor Activity.   In this context detrusor activity is interpreted from the measurement of detrusor pressure (*p* det).

Detrusor activity may be (a) normal or (b) overactive.

a.   Normal detrusor function: During the filling phase the bladder volume increases without a significant rise in pressure (accommodation). No involuntary contractions occur despite provocation. A normal detrusor so defined may be described as "stable."

b.   Overactive detrusor function: Overactive detrusor function is characterized by involuntary detrusor contractions during the filling phase, which may be spontaneous or provoked and which the patient cannot completely suppress. Involuntary detrusor contractions may be provoked by rapid filling, alterations of posture, coughing, walking, jumping, and other triggering procedures. Various terms have been used to describe these features, and they are defined as follows:

The *unstable destrusor* is one that is shown objectively to contract, spontaneously or on provocation, during the filling phase while the patient is attempting to inhibit micturition. Unstable detrusor contractions may be asymptomatic or may be interpreted as a normal desire to void. The presence of these contractions does not necessarily imply a neurological disorder. Unstable contractions are usually phasic in type (Fig. 7A). A gradual increase in detrusor pressure without subsequent decrease is best regarded as a change of compliance (see Fig. 7B).

Detrusor hyperreflexia is defined as overactivity caused by a disturbance of the nervous control mechanisms. The term *detrusor hyperreflexia* should be used only when there is objective evidence of a relevant neurological disorder. The use of conceptual and undefined terms, such as *hypertonic, systolic, uninhibited, spastic,* and *automatic,* should be avoided.

b.   Bladder Sensation.   Bladder sensation during filling can be classified in qualitative terms (see Sec. 3.1) and by objective measurement (see Sec. 5.5). Sensation can be classified broadly as follows:

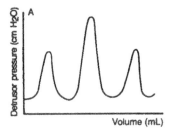

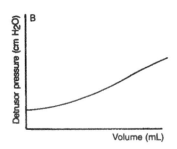

Figure 7   Diagrams of filling cystometry to illustrate (A) typical phasic unstable detrusor contraction and (B) the gradual increase of detrusor pressure with filling characteristic of reduced bladder compliance.

    a.   Normal
    b.   Increased (hypersensitive)
    c.   Reduced (hyposensitive)
    d.   Absent

c. *Bladder Capacity* (see Sec. 3.1).

d. *Compliance.* This is defined as Δ v/Δp (see Sec. 3.1).
    Compliance may change during the cytometric examination and is variably dependent on a number of factors, including the following:

    a.   Rate of filling
    b.   The part of the cystometrogram curve used for compliance calculation
    c.   The volume interval over which compliance is calculated
    d.   The geometry (shape) of the bladder
    e.   The thickness of the bladder wall
    f.   The mechanical properties of the bladder wall
    g.   The contractile/relaxant properties of the detrusor

    During normal bladder filling, little or no pressure change occurs, and this is termed "normal compliance." However, at the present time there is insufficient data to define normal, high, and low compliance.
    When reporting compliance, specify

    a.   The rate of bladder filling
    b.   The bladder volume at which compliance is calculated
    c.   The volume increment over which compliance is calculated
    d.   The part of the cystometrogram curve used for the calculation of compliance

2. Urethral Function During Storage

The urethral closure mechanism during storage may be (a) normal or (b) incompetent.

    a.   The *normal closure mechanism* maintains a positive urethral closure pressure during filling, even in the presence of increased abdominal pressure. Immediately before micturition the normal closure pressure decreases to allow flow.
    b.   An *incompetent urethral closure mechanism* is defined as one that allows leak-

age of urine in the absence of a detrusor contraction. Leakage may occur whenever intravesical pressure exceeds intraurethral pressure (genuine stress incontinence) or when there is an involuntary fall in urethral pressure. Terms such as *the unstable urethra* await further data and precise definition.

3. Urinary Incontinence

Urinary incontinence is involuntary loss of urine that is objectively demonstrable and a social or hygienic problem. Loss of urine through channels other than the urethra is extraurethral incontinence.

Urinary incontinence denotes (a) a symptom, (b) a sign, or (c) a condition. The *symptom* indicates the patient's statement of involuntary urine loss. The *sign* is the objective demonstration of urine loss. The *condition* is the urodynamic demonstration of urine loss.

Symptoms.   *Urge incontinence* is the involuntary loss of urine associated with a strong desire to void (urgency). *Urgency* may be associated with two types of dysfunction: (a) overactive destrusor function (*motor urgency*), and (b) hypersensitivity (*sensory urgency*).

Stress Incontinence.   The symptom indicates the patient's statement of involuntary loss of urine during physical exertion.

"Unconscious" Incontinence.   Incontinence may occur in the absence of urge and without conscious recognition of the urinary loss.

Enuresis.   This means any involuntary loss of urine. If it is used to denote incontinence during sleep, it should always be qualified with the adjective "nocturnal."

Postmicturition Dribble and Continuous Leakage.   These denote other symptomatic forms of incontinence.

Signs.   The sign stress-incontinence denotes the observation of loss of urine from the urethra synchronous with physical exertion (e.g., coughing). Incontinence may also be observed without physical exercise. Postmicturition dribble and continuous leakage denote other signs of incontinence. Symptoms and signs alone may not disclose the cause of urinary incontinence. Accurate diagnosis often requires urodynamic investigation in addition to careful history and physical examination.

Conditions.   *Genuine stress incontinence* is the involuntary loss of urine occurring when, in the absence of a detrusor contraction, the intravesical pressure exceeds the maximum urethral pressure.

> *Reflex incontinence* is loss of urine owing to detrusor hyperreflexia or involuntary urethral relaxation in the absence of the sensation usually associated with the desire to micturate. This condition is seen only in patients with neuropathic bladder/urethral disorders.
>
> *Overflow incontinence* is any involuntary loss of urine associated with overdistension of the bladder.

B.   The Voiding Phase

1.   The Detrusor During Voiding

During micturition the detrusor may be (a) acontractile, (b) underactive, or (c) normal.

a.   *The acontractile detrusor* is one that cannot be demonstrated to contract during urodynamic studies. *Detrusor areflexia* is defined as acontractility caused by an abnormality of nervous control and denotes the complete absence of centrally coordinated contraction. In detrusor areflexia caused by a lesion of the conus medullaris or sacral nerve outflow, the detrusor should be described as *decentralized*—not denervated, since the peripheral neurons remain. In such bladders, pressure fluctuations of low amplitude, sometimes known as "autonomous" waves, may occasionally occur. The use of terms such as *atonic, hypotonic, autonomic,* and *flaccid* should be avoided.

      b.   *Detrusor underactivity.* This term should be reserved as an expression describing detrusor activity during micturition. Detrusor underactivity is defined as a detrusor contraction of inadequate magnitude or duration to effect bladder emptying with a normal time span. Patients may have underactivity during micturition and detrusor overactivity during filling.

      c.   *Normal detrusor contractility.* Normal voiding is achieved by a voluntarily initiated detrusor contraction that is sustained and can usually be suppressed voluntarily. A normal detrusor contraction will effect complete bladder emptying in the absence of obstruction. For a given detrusor contraction, the magnitude of the recorded pressure rise will depend on the degree of outlet resistance.

2. Urethral Function During Micturition

During voiding urethral function may be (a) normal or (b) obstructive as a result of overactivity or faulty mechanics.

    a.   *The normal urethra* opens to allow the bladder to be emptied.

    b.   *Obstruction due to urethral overactivity* occurs when the urethral closure mechanism contracts against a detrusor contraction or fails to open at attempted micturition. Synchronous detrusor and urethral contraction is *detrusor–urethral dyssynergia.* This diagnosis should be qualified by stating the location and type of the urethral muscles (striated or smooth) involved. Despite the confusion surrounding "sphincter" terminology the use of certain terms is so widespread that they are retained and defined here. The term *detrusor–external sphincter dyssynergia or detrusor–sphincter dyssnergia (DSD)* describes a detrusor contraction concurrent with an involuntary contraction of the urethral or periurethral striated muscle. In the adult, detrusor sphincter dyssynergia is a feature of neurological voiding disorders. In the absence of neurological features the validity of this diagnosis should be questioned. The term *detrusor–bladder neck dyssynergia* is used to denote a detrusor contraction concurrent with an objectively demonstrated failure of bladder neck opening. No parallel term has been elaborated for possible detrusor/distal urethral (smooth muscle) dyssynergia.

    Overactivity of the striated urethral sphincter may occur in the absence of detrusor contraction, and may prevent voiding. This is not detrusor–sphincter dyssynergia.

    Overactivity of the urethral sphincter may occur during voiding in the absence of neurological disease and is termed *dysfunctional voiding.* The use of terms such as *nonneurogenic occult neuropathic* should be avoided.

    Mechanical obstruction is most commonly anatomical (e.g., urethral stricture).

    The characteristics of detrusor and urethral function during storage and micturition can be used to form an accurate definition of lower urinary tract behavior in each patient.

VII. SYMBOLS AND UNITS OF MEASUREMENT

In the urodynamic literature pressure is measured in cmH_2O and *not* in millimeters of mercury. When Laplace's law is used to calculate tension in the bladder wall, it is often found that pressure is then measured in dyne cm^{-2}. This lack of uniformity in the systems used leads to confusion when other parameters, which are a function of pressure, are computed, for instance, "compliance," (contraction force/velocity). From these few examples it is evident that standardization is essential for meaningful communication. Many journals now require that the results be given in SI units. This section is designed to give guidance in the application of the SI system to urodynamics and defines the units involved. The principal units to be used are listed in Table 1.

It is often helpful to use symbols in a communication. The system in Table 2 has been devised to standardize a code of symbols for use in urodynamics. The rationale of the sys-

Table 1   Units of Measurement

Quantity	Acceptable unit	Symbol
Volume	Milliliter	mL
Time	Second	s
Flow rate	Milliliters/second	$mL\ s^{-1}$
Pressure	Centimeters of water[a]	cmH_2O
Length	Meters or submultiples	m, cm, mm
Velocity	Meters/second or submultiples	ms^{-1}, $cm\ s^{-1}$
Temperature	Degrees Celsius	°C

[a]The SI unit is the pascal (Pa), but it is only practical at present to calibrate our instruments in cmH_2O. One centimeter of water pressure is approximately equal to 100 pascals (1 cmH_2O = 98.07; Pa = 0.098 kPa).

Table 2   List of Symbols[a]

Basic symbols		Urological qualifiers		Value	
Pressure	p	Bladder	ves	Maximum	max
Volume	V	Urethra	ura	Minimum	min
Flow rate	Q	Ureter	ure	Average	ave
Velocity	v	Detrusor	det	Isovolumetric	isv
Time	t	Abdomen	abd	Isotonic	ist
Temperature	T	External		Isobaric	isb
Length	l	stream	ext	Isometric	ism
Area	A				
Diameter	d				
Force	F				
Energy	E				
Power	P				
Compliance	C				
Work	W				
Energy per unit volume	e				

[a]Examples: pdet, max = maximum detrusor pressure; e, ext = kinetic energy per unit volume in the external stream.

tem is to have a basic symbol representing the physical quantity with qualifying subscripts. The list of basic symbols largely conforms to international usage. The qualifying subscripts relate to the symbols basic to commonly used urodynamic parameters.

BIBLIOGRAPHY

Abrams P, Blaivas JG, Stanton SL, Andersen JT, Fowler CJ, Gerstenberg T, Murray K (1986). Sixth report on the standardisation of terminology of lower urinary tract function. Procedures related to neurophysiological investigations: electromyography, nerve conduction studies, reflex latencies, evoked potentials and sensory testing. World J Urol 4:2–5; Scand J Urol Nephrol 20:161–164; Neurourol Urodynam 5:373–379.

Bates P, Bradley WE, Glen E, Melchior H, Rowan D, Sterling A, Hald T (1976). First report on the standardisation of terminology of lower urinary tract function. Urinary incontinence. Procedures related to the evaluation of urine storage—cystometry, urethral closure pressure profile, units of measurement. Br J Urol 48:39–42; Eur Urol 2:274–276; Scand J Urol Nephrol 11:193–196; Urol Int 32:81–87.

Bates P, Glen E, Griffiths D, Melchior H, Rowan D, Sterling A, Zinner NR, Hald T (1977). Second report on the standardisation of terminology of lower urinary tract function. Procedures related to the evaluation of micturition—flow rate, pressure measurement, symbols. Acta Urol Jpn 27:1563–1566; Br J Urol 49:207–210; Eur Urol 3:168–170; Scand J Urol Nephrol 11:197–199.

Bates P, Bradley WE, Glen E, Griffiths D, Melchior H, Rowan D, Sterling A, Hald T (1980). Third report on the standardisation of terminology of lower urinary tract function. Procedures related to the evaluation of micturition: pressure flow relationships, residual urine. Br J Urol 52:348–350; Eur Urol 6:170–171; Acta Urol Jpn 27:1566–1568; Scand J Urol Nephrol 12:191–193.

Bates P, Bradley WE, Glen E, Melchior H, Rowan D, Sterling A, Sundin T, Thomas D, Torrens M, Turner–Warwick R, Zinner NR, Hald T (1981). Fourth report on the standardisation of terminology of lower urinary tract function. Terminology related to neuromuscular dysfunction of lower urinary tract. Br J Urol 53:333–335; Urology 17:618–620; Scand J Urol Nephrol 15:169–171; Acta Urol Jpn 27:1568–1571.

Jasper HH (1958). Report to the committee on the methods of clinical examination in electroencephalography. Electroencephalogr Clin Neurophysiol 10:370–375.

Seventh Report: Lower Urinary Tract Rehabilitation Techniques

I. INTRODUCTION

Lower urinary tract rehabilitation comprises nonsurgical, nonpharmacological treatment for lower urinary tract dysfunction. The specific techniques are defined in this report.

Most of the conditions for which rehabilitation techniques are employed have both a subjective and an objective component. In many instances, treatment is capable of only relieving symptoms, not of curing the underlying disease. Therefore, symptoms should be quantified before and after treatment, and the means by which the physiology is altered should be clearly stated.

The applications of the individual types of treatment cited here are taken from the scientific literature and from current clinical practice. It is not within the scope of this committee to endorse specific recommendations for treatment, nor to restrict the use of these treatments to the examples given.

The standards set in this report are recommended to ensure the reproducibility of methods of treatment and to facilitate the comparison of results obtained by different investigators and therapists. It is suggested that acknowledgment of these standards, in written publications, should be indicated by a footnote to the section "Methods and Materials" or its equivalent, to read as follows:

> Methods, definitions and units conform to the standards recommended by the International Continence Society, except where specifically noted.

From J. T. Andersen (Chairman), J. G. Blaivas, L. Cardozo, and J. Thüroff, *International Continence Society Committee on Standardization of Terminology.* This article originally appeared in and is reprinted by permission of the *International Urogynecology Journal.* Neurourology and Urodynamics 11:593–603 (1992). Copyright 1992 by Wiley-Liss, Inc.

II. PELVIC FLOOR TRAINING

A. Definition

Pelvic floor training is defined as repetitive selective voluntary contraction and relaxation of specific pelvic floor muscles. This necessitates muscle awareness to be sure that the correct muscles are being used, and to avoid unwanted contractions of adjacent muscle groups.

B. Techniques

1. Standard of Diagnosis and Implementation

The professional status of the individual who establishes the diagnosis must be stated as well as the diagnostic techniques employed. Also, the professional status of the person who institutes, supervises, and assesses treatment must be specified.

2. Muscle Awareness

The technique used for obtaining selective pelvic floor contractions and relaxations should be stated. Registration of electromyographic (EMG) activity in the muscles of the pelvic floor, urethral or anal sphincter, or the anterior abdominal wall, may be necessary to obtain this muscle awareness. Alternatively or additionally, registration of abdominal, vaginal, urethral, or anal pressure may be used for the same purpose.

3. Muscle Training

It should be specified whether treatment is given on an inpatient or outpatient basis. Specific details of training must be stated:

1. Patient position
2. Duration of each contraction
3. Interval between contractions
4. Number of contractions per exercise
5. Number of exercises per day
6. Length of treatment program (weeks, months)

4. Adjunctive Equipment

Adjunctive equipment may be employed to enhance muscle awareness or muscle training. The following should be specified:

1. Type of equipment
2. Mechanism of action
3. Duration of use
4. Therapeutic goals

Examples of equipment in current use are as follows:

Perineometers and other pressure-recording devices
EMG equipment
Ultrasound equipment
Faradic stimulators
Interferential current equipment
Vaginal cones

5. Compliance

Patient compliance has three major components:

1. Appropriate comprehension of the instructions and the technique
2. Ability to perform the exercises
3. Completion of the training program

Objective documentation of both the patient's ability to perform the exercises and the result of the training program is mandatory. The parameters employed for objective documentation during training should be the same as those used for teaching muscle awareness.

C. Applications

Pelvic floor training can be used as treatment on its own, or as an adjunctive therapy, or for prophylaxis. The indications, mode of action, and the therapeutic goals must be specified. Examples of indications for therapeutic pelvic floor training are incontinence and descent of the pelvic viscera (prolapse). Examples of indications for prophylactic pelvic floor training are postpartum and following pelvic surgery.

III. BIOFEEDBACK

A. Definition

Biofeedback is a technique by which information about a normally unconscious physiological process is presented to the patient and the therapist as a visual, auditory, or tactile signal. The signal is derived from a measurable physiological parameter, which is subsequently used in an educational process to accomplish a specific therapeutic result. The signal is displayed in a quantitative way, and the patient is taught how to alter it and thus control the basic physiological process.

B. Techniques

The physiological parameter (e.g., pressure, flow, EMG) that is being monitored, the method of measurement, and the mode by which it is displayed as a signal (e.g., light, sound, electric stimulus) should all be specified. Furthermore, the specific instructions to the patient by which he or she is to alter the signal must be stated. The following details of biofeedback treatment must also be stated:

1. Patient position
2. Duration of each session
3. Interval between sessions
4. Number of sessions per day, week, or month and the intervals between
5. Length of treatment program (weeks, months)

C. Applications

The indications, the intended mode of action, and the therapeutic goals must be specified. The aim of biofeedback is to improve a specific lower urinary tract dysfunction by increasing patient awareness, and by alteration of a measurable physiological parameter. Biofeedback can be applied in functional voiding disorders in which the underlying pathophysiology can be monitored and subsequently altered by the patient. The following are examples of indications and techniques for biofeedback treatment:

> Motor urgency and urge incontinence: display of detrusor pressure and control of detrusor contractions
>
> Dysfunctional voiding: display of sphincter EMG and relaxation of the external sphincter
>
> Pelvic floor relaxation: display of pelvic floor EMG and pelvic floor training

IV.   BEHAVIORAL MODIFICATION

A.   Definition

Behavioral modification comprises analysis and alteration of the relation between the patient's symptoms and his or her environment for the treatment of maladaptive voiding patterns. This may be achieved by modification of the patient's behavior or environment, or both.

B.   Techniques

When behavioral modification is considered, a thorough analysis of possible interactions between the patient's symptoms, general condition, and environment is essential. The following should be specified:

1. Micturition complaints; assessment and quantification
   Symptom analysis
   Visual analog score
   Fluid intake chart
   Frequency/volume chart (voiding diary)
   Pad-weighing test
   Urodynamic studies (when applicable)
2. General patient assessment
   General performance status [e.g., Kurtzke disability scale (1)]
   Mobility (e.g., chairbound)
   Concurrent medical disorders (e.g., constipation, congestive heart failure, diabetes mellitus, chronic bronchitis, hemiplegia)
   Current medication (e.g., diuretics)
   Psychological state (e.g., psychoanalysis)
   Psychiatric disorders
   Mental state (e.g., dementia, confusion)
3. Environmental assessment
   Toilet facilities (access)
   Living conditions
   Working conditions
   Social relations
   Availability of suitable incontinence aids
   Access to health care

For behavioral modification, various therapeutic concepts and techniques may be employed. The following should be specified:

1. Conditioning techniques
   Timed voiding (e.g., hyposensitive bladder)
   Double/triple voiding (e.g., residual urine owing to bladder diverticulum)
   Increase of intervoiding intervals/bladder drill (e.g., sensory urgency)
   Biofeedback (see foregoing)
   Enuresis alarm
2. Fluid intake regulation (e.g., restriction)
3. Measures to improve patient mobility (e.g., physiotherapy, wheelchair)
4. Change of medication (e.g., diuretics, anticholinergics)
5. Treatment of concurrent medical or psychiatric disorders
6. Psychoanalysis or hypnotherapy (e.g., idiopathic detrusor instability)
7. Environmental changes (e.g., provision of incontinence pads, condom urinals, commode, furniture protection, etc.)

Treatment is often empirical, and may require a combination of the aforementioned concepts and techniques. The results of treatment should be objectively documented using the same techniques used for the initial assessment of micturition complaints.

C. Applications

Behavioral modification may be used for the treatment of maladaptive voiding patterns in patients when

The etiology and pathophysiology of their symptoms cannot be identified (e.g., sensory urgency)
The symptoms are caused by a psychological problem
The symptoms have failed to respond to conventional therapy
They are unfit for definitive treatment of their condition

Behavioral modification may be employed alone or as an adjunct to any other form of treatment for lower urinary tract dysfunction.

V. ELECTRICAL STIMULATION

A. Definition

Electrical stimulation is the application of electrical current to stimulate the pelvic viscera or their nerve supply. The aim of electrical stimulation may be to directly induce a therapeutic response or to modulate lower urinary tract, bowel, or sexual dysfunction.

B. Techniques

The following should be specified:

1. Access
   Surface electrodes (e.g., anal plug, vaginal electrode)
   Percutaneous electrodes (e.g., needle electrodes, wire electrodes)
   Implants
2. Approach
   Temporary stimulation
   Permanent stimulation
3. Stimulation site

Effector organ
Peripheral nerves
Spinal nerves (intradural or extradural)
Spinal cord
4. Stimulation parameters
Frequency
Voltage
Current
Pulse width
Pulse shape (e.g., rectangular, biphasic, capacitatively coupled)
With monopolar stimulation, state whether the active electrode is anodic or cathodic
Duration of pulse trains
Shape of pulse trains (e.g., surging trains)
5. Mode of stimulation
Continuous
Phasic (regular automatic on–off)
Intermittent (variable duration and time intervals)
Single sessions: number and duration of, and intervals between, periods of stimulation
Multiple sessions: number and duration of, and intervals between sessions
6. Design of electronic equipment, electrodes, and related electrical stimulation characteristics
Electrodes (monopolar or bipolar)
Surface area of electrodes
Maximum charge density per pulse at active electrode surface
Impedance of the implanted system
Power source (implants):
• Active, self-powered
• Passive, inductive current
7. For transurethral intravesical stimulation
Filling medium
Filling volume
Number of intravesical electrodes

C. Units of Measurement and Symbols

Parameters related to electrical stimulation, units of measurement, and the corresponding symbols are listed in Table 1.

D. Applications

The aims of treatment should be clearly stated. These may include control of voiding, continence, defecation, erection, ejaculation, or relief of pain. Specify whether electrical stimulation aims at

A functional result completely dependent on the continuous use of electrical current
Modulation, reflex facilitation, reflex inhibition, reeducation, or conditioning with a sustained functional result even after withdrawal of stimulation

Table 1   Parameters for Electrical Stimulation

Quantity	Unit	Symbol	Definition
Electric current	Ampere	A	1 A of electric current is the transfer of 1 C of electric charge per second
Direct (DC)			Steady unidirectional electric current
Galvanic			Unidirectional electric current derived from a chemical battery
Alternating (AC)			Electric current that phasically changes direction of flow in a sinusoidal manner
Faradic			Intermittent oscillatory current similar to alternating current (AC), (e.g., as produced by an induction coil)
Voltage (potential difference)	Volt	V	1 V of potential difference between two points requires 1 J of energy to transfer 1 C of charge from one point to the other
Resistance	Ohm	Ω	1 Ω of resistance between two points allows 1 V of potential difference to cause a flow of 1 A of direct current (DC) between them
Impedance (Z)	Ohm	Ω	Analogue of resistance for alternating current (AC); vector sum of ohmic resistance and reactance (inductive or capacitative resistance)
Charge	Coulomb	C	1 C of electric charge is transferred through a conductor in 1 s by 1 A of electric current
Capacity	Farad	F	A condenser (capacitor) has 1 F of electric capacity (capacitance) if transfer of 1 C of electric charge causes 1 V of potential difference between its elements
Frequency	Hertz	$Hz(s^{-1})$	Number of cycles (phases) of a periodically repeating oscillation per second
Pulse width	Time	ms	Duration of 1 pulse (phase) of a phasic electric current or voltage
Electrode surface area	Area	mm^2	Active area of electrode surface
Charge density per pulse	Coulomb/ area/time	$\mu C\ mm^{-2}ms^{-1}$	Electric charge delivered to a given electrode surface area in a given time (one pulse width)

Electrical stimulation is applicable in neurogenic or nonneurogenic lower urinary tract, bowel, or sexual dysfunction. Techniques and equipment vary widely with the type of dysfunction and the goal of electrical stimulation. If electrical stimulation is employed for control of a neuropathic dysfunction, and the chosen site of stimulation is the reflex arc (peripheral nerves, spinal nerves, or spinal cord), this reflex arc must be intact. Consequently, electrical stimulation is not applicable for complete lower motor neuron lesions except when direct stimulation of the effector organ is chosen.

When ablative surgery is performed (e.g., dorsal rhizotomy, ganglionectomy, sphincterotomy, or levatorotomy) in conjunction with an implant to achieve the desired functional effect, the following should be specified:

1. Techniques used to reduce pain or mass reflexes during stimulation
   Number and spinal level of interrupted afferents
   Site of interruption of afferents
   Dorsal rhizotomy (intradural or extradural)
   Ganglionectomy
2. Techniques to reduce stimulated sphincter dyssynergia
   Pudendal block (unilateral or bilateral)
   Pudendal neurectomy (unilateral or bilateral)
   Levatorotomy (unilateral or bilateral)
   Electrically induced sphincter fatigue
   External sphincterotomy

If electrical stimulation is combined with ablative surgery, other functions (e.g., erection or continence) may be impaired.

1. Voiding

When the aim of electrical stimulation is to achieve voiding, state whether this is obtained by:

Stimulation of the afferent fibers to induce bladder sensation and thus facilitate voiding (transurethral intravesical stimulation)
Stimulation of efferent fibers or detrusor muscle to induce a bladder contraction (electromicturition)

2. Continence

Electrical stimulation may aim to inhibit overactive detrusor function or to improve urethral closure. State whether overactive detrusor function is abolished or reduced by reflex inhibition (pudendal to pelvic nerve) or by blockade of nerve conduction. When electrical stimulation is applied to improve urethral closure, state whether this is by

A direct effect on the urethra during stimulation
Reeducation and conditioning to restore pelvic floor tone

3. Pelvic Pain

If electrical stimulation is applied to control pelvic pain, the nature and etiology of the pain should be stated. When pelvic pain is caused by pelvic floor spasticity, electrical stimulation may be effective by relaxing the pelvic floor muscles.

4. Erection and Ejaculation

If electrical stimulation is applied for the treatment of erectile dysfunction or ejaculatory failure, the etiology should be stated. Electrically induced erection requires an intact arterial supply and cavernous tissue, and a competent venous closure mechanism of the corpora cavernosa. Electroejaculation requires an intact reproductive system.

5. Defecation

Defecation may be obtained by electrical stimulation, either intentionally or as a side effect of electromicturition.

At present, the mechanism of action of electrically induced control of pelvic pain, erection, ejaculation, and defecation are not fully understood. The clinical applications of these techniques have not yet been fully established.

VI. VOIDING MANEUVERS

Voiding maneuvers are employed to obtain or facilitate bladder emptying. For lower urinary tract rehabilitation, voiding maneuvers may be used alone or in combination with
other techniques, such as biofeedback or behavioral modification. The aim is to achieve
complete bladder emptying at low intravesical pressures. The techniques employed may be
invasive (e.g.,catheters) or noninvasive (e.g., triggering reflex detrusor contractions, increasing intra-abdominal pressure).

　　　When reporting on voiding maneuvers, the professional status of the individual(s)
who establishes the diagnosis must be stated as well as the diagnostic techniques employed.
Also the professional status of the person(s) who institutes, supervises, and assesses treatment should be specified.

A. Catheterization

1. Definition

Catheterization is a technique for bladder emptying employing a catheter to drain the bladder or a urinary reservoir. Catheter use may be intermittent or indwelling (temporary or permanent).

2. Intermittent (In/Out) Catheterization

Intermittent (in/out) catheterization is defined as drainage or aspiration of the bladder or a
urinary reservoir with subsequent removal of the catheter. The following types of intermittent catheterization are defined:

　　1. Intermittent self-catheterization: performed by the patient himself or herself
　　2. Intermittent catheterization by an attendant (e.g., doctor, nurse, or relative)
　　3. Clean intermittent catheterization: use of a clean technique. This implies ordi-
　　　　nary washing techniques and use of disposable or cleansed reusable catheters.
　　4. Aseptic intermittent catheterization: use of a sterile technique. This implies gen-
　　　　ital disinfection and the use of sterile catheters and instruments/gloves.

a. Techniques.   The following should be specified:

　　1. Preparation used for genital disinfection
　　2. Preparation and volume of lubricant
　　3. Catheter specifications: type, size, material, and surface coating
　　4. Number of catheterizations per day or week
　　5. Length of treatment (e.g., weeks, months, permanent)

b. Applications.   Specify the indications and the therapeutic goals. Typical examples for
the use of intermittent catheterization are neurogenic bladder with impaired bladder emptying, postoperative urinary retention, and transstomal catheterization of continent reservoirs.

3. Indwelling Catheter

An indwelling catheter remains in the bladder, urinary reservoir, or urinary conduit for a period of time longer than one emptying. The following routes of access are employed:

　　Transurethral
　　Suprapubic

a. *Techniques.* The following should be specified:

1. Catheter specifications: type, size, material
2. Preparation and volume of lubricant
3. Catheter fixation (e.g., balloon (state filling volume)) skin suture
4. Mode of drainage: continuous on intermittent. For intermittent drainage specify clamping periods
5. Intervals between catheter change
6. Duration of catheterization (days, weeks, years)

b. *Applications.* The indications and the therapeutic goals should be specified. Examples of the use of temporary indwelling catheters are the following:

Suprapubic catheter: after major pelvic surgery
Transurethral catheter: to monitor urine output in a severely ill patient

Examples of the use of permanent indwelling catheters are the following:

Suprapublic: candidates for urinary diversion unfit for surgery
Transurethral: severe bladder symptoms from untreatable bladder cancer

B. Bladder Reflex Triggering

1. Definition

Bladder reflex triggering comprises various maneuvers performed by the patient or the therapist to elicit reflex detrusor contractions by exteroceptive stimuli. The most commonly used maneuvers are suprapubic tapping, thigh scratching, and anal/rectal manipulation.

2. Techniques

For each maneuver the following should be specified:

1. Details of maneuver
2. Frequency, intervals and duration (weeks, months, years) of practice

3. Applications

When using bladder reflex triggering manuevers, the etiology of the dysfunction and the goals of treatment should be stated. Bladder reflex triggering maneuvers are indicated only in patients with an intact sacral reflex arc (suprasacral spinal cord lesions).

C. Bladder Expression

1. Definition

Bladder expression comprises various maneuvers aimed at increasing intravesical pressure to facilitate bladder emptying. The most commonly used maneuvers are abdominal straining; the Valsalva maneuver and the Credé maneuver.

2. Techniques

For each maneuver, the following should be specified:

Details of the maneuver
Frequency, intervals, and duration of practice (weeks, months, years)

3. Applications

When using bladder expression, the etiology of the underlying disorder and the goals of treatment should be stated. Bladder expression may be used in patients for whom the urethral closure mechanism can be easily overcome.

REFERENCE

1. Kurtzke JF (1983). Rating neurological impairment in multiple sclerosis: an expanded disability status scale (EDSS). Neurology 33:1444–1452.

Standardization of Terminology of Female Pelvic Organ Prolapse and Pelvic Floor Dysfunction

I. INTRODUCTION

A system of standard terminology for the description and evaluation of pelvic organ prolapse and pelvic floor dysfunction, adopted by several professional societies, is presented.

The International Continence Society (ICS) has been at the forefront in the standardization of terminology of lower urinary tract function since the establishment of the Committee on Standardization of Terminology in 1973. This committee's efforts over the past two decades have resulted in the worldwide acceptance of terminology standards that allow clinicians and researchers interested in the lower urinary tract to communicate efficiently and precisely. Although female pelvic organ prolapse and pelvic floor dysfunction are intimately related to lower urinary tract function, such accurate communication using standard terminology has not been possible for these conditions because there has been no universally accepted system for describing the anatomical position of the pelvic organs. Many reports use undefined terms for the description of pelvic organ prolapse; none of the many aspiring grading systems has been adequately validated relative to either reproducibility or the clinical significance of different grades. The absence of standard, validated definitions prevents comparisons of published series from different institutions and longitudinal evaluation of an individual patient.

In 1993, an international, multidisciplinary committee composed of members of the ICS, the American Urogynecologic Society (AUGS), and Society of Gynecologic Surgeons (SGS) drafted this standardization document following the committee's initial meeting at the ICS meeting in Rome. In late 1994 and early 1995, the final draft was circulated to

From Richard C. Bump, Anders Mattiasson, Kari Bø, Linda P. Brubaker, John O. L. DeLancey, Peter Klarskov, Bob L. Shull, and Anthony R. B. Smith. Produced by the International Continence Society Committee on Standardisation of Terminology (Anders Mattiasson, chairman), Subcommittee on Pelvic Organ Prolapse and Pelvic floor Dysfunction (Richard Bump, chairman) in collaboration with the American Urogynecologic Society and the Society of Gynecologic Surgeons. *Am J Obstet Gynec* (1996) 175:10–17.

members of all three societies for a 1-year review and trial. During that year several minor revisions were made, and reproducibility studies in six centers in the United States and Europe were completed, documenting the inter- and intrarater reliability and clinical utility of the system in 240 women (1–5). The standardization document was formally adopted by the ICS in October 1995, by the AUGS in January 1996, and by the SGS in March 1996. The goal of this report is to introduce the system to clinicians and researchers.

Acknowledgment of these standards in written publications and scientific presentations should be indicated in the methods section with the following statement: "Methods, definitions, and descriptions conform to the standards recommended by the International Continence Society, except where specifically noted."

II. DESCRIPTION OF PELVIC ORGAN PROLAPSE

The clinical description of pelvic floor anatomy is determined during the physical examination of the external genitalia and vaginal canal. The details of the examination technique are not dictated by this document, but authors should precisely describe their technique. Segments of the lower reproductive tract will replace such terms as "cystocele, rectocele, enterocele, or urethrovesical junction," because these terms may imply an unrealistic certainty of the structures on the other side of the vaginal bulge, particularly in women who have had previous prolapse surgery.

A. Conditions of the Examination

It is critical that the examiner sees and describes the maximum protrusion noted by the individual during her daily activities. Criteria for the endpoint of the examination and the full development of the prolapse should be specified in any report. Suggested criteria for demonstration of maximum prolapse should include one or all of the following: (a) Any protrusion of the vaginal wall has become tight during straining by the patient. (b) Traction on the prolapse causes no further descent. (c) The subject confirms that the size of the prolapse and extent of the protrusion seen by the examiner is as extensive as the most severe protrusion she has experienced. The means of this confirmation should be specified. For example, the subject may use a small hand-held mirror to visualize the protrusion. (d) A standing, straining examination confirms that the full extent of the prolapse was observed in other positions used.

Other variables of technique that should be specified during the quantitative description and ordinal staging of pelvic organ prolapse include the following: (a) the position of the subject; (b) the type of examination table or chair used; (c) the type of vaginal specula, retractors, or tractors used; (d) diagrams of any customized devices used; (e) the type (e.g., Valsalva maneuver, cough) and, if measured, intensity (e.g., vesical or rectal pressure) of straining used to develop the prolapse maximally; (f) fullness of bladder and, if the bladder was empty, whether this was by spontaneous voiding or by catheterization; (g) content of rectum; (f) the method by which any quantitative measurements were made.

B. Quantitative Description of Pelvic Organ Position

This descriptive system is a tandem profile, in that it contains a series of component measurements grouped together in combination, but that are listed separately in tandem, without being fused into a distinctive new expression or "grade." It allows for the precise description of an individual woman's pelvic support without assigning a "severity value." Second, it allows accurate site-specific observations of the stability or progression of prolapse over time by the same or different observers. Finally, it allows similar judgments on the outcome of surgical repair of prolapse. For example, noting that a surgical procedure moved the leading edge of a prolapse from 0.5 cm beyond the hymeneal ring to 0.5 cm above the hymeneal ring denotes more meagre improvement than stating that the prolapse was reduced from grade 3 to grade 1, as would be the case using some current grading systems.

1. Definition of Anatomical Landmarks

Prolapse should be evaluated by a standard system relative to clearly defined anatomical points of reference. These are of two types; a fixed reference point and defined points that are located relative to this reference.

a. Fixed Point of Reference. Prolapse should be evaluated relative to a fixed anatomical landmark that can be consistently and precisely identified. The hymen will be the fixed point of reference used throughout this system of quantitative prolapse description. Visually, the hymen provides a precisely identifiable landmark for reference. Although it is recognized that the plane of the hymen is somewhat variable depending on the degree of levator ani dysfunction, it remains the best landmark available. "Hymen" is preferable to the ill-defined and imprecise term "introitus." The anatomical position of the six defined points for measurement should be centimeters above or proximal to the hymen (negative number) or centimeters below or distal to the hymen (positive number), with the plane of the hymen being defined as zero (0). For example, a cervix that protruded 3 cm distal to the hymen would be +3 cm.

b. Defined Points. This site-specific system has been adapted from several classifications developed and modified by Baden and Walker (6). Six points (two on the anterior vaginal wall, two in the superior vagina, and two on the posterior vaginal wall) are located with reference to the plane of the hymen.

ANTERIOR VAGINAL WALL. Because the only structure directly visible to the examiner is the surface of the vagina, anterior prolapse should be discussed in terms of a segment of the vaginal wall, rather than the organs that lie behind it. Thus, the term "anterior vaginal wall prolapse" is preferable to "cystocele" or "anterior enterocele" unless the organs involved are identified by ancillary test, two anterior sites are as follows:

Point Aa. A point located in the midline of the anterior vaginal wall 3 cm proximal to the external urethral meatus. This corresponds to the approximate location of the "urethrovesical crease," a visible landmark of variable prominence that is obliterated in many patients. By definition, the range of position of point Aa relative to the hymen is –3 to +3 cm.

Point Ba. A point that represents the most distal (i.e., most dependent) position of any part of the upper anterior vaginal wall from the vaginal cuff or anterior vaginal fornix to Point Aa. By definition, Point Ba is at –8 cm in the absence of prolapse and would have a positive value equal to the position of the cuff in women with total posthysterectomy vaginal eversion.

SUPERIOR VAGINA. These points represent the most proximal locations of the normally positioned lower reproductive tract. The two superior sites are as follows:

Point C. A point that represents either the most distal (i.e., most dependent) edge of the cervix or the leading edge of the vaginal cuff (hysterectomy scar) after total hysterectomy.

Point D. A point that represents the location of the posterior fornix (or pouch of Douglas) in a woman who still has a cervix. It represents the level of uterosacral ligament attachment to the proximal posterior cervix. It is included as a point of measurement to differentiate suspensory failure of the uterosacral–cardinal ligament complex from cervical elongation. When the location of point C is significantly more positive than the location of point D, this is indicative of cervical elongation, which may be symmetrical or eccentric. Point D is omitted in the absence of the cervix.

POSTERIOR VAGINAL WALL. Analogous to anterior prolapse, posterior prolapse should be discussed in terms of segments of the vaginal wall, rather than the organs that lie behind it. Thus, the term "posterior vaginal wall prolapse" is preferable to "rectocele" or "enterocele" unless the organs involved are identified by ancillary tests. If small bowel appears to be present in the rectovaginal space, the examiner should comment on this fact and should clearly describe the basis for this clinical impression (e.g., by observation of peristaltic activity in the distended posterior vagina, by palpation of loops of small bowel between an examining finger in the rectum and one in the vagina, etc.). In such cases, a "pulsion" addendum to the point Bp position may be noted (e.g., Bp = +5 [pulsion]; see a and b under Sec. 3.1 and for further discussion). The two posterior sites are as follows:

Point Bp. A point that represents the most distal (i.e., most dependent) position of any part of the upper posterior vaginal wall from the vaginal cuff or posterior vaginal fornix to point Ap. By definition, point Bp is at –3 cm in the absence of prolapse and would have a positive value equal to the position of the cuff in a women with total posthysterectomy vaginal eversion.

Point Ap. A point located in the midline of the posterior vaginal wall 3 cm proximal to the hymen. By definition, the range of position of point Ap relative to the hymen is –3 to +3 cm.

c. Other Landmarks and Measurements. The genital hiatus (GH) is measured from the middle of the external urethral meatus to the posterior midline hymen. If the location of the hymen is distorted by a loose band of skin without underlying muscle or connective tissue, the firm palpable tissue of the perineal body should be substituted as the posterior margin for this measurement. The perineal body (PB) is measured from the posterior margin of the genital hiatus to the midanal opening. Measurements of the genital hiatus and perineal body are expressed in centimeters. The total vaginal length (tvl) is the greatest depth of the vagina in centimeters when point C or D is reduced to its full normal position. *Note:* Eccentric elongation of a prolapsed anterior or posterior vaginal wall should not be included in the measurement of total vaginal length. The points and measurements are represented in Figure 1.

2. Making and Recording Measurements

The position of points Aa, Ba, Ap, Bp, C, and (if applicable) D with reference to the hymen should be measured and recorded. Positions are expressed as centimeters above or proximal to the hymen (negative number) or centimeters below or distal to the hymen (positive number), with the plane of the hymen being defined as zero (0). Although an examiner may be able to make measurements to the nearest half (0.5) cm, it is doubtful that further precision is possible. All reports should clearly specify how measurements were derived. Measurements may be recorded as a simple line of numbers (e.g., –3, –3, –7, –9, –3, –3, 9, 2, 2 for points Aa, Ba, C, D, Bp, Ap, total vaginal length, genital hiatus, and perineal body, respectively). Note that the last three numbers have no + or – sign attached to them because they denote lengths and not positions relative to the hymen. Alternatively, a three by three

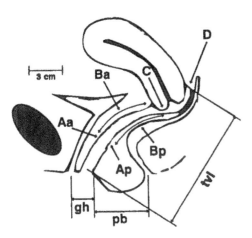

Figure 1 The six sites (Aa, Ba, C, D, Bp, and Ap), the genital hiatus (gh), perineal body (pb) and total vaginal length (tvl) used of pelvic organ support quantitation.

anterior wall	anterior wall	cervix or cuff
Aa	Ba	C
genital hiatus	perineal body	total vaginal length
gh	pb	tvl
posterior wall	posterior wall	posterior fornix
Ap	Bp	D

Figure 2 A three-by-three grid for recording the quantitative description of pelvic organ support.

"tic-tac-toe" grid can be used to organize concisely the measurements as noted in Figure 2 or a line diagram of the configuration can be drawn as noted in Figures 3 and 4. Figure 3 is a grid and line diagram contrasting measurements indicating normal support to those of posthysterectomy vaginal eversion. Figure 4 is a grid and line diagram representing predominant anterior and posterior vaginal wall prolapse with partial vault descent.

C. Ordinal Stages of Pelvic Organ Prolapse

The tandem profile for quantifying prolapse provides a precise description of anatomy for individual patients. However, because of the many possible combinations, such profiles cannot be directly ranked; the many variations are too numerous to permit useful analysis and

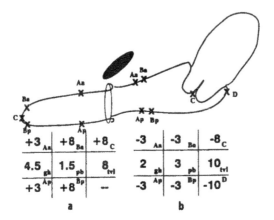

Figure 3 (a) Example of a grid and line diagram of complete eversion of the vagina. The most distal point of the anterior wall (point Ba), the vaginal cuff scar (point C), and the most distal point of the posterior wall (Bp) are all at the same position (+8) and points Aa and Ap are maximally distal (both at +3). The fact that the total vagina length equals the maximum protrusion makes this a stage IV prolapse. (b) Example of normal support. Points Aa and Ba and points Ap and Bp are all −3, as there is no anterior or posterior wall descent. The lowest point of the cervix is 8 cm above the hymen (−8) and the posterior fornix is 2 cm above this (−10). The vaginal length is 10 cm and the genital hiatus and perineal body measure 2 and 3 cm respectively. This represents stage 0 support.

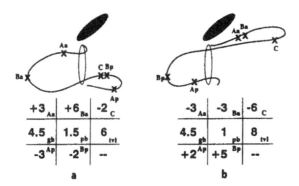

Figure 4 (a) Example of a grid and line diagram of a predominant anterior support defect. The leading point of the prolapse is the upper anterior vaginal wall, point Ba (+6). Note that there is significant elongation of the bulging anterior wall. Point Aa is maximally distal (+3) and the vaginal cuff scar is 2 cm above the hymen (C = −2). The cuff scar has undergone 4 cm of descent, as it would be at −6 (the total vaginal length) if it were perfectly supported. In this example, the total vaginal length is not the maximum depth of the vagina with the elongated anterior vaginal wall maximally reduced, but rather the depth of the vagina at the cuff with point C reduced to its normal full extent as specified in Section 2.2.1(c). This represents stage III-Ba prolapse. (b) Example of a predominant posterior support defect. The leading point of the prolapse is the upper posterior vaginal wall, point Bp (+5). Point Ap is 2 cm distal to the hymen (+2) and the vaginal cuff scar is 6 cm above the hymen (−6). The cuff has undergone only 2 cm of descent, as it would be at −8 (the total vaginal length) if it were perfectly supported. This represents stage III-Bp prolapse.

comparisons when populations are studied. Consequently, they are analogous to other tandem profiles such as the TNM index for various cancers. For the TNM description of individual patient's cancers to be useful in population studies evaluating prognosis or response to therapy, they are clustered into an ordinal set of stages. Ordinal stages represent adjacent categories that can be ranked in an ascending sequence of magnitude, but the categories are assigned arbitrarily and the intervals between them cannot be actually measured. Although the committee is aware of the arbitrary nature of an ordinal-staging system and the possible biases that it introduces, we conclude such a system is necessary if populations are to be described and compared, if symptoms putatively related to prolapse are to be evaluated, and if the results of various treatment options are to be assessed and compared.

Stages are assigned according to the most severe portion of the prolapse when the full extent of the protrusion has been demonstrated. For a stage to be assigned to an individual patient, it is essential that her quantitative description be completed first. The 2-cm buffer related to the total vaginal length in stages 0 and IV is an effort to compensate for vaginal distensibility and the inherent imprecision of the measurement of total vaginal length. The 2-cm buffer around the hymen in stage II is an effort to avoid confining a stage to a single plane and to acknowledge practical limits of precision in this assessment. Stages can be subgrouped according to which portion of the lower reproductive tract is the *most distal* part of the prolapse using the following letter qualifiers: a, anterior vaginal wall; p, posterior vaginal wall; C, vaginal cuff; Cx, cervix; and Aa, Ap, Ba, Bp, and D for the points of measurement already defined. The five stages of pelvic organ support (0 through IV) are as follows:

Stage 0. No prolapse is demonstrated. Points Aa, Ap, Ba, and Bp are all at –3 cm and either point C or D is between –tvl cm and –(tvl – 2) cm (i.e., the quantitation value for point C or D is ≤ –(tvl –2) cm). Figure 3a represents stage 0.

Stage I. The criteria for stage 0 are not met, but the most distal portion of the prolapse is more than 1 cm above the level of the hymen (i.e., its quantitation value is < –1 cm).

Stage II. The most distal portion of the prolapse is 1 cm or less proximal to or distal to the plane of the hymen (i.e., its quantitation value is ≥ –1 cm, but ≤ +1 cm).

Stage III. The most distal portion of the prolapse is more than 1 cm below the plane of the hymen, but protrudes no further than 2 centimeters less than the total vaginal length in centimeter (i.e., its quantitation value is > +1 cm but < + [tvl – 2] cm). Figure 4a represents stage III-Ba and Figure 4b represents stage III-Bp prolapse.

Stage IV. Essentially complete eversion of the total length of the lower genital tract is demonstrated. The distal portion of the prolapse protrudes to at least (tvl – 2) cm (i.e., its quantitation value is ≥ + [tvl – 2] cm). In most instances, the leading edge of stage IV prolapse will be the cervix or vaginal cuff scar. Figure 3b represents stage IV-C prolapse.

III. ANCILLARY TECHNIQUES FOR DESCRIBING PELVIC ORGAN PROLAPSE

This series of procedures may help further characterize pelvic organ prolapse in an individual patient. They are considered ancillary either because they are not yet standardized or validated or because they are not universally available to all patients. Authors utilizing these procedures should include the following information in their manuscripts: (a) describe the objective information they intended to generate and how it enhanced their ability to evaluate or treat prolapse; (b) describe precisely how the test was performed, any instruments that were used, and the specific testing conditions so that other authors can reproduce the study; (c) document the reliability of the measurement obtained with the technique.

A.   Supplementary Physical Examination Techniques

Many of these techniques are essential to the adequate preoperative evaluation of a patient with pelvic organ prolapse. Although they do not directly affect either the tandem profile or the ordinal stage, they are important for the selection and performance of an effective surgical repair. These techniques include, but are not necessarily limited to, the following: (a) performance of a digital rectal–vaginal examination while the patient is straining and the prolapse is maximally developed to differentiate between a high rectocele and an enterocele; (b) digital assessment of the contents of the rectal–vaginal septum during the examination noted in (a) to differentiate between a "traction" enterocele (the posterior cul-de-sac is pulled down with the prolapsing cervix or vaginal cuff, but is not distended by intestines) and a "pulsion" enterocele (the intestinal contents of the enterocele distend the rectal–vaginal septum and produce a protruding mass); (c) Q-tip testing for the measurement of urethral axial mobility; (d) measurements of perineal descent; (e) measurements of the transverse diameter of the genital hiatus or of the protruding prolapse; (f) measurements of vaginal volume; (g) description and measurement of rectal prolapse; (h) examination techniques for differentiating between various types of defects (e.g., central versus paravaginal defects of the anterior vaginal wall).

B.   Endoscopy

Cystoscopic visualization of bowel peristalsis under the bladder base or trigone may identify an anterior enterocele in some patients. The endoscopic visualization of the bladder base and rectum and observation of the voluntary constriction and dilation of the urethra, vagina, and rectum has, to date, played a minor role in the evaluation of pelvic floor anatomy and function. When such techniques are described, authors should include the type, size, and lens angle of the endoscope used; the doses of any analgesic, sedative, or anesthetic agents used; and a statement of the level of consciousness of the subjects in addition to a description of the other conditions of the examination.

C.   Photography

Still photography of stage II and greater prolapse may be used both to document serial changes in individual patients and to illustrate findings for manuscripts and presentations. Photographs should contain an internal frame of reference such as a centimeter ruler or tape.

D.   Imaging Procedures

Different imaging techniques have been used to visualize pelvic floor anatomy, support defects, and relations among adjacent organs. These techniques may be more accurate than physical examination in determining which organs are involved in pelvic organ prolapse. However, they share the limitations of the other techniques in this section (i.e., a lack of standardization, validation, or availability). For this reason, no specific technique can be recommended, but guidelines for reporting various techniques will be considered.

1.   General Guidelines for Imaging Procedures

Landmarks should be defined to allow comparisons with other imaging studies and the physical examination. The lower edge of the symphysis pubis should be given high priority. Other examples of bony landmarks include the superior edge of the public symphysis, the ischial spine and tuberosity, the obturator foramen, the tip of the coccyx, and the promontory of the sacrum. All reports on imaging techniques should specify the following: (a) position of the patient, including the position of her legs (images in manuscripts should be oriented to reflect the patient's position when the study was performed and should not be oriented to suggest an erect position unless the patient was erect); (b) specific verbal instructions given to the patient; (c) bladder volume and content and bowel content, including any prestudy preparations; and (d) the performance and display of simultaneous monitoring, such as pressure measurements.

2. Ultrasonography

Continuous visualization of dynamic events is possible. All reports using ultrasound should include the following information: (a) transducer type and manufacturer (e.g., sector, linear, MHz); (b) transducer size; (c) transducer orientation; and (d) route of scanning (e.g., abdominal, perineal, vaginal, rectal, urethral).

3. Contrast Radiography

Contrast radiography may be static or dynamic and may include voiding colpocystourethrography, defecography, peritoneography, and pelvic fluoroscopy, among others. All reports of contrast radiography should include the following information: (a) projection (e.g., lateral, frontal, horizontal, oblique); (b) type and amount of contrast medium used and sequence of opacification of the bladder, vagina, rectum and colon, small bowel, and peritoneal cavity; (c) any urethral or vaginal appliance used (e.g., tampon, catheter, beadchain); (d) type of exposures (e.g., single exposure, video); and (e) magnification—an internal reference scale should be included.

4. Computed Tomography and Magnetic Resonance Imaging

These techniques do not currently permit continuous imaging under dynamic conditions and most equipment dictates supine scanning. Specifics of the technique should be specified including (a) the specific equipment used, including the manufacturer; (b) the plane of imaging (e.g., axial, sagittal, coronal, oblique); (c) the field of view; (d) the thickness of sections and the number of slices; (e) scan time; (f) the use and type of contrast; and (g) the type of image analysis.

E. Surgical Assessment

Intraoperative evaluation of pelvic support defects is intuitively attractive, but as yet of unproved value. The effects of anesthesia, diminished muscle tone, and loss of consciousness are of unknown magnitude and direction. Limitations owing to the position of the patient must also be evaluated.

IV. PELVIC FLOOR MUSCLE TESTING

Pelvic floor muscles are voluntarily controlled, but selective contraction and relaxation necessitates muscle awareness. Optimal squeezing technique involves contraction of the pelvic floor muscles without contraction of the abdominal wall muscles and without a Valsalva maneuver. Squeezing synergists are the intraurethral and anal sphincteric muscles. In normal voiding, defecation, and optimal abdominal-strain voiding, the pelvic floor is relaxed, while the abdominal wall and the diaphragm may contract. With coughs and sneezes and, often, when other stresses are applied, the pelvic floor and abdominal wall are contracted simultaneously.

Evaluation and measurement of pelvic floor muscle function includes (1) an assessment of the patient's ability to contract and relax the pelvic muscles selectively (i.e., squeezing without abdominal straining and vice versa) and (2) measurement of the force (strength) of contraction. There are pitfalls in the measurement of pelvic floor muscle function because the muscles are invisible to the investigator and because patients often simultaneously and erroneously activate other muscles. Contraction of the abdominal, gluteal, and hip adductor muscles; Valsalva maneuver, straining, breath-holding; and forced inspirations are typically seen. These factors affect the reliability of available testing modalities and have to be taken into consideration in the interpretation of these tests.

The individual types of tests cited in this report are based on both the scientific literature and on current clinical practice. It is the intent of the committee neither to endorse specific tests or techniques, nor to restrict evaluations to the examples given. The standards recommended are intended to facilitate comparison of results obtained by different investigators and to allow investigators to replicate studies precisely. For all types of measuring techniques the following should be specified: (a) patient position, including the position of the legs; (b) specific instructions given to the patient; (c) the status of bladder and bowel fullness; (d) techniques of quantification or qualification (estimated, calculated, directly measured); and (e) the reliability of the technique.

A. Inspection

A visual assessment of muscle integrity, including a description of scarring and symmetry, should be performed. Pelvic floor contraction causes inward movement of the perineum and straining causes the opposite movement. Perineal movements can be observed directly or assessed indirectly by movement of an externally visible device placed into the vagina or urethra. The abdominal wall and other specified regions might be watched simultaneously. The type, size, and placement of any device used should be specified, as should the state of undress of the patient.

B. Palpation

Palpation may include digital examination of the pelvic floor muscles through the vagina or rectum, as well as assessment of the perineum, abdominal wall, or other specified regions. The number of fingers and their position should be specified. Scales for the description of the strength of voluntary and reflex (e.g., with coughing) contractions and of the degree of voluntary relaxation should be clearly described and intra- and interobserver reliability documented. Standardized palpation techniques could also be developed for the semiquantitative estimation of the bulk or thickness of pelvic floor musculature around the circumference of the genital hiatus. These techniques could permit the localization of any atrophic or asymmetrical segments.

C. Electromyography

Electromyography (EMG) from the pelvic floor muscles can be recorded alone or in combination with other measurements. Needle electrodes permit visualization of individual motor unit action potentials, whereas surface or wire electrodes detect action potentials from groups of adjacent motor units underlying or surrounding the electrodes. Interpretation of signals from these latter electrodes must take into consideration that signals from erroneously contracted adjacent muscles may interfere with signals from the muscles of interest. Reports of electromyographic recordings should specify the following: (a) type of electrode; (b) placement of electrodes; (c) placement of reference electrode; (d) specifications of signal-processing equipment; (e) type and specifications of display equipment; (f) muscle in which needle electrode is placed; and (g) description of decision algorithms used by the analytic software.

D. Pressure Recording

Measurements of urethral, vaginal, and anal pressures may be used to assess pelvic floor muscle control and strength. However, interpretations based on these pressure measurements must be made with a knowledge of their potential for artifact and their unproved or limited reproducibility. Anal sphincter contractions, rectal peristalsis, detrusor contractions, and abdominal straining can affect pressure measurements. Pressures recorded from the proximal vagina accurately mimic fluctuations in abdominal pressure. Therefore, it may be important to compare vaginal pressures to simultaneously measured vesical or rectal pressures. Reports using pressure measurements should specify the following: (a) the type and size of the measuring device at the recording site (e.g., balloon, open catheter, etc.); (b) the exact placement of the measuring device; (c) the type of pressure transducer; (d) the type of display system; and (e) the display of simultaneous control pressures.

As noted in Section 4.1, observation of the perineum is an easy and reliable way to assess for abnormal straining during an attempt at a pelvic muscle contraction. Significant straining or a Valsalva maneuver causes downward/caudal movement of the perineum; a correctly performed pelvic muscle contraction causes inward/cephalad movement of the perineum. Observation for perineal movement should be considered as an additional validation procedure whenever pressure measurements are recorded.

V. DESCRIPTION OF FUNCTIONAL SYMPTOMS

Functional deficits caused by pelvic organ prolapse and pelvic floor dysfunction are not well characterized or absolutely established. There is an ongoing need to develop, standardize, and validate various clinimetric scales, such as condition-specific quality of life questionnaires, for each of the four functional symptom groups thought to be related to pelvic organ prolapse.

Researchers in this area should try to use standardized and validated symptom scales whenever possible. They must always ask precisely the same questions concerning functional symptoms before and after therapeutic intervention. The description of functional symptoms should be directed toward four primary areas: (1) lower urinary tract, (2) bowel, (3) sexual, and (4) other local symptoms.

A. Urinary Symptoms

This report does not supplant any currently approved ICS terminology related to lower urinary tract function (7). However, some important prolapse-related symptoms are not included in the current standards (e.g., the need to manually reduce the prolapse or assume an unusual position to initiate or complete micturition). Urinary symptoms that should be considered for dichotomous, ordinal, or visual analog scaling include, but are not limited to, the following: (a) stress incontinence, (b) frequency (diurnal and nocturnal), (c) urgency,

(d) urge incontinence, (e) hesitancy, (f) weak or prolonged urinary stream, (g) feeling of incomplete emptying, (h) manual reduction of the prolapse to start or complete bladder emptying, and (f) positional changes to start or complete voiding.

B. Bowel Symptoms

Bowel symptoms that should be considered for dichotomous, ordinal, or visual analog scaling include, but are not limited to, the following: (a) difficulty with defecation, (b) incontinence of flatus, (c) incontinence of liquid stool, (d) incontinence of solid stool, (e) fecal staining of underwear, (f) urgency of defecation, (g) discomfort with defecation, (h) digital manipulation of vagina, perineum, or anus to complete defecation, (i) feeling of incomplete evacuation, and (j) rectal protrusion during or after defecation.

C. Sexual Symptoms

Research is needed to attempt to differentiate the complex and multifactorial aspects of "satisfactory sexual function" as it relates to pelvic organ prolapse and pelvic floor dysfunction. It may be difficult to distinguish between the ability to have vaginal intercourse and normal sexual function. The development of satisfactory tools will require multidisciplinary collaboration. Sexual function symptoms that should be considered for dichotomous, ordinal, or visual analog scaling include, but are not limited to, the following: (a) Is the patient sexually active? (b) If she is not sexually active, why? (c) Does sexual activity include vaginal coitus? (c) What is the frequency of vaginal intercourse? (d) Does the patient experience pain with coitus? (e) Is the patient satisfied with her sexual activity? (f) Has there been any change in orgasmic response? (g) Is any incontinence experienced during sexual activity?

D. Other Local Symptoms

We currently lack knowledge on the precise nature of symptoms that may be caused by the presence of a protrusion or bulge. Possible anatomically based symptoms that should be considered for dichotomous, ordinal, or visual analog scaling include, but are not limited to, the following: (a) vaginal pressure or heaviness; (b) vaginal or perineal pain; (c) sensation or awareness of tissue protrusion from the vagina; (d) low back pain; (e) abdominal pressure or pain; (f) observation or palpation of a mass.

ACKNOWLEDGMENTS

The subcommittee would like to acknowledge the contributions of the following consultants who contributed to the development and revision of this document: W. Glenn Hurt, Bernhard Schüssler, L. Lewis Wall.

REFERENCES

1. Athanasiou S, Hill S, Gleeson C, Anders K, Cardozo L (1995). Validation of the ICS proposed pelvic organ prolapse descriptive system. Neurourol Urodynam 14:414–415 (abstr of ICS 1995 meeting).
2. Schüssler B, Peschers U (1995). Standardisation of terminology of female genital prolapse according to the new ICS criteria: inter-examiner reproducibility. Neurourol Urodynam 14:437–438 (abstr of ICS 1995 meeting).

3. Montella JM, Cater JR (1995). Comparison of measurements obtained in supine and sitting position in the evaluation of pelvic organ prolapse (abstr of AUGS 1995 meeting).

4. Kobak WH, Rosenberg K, Walters MD (1995). Interobserver variation in the assessment of pelvic organ prolapse using the draft International Continence Society and Baden grading systems. (abstr of AUGS 1995 meeting).

5. Hall AF, Theofrastous JP, Cundiff GC, Harris RL, Hamilton LF, Swift SE, Bump RC (1996). Inter- and intraobserver reliability of the proposed International Continence Society, Society of Gynecologic Surgeons, and American Urogynecologic Society pelvic organ prolapse classification system. Am J Obstet Gynecol (submitted through the program of the Society of Gynecologic Surgeons, 1996 meeting).

6. Baden W, Walker T (1992). Surgical repair of vaginal defects. Philadelphia: Lippincott, pp 1–7; 51–62

7. See Am J Obstet Gynecol 1996, 175: Appendix 1, Part 2.

Intestinal Reservoirs

I. INTRODUCTION

In 1993, the International Continence Society (ICS) established a committee for standardization of terminology and assessment of functional characteristics of intestinal urinary reservoirs to allow reporting of results in a uniform fashion so that different series and different surgical techniques can be compared.

This report is consistent with earlier reports of the International Continence Society Committee on Standardization of Terminology, with special reference to the collated ICS report from 1988 (Abrams et al., 1988).

As the present knowledge about physiological characteristics of intestinal urinary reservoirs is rather limited relative to normal and abnormal reservoir sensation, compliance, activity, continence, and other specifications, some of the definitions are necessarily imprecise and vague. However, it was felt that this report would still be capable of stipulating the standardized assessment of intestinal urinary reservoirs and reporting the results to accumulate more information about physiological characteristics of intestinal urinary reservoirs and to establish precise definitions of normal and abnormal conditions. With increased knowledge and better understanding of intestinal urinary reservoirs, this report will have to be updated to become more specific.

It is suggested that in written publications, the acknowledgment of these standards is indicated by a footnote to the section Methods and Materials or its equivalent: "Methods, definitions and units conform to the standards recommended by the International Continence Society, except where specifically noted."

From Joachim W. Thüroff, Anders Mattiasson, Jens T. Andersen, Hans Hedlund, Frank Hinman, Jr., Markus Hohenfellner, Wiking Månsson, Anthony B. Mundy, Randall G. Rowland, and Kenneth Steven. Produced by the International Continence Society Committee on Standardization of Terminology (Anders Mattiasson, chairman) Subcommittee on Intestinal Urinary Reservoirs (Joachim W. Thüroff, chairman). *Neurourology and Urodynamics* 15:499–511 (1996). Copyright 1996 by Wiley-Liss, Inc.

II. TERMINOLOGY OF SURGICAL PROCEDURES

Up to now, when different surgical procedures for constructing an intestinal urinary reservoir are described, conflicting terminology is often used. This section defines the terminology of surgical procedures used throughout the report. These definitions may not be universally applicable to the published scientific literature to date, viewed in retrospect, but represent a standardized terminology for surgical procedures for the future.

Definitions

    Bladder augmentation is a surgical procedure for increasing bladder capacity. This may be accomplished without other tissues (e.g., autoaugmentation) or with incorporation of other tissues such as intestine (enterocystoplasty, intestinocystoplasty), with or without changing the shape of such intestine (i.e., detubularization and reconfiguration), and with or without resection of a portion of the original bladder.

    Bladder replacement—see "Bladder substitution."

    Bladder substitution (bladder replacement) is a surgical procedure for in situ (orthotopic) total substitution or replacement of the bladder by other tissues, such as isolated intestine. After subtotal excision of the original bladder (e.g., in interstitial cystitis) the intestinal urinary reservoir may be connected to the bladder neck (bladder substitution to bladder neck) and, after complete excision of the original bladder (radical cystoprostatectomy), the reservoir may be connected to the urethra as a continent outlet (bladder substitution to urethra). If indicated, the urethral closure function may be surgically supported in addition (e.g., sling procedure, prosthetic sphincter, periurethral injections). Alternatively, an orthotopically placed urethral substitute or replacement (e.g., from intestine) may be used as a continent outlet for a complete substitution of the lower urinary tract.

    Continent anal urinary diversion is a surgical procedure for continent urinary diversion utilizing bowel in continuity or isolated bowel as a reservoir and the anus as a continent outlet.

    Continent cutaneous urinary diversion is a surgical procedure for continent urinary diversion providing an urinary reservoir (e.g., from intestine and a continence mechanism, from intestine, for formation of a continent heterotopically placed [e.g., cutaneous] outlet [stoma]).

    Enterocystoplasty (bladder augmentation with intestine)—see "bladder augmentation."

    Intestinocystoplasty (bladder augmentation with intestine)—see "bladder augmentation."

III. ASSESSMENT

A. Experimental Assessment

For reporting animal studies, the principles and standards for experimental scientific publications should be followed. Species, sex, weight, and age of the animals must be stated, as well as type of anesthesia. If long-term experiments are performed, the type of treatment between the initial experiment and the evaluation experiment should be stated. Raw data should be presented and, when applicable, the type of statistical analysis must be stated. For standardization of urodynamic evaluation see Sections 4 and 5.

B. Patient Assessment

The assessment of patients with intestinal urinary reservoirs should include history, frequency–volume chart, physical examination, and evaluation of the upper urinary tract.

1. History

The history must include etiology of the underlying disease (i.e., congenital anomaly, neurogenic bladder dysfunction, lower urinary tract trauma, radiation damage, bladder cancer, or other tumors of the true pelvis) and indication for constructing an intestinal urinary reservoir (e.g., radical surgery for malignancy in the true pelvis, low bladder capacity or compliance, upper tract deterioration caused by vesicoureteral obstruction or reflux, urinary incontinence). Information must be available on the duration of previous history of the underlying disease, previous urinary tract infections, and relevant surgery.

The history should also provide information on dexterity and ambulatory status of the patient (i.e., wheelchair-bound, paraplegia, or tetraplegia). Information on sexual and bowel function must be reported for the status before applying an intestinal urinary reservoir.

The urinary history must report symptoms related to both the storage and evacuation functions of the lower urinary tract, with special reference to the technique of evacuation (i.e., spontaneous voiding with or without abdominal straining, Valsalva or Credé maneuvers, intermittent catheterization). Problems of evacuation owing to mucus production or difficulty with catheterization must be reported. Incidence of urinary infections must be reported relative to the incidence before construction of an intestinal urinary reservoir.

2. Specification of Surgical Technique

The surgical technique must be specified stating the applied type of urinary reservoir and origin of gastrointestinal segments used (e.g., stomach, ileum, cecum, transverse colon, sigmoid colon, rectum), length and shape (e.g., tubular, detubularized) of bowel segments, the technique of ureteral implantation (when applicable), and the type of the continent outlet (i.e., original urethra, functionally supported urethra, anal sphincter, catheterizable continent cutaneous outlet). If an intussusception nipple valve is applied, the technique of fixation of the intussusception (i.e., sutures, staples) should be stated.

Additional and combined surgical procedures in the true pelvis must be reported, such as hysterectomy, colposuspension, excision of vaginal or rectal urinary fistulae, or resection of rectum. Information on adjuvant treatment, such as pharmacotherapy, physiotherapy, or electrical stimulation, must be available.

3. Frequency–Volume Chart

On the frequency–volume chart the time and volume of each micturition are reported along with quantities of fluid intake. It must be stated if evacuation was prompted by the clock or by sensation. In addition, episodes of urgency and incontinence have to be reported. The frequency–volume chart can be used for the primary assessment of symptoms of urgency, frequency, and incontinence, and for follow-up studies.

4. Physical Examination

Besides general, urological, and, when appropriate, gynecological examination, the neurological status should be assessed with special attention to sensitivity of the sacral dermatomes, sacral reflex activity (anal reflex, bulbocavernosus reflex), and anal sphincter tone and control.

5. Evaluation of the Upper Urinary Tract

Evaluation of renal function and morphology must be related to the status before constructing an intestinal urinary reservoir. Studies of renal morphology can be based on renal ultrasound, intravenous pyelography, and radioisotope studies. Quantification of findings should be recorded by using accepted classifications of upper tract dilation (Emmett and Witten, 1971), renal scarring (Smellie et al., 1975), and ureteral reflux (Heikel and Parkkulainen, 1966). Renal function should be assessed by measuring the serum concentration of creatinine and, if indicated, by creatinine clearance and radioisotope clearance studies.

6. Other Relevant Studies

Reported complications of urinary diversion into an intestinal reservoir include electrolyte and blood–gas imbalance, malabsorption syndromes, urolithiasis, urinary tract infection, and development of a secondary malignancy. Follow-up evaluation should include relevant tests when applicable and indicated, and reports should state the results of such studies as serum electrolyte concentrations, analysis of blood gases; serum levels of vitamins A, B_{12}, D, E, K, and folic acid; serum levels of bile acids, urine osmolality and pH; urine excretion of calcium, phosphate, oxalate, and citrate; colonization of urine; and findings on endoscopy and biopsy of the urinary reservoir.

IV. PROCEDURES RELATED TO THE EVALUATION OF URINE STORAGE IN AN INTESTINAL URINARY RESERVOIR

A. Enterocystometry

Enterocystometry is the method by which the pressure–volume relation of the intestinal urinary reservoir is measured. All systems are zeroed at atmospheric pressure. For external transducers, the reference point is the superior edge of the symphysis pubis for bladder augmentation, bladder substitution, or continent anal urinary diversion; and the level of the stoma for continent cutaneous urinary diversion. Enterocystometry is used to assess reservoir sensation, compliance, capacity, and activity. Before filling is started, residual urine must be evacuated and measured. Enterocystometry is performed with the patient awake and unsedated, not taking drugs that may affect reservoir characteristics. In a urodynamic follow-up study for evaluation of adjuvant treatment (e.g., pharmacological therapy) of an intestinal urinary reservoir, mode of action, dosage, and route of administration (enteral, parenteral, topical) of the medication have to be specified.

   As an intestinal urinary reservoir starts to expand when permitted to store urine, time intervals between surgery for construction of the intestinal urinary reservoir, its first functional use for storage of urine and urodynamic testing must be stated. For reporting of functional characteristics of an intestinal urinary reservoir, the time interval between surgery and enterocystometric assessment must be stated to account for postoperative expansion of the reservoir.

   As several intestinal segments used in urinary reservoirs react to gastric stimuli, time interval between food ingestion and the urodynamic evaluation should be stated. Reporting of pressure–volume relations of an intestinal urinary reservoir should be obtained at standardized filling volumes or standardized pressures, which must be stated in absolute numbers.

Specify
   a. Access (transurethral, transanal, transstomal, percutaneous)
   b. Fluid medium
   c. Temperature of fluid (state in degrees Celsius)
   d. Position of patient (supine, sitting, or standing)
   e. Filling may be by diuresis or catheter. Filling by catheter may be continuous or stepwise: the precise filling rate should be stated. When the stepwise filling is used, the volume increment should be stated. For general discussion, the following terms for the range of filling rate should be used:
      i. Up to 10 mL/min is slow-fill enterocystometry ("physiological" filling).
      ii. 10–100 mL/min is medium-fill enterocystometry.
      iii. over 100 mL/min is rapid-fill enterocystometry.

Technique
   a. Fluid-filled catheter—specify number of catheters, single or multiple lumens, type of catheter (manufacturer), size of catheter, type (manufacturer), and specifications of external pressure transducer.
   b. Catheter mounted microtransducer—list specifications.
   c. Other catheters—list specifications.
   d. Measuring equipment.

Definitions
   Total reservoir pressure is the pressure within the reservoir.
   Abdominal pressure is taken to be the pressure surrounding the reservoir. In current practice it is estimated from rectal or, less commonly, intraperitoneal or intragastric pressures.
   Subtracted reservoir pressure is estimated by subtracting abdominal pressure from total reservoir pressure. The simultaneous recording of the abdominal pressure trace is essential for the interpretation of the subtracted reservoir pressure trace as artifacts of the subtracted reservoir pressure may be produced by intrinsic rectal contractions or relaxations.
   Contraction pressure (amplitude) is the difference between maximum reservoir pressure during a contraction of an intestinal urinary reservoir and baseline reservoir pressure before onset of this contraction. Contraction pressures may be determined from the pressure curves of total reservoir pressure or subtracted reservoir pressure. For assessment of functional significance of such activity of an intestinal urinary reservoir, pressure and volume must be stated for the first, a typical, and the maximum contraction. The frequency of contractions should be stated at a specified volume.
   Leak-point pressure is the total reservoir pressure at which leakage occurs in the absence of sphincter relaxation. Leakage occurs whenever total reservoir pressure exceeds maximum outlet pressure so that a negative outlet closure pressure results.
   Reservoir sensation is difficult to assess because of the subjective nature of interpreting fullness or "flatulence" from the bowel segments of the intestinal urinary reservoir. It is usually assessed by questioning the patient in relation to the sensation of fullness of the intestinal urinary reservoir during enterocystometry. Commonly used descriptive terms are similar to conventional cystometry:
      First desire to empty;

Normal desire to empty is defined as the feeling that leads the patient to empty at the next convenient moment, but emptying can be delayed if necessary.

Strong desire to empty is defined as a persistent desire to empty without the fear of leakage.

Urgency is defined as a strong desire to empty accompanied by fear of leakage or fear of pain.

Pain (the site and character of which should be specified).

Maximum enterocystometric capacity is the volume at strong desire to empty. In the absence of sensation, maximum enterocystometric capacity is defined by the onset of leakage. If the closure mechanism of the outlet is incompetent, maximum enterocystometric capacity can be determined by occlusion of the outlet (e.g., by a Foley catheter). In the absence of both sensation and leakage, maximum enterocystometric capacity cannot be defined in the same terms and is the volume at which the clinician decides to terminate filling (e.g., because of a risk of overdistension).

Functional reservoir capacity or evacuated volume is assessed from a frequency–volume chart (urinary diary). If a patient empties the urinary reservoir by intermittent catheterization, functional reservoir capacity will be dependent on presence or absence of sensation or leakage. Thus, when reporting functional reservoir capacity the following should be stated:

a. Mode of evacuation (e.g., spontaneous voiding, intermittent catheterization)
b. Presence or absence of sensation of fullness
c. Presence or absence of leakage
d. Timing of evacuation (e.g., by sensation, by the clock, by leakage)

Maximum (anesthetic) anatomical reservoir capacity is the volume measured after filling during a deep general or spinal/epidural anesthetic, specifying fluid temperature, filling pressure, and filling rate.

Compliance describes the change in volume over a related change in reservoir pressure. Compliance (C) is calculated by dividing the volume change (ΔV) by the change in subtracted reservoir pressure (ΔPs) during that change in reservoir volume ($C = \Delta V / \Delta Ps$). Compliance is expressed as milliliters per centimeter H_2O (mL/cmH_2O).

B. Outlet Pressure Measurement

Even under physiological conditions, the evaluation of the competence of the closure mechanism of a continent outlet by measuring intraluminal pressures under various conditions is considered an idealized concept. Moreover, measurements of intraluminal pressures for functional evaluation of a continent outlet do not allow comparison of results between different closure mechanisms, which are in use with different types of intestinal urinary reservoirs. In addition, similar closure mechanisms may behave differently when used in different types of intestinal urinary reservoirs.

Therefore, urodynamic measurements of a continent outlet always have to be related to symptoms of the patient as assessed by history, frequency–volume chart, and, when applicable, measurement of urine loss.

The rationale of performing outlet pressure measurements is not to verify continence or degree of incontinence, but to understand how different closure mechanisms work, which urodynamic parameters reflect their competence or dysfunction, and how their function is related to the characteristics of a reservoir.

In current urodynamic practice, intraluminal outlet pressure measurements are performed by a number of different techniques, which do not always yield consistent values. Not only do the values differ with the method of measurement, but there is often a lack of consistency for a single method—for example, the effect of catheter rotation when outlet pressure is measured by a catheter-mounted microtransducer.

Measurements can be made at one point in the outlet (stationary) over a time period, or at several points along the outlet consecutively during continuous or intermittent catheter withdrawal, forming an outlet pressure profile (OPP). OPPs should be obtained at significant filling volumes of an intestinal urinary reservoir, which must be standardized and stated.

Two types of OPP can be measured:

a. Resting outlet pressure profile—with the urinary reservoir and the subject at rest
b. Stress outlet pressure profile—with a defined applied stress (e.g., cough, strain, Valsalva maneuver).

The outlet pressure profile denotes the intraluminal pressure along the length of the closure mechanism. All systems are zeroed at atmospheric pressure. For external transducers the reference point is the level of the continence mechanism. For catheter-mounted transducers the reference point is the transducer itself. Intrareservoir pressure should be measured to exclude a simultaneous reservoir contraction. The subtraction of total reservoir pressures from intraluminal outlet pressures produces the outlet closure pressure profile.

Specify
a. Infusion medium
b. Rate of infusion
c. Stationary, continuous, or intermittent catheter withdrawal
d. Rate of withdrawal
e. Reservoir volume
f. Position of patient (supine, sitting, or standing)
g. Technique (catheters, transducers, measurement technique and recording apparatus are to be specified according to the 1988 ICS report [Abrams et al., 1988]).

Definitions
Maximum outlet pressure is the maximum pressure of the measured profile.
Maximum outlet closure pressure is the difference between maximum outlet pressure and total reservoir pressure.
Functional outlet profile length is the length of the closure mechanism along which the outlet pressure exceeds total reservoir pressure.
Functional outlet profile length (on stress) is the length over which the outlet pressure exceeds total reservoir pressure on stress.
Pressure "transmission" ratio[1] is the increment in outlet pressure on stress as a percentage of the simultaneously recorded increment in the total reservoir pressure.

---

[1]The term "transmission" is in common usage and cannot be changed. However, transmission implies that forces transmitted to the closure mechanism are generated completely by extrinsic activities. Such an assumption is not yet justified by scientific evidence. A role for intrinsic muscle activity cannot be excluded for the urethra and the

For stress profiles obtained during coughing, pressure transmission ratios can be obtained at any point along the closure mechanism. If single values are given, the position in the closure mechanism should be stated. If several transmission ratios are defined at different points along the closure mechanism, a pressure transmission profile is obtained. During "cough profiles" the amplitude of the cough should be stated if possible.

C. Quantification of Urine Loss

On a frequency–volume chart, incontinence can be qualified (with or without urge or stress) and quantified by the number, type, and dampness (damp/wet/soaked) of pads used each day. However, subjective grading of incontinence may not completely disclose the degree of abnormality. It is important to relate the complaints of each patient to the individual urinary regimen and personal circumstances, as well as to the results of objective measurements.

To assess and compare results of different series and different surgical techniques, a simple standard test can be used to measure urine loss objectively in any subject. To obtain a representative result, especially in subjects with variable or intermittent urinary incontinence, the test should occupy as long a period as possible; yet it must be practical. The circumstances should approximate those of everyday life, yet be similar for all subjects to allow meaningful comparison.

The total amount of urine lost during the test period is determined by weighing a collecting device such as a nappy, absorbent pad, or condom appliance. A nappy or pad should be worn inside waterproof underpants or should have a waterproof backing if worn over a continent stoma. Care should be taken to use a collecting device of adequate capacity.

Immediately before the test begins the collecting device is weighed to the nearest gram.

In the 1988 collated report on "Standardization of terminology of lower urinary tract functions" (Abrams et al., 1988), the ICS has offered the choices to conduct a pad test either with the patient drinking 500 mL sodium-free liquid within a short period (max. 15 min) without the patient voiding before the test or after having the bladder filled to a defined volume. Because there is a great variation in the functional capacity of different types of intestinal urinary reservoirs and because some types of closure mechanism of the outlet physiologically have a leak point and others have no leak point, it is recommended that the reservoir is emptied by catheterization immediately before the test and refilled with a reasonable volume of saline, which must be standardized and be stated in absolute numbers. A typical test schedule and additional procedures are described in the 1988 ICS report (Abrams et al., 1988). Specifications for presentation of results, findings, and statistics from the 1988 ICS report are applicable (Abrams et al., 1988).

---

anus and their intrinsic sphincter mechanisms, whereas it is unlikely to be of significance in any of the surgically constructed closure mechanisms of a continent outlet.

The terms "passive transmission" and "active transmission" have been introduced to describe different processes relative to the source of extrinsically generated forces and the mode of transmission. Passive transmission is taken to be the result of forces, which are generated by striated muscles distant from the closure mechanism (e.g., diaphragm, abdominal wall muscles) and are "passively" transmitted through surrounding tissues to the closure mechanism in the same way they are transmitted to all other intra-abdominal tissues and organs. Active transmission is taken to be the result of forces that are generated by striated muscles in direct anatomical contact with the closure mechanism (e.g., pelvic floor muscles with urethra or anus, and abdominal wall muscles with a continent cutaneous outlet), and are directly "transmitted" to the closure mechanism.

V. PROCEDURES RELATED TO THE EVALUATION OF EVACUATION OF AN INTESTINAL URINARY RESERVOIR

A. Mode of Evacuation

The mode of evacuation of an intestinal urinary reservoir varies as some patients may have a surgically constructed closure mechanism requiring catheterization (e.g., continent cutaneous urinary diversion) and some patients may have a reservoir with a physiological sphincter mechanism (e.g., bladder augmentation, bladder substitution to bladder neck or to urethra, continent anal urinary diversion), through which they may be able to evacuate urine spontaneously. However, as catheterization may also be required after bladder augmentation or bladder substitution to bladder neck or to urethra, it must be stated by what means the reservoir is emptied (e.g., spontaneous evacuation with or without Valsalva or Credé maneuvers or intermittent catheterization).

 If intermittent catheterization is necessary, whether it is performed on a regular basis or only periodically, the intervals between catheterizations must be stated.

 Measurements of urinary flow, reservoir pressures during micturition and residual urine apply only to patients with bladder augmentation or bladder substitution to bladder neck or to urethra who void spontaneously. However, as there is no volitional initiation of contraction of an intestinal urinary reservoir, spontaneous evacuation is different from voiding by a detrusor contraction.

 In patients with an intestinal urinary reservoir, evacuation is initiated by relaxation of the urethral sphincteric mechanisms or passive expression of the reservoir by abdominal straining or Valsalva or Credé maneuvers. Therefore, measurements of flow and micturition pressures must be interpreted with great caution in the diagnosis of an outlet obstruction.

B. Measurements of Urinary Flow, Micturition Pressure, Residual Urine

For specifications of measurements of urinary flow, reservoir pressures during micturition, and residual urine, the 1988 ICS report is applicable (Abrams et al., 1988). The specifications of patient position, access for pressure measurement, catheter type, and measuring equipment are as for enterocystometry (see Sec. 4.1).

VI. CLASSIFICATION OF STORAGE DYSFUNCTION OF AN INTESTINAL URINARY RESERVOIR

Dysfunction of an intestinal urinary reservoir has to be defined relative to indications and functional intentions of incorporating bowel into the urinary tract. The rationale of using an intestinal urinary reservoir is to improve or provide storage function by

 a. Reducing bladder hypersensitivity
 b. Providing/enlarging reservoir capacity
 c. Providing/improving reservoir compliance
 d. Lowering bladder pressures/providing low reservoir pressures
 e. Improving/providing the closure function of the outlet

 It is not a primary goal of surgery to maintain or provide the capability of spontaneous voiding; intermittent catheterization is required for evacuation of the reservoir in all cases of continent cutaneous diversion and in many other situations. The need to evacuate a urinary reservoir by intermittent catheterization is not considered a failure in bladder augmentation and bladder substitution to bladder neck or to urethra, even though the majority of patients may evacuate urine spontaneously.

Consequently, the classification of dysfunctions of an intestinal urinary reservoir relates to the storage phase only. Problems of storing urine in an intestinal urinary reservoir may be related to dysfunction of the reservoir or dysfunction of the outlet. The classification is based on the pathophysiology of dysfunction as assessed by various urodynamic investigations. The urodynamic findings must be related to the patient's symptoms and signs. For example, the presence of reservoir contractions in an asymptomatic patient with normal upper tract drainage does not warrant a diagnosis of reservoir overactivity unless the contractions cause urine leakage or other problems defined in the following.

A. Reservoir Dysfunction

The symptoms of frequency, urgency, nocturia, or incontinence may relate to dysfunction of an intestinal urinary reservoir and should be assessed by enterocystometry, which is an adequate test for evaluation of the pathophysiology of a reservoir dysfunction (see Sec. 4.1). Abnormal findings may relate to sensation, compliance, capacity, or activity of an intestinal urinary reservoir.

1. Sensation

Sensations from an intestinal urinary reservoir, as assessed by questioning the patient during enterocystometry, can be classified in qualitative terms. Often these symptoms are associated with contractions of the reservoir, as shown by enterocystometry or fluoroscopy. However, up to now there is insufficient information about an isolated hypersensitive state of the bowel of an intestinal urinary reservoir. If symptoms such as frequency, urgency, and nocturia are persisting after bladder augmentation or bladder substitution to bladder neck (e.g., in interstitial cystitis), they are likely to derive from remnants of the original lower urinary tract, which have not been replaced by intestine, if enterocystometry is otherwise normal.

2. Capacity and Compliance

Capacity of an intestinal urinary reservoir is determined by sensation or compliance. For definitions of reservoir capacity and compliance ($\Delta V/\Delta P$), see Sec. 4.1. Compliance describing the change in volume over a related change in reservoir pressure is likely to reflect a different physiology when determined in an intestinal urinary reservoir as compared with the urinary bladder. The calculation of compliance will reflect wall characteristics of an intestinal urinary reservoir, such as distensibility, only after a process of "unfolding" of an empty intestinal urinary reservoir has been completed and stretching of the walls begins to take place, which is different in the normal urinary bladder. Compliance may change during the enterocystometric examination and is variably dependent on a number of factors including:

    a. Rate of filling
    b. The part of the enterocystometrogram curve used for compliance evaluation
    c. The volume interval over which compliance is calculated
    d. The distensibility of the urinary reservoir as determined by mechanical and contractile properties of the walls of the reservoir

During normal filling of an intestinal urinary reservoir little or no pressure change occurs, and this is termed "normal compliance." However, at the present time there is insufficient data to define normal, high, and low compliance. When reporting compliance, specify

a. The rate of filling
b. The volume at which compliance is calculated
c. The volume increment over which compliance is calculated
d. The part of the enterocystometrogram curve used for the calculation of compliance

The selection of bowel segments, the size of bowel (diameter, length), and the geometry (shape) of a reservoir after bowel detubularization and reconfiguration determine capacity of an intestinal urinary reservoir (Hinman, 1988). For a given length of bowel, reconfiguration into a spherical reservoir provides the largest capacity. The distensibility of bowel wall, as assessed in experimental models, varies between bowel segments (i.e., large bowel, small bowel, stomach) and with orientation (longitudinal, circumferential) of measurement within a bowel segment (Hohenfellner et al., 1993). However, the relative contributions of wall distensibility (influenced by selection of bowel segments) and of geometric capacity (influenced by size of selected bowel and reservoir shape after detubularization and reconfiguration) in determining the capacity of an intestinal urinary reservoir are not yet precisely understood. Low capacity of an intestinal urinary reservoir may relate to bowel size (diameter/length) or configuration of bowel segments in the reservoir (e.g., tubular, inadequate detubularization, and reconfiguration).

3. Activity

In intact bowel segments, peristaltic contractions are elicited at a certain degree of wall distension. As a result of detubularization and reconfiguration of bowel segments in an intestinal urinary reservoir, such contractions do not encompass the whole circumference of a reservoir. Net pressure changes in the reservoir are determined by the mechanical and muscular properties of both the contracting and the noncontracting segments of the reservoir. Contractions of segments of an intestinal urinary reservoir may be observed by fluoroscopy, but may not increase subtracted reservoir pressure if the generated forces are counterbalanced by other segments of a urinary reservoir that relax and distend. Some contractile activity of an intestinal urinary reservoir is a normal finding on enterocystometry or fluoroscopy.

Overactivity of an intestinal urinary reservoir is defined as a degree of activity that causes lower urinary tract symptoms or signs of upper tract deterioration in the absence of other causes of upper tract damage, such as ureteral obstruction or reflux. Symptoms such as abdominal cramping, urgency, frequency, or leakage, may be related to reservoir activity seen during enterocystometry and thus establish the diagnosis of an unacceptable degree of reservoir activity ("overactivity"). Signs of impaired upper tract drainage may be associated with elevated subtracted reservoir pressures on enterocystometry owing to an early onset, high amplitudes, or frequency of contractions and, thus, establish the diagnosis of overactivity even if subjective symptoms are not experienced.

However, because a precise definition of normal and increased activity of a urinary reservoir from intestine is not yet established, the frequency of contractions should be reported at a specified volume and the pressure–volume relations should be stated for the following defined contractions of the reservoir:

a. First contraction
b. Contraction with maximum contraction pressure (amplitude)
c. Typical contraction

The diagnosis of overactivity of an intestinal urinary reservoir should not be made until a reasonable interval—which must be stated—has elapsed after surgery, because an intestinal urinary reservoir expands after surgery, when permitted to store urine, and because some of the reservoir activity subsides with time with an increase of capacity.

B. Outlet Dysfunction

The symptoms of incontinence or difficulties with catheterization may relate to dysfunction of the outlet of an intestinal urinary reservoir and should be assessed in terms of pathophysiology. Leakage may occur if total reservoir pressure exceeds outlet pressure so that the result is a negative outlet closure pressure as assessed by outlet pressure profiles (see Sec. 4.2). For such an event, volume and total reservoir pressure at onset of leakage (leakpoint pressure) must be stated.

Leakage may occur with a functioning closure mechanism because of an excessive reservoir pressure increase caused by contractions of the intestinal urinary reservoir (overactivity) or overdistension of the reservoir (overflow).

The definition of incompetence of a closure mechanism is different for a closure mechanism that physiologically has a leak point from that for a closure mechanism without a leak point.

A closure mechanism that physiologically has a leak point (e.g., the urethral sphincter, some types of closure mechanism in continent cutaneous urinary diversion) is incompetent if it allows leakage or urine in the absence of contraction of the intestinal urinary reservoir (overactivity) or overdistension of the reservoir (overflow) as assessed by enterocystometry (see Sec. 4.1). A closure mechanism that normally has no leak point (e.g., an intussusception nipple) is incompetent if it permits leakage of urine independent of results of enterocystometry.

BIBLIOGRAPHY

Abrams P, Blaivas GJ, Stanton SL, Andersen JT (1988). The standardisation of terminology of lower urinary tract dysfunction. Scand J Nephrol Suppl 114:5.

Emmett JL, Witten DM (1971). Urinary stasis: the obstructive uropathies, atony, vesicoureteral reflux, and neuromuscular dysfunction of the urinary tract. In: Emmett JL, Witten DM, eds. Clinical Urography. An Atlas and Textbook of Roentgenologic Diagnosis. Vol. 1, 3rd ed. Philadephia: WB Saunders, p 369.

Heikel PE, Parkkulainen KV (1966). Vesicoureteric reflux in children. A classification and results of conservative treatment. Ann Radiol 9:37.

Hinman F Jr (1988). Selection of intestinal segments for bladder substitution: physical and physiological characteristics. J Urol 139:519.

Hohenfellner M, Bürger R, Schad H, Heimisch W, Riedmiller H, Lampel A, Thüroff JW, Hohenfellner R (1993). Reservoir characteristics of Mainz-pouch studied in animal model. Osmolality of filling solution and effect of oxybutynin. Urology 42:741.

Smellie JM, Edwards D, Hunter N, Normand ICS, Prescod N (1975). Vesico-ureteric reflux and renal scarring. Kidney Int 8:65.

Standardization of Terminology of Lower Urinary Tract Function: New Report on Evaluation of Micturition

I. INTRODUCTION

This report has been produced at the request of the International Continence Society (ICS). It was approved at the 25th annual meeting of the society in Sydney, Australia.

The 1988 version of the collated reports on standardization of terminology, which appeared in *Neurourology and Urodynamics* 7:403–427, contains material relevant to pressure–flow studies in many different sections. This report is a revision and expansion of Sections 4.2 and 4.3 and parts of Sections 6.2 and 7 of the 1988 report. It contains a recommendation for a provisional standard method for defining obstruction on the basis of pressure–flow data.

II. EVALUATION OF MICTURITION

A. Pressure–Flow Studies

At present, the best method of analyzing voiding function quantitatively is the pressure–flow study of micturition, with simultaneous recording of abdominal, intravesical, and detrusor pressures and flow rate (Fig. 1).

Direct inspection of the raw pressure and flow data before, during, and at the end of micturition is essential because it allows artifacts and untrustworthy data to be recognized and eliminated. More detailed analyses of pressure–flow relations, described in the following, are advisable to aid diagnosis and to quantify data for research studies.

The flow pattern in a pressure–flow study should be representative of free-flow stud-

From Derek Griffiths, Klaus Höfner, Ron van Mastrigt, Harm Jan Rollema, Anders Spångberg, and Donald Gleason, *International Continence Society Subcommittee on Standardization of Terminology of Pressure-Flow Studies, coordinating chairman Anders Mattiasson.* Neurourology and Urodynamics 16:1–18 (1997). Copyright 1997 by the International Continence Society.

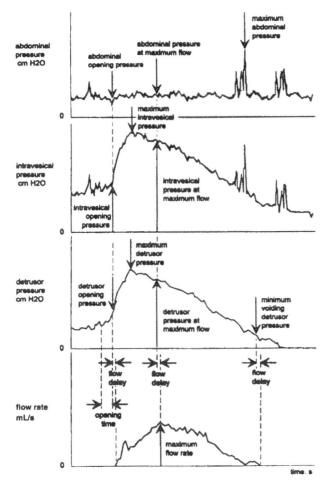

Figure 1 Diagram of a pressure–flow study with nomenclature recommended in this report.

ies in the same patient. It is important to eliminate artifacts and unrepresentative studies before applying more detailed analyses.

Pressure–flow studies contain information about the behavior of the urethra and the behavior of the detrusor. Section 2.2 deals with the urethra. Detrusor function is considered in Section 2.3.

1. Pressure and Flow Rate Parameters

Definitions. See Figure 1 and Table 2; see also Table 2 in the 1988 version of the collated standardization reports.

> *Maximum flow rate* is the maximum measured value of the flow rate; symbol: Q_{max}.
> *Maximum pressure* is the maximum value of the pressure measured during a pressure–flow study. Note that this may be attained at a moment when the flow rate is zero. symbols: $p_{abd.max}$; $p_{ves.max}$; $p_{det.max}$.

Pressure at maximum flow is the pressure recorded at maximum measured flow rate. If the same maximum value is attained more than once or if it is sustained for a time, then the point of maximum flow is taken to be where the detrusor pressure has its lowest value for this flow rate; abdominal, intravesical, and detrusor pressures at maximum flow are all read at the same point. Flow delay (see Sec. 2.1.2) may have a significant influence and should be considered; symbols: $p_{abd.Qmax}$; $p_{ves.Qmax}$; $p_{det.Qmax}$.

Opening pressure is the pressure recorded at the onset of measured flow. Flow delay should be considered; symbols: $p_{abd.open}$; $p_{ves.open}$; $p_{det.open}$.

Closing pressure is the pressure recorded at the end of measured flow. Flow delay should be considered; symbols: $p_{abd.clos}$; $p_{ves.clos}$; $p_{det.clos}$.

Minimum voiding pressure is the minimum pressure during measurable flow (see Fig. 1). It may be, but is not necessarily, equal to the opening pressure or the closing pressure. For example, the symbol for minimum voiding detrusor pressure is $p_{det.min.void}$.

2. Flow Delay

When a pressure–flow study is performed, the flow rate is measured at a location downstream from the bladder pressure measurement, so the flow rate measurement is delayed. The delay is partly physiological, but it also depends on the equipment. It may depend on the flow rate.

When considering pressure–flow relations, it may be important to take this delay into account, especially if there are rapid changes in pressure and flow rate. In current practice, an average value is estimated by each investigator from observations of the delay between corresponding pressure and flow rate changes in a number of actual studies. Values from 0.5 to 1.0 s are typical.

Definition.   *Flow delay* is the time delay between a change in bladder pressure and the corresponding change in measured flow rate.

3. Presentation of Results

Pressure–flow plots and the nomograms used for analysis should be presented with the flow rate plotted along the *x*-axis and the detrusor pressure along the *y*-axis (Fig. 2).

Specify.   The value of the flow delay that is used.

B. Urethral Resistance and Bladder Outlet Obstruction

1. Urethral Function During Voiding

During voiding, urethral function may be

    a.   Normal
    b.   Obstructive, as a result of
        i.   Overactivity
       ii.   Abnormal structure

Obstruction due to urethral overactivity occurs when the urethral closure mechanism contracts involuntarily or fails to relax during attempted micturition in spite of an ongoing

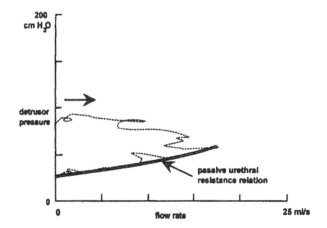

Figure 2   Plot of detrusor pressure against flow rate during voiding (broken curve), providing an indication of the urethral resistance relation (URR). The continuous smooth curve is an estimate of the passive urethral resistance relation.

detrusor contraction. Obstruction caused by abnormal structure has an anatomical basis (e.g., urethral stricture or prostatic enlargement).

2.   Urethral Resistance

Urethral resistance is represented by a relation between pressure and flow rate, describing the pressure required to propel any given flow rate through the urethra. The relation is called the *urethral resistance relation* (URR).

An indication of the urethral resistance relation is obtained by plotting detrusor pressure against flow rate. The most accurate procedure, which requires a computer or an x/y recorder, is a quasicontinuous plot showing many pairs of corresponding pressure and flow rate values (see Fig. 2). A simpler procedure, which can be performed by hand, is to plot only two or three pressure–flow points connected by straight lines; for example, the points of minimum voiding pressure and of maximum flow may be selected. No matter how the plot is made, flow delay should be considered.

A further simplification is to plot just one point showing the maximum flow rate and the detrusor pressure at maximum flow. Flow delay should be considered.

Methods of analyzing pressure–flow plots are further discussed in the following.

3.   Urethral Activity

Ideally, the urethra is fully relaxed during voiding. The urethral resistance is then at its lowest and the detrusor pressure has its lowest value for any given flow rate. Under these circumstances the urethral resistance relation is defined by the inherent mechanical and morphological properties of the urethra and is called the *passive urethral resistance relation* (see Fig. 2).

Urethral activity can only increase the detrusor pressure above the value defined by the passive urethral resistance relation. Therefore, any deviations of the pressure–flow plot from the passive urethral resistance relation toward higher pressures are considered to be a result of activity of the urethral or periurethral muscles, striated or smooth.

4. Bladder Outlet Obstruction

Obstruction is a physical concept that is assessed from measurements of pressure and flow rate made during voiding. Whether due to urethral overactivity or to abnormal structure, obstruction implies that the urethral resistance to flow is abnormally elevated. Because of natural variation from subject to subject, there cannot be a sharp boundary between normal and abnormal. Therefore, the definition of abnormality requires further elaboration.

5. Methods of Analyzing Pressure–Flow Plots

The results of pressure–flow studies may be used for various purposes—for example, for objective diagnosis of urethral obstruction or for statistical testing of differences in urethral resistance between groups of patients. For these purposes, methods have been developed to quantify pressure–flow plots in terms of one or more numerical parameters. The parameters are based on aspects such as the position, slope, and curvature of the plot. Some of these methods are intended primarily for use in adult males with possible prostatic hypertrophy.

Some methods of analysis are shown in Table 1.

Quantification of Urethral Resistance.   In all current methods, urethral resistance is derived from the relations between pressure and flow rate. A commonly used method of demonstrating this relation is the pressure–flow plot. The lower pressure part of this plot is taken to represent the passive urethral resistance relation (see Fig. 2). In general, the higher the pressure for a given flow rate, or the steeper or more sharply curved upward this part of the plot, the higher the urethral resistance. The various methods differ in how position, slope, or curvature of the plot are quantified and how and whether they are combined. Some methods grade urethral resistance on a continuous scale; others grade it in a small number of classes (see Table 1). If there are few classes, small changes in resistance may not be detected. Conversely, a small change on a continuous scale may not be clinically relevant.

Table 1   Methods of Analyzing Pressure–Flow Plots

Method	Aim	Number of p/Q points	Assumed shape of URR	Number of parameters	Number of classes or continuous
Abrams/Griffiths nomogram (1)	Diagnosis	1	n/a	n/a	3
Spångberg nomogram (10)	Diagnosis	1	n/a	n/a	3
URA (2,6)	Resistance	1	Curved	1	Continuous
linPURR (8)	Resistance	1[a]	Linear	1	7
Schäfer PURR (7)	Resistance	Many	Curved	2	Continuous
CHESS (3)	Resistance	Many	Curved	2	16
OBI (4)	Resistance	Many	Linear	1	Continuous
Spångberg et al. (10)	Resistance	Many	Linear or curved	3	Continuous + 3 categories
DAMPF (9)	Resistance	2	Linear	1	Continuous
A/G number (5)	Resistance	1	Linear	1	Continuous

[a]Schäfer uses two points to draw a linear relation, but the point at maximum flow determines the resistance grade.

Some methods result in a single parameter; others result in two or more parameters (see Table 1). A single parameter makes it easy to compare different measurements. A larger number of parameters makes comparison more difficult, but potentially gives higher accuracy and validity. If there are too many parameters, however, accuracy may be compromised by poor reproducibility.

Choice of Methods. Some methods in Table 1 are primarily intended to quantify urethral resistance. Others are intended only for the diagnosis of obstruction. Methods that quantify urethral resistance on a scale can also be used to aid diagnosis of obstruction by comparison with cutoff values. In every case an equivocal zone may be included.

Because of their underlying similarity, all of the foregoing methods classify clearly obstructed and clearly unobstructed pressure–flow studies consistently, but there is some lack of agreement in a minority of cases with intermediate urethral resistance.

One method of analyzing pressure–flow studies may be more useful for a particular purpose. In selecting a method, investigators should consider carefully what their aims are and which method is best suited to their purpose.

Identification of Optimum Methods. For a subsequent report, the International Continence Society will compare the foregoing methods with each other and may also develop new methods, with the aim of reaching a consensus on their use. The society will continue to seek better ways of clinically validating these methods. The following procedure has been chosen.

Making use of good-quality data stored in digital format, the following databases will be examined:

1. Pressure–flow studies in untreated men with lower urinary tract symptoms and signs suggestive of benign prostatic obstruction
2. Pressure–flow studies repeated after a time interval with no intervention
3. Pressure–flow studies before and after TURP
4. Pressure–flow studies before and after alternative therapeutical intervention that causes a small change in urethral resistance.

Database 1 will be used to determine which existing or new methods adequately describe the actual pressure–flow plots of male patients with lower urinary tract symptoms. Database 2 will be used to determine the reproducibility of the various methods. Database 3 will be used to determine in which groups of patients TURP significantly reduces urethral resistance, and hence, which patients are indeed obstructed. Database 4 will be used to test the various methods' sensitivity to small changes of urethral resistance.

On the basis of these analyses, the International Continence Society will attempt to identify

a. A simple and reproducible method with high validity of diagnosing obstruction
b. A sensitive and reproducible method with high validity of measuring urethral resistance and changes in resistance.

Provisional Recommendation. Pending the results of these procedures, it is recommended that investigators reporting pressure–flow studies in adult males, particularly subjects with benign prostatic hyperplasia, use one simple standard method of analysis in addition to any other method that they have selected, so that results from different centers can be compared. For this provisional method it is recommended that urethral resistance be specified by the maximum flow rate and the detrusor pressure at maximum flow (i.e., by the pair of values $[Q_{max}, P_{det.Qmax}]$. A provisional diagnostic classification may be derived from these values as follows:

    a.   If $(P_{det.Qmax} - 2*Qmax) > 40$, the pressure–flow study is obstructed.
    b.   If $(P_{det.Qmax} - 2*Qmax) < 20$, the pressure–flow study is unobstructed.
    c.   Otherwise, the study is equivocal.

In these formulas, pressure and flow rate are expressed in cmH_2O and mL/s, respectively. This method is illustrated graphically in Figure 3. It may be referred to as the *provisional ICS method for definition of obstruction*.

The equivocal zone of the provisional method (see Fig. 3) is similar, but not identical with those of the Abrams–Griffiths and Spångberg nomograms and to the region defining linPURR grade II. For micturitions with low to moderate flow rates it is consistent with cut-off values used to define obstruction in the URA and CHESS methods.

C. Detrusor Contractility During Micturition

During micturition the detrusor may be

    a.   Acontractile
    b.   Underactive
    c.   Normal

An *acontractile detrusor* is one that cannot be demonstrated to contract during urodynamic studies.

An *underactive detrusor* produces a contraction of inadequate magnitude or duration to effect complete bladder emptying in the absence of urethral obstruction. (Concerning the elderly, see later discussion.) Both magnitude and duration should be considered in the evaluation of detrusor contractility.

A *normal detrusor* in the absence of obstruction, produces a contraction that will ef-

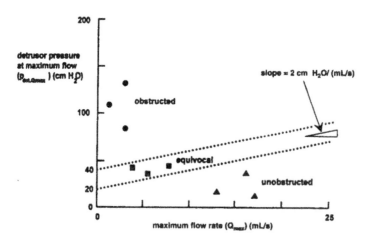

Figure 3   Provisional ICS method for definition of obstruction. The points schematically represent the values of maximum flow rate and detrusor pressure at maximum flow for nine different voids, three in each class.

Table 2   Qualifiers That Can Be Used to Indicate
Pressure and Flow Variables Relevant to Voiding[a]

Qualifiers	
At maximum flow	Qmax
During voiding	void
Opening	open
Closing	clos
Examples	
$P_{det.Qmax}$	= detrusor pressure at maximum flow
$P_{det.min.void}$	= minimum voiding detrusor pressure
$P_{ves.open}$	= intravesical opening pressure
$P_{ves.clos}$	= intravesical closing pressure

[a]When possible, qualifiers should be printed as subscripts (see foregoing).
Note that the preferred symbol for pressure is lowercase p, while the symbol for flow rate is uppercase Q.

fect complete bladder emptying. Detrusor contractility in the elderly may need special consideration.

For a given detrusor contraction, the magnitude of the recorded pressure rise will depend on the outlet resistance. In general, the higher the detrusor pressure or the higher the flow rate, the stronger the detrusor contraction. The magnitude of the detrusor contraction may be quantified approximately by means of a nomogram applied to the pressure–flow plot or by calculation.

III. ADDITIONAL SYMBOLS

Qualifiers that can be used to form symbols for variables relevant to voiding are shown in Table 2. These are additions to those in Table 2 of the 1988 standardization report.

REFERENCES

1. Abrams PH, Griffiths DJ (1979). The assessment of prostatic obstruction from urodynamic measurements and from residual urine. Br J Urol 51:129–134.
2. Griffiths D, Van Mastrigt R, Bosch R (1989). Quantification of urethral resistance and bladder function during voiding, with special reference to the effects of prostate size reduction on urethral obstruction due to benign prostatic hypertrophy. Neurourol Urodynam 8:17–27.
3. Höfner K, Kramer AEJL, Tan HK, Krah H, Jonas U (1995). CHESS classification of bladder outflow obstruction: a consequence in the discussion of current concepts. World J Urol 13:59–64.
4. Kranse M, Van Mastrigt R (1991). The derivation of an obstruction index from a three-parameter model fitted to the lowest part of the pressure flow plot. J Urol 145:261A.
5. Lim CS, Abrams P (1995). The Abrams–Griffiths nomogram. World J Urol 13:34–39.
6. Rollema HJ, Van Mastrigt R (1992). Improved indication and follow-up in transurethral resection of the prostate (TUR) using the computer program CLIM. J Urol 148:111–116.
7. Schäfer W (1983). The contribution of the bladder outlet to the relation between pressure and flow rate during micturition. In: Hinman F Jr, ed. Benign Prostatic Hypertrophy. New York: Springer Verlag, pp 470–496.
8. Schäfer W (1990). Basic principles and clinical application of advanced analysis of bladder voiding function. Urol Clin North Am 17:553–566.

9. Schäfer W (1995). Analysis of bladder-outlet function with the linearized passive urethral re-sistance relation, linPURR, and a disease-specific approach for grading obstruction: from complex to simple. World J Urol 13:47–58.

10. Spångberg A, Teriö H, Ask P, Engberg A (1991). Pressure/flow studies preoperatively and post-operatively in patients with benign prostatic hypertrophy: estimation of the urethral pressure/flow relation and urethral elasticity. Neurourol Urodynam 10:139–167.

Neurogenic Bladder Dysfunction

I. INTRODUCTION

This report has been produced at the request of the International Continence Society (ICS). It was approved at the 28th annual meeting of the society in Jerusalem.

The terminology used in neurogenic lower urinary tract dysfunction developed over the years, defined by neurologists, neurological, and urological surgeons. Because of the particular intents of each specialist, confusion exists on the various terminologies used and on their definitions. The International Continence Society did not define in detail the procedures and conditions in neurogenic lower urinary tract dysfunction. During our discussions the need for standardization of this terminology became obvious.

This report follows the earlier standardization report for lower urinary tract dysfunction (Abrams et al., 1988, 1990) and is adapted to the specific group of patients with neurogenic lower urinary tract dysfunction. Terms defined in the earlier report are marked (*) and their definitions are not repeated here. New or adapted definitions follow *the terms in italics.*

Any pertinent texts repeated from the earlier report are marked in the margin. If they are not repeated completely, this is marked by the term (abbreviated).

Recently, the International Continence Society published a dedicated standardization report on pressure–flow studies (Griffiths et al., 1997). This adapts and extends the earlier report relative to pressure and flow plots and the analysis of the results and provides a provisional standard. Some new definitions are added, some existing ones changed, and

From Manfred Stöhrer,[1]* Mark Goepel,[2] Atsuo Kondo,[3] Guus Kramer,[4] Helmut Madersbacher,[5] Richard Millard,[6] Alain Rossier,[7] and Jean-Jacques Wyndaele.[8] [1]Department of Urology, Berufsgenossenschaftliche Unfallklinik Murnau, Murnau, Germany; [2]Department of Urology, University of Essen Medical School, Essen, Germany; [3]Komaki Shimin Hospital, Johbushi, Japan; [4]Urodynamics Laboratory, Berufsgenossenschaftliche Unfallklinik Murnau, Murnau, Germany; [5]University Hospital Innsbruck, Innsbruck, Austria; [6]Department of Urology, The Prince Henry Hospital, Little Bay, Sidney, Australia; [7]Geneva, Switzerland; [8]Department of Urology, University Hospital Antwerp, Antwerp, Belgium. Produced by the Standardization Committee of the International Continence Society, A. Mattiasson, Chairman. Subcommittee on Terminology in Patients with Neurogenic Lower Urinary Tract Dysfunction, M. Stöhrer, Chairman. *Neurourology and Urodynamics* 18:139–158 (1999). Copyright 1999 by the International Continence Society.

some others no longer used. (Changed) definitions from this second report are marked differently (+).

Two more reports from the International Continence Society are in preparation and bear a relation to the present report: A general report on Good Urodynamic Practice (Schäfer et al.) and a dedicated report on Standardization of Ambulatory Urodynamic Monitoring (Van Waalwijk et al.). This document is intended to be complementary to the mentioned reports and to be consistent in particular with the recommendations in the report of Schäfer et al.

Neurogenic lower urinary tract dysfunction is lower urinary tract dysfunction caused by disturbance of the neurological control mechanisms. Neurogenic lower urinary tract dysfunction thus can be diagnosed only *in the presence of neurological pathology.*

II. CLINICAL ASSESSMENT

Before any functional investigation is planned, a basic general and specific diagnosis should be performed. In the present context of neurogenic lower urinary tract dysfunction, part of this diagnosis is specific for neurogenic pathology and its possible sequelae. The clinical assessment of patients with neurogenic lower urinary tract dysfunction includes and extends that for other lower urinary tract dysfunction.

The latter should consist of a detailed history, a frequency/volume chart and a physical examination. In urinary incontinence, leakage should be demonstrated objectively.

These data are indispensable for reliable interpretation of the urodynamic results in neurogenic lower urinary tract dysfunction.

A. History

1. General History

The general history should include questions relevant to neurological and congenital abnormalities as well as information on previous urinary infections and relevant surgery. Information must be obtained on medication with known or possible effects on the lower urinary tract. The general history should also include the assessment of menstrual, sexual, and bowel function, and obstetric history.

Symptoms of any metabolic disorder or neurological disease that may induce neurogenic lower urinary tract dysfunction must be checked particularly. Presence of spasticity or autonomic dysreflexia must be noted. A list of items of particular importance is

- Neurological complaints
- Congenital anomalies with possible neurological impact
- Metabolic disorders with possible neurological impact
- Preceding therapy, including surgical interventions
- Present medication
- Continence/incontinence (see urinary history)
- Bladder sensation (see urinary history)
- Mode and type of voiding (see urinary history)
- Infections of the lower urinary tract
- Defecation, including possible fecal incontinence (see defecation history)
- Sexual function (see sexual history)

2. Specific History

a. *Urinary History.* The urinary history must consist of symptoms related to both the storage and the evacuation functions of the lower urinary tract.
Specific symptoms and data must be assessed in neurogenic lower urinary tract dysfunction and, if appropriate, be compared with the patients' condition before the neurogenic lower urinary tract dysfunction developed.

Specify

  a. Urinary incontinence
   • Predictability of the occurrence of incontinence
   • Type of incontinence: urge incontinence*, stress incontinence*, other incontinence
   • Position or condition when incontinence occurs (supine, sitting, standing, moving, bedwetting only)
   • Control of the incontinence: medication, pads, external appliances, penile clamp, urethral plug, pessary, catheterization
   • Extent of the incontinence: pad number or weight or estimated volume per 24 hr period, frequency/volume chart*
  b. Bladder sensation*
   • Absent*
   • Specific bladder sensation (desire to void*, urgency*, pain*)
   • General sensation related to bladder filling (abdominal fullness, vegetative symptoms, spasticity)
  b1. If specific bladder sensation exists
   • Normal*, hypersensitive*, or hyposensitive*
   • Can urgency be suppressed?
   • If yes, as effective as before the neurogenic condition?
  b2. If the patient has normal bladder sensation
   • Timing and duration of the sensation
   • Ability to initiate voiding voluntarily
   • Need for abdominal straining or other triggering to initiate or sustain voiding
  c. Mode and type of voiding:
   • Voiding position (standing, sitting, supine)
   • Continuous* or intermittent flow*
   • Residual urine*
   • Initiation of voiding:
    • Voluntary voiding
    • Reflex voiding*: spontaneous or triggered (state type and area of triggering). Remark: Some patients with uncontrollable reflex voiding may use a condom urinal and a urine bag
    • Voiding by increased intravesical pressure (state mode of pressure increase: abdominal strain or Credé). Remark: Credé is contraindicated in children; also in adults when pressure exceeds 100 cmH$_2$O
    • Passive voiding by decreased outlet resistance (state mode: removal of urethral or vaginal appliances, sphincterotomy, TUR bladder neck, artificial sphincter)
    • Sacral root electrostimulation

c1. If the patient has an artificial sphincter:
- Implant date and date(s) of revision surgery
- Micturition frequency
- Cuff pressure
- Number of pump strokes
- Cuff closure time
- Continence or stress incontinence with closed sphincter

c2. If the voiding is induced by sacral root electrical stimulation
- Implant date and date(s) of revision surgery
- Location of electrodes (roots used)
- Stimulation parameters
- Micturition frequency
- Duration of voiding stimulation
- "Double voiding" stimulation

c3. If the patient empties the bladder by catheterization, residual urine is assessed to check also the effectiveness of the catheterization.

c31. *Intermittent catheterization:* Emptying of the bladder by catheter, mostly at regular intervals. The catheter is removed after the bladder is empty. The procedure may be *sterile intermittent catheterization:* Use of sterile components or *clean intermittent catheterization:* At least one component is not sterile. *Intermittent self-catheterization* is performed by the patient.
- Type, size, and material of catheter (conventional, hydrophylic)
- Use of lubricating jelly (intraurethral or on catheter only) or soaking (sterile saline, tap water)
- Disinfection of meatus

c32. An *indwelling catheter* is permanently introduced into the bladder. An external urine collecting device is used.
- Transurethral or suprapubic approach
- Type, size, and material of catheter
- Type of collecting device and associated materials (antireflux valves)
- Interval between changes of collecting device

d.   *Urinary diary* (frequency–volume chart*)

The frequency–volume chart is a specific urodynamic investigation recording fluid intake and urine output per 24-hr period. The chart gives objective information on the number of voidings, the distribution of voidings between daytime and nighttime and each voided volume. The chart can also be used to record episodes of urgency and leakage and the number of incontinence pads used.

The urinary diary is also useful in patients who perform intermittent catheterization. A reliable urinary diary cannot be taken in less than 2–3 days. The urinary diary permits the assessment of voiding data under normal physiological conditions.
- Time and volume for each voiding or catheterization
- Total volume over the period of the recording or 24-hr volume
- Diurnal variation of volumes
- *Functional bladder capacity:* average voided volume
- *Voiding interval:* average time between daytime voidings
- *Continence interval:* average time between incontinence episodes or between last voiding and incontinence (assessed only during daytime)
- The fluid intake may also be recorded

Only for patients who use catheterization it is also feasible to assess
- Residual urine
- *Total bladder capacity:* Sum of functional bladder capacity and residual urine

b. Defecation History.   Patients with neurogenic lower urinary tract dysfunction may suffer from a related neurogenic condition of the lower gastrointestinal tract. The defecation history also must address symptoms related to the storage and the evacuation functions, and specific symptoms and data must be compared with the patients' condition before the neurogenic dysfunction developed.

Specify
    a. Fecal incontinence
- Extent (complete, spotting, diarrhea, flatulence)
- Pads use (type and number)
- Anal tampons (number)

    b. Rectal sensation
- Filling sensation
- Differentiation between stool, liquid stool, and flatus
- Sensation of passage

    c. Mode and type of defecation
- Toilet use or in bed
- Frequency of defecation
- Duration of defecation
- Use of oral or rectal laxatives
- Interval between laxatives and defecation
- Use of enema (frequency, amount used)
- Antegrade continence enema (date of surgery, date(s) of revision, frequency of stomal dilation, frequency of washout)
- Initiation of defecation
  - Voluntary or spontaneous
  - After digital stimulation
  - Mechanical emptying (patient or caregiver)
  - Sacral root electrical stimulation

   c1. If the defecation is induced by sacral root electrical stimulation
- Implant date and date(s) of revision surgery
- Location of electrodes (roots used)
- Stimulation parameters
- Continuous or interrupted stimulation (interval)
- Combination with other treatment (laxatives or rectal mucosal stimulation)

c. Sexual History.   The sexual function may also be impaired because of the neurogenic condition.

Specify
MALES
    a. Sensation in genital area and for sexual functions (increased/normal/reduced/absent)
    b. Erection
- Spontaneous or inducible by psychogenic stimuli
- Mechanical or medical initiation (state method or drug)
- Sacral root electrical stimulation

b1. If the erection is induced by sacral root electrical stimulation
   - Implant date and date(s) of revision surgery
   - Location of electrodes (roots used)
   - Stimulation parameters
   - Leg clonus (absent/present)
   - If erection is insufficient: use of supportive treatment
c. Intercourse (erection sufficient or extra mechanical stimulation)
c1. If the erection is insufficient, state tumescence, rigidity, duration
d. If the patient has a penile implant
   - Implant date and date(s) of revision surgery
   - Type of prosthesis
   - Result of implantation
   - Frequency of use
e. Ejaculation
   - Natural (normal, dribbling, semen quality and appearance)
   - Artificial
      - Vibrostimulation, electroejaculation, intrathecal drugs (frequency, results)
      - Semen analysis (most recent, result)

FEMALES
a. Sensation in genital area and for sexual functions (increased/normal/reduced/absent)
b. Arousal or orgasm inducible (psychogenic or mechanical stimuli)

B. Physical Examination

1. General Physical Examination

Attention should be paid to the patient's physical and possible mental handicaps relative to the planned investigation. Impaired mobility, particularly in the hips, or extreme spasticity may lead to problems in patient positioning in the urodynamics laboratory. Patients with very high neurological lesions may suffer from a significant drop in blood pressure when moved in a sitting or standing position. Subjective indications of bladder filling sensations may be impossible in retarded patients.

2. Neurourological Status

Specify
   - Sensation S2–S5 (both sides): presence (increased/normal/reduced/absent), type (sharp/blunt), afflicted segments
   - Reflexes: bulbocavernous reflex, perianal reflex, knee and ankle reflexes, plantar responses (Babinski) (increased/normal/reduced/absent)
   - Anal sphincter tone (increased/normal/reduced/absent)
   - Anal sphincter and pelvic floor voluntary contractions (increased/normal/reduced/absent)
   - Prostate palpation
   - Descensus of pelvic organs

3. Laboratory Tests

   - Urinalysis (infection treatment, if indicated and possible, before further intervention)

- Blood laboratory, if necessary
- Free flowmetry and assessment of residual urine (mostly sonographic; by catheter in patients catheterizing or immediately preceding a urodynamic investigation). Because of natural variations, multiple estimations are necessary (at least two to three)
- Quantification of urine loss* by pad testing, if appropriate
- Imaging

  Sonography: kidneys (size, diameter of parenchyma, pelvis, calyces)
  Ureter (dilation)
  Bladder wall (diameter, outline, trabeculation, diverticulae or pseudodiverticulae)

  X-ray: cystography, excretion urography, urethrography, clearance studies, if necessary.
  Apart from the data in sonography, attention must be paid to urinary stones, spinal anomalies, reflux, bladder neck condition, and urethral anomalies.
  MRI: accordingly

III. INVESTIGATIONS

In patients with neurogenic lower urinary tract dysfunction, and particularly when detrusor hyperreflexia* might be present, the urodynamic investigation is even more provocative than in other patients. Any technical source of artifacts must be critically considered. The quality of the urodynamic recording and its interpretation must be ensured (Schäfer et al.).

In patients at risk for autonomic dysreflexia, blood pressure assessment during the urodynamic study is advisable.

In many patients with neurogenic lower urinary tract dysfunction, assessment of maximum (anesthetic) bladder capacity* may be useful. The rectal ampulla should be empty of stool before the start of the investigation. Medication by drugs that influence the lower urinary tract function should be abandoned at least 48 hr before the investigation (if feasible) or otherwise be taken into account for interpretation of the data.

A. Methods

In neurogenic lower urinary tract dysfunction, a combination of urodynamic investigations is mostly warranted. Some comments on the use of a single investigation are listed (see also Sec. 4). Urodynamic investigation should be performed only when the patient's free flowmetry and residual data are available (see Sec. 2.2.3) if the patient's condition permits these tests.

1. Measurement of Urinary Flow*

Care must be taken in judging the results in patients who are not able to void in a normal position. Both the flow pattern* and the flow rate* may be modified by this inappropriate position and by any constructions to divert the flow.

2. Cystometry*

Cystometry is used to assess detrusor activity, sensation, capacity, and compliance. As an isolated investigation this is probably useful only for follow-up studies of treatment.

3.   Leak-Point Pressure Measurement (McGuire et al., 1996)

There are two kinds of leak-point pressure measurement. The detrusor leak-point pressure is a static test and the abdominal leak-point pressure is a dynamic test. The pressure values at leakage should be read exactly at the moment of leakage.

The *detrusor leak-point pressure* is the lowest value of the detrusor pressure* at which leakage is observed in the absence of abdominal strain or detrusor contraction.

Detrusor leak-point pressure measurement assesses the storage function and detrusor compliance, in particular in patients with neurogenic lower urinary tract dysfunction, with low compliance bladder (see later) or with reflex voiding. High detrusor-leak-point pressure puts these patients at risk for upper urinary tract deterioration or might cause secondary damage to the bladder. A detrusor leak-point pressure above 40 cmH$_2$O appears hazardous (McGuire et al., 1996).

The *abdominal leak-point pressure* is the lowest value of the intentionally increased intravesical pressure* that provokes urinary leakage in the absence of a detrusor contraction. The abdominal pressure increase can be induced by coughing (*cough leak-point pressure*) or by Valsalva (*Valsalva leak-point pressure*) with increasing amplitude. Multiple estimations at a fixed bladder volume (200–300 mL in adults) are necessary.

For patients with stress incontinence, the abdominal leak-point pressure measurement gives an impression of the severity (slight or severe) or the nature (anatomical or intrinsic sphincter deficiency) of incontinence.

With the assumption that the intravesical pressure in abdominal leak-point pressure is caused only by the abdominal pressure, vaginal pressure or rectal pressure may also be used to record the intravesical pressure. This will obviate the need for intravesical catheterization.

4.   Bladder Pressure Measurements During Micturition* and Pressure–Flow Relations*

Most types of obstructions caused by neurogenic lower urinary tract dysfunction are due to urethral overactivity* (detrusor/urethral dyssynergia*, detrusor–[external]–sphincter dyssynergia*, and detrusor/bladder neck dyssynergia*). This urethral overactivity will increase the detrusor voiding pressure above the level that is needed to overcome the urethral resistance[+] given by the urethra's inherent mechanical and anatomical properties. Pressure–flow analysis mostly assesses the amount of mechanical obstruction* caused by the latter properties and has limited value in patients with neurogenic lower urinary tract dysfunction.

5.   Electromyography* (Often Combined with Cystometry/Uroflowmetry)

Depending on the location of the electrodes, the electromyogram records the function of

- External urethral or anal sphincter
- Striated pelvic floor muscles

Owing to possible artifacts caused by other equipment used in a urodynamic investigation, its interpretation may be difficult.

6.   Urethral Pressure Measurement*

Urethral pressure measurement has a limited place in the diagnosis of neurogenic lower urinary tract dysfunction. The following techniques are available:

- Resting urethral pressure profile*
- Stress urethral pressure profile*

- Intermittent catheter withdrawal (to cope with massive reflex contractions)
- *Continuous urethral pressure measurement:* the catheter sensor or opening is placed at about the point of maximum urethral closure pressure* and left there over time. This records time variations of urethral pressure and responses to various conditions of the lower urinary tract

7. Video Urodynamics

Definition. Combination of lower urinary tract imaging during filling and voiding with urodynamic measurements.

8. Ambulatory Urodynamics

An *ambulatory urodynamic investigation* is defined as any functional investigation of the urinary tract utilizing predominantly natural filling of the urinary tract and reproducing normal subject activity (Van Waalwijk, et al.). The recording of an ambulatory urodynamic investigation is comparable with Holter ECG and the patient is more or less in a situation of daily life. More detailed information on standardization of ambulatory urodynamics is found in the specific report (Van Waalwijk et al., 2000).

9. Provocative Tests During Urodynamics

- Coughing, triggering, anal stretch
- Ice water test
- Carbachol test
- Acute drug tests

10. Maximum (Anesthetic) Bladder Capacity Measurement

I The volume measured after filling during a deep general or spinal/epidural anesthetic.

11. Specific Uroneurophysiological tests

- Electromyography (in a neurophysiological setting)
- Nerve conduction studies*
- Reflex latency measurements*
- Evoked responses*
- Sensory testing*

B. Measurement Technique

1. Measurement of Urinary Flow

Specify
    0. Type of voiding
        - Spontaneous voiding: voluntary or reflex voiding
        - Triggered voiding or sacral root electrostimulation: type of triggering
    a. Voided volume
    b. Patient environment and position (supine, sitting, or standing)
    c. Filling
        i. By diuresis (spontaneous or forced; specify regimen)
        ii. By catheter (transurethral or suprapubic)
    d. Type of fluid

Technique
   a.   Measuring equipment
   b.   Solitary procedure or combined with other measurements

2. Cystometry

All systems are zeroed at atmospheric pressure. For external transducers the reference point is the level of the superior edge of the symphysis pubis. For catheter-mounted transducers the reference point is the transducer itself.

If a different type of catheter is used in follow-up cystometries the findings in Rossier and Fam (1986) may be of interest.

Specify
   a.   Access (transurethral or percutaneous)
   b.   Fluid medium (liquid or gas)

   Gas filling should not be used in patients with neurogenic lower urinary tract dysfunction.
   State type and concentration of liquid used (for example, contrast medium, isotonic saline).

   c.   Temperature of fluid (state in degrees Celsius)
   In neurogenic lower urinary tract dysfunction a body-warm filling medium is advised.
   d.   Position of patient (e.g., supine, sitting, or standing)
   Offer the patient the individually most comfortable position, particularly when voiding.
   e.   Filling may be by diuresis or catheter. Filling by catheter may be continuous or incremental; the precise filling rate should be stated.
   When the incremental method is used the volume increment should be stated.
For general discussion, the following terms for the range of filling may be used:

   i.   Up to 10 mL/min is slow-fill cystometry ("physiological" filling)
   ii. 10–100 mL/min is medium-fill cystometry
   iii. Over 100 mL/min is rapid-fill cystometry

A physiological-filling rate or alternatively a maximum-filling rate of 20 mL/min is advised in neurogenic lower urinary tract dysfunction to prevent provocation of detrusor hyperreflexia or other sequelae of faster filling. From ambulatory urodynamics data the impression arises that the mentioned filling rates should be reconsidered (Klevmark, 1997).

Technique
   a.   Fluid-filled catheter—specify number of catheters, single or multiple lumens, type of catheter (manufacturer), size of catheter
   b.   Catheter tip transducer—list specifications
   c.   Other catheters—list specifications
   d.   Measuring equipment

3. Leak-Point Pressure Measurement

Specify
   a.   Location and access of pressure sensor (intravesical—transurethral orpercutaneous, vaginal, or rectal)

b. Position of patient (i.e., supine, sitting, or standing)
c. Bladder filling by diuresis or catheter (state type of liquid)
d. Bladder volume during test, also in relation to maximum cystometric capacity*

Technique
a. Mode of leak detection (observation, alarm nappy, meatal, or urethral conductance measurement, or other)
b. Catheters—list specifications, type (manufacturer) and size
c. Measuring equipment for pressure and, if applicable, for leak detection

4. Bladder Pressure Measurements During Micturition and Pressure–Flow Relations

The specifications of patient position, access for pressure measurement, catheter type, and measuring equipment are as for cystometry (see Sec. 3.2.2).

If urethral pressure measurements during voiding* are performed, the specifications are according to those in urethral pressure measurement (see Sec. 3.2.6).

If other assessments of the relation between pressure and flow are used (e.g., stop test, urethral occlusion, condom urinal occlusion) the specifications should be equivalent, according to the technique used.

5. Electromyography

The extensive specifications in the earlier report are appropriate in a neurophysiological setting. They are condensed here for practical use during urodynamics.

Specify
a. EMG (solitary procedure, part of urodynamic or other electrophysiological investigation)
b. Patient position (supine, standing, sitting, or other)
c. Electrode placement (surface electrodes or intramuscular electrodes)
   i. Sampling site (abbreviated)
   ii. Recording electrode: location (abbreviated)
   iii. Reference electrode position
   Note: Ensure that there is no electrical interference with any other machines, for example, x-ray apparatus.

Technique
a. Electrodes
   i. Needle electrodes: type, size, material (abbreviated)
      The same holds for other types of intramuscular electrodes (e.g., enamel wire)
   ii. Surface electrodes: type, size, material, fixation, conducting medium (abbreviated)
b. Amplifier (make and specifications)
c. Signal processing (data: raw, averaged, integrated, or other)
d. Display equipment (abbreviated)
e. Storage (abbreviated)
f. Hard-copy production (abbreviated)

6. Urethral Pressure Measurement

Because of its limited place in neurogenic lower urinary tract dysfunction, the reader is referred to the earlier standardization report (Abrams et al., 1988, 1990) for the specifications.

7. Video Urodynamics

Specify imaging system (fluoroscopy, ultrasound). Further specifications according to the type of urodynamic study.

8. Ambulatory Urodynamics

Specifications according to the type of urodynamic study.

9. Provocative Tests During Urodynamics

Specify type of test, type of trigger, or drug used. Further specifications according to type of urodynamic study.

10. Maximum (Anesthetic) Bladder Capacity Measurement

Specify fluid temperature, filling pressure, filling time, type of anesthesia, anesthetic agent, and dosage.

11. Specific Uroneurophysiological Tests

Electromyography (see Sec. 3.2.5)
Nerve conduction studies, reflex latency measurements, evoked responses

Specify
   a. Type of investigation (abbreviated)
   b. Is the study a solitary procedure or part of a urodynamic or neurophysiological investigation?
   c. Patient position and environmental temperature, noise level, and illumination
   d. Electrode placement (abbreviated)

Technique
   a. Electrodes (abbreviated)
   b. Stimulator (abbreviated)
   c. Amplifier (abbreviated)
   d. Averager (abbreviated)
   e. Display equipment (abbreviated)
   f. Storage (abbreviated)
   g. Hard copy production (abbreviated)

Sensory testing
Specify
   a. Patient position (supine, sitting, standing, and other)
   b. Bladder volume at time of testing
   c. Site of applied stimulus (intravesical and intraurethral)
   d. Number of times the stimulus was applied and the response recorded; define the sensation recorded, for example the first sensation or the sensation of pulsing
   e. Type of applied stimulus (abbreviated)

C. Data

1. Measurement of Urinary Flow

- Voided volume*
- Maximum flow rate*

- Flow time*
- Average flow rate*
- Time to maximum flow*
- Flow pattern, includes the statement of continuous or intermittent voiding
- Voiding time*, when the voiding is intermittent
- *Hesitancy:* the occurrence of significant delay between the patient's voluntary initiation of micturition, as signaled, for example, by pushing the marker button on the flow meter, and the actual start of flow (note the flow delay⁺)

2. Cystometry

- Intravesical pressure
- Abdominal pressure
- Detrusor pressure
- Infused volumes at
  - First desire to void* or other sensation of filling
  - Normal desire to void* or other sensation that indicates the need for a toilet visit
  - *Reflex volume:* starting of first hyperreflexive detrusor contraction
  - Urgency
  - Pain (specify)
  - Maximum cystometric capacity (in patients with abolition of sensations, this is defined as the volume at which the investigator decides to stop filling)
  - Autonomic dysreflexia (specify)
- Compliance* $\{\Delta V/\Delta p_{det}\}$ (mL/cmH_2O) is mostly measured between (specify)
  - Reference value: detrusor pressure at empty bladder (start of filling)
  - Measurement value: the (passive) detrusor pressure:
    - At maximum cystometric capacity in patients with existing sensation and without urine loss
    - At the start of the detrusor contraction leading to the first significant incontinence in patients with failing sensation or significant incontinence
- → When a different volume range is used this should be specified in particular.

    A problem in the calculation of the compliance occurs when Δp_{det} is negative or zero: the defined calculation then gives a negative or infinite compliance. The first is physically impossible, the last gives little information. *In the compliance calculation a minimum value of 1 cmH_2O is used for Δp_{det}.* This means that the maximal possible value of the compliance will be equal to the volume range over which the compliance is calculated.

- *Break volume:* the bladder volume after which a sudden significant decrease of compliance is observed during the remainder of the filling phase (mind the distinction between passive detrusor pressure and detrusor contraction). It is yet unclear whether this observation is consistent in patients with neurogenic lower urinary tract dysfunction with or without detrusor hyperreflexia. When true, this might indicate that the detrusor is in a different state after the break volume.

3. Leak-Point Pressure Measurement

- Minimum of measured pressure for first observation of leakage

4. Bladder Pressure Measurements During Micturition
   and Pressure–Flow Relations

   - Opening time* (note the flow delay)
   - Opening pressure* (note the flow delay)
   - Maximum pressure*
   - Pressure at maximum flow[+] (note the flow delay)
   - Closing pressure[+] (note the flow delay)
   - Minimum voiding pressure[+] (note the flow delay)

All pressure values will be separately estimated for intravesical, abdominal, and detrusor pressure. They will differ not only in amplitude, but often also in timing. The detrusor pressure is generally the most important one. The maximum pressure values may be attained at a moment where the flow rate is zero (Griffiths et al., 1997).

5. Electromyography

   - Recruitment patterns,* particularly in relation to specific stimuli (bladder filling, hyperreflexive contractions, onset of voiding, coughing, Valsalva, etc.)
   - If individual motor unit action potentials are recorded: duration (ms) and amplitude (mV) of spontaneous activity, fibrillations, positive sharp waves, and complex repetitive discharges. Complexity and polyphasicity (descriptive or number)

6. Urethral Pressure Measurement

One parameter describing the contribution of the urethra to continence is the functional profile length*, the length of the urethra over which the urethral pressure exceeds intravesical pressure.

The functional profile length should reflect the length of the urethra that contributes to the prevention of leakage. In the female, this concept is straightforward, but in the male, the length of the bulbous and penile urethra will often add significantly to the functional profile length. The infrasphincteric part of the urethra, however, contributes little, if any, to continence. The functional profile length in men is thus much greater than that in women, without the associated implication that this greater length is indeed functional in maintaining continence. This functional part of the urethra probably extends down from the bladder to the junction from sphincteric to bulbous urethra, but this junction is often difficult to detect on the curve.

The contribution of the bulbous and penile urethra also show a large variance between patients and between several assessments in the same man. Therefore, a third urethral length parameter is used, the *urethral continence zone:* the length of the urethra between the bladder neck and the point of maximum urethral pressure (Gleason et al., 1974) (Fig. 1).

   - Resting urethral pressure profile:
     - Maximum urethral pressure*
     - Maximum urethral closure pressure
     - Functional profile length (not mandatory in men)
     - Urethral continence zone (not mandatory in women)
   - Stress urethral pressure profile: above parameters and
     - Pressure "transmission" ratio*
   - Intermittent withdrawal: above parameters and
     - Relaxing time before measurement is read

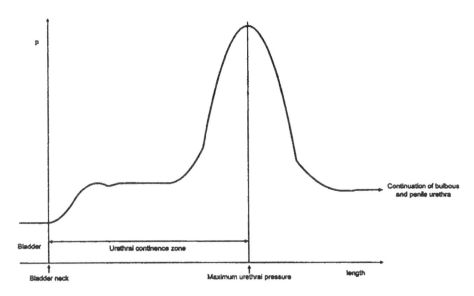

Figure 1 Schematic measurement of urethral continence zone in men.

- Continuous urethral pressure measurement. This study is probably best represented by the measured curve. Urethral pressure variations in relation to specific stimuli (bladder filling, hyperreflexive contractions, onset of voiding, coughing, Valsalva, etc.) may be described separately

7. Video Urodynamics

- According to type of urodynamic study
- Morphology
  - Configuration and contour of the bladder during filling and voiding
  - Reflux, occurrence, and timing
    - Into the upper urinary tract
    - Into the adnexa (i.e., the prostate, the ejaculatory duct)
  - Bladder neck during filling and voiding phases
- Configuration of proximal urethra during filling and voiding, urethral kinking
- Bladder or urethral descensus

8. Ambulatory Urodynamics

According to type of urodynamic study

9. Provocative Tests During Urodynamics

Response of the lower urinary tract function to the provocation. Compare with situation without provocation.

10. Maximum (Anesthetic) Bladder Capacity Measurement

Anatomical maximum volume that bladder will accommodate

11. Specific Uroneurophysiological Tests

- Electromyography (see Sec. 3.3.5)
- Nerve conduction studies
  - Latency time* (abbreviated)
  - Response amplitude* (abbreviated)
- Reflex latency measurement
  - Response time* (abbreviated)
- Evoked responses
  - Single or multiphasic response*
  - Onset of response* (abbreviated)
  - Latency to onset* (abbreviated)
  - Latency to peaks* (abbreviated)
  - The amplitude of the responses is measured in mV
- Sensory testing:
  - Sensory threshold* (abbreviated)

D. Typical Manifestations of Neurogenic Lower Urinary Tract Dysfunction

1. Filling Phase

- Hyposensitivity or hypersensitivity
- Vegetative sensations, for example, goose flesh, sweating, headache, and blood pressure increase (particularly in patients with autonomic dysreflexia)
- *Low compliance:* compliance value lower than 20 mL/cmH$_2$O
  - Cause: neural or muscular (described before as hypertonic bladder)
- *High-volume bladder:* a bladder that can be filled to far over functional bladder capacity in nonanesthetized condition without significant increase in pressure (described before as hypotonic bladder). The use of the terms excessive or very high compliance to describe this situation is discouraged, as a high value of compliance will also be measured at lower volumes when only a slight increase in pressure occurs during filling
  - Cause: neural or muscular
- Detrusor hyperreflexia, spontaneous or provoked; classified according to maximal detrusor pressure as *low-pressure hyperreflexia* or *high-pressure hyperreflexia*. Because of its clinical implications, as a practical guideline a value of 40 cmH$_2$O is proposed as cutoff value between low-pressure and high-pressure hyperreflexia (McGuire et al., 1996)
- *Sphincter areflexia:* no evidence of reflex sphincter contraction during filling, particularly at higher volumes, or during physical stress

2. Voiding Phase

- Detrusor areflexia*
- *External sphincter hyperreflexia:* involuntary activity (e.g., intermittently) of external sphincter during voiding other than detrusor sphincter dyssynergia
- Detrusor sphincter dyssynergia
- Detrusor bladder neck dyssynergia

IV. CLINICAL VALUE AND CLASSIFICATION
OF URODYNAMIC INVESTIGATION

Urodynamic investigation is needed for accurate evaluation of all patients with neurogenic lower urinary tract dysfunction. When effected in a standardized manner, it produces standardized and reproducible results (cf., Schäfer et al.). After the evaluation, its results must be summarized and evaluated:

1. Neurological background (type/duration of neurological disease or lesion) and characteristics of uroneurophysiological tests
2. Characteristics of filling function
3. Characteristics of voiding function

In the conclusive evaluation the condition of the upper urinary tract and the incontinence care in incontinent patients must also be taken into account. Core investigation of patients with neurogenic lower urinary tract dysfunction will include

1. History
2. Urine culture
3. Flow rate and postvoid residual (multiple estimations)
4. Filling and voiding cystometry

Not all urodynamic procedures are equally important in the diagnosis of patients with neurogenic lower urinary tract dysfunction. The following list is an indication of the place of each procedure in these patients.

0. Urinary diary: semiobjective quantification of the physiological lower urinary tract function. Advisable.
1. Free uroflowmetry and assessment of residual urine: first impression of voiding function. Mandatory before any invasive urodynamics is planned.
2. Cystometry: the only method to quantify filling function. Limited significance as a solitary procedure. Powerful when combined with bladder pressure measurement during micturition and even more in video urodynamics.
    Necessary to document the status of the lower urinary tract function during the filling phase.
3. Leak-point pressure measurement: detrusor leak-point pressure: specific investigation if high pressures during the filling phase might endanger the upper urinary tract or lead to secondary bladder damage. Abdominal leak-point pressure: less important in neurogenic lower urinary tract dysfunction. Useful for patients with stress incontinence.
4. Bladder pressure measurements during voiding and pressure–flow relationships: pressure measurements reflect the coordination between detrusor and urethra or pelvic floor during the voiding phase. Even more powerful in combination with cystometry and with video urodynamics. Necessary to document the status of the lower urinary tract function during the voiding phase.
    Pressure–flow analysis is aimed at assessing the passive urethral resistance relation[+] and as such of less importance in neurogenic lower urinary tract dysfunction.
5. Urethral pressure measurement: limited applicability in neurogenic lower urinary tract dysfunction.

6. Electromyography: vulnerable to artifacts when performed during a urodynamic investigation. Useful as a gross indication of the patient's ability to control the pelvic floor. When more detailed analysis is needed, it should be performed as part of a uroneurophysiological investigation.

7. Video urodynamics: when combined with cystometry and pressure measurement during micturition probably the most comprehensive investigation to document the lower urinary tract function and morphology. In this combination the first choice of invasive investigations.

8. Ambulatory urodynamics: should be considered when office urodynamics do not reproduce the patient's symptoms and complaints. May replace office (not video) urodynamics in future when all parameters from office urodynamics are available in ambulatory urodynamics too.

9. Specific uroneurophysiological tests: advised as part of the neurological workup of the patient. Elective tests may be asked for specific conditions that became obvious during patient workup and urodynamic investigations.

V. SUPPLEMENTAL INVESTIGATIONS

A. Endoscopic Procedures

Endoscopic investigation of the lower urinary tract may be necessary in a limited number of patients. The indication must be very restrictive.

B. Other Investigations to Define the Neurological Status

Specific investigations to assess the neurological status of the patient may also be necessary in individual cases.

ACKNOWLEDGMENTS

The authors used the *Manual Neuro-Urology and Spinal Cord Lesion: Guidelines for Urological Care of Spinal Cord Injury Patients* prepared by the Arbeitskreis Urologische Rehabilitation Querschnittgelähmter for the German Urological Society as a starting point for their discussions. The authors thank Dr. Clare Fowler and Dr. Derek Griffiths for valuable discussions during the production of this report.

REFERENCES

Abrams P, Blaivas JG, Stanton SL, Andersen JT. 1988. Standardization of terminology of lower urinary tract function. The International Continence Society Committee on Standardization of Terminology. Neurourol Urodynam 7:403–427; Scand J Urol Nephrol (Suppl) 114:5–19.

Abrams P, Blaivas JG, Stanton SL, Andersen JT. 1990. Standardization of terminology of lower urinary tract function. The International Continence Society Committee on Standardization of Terminology. Int Urogynecol J 1:45–58.

Gleason DM, Reilly RJ, Bottacini MR, Pierce MJ. 1974. The urethral continence zone and its relation to stress incontinence. J Urol 112:81–88.

Griffiths DJ, Höfner K, van Mastrigt R, Rollema HJ, Spångberg A, Gleason D. 1997. Standardization of terminology of lower urinary tract function: pressure–flow studies of voiding, urethral resistance, and urethral obstruction. Neurourol Urodynam 16:1–18.

Klevmark B. 1997. Ambulatory urodynamics [Letter to the editor]. Br J Urol 79:490.

McGuire EJ, Cespedes RD, O'Connell HE. 1996. Leak-point pressures. Urol Clin North Am 23:253–262.

Rossier AB, Fam BA. 1986. 5-Microtransducer catheter in evaluation of neurogenic bladder function. Urology 27:371–378.

Schäfer et al. Good urodynamic practice. In preparation.

Van Waalwijk van Doorn E, Anders K, Khullar V, Kulseng–Hanssen S, Pesce F, Robertson A, Rosario D, Schäfer W. 2000. Standardization of ambulatory urodynamic monitoring. First draft report of the standardization sub-committee of the ICS for ambulatory urodynamic studies. Neurourol Urodynam 19:113–125.

Report on Ambulatory Urodynamic Monitoring

I. INTRODUCTION

Ambulatory urodynamic monitoring (AUM) has become an established method of investigating lower urinary tract function. This report recommends uniform standards for terminology, methodology, analysis, and reporting of AUM to facilitate communication between investigators and to improve the quality of clinical practice and research. The document can be integrated with earlier reports of the International Continence Society (ICS) Committee on Standardization with special reference to the collated 1988 ICS report (Abrams et al., 1989) and the ICS recommendations on good urodynamic practice (in preparation).

AUM, in contrast with conventional urodynamic studies, frees the patient to be more independent than with fixed urodynamics apparatus. This allows the patient to perform those activities that, he or she knows from experience, will provoke troublesome urinary symptoms.

II. INDICATIONS FOR AUM

- Lower urinary tract symptoms that a conventional urodynamic investigation fails to reproduce or explain
- Situations in which conventional urodynamics may be unsuitable
- Neurogenic lower urinary tract dysfunction
- Evaluation of therapies for lower urinary tract dysfunction

From Ernst van Waalwijk van Doorn, Kate Anders, Vik Khullar, Sigurd Kulseng-Hanssen, Francesco Pesce, Andrew Robertson, Derek Rosario, and Werner Schäfer, International Continence Society Sub-committee on Ambulatory Urodynamics Studies (Ernst van Waal-wijk van Doorn, chairman, Anders Mattiasson, coordinating chairman). *Neurourology and Urodynamics* 19:113–125, (2000). Copyright 2000 by Wiley-Liss, Inc.

III. TERMINOLOGY

The terminology applied to observations during AUM should, wherever possible, be consistent with terminology used during a conventional urodynamic investigation.

An *ambulatory urodynamic investigation* is defined as any functional test of the lower urinary tract predominantly utilizing natural filling of the urinary tract and reproducing the subject's normal activity.

The terms introduced by this definition are explained further as follows:

Ambulatory refers to the nature of monitoring, rather than the mobility of the subject. Monitoring will usually take place outside a urodynamics laboratory.

Natural refers to the natural production of urine, rather than an artificial medium. Stimulation by forced drinking or pharmacological manipulation must be stated in the methodology.

Remark: The bladder may be prefilled with an artificial medium, but this is not comparable with natural bladder filling. This method of investigation needs further evaluation.

Normal activity refers to the activities of the subject during which symptoms are likely to occur. These may include maneuvers designed specifically to identify the presence of involuntary detrusor or urethral behavior or to provoke incontinence.

IV. METHODOLOGY

A. Signals

The following signals have been recorded by AUM:

- Pressure: intravesical, abdominal, urethral, intrapelvic (renal)
- Flow rate
- Micturition volume
- Urinary leakage
- Leakage volume
- Urethral electrical conductance
- Perineal integrated surface electromyography (EMG)

As examples of AUM investigations, which have been established, home uroflowmetry and ambulatory cystography can be mentioned: the first records the flow (time) signal, the latter at least records the intravesical and abdominal pressure (time) signals.

Additional information that should be recorded during any AUM investigation as event markers representing the following phenomena:

- Initiation of voluntary voids
- Cessation of voluntary voids
- Episodes of urgency
- Episodes of discomfort or pain
- Provocative maneuvers
- Time and volume of fluid intake

- Time and volume of urinary leakage
- Time of pad change

B. Signal Quality

AUM is more versatile than equivalent conventional urodynamic investigations, but for the same reasons AUM is associated with a greater risk of losing signal quality. Therefore, although all signals should be recorded as recommended in the ICS recommendations on good urodynamic practice, there are a number of cautions that apply specifically to AUM. These are described in the following.

C. Intravesical and Abdominal Pressure Measurement

Although it is possible to measure intravesical and abdominal pressures using fluid-filled lines (water or air), the use of catheter-mounted microtip transducers allows greater mobility during AUM. In the absence of continuous supervision, stringent checks on signal quality should be incorporated in the measurement protocol. At the start of monitoring, these should include testing of recorded pressures online by coughing and abdominal straining in the supine, sitting, and erect positions. The investigator must be convinced that signal quality is adequate before proceeding with the ambulatory phase of the investigation. Before termination of the investigation, and at regular intervals during monitoring, similar checks of signal quality, such as cough tests, should be carried out. Such tests will serve as a useful retrospective quality check during the interpretation of traces. The following considerations must be taken into account when using microtip transducers:

- Transducers should be calibrated before every investigation.
- The "zero point" is atmospheric pressure (there is no fixed reference point). All transducers must be "zeroed" at atmospheric pressure before insertion of the catheters.
- Water-filled pressure catheters have a fixed reference point at the upper edge of the symphysis pubis, whereas catheter-mounted microtip pressure transducers have no fixed reference point.
- Microtip transducers will record direct contact with solid material (the wall of a viscus or fecal material) as a change in pressure. The use of multiple transducers may eliminate this source of artifact.
- Under some circumstances, the pressure measured at the transducer surface will result in a discrepancy equal to the difference in vertical height between the two transducers. This can result in the estimated detrusor rest pressure being less than zero (i.e., negative) with, for instance, the patient in the supine position (Figs. 1 and 2).

D. Urethral Pressure and Conductance

The recording of urethral pressure is a qualitative measurement with emphasis on changes in pressure, rather than absolute values. The use of urethral electrical conductance to identify leakage, in association with pressure monitoring, facilitates interpretation of urethral pressure traces. Precise positioning and secure fixation of catheters are essential to maintain signal quality. The orientation of the transducer should be documented.

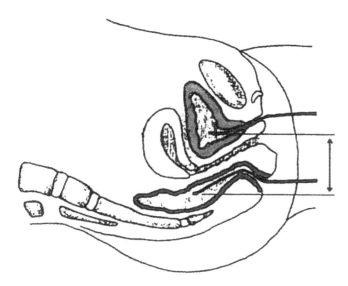

Figure 1 The difference in reference level between the vesical and rectal pressure sensor in supine position is shown schematically.

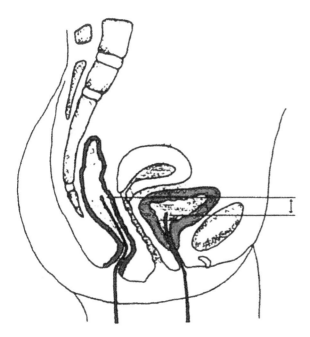

Figure 2 The difference in reference level between the vesical and rectal pressure sensor in upright position is shown schematically.

Remark: The use of multiple pressure transducers facilitates identification of movement artifact, but increases catheter stiffness and thereby deformation of the urethra during recording.

E. Catheter Fixation

As specified earlier, secure catheter fixation is essential to maintain signal quality. Methods that have been used include adhesive tape, suture fixation, and specially designed silicone-fixation devices.

F. Recording of Urinary Leakage

The method of urine leakage determination should be recorded. It should be stated whether the urinary leakage is recorded as a signal with the pressure measurements or is dependent on the subject pressing an event marker button or completing a urinary diary.

G. Instructions to the Patient

Detailed instructions for recording of symptoms, identification of catheter displacement, and hardware failure should be given to the patient. It is the recommendation of this group that such verbal instructions should be reinforced by written instructions and, in addition to the hardware built into the system, the patient is provided with a simple diary to record events. This allows the common primary aim of all urodynamics (i.e., to correlate the test outcome with symptoms).

V. ANALYSIS

A. Quality Assessment

The first step in the analysis of an AUM trace is the assessment of the quality of data recorded. The specific points that should be addressed relative to pressure measurement are as follows:

- Is the trace "active" (i.e., fine second-to-second variation in pressure), rather than a fine line?
- Is the baseline static or highly variable?
- Are the cough tests or other activities causing abdominal pressure changes that can be used for signal plausibility check, and regularly present?
- Is the subtraction adequate (e.g., minimal change in subtracted detrusor pressure with coughing)?

If the technical quality of the traces is less than perfect, then, although the investigation may yield valuable clinical information, in the context of accurate measurement, the pressure recordings must be viewed as qualitative, and further quantitative analysis can be flawed.

B. Phase Identification

Depending on the purpose of the investigation, markers must be placed to identify voluntary voids and allow differentiation of such events from involuntary events that may be associated with changes in recorded pressure. The protocol of the investigation should specifically state the point at which the markers identifying commencement and cessation of a voluntary void are placed. Analysis of the voiding phase follows the same principles and terminology used during a conventional pressure–flow investigation.

C. Events

The use of a patient diary considerably improves the detailed analysis of events occurring during AUM and is strongly recommended. The events usually recorded during AUM are identified in Section 4.1. Typical events occurring during the filling phase are detrusor contractions, urethral relaxation, and episodes of urgency and incontinence.

Remark: At least for research purposes it is strongly advized to define and validate variables for quantitative interpretation. Validation means to establish data on healthy volunteers and specific patient groups, test–retest reproducibility, interrater validity, and sensitivity to treatment modalities.

VI. CLINICAL REPORT

The report should be tailored to the urodynamic indication(s) and can include the following:
Indication(s) or urodynamic question(s), or both (*obligatory*)

- Duration of recording
- Signal and data quality description
- Fill rate, timing, method, and volume of any retrograde filling before commencing AUM
- Dose and timing of diuretics if administered
- Volume of fluid drunk during the test
- Number of voids
- Total and range of voided volumes and postmicturition urinary residual
- Episodes of urgency, urinary incontinence, and pain
- Detrusor activity during the filling phase (frequency, time, duration, amplitude, area, form)
- Pressure–flow analysis
- Results of provocative maneuvers employed during the test
- Reasons for termination of recording if prematurely terminated

VII. SCIENTIFIC PRESENTATION

To facilitate clear communication and evaluation of AUM, the following guidelines should be applied:
Description of AUM protocol, which should include

- Planned duration of recording
- Actual duration of recording
- Signal and data quality assessment
- Specification of recording device (i.e., manufacturer, type, sampling rates, events button(s))
- Catheter type, transducer, location, route, and fixation technique
- Leakage detection method or device
- Urinary flow transducer
- Protocol for diuresis
- Volume and timing of fluid drunk during test

- Dose and timing of diuretics administered
- Fill rate, timing, method, and volume of any retrograde filling before or during AUM
- Events recorded by diary or electronic markers
- Detrusor activity during the filling phase with any associated urgency, incontinence, and pain
- Pressure–flow analysis (according to ICS standards)
- Any provocative maneuvers employed during the test
- Reasons for premature termination of recording
- Presentation of urodynamic curves should include
  —Channel identification
  —Units of measurement
  —Minimum scale for pressures should be 2 mL/5 cmH$_2$O
  —Minimum scale for time should be 4 cm/min

VIII. EXPLANATORY EXAMPLES

This section aims to support this report and stimulate the further growth of use of AUM by giving examples of AUM traces with specific events. The examples with the explanatory text will also help increase one's ability to interpret AUM traces (Figs. 3–12).
     General information on traces:

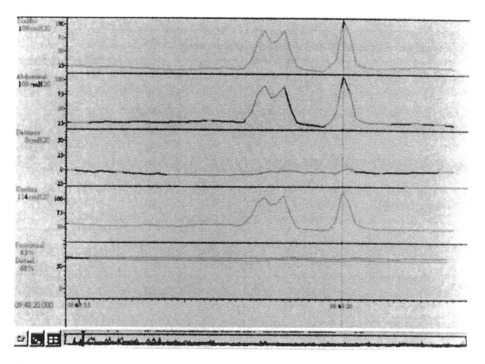

Figure 3   Typical traces of a double and single cough in supine position at 16 samples per second (x-axis, 7 s).

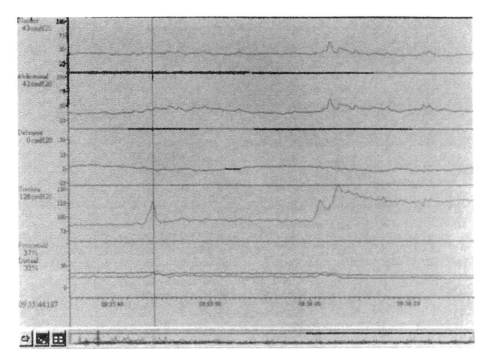

Figure 4 On the left, typical traces of a contraction of the urethral sphincter mechanism. On the right, squeezing combined with a change in position causing displacement of urethral sensor.

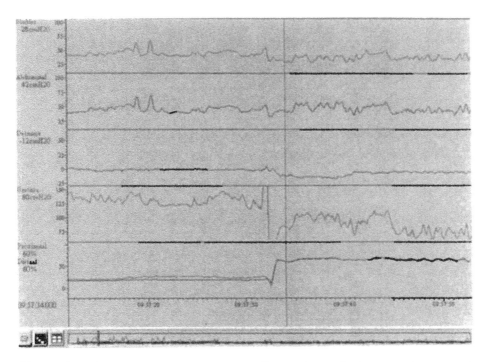

Figure 5 In the middle, typical movement artifact on the urethral pressure trace, causing sensor displacement; after the movement artifact, the urethral pressure level has decreased. The conductance signals show an increased level, indicating a displacement of the catheter toward the bladder neck.

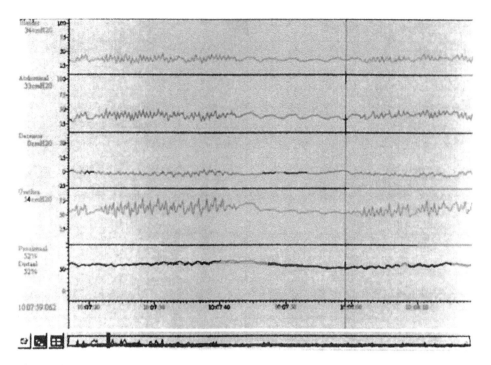

Figure 6 Typical traces show walking (first half), respiration (third quarter), walking (last quarter). The pressure waves caused by breathing can also be detected during walking. Generally, it can be stated that the pressure waves caused by respiration are affected by the type of respiration, the physical activity, and patient's stature.

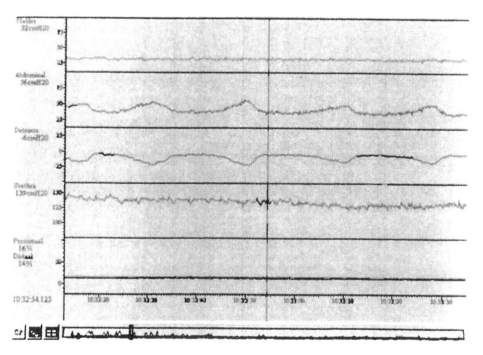

Figure 7 Typical abdominal and detrusor traces during rectal activity. Here, the patient is at rest, and hardly any effect of respiration can be detected in the traces.

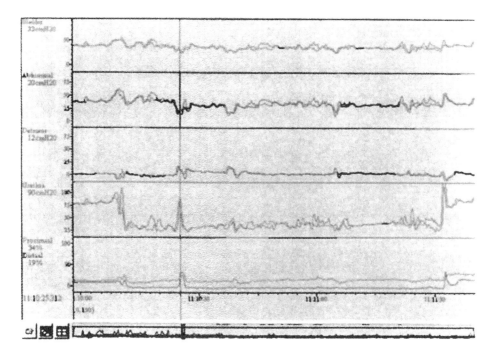

Figure 8 This example shows the traces of about 90-s duration. Because the sample rate for the pressure signals is 16 Hz, it is not possible to plot every single-sample value in the trace. The double lines represent the envelope of the pressure signals. This means that at every dot on the x-axis, the minimum and maximum pressure values of the time interval, represented by those dots, are plotted. In this plot we see a sequence of events: the patient is sitting (left), stands up (movement artifact urethra signal, and abdominal activity in the vesical and abdominal traces), walks a few steps (difference between double lines increases). At the cursor position, a "reaching" phenomenon is seen, where the urethra sensor moves shortly toward the highest-pressure region in the urethra and, at the same time, the abdomen is enlarged causing a pressure dip in the vesical and abdominal pressure signals. At 11:10:40, 11:11:10, and 11:11:25, the same kind of movement phenomenon can be seen. In between, the patient walks some steps. At 11:11:30 the patient sits again. Figure 9 shows the same events in detail.

—The analysis of AUM traces requires the ability to look at different time and signal scales. To study these examples, it is necessary to look every time at the x- and y-axes scales and the pressure ranges.

—Every example reads from top to bottom: the intravesical, abdominal (rectal), detrusor (subtracted), and urethral pressure signals followed by two urethral conductance signals (proximal and distal).

—For recording, Gaeltec microtransducer catheters (5F) and a Gaeltec MPR3 recorder are applied with the maximum sample frequency for storage set at 16 Hz.

—At the bottom of each figure, one can see which window, and where, within the complete investigation, is shown.

—Filling and voiding phases are separated by event markers (E) at the x-axis.

—Detrusor contractions are indicated by a bar under the contraction curve.

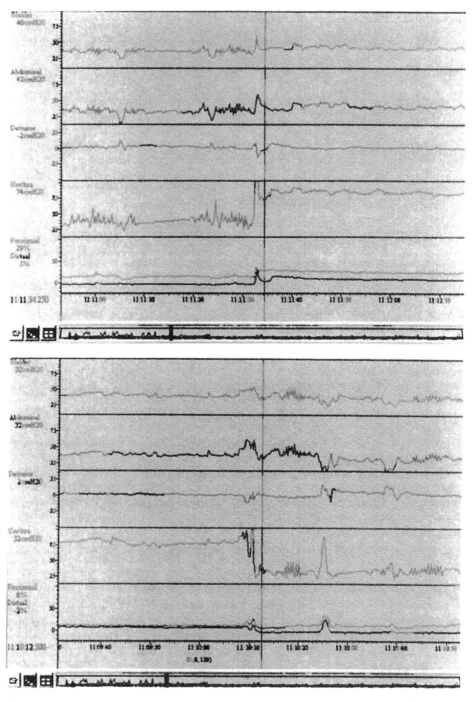

Figure 9   These traces show in detail the sequence of events described in Figure 8. Depending on the patient's activity and the signal quality, one should choose an adequate time resolution for analysis.

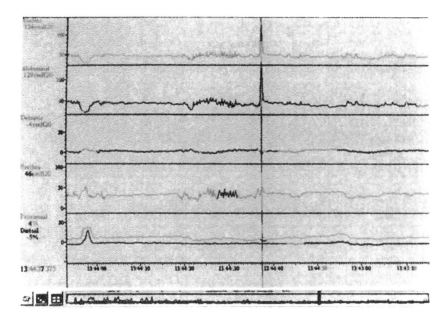

Figure 10 On the left, walking a few steps followed by a reaching movement artifact can be detected, causing a pressure dip in the vesical and rectal traces and a positive wave in the urethral pressure and conductance; at the cough pressure peak, there is decreased transmission toward the urethral sensor, owing to distal position of the urethral sensor. This interpretation is also supported by the fact that no change is seen in urethral conductance during the cough.

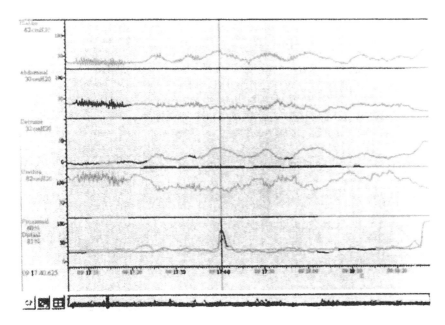

Figure 11 This example shows the most common sequence of events in a patient suffering from bladder overactivity and imperative voiding. On the left, the traces start showing walking, followed by a urethral relaxation and detrusor contractions. Then walking toward the toilet with increasing detrusor activity with a moment of urine loss (see conductance signals). Finally, the patient enters the toilet at the Event mark (bottom).

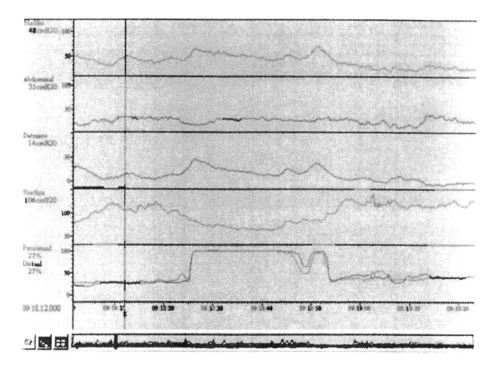

Figure 12   These traces show the continuation of the previous figure; the patient enters the toilet with detrusor activity continuing and sits down, and urethral relaxation and a voiding contraction can be seen, whereas the conductance curves show the flow phase. At the end of voiding, the urethral closure pressure recovers to the prevoiding level.

REFERENCE

Abrams P, Blaivas JG, Stanton SL, Anderson JT. 1989. The standardisation of terminology of lower urinary tract function. Scand J Urol Nephrol Suppl 114:5–19.

Outcome Studies: General Principles

I. INTRODUCTION

Scientific evaluation of the outcome of therapeutic interventions in patients is not possible without assessment both before and after the intervention. The methods and measurements used must conform to set criteria so that they may be applied to all interventions and comparisons among studies may be made. They must be valid, accurate, precise, reliable, and repeatable using a test–retest variation. Evaluations should be properly directed, such that the right variable is measured. Even though methods of intervention and evaluation may vary, certain domains of measurement should be represented and a multidimensional approach undertaken. The time scale for evaluations and interventions and the composition of the study group are important factors so that some standardization exists, enabling understanding of the results by other investigators and comparison between studies.

Unfortunately, no consensus presently exists on the way in which studies should be performed, including interventions and evaluations, nor on how the results thus obtained should be represented. The scientific basis for many methods is also frequently unclear. A recent American survey of the literature on outcome in genuine stress incontinence classified almost all of the investigations as unsatisfactory and only a few as excellent. Thus we have a dilemma between what we "know" as based on reliable scientific data, and what we "believe" based on clinical practice. This emphasizes the poor investigative technique and reporting presently in use and the need for the standardization of outcome measures.

II. STANDARDIZATION OF OUTCOME STUDIES

In 1993, the International Continence Society (ICS) set up subcommittees within the frame of the standardization committee to standardize outcome studies in patients with lower urinary tract dysfunction:

From Anders Mattiasson, Jens Christian Djurhuus, David Fonda, Gunnar Lose, Jørgen Nordling, and Manfred Stöhrer. Anders Mattiasson served as Coordinating Chairman. The other authors served as chairmen of the respective Outcome Subcommittees on Lower Urinary Tract Dysfunction: Children, Frail Elderly, Women, Men, and Neurogenic Dysfunction. *Neurourology and Urodynamics* 17:249–253 (1998). Copyright 1998 by the International Continence Society.

1. Children
2. Frail elderly
3. Women
4. Men
5. Neurogenic dysfunction

Each of these specific subcommittees was asked to make recommendations on how out-come studies should be performed in their respective fields. In this general report, common principles and outlines are discussed. These should be seen as recommendations, rather than guidelines, representing a move toward a more rational and uniform presentation of outcome studies. In the separate reports from respective subcommittees, more specific rec-ommendations are given.

III. DEFINITION OF OUTCOME MEASURES

No single measure can fully express the outcome of an intervention. It is necessary for out-come to incorporate improvement and deterioration in function, complications of the inter-vention, socioeconomic data, and the effect on quality of life. Both subjective and objective measurements should be included and bias should be eliminated where possible. It should be emphasized that frequently the perception of the patient, doctor, or therapist are at vari-ance; hence, the choice and application of measurement tool is all the more important.

An intervention might have both primary and secondary outcome objectives. The pri-mary objective might be an anatomical change (e.g., surgery), whereas the secondary ob-jective might be functional (e.g., continence).

IV. ENDPOINTS

For maximum information to be obtained, it is important that the correct endpoints are cho-sen and defined at the beginning of the study. This involves the stating of a null hypothesis, although other factors may be of importance and should be included where appropriate. Endpoints should be chosen such that they are relevant and may be incorporated into prac-tice at the end of the study. The time frame of the intervention and its expected outcome should be considered when designing a study. Long-term outcome should be measured whenever possible. Statistical expertise is vital and should be applied from the beginning of the study.

V. OUTCOME MEASURES

Directed, accurate measures are necessary to reflect the degree of change or improvement with a high degree of correlation.

The groups of measures, generally termed objective, subjective, compliance, quality of life, and socioeconomic, can also be grouped into domains of interest. The use of do-mains describes another perspective, with the interests of the involved parts weighted ac-cording to their perceived importance. Certain measurements are not easy to make because of dearth of presently available instruments and a lack of agreement about which tool is most appropriate. At present, there is also a lack of correlation between the various mea-sures mentioned.

Urinary incontinence as a symptom, a sign, and a condition is here redefined as far as the condition part is concerned. The condition "urinary incontinence" comprises the passage of urine through the urethra at an inappropriate point in time, and is thus not, as previously suggested, a part of the underlying pathophysiological process itself. Urinary incontinence is thus a consequence and not a cause, and this is valid for both the symptom, the sign, and the condition parts.

Outcome in studies of lower urinary tract function and dysfunction should be described using

Patient's observations (symptoms)
Quantification of symptoms (e.g., urine loss)
Physician's observations (anatomical and functional; compliance)
Quality of life measures
Socioeconomic evaluations.

Patient- and physician-observed measures should be considered as compulsory in all outcomes of lower urinary tract dysfunction; compliance measurements from patients and healthy volunteers should be given, and quality of life and socioeconomic data included when available. These data should be increasingly incorporated into study designs, so that the picture becomes complete.

VI.   EVALUATION AND GRADING OF OUTCOME

Although the ideal result of treatment should be cure and normalization, outcome may sometimes be better described as a degree of improvement in addition to measuring cure. Even if the elimination of symptoms is often the goal for a treatment, and thus comprises the expected outcome, some other aspects have to be considered. "Cure" usually refers to a single dimension. That a patient becomes symptom-free does not mean that the underlying pathophysiological process is completely reversed. The patient might experience normalization, but structural as well as functional changes might remain. Examples of such remaining changes could be displacement of the bladder neck, a subnormal intraurethral pressure, a hyperactive bladder, or a hyperplastic prostate. When a given treatment is directed against symptoms and not against the pathophysiological process itself, we can never expect to cure. An alternative measure could, therefore, use the terms "responders" and "nonresponders," which describe less extreme degrees of improvement than those implied by cure and normalization. However, it may be necessary to divide this into degrees of response, so that differentiation may be made between maximum responders and minimal responders who gain only small benefit from the intervention. The size of such a response should exceed the value of the test–retest variation as performed and reported by the investigators.

VII.   REPORTING OF OUTCOME STUDIES

The editors of journals, who are considering outcome studies on patients with lower urinary tract dysfunction for publication, are recommended to include a passage referring to this document in their instructions for authors.

VIII.   FUTURE DIRECTIONS

Considerable effort is needed to describe the way in which various measures correlate with each other. It may be a considerable time before final decisions can be made on what outcome means for different patient groups. This requires a multidimensional and multidisciplinary approach, including the continuous and active participation of all the members of our International Continence Society.

IX. CONCLUSIONS AND RECOMMENDATIONS

Data from five groups of measures should be represented in every scientific investigation of outcome in patients with lower urinary tract dysfunction:

- Patient's observations (symptoms)
- Quantification of symptoms (e.g., urine loss)
- Physician's observations (anatomical and functional; compliance)
- Quality of life
- Socioeconomic data.

—Measurements should be directed and accurate.
—A null hypothesis should be formulated.
—Endpoints should be defined.
—A grading of response should be measured, using the terms "responders" and "nonresponders."
—A multidimensional, multidisciplinary approach should be used.

ADDENDUM

Was the study in any part supported by commercial interest?

ACKNOWLEDGMENTS

The authors thank Drs. Andrew Fantl, Matthew Zack, and Linda Cardozo for valuable contributions to this report.

APPENDIX

Practical Points for Outcome Studies in Patients with Lower Urinary Tract Dysfunction[a]

Purpose of the study
What are the reasons for this particular study?
What do the investigators want to show?

Patient groups
Definition of patient groups
Inclusion/exclusion criteria

---

[a]Whenever an outcome study on lower urinary tract dysfunction is planned, a series of questions should ideally be considered and appropriately addressed in the manuscript at the time of submission for publication. The foregoing list serves only as a reminder. More specific information concerning the different topics is represented in the reports from the subcommittees. ICS terminology should be used wherever practicable.

Disease or disorder
Causal or symptomatic treatment?
Arrest of a process?
Reversible changes?

Intervention
Description of the intervention
Intervention related complications, morbidity, and mortality

Study design and controls
Intervention studies should have a control group and should be randomized
Define endpoints
Define response criteria
Nature of trial (e.g., double-blind, placebo-controlled, crossover)
Adverse events, dropouts

Methods of measurement
Characterization of methods, test–retest data in the hands of the investigators
Change in circumstances or procedures before and after intervention
Interindividual variation (+ differences between centers in multicenter trials)
Normal values

Statistics
Power of the study
Reason for choice of statistical method
Compliance
Statistician involved?

Time scale
Why was outcome evaluated at a particular time in relation to the intervention?
Long-term outcome?

Expected outcome
Degree of improvement
Risk–benefit analysis
Patient expectations
Quality of life effects
Socioeconomic factors

Interpretation of data
Comparison with outcome in other studies
Unexpected or adverse findings
Limitations
Clinical significance
Theoretical importance
Possible ways of improving the study
Conclusions for future investigations

Outcome Studies: Adult Female

I. INTRODUCTION

The purpose of this communication is to offer the clinical and research communities an initial attempt at incorporating outcome measurements within identifiable domains, as well as providing initial information on the reliability of those measurements most commonly used.

Scientific evaluation of the outcome of therapeutic interventions is based on assessment before and after treatment. However, the reliability of methods and measurements used in the evaluation is often poor or unclear, which makes interpretation of outcome difficult. The reliability of a test depends on the accuracy and reproducibility of the method. The diagnostic accuracy is determined by verifying test results against a reference gold standard that defines true disease status. The predictive value of a measure is considered the most important. Because it may be impossible to establish a final true diagnosis, reliability must sometimes be measured by reproducibility, which is determined by comparing results of repeated examinations of the same patient.* Reproducibility for tests where the result is given on a continuous scale may be expressed as bias with the 95% confidence limit (Bland and Altman, 1986), whereas for binary tests the kappa coefficient, which adjusts the observed agreement for expected chance agreement, is used (Gjørup, 1997).

Urinary incontinence is defined as "a condition in which involuntary urine loss is a social or hygienic problem and is objectively demonstrable." It represents a multidimensional phenomenon with wide-reaching effects that may be quantified within various areas or domains. These areas or domains include the following:

From Gunnar Lose, J. Andrew Fantl, Arne Victor, Steen Walter, Thelma L. Wells, Jean Wyman, and Anders Mattiasson. Produced by the Standardisation Committee of the International Continence Society, A. Mattiasson, Chairman. Subcommittee on Outcome Research in Women, G. Lose, Chairman. *Neurourology and Urodynamics* 17:255–262 (1998). Copyright 1998 by the International Continence Society.
*Other terms might have been chosen to denote accuracy and reproducibility. Terms such as *precision, validity, observer* or *interrater variability, observer error*, and *efficacy* have been used. At the moment it does not seem possible to establish a commonly accepted terminology. Readers of papers about reliability, therefore, in each case, must examine the author's use of the terms.

1. The patient's observations (symptoms)
2. Quantification of symptoms (e.g., urine loss)
3. The clinician's observations (anatomical and functional)
4. Quality of life
5. Socioeconomic measures

Outcome measures should be selected within the context of a specific study.

The ideal combination or measurement "in aggregate," particularly if belonging to different domains, will enhance the overall significance and value of the study results. A multidimensional approach is important, because the effect of intervention depends on the outcome measure chosen and may vary significantly among various domains and even within a certain domain.

II. DOMAIN OF SYMPTOMATOLOGY

A. Symptoms

1. General and Condition Specific

Here are included a respondent's overall opinion of the condition (incontinence) or one or more characteristics of the condition, (e.g., frequency, quantity, or magnitude). Different methods to obtain this measure include a question with a forced choice, a graded response, a statement with a Likert scale agree–disagree response, and a statement with a visual analog-graded scale response.

2. Recommendations and Comments

There is no general symptom (opinion) measure with established methodological reliability. Therefore, researchers should clearly describe their instrument and procedure and provide reliability data or indicate their absence.

III. DOMAIN OF SYMPTOM QUANTIFICATION

A. Diary (Frequency–Volume Chart)
(Larsson and Victor, 1988; Larsson et al., 1991; Wyman et al., 1988)

This entails a self-monitored record of selected lower urinary functions kept for specific time periods. Selected variables include episodes of incontinence or pad use frequency (diurnal and nocturnal), voiding and toileting frequency (diurnal and nocturnal), total voided volume, mean voided volume, and largest single void. Accuracy depends on the patient's ability to follow instructions, but is still difficult to assess because there is no gold standard against which the test result can be compared. Reproducibility depends on the parameter used and improves with an increase in the number of days that self-recording is obtained.

The highest reproducibility has been found for mean voided volume.

The circumstances under which a diary is kept should be approximate to those of everyday life, and should be similar before and after intervention to permit meaningful comparison.

1. Recommendations and Comments

A diary kept for a minimum of 3 days is recommended as an outcome measure.

B. Pad-Weighing Tests (Lose and Versi, 1992; Victor, 1990)

Pad tests can be divided into short-term tests, generally performed under standardized conditions as office tests, and long-term tests, generally performed by the patient at home during 24–48 hr.

Accuracy is difficult to assess. Reproducibility is generally poor, but improves if the circumstances are standardized as much as possible. For long-term tests, the test period should be sufficiently long.

1. Recommendations and Comments

Pad-weighing offers a potential for quantifying the degree of incontinence. For short-term tests, the experimental conditions should be described. Standardized bladder-filling volumes are generally recommended. For long-term tests, the time period should be as long as practical.

IV. DOMAIN OF CLINICIAN'S OBSERVATIONS

A. Pelvic Muscle Activity

This is the force of voluntary pelvic muscle contraction determined in direct (digital or air pressure) or indirect (surface electromyography) measures.

Accuracy is difficult to assess. Test–retest data are based mainly on correlations analysis, which is problematic to interpret.

1. Recommendations and Comments

At this time there is no conclusive information on the potential of muscle activity as an outcome measure.

Researchers should clearly describe their instrument and procedure and provide reliability data or indicate their absence.

B. Cystometry

Cystometry variables include sensation, compliance, capacity, and activity of the bladder. The investigation can be carried out in a stationary or ambulatory setting. Data obtained are method-dependent.

Accuracy is difficult to assess, because variation in various parameters is significant (Lose and Thyssen, 1996; Sørensen et al., 1988; Sørensen, 1988).

1. Recommendations and Comments

It is recommended that authors provide reproducibility data or indicate their absence.

C. Uroflowmetry

Normal female voiding produces a bell-shaped curve on uroflowmetry. Voiding dysfunctions may give rise to an intermittent or multiple peaked flow, suggesting either abdominal straining, unsustained bladder contractions, intermittent sphincter contractions, or bladder outlet obstruction.

Maximum and average flow are directly dependent on voided volume. Consequently, interpretation and comparison of flow rates require that the voided volume is taken into account. Various nomograms are available. Flow rate depends, to a lesser extent, on age and sex, whereas parity, weight, menstrual cycle phase, or menopause status do not seem to influence flow rate (Fantl et al., 1982).

A certain test–retest variation exists in terms of flow rates and pattern (Sørensen et al., 1988; Sørensen, 1988).

1. Recommendations and Comments

Uroflowmetry represents a simple initial test to assess the emptying phase of the lower urinary tract. However, researchers should describe their methodology and provide reproducibility data or indicate their absence.

D. Pressure–Flow Study

This represents the simultaneous study of urine flow and intravesical or detrusor pressure during voluntary voiding. Graphic plotting of pressure–flow data enables classification of individual patients into one of the following groups: obstructed, equivocal, or unobstructed patterns.

In patients with an irregular micturition pattern, the technique should be accomplished with simultaneous EMG recording to allow differentiation between abdominal straining, intermittent detrusor contraction, or detrusor–sphincter dyssynergia. Pressure–flow data are subject to significant test–retest variation (Lose and Thyssen, 1996).

1. Recommendations and Comments

Researchers should describe their methods and reproducibility data, or indicate their absence.

E. Electromyography

Electromyographic (EMG) recordings are performed to examine the activity (behavior) of pelvic and sphincter muscles during different maneuvers, particularly during bladder filling and voiding. This type of EMG is also called kinesiologic EMG. Both surface and intramuscular electrodes may be used for recording. Surface electrodes are more nonselective and may be used for assessing the overall behavior of the muscle bulk underlying the electrodes. Intramuscular electrodes (needle or wire) provide more selective recordings of higher quality, but reflect only the activity of a small muscle volume.

Electromyographic techniques (concentric-needle EMG, single-fiber EMG) allow acquisition of electrophysiological parameters that define a striated muscle as normal or abnormal. With concentric-needle EMG, muscle denervation and reinnervation can be assessed by recording spontaneous activity and motor unit action potentials. Single-fiber EMG reveals muscle changes caused by reinnervation by recording muscle fiber density (Flink, 1997; Vodusêk, 1996).

The reliability of EMG recordings is poorly determined.

1. Recommendations and Comments

Surface electrodes can be used to identify striated muscle activity during different maneuvers, particularly during bladder filling and voiding, and also as a biofeedback therapeutic technique.

Intramuscular electrodes can be used in the more precise studies to identify the activity patterns of individual striated muscles. Special needle electrodes are required to assess denervation and reinnervation of the pelvic floor muscles and striated sphincters.

Researchers should describe their methodology and reproducibility data or indicate their absence.

F. Nerve Stimulation

This entails neurophysiological tests involving stimulation of nervous system structures.

Electrical and magnetic stimulators are used to depolarize nervous structures (particularly the pudendal nerve and its branches, sacral roots, and the motor cortex). Recordings are obtained from both pelvic floor muscles and striated sphincters, but also from nerve structures, particularly over the somatosensory cortex. Several tests exist and can be broadly grouped into evoked potentials and reflex responses.

The reproducibility of several tests is fairly acceptable if the tests are performed under standardized conditions, but no overall accepted standards for individual tests as yet exist.

1. Recommendations and Comments

The clinical usefulness of these tests has not yet been clarified. They seem to be helpful in research. Researchers should describe their methods and their laboratories' normal values. They should indicate reproducibility data or indicate their absence.

G. Urethral Pressure Measurement

Conceptually, urethral closure pressure represents the ability of the urethra to prevent urine leakage. Technically, it represents the difference between the pressure at one given point in the urethra and the simultaneously recorded pressure in the bladder.

Measurements of urethral closure pressure may be made at one point in the urethra over a time period (continuous urethral pressure recording), or at several points along the urethra consecutively, forming a urethral pressure profile (UPP). These measurements can be made at rest or during exertion.

The results of urethral pressure measurements are highly influenced by methodological and biological factors and have significant test–retest variability. The overlap between both the static and dynamic urethral closure measurements in continent and incontinent women is significant (Lose, 1997).

1. Recommendations and Comments

Urethral pressure profile parameters are of limited value in the assessment of urethral sphincter function. Urethral pressure measurement may be useful in evaluating local pathology (e.g., diverticulum and stricture), in assessment of changes with intervention, and in therapeutic selection (e.g., intrinsic sphincter deficiency).

H. Imaging

Imaging techniques in terms of radiography, ultrasound, and magnetic resonance imaging (MRI) are used to provide morphological and functional information on the lower urinary tract and the pelvic floor. Until now, as with conventional radiology, neither ultrasound nor MRI appeared to provide conclusive and discriminatory diagnostic information. Scant information is available on reproducibility of measurement, while significant inter- and intraobserver variation in the assessment of radiography pictures has been reported.

1. Recommendations and Comments

Imaging techniques are still of limited value as outcome measures in female incontinence. Researchers should clearly describe their instrument and procedure and provide reliability data or indicate their absence.

V. DOMAIN OF QUALITY OF LIFE MEASUREMENTS

Health-related quality of life (HRQOL) is a multidimensional construct that refers to an individual's perceptions of the effect of a health condition or disease and its subsequent treatment. Primary domains of HRQOL include physical, psychological, and social functioning, overall life satisfaction and well-being, and perceptions of health status. Secondary domains include somatic sensations (symptoms), sleep disturbance, intimacy and sexual functioning, and personal productivity (e.g., household, occupational, volunteer, or community activities).

Three measurement approaches are commonly used to assess HRQOL: generic, condition-specific, and dimension-specific. Generic HRQOL instruments are designed to be used across multiple disease states or conditions, and allow for comparisons across groups by having established age and gender norms. Condition-specific instruments are designed to measure the effect of a particular disease or condition. These instruments tend to be more responsive than generic instruments in detecting treatment effects. Symptom scales are considered condition-specific; generally, these scales should include measurement of the presence of a symptom as well as its "bothersome" or "troublesome" nature. Most generic and condition-specific instruments are multidimensional (i.e., they measure more than one aspect of HRQOL). Dimension-specific instruments, in contrast, are designed to assess a single component of HRQOL, such as emotional distress. The trend in assessing HRQOL outcomes has been toward the use of a multidimensional generic or condition-specific instrument, supplemented with dimension-specific instruments, as needed (Grimby et al., 1993; Shumaker et al., 1994; Wagner et al., 1996; Naughton and Wyman, 1997).

1. Recommendations and Comments

The selection of an HRQOL instrument should be based on the purpose of the study. Descriptive or epidemiological studies should consider both generic and condition-specific instruments. Intervention studies should include a condition-specific instrument. Dimension-specific instruments should be used when more detail about a specific subdomain of HRQOL is desired. Researchers should define HRQOL as it is conceptualized for their study, clearly describe their instrument(s) and data collection, and provide reliability data if available.

It is recommended that researchers select instruments with reliability and sensitivity. In adopting HRQOL instruments, we recommend comparing results obtained in the study population with published norms. If a new condition-specific instrument will be used in a study, adequate pretesting should be done to establish its clinimetric characteristics (e.g., reliability and sensitivity).

VI. DOMAIN OF SOCIOECONOMIC COSTS

Cost-effectiveness analysis is a method to decide on the relative merits of alternative courses of action by comparing costs to achieve a given health effect. Costs can be divided into direct and indirect costs. Direct costs are all costs incurred in the routine care, diagnosis, treatment, and management of adverse consequences associated with treatment or with being incontinent, which can be assessed from the market value of goods and services. Indirect costs are those incurred as a result of being incontinent or of having to care for someone who is incontinent. These opportunity costs (e.g., time lost from enjoying leisure activity or engaging in productive effort) are more difficult to quantify and, thus, are usually not measured. If morbidity and mortality are considered, they should be converted to a monetary value.

Effectiveness is characterized as a specific health outcome (e.g., disease prevented or cured, function restored, or symptoms alleviated).

Direct costs are all costs incurred in routine care, diagnosis, treatment of incontinence, and management of adverse consequences associated with treatment or with being incontinent. Indirect costs are those incurred as a result of being incontinent or having to care for someone who is incontinent. These opportunity costs (e.g., time lost from enjoying leisure activity or engaging in productive effort) are more difficult to quantify and, thus, are usually not measured.

1.   Recommendations and Comments

The types of costs and how they are determined should be clearly articulated. Typical resource uses to be collected in a study include the following:

1. Clinician's time or service
2. Laboratory and imaging studies
3. Treatment expenses (e.g., procedural charges, medication costs)
4. Supplies (disposable and reusable products)
5. Side and adverse effects and their management
6. Travel costs to obtain health care
7. Loss of wages from receiving health care or surgery.

CONCLUSIONS

Research on lower urinary tract symptoms in adult women remains impaired by lack of standardization of outcome variables. The use of primary and secondary outcomes on different areas or domains should help overcome some of these difficulties. However, it is imperative that investigators focus attention on these issues. Studies leading to the development and standardization of outcomes should be entertained. Success in this will not only enhance knowledge of actual treatment strategies, but will also stimulate the development of new ones.

REFERENCES

Bland JA, Altman DG (1986). Statistical method for assessing agreement between two methods of clinical measurement. Lancet 1:307–310.

Fantl JA, Smith PS, Schneider V, Hurt WG, Dunn LJ (1982). Fluid weight uroflowmetry in women. Am J Obstet Gynecol 145:1017–1024.

Flink R (1997). Clinical neurophysiological methods for investigating the lower urinary tract in patients with micturition disorders. Acta Obstet Gynecol Scand Suppl 166:50–58.

Gjørup T (1997). Reliability of diagnostic tests. Acta Obstet Gynecol Scand Suppl 166:9–14.

Grimby A, Milson L, Molander U, Wiklund I, Ekelund P (1993). The influence of urinary incontinence on the quality of life of elderly women. Age Ageing 22:82–89.

Larsson G, Victor A (1988). Micturition patterns in a healthy female population, studied with a frequency/volume chart. Scand J Urol Nephrol Suppl 144:53–57.

Larsson G, Abrams P, Victor A (1991). The frequency/volume chart in detrusor instability. Neurourol Urodynam 10:533–543.

Lose G (1997). Urethral pressure testing. Acta Obstet Gynecol Scand Suppl 166:39–42.

Lose G, Thyssen H (1996). Reproducibility of cystometry and pressure–flow parameters in female patients. Neurourol Urodynam 15:302–303.

Lose G, Versi E (1992). Pad-weighing tests in the diagnosis and quantification of incontinence. Int Urogynecol J 3:324–328.

Naughton MJ, Wyman JF (1997). Quality of life of geriatric patients with lower urinary tract dysfunctions. Am J Med Sci 314:219–224.

Shumaker SA, Wyman JF, Uebersac J, McClish DK, Fantl JA (1994). Health-related quality of life measures for women with urinary incontinence: the urogenital Distress Inventory and the Incontinence Impact Questionnaire. Quality Life Res 3:291–306.

Sørensen S (1988). Urodynamic investigations and the reproducibility in healthy postmenopausal females. Scand J Urol Nephrol Suppl 114:42–47.

Sørensen S, Gregersen H, Sørensen M (1988). Long term reproducibility of urodynamic investigation in healthy females. Scand J Urol Nephrol Suppl 114:35–41.

Victor A (1990). Pad weighing tests—a simple method to quantitate urinary incontinence. Ann Med 22:443–447.

Vodusêk DB (1996). Evoked potential testing. Urol Clin North Am 23:427–446.

Wagner TH, Patrick DL, Buesching DP (1996). Quality of life of persons with urinary incontinence. Development of a new measure. Urology 47:67–73.

Wyman JF, Choi SC, Harkins SW, Wilson MS, Fantl JA (1988). The urinary diary in evaluation of incontinent women: a test–retest analysis. Obstet Gynecol 71:812–817.

Outcome Studies: Adult Male

I. INTRODUCTION

The assessment of outcome may address one or more aspects: lower urinary tract symptoms, influence of symptoms on quality of life, physical findings, and changes in urodynamics following treatment. There has been much confusion relative to nomenclature, and in this report the following terms are used:

LUTS: lower urinary tract symptoms.

QoL: quality of life; QoL can be considered to cover bothersomeness, influence on quality of life, and sexual functioning.

BPH: benign prostatic hyperplasia; this term is reserved for the characteristic histological changes associated with BPH.

BPE: benign prostatic enlargement; this term refers to documented enlargement of the gland.

BPO: benign prostatic obstruction; this term refers to obstruction documented by urodynamic studies in the presence of an enlarged gland.

BOO; bladder outlet obstruction; BOO is the generic term for obstruction.

Outcome measures will differ according to whether the investigation or trial applies to the initial development of a new therapy, or whether the study is at a later phase of evaluation of that therapy. Phase I studies examine efficacy, safety, and tolerability; are usually open and, hence, unblinded. Phase II studies are randomized controlled trials in which a ranges of "doses" of the new therapy are tested against a placebo or sham. Randomized controlled trials (RCTs) are the most important method for demonstrating the effectiveness of treatments. Phase III studies are usually RCT in format, using the regimen indicated from phase II, in comparison with placebo or a comparator, such as an equivalent drug or other therapy.

From J. Nordling, P. Abrams, K. Ameda, J.T. Andersen, J. Donovan, D. Griffiths, S. Kobayashi, T. Koyanagi, W. Schäfer, S. Yalla, and Anders Mattiasson. Produced by the Standardisation Committee of the International Continence Society, A. Mattiasson, Chairman. Subcommittee on Outcome Research in Men, J. Nordling, Chairman. These authors are the members of the ICS Male Outcome Subcommittee, A. Mattiasson, Chairman. *Neurourology and Urodynamics* 17:263-271 (1998). Copyright 1998 by the International Continence Society.

Outcome measures may be primary or secondary. Primary outcome measures are used in the power calculation needed to determine the size of any study.

During the last decade, many new treatments for BPO have been introduced, including invasive treatments, such as superficial or interstitial laser treatment, rectal or urethral heating of the prostate by microwaves, balloon dilation, temporary or permanent stents, and medical treatments such as 5-alpha-reductase inhibitors and alpha-adrenoceptor-blocking agents. The effectiveness of these treatments has been assessed in many different ways (e.g., by changes in symptoms including symptom score, quality of life, urinary flow rate, residual urine volume, prostatic volume, voiding diary, and pressure–flow parameters), or by complications, such as the number of patients going into retention. The side effects and complications of treatments have also been assessed in many different ways, so that neither the consumer (the patient) nor the treating doctor can properly compare therapies. A major reason for this is that there is no consensus on which parameters should be used to measure results of treatment. Furthermore, the tools used to measure changes are often poorly described concerning reproducibility, validity, reliability, sensitivity, specificity, and responsiveness.

The ICS report on "Standardization of Outcome Studies in Patients With Lower Urinary Tract Dysfunction" (Mattiasson et al., 1998) gives the general principles governing the present report. This report analyzes the tools used to assess the various aspects of LUTS and BPO, and on that basis gives recommendations on how to assess the outcome of treatment.

II. OUTCOME MEASUREMENTS

A. Measurement of Patient Observations and Symptoms: Assessment of Lower Urinary Tract Symptoms

From the patient's perspective, the assessment of LUTS is the most important outcome measure following therapy. To recognize the importance of the patient's view, the instruments devised over recent years have been designed for patient and *not* doctor completion. LUTS constitute the main indication for treating BPO. Scoring of severity of symptoms, therefore, is necessary to quantify the symptoms and their influence on the patient's quality of life (see following) and to register and monitor changes after treatment. Many symptom scores have been used in the evaluation of LUTS suggestive of BPO. None of them have been designed to specifically measure outcomes of treatment. None is BPE- or BPO-specific. Finally, individual symptoms may be considered separately to evaluate changes.

1. Validated Questionnaires

The following instruments have been tested for some aspects of validity and reliability.

The International Prostate Symptom Score (I-PSS) (Barry et al., 1992; Cockett et al., 1991). The I-PSS was derived from the AUA symptom score with the addition of a condition-specific quality of life question. The AUA score contains a symptom score and a bothersomeness score. The AUA symptom score was originally created by selecting seven LUTS from 15 preliminary questions based on their correlation with two global urinary bothersomeness scores and their ability to discriminate between LUTS patients and younger males < 55 years old. However, it does not contain questions related to symptoms that may develop following treatment, such as urinary stress incontinence.

The Danish Prostatic Symptom Score (DAN-PSS-1) (Hald et al., 1991; Hansen et al., 1995).   The DAN-PSS-1 contains a symptom/symptom–bothersomeness part and a sexual questionnaire part (see later). A total of 24 questions, combining symptoms and bothersomeness of symptoms, causes longer page layout and smallertype size and may be confusing, especially to aged patients. Therefore, usability among different populations and different socioeconomic groups might be lower than that of the I-PSS.

Bolognese Symptom Questionnaire for BPH (Bolognese et al., 1992).   This score system contains a symptom score, a symptom bothersomeness score, and a global urination problems question. It is an adaptation of the Boyarsky score. The Bolognese Symptom Questionnaire was constructed to assess the effect of finasteride in men with LUTS suggestive of BPO. It has otherwise not been used.

ICSmale Questionnaire (Donovan et al., 1996).   The ICSmale Questionnaire contains questions on 20 urinary symptoms, 19 of which also have an additional question to ascertain the degree of bother that they cause. This questionnaire is easy to complete. It can differentiate between men in clinical and community populations. It demonstrates reasonable agreement between relevant parts of the questionnaire and frequency volume charts when a "relatively flexible approach" is taken, but there is a very poor relation between questions assessing strength of stream and the results of uroflowmetry. It has a good internal consistency and good test–retest reliability.

2.   Unvalidated Questionnaires

The following symptom questionnaires were the first published. In general they have received no psychometric testing.

Boyarsky Score (Boyarsky et al., 1977).   The first symptom score published to assess LUTS was designed for doctor completion. It has never been validated in its original form, and is normally used in a more or less modified form.

Madsen–Iversen Score (Madsen and Iversen, 1983).   This symptom score has never been validated in its original form. It is designed for doctor completion and is often used in a more or less modified form, including weighting of symptoms by a grading system, individual to each symptom.

The Maine Medical Assessment Program (MMAP) Instrument (Fowler et al., 1988).   Little validation has been done and that only in relation to responsiveness. The MMAP was a simple questionnaire, consisting of five questions, and it was the first to be designed for patient completion.

3.   Bothersomeness of Symptoms

Another method of assessing symptoms is to ask the patient about the degree of bother each symptom causes. This approach has been used in the AUA Bother Index, the ICS*male* Questionnaire, and the DAN-PSS-1. At present, it is not known whether the bother index or the quality of life index is more responsive to therapies, or whether they measure different aspects of the effects of therapy.

4.   Sexual Function Assessment

It is now recognized that sexual function is important when assessing therapies. There are a number of instruments available, although none have been fully validated in LUTS or after therapies for BPO. The ICSsex and its derivative PROTOsex, O'Leary's Brief Sexual

Function Inventory (O'Leary et al., 1995), and DANPSS assess similar aspects of sexual function.

5. Recommendations and Comments

A validated, patient-completed symptom questionnaire must always be included in trials of therapies for LUTS and BPO to capture the patient's perspective of their condition. Ample research has illustrated that symptom questionnaires are not sex-, age-, or condition-specific. Therefore, any symptom questionnaire or score may be used to document only the presence or severity of its constituent symptoms at any point in time. However, if this limitation is appreciated, these instruments are valuable in trials of therapies for LUTS and BPO. If such a score is used, reliability and validity data should be provided, if available, or their absence indicated.

B. Documentation of Voiding Pattern

1. Urinary Diary (Frequency Volume Chart, Voiding Diary, and Bladder Diary) (Bødker et al., 1989)

A voiding diary is a self-monitored record of selected lower urinary tract functions over specific time periods. In LUTS and BPO, selected variables are often voiding or toileting frequency (diurnal and nocturnal), voided volume, and fluid intake volume. A voiding diary is essential both in the clinical work and in research to obtain semiobjective data on frequency and volume voided in particular (e.g., the average voided volume from the voiding diary provides important redundant information to judge free uroflowmetry and pressure–flow studies).

2. Recommendations and Comments

Sparse information is available concerning validation of voiding diaries in men with LUTS. If a voiding diary is used, reliability and validity data should be provided, if available, or their absence indicated. It should be emphasized that the committee considers voiding diaries to be important in the evaluation of LUTS to diagnose high diuresis or reversed day and night diuresis as the cause of frequency or nocturia.

C. Anatomical and Functional Measurements: Clinical Outcome Measures

1. Estimation of Prostate Size

Prostate size is of little interest in relation to outcome in general, because prostatic size correlates poorly with symptoms, BOO, and treatment outcome. However, where therapies aim at reducing prostate size, either by shrinkage or by tissue destruction, exact measurement of prostate size may be important. A number of methods may be used. Of the methods available, transrectal ultrasound scanning (TRUS) is the most accurate, and digital rectal examination is the easiest test, but the most inaccurate. MRI is accurate, but expensive.

From TRUS, planimetric volumetry is considered as the "gold standard" for prostate volume determination, and excellent correlation between planimetric volume and absolute volume in cadavers has been demonstrated (Jones et al., 1989; Hastak et al., 1982; Hendriks et al., 1991; Peeling, 1989). Reliability is very good (Peeling, 1989; Nathan et al., 1996). Different methods and formulas to measure and calculate prostate volume from different axes of the prostate are less accurate (Nathan et al., 1996; Bangma et al., 1996). Other, simpler formulas are used to calculate prostate volume from axial, sagittal, and coronal diameters. The accuracy of these seem sufficient for daily clinical use (Terris and Stamey, 1991). Transition zone volume and transition zone index may be a valuable supplement to whole-gland volume determination.

It has been reported that the anteroposterial diameter increases more than the transverse diameter with age, and that the shape of the prostate becomes round by transverse section (Peeling, 1989), although controversy exists (Bosch et al., 1994). Changes in microscopic features of glandular, muscle, and connective tissue content in the gland might prove to be relevant (Marks et al., 1994), and may be important in assessing some new therapies.

2.   Recommendations and Comments

If treatment intends to change prostate volume, measurements should be done before and after treatment. Timing of posttreatment testing depends on mechanism of action of the modality. The method used and its reliability and validity should be provided if available, or their absence indicated.

D.   Assessment of Bladder Outlet Obstruction

Pressure Flow Studies (pQS).   The only method of accurately diagnosing and grading BOO is pressure–flow studies with simultaneous recording of abdominal pressure, intravesical pressure, and urinary flow rate. As this is an invasive and time-consuming procedure, it will probably never be adopted as routine in all patients with LUTS suggestive of BPO. It is, however, the cornerstone of the assessment of outcome after treatments claiming to influence BOO, or to relieve symptoms because of reduction in BOO.

Urine Flow Rate.   The urinary flow rate reflects both detrusor function and outlet conditions. Because both muscle mechanics and bladder geometry depend on bladder volume, urinary flow rate increases with increasing bladder volume until a certain limit and, thereafter, decreases. This underlines the high dependence of urinary flow rates on detrusor muscle function and explains why urinary flow rate alone is of limited help in the diagnosis of outlet obstruction.

Test–retest measurements of maximum urinary flow rates have a standard deviation of about 3.5 mL/s, with a wide range (Neal et al., 1987; Grino et al., 1993). A significant overlap exists between symptomatic and asymptomatic men (Diokno et al., 1994), as well as between obstructive and nonobstructive voiding (Abrams and Griffiths, 1979). Correlation for voided volume does not change this finding.

Residual Urine Volume.   Wide intraindividual variation of residual urine volume has been demonstrated by catheter or ultrasound measurement in patients with LUTS suggestive of BPO (Bruskewitz et al., 1982; Dunsmuir et al., 1996). In the latter study, the individual variation was 42%, with a confidence interval of 55–228 mL. As poor bladder emptying may be due to either outlet obstruction or detrusor underactivity, or both, the correlation of residual urine volume with outlet obstruction alone is poor (Neal et al., 1987; Bruskewitz et al., 1982; Poulsen et al., 1994).

Cystourethroscopy.   Prostatic intraurethral protrusion and bladder trabeculation are poor indicators of bladder outlet obstruction (Andersen et al., 1980; Rosier et al., 1996). As a direct indicator of BOO after treatment, cystourethroscopy, therefore, is useless. It might in certain treatments give a clue as to why a therapy may fail (e.g., presence of the median lobe in thermotherapy).

1.   Recommendations and Comments

In research studies of outcome, pQS must be included to document the presence and degree of change in BOO.

Results should be presented as stated in the ICS 1997 standardization report on pressure–flow studies of voiding, urethral resistance, and urethral obstruction (Griffiths et al., 1997).

Change in flow rates in response to treatment is sensitive, but the degree of change is meaningless unless pretreatment detrusor voiding pressure is known. A slight decrease in outlet resistance might produce a pronounced increase in maximum urinary flow rate if outlet resistance is low before treatment; and a significant decrease in outlet resistance might produce only a small increase in maximum urinary flow rate if outlet resistance were high before treatment and an element of obstruction persists.

Posttreatment reduction of residual urine volume indicates improvement of outlet conditions and is likely to be more significant in assessing treatment response than for diagnosis. Methods used for the assessment of BOO should be stated, and reliability and validity data should be provided if available or their absence indicated.

E.   Assessment of Infuence on Quality of Life

As mentioned in the Introduction, quality of life may also include sexual function and bothersomeness of LUTS. Considerable developmental work is being undertaken to develop measurement tools within this area, but so far a widely accepted quality of life scale for LUTS does not exist. Quality of life aspects should be addressed in outcome studies.

Quality of Life Assessment.   There are numerous instruments in this everexpanding field. They can be divided into two broad categories, generic quality of life instruments and disease-specific quality of life instruments.

Generic Quality of Life Instruments.   The best-known generic instruments are the Nottingham Health Profile, the SF36, and the EuroQoL (Donovan et al., 1997). At the time of writing there is very little scientific work on the use of these instruments in men with LUTS or BPO. The aim of generic instruments is to obtain an overview of health status, and to allow comparisons between patient groups. It is unlikely that these instruments will be very sensitive to the changes following therapies, in view of the aged population with coexisting pathologies.

Disease-Specific Quality of Life Instruments.   The most commonly used instrument is the single question attached to the I-PSS. There has been concern that a single question may not adequately capture the influence of LUTS on quality of life, and therefore other instruments are being developed. The ICSQoL is part of the ICS–"BPH" Questionnaire (Donovan et al., 1997). Lukacs et al. (1994) and Girman et al. (1994) have produced disease-specific quality of life questionnaires that are currently under evaluation, and the BII (BPH Impact Index) (Barry et al., 1995) is derived from the AUA quality of life questionnaire.

1.   Recommendations and Comments

Treatment effects on quality of life are probably among the most important outcome parameters. Further research, therefore, should be done to identify the best way to measure this after treatment of LUTS suggestive of BPO.

When a QoL assessment is used, the particular method should be stated, and reliability and validity data should be provided if available or their absence indicated.

F. Socioeconomic Measurements

As health care resources are limited and both LUTS and BPO are common conditions, outcome studies must include an assessment of relative costs, at least when new treatments are introduced.

Measurement tools are under development, but are even less complete than the quality of life measuring tools. Therefore, this research area deserves much attention and might produce surprising results when properly applied (Keoghane et al., 1996).

1. Recommendations and Comments

Costs are not, strictly speaking, an outcome measure. An economic evaluation (specifically a cost-effectiveness study) should accompany any evaluation of effectiveness. Costs need to be collected from the viewpoint of the patient and society and then combined with effectiveness to give an indication of the cost-effectiveness of different treatments.

G. Treatment Complications

The treatment complications of a specific treatment must also be described and quantified in a complete outcome evaluation of any treatment. Complications, such as mortality and morbidity, must be addressed, although complications may vary considerably with different treatments. Therefore, it is not possible to give specific recommendations in this area.

H. Durability

Durability of a treatment is important. Therefore, it is essential that long-term follow-up be included in the evaluation of any new treatments. The Third International Consultation on Benign Prostatic Hyperplasia defines evaluation time into three categories: short-term, up to and including 3 months; medium-term, up to and including 12 months; and long-term, studies reporting after 12 months (Cockett et al., 1996). Issues such as treatment rate and treatment failure rate should be considered.

CONCLUSIONS

Measuring outcomes in LUTS and BPO depends on the purpose of the measurement. In the study of new treatments, all domains must be covered, meaning that those domains allegedly affected by that treatment must be investigated properly. Symptoms must be evaluated by a validated symptom score, prostatic obstruction must be evaluated by pressure–flow studies, and quality of life and cost issues should be addressed. Other critical issues are the length of follow-up and the long-term effectiveness of treatments.

In a quality assurance program, outcome could be assessed in a less ambitious way, using changes in a validated symptom score and changes in an indirect measure of outlet obstruction such as urinary flow rate or residual urine volume. However, the assessment of quality of life and costs should also be considered in such a program. In daily clinical work, the follow-up that is actually performed will depend on the resources available. A general practitioner will not have the same possibilities as a hospital clinic, and the diagnostic setup will also necessitate different methods of assessment of outcome.

A wide range of methods of evaluating outcomes in LUTS and BOO is available. The precise tools to be used will depend on the aims of the study and the type of design. Outcomes are best assessed through randomized, controlled trials, in which a new treatment or type of service is evaluated in comparison with an existing standard therapy (such as TURP), placebo, or conservative management. Within such trials, the assessment of outcome should always include measurements of LUTS (using validated questionnaires or scores), Q_{max}, residual urine and voided volume (uroflowmetry), quality of life (generic or condition-specific questionnaires or questions, sexual function), and treatment complications. All researchers should also consider including pQS, the measurement of prostate size, and an economic evaluation, particularly for trials of new treatments or services.

REFERENCES

Abrams PH, Griffiths DJ (1979). The assessment of prostatic obstruction from urodynamic measurements and from residual urine. Br J Urol 51:129–134.

Andersen JT, Nordling J (1980). Prostatism II. The correlation between cystourethroscopic, cystometric and urodynamic findings. Scand J Urol Nephrol 14:23–27.

Bangma CH. Qais A, Niemer HJ, Grobbee DE, Schröder FH (1996). Transrectal ultrasonic volumetry of the prostate: in vivo comparison of different methods. Prostate 28:107–110.

Barry MJ, Fowler FJ, O'Leary MP, et al. (1992). The American Urological Association Symptom Index for Benign Prostatic Hyperplasia. J Urol 148:1549–1557.

Barry MJ, Fowler FJ, O'Leary MP, Bruskewitz RC, Holtgrewe HL, Mebust WK (1995). Measuring disease-specific health status in men with benign prostatic hyperplasia. Med Care 334:145–155.

Bødker A, Lendorf A, Holm–Nielsen A, Glahn B (1989). Micturition pattern assessed by the frequency/volume chart in a healthy population of men and women. Neurourol Urodynam 8:421–422.

Bolognese JA, Kozloff RC, Kumitz SC, Grino PB, Patrick DL, Stoner E (1992). Validation of a symptoms questionnaire for benign prostatic hyperplasia. Prostate 21:247–254.

Bosch JL, Hop WCJ, Niemer QHJ, Bangma CH, Kirkels WJ, Schröder FH (1994). Parameters of prostate volume and shape in a community based population of men 55 to 74 years old. J Urol 152:1501–1505.

Boyarsky S. Jones G, Paulson DF, Prout GR (1977). New look at bladder neck obstruction by the Food and Drug Administration regulators. Am Assoc Genitourin Surg 68:29–32.

Bruskewitz RC, Iversen P, Madsen PO (1982). Volume of postvoid residual urine determination in evaluation of prostatism. Urology 20:602–604.

Cockett ATK, Khoury S, Aso Y, et al., eds. (1991). Proceedings of the First International Consultation on Benign Prostatic Hyperplasia. Jersey: Scientific Communications International.

Cockett ATK, Khoury S, Aso Y, et al., eds. (1996). Proceedings of the Third International Consultation on Benign Prostatic Hyperplasia. Jersey: Scientific Communications International.

Diokno AC, Brown MR, Goldstein NC, Herzog AR (1994). Urinary flow rates and voiding pressures in elderly men living in a community. J Urol 151:1550–1553.

Donovan JL, Abrams P, Peters TY, Kay HE, Reynard J, Chapple C, de la Rosette JJCH, Kondo A (1996). The ICS "BPH" study. The psychometric validity and reliability of the ICSmale questionnaire. Br J Urol 77:554–562.

Donovan JL, Kay HE, Peters TJ, Abrams P, Coast J, Matos–Ferreira A, Rentzhog L, Bosch JLHR, Nordling J, Gajewski JB, Barbalias G, Schick E, Mendes Silva M, Nissenkorn I, De la Rosette JJMCH (1997). Using the ICSQoL to measure the impact of lower urinary tract symptoms on quality of life: evidence from the ICS–"BPH" study. Br J Urol 80:712–721.

Dunsmuir WD, Feneley M, Corry DA, Bryan J, Kirby JS (1996). The day-to-day variation (test–retest reliability) of residual urine measurement. Br J Urol 77:192–193.

Fowler FJ Jr, Wennberg JE, Timothy RP, Barry MJ, Mulley AG Jr, Hanley D (1988). Symptom status and quality of life following prostatectomy. JAMA 259:3018–3022.

Girman CJ, Epstein RS, Jacobsen SJ, Guess HA, Panser LA, Oesterling JE, Lieber MM (1994). Natural history of prostatism: impact of urinary symptoms on quality of life in 2115 randomly selected community men. Urology 44:825–831.

Griffiths D, Höfner K, van Mastrigt R, Rollema HJ, Spångberg A, Gleason D (1997). Standardization of terminology of lower urinary tract function: pressure–flow studies of voiding, urethral resistance, and urethral obstruction. Neurourol Urodynam 16:1–18.

Grino PB, Bruskewitz R, Blaivas JG, Siroky MB, Andersen JT, Cook T, Stoner E (1993). Maximum urinary flow rate by uroflowmetry: automatic or visual interpretation. J Urol 149:339–341.

Hald T, Nordling J, Andersen JT, Bilde T, Meyhoff HH, Walter S (1991). A patient weighted symptom score system in the evaluation of uncomplicated benign prostatic hyperplasia. Scand J Urol Nephrol Suppl 138:59–62.

Hansen B, Flyger H, Brasso K, Schou J, Nordling J, Andersen JT, Mortensen S, Meyhoff HH, Walter S, Hald T (1995). Validation of the self-administered Danish Prostatic Symptom Score (DAN-PSS-1) system for use in benign prostatic hyperplasia. Br J Urol 76:451–458.

Hastak SM, Gammelgaard J, Holm HH (1982). Transrectal ultrasonic volume determination of the prostate—a preoperative and postoperative study. J Urol 127:1115–1118.

Hendriks AJ, Wijkstra H, Maes RM, et al. (1991). Audex Medical, a new system for digital processing and analysis of ultrasonographic images of the prostate. Scand J Urol Nephrol Suppl 137:95–100.

Jones DR, Roberts EE, Griffiths GJ, et al. (1989). Assessment of volume measurement of the prostate using per-rectal ultrasonography. Br J Urol 64:493–495.

Keoghane SR, Lawrence KC, Gray AM, Chappel DB, Hancock AM, Cranston DW (1996). The Oxford laser prostate trial: economic issues surrounding contact laser prostatectomy. Br J Urol 77:386–390.

Lukacs B, McCarthy C, Lepleqe A, Comet D (1994). Development and validation of a quality of life scale associated with health status, specific for benign hypertrophy of the prostate and including a sexuality evaluation scale. Prog Urol 4:688–699.

Madsen PO, Iversen P (1983). A point system for selecting operative candidates. In: Hinmann F, ed. Benign Prostatic Hypertrophy. New York: Springer-Verlag, pp 763–765.

Marks LSM, Treiger B, Dorey FJ, Fu YS, Dekernion JB (1994). Morphometry of the prostata: I. Distribution of tissue components in hyperplasia glands. Urology 44:486–492.

Nathan MS, Seemivasagam K, Mei Q, Wickham JEA, Miller RA (1996). Transrectal ultrasonography: why are estimates of prostate volume and dimension so inaccurate? Br J Urol 77:401–407.

Neal DE, Styles RA, Powell PH, Ramsden PD (1987). Relationship between detrusor function and residual urine in men undergoing prostatectomy. Br J Urol 60:560–566.

O'Leary MP, Fowler FJ, Lenderking WR, Barber B, Sagnier PP, Guess HA, Barry MJ (1995). A brief male sexual function inventory for urology. Urology 46:697–706.

Peeling WB (1989). Diagnostic assessment of benign prostatic hyperplasia. Prostata 114:52–68.

Poulsen AL, Schou J, Puggaard L, Torp–Pedersen S, Nordling J (1994). Prostatic enlargement, symptomatology and pressure–flow evaluation: interrelations in patients with symptomatic BPH. Scand J Urol Nephrol Suppl 157:67–73.

Rosier PFWM, de Wildt MJAM, Wijkstra H, Debruyne FFMJ, de la Rosette JMCH (1996). Clinical diagnosis of bladder outlet obstruction in patients with benign prostatic enlargement and lower urinary tract symptoms: development and urodynamic validation of a clinical prostate score for the objective diagnosis of bladder outlet obstruction. J Urol 155:1649–1654.

Terris MK, Stamey TA (1991). Determination of prostate volume by transrectal ultrasound. J Urol 145:984–987.

Outcome Studies:
Frail Older People

I. INTRODUCTION

The aim of this paper is primarily to provide a framework for investigators conducting research on incontinence in frail older people. Because it is difficult to precisely define *frailty*, the definition used in this paper is "any person over age 65 years with incontinence of urine who does not leave their place of residence without assistance of others, or a person with dementia, or a person who has been admitted to a long-term care facility." These people usually suffer from multiple medical conditions and disabilities (comorbidity), which result in them becoming homebound or institutionalized. Because they require the assistance of others to perform some or all of the most basic activities of daily living (ADLs), including bathing, dressing, toileting, and ambulating, results from younger populations or from older people without disabilities cannot necessarily be extrapolated to this population. For this population there is little validated research showing long-term efficacy of treatment for urinary incontinence.

If incontinence develops in healthy older people, its management is generally similar to the approach taken in younger individuals, except that greater caution should be taken when pharmacological intervention is being considered because of the susceptibility of older people to adverse drug reactions. This paper, therefore, does not focus on the fit older person, and in the absence of data to the contrary, the same outcome measures should be used as for adults of the same sex (Mattiasson et al., 1998). This paper deals with lower urinary tract dysfunction with a major emphasis on incontinence. Nocturia is a significant problem for older people, and the principles alluded to in this paper cover this area.

Because of the frailty of this population, all patients being considered for entry into a research protocol should be assessed for coexisting reversible or modifiable (comorbid) factors such as fecal impaction, confusional states, functional disabilities, or use of med-

From D. Fonda, N.M. Resnick, J. Colling, K. Burgio, J.G. Ouslander, C. Norton, P. Ekelund, E. Versi, and A. Mattiasson. Produced by the Standardisation Committee of the International Continance Society, A. Mattiasson, Chairman. Subcommittee on Outcome Research in Frail Older People, D. Fonda, Chairman. *Neurourology and Urodynamics* 17:273–281 (1998). Copyright 1998 by the International Continence Society.

ication that may be contributing to incontinence or might affect the outcome of the study. No patient should receive another intervention until such transient causes have been addressed. The extent of invasive testing should balance study requirements with the benefits, risks, and inconvenience to the patient.

Research in this population is difficult because of the following:

The heterogeneity of this population, resulting in difficulty in designing studies that account for comorbidity, drug use, intercurrent illness, and shorter life expectancy

Lack of standardized terminology to define and measure cure and improvement

Lack of validated research tools to measure baseline and outcome variables in the frail elderly

Lack of long-term follow-up to gauge effect, durability, and applicability of the intervention

Lack of information of the natural history of incontinence in this group

II. CONSIDERATIONS IN STUDY DESIGN

General principles in designing a study on lower urinary tract dysfunction have been published elsewhere and apply equally in this group (Mattiasson et al., 1998). The following lists some additional considerations for research in incontinence involving the frail elderly.

A. Baseline Clinical Data

The following baseline clinical data should be considered when designing a study in the frail older population. Relevant information should be included in the final report of the study's findings.

1. Descriptive Data

Type of setting of the study (e.g., home, nursing home)

Patient–staff ratio (where staff are involved in the management protocol)

Usual continence care

Direct and indirect costs of current care

Patient, family, or staff expectations

Age and gender

Description of care givers (e.g., training, qualifications)

System incentives or disincentives that may influence management options (e.g., government funding).

2. Symptoms and Investigations

Type of symptoms

Duration of symptoms

Response to prior treatment (e.g., pharmacological, surgical, behavioral)

Midstream urine for culture and sensitivities

Postvoid residual urine estimation.

3. Associated Factors

Environmental factors that might contribute to incontinence (e.g., distance to toilet, use of continence aids or appliances)

Associated comorbid conditions that might be contributing to incontinence or the effectiveness of intervention

Bowel status (e.g., constipation, incontinence)

Functional level of the patients [by use of a standardized scale such as Barthel or Katz ADL scales (Katz et al., 1963; Mahoney et al., 1965)]

Cognitive state/function of the patients [by use of a standardized scale, such as the Mini-mental Scale Examination (Folstein et al., 1979)]

Concurrent medications that could contribute to incontinence or affect outcome of treatment (e.g., sedatives, diuretics, alcohol)

Fluid intake

B. Description of Study Design

Details of study design should be provided, including methodology, recruitment, inclusion and exclusion criteria, interventions, outcome measures to be used, and statistical methods. Further information has been provided on guidelines for study design by the ICS (Mattiasson et al., 1998).

C. Outcome Data

To determine the effect of an intervention, accurate, valid, and meaningful outcome variables are needed. It is most important to define the major endpoints prior to commencing studies. Baseline diagnostic data should be gathered to characterize the patient's condition and to document the severity of incontinence (see following Outcome Measurements). The selection of an outcome variable depends on the nature of the intervention being studied (e.g., pharmacological, surgical, or behavioral). Successful short-term interventions should, wherever possible, have long-term follow-up provided (at least 12 months) to gauge more accurately their impact, durability, and relevance in this frail population.

There are age-specific influences on lower urinary tract function, and normative data are generally lacking in this frail population. In addition, test–retest reliability and sensitivity to change of the more invasive measures of lower urinary tract function are poorly documented in the frail elderly. It is, therefore, the belief of the committee that it is not appropriate to repeat invasive measures at follow-up in this frail population unless these measures are fundamental in understanding components of the intervention being studied.

The following information, which could influence outcome, should, wherever possible, be addressed and reported at time of follow-up:

Number and reason for dropouts and deaths (i.e., were they trial-related?)

Compliance issues (by patients, staff, or caregivers), such as compliance with exercise programs, toileting protocols, or drug use

Type of bladder training or toileting programs (if any)

Other intercurrent treatment not directly related to bladder function that might impinge on outcome

Medication that might affect incontinence or continence

Socioeconomic data, including effect of the intervention on the patient

Changes in caregiver or staff status or numbers

Cost of treatment

Cost–benefit data

Patient or caregiver satisfaction with the intervention
Risk–benefit data

1. Recommendations and Comments

Because comorbidity and drug use contribute to the presence and severity of continence in this population, they should be addressed or stabilized before patients are enrolled. In any research project, it is essential to clearly determine endpoints at the outset.

III. OUTCOME MEASUREMENTS

In this section, the key outcome areas are identified and recommendations are made that may be of use to researchers. In keeping with the format of the ICS Outcomes Standards Reports, outcome measurements for frail elderly people are covered under the following five headings: patient observations and symptoms; documentation of the symptoms; anatomical and functional measures; quality of life measures; and socioeconomic measures.

A. Measurement of Patient Observations and Symptoms

History alone is insufficient in diagnosing the etiology of bladder dysfunction. In the frail older person this is compounded by the age-associated decline in cognitive function and increase in depression. Caregivers may be able to provide important supplementary or supportive information. One study has recently validated a nonurodynamic-based diagnostic algorithm (Resnick et al., 1996).

1. Recommendations and Comments

Research in this group should not be based solely on patients' subjective reporting of symptoms. Patient-derived symptoms response as an outcome measure should be supplemented, where necessary, by data derived from caregivers.

B. Documentation of Urine Loss

Bladder Diaries.   Bladder diaries are simple and noninvasive and have the potential to be reliable and sensitive to therapeutic intervention, especially when completed by competent staff. However, accuracy of self-report data is always a matter of concern, and interpretation of what constitutes clinical versus statistical significance is difficult. Bladder diaries have not been validated when completed by the frail housebound or institutionalized elderly, although they may prove accurate for the cognitively intact and motivated frail older person. Bladder diaries completed by others, such as caregivers or staff (wet checks), or pad weighing, are alternatives (see following).

1. Recommendations and Comments

Bladder diaries should be a useful outcome measure for hospitalized or institutionalized older people. The usefulness of bladder diaries as an outcome measure when completed by the frail elderly or their "untrained" carers has not yet been validated.

Pad-Weighing Tests.   Difficulties with determining wetness can be overcome by weighing pads before and after specified time intervals. To standardize the pad tests, the ICS introduced the 1-hr pad-weighing test, which measures urine loss as weight gain of perineal pads under standardized conditions (Abrams et al., 1988). Only one relevant study of the 1-hr pad-weighing test in frail elderly could be identified. The 24-hr inpatient measurement of urine leakage of frail elderly patients by staff was more feasible and sensitive than the 1-hr pad test; reducibility was not directly assessed (Griffiths et al., 1991). The 48-hr home pad test with patients weighing their own pads has been reliable for quantifying urine loss in cognitively intact and reasonably independent (but not "frail") elderly incontinent women; reproducibility was not assessed (Ekelund et al., 1988).

The principal advantages in performing pad tests at home are simplicity, cost-effectiveness (as hospital personnel are not required), and the relaxed environment, which reproduces more accurately the conditions leading to incontinence when compared with the relatively unfamiliar hospital or clinic setting. It is important to provide the patient with careful written and oral instructions before attempting the test. Certain forms of handicap, such as dementia, reduced mobility, physical handicap, fecal incontinence, or defective vision, pose problems that could in some cases be compensated for by involving a caregiver in the test procedure. It should be noted that some pads leak, further reducing reliability and accuracy of this test.

2.   Recommendations and Comments

Pad-weighing offers the potential for quantifying the degree of incontinence in older patients and can be useful in the hospital setting. Further data are still required to establish its usefulness in the frail elderly, especially in those confined to home.

Wet Checks.   Wet checks consist of examining the patient at regular intervals for leakage. Such checks are a commonly used measure of incontinence in nursing home residents. At least ten clinical studies of frail incontinent elderly have been published using wet checks as an outcome measure. The exact method of determining wet or dry status is not well-described in any of the studies, while the frequency of checks varied from one to four hourly. Nonetheless, despite these limitations, wet checks appear to be a reliable means of documenting incontinence (Hu et al., 1989; Colling et al., 1992, 1995). However, in one study, when an electronic monitor was used to document incontinence, there was considerable disagreement noted with caregivers underreporting wet episodes (Colling et al., 1995). The Incontinence Monitoring Record (which is a record of whether the patient is wet on regular checking), particularly the colored form, has been shown in one study to be a reliable documentation tool when completed by nurses' aides (Ouslander et al., 1986).

Although these instruments are practical, understandable, and commonly used outcome measures, the following should be considered:

It is difficult to get ward staff to reliably check and record wetness. Hence, for research purposes, dedicated research staff may be needed to record these data.

It is sometimes difficult to correctly identify wet absorbent products now, because many of them have materials that "wick" away the moisture, making it impossible to see and even difficult to feel moisture.

Many institutes now require the use of universal precautions in handling of body fluids, which would include performing wet checks. If litmus paper is used to identify moisture, a false-negative can result unless it is placed where it is likely to pick up the urine. Conversely, a false-positive can occur when moisture from the skin shows up on litmus paper.

Wet checks are intrusive and invasive to patients, and in some cases may actually stimulate patients to void.

Absolute pad counts are not a reliable outcome measure, as it is most difficult to impose consistent criteria for changing of pads.

While the electronic monitor shows promise of increasing the accuracy of identifying wet episodes, its use has not yet been well-studied in the frail elderly and it is not yet available commercially.

3. Recommendations and Comments

The wet-check method of assessing incontinence appears to be both a practical and reliable tool to assess outcome in dependent older patients, provided attention is given to the foregoing considerations. Compliance of staff necessitates education and close supervision. The more frequent the "checking" (e.g., hourly), the more likely the data will be reliable for the actual number of wet episodes.

C. Anatomical and Functional Measurements

"Simple" Cystometry. Simple cystometry is a relatively inexpensive form of single-channel water cystometry, which can be performed without specialized equipment in an outpatient clinic, acute hospital, nursing home, or home setting. It is not so feasible and accurate in the severely cognitively impaired. The procedure is generally well-tolerated and adds little time to that needed for a postvoid residual determination by catheterization. Even though studies have shown comparability of results from simple and multichannel cystometry in an outpatient setting, this has not been demonstrated in institutional settings (Ouslander et al., 1988; Fonda et al., 1993). The major disadvantage is the lack of an abdominal pressure measurement. Adequate data on the test–retest reliability of simple cystometry do not exist. There are no data to support the usefulness of simple cystometry as an outcome measurement, nor in predicting responsiveness to various interventions or in elucidating the mechanism of action of interventions for geriatric incontinence.

1. Recommendations and Comments

Simple cystometry has not been validated as an outcome measure for research in frail patients.

Multichannel Urodynamics. The few available studies indicate that, when carefully performed, multichannel urodynamic testing of the frail elderly is feasible and safe, and reproducibly yields the same diagnosis. Fluoroscopic monitoring appears to increase its accuracy by facilitating detection of the low-pressure involuntary contractions that are more common in the frail elderly. However, compared with urodynamic evaluation of more robust individuals, testing in this population is technically more difficult to conduct, is less available, requires additional personnel, and is probably more susceptible to artifact. Furthermore, normative data are lacking for this population.

Few investigators have employed multichannel urodynamics as an outcome measure in the frail elderly. Cystometric capacity and reduced bladder sensation (both measured after therapy) have been shown to correlate with response to oxybutynin treatment (Griffiths et al., 1996). In a small study, response to prostatectomy correlated with the severity of obstruction on initial pressure–flow testing, despite persistence of unstable contractions in all patients but one (Gormley et al., 1993).

2. Recommendations and Comments

Complex urodynamic testing has not been evaluated sufficiently to determine its usefulness as an outcome measure in the frail elderly.

Pelvic Muscle Strength.   Pelvic muscle exercises may be of value in management of incontinence, either by increasing pelvic muscle strength or as a form of biofeedback. The force of voluntary pelvic muscle contraction can be determined directly (digitally or by air pressure) or indirectly (surface electromyography). For the frail elderly there are no validated data on the measurement of pelvic muscle strength as an outcome measure following teaching of pelvic floor exercises.

3. Recommendations and Comments

At present, measurement of pelvic muscle strength before and after treatment has not been validated as a useful outcome measure for frail older patients.

Ultrasound.   Estimation of residual urine is an important adjunct to investigation of older patients, especially before addition of drugs that may impair bladder emptying. Estimation of postvoid residual by a portable ultrasound device has been shown to correlate well with that measured by catheterization (Griffiths et al., 1992). Sensitivity may not be so good when volumes are greater than 200 mL as measured by catheter, in which case repeated measurements may be necessary to exclude a very high postvoid residual (Ouslander et al., 1994). Improvement in the equipment's design since this study may have improved its accuracy.

4. Recommendations and Comments

Use of ultrasound for residual urine estimation offers much potential as a convenient non-invasive research tool for frail older people, especially for drug or surgical interventions that may affect bladder emptying. Further studies are required to validate the newer portable models.

D. Quality of Life Measurements

Health-related quality of life (HRQL) is a multidimensional concept that refers to an individual's evaluation and satisfaction with his or her physical, social, and psychological health, as well as total well-being. This can be measured by a generic or condition-specific instrument. HRQL is important to measure, because a patient's life quality may improve even without change in degree of incontinence; conversely, improved continence status may not result in improved life quality. Unfortunately, few HRQL instruments have been tested for reliability, validity, and responsiveness in incontinent populations, let alone in a frail elderly population.

1. Recommendations and Comments

There is a need to develop tools to measure HRQL for frail elderly incontinent people.

E. Socioeconomic Measurements

The economic effect of continence interventions can be measured by cost, cost–benefit, and cost-effectiveness. To be of real value, all costs related to actual health expenditure should be estimated before and after the intervention. This includes those related to treatment (e.g., drugs, surgery, nursing time on bladder training) and those related to managing any incontinence (e.g., pads, skin care products, laundry, caregiver time).

Cost–benefit is even more difficult to assess, as it is unclear how to define "benefit" in this population. For example, Schnelle et al. (1995) showed modest improvement in the degree of incontinence, but at increased cost compared with usual care. It is better to be "socially continent" (dry with the assistance of pads or aids) and only occasionally disturbed by staff to change pads, or to be toileted frequently and be less wet at a greater staff cost but with a need to still wear pads?

Costs also include more nebulous areas that are borne by society as a whole rather than the health care system, such as work days lost for caregivers, effect of incontinence on the caregivers, or need for institutional care. While it is often stated that incontinence is a major factor in referral for institutional care, there are few convincing data to support this assertion.

1. Recommendations and Comments

There is a need to develop tools to help evaluate cost, cost–benefit, and cost-effectiveness for this population.

CONCLUSIONS

Research methodology for studying incontinence in the frail and housebound elderly is fraught with pitfalls. This has compromised the usefulness of past research. There is a great need for basic research to validate practical and useful outcome measures that will allow meaningful results to be obtained. In addition, an understanding is required of the importance of defining clinical, rather than statistical, significance.

REFERENCES

Abrams P, Blaivas JG, Stanton SL, Andersen JT (1988). The standardisation of terminology of lower urinary tract function. Scand J Urol Nephrol Suppl 114:5–19.

Colling J, Ouslander JG, Hadley BJ, Campbell E (1992). The effects of patterned urge response toileting (PURT) on urinary incontinence among nursing home residents. J Am Geriatr Soc 40: 135–141.

Colling J, Hadley BJ, Campbell E, Eisch J, Newman D (1995). Continence Program for Care Dependent Elderly. Final Report. NIH-NCNR-NR 01554. Bethesda, MD.

Ekelund P, Bergstrom H, Milsom I, et al. (1988). Quantification of urinary incontinence in elderly women with the 48-hour pad test. Arch Gerontol Geriat 7:281–287.

Folstein MF, Folstein S, McHugh PR (1975). Mini Mental State: a practical method for grading the cognitive state of patients for the clinician. J Psychiatr Res 12:189–198.

Fonda D, Brimage PJ, D'Astoli M (1993). A comparison of simple cystometry and multichannel cystometry in the assessment of urinary incontinence in an elderly outpatient population. Urology 42:536–540.

Gormley EA, Griffiths DJ, McCracken PN, Harrison GM, McPhee MS (1993). Effect of transurethral resection of the prostate on detrusor instability and urge incontinence in elderly males. Neurourol Urodynam 12:445–453.

Griffiths DJ, McCracken PN, Harrison GM (1991). Incontinence in the elderly: objective demonstration and quantitative assessment. Br J Urol 67:467–471.

Griffiths DJ, McCracken PN, Harrison GM, Gormley EA (1992). Characteristics of urinary incontinence in elderly patients studied by 24 hour monitoring and urodynamic testing. Age Ageing 21:195–201.

Griffiths DJ, McCracken PN, Harrison GM, Moore KEN (1996). Urge incontinence in elderly people: factors predicting the severity of urine loss before and after pharmacological treatment. Neurourol Urodynam 15:53–57.

Hu T–W, Igou JF, Kaltreider DL, et al. (1989). A clinical trial of a behavioral therapy to reduce urinary incontinence in nursing homes. JAMA 261:2656–2662.

Katz S, Ford A, Moskowitz R, et al. (1963). The index of ADL: a standardized measurement of biological and psychosocial function. JAMA 185:914–919.

Mahoney FI, Barthel DW (1965). Functional evaluation: the Barthel Index. Md State Med J 14:61–65.

Mattiasson A, Djurhuus JC, Fantl A, Fonda D, Nordling J, Stohrer M (1998). Standardization of outcome studies in patients with lower urinary tract dysfunction: a report on general principles from the Standardisation Committee of the International Continence Society. Neurourol Urodynam 17:249–253.

Ouslander JG, Urman HN, Uman GC (1986). Development and testing of an incontinence monitoring record. J Am Geriatr Soc 34:83–90.

Ouslander JG, Leach GE, Abelson S, Staskin DR, Blaustein J, Raz S (1988). Simple versus multichannel cystometry in the evaluation of bladder function in an incontinent geriatric population. J Urol 140:1482–1486.

Ouslander JG, Simmons S, Tuico E, Nigam JG, Fingold S, Bates–Jensen B, Schnelle JF (1994). Use of a portable ultrasound device to measure post-void residual volume among incontinent nursing home residents. J Am Geriatr Soc 42:1189–1192.

Resnick NM, Brandeis GH, Baumann MM, Morris JN (1996). Evaluating a national assessment strategy for urinary incontinence in nursing home residents: reliability of the Minimum Data Set and validity of the Resident Assessment Protocol. Neurourol Urodynam 15:583–598.

Schnelle JF, Keeler E, Hays RD, Simmons S, Ouslander JG, Siu AL (1995). A cost value analysis of two interventions with incontinent nursing home residents. J Am Geriatr Soc 43:1112–1117.

Technical Report: Urodynamic Equipment

I. INTRODUCTION

The two parameters that are most commonly measured in urodynamic studies are pressure and urinary flow rate. In each case a *transducer* is used to produce an electrical signal to represent these parameters in a form that can be readily recorded on chart paper or magnetic tape, displayed on an oscilloscope, or stored digitally in a computer. Another useful parameter, the *electromyogram* (EMG), is already in an electrical form. Generally, it is desirable to reproduce these parameters as "faithfully" as possible, without modifying the signal appearing at the source. This can usually be achieved by direct *amplification*. Often, however, more useful, and perhaps more readily interpretable, data can be acquired by modifying the original signal before it is eventually displayed. This, together with amplification, is referred to as *signal processing*. Interference from other physiological variables may be present in the recorded signal, appearing as if originating from the source. The recorded signals should therefore be interpreted with caution.

II. SIGNAL PROCESSORS

A typical electronic system used for measuring urodynamic parameters is shown in Figure 1, the design procedure taking into account the importance of maintaining compatibility between the various components in the overall system. Processors can be used to

1. Amplify the signal
2. Filter the signal
3. Differentiate the signal
4. Integrate the signal
5. Convert the analog signal into digital form

From *J Med Eng Technol* 11:57–64 (1987). Produced by the International Continence Society Working Party on Urodynamic Equipment. Chairman: David E. Rowan. Members: E. Douglas James, August E. J. L. Kramer, Arthur M. Sterling, and Peter F. Suhel.

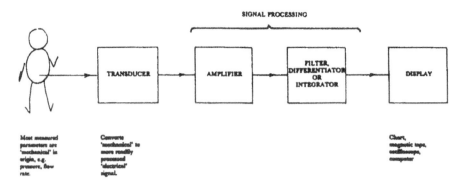

Figure 1   Typical system for measuring physiological parameters

A.   Amplification

The ideal amplifier changes the amplitude of an applied signal without distortion.

B.   Signal Filtration

Signals that change their values relative to time can be described as the sum of a number of components of different frequencies possessing different amplitudes. More rapidly changing signals contain higher frequencies. As examples, the changes that occur in bladder pressure on coughing are much more rapid compared with the slower changes that occur during detrusor activity. Other frequencies, perhaps even higher than those encountered physiologically, may also appear superimposed on the signal in the form of "noise." By limiting the frequency range of the measuring system, it is possible to reproduce signals that can adequately represent the parameter being measured, while at the same time filtering out the noise. To reproduce these rapidly changing signals, an amplifier with a frequency range of DC-15 Hz is required; however, for EMG measurements, this would have to be extended to several kilohertz (kHz).

The principle of filtering can be illustrated by reference to recordings obtained from urine flow rate meters that measure the rate at which urine is collected in an external vessel. Inevitably *mechanical noise* is introduced during this measurement, which subsequently appears as electrical noise. Without adequate filtering the recorded signal could be difficult to interpret (Fig. 2a,b). Excessive filtering not only reduces the noise further, but also prevents the important components of the signal from being recorded. The marked effects of different filters on pressure recordings are shown in Figure 3.

C.   Differentiation

Often the rate of change of a signal relative to time contains more useful information than the original signal. This information can be derived from the original signal by the process of *differentiation*. The most frequently encountered application of differentiation occurs in flow rate meters that measure the volume or mass of urine (Fig. 4a). Following differentiation (see Fig. 4b), the signal represents the volumetric or mass flow rate (see later section on "Flowmeters").

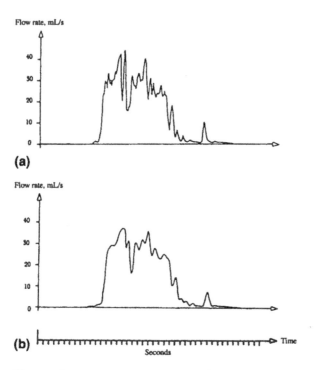

Figure 2 (a) Flow rate recording, including mechanically generated and "other" noise. (b) Following filtering the flow rate recording still contains adequate diagnostic data.

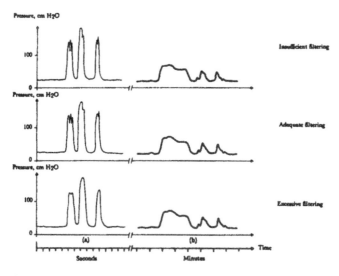

Figure 3 Coughs (rapid pressure changes) and detrusor spasms (slow pressure changes).

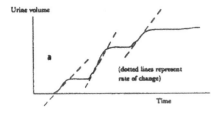

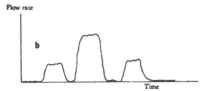

Figure 4   Differentiation: the original signal (a) representing the volume (or mass) of urine when differentiated appears as the flow rate signal (b). Integration: the original signal, now (b), when integrated represents the volume (or mass) of urine voided (a).

D. Integration

Integration, the reverse process of differentiation, is used to produce a signal to represent the area under a curve. For example, the area under the curve (see Fig. 4b) of a direct recording of urine flow rate (see section on "Flowmeters") is equivalent to the total voided volume (see Fig. 4a).

Integrating techniques also find useful application in the processing of EMG signals. In common with differentiators, integrators have characteristics that define the range over which they can be operated.

E. Analog-to-Digital Conversion

Signals representing urodynamic parameters normally appear in a continuous uninterrupted form (analog). The signals can also be approximated by a series of discrete numbers (digital). It is often useful to convert analog signals into digital form for direct presentation of numerical data, such as "the volume of urine voided" or for feeding into a computer for further processing or analysis.

III. PRESSURE TRANSDUCERS: CHARACTERISTICS AND SPECIFICATIONS

A *pressure transducer* is a device that converts an applied pressure into an electrical signal, the magnitude of which is proportional to the pressure. The pressure to be measured, for example that within the bladder, may be transmitted to an external transducer using either an open-ended or sealed, liquid or gas-filled, catheter. Alternatively, the pressure may be measured by a small transducer mounted directly on the catheter. There are four principal types of transducer: resistive (strain gauge), capacitive, inductive, and optoelectronic.

A. Units of Measurement

The SI unit of pressure is the pascal (Pa) although in urodynamics the unit cmH_2O (1 $cmH_2O = 98.07$ Pa) is still used. When parameters that are a function of pressure, for example compliance, are calculated, SI units must be used (1).

B. Important Characteristics and Specifications of Pressure Transducers

1. Pressure Range

A pressure range of 0–300 cmH$_2$O (0–30 kPa) is adequate for pressure measurements in the urinary tract and, in many cases, a range of 0–200 cmH$_2$O (0–20 kPa) is acceptable (for example, in the measurement of intravesical pressure).

2. Sensitivity

The *sensitivity* of a transducer is defined as the change in amplitude of its output signal per unit change in applied pressure. A change in sensitivity with temperature is called *sensitivity drift*. A drift of less than 0.1%/°C is desirable.

C. Linearity and Hysteresis

In an ideal transducer, the electrical output is linearly related to the applied pressure. Non-linearity is specified as a percentage of the pressure range. In addition, the output signal has a slightly different value for a given applied pressure depending on whether this is increasing or decreasing in amplitude. This effect is called *hysteresis*. It is common practice to give a combined figure for linearity and hysteresis in terms of a specified percentage deviation over a stated pressure range. A value of not more than ±1% over the range 0–100 cmH$_2$O (0–10 kPa) is acceptable.

D. Overload Pressure

Transducers can be permanently damaged by applying excess pressure. The maximum pressure that may be applied without affecting the transducer characteristics is called the *overload pressure*. Typical values are in the range of 1500–5000 cmH$_2$O (150–500 kPa). The calibration over the working range should change by less than 1% after the overload pressure is removed.

A pressure above a certain level will destroy a transducer; this is defined as the *damage pressure level*.

Note: In practice it is very easy to exceed the maximum-rated pressure if the transducer chamber is flushed out with a high resistance in the outlet (for example a fine-bore catheter or a closed tap).

E. Zero Offset

All transducers have a small electrical signal output when the applied pressure is atmospheric (or zero in the present context); this is known as the *zero offset signal*. Provided this offset is constant, no errors in measurement will be introduced because the transducer signal conditioner can be adjusted to produce a zero output. The change in the offset signal with temperature, called *zero offset drift*, is more important than the absolute value. A zero offset drift of less than 0.1 cmH$_2$O/°C (10 Pa/°C) is desirable.

F. Zero Reference Level

A transducer is normally calibrated against atmospheric pressure. In urodynamics the zero reference level is taken as the superior edge of the symphysis pubis (2). When a liquid-coupled system is used to measure pressure within the bladder, the transducer is subjected to two sources of hydrostatic pressure, which tend to cancel

1. The pressure arising from the presence of liquid in the catheter.
2. The pressure that is due to the depth of the catheter tip within the volume of urine.

With this type of system, therefore, the measurement of bladder pressure is substantially independent of the location of the tip of the catheter within the bladder. On the other hand, the pressure measured by microtip and sealed gas systems is dependent on the position of the membrane within the bladder.

Detrusor pressure is calculated by electronic subtraction of the abdominal pressure from the intravesical pressure (2). To achieve a good approximation of detrusor pressure, both abdominal and intravesical pressure should be measured with reference to the standardized zero level (superior edge of the symphysis pubis) using liquid-coupled external transducers. However, for studies involving significant patient movement (e.g., ambulatory monitoring) a liquid-filled system is unsuitable, as the zero reference may vary and major artifacts are produced from movement of the liquid in the catheter. In these cases, a qualitative assessment of detrusor pressure can be made using a microtip or sealed gas system.

G. Volume Displacement

The pressure applied to a transducer produces a movement in its diaphragm. The volume change caused by a specified pressure is called the *volume displacement* of the transducer. Typical values are in the range 0.03 mm³/100 cmH₂O–0.003 mm³/100 cmH₂O (0.03 mm³/10 kPa–0.003 mm³/10 kPa). In general, for catheters and transducer chambers filled with similar fluids, the greater the volume displacement for a given applied pressure, the lower the frequency response.

H. Frequency Response

The response of most modern transducers used for physiological purposes is more than adequate when pressure measurements are made at source. However, if the pressure to be measured is transmitted to the transducer by a liquid-filled catheter, then the dynamic characteristics of the system are limited by the dimensions and compliance of the catheter and its connections. Thus, the frequency response decreases as the internal diameter of the catheter decreases and as the length and the compliance of the coupling system increase. Because air is compressible, all air bubbles must be removed from the liquid coupling, otherwise the response will be dampened. The response of a particular system can be measured by coupling it to (1) a hydraulic sinusoidal pressure generator of variable frequency; or (2) a chamber in which the pressure can be very rapidly changed (step response).

The response required depends on the type of investigation. For example, in filling cystometry, a frequency response of typically DC-4 Hz is adequate. On the other hand, when rapid changes of pressure, which occur on coughing or during patient movement, are to be studied, a frequency response of typically DC-15 Hz is desirable.

I. Complete Pressure Measuring System

When transducers are incorporated in complete pressure measuring and display systems, further detrimental effects may be introduced. The effect on the frequency response and any additional drifts introduced by the chart recorder must be specified by the manufacturer.

IV. FLOWMETERS: CHARACTERISTICS AND SPECIFICATIONS

In urodynamic investigations a flowmeter is a device that measures and indicates the quantity of fluid (volume or mass) passed per unit time. Depending on the type of transducer used, either the *flow rate* or the *instantaneous accumulated amount* can be measured. Uroflowmeters normally indicate the *volumetric flow rate*.

A. Units of Measurement

The SI unit for volumetric flow rate is the cubic meter per second (m^3/s) and for mass flow rate is the kilogram per second (kg/s). However, the milliliter (mL) is also an acceptable unit (1), and it is conventional in urodynamic work (2) to report volumetric flow rate in milliliters per second (mL/s). The unit cubic centimeter per second (cm^3/s) should not be used.

B. Conversion of Units

The volumetric flow rate and the accumulated volume are related as follows:
Volumetric flow rate
Q = rate of change of accumulated volume (V) relative to time; i.e.,

$$Q = dV/dt$$

Similarly, accumulated volume
V = integral of the volumetric flow rate (Q) relative to time; i.e.,

$$V = \int^t Q \, dt$$

Conversion between flow rate and accumulated volume is usually performed electronically. The mass and volume of fluid are related as follows:

$$m = \rho V$$

where

m = mass of fluid
ρ = density of fluid
V = volume of fluid

The conversion between mass and volume (or between mass flow rate and volumetric flow rate) can be carried out only if the fluid density is known.
    If a particular flowmeter measures the *accumulated mass of fluid*, the volumetric flow rate is obtained from
Volumetric flow rate

Q = rate of change of accumulated mass (m) relative to time divided by the density (ρ); i.e.,

$$Q = \frac{1 \, dm}{\rho \, dt}$$

The *mass flow rate* is obtained by electronic differentiation. The volumetric flow rate is obtained by dividing the mass flow rate by the fluid density.
    Normally mass flowmeters are calibrated for water. When other liquids are used with densities significantly different from water, in particular a radioopaque medium, the instrument must be recalibrated.

C. Types of Transducer

The most commonly used uroflowmeters employ one of the following methods.

Gravimetric method: these instruments operate by measuring the weight of the collected fluid or by measuring the hydrostatic pressure at the base of the collecting cylinder. In either case, the output signal is proportional to the mass of fluid collected. Gravimetric meters, therefore, measure accumulated mass and mass flow rate is obtained by differentiation.

Electronic dipstick method: in this method the electrical capacitance of a dipstick mounted in the collecting chamber changes as the urine accumulates. The output signal is proportional to the accumulated volume and the volumetric flow rate is obtained by differentiation.

Rotating disk method: the voided fluid is directed on to a rotating disk increasing the inertia of the disk. The power required to keep the disk rotating at a constant rate is measured and is proportional to the mass flow rate of the fluid. The accumulated mass is obtained by integration.

Many other metering techniques are known including electromagnetic, ultrasonic, radioisotope, and drop spectrometry. However, these are not in general use.

D. Characteristics of Flowmeters

1. Static Characteristics

The most important static characteristic of a flowmeter is its accuracy over its usable range.

Zero offset: zero offset is the nonzero output signal of a flowmeter at zero input flow.

Linearity and hysteresis: the output signal of a flowmeter system should ideally be proportional to the input flow. In practice nonlinearity and hysteresis errors are encountered similar to those described in the section on pressure transducers.

Accuracy: the offset should be set to zero and the sensitivity control adjusted during the calibration procedure. The accuracy will then be determined by the nonlinearity and hysteresis.

It is common for manufacturers to state system accuracy only in terms of percentage full-scale error, which can be readily misinterpreted (see section on accuracy).

E. Dynamic Characteristics

Time constant (τ) is a measure of the frequency response of a system. It is defined as the time required for a system to register 63% of its final reading when subjected to a step change in input (Fig. 5). The larger the time constant, the lower the frequency response.

The time constant is increased by filtering, which can be introduced into the system mechanically or electronically. Mechanical filtering occurs primarily at the funnel. The degree of filtering is influenced by funnel design, by the location and angle at which the stream strikes the funnel and by the flow rate. The filtering effect of the funnel cannot be calculated a priori; it must be determined experimentally. Electronic filtering is designed into the system to reduce signal noise. The time constant of the electronics should be stated by the system manufacturer.

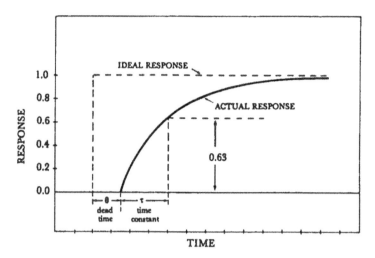

Figure 5 Typical dynamic response of a flowmeter system to a unit step change in input flow.

F. Use of Flowmeter in Pressure–Flow Studies

In many investigations urinary flow rate is measured in conjunction with bladder pressure. If the pressure events in the bladder are to be correlated with variations in the flow rate, the *dead time* between the pressure event and the flow event must be estimated.

   Dead time (θ) is the delay between the exit of the urine from the bladder and its initial registration by the flowmeter (see Fig. 5).

   Several factors contribute to the dead time:

1. The time taken for urine to traverse the urethra
2. The time taken for urine to pass from the external meatus to the flowmeter funnel
3. The time taken for urine to pass via the funnel to the transducer

G. System Specifications

1. Range

A meter with a flow rate range of 0–50 mL/s and a volume range of 0–1000 mL is adequate for clinical use. These ranges will be exceeded only in exceptional cases.

2. Time Constant

The time constant should be as short as possible. For most flowmeters on the market, a time constant of 0.75 s is needed to achieve a reasonable compromise between noise reduction and loss of meaningful temporal information. This time constant should include the contribution of both the funnel and the electronics.

3. Accuracy

For clinical purposes the measured and indicated flow rate should be accurate to within ±5% over the clinically significant flow rate range. Therefore, it is recommended that the calibration curve representing the percentage error over the entire range is made available.

The use of percentage full-scale error should be avoided, as this can be misinterpreted. For example, a flowmeter with a range of 50 mL/s and a quoted accuracy of ±5% full-scale error could have a maximum absolute error of 2.5 mL/s. If this error occurred at a flow rate of 10 mL/s, the percentage error in the measured flow rate would be 25%.

V. EMG MEASUREMENTS

Electromyography (EMG) is the recording of the electrical activity of contracting muscles and so no transducers are required. The electrical signals, however, are so minute that special amplifying techniques are needed. Consideration will be given only to the recording of EMG activity of striated muscles.

The functional contractile unit is the *motor unit*. Each motor unit while contracting has a *firing frequency* ranging from 10 to 100 discharges per second. Normal muscle activity results in the asynchronous contractions of many motor units, leading to an *interference pattern* in the EMG recording. This activity is detected by electrodes inserted into, or placed adjacent to, the muscle.

A. Electrodes

The electrical potential variations in muscle can be sensed either relative to an unchanging reference value (*monopolar approach*) or as the potential difference between two points (*bipolar approach*) in or adjacent to the muscle.

1. Monopolar

The reference value, the potential level of the extracellular fluid, is sensed by an indifferent electrode. This electrode has a greater surface area than the active electrode and is placed remotely from it. The latter may be placed on the skin in the neighborhood of the muscle (*surface electrode*) or in the bulk of the muscle (*tip electrode or coaxial needle electrode*). In the coaxial needle approach, the shaft of the needle acts as the indifferent electrode.

2. Bipolar

Bipolar surface electrodes are widely used in urodynamics; anal plug electrodes, urethral catheter electrodes, and self-adhesive electrodes on the perineum are examples. The bipolar intramuscular approach (*bipolar wire electrodes*) is less popular than the use of the coaxial needle.

B. Types of Recording

Bipolar wire and coaxial needle electrodes have sensing ranges of about 1 mm around the tip of the electrode. They register the sum of the activities of all muscle fibers within this range (*motor unit potentials*). In the sphincteric muscles bi- or triphasic potentials lasting about 7 ms are mostly recorded. The amplitudes of these potentials are dependent on the arrangement of the intermingled fibers from the various motor units relative to the electrode. With increasing contraction the discharge frequency of individual motor units and the number of asynchronously activated motor units increase, leading to a complex record of potential variation known as *interference pattern*. Parameters of this pattern are only qualitatively related to the contraction strength.

Surface electrodes register potential variations from the bulk of the muscle. These electrodes are suitable for assessing the overall behavior of large muscles. Reflex responses, sphincter activity in relation to bladder conditions, and the patient's ability to voluntarily control muscle can be checked adequately by this technique.

C. EMG Amplification

1. Characteristics

To enable the EMG to be adequately displayed, an amplifier with a wide frequency range is required. The amplifier also has special characteristics to reduce signal distortion and electrical noise.

2. Specifications

A good-quality EMG amplifier should have the following specifications:

Input impedance	Minimum of 100 megohms shunted by a maximum of 10 picofarads.
Common mode rejection ratio	Greater than 1000 (80 dB)
Frequency range	Flat characteristic from 10 Hz to 10 kHz
Voltage input range	5 μV–50 mV
Overload recovery time	Less than 100 ms
Output impedance	50 ohms

3. Artifacts

EMG recording is very sensitive to artifacts. These can be minimized by

1. Optimum positioning of electrodes and leads
2. Appropriate preparation of skin when surface electrodes are employed
3. Proper grounding of instrumentation and the use of an isolation amplifier for connection to the patient

4. Processing of EMG Signals

A variety of processing techniques are available to assist in the interpretation of EMG signals. Rectification and smoothing are often used to produce a low-frequency signal that provides information on the timing and relative strength of muscle contraction.

VI. RECORDING AND DISPLAY SYSTEMS

Electrical signals corresponding to physiological parameters can be displayed directly or stored for subsequent examination. This can be achieved in a number of ways.

1. By displaying on a screen of a cathode ray oscilloscope
2. By recording directly on to a paper chart recorder
3. By storing on magnetic tape
4. By digital storage

A. Cathode Ray Oscilloscope

Because this device can faithfully reproduce signals with a high-frequency range, it is often used to display rapidly changing physiological parameters (e.g., EMG). The displayed data can be photographed for permanency or stored for short periods (say minutes) using special *storage oscilloscopes.*

The cathode ray tube is also incorporated in video display units (VDUs) of computers and in image intensifying systems. In the latter a video mixing unit is employed to enable the registration of physiological parameters simultaneously on the same screen (video–pressure–flow–cystourethrography). The combined information can be stored on a *video tape recorder.*

B. Paper Chart Recorders

These are employed in urodynamic investigations to produce continuous visual displays of one or more parameters, usually relative to time. The basic components are

1. An electromechanical device to convert an electrical input signal to mechanical movement.
2. A writing mechanism to produce on paper a visual record of the mechanical movement (pen, ink-jet, or light beam). Recordings may be written in curvilinear or rectilinear form. Depending on the type of recorder, the paper is driven at appropriate selected speeds or held stationary as the writing mechanism operates. The parameters may be recorded relative to time (X–t recorders) or relative to one another (x–y recorders/plotters).

The frequency response of a recorder is particularly important for accurate reproduction of the signal. The following features must be taken into account when selecting a recorder:

a. Number of channels
b. Type of paper, writing principle and recording format
c. Input sensitivity and offset adjustment
d. Chart speed
e. Time and event markers
f. Writing span
g. Trace accuracy
h. Start–stop on front panel or by remote control
i. Power supply (AC or DC).

Most urodynamic signals are unlikely to contain frequency components greater than 15 Hz and can be recorded on almost any of the instruments described. For direct EMG recording, however, pen-type recorders are inadequate.

C. Magnetic Tape Recorders

Signals are stored on magnetic tape for subsequent display, processing, and analysis. Only *instrumentation tape recorders* should be used.

1. Magnetic Tape Recording Techniques

Two recording techniques are employed for analog recording, the most important being *frequency modulation* (FM) and the other the *direct mode.* The former is capable of recording signals with frequency components ranging from DC to several kilohertz. The direct mode covers the frequency range of, typically, 10 Hz–100 kHz.

In urodynamics the FM mode must be used for recording all parameters with the exception of raw EMG signals. These signals are best recorded using the direct mode.

To select a suitable instrumentation tape recorder the following features should be considered:

1. Tape speed range
2. Flutter (tape speed stability) and flutter compensation
3. Maximum input signal
4. Signal-to-noise ratio
5. Number of signal and voice channels.

D. Digital Storage

The discrete data obtained when analog signals are converted to digital form can be stored as follows:

1. On magnetic tape using the technique of *pulse code modulation* (PCM).
2. From a computer on to floppy disk, hard disk or nonvolatile *random access memory* (RAM). These techniques are known as data acquisition.

VII. ELECTRICAL SAFETY ASPECTS

Any electrical equipment used in urodynamic investigations in common with all other medical instrumentation should comply with the recommendations of the International Electrotechnical Commission (3). Prospective users of such equipment should seek advice from a suitably qualified engineer or physicist.

REFERENCES

1. The International System of Units (1973). London: Her Majesty's Stationery Office.
2. Bates P, Bradley WE, Glen E, Griffiths D, Melchior H, Rowan D, Sterling A, Zinner N, Hald T (1979). The standardisation of terminology of lower urinary tract function. J Urol 121:551–554.
3. International Electrotechnical Commission (1977). Safety of Medical Electrical Equipment. Part 1. General Requirements (IEC 601-1, Geneva).

Technical Report: Digital Exchange of Pressure–Flow Study Data

I. INTRODUCTION

To facilitate exchange of digital urodynamic data a standard file format is required. In this document an ICS standard is summarized. Its primary purpose is to enable data from pressure–flow studies to be exchanged. Enough detail is given to allow exchange of other urodynamic data. Extensions may be made as described in Section 5.

II. GENERAL DESCRIPTION OF SIGNAL STORAGE

For each pressure–flow study, urodynamic signals sampled equidistantly with an A/D converter, and other associated information, are stored in one binary MS-DOS-compatible file on a 5.25- or 3.5-in. floppy disk. The stored signals start 10 s before a detectable change in the flow rate signal and continue until 10 s after the flow rate has finally returned to the baseline. Whenever possible, all signals should be stored at the same sample rate. In this case, all signals have the same length (i.e., they contain the same number of bytes).

 The file name and extension are ABCDEFGH.ICS, where ABCDEFGH stands for a unique measurement identification string. In the case of a multicenter study requiring exchange of data, *unique* implies that this string is defined by the coordinating center. In the ICS–BPH study, for instance, this would be a number consisting of (first) three digits for center number, (next) three digits for patient number, and (finally) two digits for identification of successive measurements made on this one patient in one or more sessions.

 The file consists of a number of records of various types. In the ICSMFF proposal on which this document is partly based (see Acknowledgments), 14 different types of records are defined, numbered –1 and 1 to 13. Existing record types may not be modified, but extensions may be implemented by defining new types of record. For ICS purposes, six additional types of record, types 14 to 19, are required, and these are defined in Section 5. In addition, the structures of records of types 8 and 9 are further elaborated in Section 5.

III. VARIABLE VALUES AND TYPES

In this report, actual values for bytes or words may be given in hexadecimal notation as follows: Hex:DD for 8-bit bytes, Hex:DDDD for 16-bit words, and so on, where D stands for a hexadecimal digit.

The following variable types are used in the definitions in the following sections:

byte	:unsigned 8-bit value
word	:unsigned 16-bit value
integer	:signed 16-bit value
dword	:unsigned 32-bit value
string[N]	:N bytes including a terminating Hex:00
word[N]	:N words

IV. GENERAL STRUCTURE OF FILE AND RECORDS

Each file ABCDEFGH.ICS consists of a number of records. The number of records is not predefined. Records may be of different types, containing different kinds of data. For example, a record may contain a description of a urodynamic signal or information about the patient.

Each record starts with a descriptor containing the record type, the size of the data block in bytes, and a checksum. The descriptor is followed by the block containing the actual data (Fig. 1).

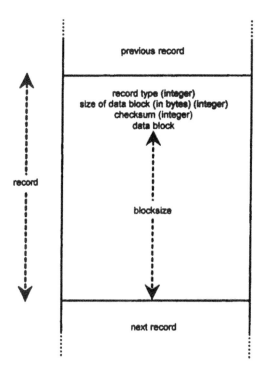

Figure 1   Schematic structure of file and records.

The record type and the block size are integers. The checksum is an integer such that the 16-bit sum of the record type, the data block size, and the checksum is zero.

V. DEFINITIONS OF RECORD TYPES

The record type defines what kind of data is contained by the data block in the record. The only constraint is that the record type is unique.

Backward compatibility is preserved by the requirement that previously defined record types may not be modified. Extensions are implemented by defining new types of record. New types of signal may be implemented by defining new signal IDs, together with signal names and units. Forward compatibility will be ensured if a user does not try to handle unknown types of record or unknown signal IDs.

A register of the types of record in use, and a register of signal IDs, signal names, and signal units, will be administered centrally by the ICS. This standard contains initial versions of the registers. Proposed extensions should be communicated to the ICS for registration.

A. Default Values

Empty fields are not permitted. Occasionally, the value for a certain field may not be available. In this case a default value should be stored (see later).

B. Signal ID (See Sec. 9: Addendum)

The following sections describe the types of record needed to implement this ICS standard. Other types are described in the document ICS Measure File Format (ICSMFF) version 1.00, dated 14.10.93 (see Acknowledgments).

VI. RECORD TYPE 8: THE MEASUREMENT MARKER RECORD

This type of record defines a marker within the measurement and an associated comment.

Record type:	8	:integer
Blocksize:	$1 + N + 1 + 4 + M$	:integer
Checksum:	$-(8 + blocksize)$	:integer
Data block:	marker type	:byte
	name	:string[N]
	signal id	:byte
	position	:dword
	comment	:string[M]

The following information should be stored in these fields:
In the field:

marker type	0 = default value
	(other types are defined in the ICSMFF document)
name	empty string as default value
	(empty string contains only the terminating Hex:00, so that $N = 1$)
signal id	as in Sec. 9: Addendum

position   the number of the sample (16-bit word) with which the marker and
                       comment are associated
comment   the comment string, terminated with Hex:00

VII.   RECORD TYPE 9: THE MEASUREMENT COMMENT RECORD

This record stores a comment. For the ICS standard it should be used to identify the patient
and the type of the measurement.

Record type: 9   :integer
Blocksize: N   :integer
Checksum: –(9 + blocksize)   :integer
Data block: measurement comment   :string[N]

The following information should be stored:

In the field:

measurement comment a free-format string, terminated with Hex:00, that uniquely identifies
                       patient and measurement for the originating center. This string would include
                       not only a patient ID (e.g., from the local hospital information system), but
                       also the relation of this measurement to a particular research study (e.g.,
                       "post-TURP investigation"). For use in a specific multicenter study, this string
                       can be specified more strictly.

VIII.   RECORD TYPE 14: THE ICS SIGNAL PROPERTY RECORD

This record type describes the properties of one stored signal, including its name, the unit
of measurement, the zero and full-scale values, and the sample rate (which, if possible,
should be identical for all signals).

Record type: 14   :integer
Blocksize: $1 + N + M + 3 * 2 + 4$:integer
Checksum: –(14 + blocksize)   :integer
Data block: signal id   :byte
    signal name   :string [N]
    unit   :string [M]
    binzero   :integer
    binsize   :word
    fullscale   :integer
    sample rate   :dword

The following information should be stored in these fields:

In the field:
signal id   as specified in Section 9: Addendum
signal name   as specified in Section 9: Addendum
unit   as specified in Section 9: Addendum
binzero   the signal value represented in the data samples field of record type
                   18 by the word 0
binsize   the full scale binary sample value
fullscale   the signal value represented in the data samples field of record type
                   18 by the full scale binary value

sample rate	sample rate specification in samples/s (Hz). The sample rate is in 16.16 format: i.e., it is a long integer, where bits 16 through 31 specify the integer part of a fixed point number and bits 0 through 15 specify the decimal part.

The following values are recommended:

—Sample rate at least 10 samples per second
—Pressure signals bipolar up to +200 cmH$_2$O with a minimum resolution of 0.5 cmH$_2$O/bit
—flow rate signal unipolar up to 50 mL/s with a minimum resolution of 0.05 mL/s/bit

Example showing how sample rate is to be specified: Suppose the rate of sampling is 512.5 Hz. Then the value to be stored in the field sample rate is the 16.16 value Hex:02008000 = 512.5 * Hex: 10000.

Example showing how binzero, binsize, and fullscale are to be used: Suppose the abdominal pressure is sampled bipolarly with a 10-bit A/D converter. Then the binary value will range from 0 to 1023. Suppose the A/D converter is configured so that this range represents the pressure range from –50 to 200 cm H$_2$O. Then the three values to be stored are:

binzero = –50
binsize = 1023
fullscale = 200

IX. RECORD TYPE 15: THE ICS PATIENT DATA RECORD

This record type contains the basic demographic data of the patient. It contains the actual text and numerical fields, plus an index table to facilitate location of a particular field. The index gives the relative position within the data block.

Record type:	15	:integer
Blocksize:	17*2+N+M+O+P+Q+R+S+T+U+V+W+X+Y+3+2	:integer
Checksum:	–(15 + blocksize)	:integer
Data block:	surname index	:word
	first name index	:word
	maiden name index	:word
	ID index	:word
	street index	:word
	housenumber index	:word
	city index	:word
	country index	:word
	postcode index	:word
	phone index	:word
	height index	:word
	weight index	:word
	sex index	:word
	comments index	:word
	birth day index	:word
	birth month index	:word
	birth year index	:word

surname	:string[N]
first name	:string[M]
maiden name	:string [O]
ID	:string[P]
street	:string[Q]
housenumber	:string[R]
city	:string[S]
country	:string[T]
postcode	:string[U]
phone	:string[V]
height	:string[W]
weight	:string[X]
comments	:string[Y]
sex	:byte*
birth day	:byte
birth month	:byte
birth year	:word[†]

*0 = male, 1 = female
[†] Birth year is expressed in full, e.g., 1895, 1995, 2005

The first name field may contain a middle or other initial in addition to the first name.

As a default, an empty string (containing only Hex:00) may be stored in any of the string fields for which information is not available or may not be disclosed because of ethical considerations. In this case the length (N, M, etc.) of the string is 1.

The index fields contain the position (in bytes) of the corresponding text or numerical field, relative to the start of the data block. Thus the value to be stored in surname index is 17 * 2; the value to be stored in first name index is 17 * 2 + N; and so on. All the index fields must be completed.

X.   RECORD TYPE 16: THE ICS SOURCE RECORD

This record type specifies the origin of the measurement. It consists of an index table together with the actual text fields.

Record type:	16	:integer
Blocksize:	10*2+N+M+O+P+Q+R+S+T+U+V	:integer
Checksum:	–(16 + blocksize)	:integer
Data block:	clinic name index	:word
	investigator name index	:word
	street index	:word
	streetnumber index	:word
	city index	:word
	country index	:word
	postcode index	:word
	phone index	:word
	fax index	:word
	comments index	:word
	clinic name	:string[N]

investigator name	:string[M]
street	:string[O]
streetnumber	:string[P]
city	:string[Q]
country	:string[R]
postcode	:string[S]
phone	:string[T]
fax	:string[U]
comments	:string[V]

The phone and fax fields should include area codes as well as local numbers.

An empty string may be stored in any of the string fields for which information is not available. In this case the length (N, M, etc.) of the string is 1.

The index fields contain the position (in bytes) of the corresponding text field, relative to the start of the data block. All the index fields must be completed.

XI. RECORD TYPE 17: ICS VOLUME RECORD

This record contains the filling volume and the residual volume.

Record type:	17	:integer
Blocksize:	4	:integer
Checksum:	−(17 + blocksize)	:integer
Data block:	filling volume	:integer
	residual volume	:integer

The following information should be stored:

In the field:

| filling volume | the calculated volume in the bladder at the beginning of the pressure–flow study (in mL). −1 = default value |
| residual volume | the volume in the bladder at the end of the study, either calculated or measured directly (in mL); if the calculated volume is negative the value zero should be stored. −1 = default value |

XII. RECORD TYPE 18: THE ICS SIGNAL VALUE RECORD

The ICS signal value record contains the actual data samples for one of the urodynamic signals. It includes a record number, allowing a signal that is too long to fit into one record to be divided such as to span several records. If the signal spans more than one record, the number of the first record should be 1 and the following records should be numbered 2, 3, and so on. If there is only one record, its record number should be 0.

Record type:	18	:integer
Blocksize:	2 + N * 2	:integer
Checksum:	−(18 + blocksize)	:integer
Data block:	signal id	:byte
record number	:byte	
data samples	:word[N]	

The following information should be stored in these fields:

In the field:

signal id   as specified in Section 9: Addendum
record number   as described above
data samples   the binary samples themselves,
                       1 word = 2 bytes = 1 sample,
                       stored in the order low byte, high byte

XIII.   RECORD TYPE 19: THE ICS MEASUREMENT DESCRIPTION RECORD

This record indicates that the file is an ICS standard file and describes the measurement's start date and time, the number of signals stored, and the number of records in the file.

Record type:		:integer
Blocksize:	1 + N + 5 + 1 + 2	:integer
Checksum:	–(19 + blocksize)	:integer
Data block:	measurement type	:byte
	name	:string[N]
	start: minute	:byte
	hour	:byte
	day	:byte
	month	:byte
	year	:byte*
	number of signals	:byte
	number of records	:word

*year is expressed modulo 100; e.g., 1995 = 95, 2005 = 05.

The following information should be stored in these fields:

In the field:

measurement type   the version number of this document, multiplied by 10 (e.g.,
                     for this version 71). Note that the version number may not
                     contain hundredths or smaller decimal fractions
name   the string "ICS standard pressure–flow study"
start   the start time and date of the measurement (if any of these are
                     unavailable, the default value Hex:00 should be stored in
                     the corresponding position: minute, hour, day, month and/or
                     year)
number of signals   the number of signals stored in this file (e.g., 3 if just intraves-
                     ical pressure, abdominal pressure, and flow rate are stored).
number of records   the total number of records stored in this file (including this
                     measurement description record)

XIV.   SIGNALS AND INFORMATION TO BE STORED:
MINIMAL SPECIFICATION AND OPTIONAL EXTENSIONS

Minimally, the following three signals should be stored in three records of type 18:

Intravesical pressure
Abdominal pressure
Flow rate

For each signal, certain associated information should be stored in a record of type 14.

Optionally, the following signals can also be stored in records of type 18, with associated information in records of type 14:

EMG envelope
Voided volume

The voided volume signal may be useful if this is the signal measured by the urodynamic system, and the flow signal is derived from it.

In addition to the signals, further information about the patient and the measurements should be stored in records of types 16, 17, and 19. Full demographic data for the patient can be stored in a record of type 15. Optionally, a free format comment can be stored in a record of type 9, and if detailed comments relating to events during the measurement are available, they can be stored in records of type 8.

XV. TYPICAL FILE STRUCTURE

Of the various record types, some are mandatory and some are optional. The structure of the file describing a particular measurement varies according to what records are stored.

The order of the records within the file is arbitrary, in principle. However, it may be convenient to place records containing easily recognizable strings near the beginning, so that the file can quickly be identified if it is accidentally renamed or misplaced. In particular, record type 19 should preferably be the first one.

Thus a typical file structure might be:

RECORD TYPE 19: ICS MEASUREMENT DESCRIPTION RECORD (identifies file as an ICS standard file)

RECORD TYPE 16: ICS SOURCE RECORD (identifies originating clinic and investigator)

RECORD TYPE 9: MEASUREMENT COMMENT RECORD (identifies patient and type of measurement)

    OPTIONALLY, RECORD TYPE 15: ICS PATIENT DATA RECORD (contains full demographic data for patient)

RECORD TYPE 14: ICS SIGNAL PROPERTY RECORD (describes properties of intravesical pressure signal)

RECORD TYPE 14: ICS SIGNAL PROPERTY RECORD (describers properties of abdominal pressure signal)

RECORD TYPE 14: ICS SIGNAL PROPERTY RECORD (describes properties of flow rate signal)

    OPTIONALLY, further records of type 14 for voided volume and EMG envelope

RECORD TYPE 18: ICS SIGNAL VALUE RECORD (contains actual intravesical pressure data)

RECORD TYPE 18: ICS SIGNAL VALUE RECORD (contains actual abdominal pressure data)

RECORD TYPE 18: ICS SIGNAL VALUE RECORD (contains actual flow rate data)

    OPTIONALLY, further records of type 18 for voided volume and EMG envelope

    OPTIONALLY, RECORD TYPE 8: MEASUREMENT MARKER RECORD

(identifies position and type of marker in data, the signal with which it is associated, and a comment)

OPTIONALLY, further records of type 8 with additional markers

RECORD TYPE 17: ICS VOLUME RECORD (contains filling volume before pressure–flow study and residual urine volume after voiding)

XVI. ACKNOWLEDGMENTS

This proposal is based partly on the ICS Measure File Format (ICSMFF) version 1.00 of 14.10.93, which was written by Michael Gondy Jensen, formerly of the Wiest Company and now of Andromeda Medical Systems, and also on an earlier proposal for a simple digital pressure–flow standard circulated by Ron van Mastrigt. Dantec Medical, Laborie Medical Technologies, Life-Tech, and Andromeda Medical Systems have agreed in principle to support a standard similar to the ICSMFF. The Life-Tech Company has agreed to support the approved ICS standard.

XVII. ADDENDUM: SIGNAL IDs

In records of types 8, 14, and 18, a signal ID of the type byte is specified. Corresponding signal names and units of the type string are required in record type 14. The following signal ID values, signal names, and units have been defined.

	Signal ID	Signal name	Unit
For intravesical pressure	1	"pves"	"cmH$_2$O"
For abdominal pressure	2	"pabd"	"cmH$_2$O"
For flow rate	3	"Q"	"mL/s"
For EMG envelope	4	"EMGenv"	"uV"
For voided volume	5	"Vvoid"	"mL"

The following are reserved for possible future use:

	Signal ID	Signal name	Unit
for p_{det} acquired independently	6	"pdet"	"cmH$_2$O"
For infused volume	7	"Vinf"	"mL"
For direct EMG signal	8	"EMG"	"uV"
For urethral pressure	9	"pura"	"cmH$_2$O"
For urethral closure pressure	10	"pclos"	"cmH$_2$O"

Additional signal IDs, signal names, and units may be introduced; proposed additions should be communicated to the ICS for registration.

Index

*Numbers in **bold** refer to ICS reports.*

Abrams–Griffiths, nomogram of, 324, 325
ACE inhibitor, 235
Acetylcholine (ACh), 10, 59, 62, 64, 208
  receptor, 682
    extrajunctional, 682
ACh (*see* Acetylcholine)
Actomyosin ATPase, 73
Acupuncture, 681
A-delta fibers, 93, 208, 545
Adenosine triphosphate (ATP), 59
Adenylate cyclase, 52, 55
Adrenoreceptors, 53, 55
Aging, 198–199
Alcock's canal, 543
α-adrenergic agonists, 489–490, 611, 653
  side effects of, 489
α-adrenergic blockers, 484, 485–486, 681
α-adrenoreceptor, 489
  supersensitivity of, 484
α-motoneuron, 75
α-motor fibers, 541
α-receptors
  central, 485
  urethral, 490
α-sarcomeric actin, 7
α-smooth muscle actin, 6, 7
α_1–receptors, 485
Alfuzosin, 485
Ambulatory urodynamics (*see* Urodynamics, ambulatory)
Anal plug, 682
Anal sphincter, 423, 541
  3–D imaging of, 391

Anaphylactic reaction, voiding cystourethrography and, 408
Anorectal manometrics, (*see* Bowel manometrics)
Antibiotics, preoperative, 629
Antibiotics, prophylactic regimen, 479, 480
Antibiotic-treated synthetic slings, 622
Anticholinergics, 137, 669
Antigenicity, tissue, 638
Anti-incontinence devices (*see also* Stress urinary incontinence), 471, 535–539
Anxiety, 680
Arcus tendineus, 18, 19, 20, 72, 111, 112, 117, 118, 195, 236, 256, 589
Arnold-Chiari, malformation of, 135
Artificial urinary sphincter (*see* Urinary sphincter, artificial)
ATP (*see* Adenosine-triphosphate)
ATPase (*see* Adenosine-triphosphatase)
ATPase, 73
Auerbach's plexus, 157
AUS (*see* Urinary sphincter, artificial)
Autologous fascia, 645–646
Autologous fat, 501–502
  complications of, 506
  contraindications for, 508
  graft survival of, 502
Autonomic dysreflexia, 227, 228, 566, 568, 570, 574, 577, 676

Baclofen, 488, 669
  intrathecal, 488, 669, 676
  side effects of, 488

Barrington's micturition center, 79, 80, 82
Barrington's nucleus, 91, 224
Bashful bladder syndrome (*see* Shy bladder)
Behavioral modification (*see also* Lifestyle interventions), **721–722**
Bellows motion, 203, 211
Benign prostatic enlargement (BPE), **808**
Benign prostatic hyperplasia (BPH), 32, 34,
    36, 160, 289, **808**
Benign prostatic obstruction (BPO), **808**
Benzodiazepines, 486–487
    side effects of, 487
β-adrenergic agonists, 487
β-adrenergic blockers, 235
β-adrenergic receptor, activation of, 544
β-adrenoreceptors, 489
Bethanechol, 12
Biofeedback, 77, 162, 449, 463–467, 647,
    679–680, **720–721**
Birth trauma, 498
Bladder, function during storage, **712–713**
    normal, **712**
    overactive, **712**
        hyperreflexic, **712**
        unstable, **712**
    sensation, **712–713**
Bladder (*see also* Detrusor)
    areflexic, 530
    augmentation, 138, 139, 140, 306, 478,
        480, 522, 528, 647, **743**
    auto-augmentation, 140, 671
    cancer, 316, 681
    capacity, 566
        Houle's formula, 144
        Koff's formula, 144
        maximum, measurement of, **771**
    compliance, 313, 315, 317, 522, 530, 555,
        611
        dynamic, 318
        static, 318
        bladder outlet obstruction and, 661–
            662
    contractility, bladder obstruction and,
        661–662
    diverticuli, 408, 477, 479, 522
    expression of, **727**
    extrophy, 137–138
    female, anatomy of, functional (*see also*
        Urethra, female, anatomy of, functional), 15–23
    hyperreflexic, 158, 530
        low pressure, **778**
        high pressure, **778**

[Bladder]
    hypersensitive, 315
    hypertonic, 158
    hyposensitive, 315
    lazy, 159, 251
    neurogenic (*see* Neurogenic bladder)
    nonneurogenic neurogenic (*see* Hinman's
        syndrome)
    overactive, pelvic floor overactivity and,
        548–549
    overworked, 317
    reflex triggering of, 727
    stone, 316, 477, 480, 521, 637, 681
    substitution, 743
    trabeculation, 36, 242, 408, 409, 477, 479
    training, 471
    transection, 670
    tumor, 637
    uninhibited contractions, 136, 137, 145,
        213, 252, 363, 366, 478, 522, 535, 549
    unstable, (*see* Bladder, uninhibited contractions)
Bladder diary (*see* Voiding diary)
Bladder neck, 358, 360, 363, 364, 368, 683
        (*see also* Urethrovesical junction)
    cuff placement around, 524–526
        suprapubic approach, 524–526
        transvaginal approach, 526
    endoscopic incision of, 484, 676
    hypermobility of, 583
    incompetence of, 367–368, 377, 385, 390
    intravaginal device and, 537–538
    narrowing of, 607
    obstruction of, 566 (*see also* Obstruction,
        bladder outlet)
    opacification of, 392–394
    position of, 408–409
    primary obstruction of, 186
    surgical reconstruction of, 605–613
        indications for, 610–612
        results of, 612–613
        types of, 605–609
    suspension (*see also* Sling surgery)
        bone anchors, 597–598
        laparoscopic, 596–597
        retropubic, 586–593
Bladder outlet obstruction (BOO) (*see* Obstruction, bladder outlet)
BMI (*see* Body mass index)
BNS (*see* Bladder neck suspension)
Body mass index (BMI), 437
Bolognese Symptom Questionnaire for BPH,
    810

Bombesin, 10
Bone anchors, 622–623, 641
   bladder neck suspension with, 597–598
BOO (*see* Obstruction, bladder outlet)
Booney's test. 256, 537
Bothersomeness, **810**
Botulinum Toxin A (BTX), 487–488, 676, 682
Bowel manometrics, 149–152, 155
Boyarsky score, **810**
BPE, (*see* Benign prostatic enlargement)
BPH (*see* Benign prostatic hyperplasia)
BPO (*see* Benign prostatic obstruction)
Brain stem, 79, 82, 206, 135, 227
   L-region, 206
   M-region, 206
Brain tumor, 315
BTX (*see* Botulinum toxin A)
Bulking agents, injection of (*see* Stress uri-
      nary incontinence, urethral injection
      and)
Burch, procedure of, 236, 587–588
   goal of, 587–588
   technique of, 588
   results of, 587

C- fibers, 93, 204, 208, 209, 669
Cadaveric fascia, 638
Cadaveric fascia lata, 646–647
Cadaveric prolapse repair and sling (CaPS),
      637
Cadaveric transvaginal sling (CaTS), 636,
      646
Calcitonin gene-related peptide, 9, 10, 208
CaPS (*see* Cadaveric prolapse repair and
      sling)
Capsaicin, 63
   intraurethral, 485
Carcinoma, endometrial, 491
Carcinoma, urethral, 416
Catecholamines, 490
Catheter, indwelling, **726–727, 766**
Catheterization, clean intermittent, 136, 137,
      140, 161, 475–481, 510, 522, 608,
      624, 676, 681, **726, 766**
   artificial urinary sphincter and, 477
   bladder outlet obstruction and, 476
   candidates for, 476–477
   candidates, evaluation of, 477–478
   catheter size and, 478
   complications of, 479–481
      calculi, bladder, 480
      epididymitis, 481
      infection, 480

[Catheterization]
      renal deterioration, 480
      trauma, urethral, 480
   cystourethroscopy and, 479
   follow-up, 479
   neurogenic bladder and, 476
   noncandidates for, 477
   preoperative, 476
   technique of, 478–479
Catheterization, intermittent self-, **766**
Catheterization, sterile intermittent, **766**
Cathode ray oscilloscope, **836–837**
CaTS (*see* Cadaveric transvaginal sling)
Cerebral atrophy, 315
Cerebral palsy, 137
Cerebral peduncles, 224
Cerebrovascular accident (CVA), 187, 195,
      247, 315, 544, 636
Cervicoplasty, 605
C-fos-immunoreactive cells, 209
Chain cystogram, 358
Chainette, 360
CIC (*see* Catheterization, clean intermittent)
Clamp motion, 203, 211
Clean intermittent catheterization (CIC)
      (*see* Catheterization, clean intermit-
      tent)
Clinical history (*see* History, clinical)
Cloaca, 140
Clonidine, 485, 679
   urethral pressure profile and, 484
Clostridium botulinum, 682
CMG (*see* Cystometrogram)
Collagen, 120
Collagen hypersensitivity, 499, 502
Collagen injection, intraurethral, 416
   complications of, 503
   contraindications for, 499
   detrusor instability and, 503
Colpocystography, 360
Colposacropexy, 238
Compliance, bladder, 313, 315, 317, 522, 530,
      555, 611
   dynamic, 318
   static, 318
Computed tomography, **737**
Condom catheter, 565, 566
Cone exercises, 449
Connexin, 50
Constipation, 137, 153, 154–157, 235, 252,
      440
   causes of, 155
   definition of, 154–155

[Constipation]
  diagnosis of, 155
  evaluation of, 155
  stress urinary incontinence and, 440
  therapy of, 156–157
Continence, electrical stimulation and, **725**
Continence, neural control of (*see* Micturition,
    neural control of)
Continence, posture evolution and, 106–107
Continence zones, 183
Contrast material, ultrasonographic, 358, 392
Contrast radiography, **737**
Corpus spongiosum, 32, 34
Corticospinal tracts, 77, 224
Cowper's gland, 134
Creatinine, nadir, 140
Crédé maneuver, 484, 676
Cryptorchidism, 141
CVA (*see* Cerebrovascular accident)
Cystocele (*see* Cystourethrocele)
Cystometrogram (CMG), 142–148, 213, 313,
    314, 315, 316, **696–698, 769, 772,**
    775, 802, 822
Cystourethrocele, 223–235
  classification of, 253–254
    Baden-Walker's, 253
    gynaecological, 253
    ICS, 254, 255
    urological, 253
  radiographic grading of, 409–410
Cystourethroscopy, 521, 587, 592, 599, 629,
    637, 640, **812**
Cytology, urine, 236

Dandrolene sodium, 487
  side effects of, 487
Danish Prostatic Symptom Score (DAN-PSS),
    810
DAN-PSS (see Danish Prostatic Symptom
    Score)
Data handling, 339–340
Data quality, 339
Defecation, electrical stimulation and, **725**
Dementia, 247
Denonvillier's fascia, 117
DESD (*see* Detrusor-external sphincter
    dyssynergia)
Detrusor activity index, 353
Detrusor-external sphincter dyssynergia
    (DESD), 136, 137, 146, 186, 196,
    223–229, 306, 319, 322, 330 360,
    661

[Detrusor-external sphincter dyssynergia
    (DESD)]
  clinical features of, 226
  complications of, 228
  definition of, 223–224
  etiology of, 226–227
    neurological, 227
    nonneurological, 227
  evaluation of, 228–229
  pathophysiology of, 226
  physiology of, 224–226
  treatment, 486–489, 565–566, 574, 580,
    661
  types of, 226
Detrusor-internal sphincter dyssynergia
    (DISD), 226, 661
Detrusor sphincter dyssynergia (DSD) (*see*
    Detrusor-external sphincter dyssyner-
    gia)
Detrusor, function during voiding, **714–715**
Detrusor, (*see also* Bladder)
  acontractile, **760**
  areflexia, 136
  compliance of, 228
  contractility, micturition and, 760–761
  decompensation, 36
  EMG of, 428
  estrogen deficiency, 316
  hyperreflexia, 36, 136, 187, 315, 316, 565
  hypertrophy, 145
  hyporeflexia, 36
  impared contractility, 322, 324
  instability, 112, 238, 241, 243, 315, 316,
    549, 584, 637
    collagen injection and, 503, 508
    de novo, 625, 637, 647
    symptoms, triad of, 242
  motor-evoked potentials of (MEPs), 429,
    433
  muscle, 36
  normal, **760–761**
  normal aging, 316
  overactivity, 340, 637, 662
  overstretched, 288
  physiology, 57–62
    after-hyperpolarization, 59
    electromechanical coupling, 60–61
    excitatory innervation, 58–59
    ion channels, 59–60
    passive membrane properties, 57–58
    pharmacomechanical coupling, 60–61
    smooth muscle relaxation, 61–62

[Detrusor]
    spontaneous activity, 58
    trabeculation, 36, 242, 408, 409, 477, 479
    underactive, **760**
    uninhibited contractions (*see also* Detrusor,
        instability), 136, 137, 145, 213, 252,
        363, 366, 671
Diabetes mellitus, 247, 476
Diaphragm, contraceptive, 537
Diaphragma urogenitale (*see also* Pelvic di-
    aphragm), 25
Diazepam, 486, 679
Diencephalon, 225
Digital rectal examination (DRE), 205, 210,
    211, 235, 253, 680
    distal sphincter mechanism, 29
Digital storage, **838**
DISD (*see* Detrusor–internal sphincter
    dyssynergia)
Distal urethral electrical conductance
    (DUEC), 277, 393
Diverticuli
    bladder, 408, 477, 479, 522
    urethral, 360, 386, 408
        saddle bag, 417
Dopamine β-hydroxylase, 10
Dorsal pontine reticular formation (DPRF),
    206
Doxapin, 161
Doxazosin, 484, 675
DPRF (*see* Dorsal pontine reticular formation)
DRE (*see* Digital rectal examination)
DSD (*see* Detrusor–external sphincter
    dyssynergia)
DUEC (*see* Distal urethral electrical conduc-
    tance)
Duhamel's procedure, 157
Dysfunction, sexual, 243
Dysfunctional elimination syndromes, 159
Dysfunctional voiding, 661, 675
Dyspareunia, 624
Dysraphism, occult, 252
Dyssynergia, detrusor–external sphincter (*see*
    Detrusor–external sphincter dyssyner-
    gia (DESD))
Dyssynergia, detrusor–internal sphincter (*see*
    Detrusor–internal sphincter dyssyner-
    gia (DISD))

Edvardsen's reflex, 544
Ejaculation, electrical stimulation and, **725**
EJPs (*see* Excitatory junction potentials)

Elastin, 120, 195
Electric conductance, 303
Electrical stimulation, 22, 467–469, **722–725**
    in children, 161
    parameters of, 468–469
Electrodes, **835**
    concentric needle, 424
    external patch, 146
    intraluminal rectal, 38
    intraurethral, 38, 424, 428
    single-fiber needle, 424
    surface, 320, 424, 464
    temporary, 684
Electromyography (EMG), 37, 122, 146, 213,
        225, 227, 228, 313, 320, 322, 386,
        705–707, 738, 770, 773, 774, 776, 803
    corpus cavernosum, 427–428, 434
    detrusor muscle, 428
    integrated, 424
    measurements, **835–836**
    urethral striated sphincter, 545, 549
    urodynamics and, 424
Electrophysiology, 423–434
    autonomic pathways, 427–434
        electromyography, 427–428
        evaluation of, 432–434
        evoked potentials, 428–429
        sacral reflexes, 430–431
    somatic pathways, 423–426
        evaluation of, 432
        evoked potentials, 424–426
        sacral reflexes, 426
        urethral sphincter, EMG of, 423–424
Embryogenesis, urinary sphincter, 1–13
EMG (*see* Electromyography)
Emotional motor system, 94–95
Encopresis, 154–157 (*see also* Constipation)
    definition of 155
Endopelvic fascia, 18, 72, 111, 117, 120, 195,
        589, 618, 626, 628
Enterocele, 235, 592
Enterocystometry, **745–747**
Enterocystoplasty, 611, 671–673, **743**
Enuresis, noctural, 157–158, 227, 245, 490,
        714
    causes, 157
Ephedrine, 489
Epididymo-orchitis, 573
Epispadias-extrophy complex, 510, 605, 610,
        611
Erectile dysfunction, 572
Erection, electrical stimulation and, **725**

Erosion, urethral, 524, 529, 531, 625–630
Estrogen, deficiency in, 198, 199, 316
Estrogen receptors, 123
Estrogen rings, vaginal, 491
Estrogens, 490–491, 498
Evoked potentials, 213, 424–426, **709–710**
    afferent pathways of, 424–425
        pudendal somatosensory, 424–425, 432
        urinary somatosensory, 428–429, 433
    auditory, 227
    cortical, 227
    efferent pathways of, 425–426
        pudendal motor, 425–426, 432
        sweat glands, 429
    somesthesic, 227
    visual, 227
Evolutionary biology, 101
Evolutionary trade-offs, 102
Examination, physical, 210–213, 235–238,
        251–259, 357, 459–460, 479, 498,
        521, 568, 574, 636–637, 652, **696,
        736, 744, 768–769, 730**
Excitatory junction potentials (EJPs), 52
External urethral meatus, 18
Extrophy, bladder, 137–138
Extrophy-epispadias complex (*see* Epispa-
        dias-extrophy complex)

Falck-Hillarp technique, 10
Fascia lata, 637, 638, 648
Fascial sling, 654
    placement of, 639–641
        abdominal and transvaginal, 639–640
        transabdominal, 639
        transvaginal (CaTS), 640–641
Fast-fatiguable striated muscle, 72
Fast-fatigue–resistant striated muscle, 72, 81
Fast-twitch fibers, 2, 20, 37, 72, 113, 447, 487
Female adult, outcome studies in, 800–806
FF (*see* Fast-fatiguable striated muscle)
FFR (*see* Fast fatigue-resistant striated mus-
        cle)
Fibril, 120
Fistula
    urethrocutaneous, 573
    urethrovaginal, 410–411
    vesicovaginal, 410–411, 625
Flap-valve mechanism, 608
Flow delay, **756**
Flow rate, urinary (*see* Uroflow)
Flowmeters, 285, **831–835**
Flow-rate-controling zone, 327

Fluid bridge test, 366
Fluoroscopy, pelvic floor, dynamic, 236
Folic acid, 135
Foramen, sacral, 684
Fourier transformation, 228
Fowler syndrome, 545
Frail older people, outcome studies in,
        817–824
Frequency chart, 262
Frequency-severity chart, 262
Frequency-urgency syndrome, 372, 379, 390
Frequency-volume chart (*see* Voiding diary)
Functional electrical stimulation, pelvic floor,
        674–675
Functional urethral length, 184, 546, 547
Fura-2, 47

G protein, 52, 55, 61
GABA (*see* γ-aminobutyric acid)
GABA interneurons, 91
γ-aminobutyric acid (GABA), 486, 488
    interneurons, 91
Gamma radiation, 638
Gating distractions, 107
    negative gating, 107
Gittes, procedure of, 594
Glutaraldehyde cross-linked collagen,
        502–503, 503–508
    disadvantages of, 502
Gore-Tex patch, 619
    vaginal placement of, 626–630
Gracile nucleus, 224
Graciloplasty, 560
Guanylate cyclase, 52
Guarding reflex, 77, 424

Hammock theory, 20, 112, 195, 236
Hammock, vaginal, 378
Health-related quality of life (HRQOL), **805,**
        823
Heritage legacy, 102
Herniated disc disease, 187, 247
Hinman's syndrome, 153–154, 159, 186, 251,
        486
Hirschprung's disease, 155
History, clinical, 210, 235–238, 241–248, 521,
        568, 574, 636, 651–652, **696, 744,
        764–768**
HIV, transmission of, 646
Hormonal replacement therapy (HRT),
        176–178
HRQOL (*see* Health-related quality of life)

HRT (*see* Hormonal replacement therapy)
Hydronephrosis, 224, 227, 228, 478, 565, 570, 575
Hyperalgesia, 204
Hypermobility, urethra, 256, 503, 626
    central protusion, 256
    lateral detachment, 256
    type II, 626
Hypothalamus, 79, 224
    paraventricular nucleus, of, 205

Ice water test, 229, 669
ICIDH (*see* International Classification of Impairment, Disability and Handicap)
ICS (*see* International Continence Society)
ICSmale Questionnaire, **810**
ICS nomogram, 328–329
IIQ (*see* Incontinence Impact Questionnaire)
IJPs (*see* Inhibitory junction potentials)
Imipramine, 161, 490
    side effects of, 490
Incontinence Impact Questionnaire (IIQ), 652
Infection, artificial urinary sphincter, 530–531
Inferior colliculus, 225
Inflammation, neural, 209
Inhibitory junction potentials (IJPs), 52
Integral theory, 21, 195, 599, 623
Intermittent catheterization, (*see* Catheterization, clean intermittent)
Internal capsule, 224
Internal pulse generator (IPG), 547
Internal sphincter, histology of, 7
International Classification of Impairment, Disability and Handicap (ICIDH), 445
International Prostate Symptom Score (I-PSS), **809**
Interval test, 277
Intestinal reservoirs, **742–753**
    assessment of, **743–745**
    evacuation, evaluation of, **750**
    storage dysfunction, classification of, **750–753**
        outlet dysfunction, **753**
        reservoir dysfunction, **751–753**
    storage, evaluation of, **745–749**
        enterocystometry, **745–747**
        outlet pressure, measurement of, **747–749**
        urine loss, quantification of, **749**
    surgical procedures, terminology of, **743**

Intinsic sphincter deficiency, treatment in female, 654–657
    devices, 654
    injectables, 655–656
    lifestyle modification and, 655
    physiotherapy, 655
    surgery for, 656–657
        artificial urinary sphincter, 656
        salvage surgery, 656–657
        slings, 656
Intinsic sphincter deficiency, treatment in male, 653–654
    artificial urinary sphincter, 654
    fascial sling, 654
    injectables, 654
    lifestyle modification and, 653
    physiotherapy, 653
    α-adrenergic agonists, 653
Intraurethral stent (*see* Sphincter stent)
Intravenous pyelography (IVP), 358, 478, 522, 568, 574
Intrinsic sphincteric deficiency (ISD), 146, 161, 185, 196–198, 298, 361, 363, 388, 535, 615, 635, 651
    causes of, 498–499
    treatment of, 651
Introital route, 363, 367
    advantages, 363
    disadvantages, 363
IPG (*see* Internal pulse generator)
I-PSS (*see* International Prostatic Symptom Score)
Ischiorectal fossa, 194
ISD (*see* Intrinsic sphincter deficiency)
Isoproterenol, 62
IVP (*see* Intravenous pyelography)
IVS (*see* Slingplasty, intravaginal)

KCO (*see* Potassium channel openers)
Kegel exercises, 444, 584
King's questionnaire, 652
Kink resistant tubing, 530
Kropp, procedure of, 608
KUB (*see* Scout film)
Kuo, stress urinary incontinence, classification of, 379

Laparoscopy, bladder neck suspension by, 596–597
L-arginine, 12
Lax vagina, 195
Lazy bladder syndrome, 159, 251

Leak point pressure (LPP), 146, 303–307,
    319, 478, 611, **770, 772–773, 775–
    776**
  bladder volume and, 304
  catheters used for, 304
  clinical applications of, 306–307
    neurogenic bladder, 306
    stress urinary incontinence (SUI), fe-
      male, 306–307
    urinary diversion, 307
    urinary incontinence, male, 307
  intraoperative, 307
  mathematical formulas for, 306
  measurement of, 306
  patient position and, 304
  technique of, 303–304
  types of, 303
    abdominal, 303, 319, 320, 314, 498,
      770
    bladder, 319
    cough, 303, **770**
    detrusor, 303, **770**
    stomal, 307
    Valsalva, 146, 303, 319, 392, 498, 510,
      653, **770**
Leak point volume, 306
Leakage, detection of, 277, 340
Lifestyle interventions (*see also* Behavioral
    modification), 437–441, 470, 653,
    655
Ligaments
  anococcygeal, 37
  Cooper's, 587, 596, 620, 622
  ileopectineal (*see* Ligaments, Cooper's)
  puboprostatic, 34, 38
  pubourethral, 18, 21, 111, 113–115, 598,
    624
  pubovesical, 34, 38, 113–115
  urethropelvic, 18, 19, 416
  uterosacral, 18
Linear passive urethral resistance relation
    (LinPURR), 325, 328
LinPURR (*see* Linear passive urethral resis-
    tance relation)
Lipomeningocele, 136, 610
Lissauer's tract, 93
Lithiasis, urinary, 226
LLP (*see* Leak point pressure)
Locus caerulus, 224
Low conus, 137
Lower motor neuron lesion, 136

Lower urinary tract dysfunction, 696,
    711–715
  classification of, **711–715**
    storage phase, **712–714**
    voiding phase, **714–715**
  clinical assessment of, **696**
    examination, physical, **696**
    frequency-volume chart, **696**
    history, clinical, **696**
Lower urinary tract symptoms (LUTS), 241,
    243, **808**
  gynecological pathology and, 246–247
  storage, related to, 243–245
    frequency, 244
    incontinence, 244–245
    nocturia, 244
    urgency, 244
  voiding, related to, 245–246
    dribble, terminal, 246
    dysuria, 246
    emptying, incomplete, 246
    hesitancy, 245–246
    intermittency, 246
    straining, 246
    stream, decreased, 246
Lower urinary tract, neurophysiologic evalua-
    tion of, **705–711**
  electromyography, **705–707**
  evoked potentials, **709–710**
  nerve conduction, **707–709**
  reflex latencies, **709**
  sensory testing, **710–711**
Lower urinary tract, rehabilitaion techniques,
    718–728
  behavioral modification, **721–722**
    applications, **722**
    definition, **721**
    techniques, **721–722**
  biofeedback, **720–721**
    applications, **720–721**
    definition, **720**
    techniques, **720**
  electrical stimulation, **722–725**
    applications, **723–725**
    definition, **722**
    measurement units, symbols, **723**
    techniques, **722–723**
  pelvic floor, training, **719–720**
  voiding maneuvers, **726–728**
    applications, **728**
    bladder expression, **727**

[Lower urinary tract, rehabilitaion techniques]
catheterization, **726–727**
reflex triggering, bladder, 727
L-region, 206
LUTS (*see* Lower urinary tract symptoms)

Madsen–Iversen score, **810**
Magnetic resonance imaging (MRI), 29, 31, 33, 107, 116–120, 227, 236, 366, 413–421, 445, 502, **737, 804–805**
cadavers, studies on, 118–120
disadvantages of, 116
dynamic, 418–420
dynamic HASTE sequence, 420
histology and, 416
living subjects, studies on, 116–118
lower urinary tract, normal and, 415–416
stress incontinence, and, 417–418
urethral abnormalities, and, 416–417
Magnetoelectric stimulation, 429
Maine Medical Assessment Program (MMAP Instrument), **810**
Male adult, outcome studies in, **808–815**
Malformations, anal rectal, 140–141
Malignant hyperthermia, 487
Marcaine, 669
Marion's syndrome, 187
Marlex mesh, 597, 619, 620–621
Marshall-Marchetti-Krantz (MMK), procedure of, 586–587
goal of, 586
results of, 587
technique of, 586–587
Measurement, symbols and units of, **715–717, 723, 761**
Mechanoreceptors, activation of, 545
Medial malleolus, 681
Meissner's plexus, 157
Memotherm®, 306
Meningomyelocele (*see* Myelomeningocele)
Menopause, 177, 198–199
MEPs (*see* Motor-evoked potentials)
Mersilene mesh, 619, 620
Met-enkephalin, 10
Micturition
bladder pressure and, **703–704**
center
brain stem, 226
pontine, 91, 92, 93, 94, 95, 97, 223, 225
sacral, 223

[Micturition]
cerebral cortex, role of, 95–96
emotional control, 95–96
somatic control, 96
control of, 202
evaluation of, **701–705, 754–761**
bladder pressure and, **703–704**
flow rate, measurement of, **701–703**
pressure–flow relation, 704
residual urine, measurement of, 705
urethral pressure during (VUPP), **704–705**
forebrain, involvement of, 94–95
motor systems, 90–93
bladder, 90, 91
external urethral sphincter, 90–91
micturition reflex, 91–93, 94
neural control of, 93–96
physiology of, 36
sensory systems, 93–94
Micturition diary (*see* Voiding diary)
Mitrofanoff's principle, 139, 656
MMAP (*see* Maine Medical Assessment Program)
MMK (*see* Marshall-Marchetti-Krantz, procedure of)
Mollard, procedure of, 606
Monti's procedure, 656
Motor-evoked potentials (MEPs), 429, 433
Motor term latencies, pudendal, 213
M-region, 206
MRI (*see* Magnetic resonance imaging)
Multiple sclerosis, 186, 223, 227, 247, 476, 544, 560, 569, 636
Muscarinic receptors, 53, 55, 59, 64
Muscle memory, 107
Muscle, smooth, 43–64, 193–194
action potentials, 51
calcium, 55, 56
cell coupling, 50, 51
contractile proteins, 56–57
myosin, 56, 73
myosin regulation, 56–57
protein kinase C, 57
thick filaments, 56
thin filaments, 56
thin-filament regulation, 57
excitatory junction potentials (EJPs), 52
hyperpolarization of, 490
inhibitory junction potentials (IJPs), 52
inner layer, 193

[Muscle, smooth]
  ion channels, 53–55
    calcium, 54
    chloride, 55
    nonselective cations, 54–55
    potassium, 54
    sodium, 53
  ionotropic action, 52
  membrane potential, 49–50
  metabotropic action, 52, 55
  middle layer, 193
  outer layer, 193
  pacemaker potentials, 51
  passive membrane properties, 50, 51
  physiology, 43–64
  receptors, 52, 53
  sarcoplasmic reticulum (SR), 55, 64, 487
  second messenger systems, 55
  space constant, 50, 51
  spontaneous activity, 52
  study methods, 44–49
    blotting techniques, 49
    cell culture, 48
    electrical conduction, 45
    flux studies, 45–47
    gene cloning, 49
    immunohistochemistry, 47
    intracellular calcium, 47
    microelectrodes, 45, 57
    molecular techniques, 45, 58
    muscle tension, 45–45
    patch clamp technique, 47, 57
    receptor density, 47
    reverse transcription polymerase chain
      reaction (RT-PCR), 49
    sucrose-gap technique, 45, 58
  time constant, 50
Muscle, striated (see also Pelvic floor)
  anterior pubococcygeus, 21
  bulbocavernosus, 74, 203, 211
  bulbospongeosus, 19, 38, 74
  coccygeus, 19, 460
  compressor urethrae, 112
  deep transverse perinea, 26, 27, 112
  external anal sphincter, 74, 19, 38, 90
  external urethral sphincter, 32, 90, 72, 73,
    75, 92, 96, 97
  fast-fatiguable (FF), 72
  fast fatigue-resistant (FFR), 72, 81
  fast-twitch (type II), 2, 20, 37, 72, 113, 447
  fatigue of, 546

[Muscle, striated]
  ileococcygeus, 118, 195, 460
  ischiocavernosus, 19, 74, 203
  levator ani, 19, 20, 37, 71, 72, 73, 111, 115,
    178, 194, 195, 203, 416, 535, 541,
    543, 546, 588
  paraurethral, 71
  pelvic floor, 71–82
    anatomy, 72
    central pathways, 79–80
    exercises, 77
    histochemistry, 72
    innervation, 74–76
    muscle types, 72–73
    physiology, 71–82
    postural changes on, responses to, 77
    reflex control, 76–79
    reflex control after injury, 80–81
    reflex effects on, arising from bladder,
      77–79
    reflex effects on, arising from urethra,
      77–79
    somatic stimulation, responses to, 77
    somatic stimuli, 76–77
    tonic activity, 75–76
  power of, 446
  primordial, 32
  puboanalis, 37
  pubococcygeus, 113, 118, 198, 460
  puboperinealis, 37, 38
  puborectalis, 37, 38, 71
  pubovesical, 113–115
  pubovesical urethral sphincter, 92, 96, 97
  pubovisceral, 120
  rectus abdominalis, 22
  slow twitch (type 1), 2, 4, 20, 37, 72, 81,
    113, 447, 487
  superficial anal sphincter, 203, 204
  superficial transverse perinea, 19,203
  transverse abdominal, 445
  transversus perinealis, 203, 543
  types of
    fast-fatiguable (FF), 72
    fast fatigue-resistant (FFR), 72, 81
    fast-twitch (type II), 2, 20, 37, 72, 113,
      487
    slow-twitch (type I), 2, 4, 20, 37, 72, 81,
      113, 487
  Wilson's, 31, 113
Myelodysplasia, 135–136, 185, 195, 223, 306,
  521, 527

Myelomeningocele, 306, 527, 610
  open, 135
Myosin, 73, 56

Nd:YAG contact laser, 565, 566, 580
Needle suspension, 593–596, 628
  goal of, 593
  nerve injury and, 595
  technique of, 593–594
    Gittes procedure, 594
    Pereyra procedure, 593
    Raz procedure, 594
    Stamey procedure, 593–594
Neobladder, orthotopic, 477
Neodymium:yttrium aluminum garnet (*see* Nd:YAG)
Nephrolithiasis, 565
Nerve conduction studies, **707–709**
Nerve entrapment, 595, 598, 638, 645
Nerve growth factor, 160, 548
Nerve injury, needle suspension and, 595
Nerve
  common perineal, 595, 640, 682
  dorsal penile, 74, 79
  femoral, 595
  genitofemoral, 595
  hypogastric, 91
  ilioinguinal, 595
  inferior rectal, 194
  inferior rectal, 9
  parasympathetic, 91, 193
  pelvic, 35, 74, 93, 187
  perineal, 9, 194
  posterior tibial, 681, 682
  pudendal, 9, 16, 35, 74, 75, 134, 187, 194,
      203, 683
    blockade of, 35
  sacral, 35, 682
  saphenous, 595
  sciatic, 595, 683
  splanchnic, pelvic, 7, 193
  sympathic, 91, 193
Neural efficiency, 102–103
Neurogenic bladder, 135, 140, 141, 145, 306,
      347, 478, 484, 527, 530, 553, 569,
      611, 673, **763–780**
  assessment of, clinical, **764–769**
    history, clinical, **764–768**
    examination, physical, **768–769**
  in children, 135, 140, 141, 145

[Neurogenic bladder]
  investigations of, **769–778**
    methods, **769–771**
    measurement technique, **771–774**
    data, **774–778**
Neurokinins A and B, 209
Neuromodulation (*see also* Neurostimulation),
      541–549, 647, 683–685
  storage, improvement by, 544–545
    urodynamic evidence of, 546
  testing of, 684
  voiding, improvement by, 545–546
    urodynamic evidence of, 546–547
Neuropeptide Y, 9, 10
Neuroplasticity, 153, 160, 202
Neurostimulation (*see also* Neuromodulation),
      541–544, 553–560, **804**
  aims of, 554–555
  future possibilities of, 560
  history of, 555–557
  indications for, 560
  mechanism of, 543–544
  modalities of, 555
    external, 557
    extradural, 558, 559
    intradural, 558, 559
  parameters of, 541
  permanent implant, 542–543
  spinal cord injury and, 558–559
  test phase of, 542
Neurourology, behavioral, 201–210
Nicotinic receptors, 64
Nitric oxide synthase, 10, 12, 74
Nitroglycerin, 669
Nocturia, 244
Nomogram, pressure–flow, 324–329
  Abrams–Griffiths', 324, 325
  ICS, 328–329
  Schäfer's, 324–328, 344
Nomograms, uroflow, 289
  adults, 289
    Backman, 289
    Bristol, 289
    Haylen, 289
    Jorgensen, 289
    Siroky, 289
    Susset, 289
    Von Garrelts, 289
  children, 289
    Szabó-Fegyverneki, 289
    Toguri, 289

Non-Fowler syndrome, 546
Nonneurogenic neurogenic bladder (*see* Hin-
    man's syndrome)
Noradrenergic neurons, 484
Norepinephrine, 10, 19, 62
Nylon cord, 620

Obstruction, bladder outlet, 316, 324, 408,
        522, 591, 675, **808**
    assessment of, **812–813**
    compressive, 327
        grades of, 328
    consequences of, 226
    constrictive, 327
        classification of, 328
    localization of, 330
    urethral resistence and, **758**
Obstruction, definition of, provisional ICS
        method for, **760**
One-repetition maximum (1RM), 446
Onuf's nucleus, 74, 79, 82, 90, 91, 92, 185,
        205
Ornade®, 490
Osteitis pubis (*see also* Osteomyelitis), 588
Osteomyelitis, 598, 624
Osteotomy, pelvic, 137
Outcome studies, **795–824**
    adult female, **800–806**
        observation, clinical, **802–805**
        socioeconomic costs, **805–806**
        symptom quantification, **801–802**
        symptoms, **801**
    adult male, **808–815**
        bladder outlet obstruction, assessment of,
            812–813
        durability, **814**
        outcome measures, clinical, **811–812**
        socioeconomic measurements, **814**
        symptoms, measurement of, **809–811**
        treatment complications, **814**
        voiding pattern, documentation of, **811**
    frail older people, **817–824**
        outcome measurements, **820–824**
        study design for, **818–820**
    general principles of, **795–799**
        definition, **796**
        endpoints, **796**
        evaluation and grading of, **797**
        outcome measures, **796–797**
        practical points, **798–799**
        reporting, **797**
        standardization, **795–796**

Overcontinence, 218
Overuse syndromes, 107
Oxybutynine chloride, 161, 669

Pad-weighing test, 275–281, 340, 536, 538,
        636, 653, **749, 802, 820–821**
    discrimination by, 276
    qualitative, 277
    quantitative, 277, **700–701**
        adults, 278–280
        children, 277
        elderly, 280
    reproducibility of, 276
    types of, 276–280
PAG (*see* Periaqueductal gray)
Pain-free window, 683
Parasympatholytics (*see* Anticholinergics)
Paravaginal defect, endopelvic, 126
Paravaginal fascia, 587
    repair of, 588–591
        goal of, 588–589
        results of, 591
        technique of, 589–591
Parkinson's disease, 187, 195, 247, 636
Passive urethral resistance relation (PURR),
        327–328, **757**
Pelvic compartments, 232
    definition of, 232
    ICS standardization of, 232–233, 236
Pelvic diaphragm (*see also* Pelvic floor,
        and/or Muscle, striated, pelvic floor),
        18, 19, 26, 29, 34, 106, 113, 195, 523,
        543
    increased awareness of, 545
    overactivity, overactive bladder and,
        548–549
Pelvic floor (*see* Pelvic diaphragm, and/or
        Muscle, striated, pelvic floor)
Pelvic floor, aging of, 175–180
    demographics, 175–176
    normal aging, 176–177
    reflex contraction of, 364
    symptoms, prevalence of, 177
    urodynamic changes, 177–179
        female, 179
        male, 178–179
Pelvic floor, connective tissue within the,
        111–129
    anatomy, 112–116
    biochemistry, 120–125
        collagen defects, 121–124
        collagen, type I/III ratio, 124–125

[Pelvic floor, connective tissue within the]
  biomechanics, 125–128
    fascia, mechanical strength of, 126–128
    joint mobility, 126–128
  heredity, 125
  histology, 112–116
    endopelvic paravaginal defect, 113
    male sphincteric complex, 115–116
    pubourethral ligaments, 111, 113–115
pubovesical muscles, 113–115
  magnetic resonance imaging (MRI),
    116–120
    cadavers, studies on, 118–120
    disadvantages of, 116
    living subjects, studies on, 116–118
Pelvic floor, infancy and childhood, 133–
    163
  anatomy, development, 134
  congenital abnormalities, 134–141
    anal rectal malformations, 140–141
    bladder extrophy, 137–138
    cerebral palsy, 137
    ectopic ureters, bilateral, 138–139
    lipomeningocele, 136
    myelodysplasia, 135–136
    posterior urethral valves, 139–140
    sacral agenesis, 136
    spinal cord injury, 137
    tethered cord, 136–137
  constipation, 154
    definition, 154–155
    evaluation, 155
    therapy, 156–157
  dysfunctional voiding, 158–163
    causes, 158–160
    therapy for, 160–163
  encopresis (see Constipation)
  evaluation, 141–152
    bowel manometrics, 149–152
    cystometrogram, 143–145
    electromyography, 146
    history, 141
    leak point pressure, 146
    physical examination, 142
    urethral pressure profile, 146–147
    urodynamics, 142–148
    uroflow-EMG, 149
    videourodynamics, 147–148
  lessons from the past, 101, 109
  noctural enuresis, 157–158
  nonneurogenic neurogenic bladder (see also
    Hinman's syndrome), 153–154

[Pelvic floor, infancy and childhood]
  urinary tract infections, 158–163
  vesicoureteral reflux, 158–163
Pelvic floor, physiotherapy of (see Physiother-
    apy, pelvic floor and/or Pelvic floor,
    re-education of)
Pelvic floor, re-education of (see also Physio-
    therapy, pelvic floor), 459–471
  physical examination, 459–460
  results of, 469–471
    anti-incontinence devices, 471
    bladder training, 471
    lifestyle interventions, 470
    physical therapies, 470
  treatment, aims of, 460
  treatment, modalities of, 460–469
    biofeedback, 463–467
    education, 461–463
    electrical stimulation, 467–469
    manual techniques, 463
Pelvic ganglia, 75, 91
Pelvic muscle, activity of, **802**
Pelvic organ prolapse, 637, 652
  cure rate of, 439
  heavy work and, 439
Pelvic pain, 205, 208, 209, 218, 541
Pelvic pain, electrical stimulation and, **725**
Pelvic trauma, 196
Penalties of evolved solutions, 103–104
Percutaneous nerve stimulation (PNS), 541
Pereyra, procedure of, 593
Periaqueductal gray (PAG), 94, 96, 97, 224
Perineal body, 19, 33, 37, 38, 134
Perineal massage, 463
Perineal route, 361
Pessaire effect, 370, 379
Pessary, 537
PET (see Positron emission tomography)
Pfannenstiel incision, 524, 589, 617
PG (see Prostaglandine)
Phenol block, 488
Phenoxybenzamine, 10, 485
Phentolamine, 184, 485, 486
Phenylpropanolamine hydrochloride, 161,
    489
  side effects of, 489
Phospholipase C (PLC), 52, 55
Photokymograph, 286
Physical examination (see Examination, phys-
    ical)
Physical therapy (see Physiotherapy)
Physiotherapy, 22, 113

Physiotherapy, pelvic floor, 443–454
  assessment, elements of, 444
  definition of, 443
  diagnosis, 444
  evaluation of, 444–446
  females and, 655
  functional electrical stimulation, 674–675
  intervention, types of, 444
  long-term results of, 452
  males and, 454, 653
  muscle training and, 446
    maintenance of, 447–448
    muscle endurance, 446
    muscle streingth, 446
    overload and, 447
    specificity of, 446–447
  planning, 444
  prevention of urinary incontinence by,
    453–454
  treatment of stress urinary incontinence by,
    448–452
    long-term results of, 452
  treatment of urge incontinence by, 452–
    453
Pippi-Salle, procedure of, 139, 608
PLC (*see* Phospholipase C)
Plexus
  pelvic, 193
  superior hypogastric, 193
PNS (*see* Percutaneous nerve stimulation)
Polyuria, nocturnal, 272
Pontine micturition center, 91, 92, 93, 94, 95,
  97, 223, 225
Pop-off mechanism, 611, 613
Positron emission tomography (PET), 92, 94,
  95, 96, 107, 206, 683
Posterior midline raphe, 33
Posterior urethrovesical angle, 360, 363, 366,
  370, 377, 385
Postvoid residual (PVR), 213, 285–291, 522,
  536, 565, 566, 574, 579, 637, 641,
  647, **812, 823**
  in aging female, 179
  in aging male, 179
  measurement of, **705**
Potassium channel openers (KCO), 60, 63–64
Pourcelot's index (*see* Pulsatility index)
Prazosin, 484, 675, 679
  side effects of, 484
Precontraction, 449
Precursor reflexes, 102
  hypersensitivity, 102
  spasticity, 102

Pressure sampling, 337
Pressure transducer, 336–337
  air-filled, 336
  liquid-filled, 336
  microtip, 296, 336
  rectal, 337
Pressure transmission ratio (PTR), 236, 238,
  297, 498, 620
Pressure
  abdominal, 311
  atrophy, urethral, 528–529
  detrusor, 311, 323
  intraurethral, 311
  intravesical, total, 311
  recording of, **739**
  voiding, 311
Pressure–flow relation, 324–329, 344, 624,
  704, 754–756, 803
  parameters of, **811–812**
  flow delay, **756**
Pressure–flow study data, digital exchange of,
  839–848
  file and records, structure of, **840–841**
  information storage, **846–847**
  record types, **841–846**
  record types, definition of, **841**
    default values, **841**
    signal ID, **841, 848**
  signal storage, **846–847**
  signal storage, description of, **839**
  types, variable, **840**
  typical file, structure of, **847–848**
  values, variable, **840**
Probe, ultrasonographic
  artefacts related to, 365–367
  endocavitary, 361, 373
  external, 360
Prolapse, genital (*see* Urethra, genital prolapse)
Prolapse, pelvic organ, **729–740**
  description of, **730–735**
    ancillary techniques for, **735–737**
    examination, **730**
    ordinal stages of, **733–735**
    quantitative, **730–733**
  pelvic floor, muscle testing of, **737–739**
  symptoms, description of, **739–740**
Prolapse, vaginal vault, 235
Prolene mesh, 599, 623
Propantheline (Pro-Banthine), 161
Prostaglandin E_1 (PGE$_1$), 10
Prostaglandin E_2 (PGE$_2$), 10, 62
Prostaglandin F_2 (PGF$_2$), 19

Prostaglandine $F_{2\alpha}$, 10
Prostate apical notch, 32, 34
Prostate size, estimation of, **811–812**
Prostatectomy, 196
Prostatic buds, 4
Prostatitis, 205
Prostatodynia, 217
Pseudodyssynergia, 146, 149, 187, 228, 486
Pseudoephedrine, 161, 489
Pseudostrain dyssynergy, 228
PTFE (*see* Teflon)
PTR (*see* Pressure transmission ratio)
Pubic ligament, 373
Pubic tubercle, 640
Pubocervical fascia, 114–115, 588
Pubovaginal sling (PVS), 584, 635
Pubovaginal spring, 537
Pudendal motor-evoked potentials, 432
Pudendal motor pathways, 425–426
Pudendal nerve block, 486
Pudendal sensory-evoked potentials, 432
Pudendal somatosensory pathways, 424–425
Pulsatility index, 393
Purinoceptors, 53, 59
PURR (*see* Passive urethral resistance rela-
    tion)
PVR (*see* Postvoid residual)
PVS (*see* Pubovaginal sling)
Pyelonephritis, 224, 228
Pyramidal tracts, 425
Pyridium, 277
Pyuria, 480

QoL (*see* Quality of life)
Q-tip test, 256, 357, 365, 366, 367, 537, 538,
    621
Quality of life, 521, 586, 652, 681, **808**
    influence of assessment on, **813**
        disease-specific, **813**
        generic, **813**
        measurements of, **823**
Questionnaires, 652, **809–810**
    disease-specific, 652

Radiation injury, 198, 521
Radical hysterectomy, 185
Radical perineal prostatectomy, 39
Radical retropubic prostatectomy, 34, 39, 115,
    184, 196, 307
    incontinence, prevalence of, 196
Radiotherapy, pelvic, 498
Raz, procedure of, 594
Rebound phenomenon, 545

Receptors
    acetylcholine, 682
        extrajunctional, 682
    anoderm, 155
    estrogen, 123, 490
    ryanodine, 55, 56, 60, 61, 64
    serotonergic, 206
Rectocele, 235, 592
Rectum, abdominoperineal resection of, 185,
    247, 432
Rectus fascia, 638, 648
Reflex
    abdominal, 257
    anal, 257
    bulbocavernosus, 142, 215, 227, 235, 252,
        257
    clitoridoanal, 257
    contraction, 22
    corticospinal, 225
    cremasteric, 257
    Edvardsen's, 544
    latencies, **709**
    loops of, 225
    micturition, 224
    precursor, 102
        hypersensitivity, 102
        spasticity, 102
    sacral
        latency of, 227
        somatosomatic, 432, 488
        viscerosomatic, 430–431, 433, 488
    secondary, 224
    sexual, 76
    spinal, 224
    spinobulbospinal, 224
    straining, 77
    urethral, 214
        continence and, 214
    urethrogenital, 76
    voiding, 225, 226
        organization of, 225
Reflux, vesicoureteral, 137, 141, 152–163,
        224, 479, 480, 522, 673
    high grade, 134
    high pressure, 140
    spontaneous resolution of, 134
Renal
    agenesis, 141
    dysplasia, 141
    scan, radioisotope, 568, 574
    ultrasonography, 478, 522
Renshaw cell, 75
Resistance, urethral, 319

Retention, chronic urinary (*see* Urinary retention, chronic)
Retrograde ureterography, 522
Retrograde urethrography, 32
Retzius, space of, 118, 586, 594
Reverse transcription polymerase chain reaction, 49
Rexed's laminae, 93
Rhabdomyosarcoma, 198
Rhabdosphincter (*see also* Striated sphincter, male), 25, 115, 186–187, 196, 543
　areflexia, **778**
　hyperreflexia, **778**
　omega-shaped, 36, 134, 194, 543
　ring-shaped, 134, 194
Rhizotomy, 559
RT-PCR (*see* Reverse transcription polymerase chain reaction)
Ryanodine receptors, 55, 56, 60, 61, 64

Sacral agenesis, 136, 252, 610
Sacral interneurons, 76
Sacrocolpopexy, 238
Sacrospinous fixation, 238
Sarcoplasmic reticulum (SR), 55, 64, 487
Schäfer, nomogram of, 324
Scout film (KUB), 408, 530
SEAPI-QMN, classification of, 307, 649, 636, 646
Sensation
　bladder, 315
　pelvic floor, 203–205
　perineum, 203–205
Sensitivity threshold, urinary, 432–433
Sensory testing, lower urinary tract, **710–711**
Serotonin, 490
Sexual abuse, 227
Sexual function, assessment of, **810–811**
Shy bladder, 104, 212, 346–347
Shy–Drager syndrome, 185
SI, units of measurement, **716**
Signet-ring, 4
Silastic mesh, 619–622
Sims' speculum, 235
Sling plasty, intravaginal (IVS), 598–599
Sling surgery, artificial material and, 615–631
　advantages of, 618–619
　artificial grafts in, 619–624
　　antibiotic-treated, 622
　　bone anchors, 622–623
　　Marlex (polypropylene), 620–621

[Sling surgery, artificial material and]
　　Mersilene (polyethylene terephthalate), 620
　　silastic, 622
　　Teflon (polytetraflouroethylene, 621–622
　　tension-free vaginal tape (TVT), 623–624
　characteristics of, 618
　complications of, 624–626
　　detrusor instability, 625
　　graft erosion, 625–626
　　infection, 619, 621, 626
　　rejection, 621
　　voiding difficulties, 624–625
　Gore-Tex patch, 626–630
　　surgical technique of, 628–629
　　suture tying, 630
　　types of sling placement, 629
　results of, 630–631
　surgical approach, 616–618
　　abdominal, 616–617
　　abdomino-vaginal, 617
　　vaginal, 617–618
Sling surgery, fascial slings and, 635–649
　complications of, 647
　evaluation for, 636–637
　　clinical history, 636
　　physical examination, 636–637
　　workup, 637
　indications for, 635
　outcomes, 644–648
　　autologous fascia, 645–646
　　cadaveric fascia lata, 646–647
　patient selection for, 635
　surgical technique of, 638–644
　tissue sources for, 637–638
Slow-twitch fibers, 2, 4, 20, 37, 72, 81, 113, 447, 487
Smooth sphincter dyssynergia (*see* Detrusor-internal sphincter dyssynergia (DISD))
Soave, procedure of, 157
Socioeconomic measurements, **805–806, 814, 823–824**
Somatostatin, 10, 208
Spectrometry, 287
Sphincter stent, 567–573, 676
　complications of, 572
　encrustation of, 570–572, 577
　epithelialization of, 570, 577
　explantation of, 572, 573, 577
　hematuria and, 573
　infertility and, 580

[Sphincter stent]
  migration of, 572, 573
  North American trial of, 568–573
    methods of, 568–569
    results of, 569–573
  placement, technique of, 567–568
  quality of life and, 578
  sphincter function and, 573
  sphincterotomy, compared to, 574–580
  tissue hyperplasia and, 570, 577
  urinary tract infection and, 572
Sphincter, thickness of, 377
Sphincterotomy, 306, 554, 566–567, 676
  complications of, 567
  quality of life and, 578
  sphincter stent, compared to, 574–580
  technique of, 566
Spina bifida, 306
Spinal cord, tethering, 135, 136–137, 141
Spinal cord injury, 137, 195, 223, 227, 306,
        521, 544, 565, 569, 610
  complete, 560
  incomplete, 560
  intermittent catheterization and, 475, 476
  neurostimulation and, 553, 555
Spinal cord tumor, 569
Spinal shock, 137, 145, 560
Spinal vascular accident, 569
Squeezing effort, 371
SR (see Sarcoplasmic reticulum)
SSRs (see Sympathetic skin responses)
Stamey, procedure of, 593–594
Standardiztion Reports, ICS, **695–848**
  list of, 691–694
  overview of, 687–689
Stent, intraurethral, (see Sphincter stent)
Straining reflex, 77
Stress urinary incontinence (SUI) (see also
        Urinary incontinence), 15, 185, 196,
        236, 241, 243, 360, 377, 498, 573,
        635, 636
  cure rate of, 439
  diet and, 439–440
  fascial biopsy in, 112
  in men, 307
  in women, 306–307
  intraurethral devices for, 538–539
  intravaginal devices for, 535–538
    external collection, 536
    intravaginal, 537–538
    occlusive, 536–537
  leak point pressure in, 306–307

[Stress urinary incontinence (SUI)]
  female, 306–307
  male, 307
  occult, 236
  pathogenesis of, 417–418
  persistent, 646
  physical exercise and, 438–439
  prevalence of, 111
  recurrent, 408, 644
    incidence of, 198
  smoking and, 439
  type II, 21
  type II,I 23, 306
  types of, 304
  weight loss and, 427–428
Stress urinary incontinence, urethral injection
        and, 497–512, 611, 647, 654, 655–656
  in children, 510
  history of, 497
  ideal substance, characteristics of, 512
  in men, 508–510
  in women, 503–508
    autologous fat, 506–508
    collagen, 503–506, 636
  mechanism of action, 498
  patient selection for, 498–499
  substances used for, 501–503
    autologous fat, 501–502
    collagen, 502–503
  technique of, 499–501
Striated sphincter, male, (see also Rhab-
        dosphincter)
  active function of, 37
  areflexia, **778**
  balloon dilation of, 566
  hyperreflexia, **778**
  in normal voiding, 36
  injury to, 38
  loop mechanism of, 36
  passive function of, 37
  protection, 38
  surgery and, 38–40
Stroke, acute hemispheric, 227
Substance P, 10, 206, 488
SUI (see Stress urinary incontinence)
Suprapontine organization, 225
Symbols (see Measurement, symbols and
        units)
Sympathetic skin responses (SSRs), 429,
        433–434
Symphysis pubis, 373
Symptom reporting, 340

Symptoms
  bowel, **740**
  local, **740**
  sexual, **740**
  urinary, **739–740**
  urodynamics in relation to, **350–351**

Tamsulozin, 485, 675
Tanagho, procedure of, 608
Tanden cuff, 529
Teflon, 497
Teflon mesh, 619, 621–622
TENS (*see* Transcutaneous nerve stimulation)
Tension-free vaginal tape (TVT), 21, 598,
    615, 623–624
Terazosin, 484, 486, 679
Terbutaline, 487
Testosterone, 74
Tethered cord syndrome, 135, 136, 141
Tetrodotoxin (TTX), 53, 58
Thyrosine hydroxylase, 10
Toilet training, 104–105
Toileting, psychological roots of, 104
Tolterodine, 161, 669
Trabeculation, bladder wall, 36, 242, 408,
    409, 477, 479
Transcutaneous nerve stimulation (TENS),
    682, 683
Transducers, pressure, **829–831**
Translabial route (*see* Introital route)
Transrectal route, 364–365
Transvaginal route, 364
  advantages, 364
  disadvantages, 364
Transverse myelitis, 223
TTX (*see* Tetrodotoxin)
TVT (*see* Tension-free vaginal tape)
Tyrosine hydroxylase, 9

UDI-6 (*see* Urogenital distress inventory)
Ultrasonography, 737 (*see also* Urethra, ultra-
    sound imaging of)
UPP (*see* Urethral pressure profile)
Upper motor neuron lesion, 136, 137
URA (*see* Urethral, resistance parameter)
Ureter, bilateral ectopic, 138–139
Ureter, obstruction of, 592
Urethra (*see also* Urinary sphincter)
  3–D reconstruction of, 386
    advantages of, 390, 391–392
  balloon dilation of, 676
  compression of, 236, 238

[Urethra]
  cross-sectional area of, 327
  development of, 32–34
  diverticula of, 412
  dynamic behavior, importance of, 214
  evaluation of function, 241–283
    examination, 251–259
    history, 241–248
    pad-weighing test, 275–281
    voiding diary, 261–273
  false passage, 477
  female
    anatomy of, functional, 15–23
    closure pressure, 20
    compliance of, 22, 179
    compressor urethra, 17, 20, 22
    continence at rest, 20
    continence during storage, 20
    continence during stress, 20
    distal sphincter, 17
    estrogen-dependence of, 15, 16
    external sphincter, 32
    extrinsic continence mechanism, 18–19
    hypermobility (*see also* Hypermobility,
      urethra), 19, 21, 256, 503, 626
    intrinsic continence mechanism, 15–17
    mucosal sealing effect, 15
    muscular synergies, 22
    pipe stem urethra, 23
    pressure, 76
  fixed, 377
  function during storage, **713–714**
  function during voiding, **715**
  functional length, 238
  hypermobility of, 19, 21, 256, 503, 626
    central protrusion, 256
    lateral detachment, 256
    type II, 626
  hyperpathic (*see also* Urinary sphincter, hy-
    pertonic), 217
    hyperreflexia (R), 217
    hypersensitivity (S), 217
    hypertonicity (T), 217
  hypersensitive, 213
  hypertonic, 460, 463
    classification of, 215
  incompetent medical treatment of, 489–491
    α-adrenergic agonists, 489–490
    estrogens, 490–491
    imipramine, 490
  kinking, 236
  low pressure, 620, 621

[Urethra]
  male
    anterior, 32
    bulbar, 32, 522, 523
    external, 29, 31, 32
    infracollicular sphincteric, 31, 32, 38
    innervation of, 34–35
    intermediate, 31
    intrinsic smooth-muscle, 31, 32
    membranous, 31, 32, 34, 38, 184
    omega shaped, 36
    pendulous, 32
    posterior, 32, 184
    prostatic, 32
    rhabdosphincter, 25
    sphincteric, 31, 32
    striated, 25–40
    supracollicular, 31, 35
  maturation, 32–34
  musculus constrictor urethrae mem-
      branaceae, 25
  normal, 196
  overactive, 196, 546
    overactive bladder and, 548–549
  physiology, 62–64
    innervation, 62–63
    ion channels, 63
    membrane potentials, 63
    membrane properties, 63
  pipe stem, 615
  position of, 411
  pressure atrophy, 528–529
  profilometry, 20
    rhabdosphincter, 17
    urethral sphincter muscle, 20
    urethrovaginal sphincter muscle, 17, 20
  proximal, lengthening of, 607
  pseudolipoma of, 506
  scarring of, 411–412
  smooth muscle, ultrasonic measurement of,
      390
  sphincter activity
    assessment of, 215
    dysfunctional prostatodynia, 217
  sphincter vesicae externus, 25, 26
  sphincter vesicae internus, 31, 32
  spinning top deformity, 152
  striated muscle, ultrasonic measurement of,
      390
  stricture disease, 477, 521, 554, 573
  unstable, 196, 204, 227, 298
  Wilson's muscle, 31

Urethra, genital prolapse and, 231–239
  classification of, 232–235
    cystocele, 233–235
    cystourethrocele, 233–235
    enterocele, 235
    rectocele, 235
    uterine descent, 235
    vault prolapse, 235
  definition of, 232–235
  diagnosis of, 236–238
    anterior compartment, 236–238
    middle compartment, 238
    posterior compartment, 238
  examination of, 235–238
  history, 235–238
  incidence of, 231, 232–235
Urethra, hyperactive, medical treatment of,
      483–489
  smooth muscle level (see also Bladder
      neck), 484–485
    α-adrenergic blockers, 484–485
  striated muscle level, 485–489
    α-adrenergic blockers, 485–486
    baclofen, 488–489
    benzodiazepines, 486–487
    α-adrenergic agents, 487
    botulinum toxin A, 487–488
    dandrolene sodium, 487
    phenol block, 488
Urethra, ultrasound imaging of, 357–396
  clinical applications of, 377–395
    delivery, 383–386
    pregnancy, 383–386
    stress urinary incontinence (SUI),
        377–383
    technology, progress in, 386–395
  color Doppler and, 393–395
  endocavitary, 358
  endourethral, 386–388
  imaging, quality of, 358–360
  methodology of, 360–365
    introital route, 363
    perineal route, 361
    transrectal, 364–365
    transvaginal, 364
  methodology, influence of, 367–377
    bearing-down, 368–370
    bladder filling, 371
    cough, 368–370
    geometric framing, 373–377
    patient's position, 367–368
    plane of, 373

[Urethra, ultrasound imaging of]
  squeezing, 371
  urethrovesical junction, localization of,
    371–372
  perineal, 236
  probe effect, 365–367
  X-ray, compared to, 359, 360
Urethral
  axis, 409
  coaptation, 395
  diverticuli, 360, 386, 408
    saddle bag, 417
  function, voiding and, 756–757
  length, 377, 388
  pulse
    ultrasonographic, 395
    urodynamic, 395
  resistance, 319, 535, **756–760**
    bladder outlet obstruction and, **758**
    plot analysis, **758–760**
    relation (URR), **757**
    urethral activity and, **757**
  resistance parameter (URA), 546, 548
  sealing, 184
    venous plexus, 184
  sphincter (*see also* Urinary sphincter)
    3–D ultrasonographic measurment of,
      388–392
  sphincterotomy, 306, 554, 566–567, 676
  stent, 521
  stricture disease, 477, 521, 554
  syndrome, 546
  valves, posterior, 139–140
    type I, 139
Urethral closure pressure (*see also* Urethral
    pressure profile), 146–147, 178–179,
    213, 236, 238
  normal, 217
Urethral plug device, 538–539
Urethral pressure profile (UPP) (*see also* Ure-
    thral closure pressure), 295–299, 363,
    366, 653, **770–771, 773, 776, 777, 804**
  α-adrenergic agonists and, 489
  clinical applications of, 298–299
  clonidine and, 484
  in children, 146–147
  estrogens and, 491
  measurements of, 297, **698–700**
    during voiding (VUPP), **704–705**
  parameters of, 297
  technique of, 295–297
  types of, 295

[Urethral pressure profile (UPP)]
  resting, 295
  stress, 295
  voiding, 295
Urethrogenital reflex, 76
Urethrography, retrograde, 32
Urethrolysis, 636, 637, 652
Urethrovesical angle, overcorrection of, 410
Urethrovesical junction (*see also* Bladder
    neck), 360
  after delivery, 383–386
  during pregnancy, 383
  hypermobility of, 621
  localization of, 371–372, 373
  mobility of, 360, 361, 367, 368, 370
    angle, defined by, 373
    distance, defined by, 373
  position of, 377
    classification, 377
    effect of surgery on, 381–383
    in continent female, 377
    in incontinent female, 377
  rotational descent of, 370
  sliding descent, 377
Urge-frequency syndrome, 205, 244,
    349–350, 541
Urge incontinence, 96, 196, 205, 541, 591
  physiotherapy, treatment by, 452–453
Urilos, 277
Urinary diary (*see* Voiding diary)
Urinary diversion (*see* Urinary reservoir, con-
    tinent)
Urinary incontinence (*see also* Stress urinary
    incontinence), 224–225, 351–352, **714**
  coital, 245
  continuous, 245
  enuresis, 157–158, 227, 245, 490, **714**
  overflow, 245, 476, 647, **714**
  postmicturition, 714
  post-prostatectomy, 36, 527
  prevalence of, 185
  prevention of, 453–454
  reflex, **714**
  stress, 245, **714**
  treatment of
    diet and, 439–440
    exercises and, 438–439
    lifestyle interventions in, 437–441, 470
    smoking and, 439
    weight loss in, 437–438
  unconscious, **714**
  urgency, 245, 244, **714**

Urinary reservoir, continent, 477, **743**
  anal, **743**
  cutaneous, **743**
Urinary retention, 541
  chronic, 205, 208, 347, 545, 584, 624
  postoperative, 476
Urinary sphincter (*see also* Urethra)
  components of, 183–185
  dysfunctional, epidemiology of, 183–187
  dyssynergia, 223–229
  dyssynergic, 186–187
  electromyography, 423–424
    analytic, 424
    dynamic, 424
  embryogenesis, 1–13
  failure, 193, 195–198
  gender-specific, 1–7
  histology
    differentiation, 6–7
    female, fetal, 2–4
    indifferent stage, 1–2
    male, fetal, 4–5
  hypertonic, 186, 201–218
  incompetent, 185–186, 193–199, 235
  innervation, 7–10
  need for, 105–106
  pelvic prolapse and, 231–239
  pharmacology, in vitro, 10–12
  pharmacology, in vivo, 12
  recording of, 213
  smooth (internal), 1, 184
  striated (external), 1,16, 17, 73, 74, 184,
    203, 204
  uninhibited relaxation of, 227, 298
Urinary sphincter, artificial, 517–532, 554,
  654, 656
  activation of, 526
    delayed, 531
  complications of, 528–532
    altered detrusor, 530
    balloon reservoir, restrictive pseudocap-
      sule of, 530
    device leak, 530
    erosion, 531
    infection, 530–531
    injuries, intraoperative, 531
    occlusion, 530
    pressure atrophy, 528–529
    risk factors for, 531
    silicone shedding, 531–532
  deactivation, 526
  history of, 517–521

[Urinary sphincter, artificial]
  operative technique, 522–526
    bladder neck cuff, suprapubic, 524–526
    bladder neck cuff, transvaginal, 526
    bulbar urethral cuff, 522–524
  patient selection for, 521–522
    cystourethroscopy, 521
    examination, physical, 521
    history, clinical, 521
    videourodynamics, 521–522
  postoperative care, 526–527
  results of, 527–528
Urinary sphincter, dyssynergic, management
  synthesis of, 661–676
  detrusor, directed to, 662–675
    pharmacological, 669
    surgical, 670–675
  urethral sphincter, directed to, 675–676
    pharmacological, 675–676
    surgical, 676
Urinary sphincter, hypertonic, 201–218, 553,
  679–685
  central nervous system and, 203–205
  examination
    clinical, 210
    physical, 210–213
  history, 210
  management of, 679–685
    acupuncture, 681
    α-adrenergic blockers, 681
    biofeedback, 679–680
    botulinum toxin A, 682–683
    catheterization, intermittent, 681
    neuromodulation, 683–685
    TENS therapy, 682
  pelvic floor sensation, 203–205
  perineal sensation, 203–205
  peripheral muscles, 208–210
  toilet-training, risks of, 202–203
  urodynamics, 213–217
    cystometry, 213
    dynamic behavior, 214, 215
    hypertonic sphincter, 215, 217
    sphincter activity, 213, 215
    urethral reflexes, 214
Urinary sphincter, incompetent (*see also* Sling
  surgery), 193–199, 553
  classification of, 195–198
    aging, 198–199
    anti-incontinence surgery, 198
    menopause, 198–199
    neurogenic, 196

[Urinary sphincter, incompetent]
  nonneurogenic, 196–198
  prostatectomy, 196
  radiation, 198
  trauma, 196
  ICS classification of, 196
  intrinsic deficiency (ISD) (see Intrinsic
      sphincter deficiency)
  pelvic floor, 195
  smooth muscle, 193–194
  striated muscle, 194
  vaginal wall, 195
  vascular component, 194–195
Urinary sphincter, incompetent, management
      synthesis of, 651–658
  clinical history, 651–652
  physical examination, 652
  quality of life, 652
  treatment of, 653–657
  urodynamics, 653
Urinary sphincter, incompetent, surgery for,
      583–600
  assessment of, 585
  bone anchors, 597–598
    complications of, 598
    goal of, 597
    results of, 598
    technique of, 597
  indications for, 583–584
  intravaginal slingplasty, 598–599
  laparoscopic bladder neck suspensions,
      596–597
    complications of, 597
    goal of, 596
    results of, 597
    technique of, 596
  needle suspensions, 593–596
    complications of, 595–596
    results of, 94–595
    technique of, 593–594
  outcomes of, 584–586
  retropubic suspensions, 586–593
    Burch procedure, 587–588
    complications of, 591–593
    Marshall-Marchetti-Krantz procedure,
        586–587
    paravaginal fascial repair, 588–591
Urinary tract infection, 152–158, 480, 527,
      577
  recurrent, 205, 212, 224, 408, 479, 613, 681
Urine loss, quantification of (see Pad-weigh-
      ing test)

Urine storage, evaluation of, 696–701
  cystometry, 696–698
  urethral pressure, measurement of, 698–
      700
  urine loss, quantification of, 700–701
Urodynamics, 213–217, 363, 364, 366, 368,
      370, 546, 569, 570, 653, 695
  in children, 142–148
    indications for, 148
  symptoms in relation to, 350–351
  ultrasound imaging and, 363, 366
Urodynamics, ambulatory, 335–354, 771,
      782–794
  analysis of, 786–787
    phase identification, 786–787
    quality, assessment of, 786
  artefacts during, 340–342
  conduct of studies on, 337–339
  future directions in, 353–354
  history of, 336–337
  indications for, 782
  interpretation of, 339
  methodology of, 783–786
    catheter fixation, 786
    conductance, 784–786
    patient instructions, 786
    pressure measurements, 784–786
    signal quality, 784
    signals, 783–784
    urine leakage, recording of, 786
  mixed urinary incontinence and, 353
  presentation, scientific, 787
  reporting of, 339–340, 787
    data handling, 339–340
    data quality, 339
    detrusor overactivity, 340
    leakage, detection of, 340
    symptoms, reporting of, 340
  studies involving
    bashful bladder syndrome, 346–347
    drug evaluation, 347–348
    female voiding, 345
    incontinence, 351–352
    male voiding, 343–345
    neuropathic bladder, 347
    patient preference, 352
    symptoms in relation to, 350–351
    urge syndrome, 349–350
    urinary retention, chronic, 347
    volunteers, asymptomatic, 342–343
  study schedule in, 337–340
  terminology of, 783

Urodynamics, equipment, 826–836
　electromyography, measurements, 835–836
　　amplification of, 836
　　electrodes, 835
　　recording, types of, 835–836
　flowmeters, 831–835
　　characteristics of, 833
　　measurement, units of, 832
　　pressure-flow studies and, 834
　　system specifications, 834–835
　　types of, 833
　　units, conversion of, 832
　pressure transducers, 829–831
　　frequency response of, 831
　　hysteresis of, 830
　　linearity of, 830
　　measurement, units of, 829
　　pressure overload of, 830
　　pressure range of, 830
　　sensitivity of, 830
　　volume displacement by, 831
　　zero offset, 830
　　zero, reference level of, 830–831
　recording systems, 836–838
　　cathode ray oscilloscope, 836–387
　　digital storage, 838
　　magnetic tape, 837–838
　　paper chart, 837
　signal processors, 826–829
　　amplification of, 827
　　conversion, analog-to-digital, 829
　　differentiation of, 827–829
　　integration of, 829
　　signal filtration, 827
Urodynamics, multichannel, 311–332, 822
　emptying, parameters of, 322–330
　filling, parameters of, 313–322
　storage, parameters of, 313–322
　　filling pressure, 315–318
　　pelvic floor EMG and, 320–322
　　sensation, 315
　　storage, 318–320
Uroflow, 213, 236, 285–291, 311, 322, 537,
　　769, 771–772, 774–775, 802–803,
　　812
　artefacts in, 290
　clinical applications of, 288–290
　　flow pattern, normal, 288–290
　differential, 289
　equipment, 286–287
　in aging female, 179

[Uroflow]
　in aging male, 178–179
　measurements of, 287, 701–703
　　continuous flow, nomenclature of, 287
　　intermittent flow, nomenclature of, 287
　nomograms, 289
　pitfalls in, 290
　technique of, 286
　variations in, 290
Uroflow-EMG, 149, 228
Urogenital aging, 176
Urogenital atrophy, 178
Urogenital diaphragm (*see* Pelvic diaphragm)
Urogenital Distress Inventory (UDI-6), 307
UroLume, 306, 521, 566
URR (*see* Urethral, resistance, relation)
Uterus, descent of, 235

Vaginal erosion, artificial sling and, 620, 621
Vaginal plug, 682
Vaginal wall, 195
Vaginitis, atrophic, 177
Vaginoscopy, 411
Valsalva maneuver, 77, 211, 235, 236, 238,
　　297, 303, 314, 360, 367, 368, 370
　bladder filling and, 371
　leak point pressure, 146, 303, 319, 392,
　　498, 510, 653
Vascularization, periurethral, 393
　bladder instability and, 393
　hormone replacement and, 393
　stress urinary incontinence and, 393
Vasoactive intestinal polypeptide (VIP), 10,
　　62
VCUG (*see* Voiding cystourethrography)
Verumontanum, 38, 139, 183, 252, 331
Vesicomyotomy, 671
Vesicoureteral reflux (*see* Reflux, vesi-
　　coureteral)
Vesicoureteral reflux dysplasia syndrome
　　(VRDS), 140
Vicryl mesh, 619
Videourodynamics, 186, 213, 237, 238, 304,
　　307, 330–332, 357, 521–522, 611,
　　771, 777
Video voiding cystourethrography (VVCUG),
　　357, 360, 392, 393
Vincent's curtsy, 141
VIP (*see* Vasoactive intestinal polypeptide)
Visual analog score, 243
Voiding, dysfunctional, 661, 675
Voiding, electrical stimulation and, 725

Voiding cystourethrography (VCUG), 357,
        358, 407–413
    abnormal bladder findings, 409–411
        cystocele, 409–410
        fistulas, 410–411
        intravesical pressure, elevated, 409
        previous repairs, 410
    abnormal urethral findings, 411–412
        diverticuli, 412
        scarring, 411–412
        urethral position, 411
    anaphylactic reaction and, 408
    indications of, 406, 410
    normal findings, 406–409
    risks of, 406
    technique of, 406
Voiding diary, 210, 213, 261–273, 461, 636,
        652, **696, 744, 766, 801, 811, 820**
    children, 264–266
    completion of, 269
    diagnostic tool, 267–269
    duration of, 267
        females, 266–267

[Voiding diary]
    interpretation of, 269–272
    normal values, 264–267
    parameters derived from, 263–264
Voiding dysfunction, classification of, 312
Voiding pressure, 570, 573, 579, 624
    high, 1
    sphincterotomy and, 570, 579
VRDS (*see* Vesicoureteral reflux dysplasia
        syndrome)
VUPP (*see* Micturition, evaluation of, urethral
        pressure during)
VVCUG (*see* Video voiding cystourethrogra-
        phy)

Washer-like effect, 194
Weight loss, urinary incontinence and,
        427–428
Wet checks, **821–822**
Writer's cramp, 683

Young–Dees–Leadbetter, procedure of,
        138–139, 510, 605–606

Printed and bound by CPI Group (UK) Ltd, Croydon, CR0 4YY

23/10/2024

01778251-0003